CLINICAL EPIDEMIOLOGY

The Architecture of Clinical Research

Alvan R. Feinstein, M.D.

1925-

Professor of Medicine and Epidemiology
Yale University School of Medicine
New Haven, Connecticut

1985

W. B. Saunders Company

Philadelphia   London   Toronto   Mexico City   Rio de Janeiro   Sydney   Tokyo

W. B. Saunders Company: West Washington Square
Philadelphia, PA   19105

1 St. Anne's Road
Eastbourne, East Sussex BN21 3UN, England

1 Goldthorne Avenue
Toronto, Ontario M8Z 5T9, Canada

Apartado 26370—Cedro 512
Mexico 4, D.F., Mexico

Rua Coronel Cabrita, 8
Sao Cristovao Caixa Postal 21176
Rio de Janeiro, Brazil

9 Waltham Street
Artarmon, N.S.W. 2064, Australia

Ichibancho, Central Bldg., 22-1 Ichibancho
Chiyoda-Ku, Tokyo 102, Japan

Library of Congress Cataloging in Publication Data

Feinstein, Alvan R.

Clinical epidemiology.

1. Epidemiology—Statistical methods.
   2. Epidemiology—Research—Methodology.   I. Title.
   [DNLM: 1. Epidemiology.   2. Epidemiologic Methods.
   WA 950 F299c]

RA652.2.M3F45 1985   614.4′072   84–10532

ISBN 0–7216–1308–X

Clinical Epidemiology: The Architecture of Clinical Research   ISBN   0–7216–1308–X

Last digit is the print number: 9   8   7   6   5   4   3   2   1

*For Miriam and Daniel,
and for a new generation*

Contents

Prologue

Since a prologue gives a writer a chance to say a few things to the reader before all the formalities begin, I want to take adantage of that opportunity.

One of the most difficult tasks in preparing this book has been to give it a suitable title. Because much of the text refers to what is enumerated and appraised when clinicians make fundamental decisions in patient care, one suggested title was *Quantification of Diagnosis, Prognosis, and Therapy*. This name was rejected because it had at least four disadvantages: it was too long; it did not indicate the full scope of the contents; it would erroneously suggest a mathematical rather than clinical emphasis; and the word *Quantitative* might scare away many of the readers for whom the book was intended.

An alternative title, which was the leading candidate for a long time, was *The Architecture of Clinical Research*. This name would properly indicate that one of the main goals of the text was to discuss the structure and function of the research published in medical literature. Despite all the instruction aimed at preparing students for their future careers in clinical practice, medical education today contains no specific courses on how to think critically about the research results that are constantly encountered by clinicians in private meetings, conferences, and public journals. Because of this omission, future clinicians are taught a great deal about how to practice medicine, but very little about how to evaluate the published evidence on which medical practice depends.

The book is intended not only to help fill that gap in medical education, but also to help guide clinicians who actually engage in research. Many medical students who never expected or wanted to be involved in research have later discovered that they were doing it as clinicians. They often participate—as investigators, collaborators, contributors, facilitators, or even subjects—in randomized trials, cohort observations, cross-sectional surveys, educational programs, or other types of clinical research. The participating clinicians are seldom prepared for these additional roles, however, because medical education seldom includes instruction on how to plan, carry out, and analyze these clinical investigative studies.

The instructional goals of the text could be implied by *architecture* and *research* in the title, but these words were transferred to the subtitle after medical students and other colleagues persuaded me that the words might be misunderstood. Some potential readers would be confused about what is meant by *architecture* (it is explained in Chapter 2), and many others might mistakenly believe that *research* referred to the laboratory-centered investigations, in molecular biology or biochemistry, that are often labeled today as "clinical research."

Another candidate title was *Quantitative Clinical Epidemiology*. This name had been used for the annual presentation of a special course in which much of the material in this book was developed and taught during the past 10 years. Although the course has been greatly enjoyed by the post-residency clinicians who attended it, they were a highly selected group. They had deliberately sought and welcomed the ideas under discussion—but a more general medical audience might not be so favorably predisposed. The combination of *quantitative* and *epidemiology* in a single phrase might evoke the adverse reactions that many clinical readers get from each term individually; and the interaction of the two terms might produce a type of intellectual anaphylaxis.

If the *Quantitative* word were dropped, the remaining title would be *Clinical Epide-*

miology—a phrase that has many different interpreters, detractors, and admirers. For some public health epidemiologists, the *clinical* prefix to *epidemiology* is an abomination that threatens further partition beyond the many ways in which epidemiology has already been divided. For other public health personnel and for some clinicians, the *clinical* prefix is a useful linguistic device that may help attract greater interest and funding for traditional epidemiologic research, while also making it more palatable to clinicians. For yet other writers, *Clinical Epidemiology* describes what happens when conventional epidemiologic research is done by someone who also takes care of patients.

Since my own approach differs from all of these and emphasizes the clinical content of the activities, the main problem anticipated for potential medical readers is the *epidemiology* part of the title. In the literal meaning of that word ($\epsilon\pi\iota$ = upon; $\delta\epsilon\mu\circ\varsigma$ = people), *epidemiology* is exactly right as a label for studies of groups of people, but the term has acquired connotations that are unappealing to many clinicians who have still not recovered from their medical school instruction in public health.

By avoiding the phrase *Clinical Epidemiology*, I could escape these problems and ambiguities, but I would have to find another title. A word I have begun to use for these activities in the past few years is *Clinimetrics*. It can refer to two types of measurement in clinical medicine. One type, discussed in Chapter 6, is the *mensuration* that occurs when rating scales and other indexes are constructed and applied to convert observed clinical phenomena into raw data. The second type of measurement produces *quantification* when the raw information is collected into groups, and when the grouped data are summarized and compared. According to the way these two types of measurement are catalogued, *clinimetrics* could be limited to the mensuration process that produces raw data for *clinical epidemiology;* or *clinical epidemiology* could be regarded as the quantification component of *clinimetrics*. The latter approach would allow *Clinimetrics* to be a suitable title for the book—but the neologism was unfamiliar, and besides, the *-metrics* suffix might be even more frightening than all the *quantitative* prefixes.

I therefore decided to reconsider *Clinical Epidemiology*. These two words were first joined (as described further in Chapter 30) when John R. Paul used the phrase as the title for his presidential address to the American Society for Clinical Investigation in 1938. Paul's goals were to expand the topics of clinical investigation and the methods of epidemiologic research. He urged clinical investigators to pay more attention to the social and community settings of disease; and he wanted the group statistics of epidemiologic research to come from careful studies of individual people.

Although generally ignored by Paul's colleagues in clinical investigation, his ideas were welcomed and developed in public health research. The new work, however, was given such names as *social epidemiology* and *community medicine,* rather than the title Paul had proposed. In 1966, when I was seeking a name for clinical research in diagnosis, prognosis, and therapy, I did not know about Paul's suggestion, almost 30 years earlier, of *clinical epidemiology*. Had I known about it at the time, I probably would have rejected the title because the work I had in mind was firmly rooted in clinical medicine, not in public health epidemiology. Although not included in the conventional interests or teaching of public health epidemiology, the intellectual territory of diagnosis, prognosis, and therapy had by then become a focus of my own clinical research for at least a decade. I had previously described some of that territory in a book called *Clinical Judgment,* but the word *judgment* was also unsatisfactory as a name for the scientific domain I was trying to christen.

As my investigative work continued along its untitled pathway, a colleague in public health epidemiology told me one day in 1967 that what I was doing—in quantitatively analyzing data for groups of people—was really *epidemiology*. I was startled by this statement because I regarded myself as a clinician. Like most clinicians, I thought of *epidemiology* as being concerned with topics in public health—but the term also had a methodologic meaning. It could denote research methods, rather than the contents of the research. As I began to realize that the literal meaning of *epidemiology* was quite appropriate for my research methods, it seemed like a good name for what I was doing. Furthermore, by adding the *clinical* prefix, I could denote the distinctive clinical focus of the activities, in much the way that other investigators had used such adjectives as *infectious disease, chronic disease, nosocomial,* or *social* to demarcate the topics pursued with their own epidemiologic methods.

During the years since I re-introduced the phrase *Clinical Epidemiology* in the clinical literature in 1968, many investigative clinicians have begun doing the kind of research I had described under that title. It has become an accepted part of the scientific territory regarded as "clinical investigation"; it has begun to develop its own scientific principles and methodologic standards; and some clinicians, occasionally to the dismay of public health epidemiologists, have even begun to use those scientific methods for studying cause-effect relationships in etiology, not just diagnosis, prognosis, and therapy. Since no choice seemed perfect for the title of this book, *Clinical Epidemiology* became the winner, in part because it was the most satisfactory of the available candidates, but mainly because of loyalty. I did not want to disappoint the many colleagues who now regard themselves as clinical epidemiologists and who did not want me to abandon the name of the child that we had jointly nourished, raised, and sustained.

I doubt that the *epidemiology* part of the title will be repugnant to a new generation of medical students, since they will probably find the research methods and clinical contents of this type of epidemiology much more exciting, appealing, and clinically pertinent than what has been traditionally taught under the epidemiologic label. As for the former medical students who are now residents, research fellows, academic faculty, or clinical practitioners, I hope they will be willing to delay whatever unfavorable first reaction they may have to *epidemiology*. It is a perfectly good word, despite the unattractive things that may have been done with it; it has been associated with some magnificent public health accomplishments; and it deserves a chance to retain its literal meaning while receiving an expanded clinical renascence in methods and topics.

When asked to indicate the potential audience for a book, most authors will usually say, "Everyone." I shall comply with this tradition. Since earlier, informal drafts of this text have already been used successfully in both undergraduate and graduate medical teaching, I belilve the book will be applicable in a course for medical students or for postgraduate physicians who want to learn to cope with the medical literature, to do patient-centered research, and to critically evaluate the claims that emerge from epidemiologic studies in clinical medicine or in public health. The text contains all the essential material, plus much more, that appeared in my now out-of-print 1977 book on *Clinical Biostatistics;* and the material has been totally revised into new clinical discussions and an integrated logical sequence that were impossible to achieve in the auto-anthology format of *Clinical Biostatistics.*

Although I have deliberately aimed at medically oriented readers and have used many clinically sophisticated illustrations and examples, I particularly want to welcome readers who are not physicians. The conventional courses in epidemiology that are attended by nurses, statisticians, sociologists, economists, hospital administrators, and other non-physicians seldom emphasize the types of topics and architecture that are pertinent for clinical medicine and scientific research. The book should help you understand the clinician's scientific ethos in epidemiologic research, and it will help fill the many clinical gaps that were left if your instruction was oriented exclusively to the topics and methods of public health epidemiology.

Since many biostatisticians and public health epidemiologists have written books explaining their viewpoints as a "primer" for clinical readers, this text can also be regarded as an act of intellectual reciprocity. The contents can act as a "primer" for non-clinical readers, explaining the scientific approach used by clinical investigators for quantitative challenges in group data of diagnosis, prognosis, therapy, etiology, and other medical topics. I hope that readers from both clinical and non-clinical domains will recognize that the two sets of "primers" are complementary rather than opposing, and that both sets can be valuable.

I realize that many public health epidemiologists and biostatisticians will not agree with everything that appears here. Some of those colleagues have already become vigorously upset by earlier versions of certain comments. Although saddened by their distress, I can only remind them that scientific investigation makes progress through the "divine discontent" that always makes us question the merits of an established *status quo*. If everything were perfect, there would be no reason for scientists to explore, change, or advance. The principle was well described by the eminent philosopher of science, Karl Popper: "If we respect truth, we must search for our errors: by indefatigable rational criticism, and self criticism." The book is conceived in that spirit, and is carried out with an additional principle of Leo Szilard: "Do not destroy what you cannot create." Although I have been critical of many established current practices, I have always tried to provide constructive alternatives.

The first six chapters of the book are relatively brief, and can readily be used in an elementary course that provides an outlined overview of the field. The next four chapters, which deal with statistics, can be used to extend that overview if no other statistical instruction will be offered elsewhere. The remaining chapters get longer and contain a more detailed discussion of what was outlined previously. Chapters 11 to 17 are particularly useful in offering a single scientific standard and architectural "model" for studies of cause-effect relationships that are now often approached with two different sets of standards and research structures. For cause-effect studies of therapeutic agents, clinicians are accustomed to the rigorous scientific demands and experimental research structures of randomized trials. For cause-effect studies of etiologic agents, epidemiologists often use a more arbitrary set of standards and various arrangements of non-experimental data. Since the basic scientific reasoning about a cause-effect relationship is the same, whether the agent be etiologic or therapeutic, the discussion in Chapters 11 to 17 provides a unified intellectual model for this appraisal, no matter what methods were actually used in the research.

Chapters 18 to 24 are concerned with the diverse alternatives that have been devised by clinicians and epidemiologists as substitute structures for the many investigative situations in which the research cannot be done with a randomized trial or long-term observational cohort study. These alternative structures, which are particularly common in epidemiologic research but which also often appear in clinical investigations of pathophysiology, produce some of the most difficult problems that confront clinicians reading the medical literature. As alternatives to the customary structure of scientific research, ecologic associations and various forms of case-control studies are methodologically alien to most medical readers—but the structures warrant careful scientific attention because they can be powerful devices for doing good (or bad) research in therapy as well as etiology of disease.

Chapters 25 to 27 are devoted to the various forms of process research used for evaluating quality in diagnostic marker tests, medical data, and clinical care. The last three chapters (28 to 30) contain additional attention to some special topics: the descriptive challenges of demarcating a "range of normal"; the majestic contributions and substantial limitations of randomized trials; and an outline of the many other types of epidemiology that have not been otherwise discussed in the text.

Although the 30 chapters have the advantage of a single author's coordination and literary style, I have had an enormous amount of help for which I am grateful to many people and institutions. The basic ideas in each chapter, as well as the "homework" exercises and answers, were originally developed for a special course given under the auspices of the Robert Wood Johnson Clinical Scholars Program at the Yale University School of Medicine. This program, which began at Yale in 1974, has joined analogous programs at other institutions as a remarkable effort, sponsored by the Johnson Foundation, to create a new breed of academic clinician. The extraordinary vision of the Foundation has been highly successful in helping produce clinicians whose research would be concerned with issues in the strategy, delivery, and policy of health care, rather than with the pathophysiologic topics that have traditionally been emphasized in academic clinical investigation.

The activities at the Yale Clinical Scholar Program have served as motivation, testing ground, source of new ideas, and detailed development for the contents of the course, and thereby, for this book. I want to thank the Yale Clinical Scholars and other course participants throughout the years for the stimulation, questions, comments, arguments, and collaboration that have brought these ideas to their current state of maturation. I also want to thank officials of the Robert Wood Johnson Foundation—particularly Dr. David E. Rogers, Dr. Leighton E. Cluff, the late Dr. Walsh McDermott, Mr. Gustav Lienhard, and Mrs. Annie Lea Shuster—for their continuing encouragement and support.

Several other institutional sources of support have been important and are gratefully acknowledged. I first began developing these ideas while working in the West Haven Veterans Administration Hospital, with whose Cooperative Studies Program Support Center I continue to be pleasurably associated. The U.S. Center for Health Services Research, now based in Rockville, sponsored many of the investigations that led to general concepts and specific examples. In more recent years, the A. W. Mellon Foundation and the Commonwealth Foundation have also provided valuable support for my activities in clinical epidemiology and in clinimetrics.

In the work that immediately preceded this book, I had many delightful collaborations with colleagues who have also joined in teaching the course from which the book is derived. Dr. Ralph I. Horwitz and I have worked together for almost a decade, and his influence has been particularly important in enhancing my appreciation of case-control studies. Dr. James F. Jekel has taught me a great deal about statistical methods of cohort analysis (in Chapter 17), and Dr. John D. Clemens originated the draft from which Chapter 27 (on quality of care) was revised. Ms. Carolyn K. Wells has constantly been an invaluable research collaborator and connoisseur of computer tactics.

Although the list would be too long if I tried to acknowledge everyone who has contributed to the diverse material contained here, I want to thank certain colleagues who have read and made helpful comments on various sections of the current text. They include all the Yale faculty members cited in the previous paragraph, as well as Drs. Robert H. Brook, John Esdaile, and Donald Mainland. They are herewith acknowledged with gratitude, but also absolved of responsibility for what has emerged.

Six persons who have not seen the text have nevertheless made particularly valuable contributions to the author's growth and morale. For more than 30 years, Dr. Paul B. Beeson has been my mentor and Dr. Robert G. Petersdorf has been a steadfast supporter. For more than 15 years, ever since I discovered I was a clinical epidemiologist, I have greatly benefited by frequent exchanges of ideas with Drs. Walter O. Spitzer and David L. Sackett. Since my earliest days in medicine, Drs. Jack L. Paradise and Jacques M. Quen have been both stimulating professional colleagues and close personal friends. This is my chance to thank these people, and many other colleagues too numerous to mention, for their friendship and for the pleausre of their company.

In the actual construction of this book, my handwritten text was converted to a superbly typed manuscript by Mary Newbury, aided (in alphabetical order) by Susan Coppola, Carrol Ludington, Elizabeth Pesapane, and Angela Voss. The drawings and other artwork were done with the greatly appreciated esthetic skills of Virginia Simon. I also want to acknowledge the staff of the publisher for their helpful suggestions in converting manuscript to published text.

To retreat into cool-headed thought, an author needs the sustenance of human warmth. It can come from friends, colleagues, and external family, but its main source is often at home. I therefore want to thank Linda M. Feinstein for her many personal contributions during the writing of this book and its predecessor, which was dedicated to her. I hope that our children, Miriam and Daniel, will accept the current dedication as the best I can do in print to thank them for granting me the gift of time, and for their other gifts of joy and love.

ALVAN R. FEINSTEIN

Chapter 1

Introduction

Since *Clinical Epidemiology* means different things to different people, the first job of a book with that title is to define itself. The word *epidemic* was originally used as a name for outbreaks of contagious disease in humans (in contrast to *epizootic* outbreaks in animals) and is derived from the Greek επι = upon and δεμος = people. *Epidemiology* is thus the study of people. More specifically, in epidemiologic studies the data refer to groups of people and the fundamental unit under observation is a person, in contrast to the animals, inanimate substances, human organs, or human fragments that are the basic materials investigated in other forms of medical research. The prefix *clinical*, which comes from the Greek κλινικος = bed, refers to sick people and to the activities conducted in the care of patients. A reasonably close etymologic definition, therefore, is that clinical epidemiology is concerned with studying groups of people to achieve the background evidence needed for clinical decisions in patient care.

With this focus of concern, clinical epidemiology contains certain important distinctions in its point of view, topics of interest, and methods of research. In point of view, clinical epidemiology represents the way in which classical epidemiology, traditionally oriented toward general strategies in the public health of community groups, has been enlarged to include clinical decisions in personal-encounter care for individual patients. In topics of interest, clinical epidemiology emphasizes issues in diagnosis, prognosis, therapy, and other distinctively clinical judgments that are usually omitted from the traditional inventory of contents in public health. In research methods, clinical epidemiology is concerned with the procedures and standards needed for scientifically rigorous studies of the complex clinical phenomena that occur in intact people. These methods are important both for the investigators who do the research and for the readers who struggle to understand and interpret the published results.

The remainder of this introductory chapter provides a historical background, describing the way in which traditional epidemiologists and traditional clinicians have migrated from their classical activities to create clinical epidemiology as a new intellectual domain in modern medical science.

1.1. THE EPIDEMIOLOGIST'S MIGRATION TO CLINICAL MEDICINE

Because epidemiology began with studies of the contagious outbreaks that were called *epidemics,* infectious diseases have been the basic source of concepts, methods, and technology in epidemiologic research. Almost all the activities of contemporary epidemiology, including its customary academic location in departments with such names as public health and preventive medicine, are derived from a heritage of infectious disease and from the pioneering role of microbiology in the evolution of medical knowledge.

In the chronology of medical science, infectious diseases were among the first human ailments that could be (1) identified during life by a specific laboratory test; (2) attributed to a demonstrable causal agent; (3) avoided by appropriate sanitation; and (4) prevented by individual treatment (with vaccination) of susceptible hosts. Infectious disease brought each of these four innovations to the study of human illness, and each innovation gave epidemiologists a focus of interest and set of research methods:

1. With bacteriologic procedures providing accurate identification of diseases, the rate of occurrence and geographic distribution of the diseases could be studied effectively.

2. The laboratory tests of bacteriology did more than identify a disease; they simultaneously demonstrated a causal agent. The ability to demonstrate causes of disease led epidemiologists to become concerned with problems of etiology not only for infections but for other diseases as well.

3. Because the community rather than the hospital was the site of study of both sanitation and the occurrence rate of disease, epidemiologists became interested in outpatient populations and in the diverse problems of public health.

4. Although sanitation helped to prevent disease in the general population of the community, vaccination provided protection to individual persons and thus advanced the conversion of epidemiology into an experimental discipline. To test new vaccines, epidemiologists had to study individual people while performing group experiments called *clinical trials* and using statistical procedures for design and analysis.

As a consequence of these different developments, epidemiology has become intellectually housed in academic sites with a wide diversity of names: hygiene, public health, preventive medicine, social medicine, community medicine, and even biostatistics. The personnel include physicians and nonphysicians with a wide variety of talents and interests. Among the nonphysicians are nurses, dentists, and veterinarians; virologists, parasitologists, and other microbiologists; geneticists, biometricians, biostatisticians, and computer experts; and people who specialize in occupational and industrial medicine, in hospital administration, and in programs of medical care. The different pursuits of these many people reflect the persistent interest of departments of epidemiology in infectious disease but also indicate a broad expansion into other clinical domains:

1. Statistical tabulations of occurrence and distribution for infectious epidemics have been extended to include rates of both mortality and morbidity, and the diseases under study, once only infectious and acute, are now also noninfectious and chronic.

2. Although causes of infectious diseases can be demonstrated by experiments in animals, the causes of chronic disease in people are not amenable to experimentation and are studied instead with statistical comparisons of data obtained from observation of naturally occurring human events.

3. Attention to community health, which previously created a challenge mainly in preventing disease with methods such as improved sanitation and nutrition, has now produced major clinical challenges in the quality, distribution, and economics of medical care.

4. The statistical procedures developed for clinical trials have been extended to include not only the prevention of acute disease in healthy persons but also the treatment as well as the prevention of chronic disease.

1.2. THE CLINICIAN'S MIGRATION TO EPIDEMIOLOGY

At the same time that classical epidemiologists have extended their boundaries from infectious disease to many other clinical territories, classical clinicians have developed many epidemiologic interests and concerns. As students of prognosis and therapy in human illness, clinicians have always been epidemiologists in the original sense of the word, but certain activities of modern clinical investigators—using statistics, studying groups of people, and delivering preventive therapy—are traditionally regarded as epidemiologic:

1. Every act of decision in diagnosis, prognosis, and therapy involves an assessment of probabilities and is thus a type of statistical exercise.

2. To make those decisions, clinicians recall their experience with previous patients, divide those patients into collections of subgroups or series, and compare the present patient with those in the various collections. These clinical subgroups and series correspond to what epidemiologists often call cohorts and populations.

3. In following the long-term outcome of treatment in chronic diseases, a clinician must leave the inpatients observed in the wards and pavilions of the hospital and must study outpatients in clinics and in community settings—the traditional locale of the epidemiologist.

4. Although clinicians do not usually regard treatment as an act of *preventive* medicine, many drugs and operations used in contemporary therapy are prophylactic rather than remedial. Their purpose is not so much to change an existing abnormality as to keep an already diseased patient from getting worse. For example, antithrombotic therapy is used not to remedy the lesion of a myocardial infarction but to prevent thromboembolic phenomena or recurrent infarction. In these prophylactic types of treatment, the goal is to prevent a more serious clinical state that does not yet exist. With this type of therapy, the clinician engages in preventive medicine—the epidemiologist's traditional concern.

1.3. THE CONTENTS OF CLINICAL EPIDEMIOLOGY

These two kinds of intellectual migration have brought many epidemiologists and clinicians into a common territory in which both groups operate, independently or in collaboration, with mutual interests and mutual techniques. As a new domain among the various divisions of contemporary medicine, clinical epidemiology is characterized neither by disease in a particular organ system (such as cardiology and endocrinology), nor by the age of the diseased subjects (such as pediatrics and geriatrics), nor by data derived from a particular form of technology (such as biochemistry and microbiology). In clinical epidemiology, any type of disease can be studied: acute or chronic, anatomically localized or diffuse, infectious or noninfectious. The subjects can be of any age: newborn or senile, young or old; and the data can be contributed by any useful technology of laboratory or bedside, ranging from electron microscopy to naked eye and from digital computer to perceptive human mind.

The distinguishing characteristics of clinical epidemiology are in its foci of investigation, its material, and its methods. The foci of investigation are topics in the occurrence, distribution, causation, diagnosis, natural history, prognosis, prevention, and therapy of disease. The unit of material in the investigation is a person rather than an animal, tissue, cell, or molecule. In some of the studies, the person will have been exposed to an agent suspected of causing a disease, and in many other studies, the person will be a patient who was treated with an agent intended to prevent or to alter a disease. The methods of investigation include techniques for identifying the characteristics of individual human hosts, for appropriately classifying those hosts and dividing them into groups, for comparing the results obtained in different groups, and for analyzing the importance of any observed differences.

The distinction between clinical and classical public health epidemiology can often be discerned by answering the question, What's in the denominator? For the various means, rates, and proportions that are examined in classical public health epidemiology, the denominator usually contains a *general population*, determined by the census counts (or sometimes by special surveys) of a particular geographic region, such as a city or nation. In clinical epidemiology, the denominator usually contains a *clinical group*, determined by studies of people with a particular clinical condition or disease.

This new definition of *clinical epidemiology* gives it a wider range of activities than those contained in previous applications of the term. When John R. Paul (in 1938 and later in 1958)[1, 2] (Fig. 1–1) originally added the word clinical to epidemiology, his goal was to extend epidemiology beyond statistical rates of disease and beyond infectious ailments alone to encompass "the circumstances under which diseases occur, where diseases tend to flourish, and where they do not." This approach—which includes environmental, occupational, cultural, and other community aspects of disease as well as the traditional studies of contagion—has sometimes been called *ecologic medicine, social medicine,* or *community medicine.* Although an obvious part of the collateral concerns of clinical epidemiology, these ecologic territories have now become generally recognized as part of the intellectual domain already under epidemiologic surveillance.

The newer usage of clinical epidemiology is intended to join the particular skills and

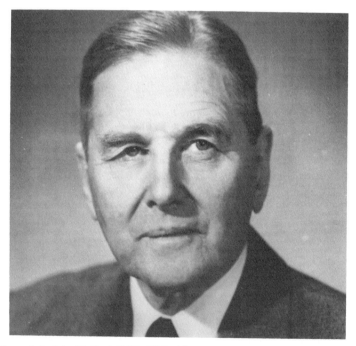

Figure 1–1. John R. Paul (1893–1971). (Courtesy of Dr. Dorothy Horstmann.)

knowledge that distinguish both the clinician and the epidemiologist. In clinical epidemiology, "clinical" preserves its connotations of human illness, and "epidemiology" preserves its connotation of groups of people. The addition of clinical sophistication to epidemiology can improve the medical interpretation of data used in studying occurrence rates and causes of disease; and the addition of epidemiologic methods to clinical medicine can help clinicians in their problems of evaluating different modes of treatment for patients. The particularly new things for the conventional epidemiologist in clinical epidemiology are the topics of clinical course and therapy for disease; the new things for the conventional clinician are the statistical organization and analysis of data from human groups.

Clinical epidemiology gets its intellectual heritage and its founding fathers from both of the "families" that it unites. The clinical heritage dates back to Hippocrates and to Thomas Sydenham, whose concern with human sickness always included an appreciation of human environment; the populational heritage dates back to John Graunt, who instigated, and to William Farr, who developed, procedures for tabulating disease rates in what is now often called *vital statistics*. Among the principal early explorers of the clinical epidemiologic domain were Pierre Ch. A. Louis (Fig. 1–2), who introduced the numerical method for investigating results of treatment; Ignaz Semmelweis (Fig. 1–3), who analyzed the results of inpatient therapy to demonstrate the iatrogenic etiology of puerperal fever; and Austin Bradford Hill (Fig. 1–4), who helped develop and popularize statistically rigorous clinical trials.

The domain of clinical epidemiology is now the site of increasingly active exploration. Within the past few decades, major advances in diagnostic tests have been followed by many studies designed to appraise old data or to obtain new data on the distribution and

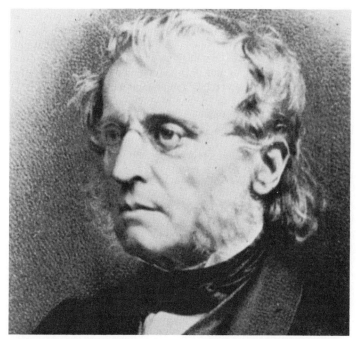

Figure 1–2. Pierre Ch. A. Louis (1787–1872). (Courtesy of Yale Medical Historical Library.)

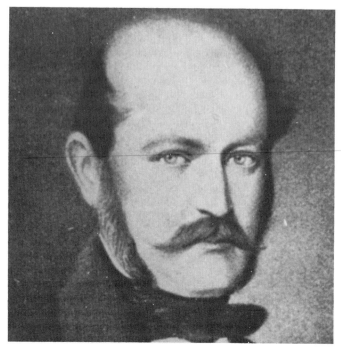

Figure 1–3. Ignaz Semmelweis (1818–1865). (Courtesy of Yale Medical Historical Library.)

clinical course of disease. Many new investigations of human populations have resulted from the search for cause in such chronic illnesses as cancer and arteriosclerosis. The causative clues obtained from these and other investigations have been followed by large-scale clinical trials, checking whether the diseases can be prevented by changes in nutrition, environment, or life style. The expansion of diagnostic technology has led to many problems in deployment of intricate machinery and evaluation of the costs and benefits of the tests. Also, the spectacular new modes of surgical and pharmaceutical therapy have produced a steady proliferation of statistical investigations of the new treatments. Even if no other reasons existed, the importance and increasing frequency of these investigations would require the delineation of clinical epidemiology as a medical domain that can provide an intellectual home for the activities.

1.4. **THE METHODS OF CLINICAL EPIDEMIOLOGY**

The topics that have just been described form the contents of the conjoint domain in which the classical epidemiologist—oriented in statistics, populations, and preventive medicine—meets the classical clinician—oriented in the artful science of diagnosis, prognosis, and care of individual patients.

Clinical epidemiology, however, can also be defined methodologically as a domain that is concerned with research involving intact human beings. The methods used in such research are necessarily different from the customary procedures used in other scientific domains. In traditional scientific concepts and teaching, research consists of experiments performed in laboratories. In a laboratory setting, the investigator can choose the animals

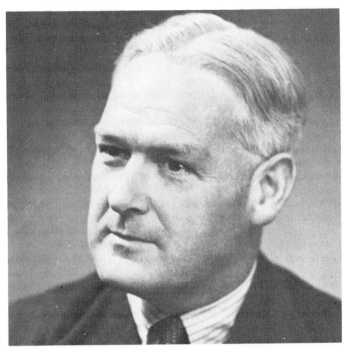

Figure 1–4. Austin Bradford Hill (1897–   ). (Courtesy of Editors, *Statistics in Medicine*.)

or inanimate substances that are the materials to be studied, divide them to form groups in any desired manner, subject them to whatever procedures have been chosen as the interventions, obtain accurate data with diverse technologic devices, and even kill (or "sacrifice") the material to verify the data and to see precisely what has happened.

These options are seldom available in research on intact human beings. Most of the data that are studied to make decisions about the etiology, distribution, diagnosis, prognosis, and therapy of human ailments come from ordinary observations, not from experiments, of events occurring during the routine activities of daily living for the people under scrutiny. The investigator does not decide who will smoke or not smoke, exercise or not exercise, breast-feed or not breast-feed. Except in the extraordinary experiments of randomized clinical trials, the investigator also does not decide who will be treated with medication, surgery, or watchful waiting, and does not choose the type of medication or surgery. All these decisions are usually made, without concern for experimental protocols, by the people under investigation and by their clinical advisors. The data used in the investigations can often come from technologic measurements of chemical and other substances, but large amounts of important epidemiologic information comes from subjective accounts of what the people under investigation (or their clinicians) have done, felt, or decided.

Because a laboratory investigator can usually conduct experiments, form groups, assign interventions, and rely on technologic information, the research can easily satisfy the fundamental scientific requirements for fair comparisons and trustworthy data. The investigator's main creative challenges, therefore, often occur in the formulation of ideas to be explored. The investigator must use imagination, verve, and insight to choose both the hypotheses that will be studied and the appropriate counterhypotheses that must be ruled out.

In research with individual persons or groups of people, however, the investigator can seldom perform experiments; the groups are usually self-selected or assigned without experimental planning; and the data are often obtained from human recollections and judgments. In these circumstances, the fundamental requirements of science are seldom easy to fulfill, and the investigator becomes creatively challenged, at a more basic scientific level, by problems in methodology itself. In the midst of information that is not acquired with the rigor of experimental planning in the laboratory, how can the investigator arrange to obtain trustworthy data and fair comparisons? How can statistical tabulations of observational information be obtained and analyzed in a manner that encourages confident belief in the results and credible acceptance? Even when an experimental clinical trial can be arranged with a group of people, the experimental plans and interpretations are inhibited by many human or clinical constraints that are not pertinent to laboratory research and that need not limit the creativity of the laboratory investigator. In the midst of these inhibitions, how can clinical investigators conduct experiments that satisfy the standards of science while answering the questions asked in clinical practice?

These scientific challenges in the performance and evaluation of human research are the main methodologic concerns of clinical epidemiology, and they will be the prime topics for subsequent discussion here.

1.5. SYNOPSIS

We can summarize the foregoing discussion by noting that clinical epidemiology is a domain of both content and methods. In content, clinical epidemiology is concerned with the etiology, diagnosis, prognosis, and care of human illnesses. The concept of *care* encompasses the strategy of therapy as well as the arrangements used to deliver therapy, and the concept of *therapy* refers to remedial or prophylactic treatment of individual patients. The methods of clinical epidemiology are intended to bring clinical sophistication and scientific rigor to the difficult challenges of investigating phenomena that occur in free-living intact people, who often cannot be studied with experimental plans.

1.6. A NOTE ABOUT THE EXERCISES

Each chapter in this book is followed by a set of exercises that can be used in any way that readers or instructors wish. The exercises were developed, and have been used for the past few years, as part of a special seminar conducted for postgraduate physicians. In that course, the written text for each chapter was read by the individual participants without any didactic lectures. The exercises provided additional illustrations and problems to challenge the reader's understanding of the subject. The written solutions to these exercises, which were turned in for review and annotation by the instructor before each class, then formed the main focus of discussion in the classroom seminars.

Suitable exercises for this type of material are not easy to create. Although many (in fact, most) of the assignments are based on events that have actually occurred in clinical or epidemiologic research, too much time would be consumed if the reader had to review a complete published report to find the particular items selected for discussion. Consequently, to allow prompt focus on the selected topic, the exercises are presented mainly as excerpts or brief summaries of the published reports. Specific references are seldom cited for these reports, because many of the exercises were chosen to depict undesirable procedures and because many other errant publications could have been selected instead.

In many ways, the exercises are the best part of the book. Medical students and practicing clinicians constantly complain about the enormous amount of memorization and the minuscule amount of thinking that is contained in medical education. These exercises are intended to make you think. Because they deliberately make use of the reader's clinical knowledge, they should give medically oriented persons the intellectual "fun" of relying on what they already know as a basis for solving problems and as a background for learning new things. The goal is to stimulate your thoughts not merely about the preceding text and the specific assignment presented in each exercise, but particularly about the challenges that regularly confront you when you read the medical literature, attend meetings where research is presented, or even do research yourself. In many instances, an exercise will reveal something you did not perceive in the text, force you to reevaluate your understanding of a particular subject, or let you see how your clinical knowledge, rather than the unfamiliar tactics of epidemiologic methods, provides the crux of the answer to many questions.

The publishers have persuaded me that answers to the exercises should be contained in the back of the book rather than issued as a separate document. Although it may be tempting, I urge you not to look at the answers until you have first thought each one through and preferably written down your solution. If this were a text on statistics, seeing the answers in advance would not quench your thought process, because you would still have the challenge of deciding what formula to use and showing that you can work your way through the calculations. Most of the exercises in this book, however, depend mainly on what you think and how you think about it. If you look at the answers prematurely, their revelation will make you miss the stimulation, the learning, and the fun.

Unlike the numerical answers that are unequivocally right or wrong for the customary exercises in a book on statistics, the answers to many of the exercises here are matters of judgment. To give the reader an idea of how someone else might answer the questions, a set of "official" answers has been prepared for each exercise. These answers, however, are merely official. They may be right or wrong, according to the judgment of the reader or the instructor. Because the goal of the exercises is to aid understanding and provide stimulation, the discussion provoked by debate about the correctness of an answer may sometimes be much more enlightening than the content or merit of the answer itself.

1.7. A NOTE ABOUT REFERENCES

To avoid repetitious listings and to save space while maintaining convenience for the reader, the bibliographic references in the text are identified in two different ways. The references are noted with sequential numbers as they appear successively within each chapter. At the end of the chapter, the numbers indicate the name of the first author and year of publication for that reference. The name of the journal is added, and sometimes letters (such as a, b, c) are appended, when needed to distinguish several references by the same author in the same year.

This end-of-chapter information will guide you to the full citation of the reference, which is listed separately at the end of the book, starting on page 738. In that section, each reference is completely identified and arranged alphabetically according to the first author. At the end of each alphabetized reference, the numbers in brackets indicate the chapter(s) in which that reference is mentioned.

EXERCISES

Exercise 1.1. In retrospective case-control studies of the etiology of a particular disease, the denominators for the compared results are obtained from a *case* group consisting of people who already have the disease and a *control* group consisting of people who do not have the disease. The members of the case group are usually chosen from patients seen at a hospital or other medical setting. The members of the control group may be chosen from patients who have other diseases or from healthy people in the community. Information about previous exposure to the suspected etiologic agent is then obtained from each member of both groups, and the rates of previous exposure are compared.

In Section 1.3 of the text, the contents of the denominator were said to provide the distinction between clinical and classic public health epidemiology. Using that distinction, which of these two domains is the proprietor of retrospective case control studies?

Exercise 1.2. Epidemiologists today engage in four types of activities that have received relatively little discussion in Chapter 1. Do you think these activities, which are described here, are part of classical or clinical epidemiology?

1.2.1. Clinics established at medical centers to give special attention to patients with occupation-associated diseases.

1.2.2. Seroepidemiologic surveys of children in different communities to analyze the results of antibodies for diverse infectious diseases.

1.2.3. Nosocomial epidemiologic studies to determine the transmission of infection to and among hospitalized patients.

1.2.4. "Detective-work" epidemiologic activities to determine the causes of such relatively new clinical illnesses as Legionnaire's disease, toxic shock syndrome, or AIDS (acquired immune deficiency syndrome).

CHAPTER REFERENCES

1. Paul, 1938; 2. Paul, 1958.

PART ONE

AN OVERVIEW OF RESEARCH ARCHITECTURE

The next five chapters contain a broad overview of the contents, methods, and results of clinical epidemiologic studies. They provide a classification for the research activities that challenge investigators who do the work and that confront readers who try to make sense of the results.

The research activities are divided into three main types: cause-effect evaluations, process evaluations, and descriptive studies. These early chapters in the text offer an outline of basic principles and standards for each type of research. The outline can be particularly helpful to a reader trying to decipher what appears in medical literature, but further details, to be presented in later chapters, are needed for a more profound or sophisticated understanding.

Chapter 2

A Classification of Medical Research

2.1. Possible Taxonomies for Medical Research
2.1.1. Eclectic Arrangement
2.1.2. Goal-oriented Arrangement
2.1.3. Group-oriented Arrangement
2.1.4. Architectural Arrangement
2.2. Basic Axes of Research Architecture
2.2.1. General Purpose: Descriptive or Comparative
2.2.1.1. Descriptive Research
2.2.1.2. Cause-Effect (Impact) Research
2.2.1.3. Process Research
2.2.2. Types of Agents: Procedures or Maneuvers
2.2.2.1. Process Procedures
2.2.2.2. Cause-Effect Maneuvers
2.2.3. Allocation of Agents: Experiment or Survey
2.2.4. Temporal Direction: Cross-Sectional or Longitudinal
2.2.5. Components of Groups: Homodemic or Heterodemic
2.3. Sequence of Presentation in Test
2.4. Synopsis

To arrive at an orderly scheme for discussing the epidemiologic methods of medical research, we need a taxonomy with which to classify the diverse activities that can take place. The candidates available as basic taxonomic choices are listed in the next section.

2.1. POSSIBLE TAXONOMIES FOR MEDICAL RESEARCH

Medical research can be classified in at least four different taxonomic arrangements, which might be labeled *eclectic, goal-oriented, group-oriented,* or *architectural.*

2.1.1. *Eclectic Arrangement*

In the eclectic approach, no specific scheme is used to classify the research. Each activity is simply cited according to the particular question that it answers. Thus, we might contemplate research projects intended to answer the following questions:

Is screening and/or the periodic health examination a worthwhile procedure?

Should we use the Salk or Sabin polio vaccine?

Are the potential medical benefits of nuclear magnetic resonance imaging worth its costs?

When a new physical finding is reported in a patient, is it really new?

Do oral contraceptive pills cause thromboembolism?

How is probability applied in genetic counseling?

Should major changes in diet be instituted to prevent atherosclerosis and, if so, at what age should these efforts begin?

Is surgery better than medical therapy for patients with coronary artery disease?

What is the best system of nomenclature for use in the diagnosis of psychiatric disorders?

Can nurse practitioners deliver a suitably high quality of primary health care?

Each of these questions can be discussed according to the type of evidence and reasoning needed to provide an answer. The discussions can then lead to more basic scientific and statistical issues in the research. The main advantage of the eclectic approach is that it provides immediate practical answers to immediate practical questions. The main disadvantage is that it does not lead to an organized, formal set of standards and procedures for either the creation or the analysis of individual projects.

2.1.2. *Goal-oriented Arrangement*

In the *goal-oriented* approach, the research is arranged according to certain goals that recur as issues to be resolved in the diverse aspects of the health sciences. Among such goals are the following:

Physiologic mechanisms

Pathophysiologic mechanisms

Risk-factor analysis

Range-of-normal determinations

Screening procedures

Diagnostic evaluations

Prognostic estimations

Pharmacokinetics

Therapeutic safety and efficacy

Quality control in data

Quality assurance in health care

This approach allows different types of research to be considered according to the general goals (and often according to the particular specialties) for which the research is employed. It has the advantage of providing a general outline within which eclectic issues can be considered. The main disadvantage is that no classification is provided for the different methods that can be used to assemble the people who compose the groups under investigation.

2.1.3. *Group-oriented Arrangement*

In the *group-oriented* approach, the research is catalogued according to the methods that created the particular composition of the groups of people under investigation. This classification would include groups organized as follows:

Randomized clinical trials

Surveys of therapy

Longitudinal cohort studies

Cross-sectional population surveys

Retrospective case-control studies

Other types of case-control studies

Hybrid arrangements of cases and controls

The group-oriented approach has the advantage of arranging the research according to the methods used for assembling the people under study. The disadvantage is that the goals of the projects are not noted.

2.1.4. *Architectural Arrangement*

An orientation toward both goals and groups can be achieved with the *architectural* classification, which will be employed here. The architectural approach is particularly powerful because the same kind of intellectual appraisal can be used to "dissect" the structure of several different types of research. An architectural arrangement also encourages the development, formation, and application of basic scientific principles and standards that are not readily perceived when the research is classified eclectically or when it is classified separately, according to goals or groups.

There are two main reasons for using the word *architecture* rather than *design* as a title for this approach. The first reason is that the word *design* has often become attached to the word *experimental* as a label for the plans of an investigation. Because most research in clinical epidemiology depends on observational data, not on experiments, the term *experimental design* is not only erroneous but can also be misleading if the premise of an experiment makes the investigator (or reader) neglect the many forms of bias that can distort the results of nonexperimental studies.

The second reason is that the word *design,* emanating from the world of art, carries no demands for reality or for function. An artist's design, like an abstract theoretic model, can be attractive and esthetically appealing, but it need not serve a real function or even correspond to any natural realities. An architect's structure, on the other hand, must have more than a design. The constructed entity must perform specific functions and must be adapted to the realities of nature. The word *architecture* is therefore used to describe the effort to create and evaluate research structures that have both the reproducible documentation of science and the elegant design of art.

2.2. **BASIC AXES OF RESEARCH ARCHITECTURE**

Before the architecture of research is discussed, the word *research* itself requires some attention. Because almost any thoughtful act of human scholarship can properly be regarded as research, the word is almost impossible to delineate, and the domain of research has almost no boundaries. A well-studied single patient, described in an enlightening case report, is an act of research; such a study (under certain circumstances) can even be the result of a designed experiment. Regardless of the purpose or structure of the work, the word *research* can properly be applied to systematic plans for discovering facts or principles in any field of knowledge. In most of the research to be considered here, the field of knowledge is clinical medicine, and the plans and discoveries refer to what is found medically in a group or groups of people.

The architecture of clinical research can be catalogued according to several separate axes of classification. Although each of these axes will be discussed later in greater detail, they are outlined in this section to help set a general framework for future discussion. The axes are based on ideas that refer to the purpose of the research, the type of agents under study, the allocation of agents, the number of temporal states, and the components of groups of data. Since these ideas must receive names to allow them to be discussed, the reader should be prepared to encounter some new terms or unfamiliar uses for old terms.

2.2.1. *General Purpose: Descriptive or Comparative*

The general purposes of research can be descriptive or comparative; the comparative purposes can be divided into evaluation of cause-effect relationships or of the quality of processes.

2.2.1.1. DESCRIPTIVE RESEARCH

Descriptive research provides collections of data that are used for purely descriptive reasons and sometimes as a background for policy decisions. No comparisons are conducted to draw conclusions about efficacy, quality, or any other accomplishments associated with the entities under study.

Descriptive studies are often used in health services research to provide information about costs and apparent needs for medical care. Thus, the individual capacity, clinical services, and expenses of maintenance might be described for the nursing homes in a particular geographic region. In clinical work, a frequently reported type of descriptive survey is a collection of data showing the spectrum of characteristics (such as age, symptoms, laboratory data, and so on) for a group (or series) of patients with a particular disease. Another kind of descriptive clinical survey is used to demarcate a range of normal for laboratory measurements or other data in a selected group of people. These descriptive clinical surveys often serve as reference background for discussions at medical conferences and for decisions about individual patients. A case report of interesting events noted in one or several patients is another commonly published type of descriptive study.

The results found in descriptive research are sometimes used later for comparative purposes. For example, the outcome of treatment A in a group of patients reported as a case series from one institution may later be compared with the results of treatment B reported in a case series from a different institution. Data assembled descriptively during the decennial census tabulations are also often used later for diverse forms of comparative research.

2.2.1.2. CAUSE-EFFECT (IMPACT) RESEARCH

In *cause-effect research,* specific comparisons are performed to draw conclusions (or obtain ideas) about the impact of a particular agent in producing certain changes. Studies of prevention, therapy, etiology, and pathogenesis of disease are almost always concerned with the effect of a causal agent.

No single word is readily available to replace the cumbersome *cause-effect* phrase as a label for this type of research. The word *analytic,* which is sometimes used by epidemiologists, has too many other connotations. The word *causal,* if used alone, may suggest research confined to etiology (i.e., cause) of disease, although studies of therapy are also concerned with the causal action, i.e., effect, of pharmaceutical substances, surgical operations, and other therapeutic interventions. If a single-word alternative is desired, perhaps the best term is *impact.* Thus, we can say that *impact research,* in contrast to the *process research* discussed in the next section, is concerned with the effects produced by an etiologic, pathogenetic, prophylactic, therapeutic, or other causal agent. In impact or cause-effect research, we focus on the changes that occur as outcomes after the intervention of the agent under scrutiny.

2.2.1.3. PROCESS RESEARCH

In *process* research, the comparison is concerned with the quality of either the product or the performance of a particular procedure. The procedure is not checked for any cause-effect impacts. We examine a product or a performance, not a change. Examples of process research for quality of a *product* are investigations of quality control in laboratory measurements; observer variability among clinicians, radiologists, and pathologists; the efficacy of diagnostic markers (such as the VDRL test for syphilis); and the construction and evaluation of new forms of clinical questionnaires and indexes. Examples of process research for quality of a *performance* are the evaluation of a physician's clinical competence and the diverse types of audit that constitute the research called *quality of care.*

2.2.2. *Types of Agents: Procedures or Maneuvers*

In both the cause-effect and process forms of comparative research, a particular agent is under investigation. In both forms of research, the basic event under scrutiny can be outlined as

$$\text{INITIAL STATUS} \xrightarrow{\text{AGENT}} \text{SUBSEQUENT EVENTS}$$

In cause-effect research, the agent is the intended or suspected cause of the effect noted as subsequent events. In process research, the subsequent events represent the performance or product of the agent under evaluation.

To have a suitable nomenclature for labeling these activities, we can use the term *agent* as a general title for the particular active entity under investigation. We can then give separate names to the agents employed in process research and in cause-effect research.

2.2.2.1. **PROCESS PROCEDURES**

For process research, the word *procedure* has already been used and seems quite satisfactory as a name for the investigated agent. With this label, the foregoing diagram would be drawn as follows for process research:

$$\text{INPUT} \xrightarrow{\text{PROCEDURE}} \text{OUTPUT}$$

The process would be represented by a combination of *procedure* and *output.* Thus, the process of measuring serum cholesterol consists of a chemical procedure that yields a numerical result for the level of serum cholesterol. The process of delivering health care for a patient with a sore throat consists of a procedure of clinical reasoning that yields a set of actions taken as diagnostic tests and therapy.

2.2.2.2. **CAUSE-EFFECT MANEUVERS**

For cause-effect research, an optimal word is difficult to find, because so many different kinds of entities can be contemplated as agents. A single word is particularly desirable for describing these entities, because the architectural model for cause-effect research provides a unified approach that encompasses both the traditional etiologic studies of epidemiology and the traditional therapeutic studies of clinical medicine.

The phrase *causal agent* is the most direct title for this idea, but it is not a single word and it could create confusion when applied to agents that do not etiologically cause disease. For example, if we want to study the prevention of poliomyelitis or the remedial treatment of congestive heart failure, it would seem strange to refer to the Sabin vaccine or diuretics as causal agents. A substitute term that might be used is *effector,* particularly because it suggests the idea of producing a change in the initial state of the recipient. A disadvantage of the word *effector,* however, is that certain agents contemplated as effectors may not actually produce an effect or change.

Of the available alternative terms, the most desirable seems to be *maneuver.* Despite the etymologic disadvantage of the meaning "to work by hand," the word maneuver does carry the connotation of an intention to produce change, and it seems generally better than either causal agent or effector. We shall therefore use *maneuver* as the name for the particular etiologic, therapeutic, demographic, or other entity that is contemplated, suspected, demonstrated, or intended to be responsible for producing a particular effect.

There are many different kinds of maneuvers, and they often lend their names to the research topics under study. The maneuver can be an allegedly noxious substance—such as atmospheric pollution, contaminated shellfish, cigarette smoking, a high-fat diet, or a slothful life style—that is believed to contribute, etiologically or pathogenetically, to development of a disease. It can also be a therapeutic entity—such as a medication, surgical operation, psychiatric technique, or physical substance (such as oxygen)—that is believed to exert a prophylactic or remedial action in disease.

The maneuver can even be a demographic attribute—such as race, gender, economic status, or educational background—that is regarded as affecting intelligence, economic achievement, or susceptibility to disease. Thus, if we state that women are more likely than men to develop urinary tract infections, the maneuver is the female gender. The maneuver can also be the personnel or fiscal system involved in purveying medical care. For example, in a clinical trial testing whether nurse practitioners are as capable as family physicians in providing primary medical care, the work of the nurse practitioners constitutes the principal maneuver under investigation.

With this concept, the basic architecture of a cause-effect study can be outlined as

$$\text{BASELINE STATE} \xrightarrow{\text{MANEUVER}} \text{OUTCOME}$$

The term *baseline state* rather than *initial state* is used here to help denote the differences, to be discussed in detail later, between the people whose initial state is contemplated for study and those who are actually entered into the research.

2.2.3. *Allocation of Agents: Experiment or Survey*

The word *experiment* is another term that is difficult to define. It is often used for any activity that is novel, regardless of whether the work has a planned comparison. For example, the first time that a newly developed drug is given to a human being, the work would probably be called an experiment, even though no controls or comparative groups are under study.

In common scientific usage, the term *experiment* is used for a planned cause-effect study in which the action of a particular maneuver is contrasted with the results of a comparative, or control, maneuver. Thus, a randomized controlled trial of therapy is an experiment; so is a physiologic study of the comparative urinary effects of saline infusion versus sulfate infusion in a healthy volunteer. The label of experiment could also be applied to a planned comparative investigation in process research. For example, to test observer variability among radiologists in the diagnosis of pulmonary embolism, we might arrange a special study in which a series of deliberately selected films are submitted (and later resubmitted) for blind, independent readings by each of the participating radiologists.

For many aspects of research architecture, the term *experiment* can be applied to a comparative study in which the investigator governs the allocation of the compared agents, assigning them according to a prearranged plan. This type of plan is used in many process studies of quality control or observer variability. In experimental research with therapeutic agents, the plan of allocation usually involves a randomized assignment of the maneuvers under comparison.

The investigator's ability to allocate the agents under comparison is one of the hallmarks that distinguishes an experiment from a *survey*. The latter term is customarily used for research projects in which the agents under comparison were not assigned according to an investigative plan. For example, in process research, data obtained under ordinary conditions of clinical practice may later be collected for an investigation of diagnostic markers. This type of study is a survey, not an experiment, because the investigator did not formally plan the strategy and sequence of arrangements for exposing each patient to the compared procedures, which are the diagnostic marker tests and the standard methods used to establish the diagnosis.

In studies of therapeutic agents, most of the published research has been conducted as surveys, not as experimental clinical trials. In regular clinical practice, treatment is assigned according to the individual patient-based judgments of the treating clinicians. At some point thereafter, an investigator may collect a series of patients who received treatment A and compare their results against those found in a series of patients who received treatment B. This type of survey has been the conventional method, before the advent of clinical trials, by which doctors evaluated the efficacy of therapy. Surveys of therapy are still commonly used today, however, and they are often the only method by which certain types of treatments can be evaluated.

Studies of etiologic agents have almost all been conducted as surveys, not as experiments, because such maneuvers as cigarette smoking, high-fat diet, and slothful living were self-selected by the recipients, not imposed by an investigative plan. Similarly, descriptive studies of natural growth and development in healthy people and of the clinical course of a disease are conducted as surveys, because the natural maneuvers were not deliberately assigned in a research plan.

2.2.4. *Temporal Direction: Cross-Sectional or Longitudinal*

The data that describe a group of people can represent observations made at one or more than one point in time for each person. For example, we can examine a group of people and summarize their average weight at the time of the examination. We can re-examine that same group of people a year later and note the average amount of weight they have gained (or lost) during the interval. We can continue re-examining these people annually for the next 10 years and determine the trend shown in their average weight during that decade. In each of these instances, the results could be reported in a single summary expression that cited average weight, average gain, or average trend. Nevertheless, despite the single summary expression, the results would cover a different number of temporal states. In the first instance, we needed to examine each patient once; in the second instance, we needed to follow the patients to note their condition at the time of a second examination a year later; in the third instance, the temporal data would extend through the initial state of each patient and a re-examined state at each annual interval in the subsequent decade.

As a name for studies in which the data for each person represent essentially one point in time for that person, we can use the term *cross-sectional*. The data in such studies do not refer to any changes that may occur subsequently. The idea of cross-sectional applies to a single temporal condition, regardless of the particular calendar dates on which the data were obtained for each person or each group. Thus, we might cross-sectionally note the presence or absence of retinopathy in members of a group of diabetic patients who were individually examined on different dates in the diabetic clinic. We also obtain cross-sectional data when we note, as a diagnostic test, a patient's response to some injected substance, such as ACTH. Although the response occurs after the ACTH injection, the data are cross-sectional because the injected substance is used to reveal the patient's condition, not to change it.

To refer to studies in which the people are followed forward in time, i.e., information regarding their condition is being obtained and analyzed at one or more subsequent occasions, the best word is *serial,* but *longitudinal* has already become well established for this purpose. Although not an optimal term, because it refers to geography rather than time and because an alternative argument could be offered for *latitudinal,* the use (or abuse) of *longitudinal* will be continued here to spare the reader any additional linguistic problems. To illustrate usage, in the first paragraph of this section the study of average weight at a single examination was cross-sectional. The studies of average weight gain and time trends in weight were longitudinal.

The word *cohort* is commonly used as a name for the group of people who are followed forward in a longitudinal study. In its original epidemiologic definition, a cohort consisted of a group of people who were all born in the same year or period of years,[1] but the word is too valuable to be so restricted. In contemporary usage, a cohort consists of a group of people followed longitudinally forward in time from some mutually common event, such as birth, entrance into college, exposure to an etiologic agent, establishment of a diagnosis, or receipt of treatment for a disease. Cohort is now used so often for this purpose that it regularly appears as an adjective, with *longitudinal studies* being called *cohort studies.*

Longitudinal (or cohort) research is usually much more difficult to do than cross-sectional research. After a single examination of each person, the investigator has the data needed for a cross-sectional study, but a longitudinal study carries the extra burden of making arrangements to follow each person and collect data at stipulated intervals thereafter. Most forms of descriptive research are cross-sectional, but descriptive studies of the natural history or clinical course of different medical conditions are longitudinal. For example, research conducted to indicate the post-therapeutic outcome of a group of patients with cancer is longitudinal; research that describes the presenting manifestations of the patients at the time treatment was instituted is cross-sectional. Some studies have both cross-sectional and longitudinal components. Thus, the spectrum-of-disease surveys that were noted earlier often contain cross-sectional descriptions of the condition of the patients on admission to the hospital, and longitudinal descriptions of what happened afterward in the patients' clinical courses.

Because cross-sectional investigations are so relatively easy to do, they are often used for cause-effect studies of the etiology of disease. For example, to investigate longitudinally whether reserpine therapy causes breast cancer, we would have to do an enormous study, assembling thousands of reserpine takers and thousands of non–reserpine takers, following both groups for many years to determine the subsequent occurrence (or nonoccurrence) of breast cancer in the two groups. To investigate this same question cross-sectionally, we could get an answer much more quickly and from much smaller groups of people. We would do a retrospective case-control study, assembling about 100 to 200 cases of people with breast cancer and a similar number of controls without breast cancer. We would ask the members of each group about their previous exposure to reserpine and then compare the rates of exposure in the two groups.

The simplicity of this case-control approach has made it highly appealing to epidemiologists interested in studying etiology of chronic disease, but the inversion of customary scientific logic in the retrospective architecture creates many problems that will be discussed later. The point to be noted now is that research studies can contain longitudinal or cross-sectional data and that cross-sectional studies are often used as a substitute for longitudinal research.

2.2.5. *Components of Groups: Homodemic or Heterodemic*

When data are summarized in a quotient, such as a mean, proportion, or rate, the numerator and denominator of the quotient may come from the same group or from different groups. In all forms of laboratory research and in all forms of research with which most clinicians are familar, the same people who are counted in the denominator are also accounted for in the numerator. For example, if we say that the one-year survival rate of a group of people is 60% (9/15), the numerator has accounted for the one-year survival status of all 15 people who appeared in the denominator: 9 were alive and 6 were dead. If we say that the group had a mean survival time of 14.7 months, everyone is also accounted for. The numerator used to calculate this mean contains the sum of values for survival time of each person, and the denominator consists of the 15 people in the group.

The name *homodemic* (i.e., the same people) refers to the type of research data in which each person who appears in a denominator is also cited in the numerator. This type of information is so expected and so common in scientific research that its absence warrants special attention. Many quotients cited in public health epidemiologic research are *hetero-demic* (different people). The same individuals who appear in the denominator are not necessarily all accounted for in the numerator. For example, when we see a statement that the mortality rate for people in the city of New Haven in 1970 was 11 per thousand, the components of this rate are a denominator of 137,707 people, determined during the census tabulation of 1970, and a numerator of 1530 deaths that were reported to the state health department. The 137,707 people who appear in the denominator are not individually accounted for in the numerator. We did not check each person's status at the end of the year and determine whether that person was alive or dead. Some of the denominator people may have moved away, so that we have no idea of their status, and some of the numerator people listed among those who died may not have been present (or alive) in New Haven when the census was taken.

The formation of a heterodemic quotient, using data from two different sources and comprising results from two different groups, is a common tactic in classical epidemiology. The tactic provides all of the general population rates of mortality, nativity, fertility, and so on, for which epidemiology is traditionally famous.

One quick way to determine whether a particular project (or set of data) is homodemic or heterodemic is to ask what is the basic unit of investigation in the research. In homodemic research, the basic unit is a person. All the pertinent data describing that person can be recorded in a single medium of storage, which can be a questionnaire, case report form, punched card, magnetic tape, or other format. The investigator assembles the results of the research by processing the data stored in the format for each individual person, and all the pertinent information under analysis is located in those individual formats.

In heterodemic research, the basic unit is a group of data collected by or submitted to commercial organizations, health agencies, or governmental institutions. These different groups of data provide numbers for the sales of products, indexes of commodity consumption, and occurrence rates of disease that are usually associated to form the heterodemic statistics. In such studies, all the pertinent information under analysis could not be recorded in a *single* format for each individual person.

2.3. **SEQUENCE OF PRESENTATION IN TEXT**

Each of the basic features just described— in purpose, agents, allocation, temporal states, and group components—could be used as the main axis on which to build a further discussion of investigative methods. Because the rest of the methodologic decisions usually depend on a project's purpose, the comparative and descriptive goals of research will be the first topics to be presented for additional discussion.

Regardless of whether a comparative study is concerned with evaluating a process or an impact, certain basic scientific principles can be stipulated for the comparison. The next chapter will be devoted to these principles, which apply to any type of comparative research.

2.4. **SYNOPSIS**

Of the diverse classifications that might be used for medical research, the architectural arrangement has the advantage of allowing the goals of the research and the component parts to be noted simultaneously. The architectural arrangements can be catalogued as follows: the purpose of the research can be descriptive or comparative; the agents under study can be processes evaluated for quality or maneuvers evaluated for cause-effect impacts; the allocated agents may be investigated in an experiment or survey; the temporal status of the observations can be cross-sectional or longitudinal; and the groups under investigation can have homodemic or heterodemic components.

Despite the different goals of process research and cause-effect research, both activities involve acts of comparison for which certain basic scientific principles can be established. The principles will be discussed in the next chapter.

EXERCISES

Exercise 2.1. For the impending 20th postgraduate reunion of college classmates, an epidemiology-oriented member of the class has obtained suitable consent to do the research studies described in the list that follows. Please classify each of these studies as cross-sectional or longitudinal and as homodemic or heterodemic.

2.1.1. From responses to questionnaires sent to all members of the class, a profile of the class will be prepared, showing current average income, marital and family status, and "happiness quotient."

2.1.2. From data on file at the college, the income status of each graduate's family when she or he began college will be related to the graduate's current income level.

2.1.3. The subjects in which each graduate began to major in college will be related to the family's income level when the graduate entered college and also to the graduate's current income level.

2.1.4. The subjects in which each graduate majored in college will be related to any deaths noted in the class since graduation.

2.1.5. The current income level of the graduates will be related to whether they actually attended the 20th reunion and also to their later presence or absence at the 30th reunion.

2.1.6. From data supplied by the college, the proportion of each appropriate class attending alumni reunions during each of the past 10 years will be obtained and will be related to the gross national product during each year.

Exercise 2.2. The material that follows contains excerpts of summaries for 11 research projects published in clinical literature. On the basis of the descriptions contained in these summaries, classify each project as impact (i.e., cause-effect), process, or descriptive; experiment or survey; cross-sectional or longitudinal; and homodemic or heterodemic.

2.2.1. *Human Placental Lactogen: The Watchdog of Fetal Distress.* Human placental lactogen measured in the last trimester of pregnancy has been used as a screening test to indicate fetal distress, neonatal asphyxia, or dysmaturity after an apparently normal pregnancy. There is a 56% chance of perinatal complications if the hormone concentration has been in the fetal danger zone (more than two standard deviations below normal) on at least one occasion.

2.2.2. *Epidemiologic Evidence for Two Types of Trigeminal Neuralgia.* Patients with trigeminal neuralgia and healthy control subjects were compared to determine whether several risk factors for trigeminal neuralgia were related specifically to the anatomic divisions of the trigeminal nerve. The vertical location of the pain was strongly related to age at diagnosis. Non-Jewish religion was primarily a risk factor for trigeminal neuralgia of the lower face (any third-division involvement), whereas non-drinking and non-smoking were risk factors for trigeminal neuralgia of the upper face (no third-division involvement). The epidemiologic evidence suggests that different etiologic mechanisms may operate for trigeminal neuralgia of the lower face and upper face.

2.2.3. *Fibrinolytic Activity and Postoperative Deep-Vein Thrombosis.* Ninety-five patients undergoing gynecologic operations were studied in a double-blind trial to assess the effects of phenformin and ethylestrenol, given for four weeks, on the incidence of postoperative deep-vein thrombosis (DVT). Forty-five patients received phenformin and ethylestrenol and 50 patients received placebo preparations. Although phenformin and ethylestrenol produced a significant shortening of the dilute blood clot–lysis time, there was no difference in the incidence of DVT in the two groups of patients.

2.2.4. *Leukocyte Electrolytes in Cardiac and Noncardiac Patients Receiving Diuretics.* In 18 patients with heart disease receiving diuretics and digitalis, the sodium and water content of leukocytes was significantly increased. The content of potassium and its concentration in cell water were significantly reduced, indicating an absolute intracellar potassium deficiency. Leukocyte sodium content exceeded potassium content in two cases. Ten patients without heart disease who were receiving diuretics had normal leukocyte sodium and water content. In this noncardiac group, leukocyte potassium content averaged 353 mEq. per kg. dry solids compared with a mean of 377 mEq. per kg. dry solids in 59 control subjects, but this difference did not achieve significance. However, a few noncardiac patients taking diuretics had very low leukocyte potassium content. The results suggest that the intracellular electrolyte abnormalities in the cardiac patients were associated more with the heart disease than with its treatment, although diuretics may increase the potassium deficiency.

2.2.5. *Are There Safer Hypnotics than Barbiturates?* The mortality associated with prescribing barbiturates and nitrazepam has been compared. Because deaths from poisoning are enumerated annually by the National Center for Health Statistics, the deaths associated with barbiturates or nitrazepam can be determined from this list. The number of prescriptions issued annually for these substances was estimated from a random sampling of pharmacists who kept special files of data. For a six-year period, the numbers of deaths in which these drugs were implicated and the death rate per million prescriptions for each drug were respectively 12,354 and 133 for barbiturates and 90 and 13 for nitrazepam. The evidence suggests that nitrazepam is a safer drug than barbiturates.

2.2.6. *Antenatal Diagnosis of Neural-Tube Defects Using Cerebrospinal Fluid Proteins.* Diagnosis of an anencephalic fetus has been confirmed by immunologic detection of β-trace protein of cerebrospinal fluid in amniotic fluid. In 75 control amniotic fluid samples, a precipitin reaction to β-trace protein could not be demonstrated. It is suggested that this method may serve as a reliable specific index of neural-tube defects.

2.2.7. *Urea Treatment of Skin Malignancies.* One hundred twelve patients with basal or squamous cell skin carcinomas were treated with urea. During the first two years, treatment consisted of injections of urea solution around the lesion, and 73% of the patients definitely benefited. In the third year, treatment was modified by combining injections of urea with scraping off and treatment of the traumatized surface with urea powder. In this way, definite benefit reached 91%. Despite very good results with the conventional therapeutic methods, urea treatment is thought to be valuable because of its simplicity, superior cosmetic results, and absence of side effects.

2.2.8. *Mortality and Anemia in Women.* Mortality over a three-year period has been related to hematocrit readings in 18,740 women examined in several hematologic surveys. There is evidence of a small increase in mortality in anemic subjects and of a distinct increase in mortality in subjects with hematocrit levels above about 46%. In the more anemic women, a higher than expected proportion of deaths were due to neoplasms, but there was a clear deficiency in the proportion of deaths due to cardiovascular disease.

2.2.9. *Variation in the Interpretation of Radiographic Change in Pulmonary Disease.* Series of chest films from five patients being treated for tuberculosis or sarcoidosis were presented in the correct chronologic sequence to a panel of five interpreters. Several weeks later, the panel read the films again, but this time the chronologic order had been reversed without the knowledge of the panel. As an earlier study had shown for pneumoconiosis, the assessment of radiographic change in tuberculosis and sarcoidosis was influenced by the assumed chronologic sequence of the serial films.

2.2.10. *Liver Scans and the Detection of Clinically Unsuspected Liver Metastases.* To determine the value of radioisotope liver imaging in the preoperative assessment of patients with treatable cancer, liver images were obtained in 46 patients with carcinoma of the large bowel who did not have hepatomegaly. At operation or necropsy, eight (17%) were proved to have hepatic metastases, and liver scans detected seven of these. The technique gave a correct answer in 44 patients, giving an overall accuracy of 95%. This evidence implies that liver imaging is useful in the preoperative assessment of patients with cancer, even if the liver is clinically normal.

2.2.11. *Plasma-Prolactin in Human Breast Cancer.* Plasma prolactin was assayed in 115 patients with breast cancer and 115 matched controls. Mean plasma prolactin levels were 6.0 ± 3.7 ng. per ml. and 5.9 ± 2.9 ng. per ml., respectively. Plasma levels in 64 members of nine families with a high frequency of breast cancer were irregularly distributed, with a mean prolactin level of 10.4 ± 8.1 ng. per ml. Statistical evaluation demonstrated that breast cancer patients and controls may be regarded as one population but that the prolactin levels in the high-risk group represent a different population ($P < 0.0004$).

Exercise 2.3. An investigator coming to you for help in planning research wants to test the idea that breast feeding in infancy helps prevent schizophrenia in later life. Without evaluating the worthiness or importance of the research, without worrying about the determinations of *breast feeding* or *schizophrenia,* and without concern for the feasibility or validity of any project you may design, name and briefly outline three different architectural structures that could be used for this research project.

Exercise 2.4. In a group of patients with omphalosis who were admitted to the clinical research center and who gave informed consent for the research, the investigators are testing the effect of a sodium sulfate infusion on renal blood flow. After baseline measurements of renal blood flow, each patient is randomly assigned to receive either a sodium sulfate infusion or a normal saline infusion. After the infusion, renal blood flow is measured again. After resting for two hours, the patient then receives another baseline measurement of renal blood flow, following which the alternative agent is infused (i.e., those who previously received sulfate get saline and vice versa). After this second infusion, renal blood flow is measured again and the investigation is concluded. Classify this research according to the format used in Exercise 2.2.

Exercise 2.5. A practicing physician, who specializes in the care of patients with diabetes mellitus, has assembled data about the effects of different forms of treatment on the patients seen in his practice. He prepared a report of his results and submitted it for publication, but the work was rejected by the *Journal of Prestigious Medicine* because the treatments were not compared in an experimental trial. Having read the description of an experiment in the fourth paragraph of Section 2.2.3, the physician now claims that his work is really experimental.

He says that he has made advance arrangements for collecting high-quality data in each patient, and he has a specific advance plan for assigning treatments. He assigns diet alone to diabetic patients who fulfill certain stipulated criteria, oral hypoglycemic agents to patients who fulfill other criteria, insulin for yet other criteria, and so on. His devoted patients accept all of his recommendations, carry them out with a high degree of compliance, and appear faithfully for his frequent examinations during long-term care. He has tabulated the data for development of vascular complications in the treated groups, and he has drawn conclusions about the merits of the treatment associated with the lowest rate of complications.

He is incensed by the rejection of his careful experimental studies and he wants you, as a clinical epidemiologist, to help compose the letter with which he will protest the unjust criticisms received from the *J. Prest. Med.* What would you advise him to do?

CHAPTER REFERENCE

1. Frost, 1939.

Chapter 3

Principles of Comparative Research

Comparison is one of the hallmarks of scientific activity, and an investigation that involves comparison is what most people think of as *research*. For cause-effect studies, the comparison is conducted when the results obtained from a particular maneuver are contrasted against those from some other maneuver, which is often called the *control*.

This is the type of comparison that is contemplated for decisions about the etiologic agents, pathogenetic mechanisms, risk factors, prognostic factors, prophylactic interventions, remedial therapy, or other maneuvers (such as health care systems) whose impact is studied in cause-effect investigations. In process research, the quality of a procedure is evaluated by comparison with either a selected *standard* or with some other performance of the same procedure. Processes are compared during investigations of observer variability, quality control in laboratory data, diagnostic and spectral marker tests, audits of clinical care, and other types of research devoted to the quality of a product or a performance, rather than to the change created by an intervention.

This chapter is concerned with four fundamental principles, applicable to both cause-effect and process research, that are used in planning comparative research, in evaluating its accomplishments, and in determining whether the results will successfully answer the questions asked by either the investigator or the reviewer. The principles refer to the basic objective of the research, the strategy of comparison, the suitability of individual components, and the similarity of compared components. The principles are merely outlined and summarized in this chapter. They will all receive extensive discussion later.

3.1. THE BASIC OBJECTIVE

In both process research and cause-effect research, the basic reasoning involves the idea that an object is acted upon by an agent, which can be called the *principal agent,* to distinguish it from any others that may be under study. The proposed action of the principal agent can be shown in the following diagram:

$$\text{INITIAL STATE} \xrightarrow{\text{PRINCIPAL AGENT}} \text{SUBSEQUENT EVENT(S)}$$

This type of diagram should be immediately familiar to readers who have already encountered its analog as a scientific "portrait" that shows the action of the agents considered in physics or chemistry. In addition to its symbolism, the diagram helps indicate that the events studied in clinical epidemiology can be approached with the same reasoning used in other branches of science.

Although the same diagram pertains to both process research and cause-effect research, the two types of research have different goals. In process research, we evaluate quality; in cause-effect research, we determine change. In cause-effect (or impact) research, we examine the subsequent events to note the change that may have occurred in the initial state of the object that received the agent. The initial object is still recognizable when the outcome is examined. Thus, after the intervention of a particular maneuver, we may want to know whether the patient was alive or dead; diseased or free of disease; feeling better or worse; or having lower or higher values for blood pressure or blood glucose.

In process research, however, the object that provides the input for the initial state completes its main job after it is entered into the procedure. What is examined subsequently as the output of the procedure may be something totally different. Thus, the input may be a specimen of serum, and the output may be a number denoting magnitude of glucose concentration; or the input may be a patient with urinary symptoms, and the output may be a series of decisions and actions carried out by a physician.

Regardless of whether the comparative research is devoted to a cause-effect impact or the action of a process, the basic objective of the research can be outlined by noting the three main components of the basic diagram: the initial state, the principal agent, and the subsequent event(s). A quick way of determining the main components of the basic objective is to answer the question, "What is being done to what (or whom) to produce what goal or result?" When the answer is given, the specifications should be clear enough to provide a reasonable idea of the three ingredients needed to draw the basic diagram. "What is being done" is the principal agent. "To what (or whom)" is the initial state of the recipient. "What goal or result" is the subsequent events.

The outline of the basic objective is somewhat analogous to the *chief complaint* that a clinician elicits when taking a history from a patient. Just as the chief complaint (when suitably stated) allows the clinician to focus on the cogent features that provoke the patient's request for medical care, the statement of the objective provides a prompt, succinct idea of what is under study in the research. Until this outline has been formally specified, neither the investigator nor the reader can clearly determine what requires attention.

For example, if an investigator says, "We want to do a study of people with headaches," the reader cannot tell whether the headaches are potentially an initial state, an agent, or a subsequent event. If the investigator says, "We want to determine what causes Reye's syndrome," we can assume that Reye's syndrome is the subsequent state for persons who were initially healthy and that one or more not-yet-specified substances will be considered as the principal causal agent(s). If the investigator's statement is "We want to determine whether surgery is better than medical therapy for patients with coronary disease," we know the initial state (coronary disease), the principal agent (surgery), and even the comparative agent (medical therapy), but we cannot complete the diagram because we do not know what subsequent event(s) will be checked for "better than." If we are told that the subsequent event is survival three years later, we have learned all three components of the objective.

Even when all of these components are known, however, we may not be sure about many important details of the research. In the project just cited, we do not yet know exactly what kind of patients will be treated (those with stable angina pectoris, unstable angina pectoris, antecedent myocardial infarction, and so on), what kind of surgery will be used (talc poudrage, tunnel implant, bypass graft), or what will constitute medical therapy (beta blockers, antiplatelet agents, anticoagulants). Nevertheless, the stated objective provides a reasonably clear general idea of what the investigator wants to do in the research. If the opening statement was "We'd like to help people with heart trouble," the idea would not be as clear, and, in fact, we really would not know what the investigator had in mind.

Similarly, if the investigator says, "We want to evaluate the accuracy of radiologists in making the diagnosis of pulmonary embolism from plain chest films," we have an excellent idea of the basic goal of the process research, and we can draw the complete basic diagram. The initial state is a plain chest film; the principal agent is a radiologist's examination of the chest film; and the subsequent event is a decision regarding the presence or absence of pulmonary embolism. With this particular stated objective, we can even have a good idea of the comparative (or standard) agent. It is a definitive diagnostic procedure to which the patient is (or was) subjected. We might not know what kinds of chest films are to be chosen for what kinds of patients, what will be the definitive diagnostic procedure, or what kind of scale will be used to express the radiologist's decisions, but the basic structure of the research is clear. We would have no idea of what is planned in the research if the investigator had said, "We want to expose the deluded overconfidence of our radiologic colleagues."

The basic objective of a research project is expected to provide an outline but not to include all the details needed to implement the outline and to describe the working plans of the research. Analogously, a patient's *chief complaint* is not expected to contain all of the details that will be assembled later in the account of the *present illness*. The outline of the research objective should have just enough information to provide a clear indication of the general target. The detailed plans that sharpen the picture of the target and provide the operating specifications for the research will be developed later.

3.2. THE STRATEGY OF COMPARISON

The basic objective of a research project in clinical epidemiology can often be formulated with relatively little scientific imagination or insight. In many instances, the three components that constitute the main question to be answered are made clearly evident by diverse issues that have already become medically prominent. For example, it takes no particular cunning to ask questions about the value of percutaneous transluminal angioplasty for patients with coronary disease, to wonder about the advantages of diagnostic images formed with nuclear magnetic resonance imaging, or to be concerned about the possible carcinogenicity of food preservatives.

A great deal of scientific insight and strategy are required, however, to choose a suitable comparative agent as the next main component of the research objective. Two different decisions are required: a selection of the particular agent(s) to be compared and a plan for allocating the principal and comparative agents to their recipients. If these two fundamental decisions are unsatisfactory, the rest of the research may be unacceptable, no matter how well the additional activities are carried out. For example, if the comparative agent for percutaneous transluminal angioplasty is medical therapy rather than surgical bypass grafting, many clinicians may reject the results of the study, claiming that the wrong question was answered. If the angioplasty is compared with bypass grafting but the comparison was conducted as a survey using routine observational data, many readers may reject the results, claiming that only a randomized experimental trial would yield scientifically credible data. These two decisions—choosing and allocating the comparative agent—are so important that they will receive extensive discussion later. The main point to be noted in the outline now is that the way in which these decisions are made, at this early stage in planning the research, can threaten the success of everything that follows thereafter.

3.2.1. *The Comparative Agent*

The choice of the comparative agent is particularly important because it determines what conclusion can be drawn in the research. Suppose we want to determine the impact of pharmaceutical agent X in the treatment of disease D. Do we compare agent X with no treatment, a placebo, or an alternative active agent? Each of these comparisons can be quite legitimate, but each will lead to different conclusions when the study is completed. If we decide to compare X with no treatment, we may not be able to tell afterward whether agent X really works or whether the physician's charisma while administering agent X was responsible for the patient's improvement. If we choose a placebo, we may not answer the more compelling questions of practitioners who want to know whether X is better than existing therapy. If we find that agent X produced results similar to an alternative "active" agent, we may wonder whether both X and the alternative agent were really effective or ineffective, because we do not know how the compared patients would have fared without active treatment.

In studying a measurement performed by process A, we can determine its agreement when compared with the result of process B, but we cannot decide about accuracy or acceptability unless process B happens to be the accepted standard. Thus, suppose we compare the diagnoses of pulmonary embolism made by two radiologists examining a series of plain films of the chest. The comparison would indicate the observer variability of the radiologists, but we could not determine how often each radiologist was right or wrong unless we had some other indication of each patient's true status for the presence or absence of pulmonary embolism.

After a comparative agent has been chosen, its action can be portrayed with the same type of diagram used for the principal agent:

$$\text{INITIAL STATE} \xrightarrow{\text{COMPARATIVE AGENT}} \text{SUBSEQUENT EVENTS}$$

3.2.2. *Comparative Diagrams*

In using the diagrams that show the research idea, we seldom have only a single person in mind. Instead, we think about the group of people (or other objects) who received the principal agent or the comparative agent. If each group is shown with the circles that are customarily used to portray "sets" in symbolic logic, the comparison would be shown more vividly as follows:

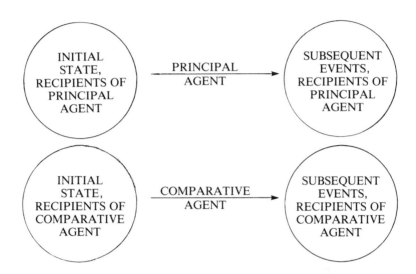

Although symbolically accurate, this type of portrait is cumbersome to use. By assuming that INITIAL STATE and SUBSEQUENT EVENTS refer to a group, rather than an individual, and by recognizing that the designated initial states and subsequent events will always be associated with the recipients of the designated agents, we can avoid the circles and the repetition of terms. The comparative diagrams can then be simplified as follows:

$$\text{INITIAL STATE} \xrightarrow{\text{PRINCIPAL AGENT}} \text{SUBSEQUENT EVENTS}$$

$$\text{INITIAL STATE} \xrightarrow{\text{COMPARATIVE AGENT}} \text{SUBSEQUENT EVENTS}$$

We can simplify things even further by assuming that the two compared groups are similar in their initial states and in the identification of their subsequent states. As discussed later, this assumption about similarity of initial states and subsequent events may not always be justified. In fact, unrecognized disparities in the compared initial and subsequent conditions are a common source of bias in comparative research. Nevertheless, for convenience in illustration, we shall make this assumption. It then allows us to use a single, simple diagram to show the comparison performed in the research:

$$\text{INITIAL STATE} \left\{ \begin{array}{c} \xrightarrow{\text{PRINCIPAL AGENT}} \\ \xrightarrow{\text{COMPARATIVE AGENT}} \end{array} \right\} \text{SUBSEQUENT EVENTS}$$

This type of basic comparative diagram, which will be used repeatedly throughout this text, offers a straightforward, easy way to cite a research project's augmented basic objective. The four items noted in the diagram indicate the three main components of the basic objective, augmented by the comparative agent.

For example, in the comparison mentioned earlier for bypass grafting versus transluminal angioplasty, the diagram could be as follows:

$$\text{CORONARY HEART DISEASE} \left\{ \begin{array}{c} \dfrac{\text{BYPASS GRAFT(S)}}{} \rightarrow \\ \dfrac{\text{TRANSLUMINAL}}{\text{ANGIOPLASTY}} \rightarrow \end{array} \right\} \text{SURVIVAL AT THREE YEARS}$$

The comparison of observer variability for two radiologists would be shown as:

$$\text{PLAIN CHEST FILMS} \left\{ \begin{array}{c} \dfrac{\text{RADIOLOGIST A}}{} \rightarrow \\ \dfrac{}{\text{RADIOLOGIST B}} \rightarrow \end{array} \right\} \begin{array}{c} \text{DIAGNOSIS} \\ \text{OF} \\ \text{PULMONARY} \\ \text{EMBOLISM} \end{array}$$

If we were comparing the diagnosis of one of the radiologists against a definitive standard, such as pulmonary arteriography, the diagram would be:

$$\text{APPROPRIATE CHEST FILMS} \left\{ \begin{array}{c} \dfrac{\text{RADIOLOGIST A}}{\text{(PLAIN CHEST FILMS)}} \rightarrow \\ \dfrac{\text{RADIOLOGIST B}}{\text{(ARTERIOGRAPHY)}} \rightarrow \end{array} \right\} \begin{array}{c} \text{DIAGNOSIS} \\ \text{OF} \\ \text{PULMONARY} \\ \text{EMBOLISM} \end{array}$$

When more than two agents are compared in the same study, the diagram can easily be augmented to show the additional comparisons. Thus, if a medically treated group were included in the previously cited comparison of treatments for coronary disease, the diagram would become:

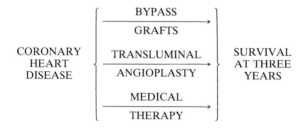

3.2.3. *Allocation of the Agents*

The allocation of the compared agents will determine whether the study is being conducted as a planned experiment or as an analytic survey of observed events. Thus, to compare agent X with standard agent Y, we can either allocate the agents in a special preplanned assignment to conduct an experimental trial, or we can analyze the results obtained when X and Y were allocated by the judgments used in the ordinary circumstances of clinical practice.

In experimental studies of therapeutic agents, randomization is the customary method used to allocate the compared agents. When randomization has occurred, it can be shown in the diagram with an additional symbol, as follows:

$$
\begin{array}{c}
\text{PRINCIPAL} \\
\text{AGENT} \longrightarrow \\[-2pt]
\text{INITIAL}\Big\} \!\!-\!\! \textcircled{R} \qquad\qquad \Big\{ \begin{array}{l}\text{SUBSEQUENT}\\ \text{EVENTS}\end{array} \\
\text{STATE} \\[-2pt]
\text{COMPARATIVE} \longrightarrow \\
\text{AGENT}
\end{array}
$$

Randomized allocation is seldom used in process research and is seldom possible in cause-effect research concerned with etiologic rather than therapeutic agents.

3.3. SUITABILITY OF INDIVIDUAL COMPONENTS

In Section 3.2.1, we briefly considered the problems produced by an unsuitable choice of comparative agent. Other major issues in suitability arise for each of the four individual components of the augmented objective: the initial state, the principal and comparative agents, and the subsequent event(s). These issues refer to the suitability with which each component was initially chosen and to the way the components were operationally specified and cogently maintained when the initial plan was implemented. Since suitability, like beauty, is often in the eye of the beholder, the brief discussion here will deal with the items that are considered rather than with criteria for making the decisions.

3.3.1. *Basic Choices*

The suitability of basic choices refers to the appropriate selection of the components included in the basic objective. The concept of *suitability* applies not only to an appropriate selection of principal and comparative agents, but also to appropriate choices of initial states and subsequent events. For example, if we decide to study the treatment of disease D in men, this selection of an initial state may make the results unsuitable for application to women. If death (or survival) is chosen as the only subsequent event to be noted, the results will not be suitable for determining relief of symptoms or other features of quality of life.

3.3.2. *Operational Detail*

When the basic plan of the research is implemented, each of the four main components must be suitably specified with details that will allow other people (investigators or readers) to recognize exactly what was done and to be able, if desired, to repeat the work. Although the achievement of suitability in operational details will be reserved for later discussion, the specification must provide such information as: exactly what kinds of patients will be admitted; how their qualifying characteristics will be identified; what mechanism will be used to conduct the randomization or to choose the people entered in a nonrandomized study; and how the subsequent events will be detected.

A suitably chosen set of basic components can often be rendered unsatisfactory by inadequate attention to operational details; conversely, the work spent in creating a splendid set of operational specifications may be wasted because the basic components are not appropriate.

3.3.3. *Cogent Maintenance*

Suitability in cogent maintenance refers to the actual conduct of the activities planned during or after administration of the compared agents. Each of the compared agents should be administered with suitable proficiency. For example, if the principal agent is an intricate surgical procedure, it should be (or should have been) performed by an appropriately skillful surgical team. If the comparative agent is a drug requiring a flexible dosage that is regulated for each recipient, the agent may lose suitable proficiency if it is given in a fixed dosage to help maintain double-blind observations. If the chest films or the viewboxes that illuminate them are of poor technical quality, the observer variability of the radiologists will not be suitably evaluated.

Another aspect of cogent maintenance refers to preservation of the group of people under investigation. For example, if large segments of the original cohort are lost to follow-up in a longitudinal study, the results found in those who remain may be seriously distorted, despite statistical efforts at adjusting the data.

A third feature of suitability in maintenance refers to the avoidance of undesirable changes in the original specifications for initial state or subsequent events when the research data are analyzed. Thus, the investigators may find, after the study is done, that the collected data about congestive heart failure were unsatisfactory. Because satisfactory information is available about usage of digitalis, however, it may then be substituted, unsuitably, to denote congestive heart failure.

3.4. **SIMILARITY OF COMPARED COMPONENTS**

A fundamental principle of scientific comparison can be expressed with the doctrine of *ceteris paribus,* i.e., all other things being equal. Thus, when we find different results in a contrast of treatment A versus treatment B, our decision that the difference is caused by distinctions in the action of the two treatments would be justified only if all other aspects of the contrast are essentially equal. To achieve these equalities, the initial states should be similar for the groups of people receiving treatments A and B; both treatments should be administered with similar proficiency; the two groups of people should be maintained with similar types of observation; and the subsequent events in both groups should be discerned with similar methods and criteria for detection.

Although an essential requirement for any scientific comparison of agents, this principle of *fairness* or *similarity in contrasts* is often neglected when evaluations are conducted. We usually concentrate on the immediate statistical results of the contrasted agents and we seldom pay close attention to similarity of initial states, similar detection of subsequent events, and similar proficiency in administration of agents when we compare three-year survival rates of medical versus surgical therapy for coronary disease or when we cite indexes of accuracy for the radiologist versus the definitive diagnostic procedure in identifying pulmonary embolism from a plain chest film.

For the conclusions to be fair, however, all of the component elements used in the basic structure of the research must also be fairly compared. This fairness requires that the basic components be chosen, identified, or utilized with reasonable similarity on both sides of the comparison. If these features of similarity are neglected or otherwise lost, the subsequent comparison of results may be distorted by bias. Agent X may yield better results than agent Y not because X is really better but because it was given to patients with better prognoses or maintained with better compliance. Radiologist A may seem more accurate than radiologist B not because of greater professional prowess but because B worked with an inferior lighting system when reviewing the films.

3.5. JUDGMENTAL DECISIONS AND SCIENTIFIC PRINCIPLES

Although the scientific principles just described can be applied to any type of comparative research, the application will affect different aspects of the way the research is interpreted, and different evaluators may apply different standards for the interpretations. These differences will occur as individual distinctions in judgment for problems in suitability and similarity, for issues in establishing policy rather than evaluating comparative research, and for the sometimes opposing approaches used by an investigator and a reviewer.

3.5.1. *Problems in Suitability and Similarity*

The problems of suitability and similarity, as outlined in Sections 3.3 and 3.4, can have two different effects on the basic credibility of comparative research. Bias in similarity leads to distorted comparison and thus affects the credibility of the comparison. Problems in suitability lead to inappropriate activities and thus affect the acceptance, pertinence, or application of the results. A study that was conducted with a magnificently fair comparison may be useless in clinical practice because the initial state, the compared agents, or the subsequent events were chosen unsuitably. A study that was perfectly suitable for issues in clinical practice may be scientifically useless because the comparisons were badly biased.

Decisions about suitability will often be judgmental rather than scientific. The decisions will reflect different beliefs about what is important and different choices of research objectives. Thus, one evaluator may believe that a particular agent is not worth testing, that a particular disease is too uncommon to warrant large expenditures of investigative energy, that data about symptoms or quality of life are too "soft" to receive serious scientific attention, or that a presumably active therapeutic agent should always be compared against an inert agent, such as placebo. A second evaluator, holding opposing beliefs about each of these issues, may reach opposite conclusions about suitability both for the research and for the basic components that might satisfy the first evaluator.

Nevertheless, the various judgments about suitability can often be aided by scientific principles. For example, if an inert agent is to be tested, its optimal composition can be determined according to scientific criteria. Certain scientific (and statistical) principles can also be used to determine whether the initial state of the particular group examined in the research is a suitable representative of the corresponding state of the population in the world beyond, to which the research results presumably will be applied.

Decisions about similarity are almost always scientific rather than judgmental. The decisions require scientific criteria for determining the similarity of the compared components and for appraising the possible effects of any dissimilarities.

3.5.2. *Scientific Evaluations and Policy Decisions*

People who must establish policy for the administrative operation of a hospital, for activities in health care delivery, or for national programs for the allocation or regulation of health care resources often complain that the available research data are inadequate for the policy decisions. The data may describe the costs, but not the risks or benefits of alternative options. The investigators may have measured survival time, but not quality of life. The technology may have been evaluated for its process role in making diagnoses, but not for its impact role in affecting the outcome of therapy.

Many of the complaints are justified, and can be eliminated or reduced with scientific improvements in the way research is designed and analyzed. Many other complaints, however, are unjustified, because the policy-making decisions require ethical, moral, or societal judgments for which scientific data and comparisons are inappropriate. No scientific evidence is pertinent to the decision about determining the exact moment at which human life begins. A set of scientific data can indicate the relative merits of different methods of performing an abortion, but the decision to make abortion legal is not a scientific issue. Similarly, a set of scientific data can indicate the methods and costs of trying to achieve a successful pregnancy in a woman who has hitherto been unable to bear a living child, and scientific data can be used to estimate the life span and anticipated earnings of that child, but only the woman (and her spouse) can decide the true value of having the baby.

Issues in policy or value judgments are often decided at a personal level by the people who are most intimately involved, and at a public level by political activity, opinion polls, religious beliefs, or regulatory authorities. Although scientific research can sometimes provide important background for these decisions, the decisions themselves often involve questions that cannot be resolved with scientific methods or comparisons. We shall return to some of these issues later, when we consider problems in deciding the value or importance of certain forms of scientific research.

3.5.3. *Investigator Vs. Reviewer: The Different Approaches*

The person who plans a research project often thinks in a manner quite different from the person who reviews the completed results. In the long run, the same scientific standards will (or should) be used for evaluating the project, but in the short run, the investigator and the reviewer will have to think differently, just as a playwright and a critic may often have different approaches to the same work.

The investigator decides that a particular topic is worth exploring; the reviewer may not agree. For example, if the reviewer believes that social, economic, or emotional problems are the most important ones to be studied, any investigation of the pathogenesis or therapy of lupus erythematosus may be deemed unimportant, no matter how well the research was done. Having chosen a topic, the investigator forms the hypothesis about what to test; the reviewer may believe that some other hypothesis is more worthy. The investigator may not be able to test the hypothesis with an experimental research structure (such as a randomized trial); the reviewer may be unconvinced by any results except those that come from an experimental structure. In using a nonexperimental research structure (such as an observational cohort, case-control, or heterodemic data study), the investigator may organize the research in a way that differs from the straightforward reasoning of the theoretical cause-effect model; the reviewer may be confused by the disparity between the theoretical model and the actual structure of the research. The investigator, after finding that the results differ from what was expected, may refer to the research as hypothesis-generating rather than hypothesis-testing; the reviewer may not regard the conclusions as a generated hypothesis until the accidental or unexpected findings have been confirmed in a separate study.

The investigator, because of problems in feasibility or mensuration, may not be able to acquire the exact data that would be most desirable. When the investigator uses various types of substitution, the reviewer may not agree that the substitutes were satisfactory. The investigator, attempting to work with the world's imperfections, may seek the enlightenment of a candle in darkness; the reviewer may be discontent with anything other than a mercury-arc beam.

For all of these reasons, the chapters that follow can be read in two different ways. One way is from the viewpoint of a reviewer of published results. For such a reader, the comments will offer helpful guides to discerning major problems in the completed work and to determining whether the conclusions are justified by the assembled evidence. A second way is from the viewpoint of an investigator, who has the more difficult task of deciding how to make the basic plans, develop their operational details, and carry out the work in a way that will convince skeptical reviewers.

For either a reviewer or an investigator, the rest of the material in this text offers certain major advantages and disadvantages. One main advantage of the architectural distinctions to be noted is that they can dissect a complex research structure into its constituent ingredients. This type of dissection has always been a major hallmark of scientific reasoning. For example, the Krebs cycle and other complex cycles contemplated in modern biochemistry provide a dissection of a metabolic pathway into each step that occurs between the initial state and the subsequent events. By noting the intermediate products, a scientific biochemist can determine what may have gone wrong in certain metabolic pathways and can develop methods for correcting the defects. Similarly, by noting the intermediate activities that occur in the conduct of research architecture, a scientific clinical epidemiologist can discern problems in the research and develop appropriate solutions.

A second advantage of the architectural distinctions is that they can be used somewhat like a *review of systems* in clinical practice. A capable clinician who has carefully noted a patient's *chief complaint* and account of the *present illness* generally gets quite a good idea of what is wrong and what to do next. Such a clinician will use the review of systems as a valuable chance for extra attention to be sure nothing important has been overlooked. For an inexperienced clinician, however, the review of systems is invaluable because it provides directions for what to do if he is uncertain about topics in soliciting the present illness or if the patient does not volunteer all the cogent information. The architectural points to be noted can thus be used somewhat like a check list, to appraise the status of each system encountered in the research.

The availability of such a check list, however, can also be a substantial disadvantage or major hazard for readers who are not adept at the type of perceptive reasoning that calls for distinguishing a forest from the constituent groves, trees, leaves, and chlorophyll. While contemplating all the details of all the activities that can occur (and go wrong) in a research project, the reader may lose track of what is important and what is trivial. Similarly, since a carefully detailed review of systems will usually yield many positive responses even if the patient is in perfect health, the evaluating clinician must determine when a positive response indicates an important problem and when it is within the range of healthy vicissitudes. No research project can be perfectly conceived, conducted, or analyzed; imperfections can readily be found if enough items are checked. The crucial issue is to decide which imperfections are important and which are not. Unless an investigator makes these decisions effectively, minor flaws may be magnified and may create fears that inhibit the pursuit of otherwise worthwhile research. Unless the reviewer uses the architectural principles wisely, important contributions may be rejected because of minor blemishes.

Although no definitive guidelines can be offered for the challenge of distinguishing major from minor defects, certain basic principles can be listed:

1. As John Tukey[1] has said, "Better an approximate answer to the right question than an exact answer to the wrong question."

2. If a particular research component is unsuitable, is it so unsuitable that the entire project becomes valueless? For example, if a randomized trial of medical versus surgical treatment for coronary disease is conducted in a group consisting of male veterans, the results may still be quite pertinent to many aspects of evaluating the two treatments in persons who are not male veterans. On the other hand, the overall results may become valueless if most of the people allocated to surgery refused to have it done or if most of the patients assigned to medical care later had surgery.

3. If a bias has occurred in the similarity of compared components, can the bias be responsible for destroying the distinction attributed to the compared agents? If so, what is a plausible mechanism by which the bias might act? For example, suppose we discover that in a nonrandomized comparison of medical versus surgical treatment for coronary disease, the average level of education was substantially lower in the medical group than in the surgical group. There is clearly a difference in the educational level of the two groups, but unless we can propose a mechanism by which educational level alone could cause a substantial difference in the results of treatment, the difference might be unimportant. On the other hand, if the members of the medical group were deemed inoperable because they were much older and sicker than the operable patients, this bias might vitiate any apparent superiority found in the results of the surgically treated group.

3.6. SUBSEQUENT SEQUENCE OF PRESENTATION

An alert reader will have noted that the ensuing text can now go in several directions. Having just discussed principles of comparative research, we could turn next to descriptive research. Alternatively, we could extend the discussion of comparative research to focus on further distinctions of either process studies or cause-effect studies.

The author's choice is to go next to cause-effect studies, because they are often the most important, exciting, and controversial types of clinical epidemiologic research. Also, many of the principles stipulated for the details of cause-effect research will be pertinent when we later turn to studies of process and of purely descriptive phenomena.

3.7. SYNOPSIS

For the comparative reasoning used in either process or cause-effect research, four scientific principles can be applied:

1. The basic objective of the research is specified by noting the principal agent under study, the initial state upon which the agent acts, and the subsequent events that follow.

2. The comparative agent must be carefully chosen to answer the particular question asked in the research, and its method of allocation (by designed experiment or by personal judgment) must be acceptable. A simple diagram, resembling those used in other scientific activities, can be drawn to show the four main components that indicate the basic objective and comparison conducted in the research.

3. Each of the four individual components must be suitably chosen for its selected role, suitably specified in operational details, and cogently maintained during the actual conduct of the research.

4. To allow observed distinctions to be ascribed to inherent differences in the compared agents, all other components of the comparison should be similar. These similarities include the initial states of the compared groups, the proficiency with which the agents are administered, and the observation and discernment of subsequent events.

Decisions about appropriate similarity can usually be made with scientific criteria, but appraisals of suitability will often rest on the judgments of the people who plan or evaluate the research. Judgmental decisions, rather than scientific criteria or evidence, will also often be needed for policy issues that involve ethical, moral, or societal values.

Although the principles discussed in this and in subsequent chapters can provide a valuable dissection of the main ingredients and intermediate steps involved in a complex research project, people who use these principles as a check list must be careful to distinguish important problems from the minor imperfections that are inevitable in all scientific research.

EXERCISES

Exercise 3.1. Before a research objective can be implemented with plans for the actual research, the three main components must be clearly outlined. For example, a client who says, "I am seeking truth" can be admired and applauded but cannot be helped to construct a research design unless the consultant has a better idea of the particular topic whose truth is to be revealed and the particular goal of the quest.

The list that follows contains a series of statements of research proposed by people who have come to you for consultation in planning an investigation. When you try to outline the basic objective of the research by noting the initial state, the principal agent, and the subsequent state in each proposal, you may find that some of the proposals are not adequately described. What problems, if any, do you see in each of the following statements?

Note that we are not concerned here with the feasibility of the research, with any details of its implementation, or with the choice of a comparative maneuver. We merely want to get a reasonable idea of what the investigator has in mind. For example, if the investigator says he wants to appraise the influence of parental love on a child's intelligence, you know what he wants to determine. You need not be concerned now about how to measure parental love or intelligence. On the other hand, if the investigator wants to determine whether children are affected by parents, you do not know what is going to be asked or sought in the research. Your first questions would therefore be, What aspect of parents is supposed to have an effect, and what aspect of children is supposed to be affected?

3.1.1. We want to find out whether schizophrenics have unusual family backgrounds.

3.1.2. Is radical surgery superior to simple surgery for patients with breast cancer?

3.1.3. Is a test of carcinoembryonic antigen (CEA) an acurate method of making the diagnosis of colonic cancer?

3.1.4. Are there any peculiar changes in the serum of patients with diabetes mellitus?

3.1.5. Is smoking marijuana harmful?

3.1.6. Should the sale of marijuana be made legal?

3.1.7. We want to do a cost-benefit analysis of the new diagnostic technology, nuclear magnetic resonance imaging.

3.1.8. Are infant mortality rates related to individual socioeconomic status and general national prosperity?

3.1.9. We want to develop a better index for assessing health.

3.1.10. We want to determine the reliability of our surgical pathologist in interpreting specimens.

3.1.11. What is the optimum dose of the new drug, Excellitol?

3.1.12. We want to determine the effect of Excellitol on menstrual cramps.

3.1.13. Is the cost of renal dialysis worth its benefits?

Exercise 3.2. In the proposals that follow, the four parts of the basic outline (initial and subsequent states, principal and comparative maneuvers) are clearly stated. Ignoring all issues of feasibility or implementation of details, what major problems in basic objective, strategy of comparison, suitability of components, or similarity of components do you discern for the conclusions that might be drawn from the following research proposals?

3.2.1. We want to show that survival rates in cancer have been substantially improved by modern chemotherapeutic agents. We shall compare the survival rates for a current series of patients with the survival rates noted two decades ago in patients with similar cancers.

3.2.2. We want to determine the impact of computerized tomographic (CT) scans of the head on the care of patients admitted with stroke. We shall compare survival rates of patients with stroke in hospital A, which does not have such a scanner, with the rates found in hospital B, where the scanner is regularly used.

3.2.3. The therapeutic potency attributed to chicken soup is a myth that needs to be tested. For this test, we plan to monitor the offices of a collaborating consortium of practitioners. Whenever patients appear with the types of upper respiratory infections and malaise that are often treated with chicken soup, we shall perform a randomized trial, comparing symptomatic relief in the results of chicken-soup therapy with those of alternative forms of treatment.

CHAPTER REFERENCE

1. Tukey, 1962.

Chapter 4

An Outline of Cause-Effect Evaluations

Perhaps the most difficult challenge in modern clinical epidemiology, and the source of some of its most notorious controversies, is the evaluation of cause-effect relationships. The evaluations are used to decide that a suspected etiologic agent may be causing disease, that a protective agent may be preventing disease, or that therapeutic agents may be beneficial or harmful or both.

The challenge is not at all new. It occurred in the days of antiquity, when Hippocrates, Galen, and their colleagues analyzed the etiologic roles of water, air, and deranged humors, and the therapeutic roles of bloodletting, blistering, purging, and puking. The challenge occurs today when medical journals, newspapers, television, and other media regularly announce either the indictment of industrial toxins, atmospheric pollutants, nutritional inadequacies, and adverse drug reactions, or the latest miracles attributed to pharmaceutical substances, organ transplants, surgical reconstructions, and healthy life styles.

For several millenia in medical history, cause-effect evaluations were carried out without the formal use of data. Authorities observed, reasoned, and decided, then offered their pronouncements unimpeded by a demand for experimental or any other organized form of documentary evidence. Today, the pronouncements are almost always accompanied by the quantified documentation that is sought by scientists, required by regulatory agencies, and solicited by the public. Because of the technologic and other changes that now provide organized evidence, the challenge of evaluating cause-effect relationships has been substantially altered. The evaluator must now struggle with statistical decisions about the quantitative attributes of the evidence and with scientific decisions about its quality.

This chapter is concerned with the reasoning used in those scientific decisions. We shall develop an intellectual model, outlining the architectural constituents of cause-effect reasoning, that pertains to any of the etiologic, therapeutic, or other types of agents appraised in impact research. The reader should bear in mind that the model is intellectual:

it refers to the way in which we *think* about the research. The research itself may have been conducted with investigative structures whose architecture is substantially different from what is outlined in the model. Thus, the architecture of a randomized trial and an observational cohort study can readily be portrayed in the exact format of the intellectual model, but the use of these two research structures may have been thwarted by ethical, logistic, or other difficulties. Instead, the investigators may have conducted the cause-effect research using cross-sectional surveys, heterodemic arrangements, or other structures that differ drastically from the architecture shown in the intellectual model.

These differences between the intellectual reasoning and the actual structures of cause-effect research are often a source of confusion or bewilderment to scientists who do not appreciate the pragmatic human constraints that create major limitations in clinical epidemiologic research. In traditional research activities, a scientist can regularly perform laboratory experiments on animals or inanimate substances, and is accustomed to using research structures that correspond exactly to the intellectual model with which the research is interpreted. A clinical epidemiologist, however, can seldom use people as the subjects of the precise experiment that is desired, and is often forced to rely on alternative research structures containing data arranged in orientations quite different from the customary pathway of scientific thought.

Regardless of what type of research structure provides the documentary evidence, however, the scientific question about a cause-effect relationship remains the same, and the answer requires the same scientific reasoning. The intellectual model used in that reasoning is the topic discussed in the rest of this chapter. The purpose is to note the model and to outline its main constituents. The constituents will receive detailed consideration later, in Chapters 11 to 17.

4.1. NOMENCLATURE, SYMBOLS, AND DIAGRAMS FOR THE COMPARISON OF MANEUVERS

In Chapter 3, we considered a basic architectural model, applicable to any type of comparative research, in which the main components were named as *initial state, subsequent event(s),* and *principal and comparative agents.* To distinguish the issues of cause-effect research from those of process research, each of these components will be given different names for each of the two types of research. The names to be used are as follows:

	Name of Initial State	Name of Agent	Name of Subsequent Event(s)
Cause-effect research	Baseline state	Maneuver	Outcome
Process research	Input	Procedure	Output

Thus, in process research, we consider the *output* of a *procedure* acting on the *input.* In the cause-effect research discussed in this chapter, we consider the *outcome* that follows a *maneuver* imposed on a *baseline state.*

In Chapter 3, we also developed a diagram that could be used to show the basic architectural model of any type of comparative research. To be sure the concepts are clear, the diagram will be redeveloped here using cause-effect nomenclature and will then be expanded to include some additional distinctions.

When we examine the outcome of a maneuver in a particular person, the basic model for the change is

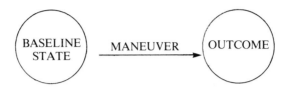

For a group (or set) of people, the diagram would be

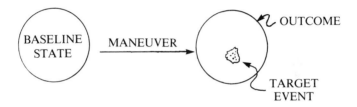

If we look for a specific target event in the outcome state, such as death or development of myocardial infarction, we would search for the subset of people in whom the event occurred. The diagram would be

If we look for a change in dimensional or ordinal data, such as a rise in hematocrit level or a fall in a pain score, we would observe the original and subsequent value in everyone. The diagram would be

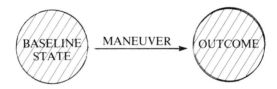

To simplify the symbolism and to avoid drawing all the circles and shadings, the simple diagram of

will be used hereafter to represent the group under study, not just an individual person.

Whenever a maneuver is intended to produce (or is suspected of producing) a change, the reasoning follows a sequence of cause → effect. Because the effect follows the cause, if one event is noted to follow another in human activities, the observed sequence creates a major intellectual hazard, which is customarily stated in Latin as *post hoc, ergo propter hoc* (after this, therefore because of this). With *post hoc* reasoning, we conclude that event A, which preceded event B, also caused event B. For example, we may see an eclipse of the sun. We then beat on a drum. The eclipse disappears and the sun is restored. We conclude that our drum beating restored the sun. Alternatively, we encounter a patient with fever and chest pain. We apply leeches to the site of the pain. The next day the temperature is normal and the chest pain is gone. Therefore, the leeches cured the ailment.

A prime distinction of scientifically planned cause-effect research is the effort made to avoid the hazard of *post hoc* reasoning. The most important mechanism is the use of a comparative maneuver, which is often called a *control*. The outcomes noted in the group who received the principal maneuver are compared with the outcomes noted in the *control group*, who received the comparative maneuver. If the two sets of results are impressively different (and if all other factors are equal), the evidence suggests that the principal maneuver actually accomplished the effect proposed for it.

The procedure can be shown schematically as follows:

$$\begin{array}{c} \text{BASELINE} \\ \text{STATE} \\ \text{(Group A)} \end{array} \xrightarrow[\text{MANEUVER}]{\text{PRINCIPAL}} \text{OUTCOME}$$

$$\begin{array}{c} \text{BASELINE} \\ \text{STATE} \\ \text{(Group B)} \end{array} \xrightarrow[\text{MANEUVER}]{\text{COMPARATIVE}} \text{OUTCOME}$$

This diagram immediately shows a source of trouble. In order to test the maneuvers, we had to assemble two groups, A and B. If differences in the subsequent states of groups A and B are to be attributed to differences in the compared maneuvers, we must be sure that groups A and B are reasonably similar in their baseline states. Otherwise, the subsequent differences in outcome may be due to the baseline differences, not to the action of the maneuvers.

The demonstration that two compared groups are reasonably similar in their baseline states is often difficult and offers many creative challenges that will be discussed at greater length in subsequent sections. For the moment, we shall assume that the main group we wanted to study has been equitably divided into the two subgroups exposed to the compared maneuvers. The diagram would then be

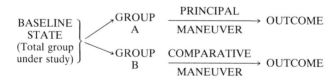

If randomization is (or was) used to allocate the maneuvers that produced this division, the designation of a total group under study and of the two compared groups can be omitted. The diagram can be shown as

$$\begin{array}{c} \text{BASELINE} \\ \text{STATE} \end{array} - \textcircled{R} \Big\langle \begin{array}{l} \xrightarrow[\text{MANEUVER}]{\text{PRINCIPAL}} \text{OUTCOME} \\[2em] \xrightarrow[\text{MANEUVER}]{\text{COMPARATIVE}} \text{OUTCOME} \end{array}$$

To initiate cause-effect reasoning, however, we want a diagram that outlines the objective of the research by showing the four basic structural elements, without regard to the allocation mechanism. The fundamental diagram for comparing the impact of cause-effect maneuvers thus becomes shortened to the same arrangement shown in Chapter 3:

$$\text{BASELINE STATE} \left\{ \begin{array}{c} \dfrac{\text{PRINCIPAL}}{\text{MANEUVER}} \longrightarrow \\ \dfrac{\text{COMPARATIVE}}{\text{MANEUVER}} \longrightarrow \end{array} \right\} \text{OUTCOME}$$

Although the diagram refers to groups, the baseline state and outcome are usually designated for entities observed in the individual people under investigation. Thus, the baseline state would best be labeled as "coronary heart disease" rather than "group of people with coronary disease." The outcome is also best labeled according to the particular target event or variable under observation for individual people, not for groups and not for changes that may be calculated from the data. Thus, an appropriate label would be "survival at 3 years" rather than "3-year survival rate"; and "hematocrit" rather than "mean hematocrit" or "mean fall in hematocrit." If the data are collected in a special format for each person, the baseline state should be labeled with the name of the particular condition that allowed people into the study; the outcome should be labeled with the particular variable or condition that was recorded to determine what had happened to each person. This strategy of labeling will pertain to all diagrams for homodemic research. The labels will differ for heterodemic studies, because individual people are not under observation in the baseline and outcome states.

The diagram can serve as a basic intellectual model for any type of cause-effect reasoning. The model can also be used for outlining the *structure* of forward-directed studies, in which the people under observation are followed as a cohort from baseline state through imposition of maneuvers to the occurrence of outcomes. This type of cohort research is called a *clinical trial* when the maneuvers are imposed with an experimental plan, or an *observational cohort* when the maneuvers are imposed under ordinary circumstances, being self-selected by the recipients, chosen by clinical judgments of practicing physicians, or occurring as natural phenomena. When either type of cohort research is under discussion, the intellectual model and the actual structure of the research will be similar. For other forms of cause-effect research, the actual structure of the investigation will differ from the conceptual model with which the results are interpreted. A different set of diagrams, to be discussed later, will be needed to show the structures used in such research.

4.2. PROBLEMS IN BIAS

In Chapter 3, we considered the issues of suitability and similarity that determine whether a comparative study will give an effective, undistorted answer to the question asked in the research. In cause-effect studies, the problems of achieving similarity in the compared components are particularly thorny. When the compared components are not sufficiently similar, the comparison is said to be *biased*. The biases, which arise because of vicissitudes in the world of reality or in the investigator's planning of the research, can occur at four different locations in the cause-effect pathway. The consequences are called *susceptibility bias, performance bias, detection bias,* and *transfer bias.* These biases are outlined in the next sections and will receive extensive consideration later in the text.

4.2.1. *Susceptibility Bias*

Susceptibility bias occurs if the compared maneuvers are received by groups whose collective baseline states have distinctly different prognostic expectations for the subsequent occurrence of the outcome event. A prime role of randomization in experimental research is to prevent bias when the compared maneuvers are allocated. For example, if therapy is assigned according to the judgments of practicing clinicians, patients with better prognoses may be chosen to receive treatment A and those with worse prognoses may be given treatment B.

A simple example of this problem occurs in evaluating the results of treatment for cancer. Surgeons ordinarily decide about "operability" by requiring that the patients have both localized cancers and a general condition healthy enough to tolerate the surgery. Such patients will have better prognoses, even if surgery is not performed, than the patients with nonlocalized cancers, major co-morbidity, or both, who are deemed inoperable and assigned to nonsurgical treatment. The post-therapeutic results found in these operable patients may then be compared, however, with the results found in the inoperable patients who received chemotherapy or radiotherapy. The situation can be diagrammed as follows:

OPERABLE PATIENTS
(Localized cancers and $\xrightarrow{\text{SURGICAL TREATMENT}}$ OUTCOME
no major co-morbidity)

INOPERABLE PATIENTS
(Nonlocalized cancers or $\xrightarrow{\text{NONSURGICAL TREATMENT}}$ OUTCOME
major co-morbidity or
both)

The bias of this comparison is immediately evident from the diagram. The two groups of patients have major baseline differences, before therapy, that create susceptibility bias for development of such outcome events as death or unimpaired functional capacity. The bias is commmonly overlooked, however, when results are ascribed only to therapy, with survival rates being compared for surgical and nonsurgical forms of treatment.

Differences in prognostic susceptibility to the outcome event can also occur when the maneuver is an etiologic agent, self-selected by its recipients or imposed without medical intervention. For example, the "healthy worker effect" is the name often given to a susceptibility bias whose discovery surprised and startled occupational epidemiologists. To test the deleterious effects of occupational toxins, the survival rates of a group of workers exposed to such toxins were compared with survival rates in the general population. The investigators were stunned to find that the exposed workers had substantially *higher* rates of survival. An explanation, which involved the role of susceptibility bias, became apparent when the investigators realized that health status is usually checked carefully before workers are allowed to undertake dangerous jobs. Compared with the rest of the general population, the exposed workers were substantially healthier at baseline, before the exposure began. The diagram for the comparison is as follows:

PARTICULARLY
HEALTHY $\xrightarrow{\text{EXPOSURE TO INDUSTRIAL TOXINS}}$ SURVIVAL
WORKERS

GENERAL $\xrightarrow{\text{NO SPECIFIC EXPOSURE}}$ SURVIVAL
POPULATION

Thus, although the industrial toxins may have had some adverse effects, the adversities could not overcome the major survival advantages that susceptibility bias had given the healthy workers.

Another potential issue in susceptibility bias occurs with such self-selected maneuvers as a healthy life style. People who decide to live this way may be otherwise destined at baseline—by virtue of psychic, constitutional, or clinical features—to survive longer than people who do not choose (or manage) to live healthfully.

By removing judgmental decisions when the compared maneuvers are assigned or selected, randomization removes the allocation bias that can produce susceptibility bias. Nevertheless, because of occasional caprices of fate during the randomized "luck of the draw," a randomization can create susceptibility bias if important prognostic factors become distributed in a disproportionate manner among the compared groups. Because susceptibility bias can occur with or without randomization, the methods of detecting, analyzing, and adjusting for susceptibility bias are important principles of research architecture, regardless of the mechanism used for allocating the compared maneuvers. Because susceptibility bias affects the composition of the compared groups, its location in the cause-effect model can be shown as follows:

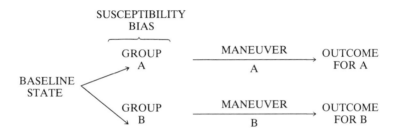

4.2.2. *Performance Bias*

Performance bias arises if the compared maneuvers did not receive similar proficiency in the way they were administered. For example, the comparison of simple surgery versus radical surgery is unfair if the simple surgery is performed by a medical student and the radical surgery by an expert.

The proficiency of a nonsurgical maneuver may depend on such features as dosage schedule, compliance, and regulation of an associated variable. Thus, hypoglycemic therapy for prevention of diabetic vascular complications cannot be fairly compared if the oral agents produce excellent regulation of blood sugar and the injectable agents are poorly regulated. Two oral regimens for treatment of hypertension are unfairly compared if one is maintained with excellent compliance and the other is not.

Performance bias can also arise from the additional maneuvers that may augment the main maneuvers under comparison. Suppose that patients with advanced cancer who are receiving chemotherapeutic agent A also receive supportive treatment with blood products, antibiotics, and steroids, but that no supportive treatment is used for patients receiving chemotherapeutic agent B. A comparison of results for agents A and B would be unfair if the contributions of the supportive treatment were ignored.

If the maneuver requires a particular form of human capability—as in surgery, psychotherapy, or certain forms of physiotherapy—the skill of the performer is an important determinant of proficiency. Thus, if a supremely skilled Freudian analyst is compared with an unskilled behavioral therapist, the result is not a fair comparison of Freudian versus behavioral therapy.

The location of performance bias in the architectural model can be shown as follows:

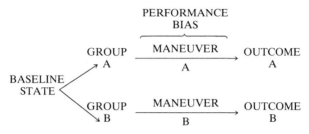

4.2.3. *Detection Bias*

Detection bias arises if the outcome event is detected unequally in the two groups. The detection of an outcome involves three different activities: surveillance of the group members to discern events that require diagnostic testing; ordering and performance of the diagnostic tests; and interpretation of the evidence obtained in the tests. Substantial inequalities in any of these three activities—surveillance, diagnostic testing, or diagnostic interpretation—can lead to detection bias.

For example, patients receiving treatment A, which requires careful regulation of dosage, may be kept under much closer medical supervision than patients receiving treatment B, which can be given in fixed dosage, without monitoring. The increased medical supervision of group A may then lead to increased detection and diagnosis of intercurrent ailments that may escape recognition in group B. If treatment C produces a clinical side effect (such as dyspepsia) that is unrelated to the main outcome event, the side effect may evoke additional diagnostic testing (such as cholecystography), which reveals a symptomless disease (such as silent gallstones) that may be undetected in patients receiving treatment D, which may produce other side effects (such as tachycardia), but not dyspepsia. The increased number of gallstones detected in patients receiving treatment C may then be fallaciously ascribed to the treatment.

The most easily recognized form of detection bias occurs during the subjective activities in which symptoms are perceived, reported, and interpreted by both patients and clinicians. The subjective sensations that are regarded as symptoms may be discerned and designated in different ways if the patient or clinician knows that a placebo is being used rather than an active agent (or vice versa). To prevent this type of bias, the maneuvers in experimental studies are commonly administered with double-blind procedures whenever possible.

In the architectural model for cause-effect research, detection bias occurs in the following location:

DETECTION
BIAS

GROUP   MANEUVER   OUTCOME
A   A   A
BASELINE
STATE
GROUP   MANEUVER   OUTCOME
B   B   B

4.2.4. *Transfer Bias*

Although the basic intellectual model may show what transpired in nature and in the evaluator's reasoning, the model does not show what actually happened in the research.

The baseline states, maneuvers, and outcomes under consideration do not become research data until the groups and the necessary information have been collected by the investigator. After the outcome has already occurred in the medical itinerary, members of the original cohorts may be lost, excluded, or transferred in various ways to produce *transfer bias* in the groups that are collected for the actual comparison of results.

For example, if treatment A often produces a prompt cure of the treated condition, the cured recipients may drop out of the study, becoming lost to follow-up, leaving only the patients with relatively poor responses available for collection of results. If the investigator is unaware of the reasons for the losses, he may assume that the maintained patients resemble those who were lost. Treatment A will then be unfairly compared because of the transfer bias that has distorted the collected results.

An analogous form of transfer bias, with opposite effects, occurs when surgeons report postoperative results in patients who are available for follow-up. Thus, a particular operation may be cited as having an 80% success rate because favorable outcomes were noted in 40 of the 50 patients whose subsequent course was evaluated after they left the hospital. What may have been omitted from the data, however, was an account of 30 patients who died postoperatively and never left the hospital. With this additional group included as failures, the success rate would drop to 50% (40/80).

Transfer bias is relatively easy to discern and adjust if the research is conducted as an experiment in which the investigator identifies all members of the initial groups and keeps track of what happened to them thereafter. If the research is based on observational data, however, the bias may be more difficult to find and to counteract. For example, suppose an investigator wants to compare the results of treatment A and B in the cohort of patients who received therapy for Disease D 5 years ago. Checking a diagnostic registry maintained at the medical center, the investigator finds the names of all people noted to have had that disease 5 years ago. When the patient's records are delivered before the start of the research, the investigator discovers that 10% of the solicited records were not obtained and are marked "missing from file." If the missing records are a random sample of the rest, their absence may not create a problem; but suppose another investigator—unbeknownst to the first investigator or to the medical records librarian—has sequestered the records of all patients who developed a severe complication after treatment A. The absence of those records will substantially distort the results noted in the remaining patients who received treatment A, and the transfer bias may lead the investigator to the false conclusion that treatment A was remarkably innocuous.

Problems of transfer bias can also be produced by the investigator's decisions about whom to include or exclude in the compared groups, particularly when the research is conducted with the case-control structure discussed later.

Transfer bias enters the architectural diagram in the following location:

4.3. **PROBLEMS IN SUITABILITY**

The problems just cited produce biases that can lead to unfair comparison of results for the contrasted maneuvers. Even if the comparison is fair, however, the results may be unacceptable to the medical community because they focus on the wrong target or they cannot be generalized. The targets at which the research is aimed and the ensuing generalizability of results depend on issues of suitability in the main components of the research. Results often cannot be generalized, or they may be regarded as misdirected, because of an unsuitable selection of baseline states or outcome events, or because of inadequate proficiency in one or both of the compared maneuvers.

4.3.1. *Unsuitable Focus*

The problems of unsuitable focus do not require a special diagram and they are not issues in biased comparison. They arise if the research has been directed at the wrong target or conducted in a way that answers either the wrong question or a question whose answer is not pertinent for clinical or epidemiologic decisions.

These problems, which were briefly discussed in Chapter 3 and which will be covered more extensively later, arise if the baseline state, compared maneuvers, or selected outcomes do not represent what was needed to answer the basic question that presumably evoked the research. For example, a comparison of intelligence in group A versus group B may be unsuitable if intelligence is defined by the ability to knit a sweater, lift a 200-lb. weight, or score well in a television quiz show. A comparison of patients who had simple mastectomy versus radical radiotherapy for localized breast cancer will be unsuitable for answering questions about the relative merits of a simple lumpectomy.

4.3.2. *Distorted Assembly*

The four types of bias discussed in Section 4.2 create a distorted comparison *within* the cause-effect model of reasoning. Although all other things should be kept equal except the distinctive action of the compared maneuvers, these four biases act at the cited locations to create inequalities that may make the comparison unfair or distorted.

Regardless of how well that internal comparison has been conducted, however, a problem of unsuitability may arise when the results of the research are extrapolated or generalized externally to the world that lies beyond the particular groups under study. This problem occurs if the investigated groups are a distorted assembly of the people they are supposed to represent.

This type of distortion is commonly produced by decisions made during the complex itinerary that brought people from their anonymous existence at home to their exalted status as statistical units in a research project. A person's decision to see a particular physician, the physician's decision to refer the patient to a particular hospital, the house officer's decision to send the patient to a particular clinical service, the attending physician's decision to order a particular work-up, the medical records room's decision in having the capacity to retrieve the patient's record, and the investigator's decision about criteria for admitting the patient to the baseline group under investigation—all these decisions can substantially alter the composition of the baseline group so that it does not suitably represent the real-world group for whom the research results are intended.

For example, to remove the variability of race, gender, age, clinical complexity, co-morbidity, co-medication, and compliance from the comparisons conducted during a randomized trial of maneuver A versus maneuver B for coronary artery disease, the investigators may admit only a diagnostically "pure" group of patients. They may be white men, ages 45 to 50, with stable angina pectoris, no other clinical manifestations of coronary disease, no associated diseases, and no associated medications other than the allocated regimen, who have been screened to demonstrate their cooperation in complying with the prescribed protocol of the study.

The trial may then provide a splendid comparison of maneuvers A and B in this pure population, but the results may not be pertinent for the impurities that are constantly found in the intended population that is treated in clinical practice. A practitioner, on reading the results of the trial, may not be able to apply them when deciding whether to prescribe maneuver A or B for an elderly black woman with unstable angina pectoris, who is receiving insulin for diabetes mellitus and diuretics for hypertension and who often fails to take her medications.

The unsuitable generalization that can be caused by distorted assembly is depicted as follows:

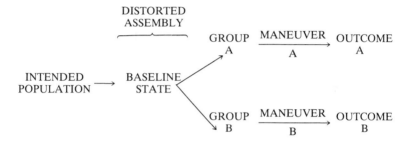

4.4. A WORD OF WARNING

The architectural model just described is a powerful intellectual mechanism for analyzing scientific issues in suitability and similarity for any type of research or collection of data having cause-effect implications. The model can guide the reader's thoughts in deciding whether the collected evidence provides a credible answer to the question(s) under consideration.

The research itself, however, may sometimes be conducted with structures that differ considerably from the constituents noted in the model. Because randomized trials and observational cohort studies are constructed with the same format as the model, research performed with either one of these cohort structures will be relatively easy to evaluate. A reader looking for baselines states, maneuvers, and outcome events will readily find them in the published data and can promptly begin to appraise their quality.

In other types of research, however, there may be a major disparity between the intellectual model of the reasoning and the structural format of the research. This problem will sometimes arise in traditional clinical investigations and will always occur in epidemiologic research when case-control studies, cross-sectional surveys, or heterodemic data are used to evaluate etiology of disease, adverse results of therapeutic agents, or other cause-effect relationships. In these situations, a reader trying to understand what was *done* in the research will have to examine alternative architectural structures that greatly deviate from the straightforward intellectual model of cause-effect reasoning. Amid those alternative structures, which will receive extensive discussion in Parts IV and V of this text, the reader may sometimes have difficulty finding an account of baseline states or the other main constituents of scientific evaluation. The intellectual model can still be used, of course, to decide whether the research has accomplished its mission and supported its conclusions.

Many mental gyrations may be needed, however, before the structural constituents of the actual data can be recognized and transferred into the intellectual constituents of the reasoning. Furthermore, the alternative research structures provide many opportunities to introduce forms of bias or other problems that have not yet been described.

4.5. SYNOPSIS

The intellectual model used to evaluate the scientific quality of cause-effect research contains a comparison of results in the outcome that follows the imposition of compared maneuvers on baseline states. The comparison may be unfair if the compared basic components are disparately affected by *susceptibility bias* in the baseline state, by *performance bias* in the administration of maneuvers, by *detection bias* in the discernment of outcome events, and by *transfer bias* in the groups subsequently collected for the study.

Some parts of the project or all of it may be deemed unacceptable if the individual basic components were not suitably chosen to answer the questions asked in the research. An important source of unsuitability, often called *distorted assembly*, refers to problems in the external generalization of the research, rather than to unequal internal comparisons. Distorted assembly arises when the group of people who enter a study is so constrained by the admission criteria that the group does not suitably represent the outside-world population for which the research results are presumably intended.

The principles just cited can be added to the features previously noted for evaluation when a completed project receives a critical *review of systems*. The ideas will also be valuable, as discussed later, when a project is being planned, implemented, and conducted.

In full regalia, the complete intellectual model for cause-effect research and the location of the attendant major problems are shown as follows:

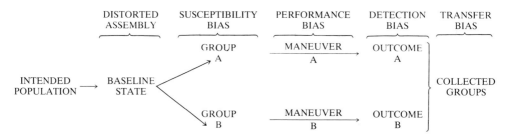

EXERCISES

Exercise 4.1. The list that follows contains six questions to be answered in research projects. For each research question, draw a single schematic diagram (as shown at the end of Section 4.1) for the baseline state of the entities under observation, the principal maneuver, the comparative maneuver (when pertinent), and the particular target event you would seek in the outcome.

    4.1.1. Does cigarette smoking cause cancer of the bladder?
    4.1.2. Does breast-feeding reduce the occurence of infections in an infant's first two years of life?
    4.1.3. Does vasectomy ensure that motile sperm will not be ejaculated?

4.1.4. Are the costs of health care lower with prepaid group practice than with fee-for-service group practice?

4.1.5. Is steroid therapy useful in the treatment of chronic active hepatitis?

4.1.6. What are the costs of maintaining elderly people in nursing homes?

Exercise 4.2. For each project listed in Exercise 4.1, what might be a source of susceptibility bias if the project was not conducted as a randomized trial?

Exercise 4.3. An anesthesiologist believes that a new anesthetic agent, X, causes changes in blood urea nitrogen. He proposes to obtain a BUN measurement in each patient before and after X is administered. When asked about a control group, he replies that none is necessary because the patients will act as their own controls. Is he correct? If not, why not?

Exercise 4.4. Here are five research projects that can produce (or have produced) controversial or misleading results because of problems arising from bias or unsuitability. See if you can identify the major type of bias or unsuitability that led to the main problem. (There is no need here to engage in a profound review of all aspects of the research and no need to engage in a series of "buckshot" critiques, citing all possible flaws. Try to "aim at the jugular," picking out the one flaw that you think was "fatal.")

4.4.1. In New York City, the death rate for pneumococcal meningitis treated with adequate doses of penicillin was found to be 40% at the municipal Bellevue Hospital and 15% at the "carriage-trade" New York–Cornell Medical Center. If the physicians are equally competent and the penicillin is equally potent at both institutions, what might account for the discrepancy?

4.4.2. In randomized trials conducted cooperatively at Veterans Administration hospitals shortly after the introduction of surgical bypass therapy, the surgical treatment showed no superiority over medical therapy for patients with coronary heart disease, except in a subgroup of patients with disease of the left main coronary artery. Despite this demonstration, the results have not been accepted by most surgeons and cardiologists, and bypass operations continue to be performed in patients with non-left-main disease. Assuming that the motivation is scientific rather than fiscal, why do you think the results of this trial have not received widespread acceptance?

4.4.3. We want to determine whether the elimination of written tests or other examination procedures will improve the ability of students to learn medicine. The students at our medical school will be given no midterm, final, or other examinations in any of their courses. At the end of their first two years, however, the students will be required to take the National Board examinations that are given optionally at the end of the second year to medical students throughout the country. Passage of these examinations, which is customarily used as a prerequisite for licensure, will be demanded of our students before they can advance to clinical training, and the grades will be used for ranking them in class standing. To let us know how well our educational program is working, our students' performance in these National Board examinations will be compared with the performance of students at other schools that employ regular testing procedures at the conclusion of each academic course.

4.4.4. An epidemic of retrolental fibroplasia (RLF) occurred, mainly at major academic medical centers, causing blindness in many premature infants born during the years 1947 to 1957. The cause of the epidemic was later found to be high concentrations of oxygen, delivered via specially constructed incubators, that were routinely given to premature infants in the hope of averting (or, sometimes, treating) the respiratory distress syndrome that commonly occurs in "premies." Several years after the epidemic began, the oxygen was accused as a causal agent when the results of observational cohort surveys showed a higher rate of RLF in premature infants treated with than in those treated without high-dose oxygen. The results of these surveys were disregarded or dismissed, however, because of the results found at a single institution, the New Orleans Charity Hospital (a teaching branch of Tulane University Medical School). At Charity Hospital, high-dose oxygen had been used routinely for many years in premature infants, but the occurrence rate of RLF was quite low. This finding was interpreted as exonerating the use of oxygen, and the RLF epidemic continued for several more years until the "guilt" of oxygen was finally demonstrated in a randomized controlled clinical trial. Later, during a retrospective review of the diverse problems that allowed this academic epidemic to be perpetuated for so long, a major fallacy was discovered in the exonerating evidence originally acquired at Charity Hospital. What do you think this fallacy might have been?

4.4.5. In a randomized clinical trial, patients with adult-onset diabetes mellitus who had demonstrated an ability to remain free of ketosis without insulin were assigned to one of five different regimens, four of which were hypoglycemic agents. The regimens were: an oral placebo, a fixed daily dose of oral phenformin, a fixed daily dose of oral tolbutamide, a fixed daily dose of injected insulin, and a variable daily dose of injected insulin. The dose of the flexible insulin regimen was frequently adjusted for each patient's apparent needs. At the end of the study, the rates of mortality and vascular complications were not substantially higher in the placebo group than in any of the groups receiving the other four treatments. The investigators concluded that it is not worthwhile to try to maintain excellent regulation in the control of blood glucose for diabetic patients. Many practicing diabetologists have rejected this conclusion. What do you think is the main reason for the rejection?

Chapter 5

An Outline of Process Evaluations

With the increasing costs and technologic complexity of medical care, people have become increasingly concerned with evaluating its quality. Are individual practicing clinicians doing a good job? Are individual hospitals providing satisfactory services? Are expensive new devices, complicated surgical operations, and powerful but dangerous drugs worth their costs and risks?

The investigators who began trying to answer these questions soon found that perfect scientific answers were not attainable. If the perfect answers were sought from randomized controlled trials, the evidence was either not available or impossible to obtain. For many of the questions, randomized trials had not yet been conducted, and for many other (perhaps most) questions, randomized trials would never be conducted, because the trials themselves would be either unethical, unfeasible, or too costly.

If the answers, although less than perfect, came from observational studies, the investigators found that the observational evidence was often inadequate for the needs of the research. In many circumstances, no evidence was available, because studies had not been done to evaluate the merits of alternative forms of management for *each* of the diverse conditions encountered in a clinician's daily practice or in a hospital's services. In other circumstances, the evidence that was available was not pertinent for certain issues or was highly controversial. Even when pertinent and undisputed, the evidence was still likely to be unsatisfactory because it dealt mainly with the evaluation of a single maneuver aimed at a single outcome, whereas the totality of patient care contains many maneuvers and many outcomes.

For all these reasons, investigators who wanted to evaluate the quality of medical care could not do so with cause-effect research models. There were too many interventions to be considered as principal or additional maneuvers, too many outcomes to be assessed and classified, and too many uncertainties about how to obtain the data, arrange the comparisons, and analyze the results. Instead of evaluating the impact of medical care, investigators therefore began to focus not on what had happened to the patients but on what the clinicians had done. If standards were established to indicate what constituted good clinical practice, the quality of an individual clinician's care could be assessed by comparing its performance with those standards. The term *process research* was used to distinguish such evaluations from more conventional investigations that emphasized the *outcome* rather than the procedures of care.

Although originally applied to evaluations of quality in clinical care, the term *process research* is also pertinent for many other investigative activities. These activities occur whenever the research is concerned with evaluating the quality of a process rather than with determining the changes produced in a cause-effect relationship. The process may

Table 5–1. NOMENCLATURE AND EXAMPLES OF PROCEDURES COMPARED FOR AGREEMENT IN PROCESS RESEARCH

Name of Process Research	Procedure A	Procedure B
Quality control in laboratory data	Result of serum sodium test in laboratory A	Result of serum sodium test in laboratory B or in reference laboratory
Observer variability	Decision regarding histologic type of cancer, pathologist A	Decision regarding histologic type of cancer, pathologist B
Diagnostic marker	Positive or negative result of serum test for cancer	Definitive diagnosis regarding presence or absence of cancer
Spectral marker	Result of serum test denoting whether cancer is localized or disseminated	Definitive evidence regarding anatomic spread of cancer
Prognostic marker	Predictions made by index regarding survival of individual patients or groups	Actual survival of individual patients or groups
Audit of quality in medical care	Activities conducted by clinician under evaluation	Standards or criteria established for *good* care
Examinations given for medical licensure	Answers to questions in the examination given by candidate	"Correct" answers given by authorities

accomplish such jobs as generating a substance, creating an item of data, establishing an identification, executing a task, or delivering a service. Thus, the result of a process is under investigation when we compare data that emerge from two different methods of measuring serum sodium levels or from the interpretation given by two different pathologists to the same tissue specimens. The performance of a process is also investigated when we check a practitioner's compliance with accepted standards of patient care or verify the ability of a diagnostic test to provide correct identification of a particular disease.

The main focus of process research is different from that of cause-effect research, in which the changes produced by the principal maneuver are contrasted with those of the comparative (or control) maneuver. In process research, the focus is on agreement. The quality of the process is evaluated by the degree to which its results agree with either an established standard or with some other performance of the same process.

Table 5–1 shows the names given to different types of process research, together with examples of the types of procedures that might be compared in the research. In this table, the procedures marked *A* would be checked for their agreement with the established standards or alternative performances cited in the procedures marked *B*. Because certain basic principles are pertinent to all of these other activities, as well as to evaluating quality of care, the entire group will be presented under the title of *process research*. The rest of this chapter is concerned with merely outlining those principles. Many additional details will be presented in Part Six, where certain individual types of process research receive further discussion.

5.1. BASIC STRUCTURAL ELEMENTS

The basic structure of a process evaluation can be shown as

$$\text{INPUT} \xrightarrow{\text{PROCEDURE}} \text{OUTPUT}$$

In this diagram, the *input* represents what is exposed to the procedure, and the *output* represents either the product that emerges or the way in which the procedure was performed. Thus, if the process is intended to evaluate cardiac size, the input may be a roentgenogram of the chest; the procedure is a radiologist's examination and interpretation of the film; and the output is the particular expression that describes cardiac size. If the process is intended to evaluate a certain aspect of quality of care, the input may be a patient (or a case report of a patient) with urinary symptoms; the procedure is a clinician's examination and reasoning; and the output is a selected set of diagnostic and therapeutic plans. Although many processes occur as an integral combination of *procedure* and *output*, the two entities have been deliberately separated here to facilitate the architectural analysis of the research.

The same substance or event can be studied in several different forms of process research. For example, a collection of roentgenograms of the chest can be used to check the technical quality of the films, to study observer variability among radiologists, to determine the accuracy of plain films in demonstrating pulmonary embolism, to appraise the next step each film evokes in a clinician's plan of care, or to test the interpretations of the films by candidates for specialty-board certification in radiology.

For most of the comparisons conducted in process research, the *principal procedure* is the entity being tested or checked, and the *comparative procedure* is a definitive or reference procedure that serves as the standard result. The architectural diagram is shown as

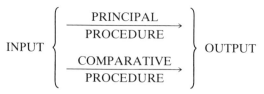

The standard result can be determined from a repeat performance of the same procedure, from a definitive procedure, or from criteria established by an accepted authority. Thus, in the examples cited in the preceding paragraph, criteria would be used to check the technical quality of roentgenograms or to appraise the next step chosen in a plan of care; a set of pulmonary angiograms from the same patients might provide the definitive standard for the detecting the presence of pulmonary embolism; and the correct answers in the board-certification test might be supplied as the consensus of a panel of radiologists interpreting the same set of films.

An exception to this arrangement occurs in circumstances in which a definitive standard is not readily available. Thus, we might want to test the observer variability of two radiologists in determining cardiac size from the silhouette seen in an ordinary roentgeno-gram, without any definitive evidence available from other procedures to denote the actual size of the heart. A definitive standard would also be absent if we were testing observer variability among histopathologists, unless one of the pathologists was given the deified status of ultimate authority. Similarly, if someone has developed a new scale for measuring anxiety, we can compare it with the results obtained from existing scales for the measure-ment of anxiety, but a definitive standard may not be available.

To indicate that the procedures under evaluation may not always be designated as *principal* and *comparative* (or *standard*), the most general way of drawing the architectural diagram for process research is

$$\text{INPUT} \left\{ \begin{array}{c} \dfrac{\text{PROCEDURE}}{\text{A}} \longrightarrow \\[2ex] \dfrac{\text{PROCEDURE}}{\text{B}} \longrightarrow \end{array} \right\} \text{OUTPUT}$$

The four principles listed in Chapter 3 can be applied in process research, although their application will be somewhat different from that used in Chapter 4 for cause-effect research. The principles refer to basic objective, strategy of comparison, suitability of components, and similarity of components.

5.2. THE BASIC OBJECTIVE

The first step in process research, as in any other type of research, is to determine the objective. Unless the goal is clearly indicated, the research may aim at the wrong target or may yield defective results.

For example, when the methods of different laboratories are studied for their agreement in certain chemical measurements, the ultimate goal is to reduce or remove the disagreements. The studies are therefore designed in a manner that allows the participants to discern sources of variability in the methods and to try thereafter to correct the defects. Because the removal of the variability improves the quality of the work, the name often given to this type of research is *quality control*. In contrast, investigations of the analogous disagreements that occur among clinicians, radiologists, and pathologists are usually called, and conducted merely as studies of, *observer variability*. After the intraobserver or interobserver disagreements have been noted and expressed in a quantitative index, improvements are seldom developed to reduce the disagreements. If the purpose is to remove rather than merely to quantify variability, the main goals of the research are not being met.

Other examples in which the designed research does not accomplish the desired goal can be noted in many current evaluations of the contributions of such recent informational technology as radionuclide scans, computerized tomographic scans, and new types of endoscopy. In many appraisals, the new technologic information is checked for its value in diagnosis alone, without regard to the prognostic, therapeutic, and other clinical decisions (beyond diagnosis alone) for which the data are used. A study that evaluates only the diagnostic role of the data will give a constricted, inadequate report of the complete contributions of the technologic procedures.

These disparities between the desired goal and the actual architecture of the research can be avoided if the objectives are clearly specified and appropriately aimed. Such specifications and aims are essential for effective decisions about the strategy of comparison and the suitability of components.

5.3. THE STRATEGY OF COMPARISON

Just as the selection of a suitable control group is crucial for good design in cause-effect research, the choice of a suitable type of comparison is essential for well-designed process research. The decision involves selecting both the type of comparison to be performed and the comparative procedure.

The type of comparison done in the research can be aimed at determining either *consistency* or *conformity*. Consistency refers to the agreement of two processes in situations (such as studies of observer variability) in which neither process is assumed to be correct or definitive. Conformity refers to the agreement of a principal process with the reference process that has been established as the standard.

5.3.1. *A Digression About Nomenclature*

The choice of names for describing different types of agreement is itself a matter of dispute. The idea of *consistency* is sometimes cited as *reliability, reproducibility,* or *repeatability*. The term *reliability* seems unsatisfactory because it implies confidence and trust beyond whatever is noted as agreement. For example, two observers who both refer to *rain* as *snow* are consistent in their agreement, but neither one would be a reliable weather reporter.

The word *consistency* also seems preferable to *reproducibility* and *repeatability*, both of which tend to refer to results obtained when the same procedure is reapplied to the same specimen by the same performer. Because the same procedure may not always be reapplied by the *same* performer, this implication of intraobserver assessment makes both of these words less desirable than *consistency* for describing agreement between (as well as within) different procedures or performers. The term *precision*, which statisticians sometimes use to indicate agreement, is misleading, because most scientists regard *precision* as the amount of detail contained in an observation. Thus, two measuring systems that yield 3.1 as the value of π are consistent but not as precise as a system that yields 3.14159. A measurement system that produces 5.7312806 as the value of π may be very precise, but the result is wrong. For all of these reasons, *consistency* is probably the best term for indicating agreement in circumstances where a standard does not exist.

The idea of *conformity* with a standard is sometimes cited as *accuracy, correctness,* or *validity*. *Accuracy* is a quite acceptable term when the process yields an item of data—such as a serum sodium concentration, a diagnostic identification, or a prognostic prediction—that can be verified against the "true" result obtained with the standard. The term *accuracy* is unsuitable, however, when a process is assessed not for a product but for quality in performance. Thus, we might describe quality of clinical care as *good* or *excellent* but not as *accurate*. Besides, some scientists, confusing *accuracy* with *precision*, may use *accuracy* to refer to the amount of detail in the observation.

The term *correctness* would be satisfactory except for its implication that the standard is "truth" rather than an arbitrarily established benchmark or guideline. Many of the standards established as correct in quality of care today may be regarded as incorrect next year. Another candidate term, *validity*, has so many connotations and has been prefixed with so many confusing adjectives (*face validity, concurrent validity, construct validity, predictive validity*, and so on) that its specificity of meaning has been lost. Besides, some investigators might argue that *validity* is not appropriate for process research and should be used only when cause-effect outcomes have been studied. Hence, the word *conformity* seems best for denoting agreement with an arbitrarily designated standard.

5.3.2. *Problems in Choosing a Standard*

To evaluate consistency, the comparison is easily planned, because none of the compared procedures need be chosen as a standard. The evaluation of conformity, however, requires the use of a definitive standard, which may be unavailable or difficult to choose. In some of the instances noted earlier, such as the measurement of anxiety, no definitive process exists for identifying the measured entity. In other circumstances, the entity selected as the standard may itself be measured inconsistently. For example, the results found on a coronary arteriogram often serve as the standard for determining the diagnostic accuracy of an exercise stress test, but considerable observer variability may exist in the interpretation of a coronary arteriogram.

In yet other situations, the acquisition of a standard result may not always be convenient or feasible. For example, suppose we wanted to evaluate the accuracy of barium enema findings in making the diagnosis of appendicitis. In a patient with classic clinical symptoms and a positive barium enema result, surgery will often be performed to remove the appendix and allow the pathologic examination that serves as the standard. If the patient has atypical symptoms and negative barium enema results, surgery will seldom be performed; therefore, no standard will be available to verify that appendicitis is absent. If the research is confined only to patients for whom the standard result is available, the analysis may contain the distortions noted later in Section 5.4.3. If the research is abandoned because the standard results are often missing, the procedure remains unevaluated.

One way out of this dilemma is to change either the standard or the objective of the research. For example, the definitive decision about whether a patient had appendicitis might be altered to depend on the patient's subsequent clinical course rather than on the current state of health, sickness, or tissue. Alternatively, the goal of the diagnostic marker study might be altered to aim at a management decision, such as whether to operate surgically, rather than at a diagnostic decision, such as whether the patient has appendicitis. The value of the barium enema could then be appraised according to the successful or unsuccessful results of the clinical course that followed the management decision.

5.3.3. *The Choice of Judges and Criteria*

In many process evaluations, the standard is established as a set of criteria or a scoring process determined by a selected judge or judges. The choice of timing, judge, and criteria for these standards can create major problems in studies of the quality of health care services.

If the evaluation is planned before the services occur, a set of *explicit* criteria can be developed for rating each type of activity under scrutiny. If the evaluation takes place afterward, with the services checked from medical records or other archival data, explicit criteria can also be developed, but sometimes the evaluations may use *implicit* criteria to give each case a rating of **excellent, good, fair,** and so on. Because the implicit criteria are not formally stated and are developed and applied *ad hoc* for each case under evaluation, the criteria may contain many inconsistencies.

A separate problem in creating criteria deals with the choice of judges. Who should set the standards for medical care—academic professors, community practitioners, patients' ombudsmen, or some other group? How do we decide that the chosen standards, regardless of source, are both desirable and feasible? How do we modify the standards if they are too rigid or too restricted for the nuances encountered in individual cases? Because unanimous agreement will seldom be achieved in the answers to these basic questions, research concerned with quality of care will often be controversial, not because the work was badly executed but because of conflict over the choice of standards in the basic architecture.

5.4. SUITABILITY OF COMPONENTS

Although the input, procedures, and output of a process must each be suitably chosen, each of these main components contains its own constituent components.

5.4.1. *Suitability of Input*

The suitability of input depends on the individual units that receive the procedure, the scope of spectrum in the groups, and the avoidance of biased spectrums.

5.4.1.1. INDIVIDUAL UNITS

The individual unit subjected to a procedure is usually a person or a specimen. Unless these units are suitably chosen or prepared, the process will not be properly evaluated. For example, the serum collected for a chemical measurement should be (if necessary) obtained under fasting conditions, removed without prolonged venous stasis, separated without hemolysis, and either promptly processed or stored under conditions that do not alter the chemical substance's stability or reactivity. The radiographic films or histologic slides used for studies of observer variability should be chosen for their good technical quality (unless the study is concerned with the decisions made for poor quality specimens). If delivery of a service is being evaluated, each recipient should be suitably eligible to receive that service.

The suitability of individual units thus requires a set of *eligibility criteria,* analogous to the *admission criteria* used in cause-effect research, that specify the prerequisite condition of individual units entered in a process evaluation. These criteria serve three roles: they help the investigator be consistent in choosing admissions to the study; they allow the reviewer to appraise the suitability of the input; and they provide some of the many directions needed by an investigator who wants to repeat the research.

5.4.1.2. SCOPE OF SPECTRUM IN GROUPS

The individual units admitted as input to a study will form the spectrum of the group for which the results are reported. This spectrum should be broad enough to cover the scope of the phenomena under investigation and to provide a suitable challenge to the procedure. For example, unless specimens with particularly high and low values are included, a process for measuring serum cholesterol levels may be mistakenly regarded as fully satisfactory because it produced excellent results for the levels that commonly occur in the middle zone. The process may yield quite erroneous results, however, for the uncommon levels found at the extremes. A similar problem occurs in the evaluation of diagnostic marker tests if a broad, challenging spectrum is not used for both the diseased and nondiseased groups entered in the study.

The demand for a suitably challenging spectrum in the processed objects is also pertinent in research concerned with performance of a service. For example, if the process of health care delivery is being contrasted in nurse practitioners and in family physicians, the comparison is inadequate unless the spectrum of patients' conditions includes some unusual, difficult problems in clinical judgment. These problems may not occur frequently in family practice, but their management is one of the main challenges that helps distinguish a suitably skillful practitioner.

To find a suitable spectrum, the investigator may need special techniques of assembling the individual units under investigation. If assembled in retrospect, the group may be so highly selected that it does not represent the true proportions of what would ordinarily be encountered in the spectrum. For example, in most diagnostic marker studies, the number of control (nondiseased) patients is usually about the same as the number of patients with the disease under scrutiny. Because the proportionate prevalence of the disease is almost always much higher in the studied groups than in the general population, the predictive accuracy calculated from the results will be erroneous when the test is used later for screening purposes.

On the other hand, if the group under study represents a consecutive series of instances in which the marker test was applied, the prevalence of the tested conditions may not be distorted, but the assembled patients may not represent enough unusual cases to provide a full spectrum of challenges. For these reasons, the group selected for investigation is probably best chosen as a combination of a consecutive, unselected series of cases, augmented by specially selected groups to complete the scope of the spectrum.

5.4.1.3. REPRESENTATIVE AND BIASED SPECTRUMS

Two other problems of spectrum, which are particularly prominent in evaluations of diagnostic marker tests, produce difficulties analogous to the transfer biases and distorted assemblies noted as a hazard in cause-effect research.

The first problem occurs if people who have indeterminate data for a particular diagnostic marker test, or who have inconclusive results in the standard used for diagnosis of the associated disease, are omitted from the group chosen for the evaluation. The elimination of such people is an attractive way of avoiding difficulties in analysis of the data, but their transfer out of the appropriate total spectrum can lead to a distorted evaluation of the merits of the diagnostic test. This phenomenon was illustrated in a demonstration[1] of the "tip of the iceberg" that is commonly used for evaluating exercise stress tests in the diagnosis of coronary disease.

The second problem occurs, as suggested in Section 5.3.2, if an inconvenient or invasive standard test is ordered mainly in response to positive or negative results in the diagnostic marker test. The group assembled for the evaluation will be flawed by a "work-up" bias that may misrepresent the true value of the test. For example, in an asymptomatic patient with a negative stress test, a coronary arteriogram is seldom ordered to provide a standard result for the true state of coronary vasculature. Because the arteriogram is ordered predominantly for patients with positive stress tests and because people will be entered in an evaluation study only if they have had both the stress test and the arteriogram, the resulting spectrum will no longer represent the true results obtained with the test in customary clinical practice. As demonstrated in Chapter 25, the nosologic sensitivity of the test will be falsely elevated and the nosologic specificity will be falsely lowered.

5.4.2. *Suitability of Procedures*

The suitability of a procedure depends on three components: the setting in which the procedure is performed; the instruments, materials, or other equipment used by the human performer; and the attributes that are inherent either in the performer or in the interplay between performer and equipment.

5.4.2.1. THE SETTING

The setting refers to the particular environment and associated milieu in which the process takes place. An unsuitable setting, such as a distracting noisy room, can obviously affect the quality of a person's performance. The role of the setting is particularly important in appraising the quality of health care, because the setting may be used in a way analogous to that of an ancillary maneuver in cause-effect research. For example, certain features of the nursing and administrative staff of a particular health program may greatly facilitate (or impede) its operation, but these features of the setting will be improperly ignored if the quality of care in the program is evaluated only in terms of appraisal of the work done by the physicians. These features of the setting are sometimes called *structure* in health care research.

5.4.2.2. THE METHODS

Although the terms *equipment* and *performer* might best serve to label the other two components of a procedure, the corresponding words *method* and *observer* have already been well established for this purpose. To avoid any new problems in nomenclature, *method* will be retained to refer to the instruments, materials, or other equipment used in a procedure, and *observer* will be used to refer to the performer. The events produced during the combined action of equipment and performer are often called *observer/method variability*. As an example of the distinctions and problems, a clinician who has excellent hearing and excellent auscultatory techniques may use a stethoscope that has been acoustically tested and found to be perfect, but the earpieces may fit so poorly that the total performance is impaired.

To be suitable, the methods under study should be carried out under conditions that ensure proper function. These conditions might include such features as calibration of equipment and use of stable reagents. If the method consists of a questionnaire or some other intellectual instrument, the instrument should have a clearly specified format and appropriate instructions for its application.

The criteria involved in process research can be divided into at least two types: the *procedural criteria* that deal with basic activities in performing a task or operating an instrument, and the *conversion* (or *pre-output*) *criteria* that convert the results of the basic operations into the final service or product. For example, in a chemical measurement of cholesterol, the procedural criteria would provide guidelines for mixing reagents and for using the equipment involved in producing the basic entity, such as a voltage reading, that is ultimately observed. The conversion criteria would indicate the way in which this observed entity becomes transformed to a final reading, such as *serum cholesterol = 180 mg./dl.* In many processes, the output result is expressed as an index formed from the interpretation or aggregation of contributory elements. For such activities, which occur in the use of a questionnaire (or examination test), the procedural criteria would indicate the way in which the individual questions are to be answered and then scored as contributory elements. The conversion criteria would show the method by which the individual scores are arranged into the output index that is the final score.

Perhaps the most common source of unresolved problems in observer/method variability today is the absence of separate criteria for the two different acts that occur during the formation of the output: the basic procedural acts of observation with which the contributory elements are noted, and the subsequent acts of conversion with which these elements are interpreted or aggregated to form the output index. If specific criteria for these two separate acts are absent or inadequate, the process under investigation will inevitably be performed without consistency.

Thus, when two auscultators disagree about whether an adolescent's heart murmur is physiologic or due to mitral regurgitation, the source of disagreement may be the procedural criteria for noting such observational elements as *Grade 3/6, blowing, transmitted to axilla, loudest at apex,* and so on, or the conversion criteria for deciding whether the aggregate of the observed elements should be designated as *physiologic* or *mitral regurgitation.* Two observers who use the same procedural criteria may differ in conversion criteria, and vice versa. Unless both sets of criteria are specifically recognized and appropriately applied, the source of disagreement in the output cannot be determined and removed.

5.4.2.3. **THE OBSERVERS**

The understanding and basic skill of the observer (or performer) is essential for the proper use of any instrument. If the instrument is a questionnaire, algorithm, or protocol that is to be disseminated for general usage, pilot studies should first be performed to determine that the users know what to do. For example, the consistency of the performers improved substantially when the wording of the questions was revised in an instrument designed for operational identification of adverse drug reactions.[2] By checking that the performers understood the method, the investigators were able to improve the associated instrument.

5.4.3. *Suitability of Output*

This aspect of suitability occurs last in this sequence of presentation, because *output* appears at the far right side of the diagram illustrating the architecture of process research. Nevertheless, because the acceptability of the basic objective usually depends on a suitable choice of output, its selection is often a crucial first step in the research. For this reason, the designer of a process evaluation is sometimes well advised to follow the aphorism "Begin at the end." After choosing an appropriate focus and scale of expression for the output, the investigator can then work backward to make appropriate selections for input and procedures.

5.4.3.1. **FOCUS OF THE OUTPUT**

If the process yields a product, what particular features of the product should be assessed? For example, if several different chemical procedures can be used to develop the films of a roentgenogram, what attributes of shadow, texture, and so on should be examined to rate the quality of the films? What are the attributes to be scored when an essay is written as an answer to an examination question? If the process consists of a performance, what aspects of the performance will be chosen for grading? Unless these questions about the focus of the output are suitably answered, the research may be distracted or distorted from its principal goals.

For example, the modern approach to educational testing has been severely criticized for the exclusive use of multiple-choice questions and the elimination of essays that would indicate a candidate's creativity, compositional skill, and ability to synthesize information. One main problem in using essays for examinations is the logistic difficulty of achieving a uniform (or automated) procedure for grading. A more cogent problem, however, is intellectual—the failure to establish a set of attributes and criteria that will allow the essays to be graded by human readers in a consistent and unbiased manner.

Many other activities in process research have been distorted by analogous failures to cope with major intellectual challenges in choosing, expressing, and grading a suitable focus for the output. The problems are particularly evident in current processes concerned with certifying the competence of clinicians or appraising the quality of hospital care. The foci of the research (cognitive knowledge, length of patient stay in hospital, ordering of therapeutic agents, etc.) are usually chosen for the ease with which the investigators can rate the output, not for their pertinence in what patients or practitioners would regard as good quality of clinical care.

5.4.3.2. SCALAR EXPRESSION FOR THE OUTPUT

A scale of expression for the output is easily chosen when the result is cited, like a chemical measurement, in precise dimensional data. The situation becomes much more difficult when the scale must reflect contributions from many different observations. How should we combine the different elements that might be rated in clinical care, and what criteria should be used for expressing each of the final possible ratings, such as **excellent, good, fair,** etc.? How much disparity between two radiologists interpreting a chest film will be regarded as **no, mild, moderate,** or **major** disagreement? How many categories should be used for expressing the different gradations of disagreement?

The answers to these and other questions about the scale of expression for the output are often crucial determinants in the success of the research. For example, suppose the output of a study of observer variability or a diagnostic marker test represents a basically dichotomous choice, such as *pass-fail, agree-disagree, normal-abnormal, or diseased-nondiseased*. The number of categories in the final scale of expression and the availability of an indeterminate middle category can greatly affect the likelihood that different methods or observers will produce similar results when using the scale. Thus, the chances of agreement will differ according to whether a scale has an even number of categories—such as *strongly agree, mildly agree, mildly disagree,* and *strongly disagree*—or an odd number of categories that includes a *no opinion* category in the middle rank.

Agreement will also depend on whether a scale is "coarse" or "fine." Thus, a coarse dichotomous scale such as *normal* or *abnormal* may be expanded to a finer ordinal scale with grades such as *definitely normal, probably normal, slightly abnormal, moderately abnormal,* and *very abnormal*. The finer gradings in the expanded scale of categories may enhance the designation of degrees of agreement or disagreement, but the inclusion of too many categories may exceed the observer's ability to discriminate among the gradations.

5.5. SIMILARITY OF COMPONENTS

Each of the main distinctions just described in suitability of components has a counterpart in similarity.

5.5.1. *Similarity of Input*

Because the same unit is usually subjected to each of the procedures under comparison, the input should usually be the same for each procedure. A problem will arise, however, if the unit's condition is unstable (such as a specimen of serum that has not been properly maintained) or is altered by performance of the first procedure.

For example, if we want to compare observer variability when a patient's history is taken by two different examiners, the patient's clinical state may change between one session and the next, or the stimuli of the first examination may evoke reflections that alter the information the patient supplies to the second examiner. As another example, the loudness and transmission of a cardiac murmur may differ from one auscultation to the next if the patient's temperature or degree of cardiac compensation has changed during the interval. Unless adequate provision is made for these variations in the input state of the processed objects, the disagreement attributed to the process may be falsely high.

The similarity of groups is particularly important when two procedures are compared without the same individual items of input being used for each procedure. For example, suppose we want to compare the accuracy of staging systems A and B in predicting the outcome of patients with a particular disease. If the results of system A, applied to patients at hospital X, are different from those of system B, applied to patients at hospital Y, we would need to worry about the possibility that the differences arise not from the two staging systems but from unrecognized differences in the groups of patients assembled at the two hospitals.

5.5.2. *Similarity of Procedures*

Although the need for similar settings is obvious, the two settings under comparison may have subtle differences that can affect the results. For example, suppose we compare the clinical decisions made by the house staff of hospital A and hospital B in managing patients who come to the emergency room with the same type of ailment. Although the compared groups of patients might be similar, the performance of the house staff may be affected by the availability and excellence of the consultants who were on call to provide advice at the two emergency rooms.

An important problem in the evaluation of procedures can arise if the concomitant effects of the two separate sources of variability—in methods and observers—are over-looked. A process that seems mainly method-oriented, such as laboratory measurement of a chemical substance, may be evaluated without regard to the skill of the technician who operates the equipment. Conversely, a process that seems mainly observer-oriented, such as a physician associate's work in using a flow chart (or instructional protocol) for managing patients, may be appraised without attention to the quality of instructions in the algorithm itself.

When two processes are contrasted, the investigator should clearly specify whether the main focus of the research is the total procedure (i.e., method plus observer), the method alone, or the observer alone. If the main focus is the method or observer alone, the investigator should select the other procedural component in a way that reduces or eliminates its variability. The variations produced by the complementary component of a procedure can be a major, neglected source of inequality in comparison when the other component is evaluated.

5.5.2.1. **SIMILARITY OF METHODS**

In a study intended to contrast method A with method B, each method should be used either by the same observer or by observers having equal degrees of proficiency. If observer A is a neophyte and observer B is a skilled professional, this distinction in skill, rather than differences in the methods, may be responsible for the differing results that emerge when method A is compared with method B. Another important feature of equality in comparison is the determination that both methods are being used with appropriately similar procedural criteria and conversion criteria.

5.5.2.2. SIMILARITY OF OBSERVERS

The results of process research can be seriously biased if double-blind techniques are not used when needed. If the investigation deals with variability in an observer-oriented procedure, the need for appropriate blinding is obvious. This need is equally important but may sometimes be neglected if the investigated procedure seems method-oriented.

The consequences can produce major problems in studies in which the results of a diagnostic marker test are compared with the true diagnosis that represents the result of the reference standard test. If the procedures involve subjective interpretation, *test-review bias* can arise if the diagnostic marker test is interpreted by an observer who already knows the results of the standard, and *diagnostic-review bias* can arise if the results of the marker are known when the decision is made about the standard.

For example, when introduced several decades ago, the nitroblue tetrazolium (NBT) test was reported to have a high degree of accuracy as a diagnostic marker for bacterial infection. The test was enthusiastically accepted and received widespread usage until it was later abandoned because of a poor degree of accuracy. The source of the problem turned out to be the requirement for subjective interpretation of microscopic evidence in the test. In subsequent studies, when the observer who interpreted the slides was kept unaware of the simultaneous results in the standard procedure, the accuracy of the NBT test was substantially reduced.[3]

This type of bias can commonly arise when tests are performed in ordinary clinical practice, because of the information exchanged between the observers who subjectively interpret the compared procedures. Thus, the interpretation of a coronary arteriogram may be altered if the radiologist knows the results of a preceding exercise-stress test. Conversely, the interpretation of an exercise-stress test may be altered if the cardiologist knows the results of the coronary arteriogram. To reduce or eliminate these sources of bias, an observer can receive the minimum background information (such as age, gender, and perhaps clinical manifestations) needed for performing a procedure but should be kept unaware of what was previously concluded in other procedures or in previous interpretations of the same procedure. If the background information cannot be made free of prejudicial content or data, the information should be truncated appropriately or withheld entirely from the research study.

5.5.3. *Similarity of Output*

To qualify as similar components for comparison, two outputs should be aimed at the same focus and expressed in the same scale.

5.5.3.1. SIMILAR FOCUS

If the output being evaluated is a particular product—such as a chemical measurement, interpretation of cardiac size, or choice of a diagnostic title—the focus of the compared procedures can easily be identified and established as similar for both procedures. However, if the output is the performance of a task, the compared procedures may not necessarily aim at the same focus. For example, a clinician making decisions about the clinical care of a patient may not necessarily have the same goals as the auditors who evaluate the quality of the care or the certification board examiners who rate the clinician's competence.

The problem of disparate focus is particularly likely to occur when standards of performance are not described in explicit detail. If the different observers who act as the standard auditors or examiners use only implicit (i.e., unexpressed) criteria, the evaluation activities may become inconsistent. In deciding about quality of care, one auditor may emphasize the details of the information recorded to describe the patient's problems; another may emphasize the choice of diagnostic tests; a third may focus on the choice of therapeutic agents; and a fourth may examine the arrangements made for follow-up care. To avoid these inconsistencies, the focus of evaluation may be shifted to a different target that is easier to identify and appraise explicitly. Thus, the focus of quality of care may be converted to the duration of the patient's stay in the hospital, and a clinician's competence may be evaluated not from the actual care of patients but from performance on a written, multiple-choice examination.

The shift of focus solves the problem of consistency when performance is evaluated, but may create an even greater problem in suitability. The duration of a patient's hospitalization or the results of a clinician's performance in a multiple-choice examination may no longer be suitable as outputs for evaluating either the quality or competence of care.

5.5.3.2. COMMENSURATE SCALES OF EXPRESSION

For proper assessment of agreement, the output of the two products must be expressed in a similar scale of expression. For example, if one observer cites the age of people as either *young* or *old*, and another observer uses the categories of *young, middle-aged,* or *old*, we can see a general trend in their ratings, but we cannot determine how closely they actually agree. What is required, therefore, is that the two observers express their results in commensurate scales, having exactly the same type and number of available categories. Thus, if a diagnostic marker test is cited in a three-category scale as *positive, uncertain,* or *negative,* and if the standard of diagnosis is cited in a two-category scale as *positive* or *negative,* the exact agreement of the two procedures cannot be established.

5.6. SYNOPSIS

Process research is concerned with the agreement noted in the quality with which two (or more) procedures convert an input to an output. The individual unit of input can vary from a specimen of blood to a patient seeking clinical care, and the output can vary from a tangible product—such as a measurement of cholesterol or a diagnostic marker test for coronary disease—to the performance of a task, such as the activities delivered in patient care. The agreement of two procedures can be checked for consistency alone or for conformity, if one of them serves as the reference standard. The basic objective of the research should be outlined in a way that allows it to achieve the desired goal, and the comparative procedures should be chosen so that the reference standard, when used, is both acceptable and available for its definitive role.

The adequacy of the evaluative comparison requires suitability and similarity for all of the basic components that form the input, procedures, and output. To be suitably chosen, the input components should fit the goals of the research, receive specified eligibility criteria, and contain a spectrum broad enough to be challenging. The spectrum should be adjusted to avoid the bias produced if the decision to order one of the procedures depends on the results noted in the other. The procedures should be performed in a suitable setting, with properly trained observers using properly checked methods. The *procedural criteria* for performing a task or using an instrument should be separated from the *conversion criteria* with which the basic results are interpreted. The output should be focused on the goal of the research and cited in appropriate categories of expression.

The comparison may be biased if the individual units of input for each procedure are not similar or if they produce disparate groups; if the compared settings are sufficiently different; if different methods are compared by observers of dissimilar competence; or if the observers using each method are not suitably blinded to previous results. The comparisons will be conducted inconsistently if explicit criteria are not used to specify the focus of the output, and agreement of the processes will be difficult to evaluate if commensurate scales are not used to express the results.

EXERCISES

Exercise 5.1. You want to study the *accuracy* (not variability alone) of the processes that follow. A definitive standard result will often be unavailable if an invasive procedure, such as catheterization or surgery, is routinely required to provide the data or if the standard requires a unique human judgment. What can you do to provide a standard result for use in these evaluations?

5.1.1. Radionuclide scans for diagnosis of acute cholecystitis
5.1.2. Radionuclide scans for grading left ventricular function
5.1.3. Histopathologic diagnosis of cellular types of lung cancer
5.1.4. Serum amylase test for diagnosis of acute pancreatitis

Exercise 5.2. You want to review the medical records of patients at your hospital to perform an audit of the quality of clinical care delivered by the practicing clinicians. Because you cannot establish explicit criteria for evaluating every clinical challenge that might be encountered, how can you narrow the focus of the study to allow a consistent approach?

Exercise 5.3. What important aspects of clinical care would be either evaluated ineffectively or excluded from attention because you chose medical records for the audit proposed in Exercise 5.2?

Exercise 5.4. A group of clinicians has joined together to offer the public a Clinitol Plan for providing superior medical care. The clinicians want to demonstrate its superiority over conventional care by performing a set of evaluations that can justify the conclusions that follow. The goal of the research is to show better results for Clinitol in each of the cited phenomena when patients receiving the Clinitol Plan are compared with patients receiving conventional care. Without regard to the logistics or feasibility of carrying out the research to test each hypothesis, classify each conclusion as being a cause-effect or process evaluation:

5.4.1. Patients with similar clinical conditions recover sooner.
5.4.2. The total cost of care is lower.
5.4.3. Dosages and indications for prescribed treatments are more likely to agree with the guidelines established by the American Medical Association.
5.4.4. Patients are more likely to comply with the prescribed therapeutic regimens.
5.4.5. Patients are more satisfied with the care they receive.
5.4.6. Clinicians are more satisfied with their professional style of practice.
5.4.7. Clinicians have an easier time keeping up-to-date.
5.4.8. The improved activities in screening and periodic health examinations allow diseases to be detected more often at an early stage.

Exercise 5.5. For each of the eight research goals cited in Exercises 5.4.1 to 5.4.8, name at least one major precaution that should be taken to avoid major bias or other inadequacies in the results when the two types of care are compared.

CHAPTER REFERENCES

1. Philbrick, 1982; 2. Kramer, 1979; 3. Ransohoff, 1978.

Chapter 6

An Outline of Descriptive Studies

Every collection of data is really a descriptive study, regardless of what is done thereafter with the data. In the activities of Chapters 3 to 5, collections of descriptive data were compared to reach decisions about cause-effect relationships or the quality of processes. In the activities to be discussed now, collections of descriptive data can be used to answer questions regarding such policy decisions as whether to build additional hospitals, add new medical schools, change the fiscal mechanisms for reimbursing the costs of care, or legalize the sale of marijuana.

Descriptive data can also provide useful information about the state of current events or about the consequences of previous events or policy decisions. For example, we might like to know whether more women are becoming physicians today than previously. Has there been a change in the physician-to-patient ratio in rural areas or in places where people are poor? Are current hospital facilities being fully utilized?

Descriptive information is also useful in case reports that alert practicing clinicians to a new benefit or hazard of treatment or to some other interesting point in the etiology of disease or the management of patients.

Because collections of data are used for both comparative evaluations and direct descriptions, the acquisition of data is fundamental to any type of research.

6.1. THE TWO TYPES OF MEASUREMENT

The act of obtaining data is often called *measurement*—a word that is ambiguous because it can refer to two different activities: mensuration and quantification.

Mensuration is the process of acquiring raw data by converting an observed entity into a descriptive statement. *Quantification* is the process of collecting a group of descriptive statements and expressing them in a numerical summary. For example, in examining a group of people, we engage in mensuration when we note and record each person's gender and blood pressure; we engage in quantification when we say that the group contains 11 men and 9 women and that the group's mean systolic pressure is 120.5 mm. Hg. Mensuration thus refers to the act of obtaining individual items of data for individual people; quantification refers to the act of collecting the individual data into groups and summarizing the contents of the collection.

Both types of measurement produce the basic data used in research, regardless of whether the research is descriptive or comparative, but the activities of mensuration are exclusively phenomena of science, whereas the activities of quantification are both statistical and scientific. Mensuration is a scientific procedure that converts observed phenomena into the raw data for each person. Quantification contains a statistical component, consisting of the numerical expressions used to summarize groups of data, and a scientific component, consisting of the decisions made about which groups to collect and compare.

This chapter is concerned with basic scientific issues involved in mensuration and quantification. The next few chapters contain an outline of the statistical expressions used to summarize data.

6.2. THE PROCESS OF MENSURATION

Of the many processes that occur in scientific research, mensuration is obviously basic. None of the events and phenomena that come under scientific scrutiny can be analyzed or discussed until they are converted into data, and the analyses and discussions are not scientific unless the data are trustworthy. To give scientific credence to a mensurational process, we want to have confidence in the quality of the data and we want to be able to verify that our confidence is justified.

The data entered into a research analysis are often transformed from the raw expressions in which they were originally cited. For example, a patient whose age was recorded as **68 years** may enter the data as **old**. The analytic category of **angina pectoris** may be used for someone whose basic data were recorded as *location of chest pain:* **substernal;** *mode of provocation:* **exertion;** and *mode of relief:* **rest.** The analytic category

Apgar score 8 may be used as a composite index for five different attributes that originally expressed the condition of a newborn baby.

When raw primary data are converted into secondary expressions (such as **old** or **angina pectoris**) and composite indexes (such as **Apgar score 8**), the transformation is an act of clinimetrics,[1] involving separate analytic processes and criteria. Our main concern in mensuration now is the observational processes that produce the raw primary data. Thus, during the conversation conducted as part of history-taking, a patient may say "I get a squeezing sensation here (pointing to the center of his chest) when I walk uphill, but it disappears when I stop." The mensurational process is what converts this observation to the raw primary data of *location of chest pain:* **substernal;** *mode of provocation:* **exertion;** and *mode of relief:* **rest.**

6.2.1. *The Concept of Mensuration*

The concept of scientific mensuration is sometimes inappropriately restricted to information expressed in dimensional numbers, such as *age, height, weight, serum cholesterol level,* or *white blood count.* In fact, however, a type of mensuration occurs when *gender* is cited as **male** or **female;** when *cardiac size* is reported as **normal, slightly enlarged, moderately enlarged,** or **massively enlarged;** or when a person's religion is listed in a category such as **Protestant, Catholic, Jewish, Mohammedan, Buddhist,** or **Other.** The requirement for a scale of measurement is that it contain a consistent, distinctive rule for assigning categories. The *consistent* rule enables the same category to be assigned to the same thing under the same conditions; without this rule, we could select categories randomly. The *distinctive* rule allows different categories to be assigned to different things or to the same thing under different conditions; without this rule, we could achieve consistency by giving everything exactly the same label.

Once we recognize that scientific mensuration requires consistent and distinctive categories, although the categories need not be dimensional expressions, we are ready to proceed to the challenges involved in the mensurational process.

6.2.2. *Constituents of Mensuration*

As noted in Chapter 5, the production of data always requires a mixture of human observer and instrument. Even if the instrument is fully automated—such as certain modern clinical procedures that receive a specimen, do the chemical transformations, and print out the measured result—a human observer must note the result and decide that it is, in fact, an item of data. Although most biologists generally think of an instrument as a mechanical apparatus, the word *instrument* is regularly used for other kinds of apparatus that help provide data. In particular, a questionnaire, scaling system, or other format that solicits or "captures" data in an organized manner is often called an instrument. For people accustomed to the technologic devices that generate laboratory data, the term *instrument* may seem strange when applied to a questionnaire or written format, but the latter two devices are quite appropriately labeled with this title, because each of them also serves as an apparatus that helps provide data.

Because of these distinctions, the instruments involved in a mensurational process can be as diverse as a spectrophotometer, a question-and-answer sheet, or a person. The input for the process is the source entity; the procedure consists of an observer-recorder using an instrument; and the output is the result. Thus, a laboratory technician (observer-recorder) may use a spectrophotometer (instrument) to measure the molybdenum concentration (output) in a patient's serum (input). A clinician (acting as observer-recorder and instrument) may interview a patient (input) to take and record a medical history (output).

The mensurational process can become quite complicated because of the different ways in which it is carried out. Thus, if a patient fills out a questionnaire about himself, the act of completing the questionnaire instrument is the procedure, and the patient is both the input source and the observer-recorder. If the spectrophotometer produces a printed numerical result rather than a level on a dial that is read by a person, the array of equipment becomes both the procedure and the observer-recorder.

6.2.3. *Production of Data*

A major problem in medical research today is the absence of suitable attention to data. In the midst of an elaborate statistical and electronic technology for processing, tabulating, analyzing, and drawing conclusions from data, relatively little emphasis has been placed on the fundamental issues that are involved in obtaining, specifying, and expressing the data. What is generally overlooked is the realization that data are human artifacts, produced by a deliberate process in which an observed entity is described and categorized.

The ingredients and sequence of the mensurational components depend on the kind of entity under observation and the kind of data selected for expression. The table that follows contains an outline of some of the diverse ways in which the components are employed.

(Source) Observed Entity	Component #1	Observational Expression	Component #2	Citation of Data
Serum	Chemical isolation	Cholesterol	Assessment of magnitude	Serum cholesterol value
Electron micrograph	Selection of certain squiggles	Thin, cylinder-shaped	Designation criteria	Microtubules
Patient's activities	Notices intra-thoracic sensation	Describes sensation	Clinician hears and summarizes patient's statement	Chest pain
Patient's chest pain	Clinician asks more questions or patient gives more description	Substernal, pro-voked by exertion, relieved by rest	Designation criteria	Angina pectoris
Patient's abdomen	Examined by clinician	Mass in right upper quadrant below ribs, moves with in-spiration	Designation criteria	Palpable liver

At least two different components were involved in each of these activities. The first consisted of observing a larger entity and choosing (or isolating) more specific elements for focus in the description. The second consisted of converting each description into data, using criteria for designating a category. These two components actually comprise four different activities:

1. A focus is selected for specific observational attention.
2. Further observational details are acquired.
3. The details are subjected to a set of criteria.

4. The criteria convert the details into a cited category of expression.
The quality of a mensurational process will depend on the quality of these four activities in recognizing the focus, describing the observations, applying the criteria, and expressing the categories.

6.3. SCALES OF EXPRESSION

Just as a clinician who is diagnosing a patient's ailment must have a list of diagnostic categories from which to choose, a mensurational process achieves its output by choosing the particular entity that is to be described and by expressing the description in a category selected from an available scale.

This section contains an account of the nomenclature used for these activities and a classification of the different types of scales in which measurements are expressed. The excursion into a taxonomy of scales may seem somewhat dreary, but the taxonomy has several important roles: (1) the decision regarding how closely two measurements agree requires attention to the scope of categories available for disagreement; (2) the creation of new scales to describe important but neglected clinical phenomena requires a knowledge of the structures that can be used for the output; and (3) the statistical expressions discussed in Chapters 7 to 10 often depend on the characteristics of the scale whose data are being summarized.

In the taxonomy of mensuration, the term *variable* is regularly used for the particular entity or type of data that is being measured. A person's age, height, gender, occupation, symptoms, diagnosis, and family support system can each be expressed as a variable. The individual citation for that person is chosen from a series of categories that constitute the *scale* for that variable. Thus, *gender* is a variable expressed in a scale whose customary categories are **male** and **female.** The variable *age in years* is expressed in a scale whose customary categories are **1,2,3, . . . ,95,96, ...** (The ". . ." marks refer to items that have been omitted.) The categories chosen to describe a particular person are called the *values* of the variable for that person. A particular patient might have the values of **female** for *gender* and **43** for *age in years*.

6.3.1. *Classification of Scales and Variables*

Variables are often classified according to the types of scales in which they are expressed, and several schemes of classification can be used.

6.3.1.1. NOMINAL (UNRANKED) SCALES

One basic taxonomic distinction in data depends on whether the adjacent categories in the scale can be ranked according to a progressively (or "monotonically") ascending or descending magnitude. The categories of the scale have such a monotonic order for *age in years* but not for *gender*. When the adjacent categories cannot be ranked, the variables (and scales) are called *nominal*. In addition to *gender*, such variables as *occupation, religion, diagnosis*, and *place of birth* are nominal.

6.3.1.2. DIMENSIONAL AND ORDINAL SCALES

Ranked variables can be divided according to the magnitude of the interval between adjacent categories. In a *dimensional* scale, this interval can be specifically measured and is of equal magnitude between each pair of adjacent categories. Thus, *age in years* has a dimensional scale. The interval between **2** and **3** is the same size as the interval between **95** and **96.** If the interval between adjacent categories has been created arbitrarily and is not measurably equal, the scale is *ordinal.* Many clinical phenomena are expressed in arbitrarily created ordinal scales. They include such categories as **mild, moderate,** and **massive** for cardiac enlargement and the categories **0, 1+, 2+, 3+,** and **4+** that are often used to express such variables as *briskness of reflexes, amount of glucose in urine,* or *severity of illness.*

Because of the equi-interval characteristic, dimensional scales are sometimes called *interval scales,* especially by psychologists and sociologists, but the term *interval* is confusing for clinicians because of its common medical usage to refer to a duration of time. Statisticians sometimes use the term *continuous* in reference to dimensional variables, but not all dimensional variables are expressed in the finer and finer units with which a continuous variable can be measured. For example, *serum sodium level* is a dimensional variable that is continuous. If the measuring apparatus permitted, we could express the result of serum sodium as **137, 137.3, 137.25, 137.248,** and so on. *Age* could also be cited in a way that makes it a continuous variable. *Number of children* and *number of previous pregnancies,* however, are dimensional variables that are not continuous. They are expressed in discrete integer categories as **0,1,2,3,4, ...**

Ordinal variables are most commonly cited in a scale containing a limited number of grades, such as **excellent, good, fair,** and **poor,** or **0, 1+, 2+, 3+,** and **4+.** Occasionally, however, an ordinal scale can have an unlimited number of ranks. For example, for the variable called *class standing* at an academic institution, the members of the class are ranked from *1* to *n,* where *n* is the number of members in the class. A similar unlimited ordinal ranking is prepared by participants in the national matching plan, in which medical students seek house staff positions.

6.3.1.3. **QUASI-DIMENSIONAL SCALES**

Certain ranked scales are constructed in a manner that makes them seem dimensional, but they do not strictly fulfill the demand for a measurably equal interval between adjacent categories. Such quasi-dimensional scales can be created in two different ways.

In the first approach, the scale is created as a composite score derived by adding components from other scales that were not dimensional. For example, the *Apgar score* may seem dimensional because it is expressed on a scale of **0,1,2, . . . ,9,10.** The score is formed, however, as a sum of ordinal ratings, each having the arbitrary values of **0, 1,** or **2,** that are assigned to five different variables that are the component elements of the score. Similar quasi-dimensional scales are produced when the final score in a certifying examination is obtained by adding the arbitrary nondimensional grades given to a candidate's performance in different parts of the examination.

A second method of obtaining quasi-dimensional data is an intriguing procedure called a *visual analog scale.* The observer is asked to place a mark on a measured line that lies between two extreme values. The location of the mark can then be measured and the result used as a quasi-dimensional value. For example, to measure the severity of pain, we might ask a patient to place a mark, such as an "X" or a "|," on the following line:

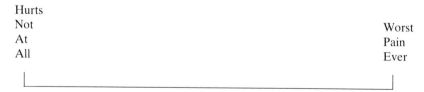

Because the line is 100 mm. long, the mark placed by the patient could be measured to indicate something like 35 quasi-dimensional mm. units of pain.

6.3.1.4. **BINARY (DICHOTOMOUS) SCALES**

A special subset of scales for ordinal variables is the *binary* or *dichotomous* scale used to denote the existence of a particular attribute as **yes** or **no, present** or **absent, normal** or **abnormal, positive** or **negative.** Such scales can be used to express simple phenomena, such as *presence of chest pain* or *result of CEA test.* The scales also can cite the results of more complex decisions, such as fulfillment of *Jones criteria for diagnosis of acute rheumatic fever.* The ordinal characteristic of these binary scales becomes apparent if we expand the categories of expression. Thus, a dichotomous scale for existence can be expanded into **definitely present, probably present, uncertain whether present** or **absent, probably absent,** and **definitely absent.**

Any measurement produced by a mensurational process can be expressed in one of these four types of scales. In order of ascending ability to provide ranked magnitudes, the scales are: nominal, binary, ordinal, and dimensional.

6.3.2. *Composite Scales and Variables*

Many medical data are cited in scales that are constructed as *composite variables,* containing discrete contributions from two or more other variables. A composite variable, which is often identified by such names as *index, scale, factor, score, system,* or *stage,* has its own scale of categories, derived from the way in which the constituent elements were arranged. They are often added together, as in the *Apgar score* described earlier, but they can also be formed as clustered categories, as in the groupings **I, II,** and **III** that form the scale that is called the *TNM system for staging cancer.* The term *multidimensional scale* (or *index*) is sometimes used for composite variables, particularly if all the constituent elements are expressed numerically. The *Dow-Jones Index* of stock market activities is a well-known nonmedical multidimensional scale.

6.3.3. *Constituent States*

Most scales of expression are *single-state indexes.* They refer to a condition noted at a single state in time. Certain other scales may emerge from the comparison of results in two single-state indexes. These two-state comparisons, which are often called *transition indexes,* may be expressed in such categories as **+10.3, −8.7, better, larger, same, rise,** or **improved.** Certain other scales require a consideration of more than two states, as in the decision to list the variable *glucose tolerance curve* as **normal** or **abnormal.**

6.4. **EVALUATING A MENSURATIONAL PROCESS**

A mensurational process can be evaluated for its operational performance, for the results of a single measurement, or for the results of a group of measurements.

6.4.1. *Operational Identification*

A great cook may be able to work entirely by memory, experience, and intuition, but, unless the procedures and ingredients are recorded in a carefully stated recipe, no one else can prepare the same product. Similarly, a process of measurement must be *operationally identified* with an account of the set of conditions, the constituent elements, and the sequence of activities that produce the result, called the *measurement.* Unless a satisfactory operational account is provided, the process will be difficult to evaluate and impossible to improve if later evaluations show that the results are inappropriate, inconsistent, or inaccurate.

One of the greatest difficulties in clinical epidemiology today is the absence of operational identifications for most of the important entities under consideration. A reader who doubts this assertion is invited to contemplate the existing operational identifications (or absence thereof) for the conditions that are diagnosed as diseases; as complications or drug reactions; as risks, benefits, and costs; and as satisfactions with either life or health care. These entities can all be described in the ordinary sense of a definition, but very few of them have received operational identifications.

For example, what are the operational diagnostic criteria used to decide that a patient's death was caused by his myocardial infarction rather than by his metastatic cancer; that a patient's nausea is due to an adverse drug reaction; or that a pulmonary embolism was caused by pulmonary artery catheterization rather than by the congestive heart failure for which the catheterization was performed? What are the operational criteria for deciding that a patient was helped by a particular treatment or that the treatment carries a high risk? What criteria are used to explore the complex financial activities of a modern hospital and to determine the actual costs of performing a particular diagnostic or therapeutic procedure?

The difference between an ordinary *definition* and an *operational identification* is an essential scientific distinction that is often misunderstood or neglected. For example, we can define blood glucose as the concentration of a monosaccharide hexose, $C_6H_{12}O_6$, that is contained in a quantity of whole blood, but this definition will not allow us to measure blood glucose. To perform the measurement, we would need an operational identification that provides all the instructions and sequential directions for conducting an accepted laboratory method, such as the Folin-Wu procedure. The directions would start with something like "Transfer 2 ml. of copper tartrate to 2 ml. of whole blood in a Folin-Wu tube" and would go on through a series of steps ending in something like "Mix and make color comparison in a spectrophotometer." We would also need a separate set of directions to tell us how to operate the spectrophotometer.

These operational instructions can be supplied as ordinary descriptions or in the form of an algorithm, protocol, or flow chart. As long as these instructions remain absent for so many important mensurational processes, however, vast amounts of basic epidemiologic data will continue to lack the fundamental quality demanded in other forms of modern scientific research. Without an account of how the information is created, it cannot be properly checked for its suitability, accuracy, precision, or consistency.

6.4.2. *Results of a Single Measurement*

A single measurement can be appraised according to three of the same principles noted earlier for process research: suitability, conformity, and scope. The *suitability* of a measurement refers to its *qualitative* accuracy in being correctly aimed at the entity that is the focus of assessment; the *conformity* refers to its *quantitative* accuracy in reporting the *magnitude* or *rating* of that entity; and the *scope* refers to the *precise details* that allow the measurement to be usefully employed for its immediate or subsequent purposes.

6.4.2.1. **SUITABLE FOCUS**

A measurement process is suitable if it really indicates the entity that it allegedly measures. For example, 4.2 mm. might be an operationally defined, quantitatively correct measurement of pupil size, but the measurement might not be a suitable expression of *anxiety*. Similarly, a serum cholesterol level of 249 mg./dl. might be accurate as a measurement but would not be a suitable index of diagnosis of coronary artery disease. A staging system that divides Hodgkin's disease into one group of lesions above the diaphragm and another group below the diaphragm might be suitable for demarcating the anatomic distribution of the disease but not for making subtle prognostic distinctions.

The problem of obtaining suitable measurements is particularly pertinent in modern medicine, in which so many data exist as surrogate or proxy variables (substituting *pupil size* for *anxiety,* or *survival time* for *quality of life*). The substitutions also occur as a group of individual judgments, such as the decision that *tumor regression* is an effective measurement of the accomplishments of chemotherapy or that *infant mortality rate* is a satisfactory measurement of achievement by a nation's health care system. The use of surrogate contrived variables is also inevitable for measuring intangible attributes, such as the I.Q. test scores that allegedly measure intelligence. In all of these situations, the issue of suitability of the measurements is often neglected, probably because the issues are difficult, often controversial, and not amenable to easy solutions.

The problem of suitability also arises in certain aspects of chemical measurement. Several different laboratories may all arrive at the same quantitative result when they use a particular procedure for measuring blood glucose, but the measurement may be incorrect because the chemical techniques have not isolated glucose and are actually measuring a combination of glucose plus galactose. This issue has sometimes been raised by opponents of technologic procedures in which a single machine performs multiple chemical tests simultaneously. The argument is that the substances being measured are not always isolated correctly. Thus, the different magnitudes of serum bilirubin at successive measurements may be correctly related to one another and can be used effectively to show changes in the patient's hepatic function, but the actual individual levels of serum bilirubin may be wrong.

6.4.2.2. ACCURACY OF RATING

Section 5.3.1 contained a discussion of why *conformity* is a better word than *accuracy* for denoting agreement with the output of a standard process. When the process produces a direct mensuration of data rather than a judgment about quality of care, however, *accuracy* can be retained because it is used so often to denote this type of agreement. In its most common application, *accuracy* has a quantitative meaning, referring to the closeness with which the magnitude of a measurement approximates the value produced by a standard process that yields the correct result. In a stricter sense, however, *accuracy* refers to agreement in using the categories of a scale, and the scale need not be expressed in dimensional terms. Thus, someone who categorizes a baby girl as *male* is inaccurate.

The assessment of accuracy in rating requires the existence of an authoritative standard against which the observed measurement can be checked. This standard measurement can be established by general agreement (sometimes called consensual validation) or by an alternative measurement provided by a reference source, which can be some other measurement procedure or even the opinion of a selected expert. Thus, a chemical measurement can be compared against the result obtained with a reference method or reference laboratory. A diagnosis of schizophrenia might be regarded as correct if it is confirmed by a professor of psychiatry.

If an authoritative standard does not exist and cannot be created by some of the tactics described in Section 5.3.2, accuracy cannot be determined. For example, suppose an investigator decides that a patient's response to treatment of congestive heart failure is *excellent* if peripheral edema has disappeared, although the patient remains dyspneic. We might dispute this decision and be reluctant to accept it, but we cannot argue that it is inaccurate unless we can point to some standard rating scale with which it disagrees. As noted earlier (in Section 5.3.2), accuracy can be readily determined for dimensional measurements but may be much more difficult and sometimes impossible to appraise for nondimensional categories. Who is to be used as the ultimate authority for the mensurations indicating that a particular tumor is *adenocarcinoma,* that a particular clinician is *highly competent,* or that a particular technologic agent is *cost-effective?*

6.4.2.3. SCOPE OF DETAIL

The scope of detail in a measurement is particularly important in descriptions of clinical phenomena, because the details are needed when criteria are applied for such acts as designation and categorization. The amount of detail often determines whether the measurement will be useful when employed for additional purposes beyond those that are immediately evident. For example, if told that two candidates have each achieved 50% of the vote in an election, we could not determine the victor until the scope of detail in the measurements was expanded to 50.1% and 49.9%. Similarly, the expression "substernal pressure, provoked by exertion, relieved by rest" is satisfactory for allowing the designations *chest pain* and *angina pectoris,* but "substernal pressure" alone is not precise enough to allow more than *chest pain.* The details that allow a designation of *angina pectoris* might not have enough scope to allow a rating of *anginal severity.*

This attention to scope of detail is a common scientific concern that is often overlooked in many statistical assessments of mensuration. In fact, there is no statistical word for indicating that a measurement contains a satisfactory amount of detail. The customary scientific term for this attribute is *precision,* but statisticians usually apply this term for a different purpose, referring to the reproducibility or consistency of a measurement process. In its common scientific definition, the precision of an instrument depends on the significant digits of measurement that it provides. An instrument that can measure 3.14159 is more precise than one that can measure only 3.14. In dimensional data, each digit represents a different variable of measurement. Thus, in 3.14, the 3 represents *units,* the 1 represents *tenths,* and the 4 represents *hundredths.* Similarly, the precision of detail in a measurement such as "substernal pressure, provoked by exertion, relieved by rest" could be demonstrated numerically if the result were coded for expression in symbolic digits such as 925, where 9 represents *location,* 2 represents *mode of provocation,* and 5 represents *mode of relief.*

6.4.3. *Results of Repeated Measurements*

Although focus, accuracy, and scope can be checked for a single isolated measurement, perhaps the most important attribute of scientific quality cannot be determined until several measurements are available to show that the mensurational process consistently achieves a closely similar result when repeated.

The repetition can be attempted on the same entity, using the same or another mensurational procedure, provided that the entity is itself preservable and unchanged by the measurement process. This type of repetition, however, may not always be possible. A biologic or chemical substance may deteriorate in a stored specimen. A patient's clinical condition may change from one examination to the next. A clinician who has taken a specialty board certification examination cannot be retested with the same written set of questions. For this reason, the consistency of certain measurement processes may not always be demonstrable by direct repetition. Nevertheless, with suitable ingenuity, investigators can often develop plans to check the process for interobserver variability, intraobserver variability, or both.

A separate issue in checking for consistency is the decision about what constitutes a disagreement. How large can a disparity be without being a real disagreement? For example, we would have few doubts about the consistency of a measurement process that reports **137.3** and **137.4** for two measurements of the level of serum sodium in the same specimen. We might be reluctant to trust anything about the process, however, if the two results were cited as **137.3** and **127.4**. This issue will be reserved for a discussion of observer variability in Chapter 26.

6.4.4. *Decisions About Quality*

The four attributes that have just been cited are the prime features that determine scientific quality when a measurement process is evaluated according to principles discussed in Chapter 5 and in Part VI. The measurement should yield results that are consistent and that have an appropriate scope of precision in detail. If a standard is available, the results should be tested for accuracy. Above all, the results should have a suitable focus.

The latter attribute, which is sometimes called *face validity,* is often overlooked in many statistical assessments because, unlike consistency and accuracy, it cannot be calculated from the data and given a numerical citation. The suitability of focus must be evaluated with principles that are probably best called "scientific common sense." No matter how precise, consistent, and accurate, a measurement of temperature is unsuitable as an index of anxiety or intelligence. The duration of hospitalization is by itself not suitable as an index of quality of clinical care. A question about the lifetime batting average of Joe DiMaggio is not a suitable item in a specialty board certification examination in hematology, even if the results of the question show an excellent separation between competent and incompetent hematologists.

The problems created by an unsuitable focus of mensuration will appear repeatedly in subsequent discussion.

6.5. EVALUATING A GROUP OF DATA

Although the word *group* usually refers to a collection of persons, a group of data can be assembled in several different ways. The most common basic elements are individual people, with the group of data created by single measurements of the same individual variable (or variables) in each person. Thus, we might have a collection of data containing the height, weight, age, and gender for each member of the group. A single person, however, can be the source of a group of data whose basic elements are different variables or different occasions. Thus, the results of a patient's laboratory tests on admission to a hospital form a group of data (often called a *profile*). The patient's daily values for temperature or for blood pressure would form a group of data that show the results of a single variable on different occasions.

Finally, a group of data can depend on different procedures of mensuration. Thus, for a study of observer variability, we might use the group of data formed by the interpretations given to the same set of roentgenograms by each of four different radiologists. The basic axes for forming a group of data can thus be persons, variables, occasions, and observers. For most of the ensuing discussion in this chapter, the groups depend on the variables noted in a collection of persons.

Many problems in the appraisal of group data occur not in the group but in the basic data. The information itself may be so unreliable that the results have little or no credibility. This type of problem often arises, for example, when death certificate data are used to infer changes in the occurrence rate of different diseases. On the other hand, assuming that the basic raw data are acceptable mensurations of individual variables, certain additional attributes—not present in individual variables—occur when information is assembled into a group. This section is concerned with the attributes that are distinctive to such an assembly.

6.5.1. *Collection of a Group*

The same type of specifications needed to describe the operations of a mensurational process are also needed to describe the process by which a group was collected. This process contains two distinct components, which involve first the solicitation of potential candidates and then the acceptance of the actual members of the group.

6.5.1.1. **SOLICITATION OF POTENTIAL CANDIDATES**

If the group consists of different people, the investigator should describe the mechanisms that were used to attract those people or to have them referred for consideration. If the people were obtained from an archival source of data, such as medical records, the people have already gone through a solicitation or referral process that led them to the site where the archives were assembled. The investigator then imposes an additional solicitation that leads to the retrieval and review of those records. If the group consists of a series of different specimens—such as the films, slides, or forms that might be tested in a study of observer variability—how were those specimens found and identified?

6.5.1.2. **CIRCUMSCRIPTION OF AVAILABLE CANDIDATES**

After the potential candidates have been solicited, they are evaluated for acceptance into the group. During this process, the available candidates are circumscribed according to various criteria that determine whether they are satisfactory or unsatisfactory for inclusion in the group.

These two activities in soliciting and circumscribing the contents of a group can create many problems, some of which have already been discussed and many others that will be considered later. Unless a full description of both activities is provided, neither the investigator nor the reviewer can determine whether major problems are present in a group of data and what the consequences may be.

6.5.2. *Spectrum of a Group*

The contents of a group form a spectrum that can be considered for its apportionment, representativeness, and scope.

6.5.2.1. **APPORTIONMENT**

The apportionment of a spectrum indicates the proportionate distribution of a group. Does it contain 90% men and 10% women, or vice versa? Are the people mostly sick or mostly healthy? What is their age distribution?

The attributes chosen to demonstrate apportionment are particularly important. They are used, as noted in the next two sections, to determine the representativeness and scope of the group. They are also used for internal analysis of the group and for external comparisons.

For internal analysis, a group is often divided into subgroups that are more homogeneous than the total group. For example, mortality rates may be cited not just for an entire group but separately for men and women or for people of different age levels. If we want to know the average amount of care required by patients in a nursing home, the results would be more meaningful if the data are presented for patients divided according to different levels of functional impairment.

For external comparison, the results found in one group are contrasted with results found in another. Because this comparison can be unfair or misleading if the two groups do not have a similar apportionment, a standard mechanism for avoiding or reducing the distortion is to compare results in relatively homogeneous subgroups. Thus, the results of chemotherapy A versus chemotherapy B for a particular cancer would be contrasted not in heterogeneous mixtures of all patients with that type of cancer, but in the more homogeneous subgroups demarcated as TNM Stages I, II, and III.

6.5.2.2. REPRESENTATIVENESS

The events that occurred when a group was being collected may alter its contents so that the assembled data do not adequately represent the actual group itself or similar groups elsewhere. If the group is collected as a result of a public call for volunteers, the people who choose to volunteer may be different from those who do not. The patients with disease X at a particular medical setting may be different in age, severity of disease, and co-morbidity from other patients with that same disease. The criteria used to include or exclude the available candidates may also alter the contents of the group so that it does not represent the spectrum of available candidates.

For these reasons, a thorough description of a group will include not only its actual contents but an indication of the potential candidates who were not obtained or who were obtained but deliberately excluded. In many instances, this description may merely enumerate the unobtained members. Thus, the investigator may report that 100 people were solicited, of whom 60 volunteered, and 30 were actually accepted for the study. In other instances, to demonstrate that the assembled group truly represents its parent group or analogous groups elsewhere, the investigator may compare the apportionment of the spectrum of accepted and unaccepted candidates, or the spectrum of the various groups under consideration.

6.5.2.3. SCOPE

This attribute, which refers to the extensiveness or completeness of the data, has both qualitative and quantitative components.

6.5.2.3.1. *Qualitative Scope*

The qualitative scope of a group refers to the extensiveness of the characteristics it includes. Does the collection of variables include all of the ones that are pertinent and desirable? For example, do the collected data indicate survival times and birth rates but not what we also wanted to know about socioeconomic difficulties or quality of life? Does the collection of people include the uncommon persons who provide some of the most important problems or challenges for whatever activity is being considered? For example, an apparatus that performs automated electrocardiography might have a perfect score for diagnostic accuracy in a group containing 100 healthy people, but this spectrum of patients might not include any arrhythmias or other complexities that produce a substantial challenge to the apparatus.

6.5.2.3.2. *Quantitative Scope*

If the spectrum is intended for complete enumeration, rather than representation, have all of the appropriate members of the spectrum been found and counted? The problem of quantitative scope regularly occurs in traditional epidemiologic data that supply counts of populations, births, and deaths. For example, it is often alleged that census data produce excessively low counts of the number of young black men in U.S. urban regions. Before the effective development (at least in technologically advanced countries) of a national system for filing official certificates of birth and death, investigators could not be assured that all of the births and deaths were actually being enumerated.

6.6. SOURCES AND ADDITIONAL USES OF DESCRIPTIVE DATA

The most traditional descriptive study in medical research is a report of an individual case or of several cases. Such reports are usually intended to provide information about new diagnostic or therapeutic procedures, warnings about adverse effects of such procedures, diagnostic hints, suspicions of etiologic or pathogenetic mechanisms, or epidemiologic or pathologic curiosities. The reports usually contain straightforward descriptions of the observed data for each case, without any quantitative summaries of the information.

6.6.1. *Spectral Studies*

A collection of case reports can become quantitative when a large series of patients (rather than one or a few) is assembled and studied for one or more of the foregoing purposes. Such collections have been traditionally used to show the quantitative spectrum of a particular disease or manifestation.

An example of such a *spectral study* would be a report stating that among patients with disease D, 20% have symptom X, 40% have symptom Y, and 55% have symptom Z. The different variables cited in the spectral studies may refer to demography, symptoms, physical signs, paraclinical data, therapy, and clinical courses for patients with the selected disease. The reports are regularly consulted by clinicians who want to know more about a disease, particularly when preparing to discuss it during "rounds" or some other public occasion. Reports of these clinical spectrums regularly appear in such publications as *Medicine, Quarterly Journal of Medicine, Pediatrics,* and *Journal of Chronic Diseases.* Epidemiologic journals regularly contain reports of the potential etiologic spectrums noted in the microbial, nutritional, or environmental data of patients with a particular disease.

6.6.2. *Agencies, Bureaus, and Other Collectors*

The spectral studies just discussed, and many other descriptive investigations to be noted later, are conducted in an *ad hoc* manner. The investigator chooses a particular group of people for the project and arranges to collect the desired data from those people directly. In many situations, however, the investigator may augment the research data or even get the data exclusively from results obtained in work performed routinely at various private or public agencies, and published in tabulations issued by those agencies.

Perhaps the most common type of quantitative descriptive publication is a collection of statistical data about the occurrence and distribution of various vital phenomena, such as birth, marriage, disease, migration, or death. Descriptive data of this type are, in fact, responsible for the word *statistics.* Several centuries ago, as the rulers of various states or nations began to seek information about the population and commerce of their states, the people who became the collectors of such information were originally called *statists.* The data they collected and enumerated were called *statistics.* Only in the past two centuries, after methods of mathematical aggregation and probability were developed, did the word statistics begin to acquire its additional meaning as a set of procedures for analyzing data and drawing inferential conclusions.

A fundamental source of data in modern statistical tabulations is the national *census bureau* of each country. At periodic intervals (every 10 years in the U.S.), a national census is taken to enumerate the individual persons in each geographic region as well as their age, gender, race, and other demographic attributes. This information can be used for many descriptive purposes, but its fundamental job in epidemiology is to provide the denominators needed to calculate rates of occurrence when the numerator data regarding deaths, births, marriages, and so on are supplied by such sources as regional or state health departments. An excerpt of data obtained from the Census Bureau is shown in Table 6–1.

Another basic source of epidemiologic data is an agency called the *National Center for Health Statistics* in the U.S. and the *Bureau of Vital Statistics* in other countries. This agency collects the denominator information from the Census Bureau and the numerator information from regional health departments, and then puts the data together to issue annual tabulations of birth rates, death rates, marriage and divorce rates, etc. for the entire country as well as for individual regions (such as each of the 50 states). The National Center for Health Statistics also performs many other descriptive services. It regularly conducts special surveys that are published in grouped series under the general title of *Vital and Health Statistics*. Because the pamphlets for each series have covers with distinctively different colors, the documents are often called the *Rainbow Series*. Familiarity with these documents can be a useful item in an epidemiologist's tool chest. An excerpt of data from tabulations issued by the National Center for Health Statistics is shown in Table 6–2. An example of data issued from the Census Bureau, via state agencies, is shown in Table 6–3.

In addition to these documentary sources, many medically valuable types of descriptive tabulations are contained in the annual reports of a hospital's activities and in documents issued by agencies (such as insurance companies) that pay for costs of medical care. When certain substances undergo investigation as etiologic factors of disease, the investigators may begin with descriptive tabulations issued by appropriate commercial organizations to show annual figures regarding sales of cigarettes, consumption of alcohol, prescription of pharmaceutical agents, etc.

Because the voluminous data are seldom enthusiastically received by the editors of medical journals, these descriptive tabulations rarely appear in conventional medical literature. They are usually issued in separate publications and documents. In addition to the publications already cited, an enormous amount of useful descriptive information is issued annually by the Bureau of the Census in a book called *Statistical Abstract of the United States*. Analogous publications exist in other countries.

Table 6–1. RESIDENT POPULATION OF THE UNITED STATES FROM 1900 TO 1980

| | Population in Millions | | | Per Cent of Total Population | |
Year	*Total*	*White*	*Nonwhite*	*White*	*Nonwhite*
1900	76.0	66.8	9.2	87.9	12.1
1910	91.9	81.7	10.2	88.9	11.1
1920	105.7	94.8	10.9	89.7	10.3
1930	121.7	110.3	11.4	90.6	9.4
1940	131.7	118.2	13.5	89.7	10.3
1950	150.7	134.9	15.8	89.5	10.5
1960	178.5	158.5	20.0	88.8	11.2
1970	203.2	178.1	25.1	87.6	12.4
1980	226.5	194.8	31.7	86.0	14.0

From *Statistical Abstract of the United States 1982–1983*. Bureau of the Census, U.S. Dept. of Commerce, 1982.

Table 6–2. ENUMERATION OF MORTALITY FROM SELECTED CAUSES, UNITED STATES, 1900–1975

Cause	1900	1910	1920	1930	1940	1950	1960	1970	1975
All causes	1,308,134	1,356,528	1,382,892	1,393,352	1,417,288	1,452,454	1,711,982	1,921,031	1,892,879
All diseases of circulatory system, including heart disease	115,206	171,599	200,796	293,045	413,968	745,074	923,635	1,007,984	971,047
Diseases of the heart	104,553	146,834	169,814	263,630	385,133	535,629	661,712	735,542	716, 215
Cancer	48,700	70,414	88,793	119,877	158,398	210,733	267,627	330,730	365,693
Rheumatic fever	4033	5729	4046	3077	1712	1959	—	—	—
Syphilis	2054	4898	9476	10,831	18,960	7568	2945	461	272
Leukemia	761	1479	2023	2585	4872	8845	12,725	14,492	14,754
Alcoholism	4033	5082	1065	4303	2502	2267	—	—	—
Influenza	20,317	13,122	75,059	23,877	20,145	6597	7872	3707	4277
Diphtheria	30,666	19,498	16,289	6031	1448	410	—	—	—
Pneumonia	133,469	130,940	145,646	101,661	72,286	40,523	58,931	59,032	51,387
Tuberculosis, all types	147,927	142,121	120,413	87,508	60,436	33,959	10,866	5217	3333
Accidents	48,973	78,083	75,591	99,077	96,909	91,249	93,806	114,638	103,030

From "Vital Statistics Rates in the United States, 1900–1940" by F. E. Linder and R. D. Grove, Washington, D.C., U.S. Government Printing Office, 1947, and "Vital Statistics of the United States:" 1950, Vol. I; 1960, Vol. I; 1970, Vol. II; 1975, Vol. II, Public Health Service, U.S. Dept. of Health, Education, & Welfare.

Table 6–3. RATES OF SERIOUS CRIMES* KNOWN TO POLICE, 1980

	Total Number of Crimes	Rate Per 100,000
Meriden, Connecticut	3529	6245
Miami, Florida	182,164	11,582
Midland, Texas	3418	4153
Milwaukee, Wisconsin	74,595	5355
Minneapolis–St. Paul, Minnesota	129,244	6133
Mobile, Alabama	32,298	7341
Modesto, California	20,236	7617
Monroe, Louisiana	7427	5454
Montgomery, Alabama	16,244	5947
Muncie, Indiana	5827	7864
Muskegon, Michigan	6035	14,895
Nashua, New Hampshire	4413	6507
Nashville-Davidson, Tennessee	34,886	7718
Nassau-Suffolk, New York	133,427	5124
New Bedford, Massachusetts	6217	6318
New Britain, Connecticut	1233	1674
New Brunswick, New Jersey	4542	11,018
New Haven, Connecticut	17,834	14,178

*Includes murder and non-negligent manslaughter, forcible rape, larceny, robbery, aggravated assault, burglary, and motor vehicle theft.

From U.S. Bureau of the Census. State and metropolitan area data book 1982. Washington, D.C., U.S. Government Printing Office, 1982.

6.6.3. *Comparative Use of Descriptive Data*

The information contained in a descriptive study can be regarded as purely expository data, but it is also often used for analytic comparisons. For example, someone might analyze the data in Table 6–1 to reach the conclusions that (1) the general financial depression that occurred in the U.S. during the decade beginning in 1930 also depressed the rate of population growth, and that (2) after the depression was over, the nonwhite population grew at a faster rate than the white. The data in Table 6–2 can be interpreted to indicate that the number of deaths due to tuberculosis had been decreasing long before the introduction of antibiotics during 1940–1950 but that deaths from pneumonia have paradoxically increased since that time. Furthermore, the disease whose lethal numbers have proportionately risen most dramatically since 1900 is leukemia. The data in Table 6–3 might lead to the conclusion that New Britain, Connecticut, has an extraordinarily low rate of serious crimes, and that New Haven has a relatively high rate, but not as high as that of Muskegon, Michigan.

With such arrangements and interpretations, an investigator can regularly convert a collection of passive descriptive data into an active comparative project. The use and abuse of these heterodemic investigations is discussed in Chapter 24.

6.7. SYNOPSIS

Any collection of data represents a descriptive study. The measurements that provide the descriptions are performed with two different processes: the *mensuration* that converts observed phenomena into the statements that constitute the primary or transformed raw data, and the *quantification* that provides summaries of the raw data collected for a group of persons, variables, occasions, or observers.

The mensurational process involves selecting a focus of observation, adding observational details, and subjecting the details to criteria that convert them into categories of a scale of expression. The scales of expression need not be dimensional. Many important phenomena are measured in scales whose categories are ordinal, binary, or nominal. The quality of a process of mensuration is evaluated according to its suitability in focus, accuracy of rating, precision of detail, and consistency in repeated performances. The evaluations require the process to be operationally identified rather than merely defined. When raw data are collected into a group, the group should be clearly identified for the mechanisms used to solicit and circumscribe the accepted members. The spectrum of the group should be described and can be evaluated for its apportionment, representativeness, qualitative scope, and quantitative scope.

Descriptive studies can appear as individual case reports, as collections of cases that are presented to show the clinical or etiologic spectrum of a disease, or as populational data for rates of death, birth, marriages, and other demographic phenomena. In the United States, the Census Bureau, state health departments, and the National Center for Health Statistics are prime sources of descriptive data, but other useful information can be obtained from hospitals, insurance agencies, and commercial organizations.

Although descriptive data are usually assembled for purely informational purposes or as background for policy decisions, the information is often applied in the comparative analyses to be discussed later.

EXERCISES

Exercises 6.1 through 6.6 are intended to make you think about the mensurational process by which an entity is observed and converted into data. The exercises all deal with this process, but they do not necessarily require answers that employ the specific concepts or jargon used in the text. The objective is for you to consider the entities that are actually observed and the components of the actual observational process that produces the mensurational result.

Exercise 6.1. In the automation of electrocardiographic, electroencephalographic, or other technologic procedures that produce graphic tracings and images, the basic phenomena are observed and directly interpreted by a machine, without human intervention. Name the particular characteristics of the observed entity that have allowed the automated (computerized) interpretation of electrocardiograms to be achieved much more easily than automated interpretation of electroencephalograms, differential white blood cell counts, or chest x-rays.

Exercise 6.2. Computerized electrocardiography has not been particularly successful for diagnosis of major arrhythmias or for comparison of successive tracings. What aspects of the measurement process do you think are responsible for these two problems?

Exercise 6.3. Two physicians have just auscultated the heart of a 10-year-old girl. One doctor says the girl has *mitral regurgitation*; the other says she has a *normal heart*. Name several aspects of the mensuration process that may be responsible for the disagreement. How would your answer differ if the diagnoses were *aortic regurgitation* versus *normal heart?*

Exercise 6.4. Name five different potential sources of error in a reported measurement of a particular patient's serum cholesterol level.

Exercise 6.5. What defects have been created in the observational process that converts an observed entity to a described entity when the findings of a physical examination are reported in the following terms?

The patient looks anemic.
The patient smells uremic.
The murmur sounds like mitral regurgitation.
The chest pain is pleuritic.
The skin is dehydrated.
The liver is enlarged.

Exercise 6.6. Give an example of an observational (or measurement) process yielding data that are:

> **6.6.1.** Consistent and precise but not accurate
> **6.6.2.** Consistent and accurate but not precise
> **6.6.3.** Accurate and precise but not consistent

The data should preferably be expressed in a nondimensional scale, but dimensional data can be cited if you cannot think of any other examples.

Exercise 6.7. If you evaluate the quality of individual measurements and of groups, what are some of the major sources of error that you might suspect for the tabulations presented in:

> **6.7.1.** Table 6–1
> **6.7.2.** Table 6–2
> **6.7.3.** Table 6–3

Exercise 6.8. The ten summaries that follow contain the titles and abstracts of descriptive case reports recently published in medical journals. Classify the purpose of each of these reports according to the goals cited in the first paragraph of Section 6.6. (All that is needed here is a brief categorization, e.g., "6.8.11.: New therapeutic procedure." In classroom usage, the results of individual categorizations can provide an interesting illustration of observer variability.)

> **6.8.1. Coincident Salmonella infections and ulcerative colitis: problems of recognition and management.** The diagnostic combination was recognized late in three of five cases of coincident salmonellosis and ulcerative colitis. If corticosteroid therapy is given for the colitis, then simultaneous systemic antibiotic cover is advisable once the combination is recognized. During corticosteroid therapy alone, one of the five patients died from Salmonella septicemia due to a usually noninvasive organism.
> **6.8.2. Diabetes mellitus associated with epidemic of infectious hepatitis in Nigeria.** Nine cases of diabetes mellitus, all with classic symptoms and signs, were noted after an epidemic of infectious hepatitis swept through eastern Nigeria. A few months after treatment, the diabetes completely disappeared. Corticosteroid-glucose tolerance tests for four patients were normal 12 to 30 months after remission of the diabetes. The remaining five patients were lost to follow-up after the remission. The infectious hepatitis virus may have damaged pancreatic islet cells, causing an acute remittent form of diabetes mellitus.
> **6.8.3. Reversible encephalopathy possibly associated with bismuth subgallate ingestion.** Four patients who had undergone abdominoperineal resection for carcinoma of the colon and who had been taking oral bismuth subgallate developed a stereotypical recurrent and

reversible neurologic syndrome, characterized by confusion, tremulousness, clumsiness, myoclonic jerks, and an inability to walk. Symptoms regressed when the intake of bismuth was stopped. Despite extensive investigations, including autopsy in one patient, no alternative cause could be found. The encephalopathy in these four patients may have been due to their bismuth subgallate ingestion.

6.8.4. Subungual malignant melanoma: difficulty in diagnosis. Subungual malignant melanoma developed on both great toes of a 61-year-old woman. For two years the lesions had been diagnosed and treated as ingrowing toenails. The difficulty in clinical diagnosis is illustrated by the description of three other patients with subungual malignant melanoma. The tumor should be considered as a possible cause of any persistent abnormality of the nail bed or the nail itself, especially if it is pigmented.

6.8.5. Aspirin and anemia in childhood. Chronic aspirin ingestion in childhood is not uncommon, often goes undetected, and may cause serious anemia due to occult blood loss. Five cases are described.

6.8.6. *Haemophilus influenzae* meningitis in adults. Although common in children, *Haemophilus influenzae* meningitis is rarely seen in adults. Four of eight cases seen in the past 5 years were in patients older than 20 years of age. In each case there was difficulty in identifying the organism in the Gram-stained film of the cerebrospinal fluid sediment.

6.8.7. Lethal neonatal deficiency of carbamyl phosphate synthetase. A male infant, who appeared normal at birth, manifested hypothermia, irritability, and hypertonia 24 hours after beginning protein feedings. Increasing rigidity and coma ensued, and the child died at 75 hours of age. A male sibling had also died with an identical clinical picture. Laboratory studies on the proband demonstrated a blood ammonia level of 1480 μg. per 100 ml. (normal <150 μg. per 100 ml.). Assay of the urea cycle enzymes in liver obtained at autopsy revealed selective deficiency of carbamyl phosphate synthetase activity, with normal activity of the other four urea cycle enzymes. Deficiency of this enzyme must now be added to the causes of lethal hyperammonemia in the newborn.

6.8.8. A case for venom treatment in anaphylactic sensitivity to Hymenoptera sting. When anaphylaxis developed after a honeybee sting, a child of a beekeeping family was treated with the conventional therapy, whole-(insect)-body extracts, for 9 months, but a second sting caused anaphylaxis again. Because a sister had died under similar circumstances, he was immunized with 1.4 mg. of honeybee venom over a 2-month period; the last two doses were 100 μg (~ two bee stings). After this immunization, his sensitivity to venom decreased, his blocking (IgG) antibody level increased 300 times beyond the former level, and he tolerated a honeybee sting without reaction. Venom immunization may be the treatment of choice for Hymenoptera sensitivity.

6.8.9. Esophageal apoplexy. Three cases of spontaneous bleeding into the wall of the lower esophagus with submucosal hematoma formation are described. The presenting symptom was severe, constant pain behind the lower part of the sternum and in the lower part of the posterior chest. The patients were all women in the seventh decade of life and all seemed to have disordered function of the lower esophagus and cardia. Despite the dramatic presentation, conservative treatment was sufficient in all cases.

6.8.10. Polymyalgia rheumatica and liver disease. In a case of polymyalgia rheumatica, liver biopsy revealed portal inflammation, liver cell necrosis, and a granuloma. Because liver function tests returned to normal after treatment with steroids, and because other investigations of liver disease were negative, the biopsy findings were probably due to the polymyalgia rheumatica rather than a second coincident liver disease. Polymyalgia rheumatica may be another rare cause of liver granulomas.

Exercise 6.9. The medical literature has sometimes been criticized for its scientific defects because control groups are often absent and because the experimental method is seldom employed in the reported projects. The 10 projects whose summaries you read in Exercise 6.8. were not conducted as experiments and involved no control groups. What justifications (if any) would you offer for or against the policy of publishing such papers? (You may refer to any of the individual projects that you wish to cite in your argument.)

CHAPTER REFERENCE

1. Feinstein, 1983.

PART TWO

AN OUTLINE OF STATISTICAL STRATEGIES

Because an escape from the throes of mathematics may have been one of the great appeals of studying health and illness, many readers of this book will not welcome a set of chapters dealing with statistics. Before skipping those chapters in quest of more comfortable topics, however, such readers are urged to pause for a few words of reassurance and caution.

The reassurance is that the quantitative issues to be discussed should be relatively easy to comprehend. They deal mainly with *descriptive* statistical expressions, such as the means, proportions, rates, and trends that readers have frequently seen and understood in daily life. Some of the descriptive expressions become more formal, fancy, and formidable during their roles in summarizing medical data, but the basic principles should be familiar to anyone who can understand statistics describing the performance of teams in a sporting event, the rise or fall of a stock market index, or a trend in the rate of inflation.

When we turn from descriptive summaries to decisions about probability, the mathematics can become more complicated, but there is no need to become fixated on the mathematics. The P values, confidence intervals, and other inferential statistical terms that often assail a reader of medical literature can be understood without any profound attention to mathematics; and the basic ideas should not be too difficult for anyone who has tried to estimate the chances of filling an inside straight in poker, tossing a seven with dice, or having an airplane flight canceled on a rainy day.

If these reassurances do not make you enthusiastic about continuing, perhaps a word of warning will be more persuasive. The warning is that people who do not learn about statistical strategies will be deprived of a crucial intellectual mechanism for evaluating medical literature. As the main output of most research activities, statistical expressions and analyses will often be the first thing a reader sees in a set of published results. If too confused, flustered, or awed by the exterior statistical package, the reader may fail to look inside the package to find the underlying architectural distinctions that determine whether the results really warrant credibility and acceptance. These architectural distinctions can be readily comprehended by someone with a scientific background in health and human illness, but a reader who is scared off by the unknown may not reach the known. To prevent this mental penetration from being thwarted by the statistical packages in which the substance of research may be wrapped, a reader needs to be able to get through the numerical exteriors. This ability can be improved by "biting the bullet" and continuing with the next four chapters.

Statistical Indexes for a Spectrum of Data

Every group of data contains a spectrum of results for the variables that have been observed in that group. If the group is small enough, each of the individual items of data can be shown, and we can see everything directly. If the group is large, however, the individual items may occupy too much space to be published, and the time needed to examine all of them may be prohibitive. Besides, regardless of whether the total volume of data is large or small, the information will not make sense unless we find a suitable way of summarizing it.

For example, suppose we want to determine how well our soccer* team has performed this year. We can look at the scores of each individual game the team has played throughout the season against every other team in the league. After reviewing the scores of each game with each opponent, we could note whether our team won, lost, or tied that game. When this review is finished, however, we will not know how well the team has performed unless we compile a summary statistic, consisting of the team's total number of wins, losses, and ties. This summary will indicate what the team has done, but we will not know how *well* it has done unless we engage in another statistical act, achieved by assembling the same summary for the performance of all other teams in the league. When we arrange the teams according to the values found in the summary index, we can determine their standing and reach our conclusion.

These two activities demonstrate the two main purposes of summarizing a spectrum. In one instance, we indicate its internal composition. This type of descriptive information would be used not only in sports but also by a political analyst who wants to know the way a group will vote, by a marketing analyst who wants to appeal to a group's purchasing preferences, or by a health care planner who needs to determine the age of a population or the types of medical facilities available in a particular region. In the second instance, we perform an external comparison, contrasting the results of the spectrum against those of some other spectrum. This type of contrast might be used to rank the teams in a sports event or to compare the effects of several treatments.

The indexes to be discussed in this chapter provide univariate summary expressions for the data contained in the spectrum of a single variable. Statisticians often use the word *distribution* to describe a collection of data, but the term *spectrum* is scientifically more familiar. It is also scientifically more useful, because the same word, *spectrum*, can often be employed for both the architecture of the research and the statistical expression of results.

7.1. **THE CONCEPT AND SCOPE OF A UNIVARIATE SPECTRUM**

Suppose we have assembled the data shown in Table 7–1 for the age, birthplace, severity of illness, and 3-year survival status for each of 20 people. We might have collected the data of these four variables to determine the relationship between age and severity of illness or between birthplace and survival, but before doing anything else, we want to see what the data show for each variable individually. The univariate spectrum of each variable contains the group of values that have been observed for that variable.

To summarize a univariate spectrum, we can begin by counting the frequency with which each value appears in the results. The scope of the spectrum can then be shown by listing the number of people with each value in a set of appropriate "containers." The

---

*My favorite sport for statistical illustrations is baseball, but in deference to readers who are not American, I shall use something else. In deference to American readers, however, I shall label as *soccer* what the rest of the world usually calls *football*.

Table 7–1. HYPOTHETICAL DATA FOR FOUR VARIABLES IN 20 PEOPLE

Person's Identity	Severity of Illness	Age	Birthplace	Status 3 Yrs. Later
1	Mild	47	Canada	Alive
2	None	50	Brazil	Alive
3	Mild	63	Canada	Alive
4	Moderate	49	U.S.	Dead
5	Mild	51	Costa Rica	Dead
6	Moderate	48	U.K.	Dead
7	Severe	54	U.S.	Dead
8	None	53	U.K.	Alive
9	Mild	51	U.S.	Dead
10	Moderate	50	France	Alive
11	Mild	51	U.S.	Alive
12	Severe	82	U.S.	Dead
13	None	53	Spain	Alive
14	Moderate	50	U.S.	Alive
15	Severe	59	Canada	Dead
16	Mild	52	Canada	Alive
17	None	48	U.S.	Dead
18	Moderate	61	Germany	Dead
19	Severe	55	U.K.	Alive
20	None	49	U.S.	Alive

numbers that are put in each container can be found by tallying the individual values as we go down the list in Table 7–1 or by making a direct count of all the people with each value.

For the binary data of survival status, the ordinal data of illness severity, and the dimensional data of age, we can set up the containers in an adjacent linear arrangement. For the two categories of survival status, the arrangement would be:

DEAD	ALIVE
9	11

For four categories of severity of illness, the ascending linear order in the adjacent arrangement would be:

NONE	MILD	MODERATE	SEVERE
5	6	5	4

For the linear array of dimensional categories of age, we can set up an appropriate container for each value, or we might consolidate all values above 55 into a single group as follows:

47	48	49	50	51	52	53	54	55	>55
1	2	2	3	3	1	2	1	1	4

Since birthplace contains nominal data, which cannot be ranked, we cannot use a linear pattern of adjacent arrangements. Instead, we can show the containers as a set of nonranked circles. Furthermore, for those countries that appear only once in Table 7–1, we might establish a container called "Other." With this technique, the spectrum for birthplace might be shown as follows:

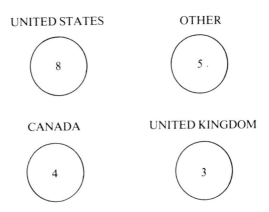

7.2. THE BASIC TACTICS: SUMS, QUOTIENTS, AND RANKS

The displays in Section 7.1 are a first step in summarizing the contents and scope of a univariate spectrum. For the remaining activities, we make use of three basic tactics: forming sums, calculating quotients, and determining ranks. The tactics and the associated symbols are described in this section.

7.2.1. *Sums*

A sum can be formed by adding individual units or individual values.

7.2.1.1. FREQUENCY COUNTS

A frequency count is the most common quantitative expression in descriptive statistics. The tactic is constantly used to determine N, the total number of members in a group of data, and to indicate the constituent subgroups as n_1 for subgroup 1, n_2 for subgroup 2, and so forth. As a general symbol, we can let n_i represent the number of people in subgroup i. Using Σ to represent the act of addition, we can state that N $= \Sigma(n_1 + n_2 + n_3 + n_4 + \cdots)$. To simplify this expression and to show the scope of the addition, we can write $N = \sum_{i=1}^{m} n_i$, where m = the number of sub-groups. Because we almost always add *all* the subgroups, the extra notation is usually omitted from the Σ sign, and we can write simply that $N = \Sigma n_i$.

For example, for the severity of illness shown in Section 7.1, the subgroups are $n_1 = 5$, $n_2 = 6$, $n_3 = 5$, and $n_4 = 4$. The total of 20 people is $N = 20 = 5 + 6 + 5 + 4$. If the frequency counts for our soccer team show that it has won 37 games, tied 9, and lost 17, we can say that $n_1 = 37$, $n_2 = 9$, and $n_3 = 17$. The total number of games will be $N = \Sigma(37 + 9 + 17) = 63$.

7.2.1.2. **ADDITIVE AMOUNTS**

For nominal, dichotomous, and ordinal variables, the individual values such as **dead,** **moderate,** and **Brazil,** cannot be added. For dimensional variables, such as age, however, the individual amounts of each value have mathematical attributes that allow addition and other arithmetical activities, such as multiplication.

The symbol X is regularly used to show the observed value of an individual item of data in a collection. Appropriate subscripts are appended to denote the individual items. For example, for the age of person 1 in Table 7–1, $X_1 = 47$. For person 2, $X_2 = 50$; for person 15, $X_{15} = 59$. Using X_i to represent any one of the values, their total sum, from the first to the Nth person, would be $\sum_{i=1}^{N} X_i$. This would be $\Sigma(47 + 50 + \cdots + 59 + \cdots + 49) = 1076$. With the convention that all values are being included, we can omit the extra notation around the Σ sign and simply write ΣX_i for this sum.

When the individual data have been grouped into the spectrum shown in Section 7.1, we could also let the X_i symbols represent different values for recurrent items of data. We can then use f_i to represent the frequency count for each subgroup having the value of X_i. For example, in the spectrum of age, the value of 47 occurs once, 48 occurs twice, 49 occurs twice, 50 occurs three times, and so on. We can symbolize these items as $X_1 = 47$, $f_1 = 1$; $X_2 = 48$, $f_2 = 2$; $X_3 = 49$, $f_3 = 2$; $X_4 = 50$, $f_4 = 3$; and so on. With this convention, the sum of values would be written as $\Sigma f_i X_i$ and calculated as $(1 \times 47) + (2 \times 48) + (2 \times 49) + (3 \times 50) + \cdots$. Because the ">55" value for the highest four numbers is not precise, we would return to their actual values for this addition. The sum of values would be $(1 \times 47) + (2 \times 48) + (2 \times 49) + \cdots + (1 \times 63) + (1 \times 82)$. Because the f_i values represent the frequency of individual values, the total frequency of these occurrences will be the size of the group; therefore, $N = \Sigma f_i$.

The tactic of obtaining a summed amount by adding the products of frequency counts and individual values is particularly helpful when certain individual values occur repeatedly. For example, suppose our soccer team is given a point-credit score of 2 points for a win, 1 point for a tie, and 0 points for a loss. To determine the total point score, we can add up the results for each game as $2 + 0 + 2 + 2 + 1 + 2 + 1 + \cdots$. Alternatively, for the 37 victories, 9 ties, and 17 defeats, we can find the total as $(37 \times 2) + (9 \times 1) + (17 \times 0) = 83$.

In these symbols, f_i represents the frequency of each value, and n_i represents the number of members in a subgroup. Ordinarily, if each member of the total group is represented by a single value in the data, $\Sigma f_i = N$ and $\Sigma n_i = N$. In some instances, such as repeated measurements of blood pressure for individual people, Σf_i will represent the total number of measured values, and it will exceed N, the number of people.

7.2.2. *Quotients*

To compare groups of data that have different numbers of members, we need a method of standardizing the results obtained with frequency counts and additive values. We obtain this adjustment by expressing the results in quotients having the denominator of N, the size of the group under consideration. These quotients create the *proportions* and *means* that are the most popular form of descriptive statistical indexes. A third type of quotient, called a *rate*, is often constructed for the sums found in two different groups.

7.2.2.1. **PROPORTIONS**

In the spectrum of survival status in Section 7.1, we saw that 6 of the 20 people were alive three years later. If some other group had 17 survivors among 45 people, we would have difficulty comparing the two sets of results, because the groups have different sizes. The comparison becomes easy, however, if we express the two survivals as a proportion of 6/20 = 0.30 for the first group, and 17/45 = 0.38 for the second. Similarly, our soccer team's performance may be easier to interpret if we say that it has won 37/63 = 0.59 of its games. Because expressions such as "thirty-eight hundredths" or "fifty-nine hundredths" are awkward, they are regularly multiplied by 100 and expressed as percentages, such as 38% or 59%.

The symbol p_i is regularly used to represent a proportion or percentage. It is determined as $p_i = n_i/N$. For dichotomous data, the complementary proportion is $q_i = 1 - p_i = (N - n_i)/N$. Thus, for a survival proportion of 0.30, the mortality proportion is 0.70. For a survival percentage of 38%, the mortality percentage is 62%.

Our soccer team has $p_1 = 59\%$ for victories, $p_2 = 9/63 = 14\%$ for ties, and $p_3 = 17/63 = 27\%$ for defeats. When a total collection is divided into its spectral proportions, they should add up to 1 (if expressed in proportions) or to 100%. For our soccer team, $\Sigma p_i = 1$, because $59\% + 14\% + 27\% = 100\%$, but the sum of constituent proportions may sometimes be a little above or below 1 (or 100%) because of rounding in the individual calculations. (For example, suppose a group of 60 people has six subgroups, each containing 10 persons. The percentage of the total group in each of these subgroups is 10/60 = 16.666 . . . %, which would be rounded to 17%. When we add the six values of 17% for each subgroup, the total is 102%.)

7.2.2.2. MEANS

The most famous quotient in descriptive statistics is the mean, which is symbolized as $\bar{X}$ and calculated as $\bar{X} = \Sigma X_i/N$. Because the i subscript is readily understood, it is often omitted, and the mean is cited as $\bar{X} = \Sigma X/N$.

For the ages that were added in Section 7.2.1.2, the mean is 1076/20 = 53.8. For our soccer team's point-credit score, the mean per game is 83/63 = 1.32.

7.2.2.3. RATES

In its customary scientific meaning, a *rate* is the quotient obtained by dividing measurements of two different entities. Thus, velocity is the rate of speed obtained when a measurement of the distance traveled is divided by a measurement of the time consumed for the travel. The word *per* is often inserted between the two different units of measurement, so that we can describe velocity as *kilometers per hour*. The rate of an automobile's gasoline consumption is often expressed as *miles per gallon*.

In epidemiologic data, the word *rate* is most appropriately used for the quotient obtained by dividing frequency counts for two *different* groups. Thus, to form an annual mortality rate, we obtain the denominator from a census count that is used to estimate the total number of people living in a particular region. We obtain the numerator from another source, which gives the frequency count of inhabitants who died during a particular year. A rate in two differently counted groups would be shown as N_1/N_2. This expression differs from the n_i/N that we used to represent a proportion of a particular subgroup, n_i, within a total group, N.

Although regularly applied to the heterodemic quotient formed by the frequency counts of two different groups, the word *rate* is often misused and is applied to the homodemic spectral *proportion* that is produced when the numerator is a counted subset of the same people counted in the denominator. Thus, for the six persons who were alive three years later among the group of 20 listed in Table 7–1, the value of 6/20 = 30% really shows the proportion who have survived but is generally called a *survival rate*.

Another use of *rate* is to express results in which the denominator is an entity containing a mixture of persons and durations. Suppose we have followed 100 patients for different lengths of time: 10 were followed for one year, 60 for two years, and 30 for three years. Calculating the follow-up period as $(10 \times 1) + (60 \times 2) + (30 \times 3)$, we can call it 220 *person-years*. If during that period we found that 38 streptococcal infections had developed, we can cite the result as an *attack rate* of 38/220 or 17.3 per 100 patient-years.

These two additional but incorrect uses of the word *rate* are now so widespread that attempts to alter the process are futile. In fact, the abuse will be continued at various places in this text, particularly when familiar phrases such as *survival rate* are used instead of the correct but unfamiliar *survival proportion*.

The main point to be noted now is that most clinical usages of the word *rate* refer to proportions calculated when a single homodemic spectrum is divided into constituent subgroups, whereas most classical epidemiologic rates are heterodemic quotients of total counts for two spectrums. The scientific consequences of this distinction will be discussed in Chapter 24.

An additional quotient, called a *ratio*, is often determined when one rate (or proportion) is divided by another. Because this type of quotient is constructed to compare two rates (or proportions), the construction will be discussed further in Chapter 8.

7.2.3. *Ranks*

Ranks can be used externally to compare the magnitude of results for two or more groups, or internally to arrange and demarcate the spectrum of data within a single group.

7.2.3.1. EXTERNAL COMPARISONS

The way we determine our team's standing in the soccer league is by ranking the teams according to an index of spectrum in their results. One reason for using a proportion rather than frequency count of victories for this index is to avoid unfair rankings if the teams have played different numbers of games. For example, our team has fewer victories in its 63 games than another team whose current record is 38 wins, 10 ties, and 18 losses, but the other team has played 66 games and has thus had three more chances to win. If our team wins its next three games, it will have a better record. Therefore, if we want to compare the two teams now, the proportion of victories would be a better index than the frequency count. Because the other team's proportion of victories is 38/66 = 58%, it currently would be ranked below our team.

Another index that might have been used for this external ranking is the mean point-credit score. This index for our team was 83/63 = 1.32. For the team with a record of 38 wins, 10 ties, and 18 losses, the index would be $[(38 \times 2) + (10 \times 1) + (18 \times 0)]/66 = 86/66 = 1.30$. In rank according to this index, our team would still be slightly ahead.

7.2.3.2. INTERNAL DEMARCATIONS

A different role of ranking is in the internal organization and demarcation of a spectrum of data. This type of arrangement was used to prepare the containers shown for *severity of illness* and *age* in Section 7.1. When ordinal or dimensional data are placed in an ascending or descending order of magnitude, certain positions in the spectrum can be demarcated according to the ranks, and the spectrum can be described according to the values of data that occupy those positions.

For example, in our collection of 20 items of data, each item occupies 1/20 or 5% of the entire spectrum. The first five items occupy 25% of the collection, the first 10 items occupy 50% of the collection, and so on. For the 63 games played by our soccer team, the result of each game (as a win, tie, or loss) occupies 1/63, or about 1.6% of the collection.

Selected sites in the ranks of occupation can be demarcated and called *percentiles* or *fractiles*. The *median* is the name given to the particular rank that occurs midway in the collection, separating the upper half from the lower half. In our array of 20 values for age, the lower 10 values occupy the lower 50% of the collection, and the upper 10 values occupy the upper 50%. The median would occur midway between them. Because the 10th ranked value is 51 and the 11th ranked value is also 51, the median would be 51. In the array of 20 values for severity of illness, the 10th and 11th ranked values are both **mild,** and so the median is **mild.**

The determination of a median is easy if N is an odd number. The median occurs at the value whose rank is $(N+1)/2$. Thus, for the 63 games of our soccer team, the median value has the rank of $64/2 = 32$. Because the team had 37 wins, the median would be **win.** If N is even, the median is arbitrarily placed midway between the rank of $N/2$ and $(N+2)/2$. If those two ranks have the same values, as in the *age* and *severity of illness* of our 20 people, there is no problem. If the ranks have different values, the median is taken as the average of the two. Thus, if the 10th ranked age had been 51 and the 11th ranked age had been 52, the median would have been 51.5.

Because the median occupies the 50th percentile, it passes through the middle rank of the data when N is odd. For example, in our collection of 63 soccer game results, the ranked entries from 1 to 31 occupy the lower 49.2% ($= 31 \times [1/63]$) of the collection, and the ranked entries from 32 to 63 occupy the upper 49.2%. The 50th percentile thus passes through the mid-ranked 32nd entry, with its 1.6% of the collection. The term *lower quartile* is used for the item of data that occurs at the 25th percentile, and *upper quartile* is used for the item that occurs at the 75th percentile. In the collection of 20 items for age, the lower quartile is midway between the 5th and 6th ranks; the upper quartile is midway between the 14th and 15th ranks. In the collection of 63 items for our soccer team, the lower quartile is the 16th ranked item, which would be a **loss,** and the upper quartile is the 48th ranked item, which would be a **win.**

We shall later return to the important role of percentiles in summarizing a spectrum of data.

7.2.3.3. MANAGEMENT OF TIED RANKS

When ordinal data are given unlimited ranks, as in a rating of students for a class standing, the arrangement of ascending ranks is easy. When ordinal data occur as a limited set of grades, such as **none, mild, moderate, severe** or as **win, tie, loss,** the ranking is somewhat tricky, because many members will have the same grade.

With our soccer team, for example, 17 items compete for the lowest rank of **loss,** nine compete for the next rank of **tie,** and 37 compete for the highest rank of **win.** For the descriptive purposes of finding medians, lower quartiles, or other percentiles, this tied-rank situation creates no major difficulties, and we easily found the appropriate values, as noted in Section 7.2.3.1, by counting the ranked location of each item of data. Thus, in the 63 games played by our soccer team, the value at the 5th rank is **loss,** the value at the 10th rank is **loss,** the value at the 15th rank is **loss,** the value at the 20th rank is **tie,** the value at the 60th rank is **win,** and so on. In certain statistical tests discussed in Chapter 9, however, each ranked entity must be identified with a specific value for its rank.

This problem in tied ranks is managed by giving the tied entities the average value of the lowest and highest ranks for which they are tied. For example, our soccer team's 17 losses, which are tied for ranks 1 to 17, would each be given the ranking of $(1+17)/2 = 9$. The nine ties, which all compete for ranks 18 to 26, are each ranked as $(18+26)/2 = 22$. The 37 wins, which are tied for ranks 27 to 63, are each ranked as $(27+63)/2 = 45$. [You can check the accuracy of these calculations by recalling that the sum of a set of consecutive numbers from 1 to n is $(n)(n+1)/2$. Because the sum of ranks should be the same for the original values as for the ties, we can note that the sum of the ranks from 1 to 63 is $(63)(64)/2 = 2016$ and that $(17 \times 9)+(9 \times 22)+(37 \times 45)$ also equals 2016.]

7.3. BASIC GOALS FOR SPECTRAL INDEXES

In summarizing a univariate spectrum, we can have at least three different goals. The first goal is the simple descriptive purpose of seeing what the spectrum contains. The second goal is an internal comparison, within the spectrum, to see whether its contents are relatively homogeneous or heterogeneous and whether any of its members are unusual or extraordinary. The third goal is an external description, which will be used to represent the results of the spectrum for comparison with results from other spectrums.

Thus, when we looked at our team's performance in the soccer league, we examined two separate spectrums. First, we looked at the internal contents of the team's individual spectrum, which was summarized with a listing of its total wins, ties, and losses. We might have given more attention to the internal contents of this spectrum, but we did not do so with our soccer team, because its record of 37 wins, 9 ties, and 17 losses did not seem particularly outstanding. An internal spectrum that might have been more exciting and more likely to elicit comment about the unusual results would have been a record such as 62 wins, 0 ties, and 1 loss. An unusual internal feature of the age spectrum in Table 7–1 is the 82-year-old person, who seems somewhat out of place in comparison with the substantially lower ages of the rest of the people in that spectrum.

Although not particularly important as an act of statistical description, the search for unusual items in a spectrum is a crucial activity when we later engage in the inferential reasoning used for probabilistic comparisons of spectrums. The entities that are the unusual or uncommon members of certain theoretically created spectrums become the source of decisions about probabilities and statistical significance.

After examining our team's internal spectrum of performance at soccer, we compared it externally by constructing a new, additional spectrum—usually called a list of team standings—in which our team's results were ranked in comparison with the results of other teams. A key decision in this step was the choice of an index to represent our team's performance. We could have used the number of victories, the proportion of victories, or the mean point-credit score per game.

The examples just cited help demonstrate that our goals in internal and external summaries for the data of a spectrum are to do the following things:

1. Choose a single central index that will adequately summarize the spectrum and also represent it for comparison with other spectrums.
2. Determine the scope of the spectrum.
3. Determine whether the contents of the spectrum have any unusual attributes.
4. Determine how well a single index serves to represent the spectrum.

The first two sets of decisions provide the summary indexes for external description of the spectrum. The second two sets of decisions deal with the internal distinctions of the spectrum and the adequacy of the external indexes. These four decisions are essential for all the statistical activities to be discussed in the rest of this chapter and in Chapters 8, 9, and 10. The external summary indexes will be used in Chapters 8 and 10 to represent each spectrum when we contrast the results of two or more spectrums. The unusual distinctions of a spectrum and the adequacy of the external indexes will have important roles in the statistical significance considered in Chapter 9.

The remainder of this chapter contains the background preparation for these coming attractions. The external descriptive indexes are discussed in Section 7.4, the internal composition of a spectrum in Section 7.5, and the suitability of a central index in Section 7.6. Because the methods of making the four basic decisions depend on the scale of expression for the data, the decisions will be considered separately for each of the four main types of scale.

7.4. **EXTERNAL DESCRIPTION OF A SPECTRUM**

To arrive at a general description of a spectrum, we need an idea of its scope and of the magnitude of the values it contains. For example, suppose we have measured the length of each member of a group of objects. Are these values in the general region of 6 cm., 60 cm., 600 cm., or 6000 cm.? Are we talking about the length of a human body, of a ship, or of the distance between two cities? Because magnitudes can be cited on a line of numbers extending from minus infinity to plus infinity, a summary index of magnitude should show us approximately where our spectrum is located on that line. For this reason, the term *index of location* is often used for the index of magnitude.

Thus, when we say that a soccer team has won 59% of its games, we have a single index that locates the spectrum of its performance. A value of 13% or 91% would place the performance in a different spectral location. Similarly, if we say that the players on the team have an average age of 34.1 years, we get an idea of the spectral location of the group's age. The players are (at least on average) neither children nor octogenarians.

The *index of scope* should indicate how far the spectrum of the variable extends. For example, the index of location may tell us that the team has won 59% of its games, but it does not indicate whether the remaining 41% of the games were all lost, all tied, or some of both. To know from an index of location that the soccer players have an average age of 34.1 does not tell us whether all of them are between 32 and 36 years old or whether the age range extends from 12 to 67.

The selection of these two indexes—for location and scope—is discussed in the rest of this section.

7.4.1. *Indexes of Location (Central Indexes)*

The indexes used to show the location of a spectrum will depend on the type of scale used in the data.

7.4.1.1. NONDIMENSIONAL DATA

Nominal data are summarized by citing the proportions occupied by each category (or subgroup) in the data. If a single category must be chosen to represent the group, it is usually the one with the highest proportion. For example, the spectrum of birthplaces in Table 7–1 and Section 7.1 could be summarized with the statement that 8/20 = 40% of the people were born in the United States. The rest of the spectrum would consist of 20% born in Canada, 15% born in the United Kingdom, and 25% born in "Other."

Binary data are summarized with either one of the two complementary proportions. Thus, the survival status of the 20 people in Table 7–1 can be cited either as a survival rate (or proportion) of 30% or as a fatality rate of 70%.

Ordinal data can be managed in three different ways. The first, which is probably the clearest and most universally accepted, is to avoid choosing a single index of location. Instead, the proportions are cited for each subgroup of data. Thus, the *severity of illness* for the 20 people in Table 7–1 could be cited as **none**, 25%; **mild**, 30%; **moderate**, 25%; and **severe**, 20%. A second approach, which involves making a single choice of location, is to cite the subgroup with the largest proportion in the spectrum (e.g., **mild**, 30%). Alternatively, the single choice might be the median value, which in this case is also **mild**.

A third technique, which is often used although not universally acceptable, is to "dimensionalize" the ordinal grades by assigning arbitrary numerical values to them. This was the tactic used earlier when we gave the soccer team 2 points for a win, 1 point for a tie, and 0 points for a loss, and determined a mean value of 1.32 point-credits per game. The arbitrary dimensional values permit a mean to be calculated and used as a single index of location for ordinal data. Similarly, for severity of illness, we could assign arbitrary scores of **0** for none, **1** for mild, **2** for moderate, and **3** for severe. The mean score for severity of illness in our 20 people would then be $[(5 \times 0) + (6 \times 1) + (5 \times 2) + (4 \times 3)]/20 =$

28/20 = 1.14. The arguments that can be offered both for and against the statistical propriety of this pseudo-dimensional procedure are beyond the scope of this discussion.

7.4.1.2. **DIMENSIONAL DATA**

Because dimensional data have a greater mathematical richness than the other three types of data, a much larger set of options is available.

The citation of proportions for each category of dimensional data is usually undesirable, because too many categories would have to be cited. Sometimes, however, a data analyst may dichotomize dimensional data and cite the results as proportions. Thus, if anyone above age 50 is regarded as "old," the spectrum of age in our 20 people could be summarized with the statement that 12/20 = 60% of the group was **old**. Occasionally, dimensional data are ordinalized and cited as proportions for ordinal categories. For ages in our group of 20 people, this result would be **47–49**, 25%; **50–52**, 35%; **53–55**, 20%; and >55, 20%. This type of ordinalization is used when histograms or frequency polygons are drawn to show the proportions of the spectrum at consolidated categories of dimensional data.

The most common tactic used for dimensional data, however, is to cite location with an index of central tendency. Both the mean and the median can claim this role of *central index*. The median is central because it occurs midway in the ranked array of data; the mean is central because it divides the group of data into two weighted zones that are equally balanced, with half the sum of weights occurring in the deviations on one side of mean and half on the other. For example, suppose we calculate the mean age of five soccer players who are 22, 23, 25, 26, and 29 years old. The formula $\Sigma X/N$ yields $(22+23+25+26+29)/5 = 25$ years as the mean. The respective deviations of each player from the mean, calculated as $X_i - \overline{X}$, are -3, -2, 0, $+1$, and $+4$. The sum of the negative deviations (-5) exactly equals the sum of positive deviations $(+5)$.

The mean can sometimes be misleading if one or several members of a relatively small group are "outlyers," who differ substantially from the others. For example, suppose one magnificent sexagenarian, still active and vigorous at age 67, plays goalie on a soccer team of teenagers. The other 10 members of the team are ages 12, 13, 13, 13, 14, 14, 14, 14, and 15 years old. The mean age of this team of 11 people will be 18.5 years—a result that is misleading because it suggests that most members of the team are much older than they really are. In addition, no one on the team is actually 18.5 years old or even comes within 3 years of it.

To avoid this type of problem, the *median* has increasingly been preferred as a central index. In the cited group of 11 players, the median would be the 6th ranked age (from either end): 14 years. As the mid-ranked central value in the group, the median has several other desirable attributes. It can express results for a longitudinal study that is incomplete. For example, suppose we are following the course of seven patients with advanced cancer. We find that death occurred in six patients at 3, 6, 8, 9, 11, and 12 months after treatment, but the seventh patient is still alive. We cannot calculate a mean survival time for this group until the seventh patient dies, but the median survival will be 9 months, no matter how long that last patient lives. A second advantage of the median is that it can avoid some of the peculiar fractions that occur when means are calculated for dimensional data that are integers. Thus, if a statistical report says that the average family today has 2.63 children, the reader may wonder about the status of the 0.63 fraction of a child.

The main advantages of the mean are that it is a standard ingredient (as noted later) of the formulas used for inferential statistics, and that, in the days before programmable hand-held electronic calculators, the mean was easier to compute than the median.

7.4.1.3. THE GEOMETRIC MEAN

Of several other indexes (the mode, harmonic mean, etc.), that can be used to express central tendency in dimensional data, the only one that is regularly used in medical research is the *geometric mean*. It is particularly pertinent when data are cited in exponential powers of a particular number that serves as the base for the values. Thus, bacterial counts are often expressed in powers of 10, with values such as 2.7×10^3, 8.7×10^5, 9.8×10^6, and so on. Antibody titers may be cited as the reciprocals of tube dilutions that are expressed in powers of 2 such as 1:8, 1:16, 1:512, and 1:1024. Although such measurements are expressed on a dimensional scale, the intervals between the main adjacent categories of the scale are equal in their exponential rather than incremental changes. The additive mean that is calculated for a series of exponential values will therefore be dominated by the largest of the numbers. Thus, the additive mean of 2.7×10^3, 8.7×10^5, and 9.8×10^6 is 3.6×10^6.

To avoid this problem, the geometric mean is calculated as the *nth root* of the *product* of the values in the data. In symbolic terms, a Π sign is the multiplicative equivalent of the Σ sign used for addition, and the 1/n exponential (or $\sqrt{}$) symbol is used to show the act of taking an nth root. Thus, the geometric mean is shown as

$$\text{G.M.} = (\Pi X_i)^{1/n}$$

For the three values under discussion here, the geometric mean is $[(2.7 \times 10^3)(8.7 \times 10^5)(9.8 \times 10^6)]^{1/3} = [2.30202 \times 10^{16}]^{1/3} = 2.84 \times 10^5$.

In the days before hand-held electronic calculators could easily compute n^{th} roots (using a function key usually marked y^x), the geometric mean was difficult to calculate directly. Instead, the observed values were transferred to logarithms, which could be added. The mean of the added logarithms, which was called the *log mean*, could then be transformed (if desired) to the geometric mean by finding its antilog, as $10^{\log\ mean} =$ geometric mean. For the three numbers mentioned in the previous paragraph, the respective logarithms are 3.43, 5.94, and 6.99. The log mean is 5.45, and $10^{5.45} = 2.84 \times 10^5$, which is the same as the geometric mean.

The word *mean* appears in both the additive mean, depicted with Σ, and the multiplicative (or geometric) mean, depicted with Π. When the word *mean* is used alone, however, it always refers to the conventional additive (or arithmetical) mean. When the multiplicative model is used, the result is called the *geometric mean*.

7.4.2. Indexes of Scope (Dispersion)

Nondimensional data seldom require special indexes of scope, because the scope of the spectrum is demonstrated when proportions are cited for the categorical constituents of the spectrum. For dimensional data, however, the scope of the spectrum is an important attribute that can be summarized in several different ways. The statistical expressions used for this purpose are often called *indexes of scope, spread,* or *dispersion*.

7.4.2.1. RANGE

The simplest index of dispersion for dimensional data is the *range*, which shows the spread between the highest and lowest values in the dimensional spectrum. In the 20 people of Table 7–1, the range of age was 35, extending from 47 to 82. The team of 11 soccer players noted in Section 7.4.1.2 had an age range of 55, from 12 to 67.

The trouble with range is that it gives no idea of the density (or compactness) of the data. In the latter example, we would not know whether the players are evenly spread in age along the spectrum from 12 to 67 or whether most of them are ages 24 to 26, with one outlyer at 12 and another outlyer at 67. Similarly, in Table 7–1, all but one of the people was less than 64 years old and most of them were below 55, yet the range extended to age 82.

The main mechanism that can be used to avoid this problem is to demarcate an inner zone of data, thus eliminating the outlyers. The size of the inner zone depends on the analyst's choice. For different purposes, the inner zone can occupy the middle 50%, 80%, 95%, or other proportions of the collected data.

7.4.2.2. **INNER-PERCENTILE RANGES**

The inner zone of data in a dimensional spectrum can be determined in at least two different ways: by ranking or by computing and inferring.

The ranking technique makes use of percentiles. Thus, the *interquartile* range is an inner 50% zone of data that extends from the 25th percentile, which is the *lower quartile*, to the 75th percentile, which is the *upper quartile*. For example, in the team of 11 soccer players in Section 7.4.1.2, the lower quartile is at age 13, the upper quartile is at age 14, and so the interquartile range is 1. For the 20 people in Table 7–1, the lower quartile is at 49.5, and the upper quartile is at 54.5. The interquartile range is 5.

Of the other inner percentile ranges, the most useful is the *inner 95-percentile range*, which is symbolized as ipr_{95}. It extends from the 2.5 percentile point to the 97.5 percentile point. The ipr_{95} is important, because it corresponds to the inner 95% zone of data that can be demarcated with the standard deviation technique described in the next section. For sets of data containing only 11 or 20 members, the 2.5 and 97.5 percentile points occur within the first and last members of the ranked spectrum, and so the ipr_{95} for small groups is usually the same as the range.

Henrik Wulff,[1] recognizing that a 2.5 percentile point occurs 1/40 of the way through the data, has proposed the word *quadragintile* for the lower and upper 2.5 percentile points. If you like or prefer this term, the ipr_{95} can be called the *quadragintile range*.

7.4.2.3. **STANDARD DEVIATION**

Another way to define an inner zone is by computing and inferring. The process depends on a statistical entity called the *standard deviation*. It represents an approximate average of the amount by which each item of data, X_i, deviates from the mean, $\overline{X}$. If we simply took a direct average of these deviations as $\Sigma(X_i - \overline{X})/N$, the result would always be zero. Instead, we could work with the absolute value of the deviations, regardless of sign, and get $\Sigma \mid X_i - \overline{X} \mid /N$—but the process is cumbersome. Consequently, for mathematical convenience, we square the deviations, add them, get an average, and take its square root.

The process produces several intermediate entities that are useful enough (for other purposes) to have been given specific names. First, we find and square each deviation from the mean as $(X_i - \overline{X})^2$. We then add these deviations to get the *deviance*, which is symbolized as $S_{xx} = \Sigma(X_i - \overline{X})^2$. [The two x subscripts on the S indicate that the deviance is calculated from $(X_i - \overline{X})(X_i - \overline{X})$. Later in Section 10.2.1, we shall meet an entity called *co-deviance* that is calculated for two variables, X and Y, as $S_{xy} = \Sigma(X_i - \overline{X})(Y_i - \overline{Y})$.] The univariate deviance is divided by either N or N−1 to form its average, which is called the *variance*. The *standard deviation* is the square root of the variance.

The decision to divide the deviance by N or by N−1 depends on whether the result will be used descriptively, to show the scope of data, or inferentially, to calculate a P value, standard error, or confidence interval. For purely descriptive purposes, we divide by N. For inferential purposes (as discussed in Chapter 9), the observed group of data becomes regarded as a sample from a larger population, and we divide by $N-1$. The division by $N-1$ will be used here because most modern electronic calculators employ $N-1$ for computing standard deviations. (If N is relatively large, the distinction between N and $N-1$ is trivial.)

Thus, the formula for calculating the standard deviation, s, is

$$s = \sqrt{S_{xx}/(N-1)} = \sqrt{\Sigma(X_i - \bar{X}_i^2)/(N-1)}$$

If you are actually going to do this calculation, rather than having a calculator accept the numbers and produce the result, the computation of S_{xx} is easier if you work with the alternative formula

$$S_{xx} = \Sigma X_i^2 - [(\Sigma X_i)^2/N]$$

For example, consider the five soccer players mentioned in the third paragraph of Section 7.4.1.2, who had a mean age of 25 and deviations from the mean of -3, -2, 0, $+1$, and $+4$. In this instance, the computation of S_{xx} is easy. As the sum of squared deviations, it will be $S_{xx} = 9+4+0+1+16 = 30$. The variance, obtained with $N-1 = 4$, is $30/4 = 7.5$, and the standard deviation is $\sqrt{7.5} = 2.74$. If we had not previously calculated the individual deviations from the mean, the deviance could be found as follows: $\Sigma X_i^2 = 22^2 + 23^2 + 25^2 + 26^2 + 29^2 = 3155$. $\Sigma X_i = 22+23+25+26+29 = 125$, and $(\Sigma X_i)^2/N = (125)^2/5 = 3125$. Then $\Sigma X_i^2 - (\Sigma X_i)^2/N = 3155 - 3125 = 30$, which is the same result obtained from $\Sigma(X_i - \bar{X})^2$.

The great virtue of the standard deviation is that an inner zone calculated as $\bar{X} \pm 1.96s$ will span 95% of the data—provided that the spectrum of dimensional data is distributed around the mean in the symmetrical bell-shaped pattern that is called *Gaussian*. Because the "1.96" is easily remembered as "2," a reader who sees values for the mean and standard deviation of a spectrum of Gaussian data can quickly get an idea of the scope of the spectrum. The inner 95% zone is found with a mental calculation that gives the boundary values as $\bar{X}-2s$ and $\bar{X}+2s$.

This approach to an inner 95% zone is so appealing that most people forget how often it is misleading because the data do not have a Gaussian pattern. For example, with the team of five soccer players whose ages have a mean of 25 and a standard deviation of 2.74, the values of $\bar{X}-2s$ and $\bar{X}+2s$ produce an inner 95% zone that extends from 19.52 to 30.48. This zone is larger than the actual range of the data, which extended only from 22 to 29. (If we calculated the variance with N, rather than $N-1$, the standard deviation would be $\sqrt{6} = 2.45$, and the inner 95% zone would be somewhat better, extending from 20.1 to 29.9.) For the 20 people in Table 7–1, the mean age was 53.8, and the standard deviation was 7.9. The inner 95% zone, calculated as $53.8 \pm (2)(7.9)$, extends from 38.0 to 69.6 and goes far below the lowest value (47) in the spectrum. The problem is not helped if we divide the deviance by N rather than $N-1$. If calculated with $N = 20$, rather than $N-1 = 19$, the standard deviation would drop slightly to 7.7, and the boundaries of the 95% zone would be about the same.

Beyond this problem, the standard deviation can sometimes produce a peculiar or impossible inner 95% zone in data that have distinctive outlyers or other non-Gaussian patterns. Thus, for the soccer team of 11 players cited in Section 7.4.1.2, the mean age is 18.45 years, and the standard deviation is 16.12. The inner 95% zone calculated from this information has an upper border of 50.69 years, but the lower border is an impossible -13.79 years.

For all these reasons, the standard deviation, although constantly used inferentially to calculate tests of statistical significance, has no *external descriptive* advantages except literary economy. It allows the central tendency and scope of a spectrum to be expressed in three symbols: $\overline{X} \pm s$. This economy has made those three symbols a popular statistical expression in scientific literature, but the statistical economy has its scientific costs. The mean, $\overline{X}$, will often misrepresent the central tendency of the data and is best replaced by the median. The inner 95% zone calculated with a standard deviation will often be peculiar or impossible, and is best determined using the 2.5 and 97.5 percentile values as an ipr_{95}.

7.5. INTERNAL COMPOSITION OF A SPECTRUM

When we examine the internal composition of a spectrum in search of unusual attributes, the idea of *unusual* or *heterogeneous* can be determined either by biological or by statistical reasoning. For example, if we say that each member of a spectrum weighs 4 kg., the spectrum is statistically homogeneous in weight. Biologically, however, the spectrum may be quite heterogeneous, consisting of newborn infants, small dogs, and large fish. If we say that each of four groups in a spectrum occupies 25% of the spectrum, the spectrum has an equiproportional or uniform distribution. Biologically, however, if the spectrum contains 50 men, 50 women, 50 children, and 50 fish, we would wonder what the fish are doing in the total group.

Although our attention is here concerned with statistical descriptions of a spectrum's contents, a reader should bear in mind that the statistical distinctions will often fail to denote important features that can be discerned only with logical or biological rather than mathematical reasoning.

7.5.1. *Nondimensional Spectrums*

The composition of a nondimensional spectrum is evident from the proportions contained in each category. An inspection of those proportions will indicate which categories are common or uncommon.

In a nominal spectrum, such as birthplace in Table 7–1, we can sometimes concentrate on the individual uncommon members, such as *Brazil* and *Costa Rica,* or we may consolidate the uncommon categories into an *Other* group for further analysis.

In a dichotomous spectrum, such as survival status, the composition of the spectrum is evident from either of the two proportions (for alive or dead), and its internal attributes usually receive no further attention.

An ordinal spectrum is usually evaluated according to the way it is scaled. If the individual categories are assigned arbitrary dimensional values, like the point-credit scores given to the soccer team, the spectrum can be analyzed in the manner used for dimensional data. If the ordinal categories are preserved as categories, their proportionate occurrence can be reviewed in the manner used for nominal data.

7.5.2. *Dimensional Spectrums and Standardized Variables*

The strategies used to evaluate the internal composition of a dimensional spectrum are both complicated and important. They are complicated because the spectrum usually contains too many individual dimensions for each one to be cited as a spectral proportion, and besides, the individual proportions would not denote the spectral location of the dimensional values. The strategies are important because they will be used not only now for deciding about unusual descriptive features of a spectrum, but also later for decisions about probabilities and chance.

Another aspect of the complexity arises because dimensional variables are expressed in arbitrarily selected units of measurement. *Age* can be cited in months or years; *height*, in inches or centimeters; *weight*, in pounds or kilograms; *serum sodium concentration*, in milligrams or millimoles per deciliter. Although the univariate spectrum of age, height, weight, or serum sodium concentration should be the same, regardless of which units are chosen for the measurement, the indexes of location and dispersion for each spectrum will differ according to the choice of units. These differences will create difficulties if we want to compare certain features of spectrum for two different variables. Furthermore, in certain multivariate analyses that are discussed later, the importance of a particular variable can be indicated by the coefficient attached to it, but the magnitude of this coefficient will be arbitrarily altered by the choice of the units in which the variable is measured.

7.5.2.1. **THE STANDARDIZED Z-SCORE**

A helpful tactic in dealing with all of these problems is to convert the values of a dimensional variable into a standardized form that makes them independent of the units of measurement. If the individual values of a group are cited as X_i, with $\overline{X}$ and s representing the mean and standard deviation of the spectrum, the standardized expression is

$$Z_i = \frac{X_i - \overline{X}}{s}$$

This formula says that we form Z_i by determining how greatly a particular value of data deviates from the mean and then dividing this individual deviation by the standard deviation of the group. For example, for the five soccer players whose ages were 22, 23, 25, 26, and 29, the group had a mean of 25 and a standard deviation of 2.74. To convert these ages to standardized variables, the value of Z_1 would be $(22-25)/2.74 = -1.09$. The value of Z_2 would be $(23-25)/2.74 = -0.73$. The remaining values are $Z_3 = 0$, $Z_4 = 0.36$, and $Z_5 = 1.46$.

This standardized transformation, which is sometimes called a *Z-score*, has several appealing virtues. It immediately indicates whether the magnitude of a particular item of data is above or below the mean and how greatly it differs from the mean. The Z-scores are also dimension-free, because they are expressed in relation to the standard deviation of the variable. A third merit of Z-scores, which will not be appreciated until later, is that the spectrum of a set of Z-scores has a mean of 0 and a standard deviation of 1.

The virtues of Z-scores can be used in at least three different ways. One common usage is in educational testing, where Z-scores are regularly employed to "grade on a curve" and to express results that can be compared for a student's performance in several different subjects (e.g., French literature, African geography, South American history), regardless of the particular units in which the individual tests were originally graded. The second usage, which will be described later, is in standardizing the variables (or the coefficients) of a multivariate analysis, so that all coefficients can be directly compared.

The third usage of Z-scores is in the interpretation of individual values of data. The Z-score provides a standardized method of determining how unusual a particular item of data may be. This unusualness, as discussed in the next section, can help us make decisions about items in a spectrum and also, as noted in Chapter 9, about variations that may occur by chance alone. The discussion that follows in Sections 7.5.2.2 and 7.5.2.3 is intended not only to help with decisions about unusual or uncommon members of a spectrum but also to prepare the reader for subsequent material, in Chapter 9, about statistical inferences based on probability.

7.5.2.2. UNCOMMON MEMBERS OF A SPECTRUM

When we summarized a spectrum of nondimensional data, the proportionate occurrence of each value immediately told us which members of the spectrum were uncommon. In a dimensional spectrum, however, these proportions of occurrence are seldom calculated. Furthermore, for dimensional data, the idea of *uncommon* generally refers to the magnitude of the item of data rather than its relative frequency of occurrence. We think of the uncommon or unusual members of the spectrum as those whose values are most distant or deviant from the central index.

An obvious way of finding the members with very high or very low values in a dimensional spectrum is to rank them and note their percentile locations or their positions at opposite ends of the spectrum. This process will identify the extreme members of the spectrum but will not indicate how greatly they deviate from the mean. Even if we subtract their values from the mean, the deviations will be absolute rather than standardized magnitudes. To indicate a standardized magnitude for uncommonness, we can use the Z-score technique. The formula listed for Z_i in Section 7.5.2.1 allows us to express any item of data in a spectrum as

$$X_i = \overline{X} + Z_i s$$

If the item is close to the mean, Z_i will be small. If the item is far from the mean, Z_i will be large, with its positive or negative sign indicating the side of the mean on which it lies.

To illustrate this process, consider the data for age in Table 7–1. The original values of the data tell us relatively little until they are arranged in the spectrum shown in Section 7.1. By noting that the spectrum has a mean of 53.8 and a standard deviation of 7.9, we can convert the data into Z-scores as follows:

Original Value	Z-Score
47	−0.86
50	−0.48
63	1.16
49	−0.61
51	−0.35
48	−0.73
54	0.03
53	−0.10
51	−0.35
50	−0.48
51	−0.35
82	3.57
53	−0.10
50	−0.48
59	0.66
52	−0.23
48	−0.73
61	0.91
55	0.15
49	−0.60

The standardized Z-scores immediately tell us several things that were not apparent in the original data. First, the spectrum is not symmetrically distributed around the mean. The Z-scores are negative for 14 items and positive for only six. In a symmetric distribution, we would expect about equal numbers of positive and negative Z-scores. Second, 11 items of data are relatively close to the mean, having absolute Z-scores below 0.5. Another seven items are reasonably close to the mean, with absolute Z-scores between 0.5 and 1.0. Of the remaining two items, one has a Z-score of 1.16 and the other, 3.57. The 3.57 value is particularly striking. We may originally have thought that the 82-year-old person was unusual in this group, but the Z-score adds a quantitative confirmation of that belief.

Similarly, for the team of 11 soccer players described in Section 7.3.1.2, the 67-year-old goalie was obviously unusual in age. Because the team had a mean of 18.45 and a standard deviation of 16.12, we can quantify that unusualness by noting that the goalie's Z-score is 3.01. By contrast, the youngest player on the team (at age 12) had a Z-score of -0.40 and the next oldest player (at age 15) had a Z-score of -0.21.

7.5.2.3. Z-SCORES AND RELATIVE FREQUENCIES IN A GAUSSIAN SPECTRUM

Perhaps the most remarkable feature of Z-scores occurs when they are calculated for a spectrum of data whose relative frequencies form the cocked-hat or bell-shaped symmetric curve that is called a *Gaussian distribution*. For this type of curve, about 68% of all the data in the spectrum are located in the range between $Z = -1$ and $Z = +1$, and 95% of the data are in the range between $Z = -1.96$ and $Z = 1.96$. If we decide that this inner 95% zone represents the common members of the data, the uncommon members will be located in the lower 2.5%, where $Z < -1.96$ and the upper 2.5% where $Z > 1.96$.

Thus, the Z-score for a Gaussian distribution can immediately tell us not only the standardized magnitude of deviation for an item of data, but also its position in a zone of relative frequency. Each value of Z separates the distribution into two zones containing a corresponding proportion of the distribution. The distinctions are shown in Figures 7–1 and 7–2.

In Figure 7–1, Z is given a single value, such as 1.96, which separates the distribution into two parts, with 2.5% of the distribution lying above the Z value, and 97.5% below it.

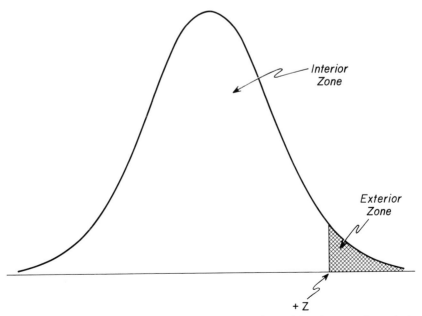

Figure 7–1. Division of a Gaussian spectrum into exterior and interior zones by a single value of Z ("one-tailed" arrangement).

In Figure 7–2, Z is marked symmetrically with the two values of +1.96 and −1.96. They separate the distribution into three parts, which form two zones. The inner zone, lying between the values of −1.96 and +1.96, contains 95% of the data. The outer zone contains 5% of the data, with 2.5% lying below −1.96 and 2.5% above +1.96.

For example, although the spectrum of age in Table 7–1 is not Gaussian, we noted in Section 7.4.2 that 11/20 = 55% of items in the data were in the zone from Z = −0.5 to Z = 0.5. If we use Z = ±1 to demarcate an inner zone, it contained 18/20 = 90% of all the values. An inner zone formed by Z = ±1.96 contained 19/20, or 95%, of the values in that spectrum.

7.5.2.4. **PROBABILITY VALUES & THE PARTITIONING ROLES OF A Z-SCORE**

In the foregoing discussion, we could think of a Z-score as producing a single boundary or a symmetric double boundary for the items contained in a spectrum. The single boundary divides the spectrum into two parts. The double boundary divides the spectrum into three zones: an inner zone and its two surrounding outer zones. The parts or zones of the spectrum that are exterior to the Z boundary are called its *tails*. Thus, for our 20 items of age in Section 7.5.2.2, if we choose Z = 0.5 as a one-tailed boundary, the exterior tail contains four items of data. They are the values for which Z = 1.16, 3.57, 0.66, and 0.91. If we choose Z = 0.5 as a two-tailed boundary, the exterior zone contains nine items. They include the four items just cited for the upper zone plus the items in the lower zone where Z = −0.86, −0.61, −0.73, −0.73, and −0.60.

As a one-tailed boundary, Z = 0.5 divides the spectrum into two parts with 4/20 = 20% of the items having a value above Z = 0.5 and 80% of the items being below it. As

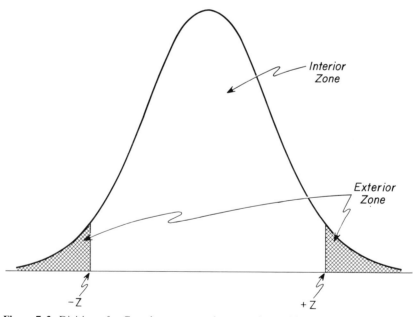

Figure 7–2. Division of a Gaussian spectrum into exterior and interior zones by positive and negative locations for a single value of Z ("two-tailed" arrangement).

a two-tailed boundary, $|Z| = 0.5$ divides the spectrum into three zones. The two exterior zones contain $9/20 = 45\%$ of the spectrum. The interior zone, with items having $|Z|$ values <0.5, contains $11/20 = 55\%$ of the spectrum.

If we happen to be dealing with a Gaussian curve, the mathematical shape of the curve lets us know the relative frequencies of items in the partitioned spectrum as soon as we know the value of Z. Table 7–2 shows this relationship for a Gaussian spectrum. For example, in a Gaussian spectrum, we would expect about 31% (actually 0.3085) of the values to exceed a one-tailed $Z = 0.5$ and about 62% (actually 0.617) to exceed a two-tailed $|Z| = 0.5$. In our observed non-Gaussian spectrum of age, the corresponding results were 25% and 45%.

This correspondence between Z-scores and relative frequencies in the spectrum has another valuable role. Suppose we intend to select one member randomly from the spectrum. The relative frequencies will tell us the chances of choosing someone with any designated value of Z. Thus, for the 20 people in Table 7–1, the chance of choosing someone with a two-tailed $|Z|$ value above 0.5 was 45%. The chance of choosing someone with a one-tailed Z value above 0.5 was 20%. In the Gaussian distribution shown in Table 7–2, the chance of choosing someone with a $|Z|$ value above 0.5 is 62%. The one-tailed chances for $Z \geqslant 0.5$ are 31%. The one-tailed chance for $Z \geqslant 1.645$ is 0.05. The two-tailed chance for $|Z| \geqslant 1.96$ is 0.05. The chance of getting someone in the interior zone where $|Z| < 1.96$ is 0.95.

As we shall see in Chapter 9, the term *P value* is used for the relative frequencies that denote the random chances of getting Z values in the designated exterior zones of a spectrum.

7.5.2.5. Z-SCORES AND COMPRISING INTERVALS

A Z-score can do yet another helpful thing. Suppose we do not know the mean of a Gaussian spectrum, but we know the value of s (the standard deviation) and we know the value of X_i for a single member of the spectrum. To estimate the mean of the spectrum, we can use the Z-score strategy to calculate a comprising interval in which the mean is likely to be located.

The principle works as follows. In a Gaussian distribution, the values of Z can be used

Table 7–2. RELATIVE FREQUENCIES IN A GAUSSIAN SPECTRUM

Value of Z	One-Tailed Partition Below Z	Above Z	Two-Tailed Partition Interior Zone	Exterior Zones
0	0.5	0.5	0	1
0.5	0.6915	0.3085	0.383	0.617
1.0	0.8415	0.1585	0.683	0.317
1.5	0.933	0.067	0.866	0.134
1.645	0.95	0.05	0.90	0.10
1.96	0.975	0.025	0.95	0.05
2.0	0.977	0.023	0.954	0.046
2.24	0.9875	0.0125	0.975	0.025
2.5	0.994	0.006	0.988	0.012
2.576	0.995	0.005	0.99	0.01
3.0	0.99865	0.00135	0.9973	0.0027
3.29	0.99995	0.0005	0.999	0.001

to create zones around the mean containing a specified proportion of the data. Thus, as shown in Table 7–2, if $Z = 0.5$, a zone of $0.5s$ surrounding the mean contains 38% of the data. If $Z = 1.0$, a zone of $1.0s$ around the mean contains 68% of the data. If $Z = 1.96$, a zone of $1.96s$ around the mean contains 95% of the data. In a Gaussian distribution with a mean of 53.8 and standard deviation of 7.9, 95% of the data would be located in the zone of $53.8 \pm (1.96)(7.9)$. This zone runs from 38.32 to 69.28.

We determine the size of this zone by our choice of a value for Z_α. The subscript α is used to indicate the preselected value of Z, and $1 - \alpha$ represents the size of the corresponding interval. If we want to include 95% of the data, then $1 - \alpha = 0.95$, and $\alpha = 0.05$. If we start with a single value of X_i, a zone of $Z_\alpha s$ placed around X_i will have a chance of $1 - \alpha$ of containing the mean. Thus if $Z_{0.32} = 1.0$, the zone has a 68% chance of containing the mean, and if $Z_{0.05} = 1.96$, the chance is 95%. Consequently, if we know that the distribution has a standard deviation of 7.9 and we are told that one value in the distribution is 63.8, we can construct the 95% comprising interval of $63.8 \pm (1.96)(7.9)$. This interval, which runs from 48.32 to 79.28, will have a 95% chance of including the true mean of the distribution. (Strictly speaking, the foregoing statement is not exactly correct. The exact statement is that the true mean will be included in 95% of comprising intervals calculated in the cited manner. Except for the risk of distressing a pedant, however, we will not get into trouble by thinking that the single comprising interval has a 95% chance of including the mean.)

The process of estimating the location of a mean by using a single item of data, a standard deviation, and a Gaussian Z-score does not seem very useful at the moment. After all, if we have a set of data and know the standard deviation, we are certainly likely to know the mean, and we would not need to estimate its location. The estimation process will become important later in Section 7.6, however, when we want to make decisions about the mean in a parent population by using the mean value found in a sample of data.

7.6. SUITABILITY OF A CENTRAL INDEX

When we chose a central index in Section 7.4.1.2, we thought about such candidates as the mean, median, and geometric mean, and we picked the one that seemed most suitable for the type of data under consideration. The choice was made intuitively, without any quantitative guidelines.

In many other circumstances, however, when we plan to use the central index externally, we may want or need a quantitative indication of how well the index does its job in representing the spectrum. These external representations occur when we compare two (or more) spectrums by contrasting their central indexes. Thus, we might compare the results of group A versus group B by examining the mean values in the two groups. Another type of external representation occurs when we use a single group as a *sample* for estimating what would be found in a larger population.

The internal characteristics of a spectrum become valuable for these goals. With appropriate combinations of the internal attributes of the spectrum, we can get reasonably good ideas about the external function of the central indexes.

7.6.1. *Index of Relative Dispersion*

Suppose we wanted to contrast the central indexes for group A versus group B. Before doing this comparison, we might want to know how well each central index fits the data of the spectrum it represents. If the data are relatively compact, with a small scope or dispersion, the index of central tendency is a good representative. If the data are diffusely spread in a wide spectrum, the index of central tendency may be the best single choice we can find, but it cannot do a very good job. For example, suppose we know that the standard deviation of a set of data is 4. If the mean is 250, the data set is quite compact. If the mean is 2, the data are quite dispersed.

The simplest way to get an idea of the compactness or relative dispersion of a set of data is to divide the index of scope by the index of central location. Because several different indexes can be used for scope and several others for location, a great many possibilities exist for calculating this *index of relative dispersion*. Of those possibilities, the only one that is commonly employed is called the *coefficient of variation*. It is calculated as $s/\overline{X}$: the standard deviation divided by the mean. Thus if $s = 4$ and $\overline{X} = 250$, the coefficient of variation (c.v.) is $4/250 = 0.016$. If $s = 4$ and $\overline{X} = 2$, the c.v. is $4/2 = 2$. The smaller the value of c.v., the more compact is the data set and the better will the mean represent the total group.

Another index of relative dispersion is called the *quartile deviation*. It is calculated as the semi-interquartile range divided by the median. Although often used in sociology, this index seldom appears in medical research.

No general standards have been established for making the decision that the index of location provides a good fit for the data. If the standard deviation is at least as large as the mean, i.e., $s/\overline{X} \geq 1$, the fit cannot be very good. Consequently, $s/\overline{X}$ should be <1 to denote a good fit, and the smaller the value of $s/\overline{X}$, the better the fit.

When two spectrums are *not* well fit by their central indexes, we can go ahead and compare them anyway—because there is no alternative if we still want to do the comparison—but some sort of caution needs to be imposed. The caution is provided, as we shall see in Chapter 9, by tests of statistical significance. When a central index does not fit well, the spectrum will have high variance, and high variance is a deterrent to achieving statistical significance.

7.6.2. *Stability of a Central Index*

We would like a central index not only to fit the data well but also to be relatively stable. The stability or fragility of a central index depends on N, the size of the group from which it is derived. For example, consider the proportion 0.25 as a central index for a group of binary data. This index can come from a group having four members, so that $0.25 = 1/4$; it can also come as 20/80 from a group having 80 members.

To demonstrate the fragility of 1/4 versus 20/80, let us arbitrarily remove one person from each group and see what happens to the index. According to the characteristics of the removed person, the central index for the reduced spectrum of 1/4 will be either 0/3 or 1/3. Thus, with a loss of only one person from the spectrum, the proportion of 0.25 can be altered to 0.00 or to 0.33. The spectrum of 20/80 is much more stable, however, because a similar loss of one person would make it vary only between $19/79 = 0.241$ and $20/79 = 0.253$.

A similar analysis of fragility can be undertaken if we arbitrarily remove one person from the spectrum of 20 values for age in Table 7–1. If we take out the 47-year-old person, the reduced mean becomes 54.2. If we take out the 82-year-old person, the reduced mean becomes 52.3. For any other removals, the reduced mean will vary between 52.3 and 54.2. This degree of variation around the observed mean of 53.8 is much less than the fragility noted for the proportion of 1/4. In the survival spectrum of Table 7–1, the survival rate was $11/20 = 55\%$. With the arbitrary removal of one person, this rate could vary from $11/19 = 58\%$ to $10/19 = 53\%$.

The technique of seeing what happens when one person is removed from the spectrum is one method of showing the relative fragility of a central index. A more conventional statistical approach is to use the *standard error* of the mean as described in the next section.

7.6.3. *The Standard Error*

In the foregoing discussion, we examined the relative stability (or fragility) of a central index by seeing what happened if one person were arbitrarily removed from the spectrum of data. The traditional statistical approach is to appraise fragility by using an entity called the *standard error*. The concept of a standard error is often hard to understand because it involves a flight into an imaginary mathematical world of repetitive sampling from a hypothetical population. As we begin that flight, fasten your seat belt.

Suppose we had a huge population of data having μ as its mean and σ as its standard deviation. These values of the mean, standard deviation, or other statistical attributes of the population are called its *parametric values,* or *parameters.* They are the values that are estimated when we take samples from the population. Now suppose we took a random sample of N members from that population and we calculated $\bar{X}$ as the mean of that sample. Now suppose we took a second random sample of N members and calculated its mean. To distinguish the two means, we can call the first one $\bar{X}_1$ and the second one $\bar{X}_2$. We now continue, taking a third sample of N members and obtaining its mean, $\bar{X}_3$. We do the same thing again to get a fourth sample, with its mean, $\bar{X}_4$. (If the parent population is big enough, we need not return each sample when we have finished calculating its mean. Otherwise, we return or replace each sample before taking the next one.) If we continue this sampling process over and over, we would get a series of mean values $\bar{X}_1, \bar{X}_2, \bar{X}_3, \bar{X}_4, \bar{X}_5$, and so on for a series of samples, each containing N members.

These values of the means would constitute a group of data. The group would have a mean of its own and a standard deviation of its own. With some mathematics that the reader will be spared, it can be shown that the mean of this group of means would approach μ, which is the *parametric* mean of the parent population, and the standard deviation of the group of means would approach $\sigma/\sqrt{N}$, where σ is the *parametric* standard deviation.

All this activity seems very theoretical, and it is, but it has a pragmatic application. If we have a single group of data, with mean $\bar{X}$ and standard deviation s, we can regard the group of data as a random sample from a larger population. We can use s to estimate the value of σ in that larger population. If we then calculate $s/\sqrt{N}$, we will have an estimate of the standard deviation that would be found in a group of means taken from the larger population. This value of $s/\sqrt{N}$, which is called the *standard error of the mean* and is symbolically written as $s_{\bar{x}}$, could then serve as an index of the fragility of the mean.

7.6.3.1. ILLUSTRATIONS OF STANDARD ERROR

For dimensional data, the standard error of the mean is directly calculated from the standard deviation, s, and the size of the group, N. Thus, for the spectrum of 20 values of age in Table 7–1, the mean was 53.8 and the standard deviation was 7.9. The standard error of the mean would be $s_{\bar{x}} = 7.9/\sqrt{20} = 1.77$.

For data expressed in proportions, the standard deviation of the proportion p is $\sqrt{pq}$, and the standard error of the proportion is $\sqrt{pq/N}$. This formula lets us know why 0.25 was a fragile value in Section 7.6.2 when obtained from 1/4 and relatively stable when obtained from 20/80. With 1/4, the standard error of the proportion is $\sqrt{(0.25)(0.75)/4} = 0.217$. With 20/80, the standard error is $\sqrt{(0.25)(0.75)/80} = 0.048$.

7.6.3.2. INTERPRETATION OF STANDARD ERROR

The values of s and $s_{\bar{x}}$ have a distinct correspondence beyond the mere calculation of $s_{\bar{x}} = s/\sqrt{N}$. As the standard deviation of items in the data, s serves as an index of dispersion for the data. As the standard error of the mean, $s_{\bar{x}}$ is an index of dispersion for a series of hypothetical means taken as samples from a larger parent population. Because small values of s imply a compact distribution of data, small values of $s_{\bar{x}}$ imply a compact spread of possible values for the mean. Because $s_{\bar{x}}$ is calculated as $s/\sqrt{N}$, it is not surprising that $s_{\bar{x}}$ will become small with large sizes of N. The larger the size of the group, the more stable is its mean.

Another important point to bear in mind about $s_{\bar{x}}$ is that it is an inferential, not a descriptive, index. It does not describe the scope of data observed in a group. It provides an estimate of fragility for the mean of the data. We can use that estimate, as noted shortly, to calculate a special zone called a *confidence interval,* but the standard error does not describe the collection of data. The standard error is often used improperly for descriptive purposes on graphs or bar charts where the mean is marked and surrounded by small flanges, such as $\vdash\!\bullet\!\dashv$, which show a surrounding zone of one standard error on either side of the mean. Because the value of $s/\sqrt{N}$ will always be smaller than s, the zone between the flanges will always be smaller and look more compact than the zone that would be produced descriptively as $\bar{X}\pm s$. The result is a distorted portrait of the data, because what is being described as $\bar{X}\pm(s/\sqrt{N})$ is an indication of the fragility of the mean, not an indication of scope for the spectrum of data.

7.6.4. *Confidence Intervals for a Central Index*

Everything we have discussed so far was devoted to describing a group of data, regardless of how the group was obtained. Another fundamental role of statistical activity, however, is to make inferences rather than mere descriptions. The inferential work occurs when we acquire a group deliberately as a *sample,* randomly drawn from a larger parent population. The purpose of the sampling and the inference is to estimate the parameters of the parent population.

In the customary statistical notation for this process, we use Roman letters, such as $\bar{X}$, s, and p, for the mean, standard deviation, or proportion observed in the sample. We then use the corresponding Greek letters, μ (mu), σ (sigma), and π (pi), respectively, for the parametric values in the parent population.

This type of inferential sampling seldom occurs in medical research. Almost all the groups studied in medical research were assembled as collections of people who were conveniently available to the investigator. Inferential sampling is commonly done, however, for political polls, marketing analysis, and other social science activities. Although the inferential reasoning for a single sample or group may not seem pertinent for medical work, the strategy will become important later on, in Chapter 9, when it becomes applied for stochastic contrasts of the results in two (or more) groups.

7.6.4.1. ESTIMATING μ, σ, OR π

When we have a single sample of data, we can use the results immediately to estimate the population parameters. With mathematical proofs that are not shown here, it can be demonstrated that a population proportion, π, is best estimated from the proportion, p, found in the sample. The mean, μ, is best estimated from the $\bar{X}$ in the sample and the standard deviation, σ, from s in the sample. (The reason for calculating s with $N-1$ rather than N is that the $N-1$ calculation usually gives closer estimates of σ.)

This process will give us estimates of the populational parameters, but we have no idea of how accurate those estimates might be. Thus, if the proportion of 0.25 comes from 20/80, we might be much more confident that the parameter is actually 0.25 than if the sample size is 4, with the sample proportion being 1/4. What we need, therefore, is a mechanism for indicating the confidence that can be given to the estimate derived from the sample.

7.6.4.2. ROLE OF THE STANDARD ERROR

If you recall what was done in Section 7.6.3, we obtained the standard error from a process of repetitive hypothetical sampling. We found a special group containing individual items that were sample means, and the standard deviation of that group of means was the standard error. Its value was $\sigma/\sqrt{N}$, and we could estimate it as $s/\sqrt{N}$.

Now recall what was done in Section 7.5.2.5, when a comprising interval was calculated. For a single item of data, X_i, from a Gaussian distribution having standard deviation s, we could determine a comprising interval for the mean as $\overline{X} = X_i \pm Z_\alpha s$. We now apply this same principle in our current situation, where we have a single item of data, $\overline{X}$, as the observed mean in a potential collection of means having $s_{\overline{X}}$ (the standard error) as their standard deviation. If the hypothetical collection of means has a Gaussian distribution, we could use this tactic to determine a comprising interval for μ. The interval would be $\mu = \overline{X} \pm Z_\alpha s_{\overline{X}}$.

7.6.4.3. ROLE OF THE CENTRAL LIMIT THEOREM

The demonstration that a collection of repetitively sampled means (or proportions) has a Gaussian distribution is provided by the *Central Limit Theorem*, which we shall accept here without showing the pages of higher mathematics required for a proof. According to this theorem, which is regarded as one of the most important in all of mathematical statistics, we obtain a Gaussian distribution when we assemble a collection of repetitively sampled means (or proportions) from a parent population. The remarkable thing about the theorem is that the distribution of the parent population is unimportant. It can be rectangular, U-shaped, J-shaped, or any other shape. The *means* of the samples taken repetitively from the distribution will have a Gaussian shape.

7.6.4.4. CALCULATION OF THE CONFIDENCE INTERVAL

With the reassurance that a Gaussian strategy can be applied, we can proceed to use it. We choose a level of Z_α for the confidence that we want in the calculation, and we then calculate a *confidence interval* around the sample mean as $\overline{X} \pm Z_\alpha s_{\overline{X}}$. We now call it a *confidence interval* rather than a *comprising interval,* because it is calculated from a mean rather than from a single item of data in a sample and because it is used to estimate μ, the populational parametric mean. According to this estimate, μ has a chance of $1-\alpha$ of lying in the interval spanned between $\overline{X} - Z_\alpha s_{\overline{X}}$ and $\overline{X} + Z_\alpha s_{\overline{X}}$.

7.6.4.5. ILLUSTRATION OF CALCULATIONS AND INTERPRETATION

Consider the 20 people in Table 7–1 who had a mean age of 53.8, with a standard deviation of 7.9. If these people were randomly sampled from a larger population, the true mean of that population has a 95% chance of being located in the interval

$$53.8 \pm 1.96(7.9/\sqrt{20})$$

This interval is 53.8 ± 3.46 and extends from 50.3 to 57.3.

In Table 7–1, the survival rate was $11/20 = 55\%$. If we wanted a 99% confidence interval around this rate, we would want to have $1-\alpha = 0.99$, and so we need to find $Z_{0.01}$. In Table 7–2, $Z_{0.01} = 2.576$. We therefore calculate the 99% confidence interval as

$$0.55 \pm 2.576 \sqrt{(0.55)(0.45)/20},$$

which is 0.55 ± 0.287. The confidence interval would run from 26.3% to 83.7%.

This result shows that the confidence interval, although calculated for statistical inference from a central index, is also a useful way of describing the fragility of the index. Thus, the value of 55%, when obtained from the numbers 11/20, is a fragile proportion. Its true value, with 99% confidence, can run from 26.3% to 83.7%. For a less confident interval, we could calculate it with 95% rather than 99% confidence. When $1-\alpha = 0.95$, $\alpha = 0.05$ and $Z_{0.05} = 1.96$. The 95% confidence interval would be $0.55 \pm 1.96 \sqrt{(0.55)(0.45)/20}$, which is 0.55 ± 0.216. The 95% confidence interval would be smaller than before, but still quite large. It would run from 33.4% to 76.6%.

The value of the standard error, $s_{\bar{x}}$, is a good indication of the fragility of a central index because the confidence interval is calculated as $\bar{X} \pm Z_{\alpha}s_{\bar{x}}$. A small value of $s_{\bar{x}}$ will yield a tight confidence interval and suggest that the $\bar{X}$ value is a close estimate of the true mean.

Thus, in Section 7.5.2.6, when $s_{\bar{x}}$ was $7.9/\sqrt{20} = 1.77$, the confidence interval around 53.8 went from 50.3 to 57.3. On the other hand, if the standard deviation of the data were 1.4 rather than 7.9, the standard error would be $1.4/\sqrt{20} = 0.31$. The confidence interval around 53.8 would go from 53.2 to 54.4, and the value of 53.8 would seem less fragile. Consequently, although the ratio of $s/\bar{X}$ may be used to indicate the coefficient of variation with which the mean represents the data, the ratio of $s_{\bar{x}}/\bar{X}$ can be viewed as denoting the fragility of the mean itself. In fact, as we shall see in Chapter 9, the inverse of this ratio—$\bar{X}/s_{\bar{x}}$—is an excellent index of stochastic or probabilistic variation in a group of dimensional data.

7.7. SYNOPSIS

All the indexes discussed so far refer to the spectrum of a single variable in a group of data. Because the group of data can contain several variables, we might also want to examine the relationships among two or more variables—but a reader who has come this far deserves a rest. The relationships among variables will be saved for the statistical indexes of association discussed in Chapter 10. The univariate spectral indexes that have just been discussed can be summarized as follows:

Statistical quantification uses three basic tools: *sums,* obtained as frequency counts or added amounts; *quotients,* obtained when one sum (or quotient) is divided by another; and *rankings,* which can be applied for external comparisons of spectral indexes or for internal comparisons of data within a spectrum. Quotients can be formed as a *mean,* which is an added amount divided by a frequency count; a *proportion,* which is the frequency count of a subgroup divided by the count of the total group; or a *rate,* which is classically a division of frequency counts for two different groups.

The spectrum (or distribution) of a single variable in a group of data is summarized by citing a central index of magnitude for the data and an index of scope (or dispersion). For dimensional data, the median is often preferable to the mean as a central index, and an inner percentile range is often preferable to the standard deviation for denoting dispersion. The geometric mean may be the best central index when the dimensions are expressed in exponential powers of a selected base. A nondimensional variable is summarized with the proportions occupied by the relative frequencies of each category.

The internal attributes of a dimensional spectrum are often best demonstrated by transforming the items of data to Z-scores, which indicate each item's magnitude of standardized deviation from the mean. For a Gaussian distribution, each Z-score also demarcates specific zones of relative frequency for the data.

An index of relative dispersion, such as the coefficient of variation, will show the effectiveness with which a central index represents the data in the spectrum. The standard error can be calculated to indicate the stability of the central index or to form a confidence interval, using a selected value of Z_α, that shows the zone of likely location for the populational parameter estimated from the central index.

EXERCISES

Exercise 7.1. Here is a summary of a patient's medical record: "The patient is a 32-year-old farmer who lives with his wife and two children in Cheshire, Ct. His chief complaint is fever for the past 3 months. His white blood count was 8700 and urinalysis was normal." Make a list of all the variables that can be noted in this descriptive account. For each variable, name the type of scale that was used to express the result, cite the particular value associated with this patient, and cite the index expressions you would use for summarizing the results of analogous data assembled for the same variables for a group of patients. Please use the following format:

Name of Variable	Type of Scale	Value for This Patient	Summary Indexes
Age (yrs.)	Dimensional	32	Mean and standard deviation (or median and ipr_{95})
•	•	•	•
•	•	•	•
•	•	•	•

Exercise 7.2. A group of patients on a medical ward have the following values for fasting blood sugar: 62,78,79,80,82,82,83,85,87,91,96,97,97,97,101,120,135,180, 270,310, and 400. Calculate or demonstrate the following indexes for these data: mean, median, geometric mean, range, standard deviation, coefficient of variation, inner 90-percentile range, standard error of the mean, 95% confidence interval for the mean.

Exercise 7.3. What indexes would you prefer for summarizing the central tendency and spread of the data in Exercise 7.2? (State the reasons for your choice.)

Exercise 7.4. The results of a clinical trial are presented in a two-way table as follows:

	Number of Patients Who Received:		
Outcome	Treatment A	Treatment B	Treatment C
Success	40	70	50
Failure	320	280	295

7.4.1. Classify the scales used for the variables displayed in this table.
7.4.2. What proportion of patients received treatment A?
7.4.3. What is the proportion of patients who were successful when receiving treatment C?

7.4.4. If you had to give a single index for the success achieved in this entire trial, what would you choose?

Exercise 7.5. A poll taker has been asked to conduct a poll to reassure the leaders of a political party that they will win the next election. They want the confidence interval to be 97.5% for this reassurance. They believe that about 55% of the voters are currently in favor of their party. What sample size is needed for the poll to be able to provide the desired reassurance?

Exercise 7.6. In the certifying examination of the American Board of Omphalology, the candidates receive a total raw numerical score based on right and wrong answers to the questions. For psychometric (that's a fancy word for educational test-ology) purposes, the board wishes to transform all these results so that the group of candidates will have a mean score of 500, with a standard deviation of 100. How would the board alter the individual raw scores to accomplish this goal?

Exercise 7.7. According to the spectrum of results in a hospital laboratory, serum chloride has a Gaussian distribution with a mean of 101.6 and a standard deviation of 5.2.

7.7.1. What is the probability of finding a patient whose chloride value is >114?

7.7.2. What inner range of chloride values will include 90% of patients?

7.7.3. What proportion of patients can be expected to have chloride values lower than 88.6?

Exercise 7.8. A hospital laboratory reports that its customary values in healthy people for serum licorice concentration have a mean of 50 units with a standard deviation of 8 units. From these values, the laboratory calculates its range of normal as $50 \pm (2)(8)$, which yields the interval from 34 to 66. In the results sent to the practicing physicians, the laboratory says that 34–66 is the 95% confidence interval for the range of normal. What is wrong with this statement?

CHAPTER REFERENCE

1. Wulff, 1976.

Statistical Indexes of Contrast

Although seldom discussed in textbooks of statistics, indexes of contrast are probably the most valuable summary expressions used in science. These are the numbers we think about when we decide that a distinction is quantitatively important. We seldom recognize the specific indexes used for the decisions, because the acts of contrast are often performed mentally, without specific calculations.

We do those quantitative mental comparisons when we decide that a child has grown much taller since last seen or that a person has lost a great deal of weight. A simple ranking of magnitudes would suffice to show that one height or weight is larger than the other and that a gain or loss has occurred, but the comparison acquires a judgmental component when we say "much taller" or "a great deal of weight." To use those phrases, we had to make a decision about how much is "much" or "a great deal."

This chapter contains a discussion of what we think about and how we use the information when we compare two quantities and decide that the distinction between them is important or trivial. Although quantitative importance is constantly determined when data are evaluated, the constituent elements of the process are seldom formally identified. A few of those elements have become prominent in recent years, however, and have received formal citations. To determine the sample size needed for a clinical trial, the investigator must often begin by specifying an *expected proportionate improvement* in the group receiving the principal treatment. In discussing the alleged etiologic role of various agents in producing disease, epidemiologists often refer to an *incremental risk*, a *risk ratio*, or an *odds ratio*. The ideas contained in the italicized terms all arise from indexes of contrast.

8.1. INDEXES AVAILABLE FOR CONTRASTS

An index of contrast is used to summarize a comparison of the spectrums in two sets of data. Let us assume that A represents the result—it can be a mean, median, proportion, or rate—that summarizes data for group A; and that B represents the corresponding result for group B. To make things concrete, let us say that A is 19.2 and B is 8.7. These two numbers can be compared to yield six different indexes of contrast. There are two *increments*, two *ratios*, and two *proportionate increments*. The rest of this section is concerned with the way those six values can be reduced to the two that are the essential indexes of contrast.

The two increments can be created as $A - B$ or as $B - A$. Thus, for 19.2 and 8.7, the available increments are 10.5 and -10.5. (To avoid having to use two words, *increment* and *decrement*, for positive and negative values, *increment* will be employed here for whatever occurs as the result of subtracting two numbers.) The two ratios are A/B and B/A. In this case, they are $19.2/8.7 = 2.21$ and $8.7/19.2 = 0.45$. The two proportionate increments refer to the relative magnitude of each increment in reference to its starting point. Thus, the proportionate increments are $(A - B)/B$ and $(B - A)/A$. In this instance, the proportionate increments are $10.5/8.7 = 1.21$ and $-10.5/19.2 = -0.55$. Proportionate increments are regularly multiplied by 100 and expressed as percentages. Thus, the two foregoing proportionate increments are 121% and -55%.

Some simple algebra can show that the proportionate increments and ratios are mutually redundant, because the ratio equals the corresponding proportionate increment minus one. Thus, $(A - B)/B = (A/B) - 1$. Consequently, if we know the ratio, we can always find the proportionate increment and vice versa. This redundancy allows us to reduce the six possible expressions to four if we eliminate either the ratios or the proportionate increments. We can eliminate either one; but to allow us to proceed, let us keep the ratios. (The reader should bear in mind that *proportionate increment* could replace the *ratio* wherever a *ratio* appears in the ensuing discussion.) We are now left to choose among $A - B$, $B - A$, A/B, and B/A.

In any comparison, we usually have something in mind as the baseline. It can be a pretreatment value or the result found in a control or standard group. If we let B represent the baseline value, we will want to know the contrast of A versus B. The indexes will then be reduced to two: $A - B$ and A/B.

8.2. THE NEED FOR TWO INDEXES

Just as we needed two indexes—magnitude and scope—to summarize a univariate collection of data, we also need two indexes—increment and ratio—to summarize a contrast of two spectrums.

When we decide that a particular distinction is quantitatively impressive, the decision is usually based on a simultaneous appraisal of both the increment and the ratio. Thinking about the ratio alone can be misleading because we can sometimes find high ratios with trivial increments. For example, suppose the control group of people in a study of weight reduction loses a mean of 0.2 kg. and the actively treated group loses 0.6 kg. The ratio here is impressive: The actively treated group lost three times as much weight as the controls; but the increment of 0.4 kg. shows that the distinction is trivial. Conversely, we can sometimes find impressive increments for trivial ratios. Thus, a value of 5 kg. would seem substantial as the increment in the means of two similar groups in a weight reduction program. If both groups were massively obese, however, and were incarcerated so that the active group lost a mean of 60 kg. and the control group lost 55 kg., the ratio of 1.1 (= 60/55) would not be impressive.

The need to look at two indexes of contrast is particularly important when we consider epidemiologic data about risks of disease. Suppose cancer of the thyroid is reportedly found in 4 of 10,000 people who drink tea and in 1 of 10,000 people who do not drink tea. The two rates of 0.0004 and 0.0001 form a ratio of 4, which might be an impressive item of evidence in the proposal that tea drinking causes cancer of the thyroid. The incremental risk of 0.0003, however, might seem small enough so that devoted tea drinkers might not want to discontinue their favorite beverage.

8.3. THE PROBLEM OF PERCENTAGES OF PERCENTAGES

An important problem in evaluating contrasts occurs when proportional increments create percentages of percentages. Suppose the failure rates in a particular trial of therapy are 31% for the control group and 28% for the treated group. The treatment will have lowered the failure rate by an increment of 3%. If the result is expressed as a proportionate increment, however, the treated group's result is $3/31 = 0.097 = 10\%$ lower than that of the control group. Thus, if the investigators state that results in the treated group were "10% better" than in the controls, we cannot tell whether the 10% is a proportional increment or a direct increment. If the 10% increment were a direct reduction in fatality rate, the treated group's result would fall to 21% and would be much more impressive than 28%, which was actually observed.

This distinction is particularly vital when the planners of a clinical trial choose a quantitatively important difference. Suppose they want the actively treated group to have a proportionate improvement 25% better than that of the control group. If the "improvement" here is based on mortality rate and if mortality in the control group is 8%, the treated group's mortality would have to be 6%, which is 25% lower than 8%. As we shall see later (in Chapter 9), the sample size needed for statistical significance is calculated according to the direct rather than the proportionate increment. Consequently, an enormous number of patients will be needed in this trial to show that a direct increment of 2% is more than a chance phenomenon.

8.4. QUANTITATIVE AND CLINICAL CONSIDERATIONS IN THE MAGNITUDE OF "IMPORTANCE"

Although both the increment and the ratio (or proportionate increment) must be evaluated to decide the impressiveness (or quantitative significance) of the distinction noted in a contrast of two numbers, no precise magnitudes can be cited for the boundaries that define "importance." The importance of a distinction will obviously increase with increasing values of both the increment and the ratio, but certain decisions will often depend on the biologic or clinical content of the contrast, rather than on the numerical magnitudes alone.

For example, suppose 2% is the incremental difference in success rates for treatment A versus treatment B. This increment may not seem impressive if success is defined as "total relief of headache within 4 hours after taking medication." The increment may be quite impressive, however, if it refers to "absence of postdelivery complications in babies with breech presentations." In different examples, the two proportions of $38/63 = 0.603$ and $37/63 = 0.587$ are unimpressive for their increment of 0.016 and ratio of 1.03; yet the distinction may be enough to decide which team wins the soccer championship of the league. An increment of 0.0025, i.e., 0.25%, may seem trivial but can lead to major effects in the stock market if it represents a change in the prime lending rate.

8.4.1. *Decisions About Rankings*

The foregoing examples help illustrate the many attributes that must be considered when quantitative decisions are made about importance. The first step is to decide whether the quantitative distinctions are to be ranked or rated. For a ranking, decisions are easy. Whichever magnitude is larger or smaller is the "winner" according to the desired specifications of high or low scores for success.

The only caveat in a ranking is that N be large enough to keep the value or score from being too "fragile" for serious consideration. For example, a soccer team that has won 75% of its games has outranked another team that has won 74% of its games. If the 74% comes from 48/65 and the 75% comes from 3/4, however, we might regard the 3/4 as being too fragile to warrant comparison. The team that has played only 4 games might be regarded as ineligible for the compared rankings.

8.4.2. *Internal Decisions for Rating Importance*

Aside from the caveat about group size, decisions are easy when two magnitudes are merely ranked. The real problems arise when the quantitative distinction must be rated (or graded) as large or small, important or trivial.

The decision can sometimes be made internally, merely from the two quantitative indexes of contrast, if they are both impressive or unimpressive and if there are no external considerations that affect the decision. For example, if the success rates in a clinical trial are 68% for treatment A and 17% for treatment B, the ratio of 4 and the direct increment of 51% are obviously both impressive. If the rates are 13.50% for A and 13.25% for B in some other circumstance, the increment of 0.25% and the ratio of 1.02 are both quantitatively unimpressive. In the latter instance, however, we might think about the external clinical considerations before deciding that the distinction was trivial. Thus, if 13.50% and 13.25% referred to values of the prime lending rate for a national bank, the external considerations might make us decide that the distinction was important, despite its relatively low magnitudes for ratio and increment.

Even when both indexes of contrast seem impressively high, a consideration of external phenomena may modify the decisions about importance. For example, in the clinical trial noted in the previous paragraph, suppose that success was defined as "increase of at least 10 ml. in maximum breathing capacity." Despite the impressive quantitative distinction in the success rate for treatment A, we might conclude that the distinction was not clinically important because the criterion for success was relatively trivial.

Consequently, decisions about the quantitative importance of a distinction are regularly affected by factors external to the two indexes of contrast. When the two indexes are similar in suggesting that the distinction is important or unimportant, the decision can sometimes be reversed by the external factors. When the two indexes are not similar—i.e., the ratio seems important, but the increment seems trivial or vice versa—the external factors may be the main mechanism used for reaching a decision.

8.4.3. *External Considerations for Rating Importance*

The external considerations in appraising ratios and increments usually involve two quantitative decisions and one qualitative judgment. The quantitative decisions rest on the relative frequency of general occurrence of the agent and the condition under study. The qualitative judgment rests on the medical importance of the condition.

For example, a drop in a failure rate from 10% to 7.5% does not seem particularly impressive as a ratio of 1.3 and increment of -0.025. Qualitatively, the decline may seem more important, however, if it refers to a 30-day mortality rate for a particular clinical condition. If the clinical condition is quite uncommon, the decline may still not be impressive. If the condition is a common event, such as acute myocardial infarction, the result may be quite impressive if converted to number of lives saved rather than mortality-rate increments.

The quantitative concept of prevalence was also used to decide that a change of 0.25% was important in the prime lending rate. As an individual increment or ratio, the change was unimportant. When multiplied by the amount of money that would be affected, the result became impressive. Even without this quantitative distinction, however, the change of 0.25% might be perceived qualitatively as important if it marked an alteration in the trend of a nation's fiscal policy.

The quantitative occurrence of exposure may be important if a commonly used agent—such as coffee, tea, or aspirin—has a risk associated with it. The incremental magnitude of the risk may seem quite small, but the total number of cases may become impressive if large numbers of people are exposed. For example, as noted in Section 8.2, suppose the rate of thyroid cancer is indeed 0.0004 in tea drinkers and 0.0001 in non–tea drinkers. The rate of incremental risk, 0.0003, may not be frightening to individual tea drinkers. A society that contains 10,000,000 tea drinkers, however, can expect to have 4000 cases of thyroid cancer, of which 3000 would be attributable to the tea drinking.

This distinction between the individual risk and the societal or public health risk often determines the way that importance is judged for clinical or public health decisions. For clinical practitioners and patients, the decision often depends on the individual internal magnitudes of ratios and increments. For public-health policy makers, the decision often involves external considerations of prevalence and total societal burden. Because the external considerations will often produce decisions opposite to those determined from internal considerations alone, conflicting evaluations can regularly be expected. Thus, individual people who like drinking tea and who do not feel threatened by its incremental risk of 0.0003 may be appalled by the policy zealots who want sales of tea to be discontinued or heavily taxed in an effort to eliminate the 3000 extra cases of thyroid cancer in the general community.

Because there are no right or wrong answers to these conflicts and because a reasonable justification can be offered for both policies, the main point to be noted now is simply that quantitative importance can be discerned by inspecting both an increment and a ratio and by then considering their external connotations. For data expressed in proportions, most people would probably regard a direct increment of 0.10 as significant, regardless of the associated ratio. Smaller increments in proportions may become significant if the associated ratio is large enough. The value for "large enough" will often depend on where the direct increment is located in the scale of proportions. For example, a change in the improvement rate from 1% to 4% may become regarded as significant because the ratio is 4, but a change from 81% to 84% may be regarded as trivial.

If the contrast involves external considerations that affect medical importance, these external considerations may allow quantitative significance to be declared when the increments and ratios are both relatively small. Thus, a decline in mortality rate from 10% to 7.5% may be regarded as significant, despite its relatively small values for increment and ratio.

The exercises at the end of the chapter contain some challenges that will allow you to use your own beliefs and demarcations for quantitative significance.

8.5. **THE CONTRAST OF COMPLEMENTARY RATES**

One of the most common statistical displays for clinical epidemiologic data is a fourfold table. It contains two variables, each expressed dichotomously. They often represent presence or absence of a particular maneuver and presence or absence of a particular outcome event. Thus, we might examine a fourfold table to inspect the success rates for treatment A versus treatment B or the occurrence rates of thyroid cancer in tea drinkers and non–tea drinkers. These fourfold tables can become statistically quite complex, because an apparently simple contrast of *two* rates (or proportions) actually produces a table containing *nine* numbers, which can then be expressed with diverse statistical indexes.

For example, suppose we want to contrast the success rates of 22% for treatment A and 14% for treatment B. We can immediately say that A was better by an increment of 8%, by a ratio of $22/14 = 1.57$, and by a proportionate increment of 57% ($= 8\%/14\%$). Looking at the actual numbers that produce the original percentages of success, we find that they represent proportions of 11/49 for A and 7/50 for B. We can now construct the following table:

| Treatment | Number of Patients | | Total |
	Success	*Failure*	
A	11	38	49
B	7	43	50
Total	18	81	99

These nine numbers contain the four interior cells that are the basic elements of the fourfold table. They also contain the marginal totals for each dichotomous category of the two main variables. Finally, they show N, the grand total.

8.5.1. *Paradoxical Contrasts*

Because the rates or proportions that express the results of a fourfold table are complementary, we can encounter some striking paradoxes if we form ratios from the complementary rather than the original rates.

Thus, for the success rates of 22% for treatment A and 14% for treatment B, the ratio was 1.57 and the proportionate increment was 57%. On the other hand, if we look at the complementary failure rates—78% for A and 86% for B—the increment of 8% retains the same absolute value, but the other relative superiorities of treatment A become strikingly changed. The ratio of 78/86 is 0.91 and the proportionate incremental reduction will be 9%, which can be calculated either as $0.91 - 1$, or as $-8\%/86\%$.

We are thus left with a paradox. For exactly the same set of data comparing the results of two treatments, A is proportionately 57% better than B if we look at success rates but only 9% better if we look at the complementary failure rates. The distinction can easily be shown algebraically if we use the symbols p for the success rate and $q = 1-p$ for the complementary failure rates. The incremental difference in results will have the same magnitude because $p_A - p_B$ gives exactly the opposite magnitude of $q_A - q_B$, which is $1 - p_A - (1 - p_B) = -(p_A - p_B)$. The ratios and proportionate increments will usually have different magnitudes, however, because p_A/p_B is not the same as $q_A/q_B = (1 - p_A)/(1 - p_B)$.

The paradox is also important when we contemplate sample sizes and accomplishments in a clinical trial. Thus, in the example cited earlier, the results in the treated group will be proportionately 25% better than in the control group if mortality is reduced from 8% to 6%. This proportionate distinction will be much less impressive if the results are expressed for the same increment in the complementary survival rates, which change from 92% to 94%.

8.5.2. *Contrasts Based on Alternative Marginal Totals*

Once the fourfold table is established, we might decide to perform our contrast by using the other set of marginal totals as denominators. Instead of contrasting the success rates (or failure rates) for treatment A versus treatment B, we might contrast the proportion of patients who received treatment A (or treatment B) for those who succeeded versus those who failed. The proportion of successes who received treatment A was 11/18 = 61%. The proportion of failures who received treatment A was 38/81 = 47%. This contrast produces an increment of 14%, a ratio of 1.30, and a proportionate increment of 30% [= (61% − 47%)/47%]. The corresponding proportions of successes and failures who received treatment B are 39% and 53%. For this contrast, the increment is − 14%, the ratio is 0.74, and the proportionate increment is − 26%.

The proportions used for the alternative basic expressions here seem peculiar and would probably be rejected as a method of expressing the results of treatment. Because the basic groups in this study were determined by the assignment of treatment, the treatment groups would be expected to form the denominators of the spectrum in which results are cited. Nevertheless, the alternative denominators are available and could be used if the investigator insisted. In certain circumstances, as described later when we come to cross-sectional research, there may be no way of knowing which set of denominators is most appropriate for the contrast of proportions.

8.5.3. *The Odds Ratio*

The results for the fourfold table we have been considering can be expressed in a different kind of index called the *odds ratio*. The *odds ratio* is based on the same strategy that forms the odds offered in a gambling casino. The first step is to determine odds for a particular event. If we toss a single six-sided die, there is one chance in six of getting a *3*. There are five chances in six of not getting it. When these two chances are divided, we get $(1/6) \div (5/6)$, or 1/5. The odds of getting a *3* are thus 1:5 in favor, and 5:1 against. In general, if the chances of an occurrence are r/n in favor, and $(n−r)/n$ against, we can omit the longer division of $(r/n) \div [(n−r)/n]$ and simply cite the odds as either $r/(n−r)$ in favor or $(n−r)/r$ against. We can therefore determine the odds by looking at the two components that form n, without including n itself.

For example, in the fourfold table under consideration, if we consider patients who were successful, the odds were 11 to 7, or 11/7 = 1.57 that treatment A had been used. Among failures, the odds for use of treatment A were 38/43 = 0.88.

Once we have the odds for each of two contrasting events, we form the *odds ratio* by dividing the two sets of odds. Thus, when we divide 1.57 by 0.88, we would get 1.78 as an odds ratio for the favorable effect associated with treatment A.

The odds ratio has the advantage of giving the same result if calculated horizontally rather than vertically. Thus, if we had formed a denominator ratio after vertically noting the proportion of successes and failures who used treatment A, we would get (11/18)/(38/81) = 1.30. When we horizontally calculated a ratio of success rates, using the totals of the data as denominators, the results for A/B are (11/49)/(7/50) = 1.60. If the horizontal calculation, however, is done as an odds ratio rather than as a denominator ratio, we get 11/38 = 0.289 for the odds of success in a user of treatment A and 7/43 = 0.163 for the odds of success in a user of treatment B. The odds ratio of 0.289/0.163 = 1.78 and is the same as the value obtained earlier with the vertical calculation.

The distinction is easy to see if we list things algebraically as follows:

	Number of Patients		
Treatment	*Success*	*Failure*	**Total**
A	a	b	a+b
B	c	d	c+d
Total	a+c	b+d	N

The horizontal denominator ratios for proportion of success in the two treatments are a/$(a+b) \div c/(c+d)$. The vertical denominator ratios for proportionate use of treatment A in the failures and successes are a/(a+c) $\div$ b/(b+d). The corresponding odds ratios are (a/b) $\div$ (c/d) horizontally and (a/c) $\div$ (b/d) vertically. For either odds ratio, the result is ad/bc. Because this result is achieved by multiplying the diagonal products of the fourfold table and then dividing, the odds ratio is sometimes called the *cross-product ratio*.

The odds ratio is almost never used in research concerned with prognosis and therapy of clinical groups, because clinicians usually prefer a direct comparison of the rates of success. Because of certain mathematical properties discussed in Chapter 20, however, the odds ratio is particularly popular for case-control studies of etiology of disease.

8.6. EXPRESSIONS AND CONTRASTS FOR RISKS

In classic epidemiologic nomenclature, the term *risk* is regularly used to represent the *rate of occurrence* of a particular disease. This rate is often determined from a quotient in which the denominator represents the count of a general population inhabiting a particular geographic region, such as a city, county, state, or nation. The numerator is the count of certain events such as births, deaths, or reported cases of disease that have occurred in that region. For example, suppose that during a particular year, in a region containing 1,793,000 people, there were a total of 17,120 deaths, of which 589 were attributed to pneumonia. The annual total mortality rate in that region would be 17,120/1,793,000 = 0.009548 and the cause-specific mortality rate for pneumonia would be 589/1,793,000 = 0.0003285. To avoid the cumbersome array of zero digits after the decimal point, total mortality rates are usually multiplied by 1000 and cause-specific rates by 100,000. Thus these rates would be cited, respectively, as 9.5 per thousand (or "$\times 10^{-3}$") for total mortality and 33 per hundred thousand (or "$\times 10^{-5}$") for mortality attributed to pneumonia.

8.6.1. *Incidence and Prevalence*

A great deal of fuss is often made about the distinction between rates of *incidence* and *prevalence*. Incidence rates represent longitudinal events, noted in the follow-up of a cohort. Prevalence rates represent cross-sectional events, noted at a single point in time for the state of the group under study. Thus, if we were able to determine on a single day in this region that 339 people had pneumonia, the prevalence of pneumonia would be 339/1,793,000 = 0.000189 = 19 per hundred thousand. The mortality rate for pneumonia is obviously an incidence rate.

Although incidence and prevalence rates are constantly used in public health epidemiology, the actual calculations are seldom exactly correct, because the individual members of the group are almost never directly examined and followed. The rates are usually determined heterodemically, from two different sources. Furthermore, the rates cited as *incidence* for events other than death seldom represent a true incidence. Thus, the cancers newly reported to a regional tumor registry may be a mixture of "prevalence cases" detected through a screening program and "incidence cases" detected in people who were previously examined and found to be free of the cancer. Nevertheless, the mixture of newly reported cases in a particular year is often cited as an incidence rate. The term *occurrence rate* can be used as a noncommittal term that avoids some of these ambiguities.

8.6.2. *Contrasts of Risks*

Suppose we have performed a large cohort study in which almost 70,000 people were examined to find the relationship between thyroid cancer and tea drinking. The results show the following:

Exposure	Number with Disease (Thyroid Cancer)	Number Without Disease (No Thyroid Cancer)	Total
Tea drinkers	19	49,731	49,750
Not tea drinkers	2	19,862	19,864
Total	21	69,593	69,614

From these data, we would say that the risk of thyroid cancer in non–tea drinkers is $2/19,864 = 0.0001$, or 1 per 10,000. The risk of thyroid cancer in tea drinkers is $19/49,731 = 0.0004$. From these two values, we can calculate an entity called the *incremental risk*. It is simply the increment of $0.0004 - 0.0001 = 0.0003$. We can also calculate an entity that goes under two names, according to the whim of the user. It is called the *risk ratio* or the *relative risk*. It is simply the ratio of $0.0004/0.0001 = 4$. Although the terms *incremental risk, risk ratio,* and *relative risk* are commonly used in epidemiology, we now see that they represent simply the indexes of contrast for two proportions or rates. The word *risk* appears in the phrases via the epidemiologic custom in which occurrence rates of adverse events, such as disease or death, are called *risks*.

Note that our efforts to obtain the value of the risk ratio (or relative risk) for the development of thyroid cancer in tea drinkers required obtaining data for about 70,000 people. The advantage of the odds ratio, as we shall see in Chapter 20, is that it allows the risk ratio to be approximated from the much smaller number of people investigated in a case-control study.

8.7. ADJUSTMENT OF OCCURRENCE RATES

The comparison of occurrence rates often requires an adjustment for problems that can occur in denominators or numerators of the data.

8.7.1. *Disparate Composition of Denominators*

Suppose we compare the mortality rates in Arizona and Connecticut. Because Arizona is well known for its "healthy" climate, we may be shocked to find that its mortality rate is substantially higher than Connecticut's. The shock may disappear when we discover that Arizona's population is substantially older than Connecticut's, mainly because so many elderly people have retired and moved to Arizona.

The problem here is thus a variant of the susceptibility bias discussed earlier in Section 4.2.1. To prevent the unfair comparison of denominators that have a disparate prognostic composition, we can examine the mortality rates in each region for groups stratified at ages 21–30, 31–40, 41–50, 51–60, 61–70, and so on. We can then standardize the results in the two regions to give a fair comparison. This standardization procedure, which can be done in the several ways discussed in Chapter 20, is responsible for such epidemiologic phrases as *age-adjusted* or *age-sex–adjusted* rates.

8.7.2. *Losses in Numerators*

In a longitudinal study, numerator problems will arise if various members of the cohort become lost to follow-up. We will be able to count these lost persons in the denominator, but we do not know how to count them (as alive or dead, success or failure, etc.) in the numerator. The method of managing these problems is derived from the estimations of life expectancy that were developed by demographers and insurance company actuaries. The adjustment process, which is sometimes called *life-table analysis* or *actuarial analysis*, will be discussed in Chapter 17.

8.8. SYNOPSIS

For a descriptive contrast of two groups, the central indexes for each group can be subtracted to form an increment, divided to form a ratio, or arranged as a proportionate increment. Because one group is used as a base or control for the other and because the proportionate increment and ratio are mutually convertible, most contrasts can be expressed with two indexes: an increment and either a ratio or a proportionate increment. The proportionate increment can be difficult to interpret if it is expressed as a percentage and if the two central indexes under comparison are also percentages.

Although the quantitative impressiveness of a contrast depends on the increment and ratio, the decisions about the importance or clinical significance of the results involves external considerations of the total situation and the purpose of the contrast.

When complementary events, such as life and death, are expressed as the complementary rates, p and q = 1 − p, major paradoxes can arise because the ratios and proportionate increments will differ if the comparisons are based on p or q.

In epidemiologic custom, the term *incidence* is used for the rate of subsequent occurrence of a new event, during a specified time interval, in people who were initially free of that event. *Prevalence* is used for the rate of cross-sectional occurrence of the event at a single point in time for the people under observation.

The *incremental risk* and *risk ratio* (or *relative risk*) expressions that commonly appear in epidemiologic literature are simply increments and ratios for a comparison of the occurrence rates of disease in people exposed and not exposed to a suspected etiologic agent. The *odds ratio* is especially popular for approximating the risk ratio from data of the relatively small groups investigated in case-control studies of etiology.

To avoid problems of susceptibility bias, occurrence rates are often adjusted for denominator disparities in age and gender. To compensate for missing members who are lost to follow-up, incidence rates in a cohort are regularly adjusted with life-table or actuarial analyses.

EXERCISES

Exercise 8.1. Here is an opportunity for you to indicate what you mean by quantitative significance (and for the class convener to note observer variability in the decisions).

You have been asked to choose a specific boundary point for the result of the treated group that will allow each of the quantitative contrasts stated below to be regarded as important or worthwhile. What boundaries would you choose for each decision? If you used specific increments, ratios, or other quantitative criteria for making the decisions, please indicate what they were.

8.1.1. The success rate of the active treatment is substantially better than a placebo success rate of 45% in reducing manifestations of acne.

8.1.2. The 1-year mortality rate of the treated group is substantially better than the 12% noted in the placebo group.

8.1.3. Short-term pain relief has been rated on a scale of **0** to **3**, with **0** = no relief and **3** = complete relief, and the scores are used as quasi-dimensional data. The actively treated group had a mean rating that was quantitatively better than the mean rating of 1.3 for the placebo group.

8.1.4. The rate of endometrial carcinoma in postmenopausal women who do not use estrogens is 0.001. What rate, if correctly associated with estrogens, will alarm you enough to make you want to stop estrogen treatment in a patient whose distressing menopausal syndrome is under excellent control?

Exercise 8.2. In the UGDP randomized trial of hypoglycemic therapy for patients with diabetes mellitus, the following frequency counts were noted for the outcome of patients after they had been followed for 5 years.

Treatment	Deaths Attributed to Cardiovascular Causes	Deaths Attributed to Noncardiovascular Causes	Alive	Total
Placebo	10	11	184	205
Tolbutamide	26	4	174	204
Total	36	15	358	409

What indexes or expressions would you use to contrast the results of placebo and tolbutamide?

Exercise 8.3. In the first case-control study that described an alleged relationship between reserpine and breast cancer, the investigators assembled 150 cases of breast cancer and matched eight controls for each case. After each patient was checked for antecedent usage of reserpine, the results were as follows:

	Breast Cancer Cases	Control Patients Without Breast Cancer	Total
Users of reserpine	11	26	37
Nonusers of reserpine	139	1174	1313
Total	150	1200	1350

8.3.1. What indexes would you use to express the risk of breast cancer in reserpine users versus nonreserpine users?

8.3.2. What is the incremental risk of breast cancer in users of reserpine?

Exercise 8.4. Exercise 7.4 contained a table showing results of a clinical trial. Please answer the following questions for that table.

8.4.1. Is the proportion of patients who received treatment A a rate of prevalence or incidence?

8.4.2. Is the proportion of patients who were successful with treatment C a rate of prevalence or incidence?

8.4.3. What are the odds that a particular patient in that trial received treatment B?

8.4.4. Is the answer to 8.4.3 a prevalence or an incidence?

8.4.5. Assume that treatment A is the standard treatment. What is the risk ratio for *failure* with treatment B? What is the risk ratio for *success* with treatment C?

8.4.6. Still assuming that A is the standard treatment, what are the odds ratios for failure with treatment B and for success with treatment C?

Exercise 8.5. In an analysis of 273 cases of omphalosis at an academic medical center, the patients' age in years was distributed as follows:

<40:	10	*(4%)*
40–49:	17	*(6%)*
50–59:	141	*(52%)*
60–69:	72	*(26%)*
≥70:	33	*(12%)*

The authors concluded that omphalosis occurs predominately in middle-aged people (in the age group 50–69). Do you agree with this conclusion? If not, why not?

Chapter 9

Stochastic Contrasts

In addition to the quantitative distinctions discussed in Chapter 8, a statistical contrast has another important mathematical attribute. Suppose a well-designed, well-conducted randomized trial has produced success rates of 75% for new treatment A and 33% for old treatment B. These distinctions are quantitatively significant, because the direct increment is 42% and the ratio is 2.3, and there are no complaints about the structure of the research. Are we ready to conclude that treatment A is better than treatment B?

Before reaching this conclusion, we need to look at the size of the groups. Suppose you discover that treatment A was given to only four patients and treatment B to only three. The values of 75% versus 33% came from a contrast of 3/4 versus 1/3. Because both these proportions are very fragile, you would now probably be quite reluctant to accept the conclusion. The group sizes are too small for the observed distinction to be convincing. On the other hand, if the 75% versus 33% contrast came from such numbers as 225/300 versus 100/300, you would have no problem in accepting the stability of the proportions. The distinction of 225/300 versus 100/300 would be convincing by what Joseph Berkson has called the *traumatic interocular test*: the result hits you between the eyes.

In the two instances just cited, both pairs of contrasts could readily be evaluated with sheer intuition. For the same comparison of proportions—75% versus 33%—intuition alone could persuade us that the contrast of 225/300 versus 100/300 had numbers large enough to be convincing and that 3/4 versus 1/3 was too small. Intuition might continue to help us as these extremes become less dramatic. For example, still keeping the contrasted proportions as 75% versus 33%, we might remain persuaded by 45/60 versus 20/60 and unpersuaded by 6/8 versus 2/6. At some point, however, intuition might begin to fail. What decision do we make, for example, if the results are 15/20 versus 6/18? Are these proportions too fragile or are they stable enough to be taken seriously?

The role of tests of statistical significance is to remove intuition from these decisions about numerical fragility and to provide mathematical probabilities and criteria for the judgments. The statistical procedure is often called *hypothesis testing,* but the latter term has too many important scientific uses to be assigned an exclusively mathematical role. Because the word *stochastic* refers to random variables, and because the statistical procedure is concerned with the role of random chance in quantitative contrasts, the term *stochastic contrasts* will be used here to describe the activities.

In the traditional nomenclature of these procedures, an impressive distinction is called *statistically significant.* This term is highly ambiguous, however, because it does not differentiate between two types of significence in statistical data: the *quantitative significance* discussed in Chapter 8 and the *probabilistic significance* that is under consideration in a stochastic contrast. To eliminate this ambiguity and to avoid the tongue-twisting pronunciation of "probabilistic," the term *stochastic significance* will be used throughout this text for impressive distinctions in a stochastic contrast. If you are uncomfortable with the new phrase or if you fear being misunderstood by someone who prefers the traditional ambiguity, you can think of *stochastic significance* as being what is usually called *statistical significance,* or you can revert to the conventional term. The differences between quantitative and stochastic significance will be particularly emphasized, however, when the interpretation of results is discussed in Section 9.5.

Stochastic contrasts can be done with at least two distinctly different procedures. The traditional *parametric* procedure is relatively difficult to understand because it involves mathematical assumptions and inferences that are unfamiliar to most medical readers. The less traditional *nonparametric* technique is much easier to comprehend because the results emerge from direct permutations of the observed data. Although both procedures will be discussed, we shall begin with the simpler nonparametric approach, using permutations of the observed data.

9.1. COMMENT TO THE READER

You are hereby warned that this is a long chapter. It contains a survey of ideas and tactics that occupy complete textbooks of statistics and that are usually taught in one or two semesters of classroom instruction. According to those standards, however, the chapter is short. I hope that the relative length will acquaint you with many useful things that you might not otherwise get to know, and that the relative brevity will entice you to read through it.

Medical readers who approach this type of writing must bear in mind that mathematical ideas cannot be read with the same speed as biologic assertions. Although I have tried to make the writing as clear as possible, the material contains concepts to be grasped, rather than facts to be memorized. You may often have to stop and digest, rather than gulp and race. In many circumstances, you may want to use a calculator to check certain statements, or a pencil and paper to work out others. If you are willing to make those extra efforts, which are above and beyond the call of duty for perusing the traditional contents of medical literature, I believe (and hope) you will grasp the basic ideas and principles and will thereby be well prepared for the stochastic onslaught that awaits you in medical literature.

Since I have not tried to insert any "intermissions" in the chapter, readers can go along at their own pace, and instructors can decide how to break the bulk into digestible units. A few "homework" exercises have been inserted at the end of the chapter, but I have avoided using problems requiring a mastery of complex calculational formulas. Instructors who want to emphasize some of these calculations can readily find (or create) suitable exercises.

9.2. STOCHASTIC CONTRASTS VIA RANDOM PERMUTATIONS

In examining the success-rate contrast of 3/4 for treatment A versus 1/3 for treatment B, we decided by intuition that the distinction was too "chancy" to be accepted. To quantify this intuition, we can use a random permutation process in the following manner:

Let us assume that treatments A and B are equivalent. If so, each of the seven people treated in those two groups should have exactly the same result regardless of whether they were treated with A or with B. Let us now individually identify those seven people. The letters *t, u, v,* and w will be used for the four persons who received treatment A; and the *t, u,* and *v* are put in italics to denote the three persons who were successful. The letters *x*, y, and z are used for the three persons who received treatment B, with *x* representing the one success in that group.

9.2.1. *Rearrangements of the Observed Results*

In the observed results, the seven people were divided so that four went into one group and three into the other. It so happened that *t, u, v,* and w went to treatment A and *x*, y, and z to treatment B. There are many other ways in which these seven people could have been arranged, however, while still putting four into one group and three into the other. Furthermore, if the two treatments are equivalent, each person should have exactly the same result (success or failure) regardless of the assigned treatment.

Let us therefore examine all of the possible ways in which these seven persons might have been arranged while still having four in one group and three in the other. For each arrangement, we can see what the success rates would have been for treatments A and B, and we can calculate the incremental difference in those rates. The 35 possible arrangements and the associated calculations are shown in Table 9–1.

Table 9–1. SUCCESS RESULTS FOR SEVEN PEOPLE ARRANGED IN ALL POSSIBLE COMBINATIONS OF TWO GROUPS, WITH FOUR PEOPLE IN ONE GROUP AND THREE IN THE OTHER

Identification of Arrangement	People in Treatment A	People in Treatment B	Success Results for: A	B	Percentage Difference of A − B
1	t,u,v,w	x,y,z	3/4 (75%)	1/3 (33%)	42%
2	t,u,v,x	w,y,z	4/4 (100%)	0/3 (0%)	100%
3	t,u,v,y	w,x,z	3/4 (75%)	1/3 (33%)	42%
4	t,u,v,z	w,x,y	3/4 (75%)	1/3 (33%)	42%
5	t,u,w,x	v,y,z	3/4 (75%)	1/3 (33%)	42%
6	t,u,w,y	v,x,z	2/4 (50%)	2/3 (67%)	−17%
7	t,u,w,z	v,x,y	2/4 (50%)	2/3 (67%)	−17%
8	t,u,x,y	v,w,z	3/4 (75%)	1/3 (33%)	42%
9	t,u,x,z	v,w,y	3/4 (75%)	1/3 (33%)	42%
10	t,u,y,z	v,w,x	2/4 (50%)	2/3 (67%)	−17%
11	t,v,w,x	u,y,z	3/4 (75%)	1/3 (33%)	42%
12	t,v,w,y	u,x,z	2/4 (50%)	2/3 (67%)	−17%
13	t,v,w,z	u,x,y	2/4 (50%)	2/3 (67%)	−17%
14	t,v,x,y	u,w,z	3/4 (75%)	1/3 (33%)	42%
15	t,v,x,z	u,w,y	3/4 (75%)	1/3 (33%)	42%
16	t,v,y,z	u,w,x	2/4 (50%)	2/3 (67%)	−17%
17	t,w,x,y	u,v,z	2/4 (50%)	2/3 (67%)	−17%
18	t,w,x,z	u,v,y	2/4 (50%)	2/3 (67%)	−17%
19	t,w,y,z	u,v,x	1/4 (25%)	3/3 (100%)	−75%
20	t,x,y,z	u,v,w	2/4 (50%)	2/3 (67%)	−17%
21	u,v,w,x	t,y,z	3/4 (75%)	1/3 (33%)	42%
22	u,v,w,y	t,x,z	2/4 (50%)	2/3 (67%)	−17%
23	u,v,w,z	t,x,y	2/4 (50%)	2/3 (67%)	−17%
24	u,v,x,y	t,w,z	3/4 (75%)	1/3 (33%)	42%
25	u,v,x,z	t,w,y	3/4 (75%)	1/3 (33%)	42%
26	u,v,y,z	t,w,x	2/4 (50%)	2/3 (67%)	−17%
27	u,w,x,y	t,v,z	2/4 (50%)	2/3 (67%)	−17%
28	u,w,x,z	t,v,y	2/4 (50%)	2/3 (67%)	−17%
29	u,w,y,z	t,v,x	1/4 (25%)	3/3 (100%)	−75%
30	u,x,y,z	t,v,w	2/4 (50%)	2/3 (67%)	−17%
31	v,w,x,y	t,u,z	2/4 (50%)	2/3 (67%)	−17%
32	v,w,x,z	t,u,y	2/4 (50%)	2/3 (67%)	−17%
33	v,w,y,z	t,u,x	1/4 (25%)	3/3 (100%)	−75%
34	v,x,y,z	t,u,w	2/4 (50%)	2/3 (67%)	−17%
35	w,x,y,z	t,u,v	1/4 (25%)	3/3 (100%)	−75%

9.2.2. *Summary of Distinctions in the Rearrangements*

When we summarize the results of Table 9–1, we find that one of the 35 arrangements would have produced a success-rate incremental difference of 100% in favor of treatment A and 12 arrangements would have produced a difference of 42%. Treatment B would have been better by 17% in 18 of the arrangements and better by 75% in four arrangements. Table 9–2 contains a summary of the results of Table 9–1, together with appropriate identifications of each arrangement in Table 9–1. As shown in Table 9–2, if we happened to pick any one of those 35 arrangements randomly, the chances would have been 1/35 = 0.029 of getting the one in which A was better by 100% and 12/35 = 0.343 of getting one of the arrangements in which A was better by 42%.

Table 9–2. SUMMARY OF RESULTS OF TABLE 9–1.

Type of Outcome	Identity of Arrangements Where This Outcome Occurs	Random Probability of Achieving This Outcome
A is 100% better than B	2	$p_1 = 1/35 = 0.029$
A is 42% better than B	1,3,4,5,8,9,11, 14,15,21,24,25	$p_2 = 12/35 = 0.343$
B is 17% better than A	6,7,10,12,13,16, 17,18,20,22,23,26, 27,28,30,31,32,34	$p_3 = 18/35 = 0.514$
B is 75% better than A	19,29,33,35	$p_4 = 4/35 = 0.114$
		Total $= 1.000$

Thus, if the two treatments are equivalent, random fate alone would give us a chance of $0.029 + 0.343 = 0.372$ of obtaining a result at least as large as the difference we observed in favor of A. If we did not care whether A was better than B and we simply wanted to know the random chance of getting a difference that equals or exceeds 42% in either direction, we would augment the value of 0.372 by the value of $4/35 = 0.114$ for the four arrangements in which B exceeded A by 75%.

Therefore, by random fate alone, treatment A would exceed B by at least 42% in about 0.37 of the random selections, and a success rate increment of at least 42% in the two treatments would occur in about 0.48 of the selections. These calculated results provide quantitative confirmation for our intuitive decision that the contrast of 3/4 versus 1/3 was "chancy." The probabilities are quite high (0.37 or 0.48) that the observed distinctions or even larger ones could occur by chance alone if the two treatments are equivalent.

We thus have a quantitative basis for the conclusion that the distinction of 3/4 versus 1/4 is *not* stochastically significant. On the other hand, if the observed results had been 4/4 for treatment A and 0/3 for treatment B, we might have also thought intuitively that the numbers were small and "chancy." Nevertheless, the quantitative display in Table 9–2 shows that this distinction has a chance of only 0.029 of arising by random fate if the two treatments are equivalent. The 0.029 chance of random occurrence might seem small enough and remote enough to make us conclude that the difference of 4/4 versus 0/3 *is* stochastically significant.

9.3. GENERAL PRINCIPLES OF STOCHASTIC DECISIONS

What we have just done illustrates the basic principles of making decisions about stochastic significance. The process always involves six separate steps: (1) forming a null hypothesis; (2) choosing a test statistic; (3) examining the distribution of the test statistic under the null hypothesis; (4) choosing a two-tailed or one-tailed examination of the exterior probabilities; (5) choosing a boundary for the rejection zone; and (6) forming a concluding decision to reject or concede the null hypothesis. These six steps are discussed in the rest of this section.

9.3.1. *Forming a Null Hypothesis*

The null hypothesis is the original assumption that we intend to reject when we declare that a distinction is stochastically significant. In the instance just cited, the null hypothesis was that treatments A and B were equivalent. It illustrates the most common situation in which, wanting to show that an observed difference is significant, we make the opposite assumption, i.e., that there is no difference in the groups that are the source of the observed distinction. In other situations, however, as noted in Section 9.6.4, we may want to conclude that the observed distinction is trivial. In such a situation, we begin with the null hypothesis that a major difference exists.

9.3.2. *Choosing a Test Statistic*

In Section 9.1 and Table 9–1, the statistic whose distribution we examined under the null hypothesis was the difference in success proportions of the two groups. In other types of statistical procedures, the test statistic might be a difference in the means of the groups, in certain attributes determined from the ranks of the data, or in special mathematical entities that are calculated from the data.

The names given to the stochastic procedures and the mathematical strategy they employ depend on the entity used as a test statistic and on the way its null hypothesis distribution is determined. In *parametric* procedures, the test statistics are specially calculated entities that are named with such symbols as Z, t, X^2, and F; their null hypothesis distribution is determined from certain assumptions about the parameters, i.e., the true means or proportions, of a large hypothetical population from which the observed groups are regarded as samples. In *nonparametric* procedures, the null hypothesis distributions are determined directly from the observed data, rather than from assumptions about a parameter in a hypothetical population.

With a random permutation test, as shown in Tables 9–1 and 9–2, the nonparametric distributions depend on the actual values observed in the research data. With other types of nonparametric tests, the distributions depend on permutations of values for a test statistic obtained from ranked magnitudes in the observed data. Nonparametric tests are usually christened with eponymic titles. The names *Fisher* and *Pitman-Welch* are used for permutations of the observed data, and such names as *Mann-Whitney* and *Wilcoxon* are given to permutations of ranks.

9.3.3. *Examining the Distribution of the Test Statistic*

In Table 9–1, we inspected the distribution of the test statistic, i.e., the difference in success-rate proportions for treatments A and B, under the null hypothesis. The results of this distribution were summarized in Table 9–2.

Because the construction and summarization of these distributions is a tedious job, the process can be expedited in various ways that will be described in ensuing sections. For many procedures—both parametric and nonparametric—a distribution need not be constructed. Instead, we can use special tables that associate each calculated value of the test statistic with a P value for its exterior probabilities. The need to look things up in such a table can be eliminated when the statistical procedure is done with a computer program that presents the P value along with the calculated value of the test statistic.

9.3.4. *Choosing One-Tailed or Two-Tailed Zones for Exterior Probabilities*

The *exterior probability* of an observed result is the random chance, under the null hypothesis, of obtaining a result that is as large as what was observed, or even larger. This exterior probability is called a *P value*. It can go in the same direction as the observed results or in both directions. Thus, in Table 9–2, the P value for randomly obtaining a difference of 42% or higher in favor of treatment A was $0.029 + 0.343 = 0.372$. A P value confined to the same direction as the observed distinction is called *one-tailed*. The distinction would be expressed symbolically as $(A - B) \geqslant 42\%$. To determine the P value for obtaining a difference of 42% or higher *in favor of either treatment,* we added 0.114 to the previous probability, to account for the situation in which $B - A$ exceeded 42%. Thus, the *two-tailed* P value was 0.486. The two-tailed distinction would be expressed as $| A - B | \geqslant 42\%$.

(If the last part of Chapter 7 was not too traumatic, you may recall that Section 7.5.2.4 contained an analogous discussion of one-tailed and two-tailed partitions for a spectrum, except that we were thinking about Z values rather than P values. In the one-tailed situation, the exterior zones at one end of the spectrum had positive values of Z that were as large as the chosen boundary value or even larger. In the two-tailed situation, we considered the exterior zones at both ends of the spectrum, where the absolute values of Z, regardless of positive or negative signs, equalled or exceeded the boundary value. We shall soon meet the Z procedure again, because it provides a *parametric* approach for obtaining P values in tests of stochastic significance.)

The decision about whether to use one-tailed or two-tailed values of P is a matter of scientific policy rather than mathematical strategy. If we have no idea of whether treatment A is (or should be) better than treatment B, the bilateral (i.e., two-tailed) P value should be used. On the other hand, if we expect A to be better than B because B is a placebo and A is active treatment, our interest in P values would be one-tailed. If the results turned out to be better for B than for A, we would either want to repeat the study or test a new treatment. We would not seek stochastic support for the superiority of placebo.

Investigators who are eager to show a stochastically significant difference often prefer to use a one-tailed rather than a two-tailed interpretation because the one-tailed procedure produces lower P values, which are therefore more likely to be significant. If the unilateral direction of the research hypothesis is clearly stated beforehand, a one-tailed interpretation of P values seems justified. In many instances, however, investigators do not state their hypothesis beforehand. Instead, the P value is determined after the research is completed, and it is then interpreted as one- or two-tailed according to a hypothesis that emerges from the data. To thwart this type of impropriety, many statisticians insist that all P values be interpreted as two-tailed. Although appropriate if an advance hypothesis has not been specified, this demand may be too rigid and scientifically counterproductive if the investigator, in planning the study, has clearly indicated the unilateral direction of the anticipated distinction.

9.3.5. *Choosing a Rejection Boundary*

If you recall your elementary school geometry, you may remember that theorems were proved by a method analogous to establishing and then rejecting a null hypothesis. In geometric reasoning, we would establish a hypothesis contrary to the conclusion we wanted to reach. The "proof" would then contain assertions and reasoning to demonstrate that this hypothesis led to a consequence that is impossible (i.e., $P = 0$). We would then reject the original hypothesis and accept its opposite, i.e., the conclusion we wanted to reach.

The reasoning in a stochastic contrast is quite similar, except that P values never reach zero. In the arrangement of the mathematical reasoning, all magnitudes of distinction have a chance of occurring, even though the chance for certain distinctions may be infinitesimal. Because we will not have P values of 0 to let us reach the unequivocal rejection decision we could get in geometric proofs, we need to establish a boundary that will let the stochastic decision occur. This boundary is called the α *level* or the *rejection zone*. If the observed P value (at the one- or two-tailed level of interpretation) is at or below the level of α, we decide to reject the null hypothesis. When the null hypothesis is rejected, the observed distinction is declared to be *stochastically significant.*

Thus, in the data of Table 9–2, we thought about rejecting the null hypothesis when P was 0.029 but not when P was 0.372. We had therefore set our α level to lie somewhere between 0.029 and 0.372. The choice of the actual boundary value for α is a completely arbitrary act of judgment. It can be set at 0.3, 0.2, 0.1, 0.05, 0.02, 0.01, or at any other desired level. As a matter of convenience and custom, however, the usual level of α is 0.05, thus leading to the frequent statement in medical literature that "the result is statistically significant at $P \leq 0.05$." If we choose α to be 0.05, the observed difference of 4/4 versus 0/3 would be stochastically significant. If we choose α to be 0.02, the significance would vanish.

The particular act that established α as 0.05 was an arbitrary policy decision by Sir Ronald Fisher. He noted that 95% of the data in a Gaussian distribution was contained in the zone formed by boundaries drawn at 1.96 standard deviations around both sides of the mean. Because the 1.96 could easily be remembered as "2," an inner zone of $\bar{X} \pm 2s$ would encompass 95% of the data. The exterior 5% zone that was formed at the two tails of the Gaussian distribution would then be regarded as uncommon, unusual, or extraordinary. Applying this tactic to a particular observed value, X_i, Fisher could readily determine if it was a conventional or unconventional member of the spectrum. The unconventional members, i.e., those in the unusual 5% zone, could then be regarded as aliens who probably did not really belong in that spectrum.

The choice of a 0.05 level for α is a reasonable way of allowing the stochastic reasoning to proceed, but it has the same false-positive hazards as any diagnostic test. With α set at 0.05, a false-positive conclusion will occur in about 1 of 20 rejection decisions for a null hypothesis that is actually true. Contrary to the conclusion, the alien value on that occasion really belongs to the spectrum of results that are possible with a correct null hypothesis.

This false-positive risk occurs whenever a null hypothesis is rejected. If we reject at a chosen level of α or at an observed level of P, the risk of a false-positive (or *Type I*) error is α or P. The stochastic chance of correctly rejecting the null hypothesis will be $1 - \alpha$ or $1 - P$.

9.3.6. *Forming a Conclusion*

In a geometric proof, when we rejected the null hypothesis, we drew the opposite conclusion. The same process takes place when we reject a stochastic null hypothesis. If the null hypothesis is that the two treatments or the two population parameters are equivalent, our rejection leads to the decision that they are not equivalent. We then conclude that they are stochastically different, i.e., significant.

A problem arises, however, when the observed value of P *exceeds* the selected boundary of α. In this situation, we cannot reject the null hypothesis—but can we accept it? When $P > \alpha$, have we proved that the two treatments are equivalent? The answer to this question is: no. We have not proved that the two treatments are equivalent. If we wanted to prove equivalence, we would have to calculate a different type of P value, discussed later in Section 9.7. Therefore, when $P > \alpha$, we concede the null hypothesis rather than accepting it. We can state that the observed distinction is *not stochastically significant*, but we cannot state that it is *stochastically insignificant*. In fact, as we shall see later, when we concede the null hypothesis, we take the chance of committing a false-negative (or *Type II*) error. The observed results might emerge from groups having major distinctions that we have stochastically failed to detect.

9.4. AN OUTLINE OF STOCHASTIC PROCEDURES

Sections 9.2 and 9.3 should provide a reasonably good outline of what takes place in a stochastic test and what makes a P value become regarded as significant or nonsignificant. Because statistical methods are not the main focus of this book, readers who want to know a great deal more about the actual test procedures should look for details elsewhere.

For readers who want to know a bit more without pursuing all the details, however, the subdivisions of this section contain an annotated inventory of some of the most popular and valuable stochastic tests. Readers who want to skip this inventory should go directly to Section 9.5, which discusses the interpretation of the tests' results. Before you take that leap, however, please have a look at Section 9.4.1. It is particularly worth examining because it provides a reasonably detailed discussion of random permutation tests. These tests are seldom emphasized in most statistics books because the calculations are so extensive. In the days before digital computers and programmable hand-held electronic calculators, random permutation tests were abhorred because they were a computational nuisance. The parametric and nonparametric ranking tests were preferred and achieved their current popularity mainly because they were more convenient and easy to calculate.

For a medical reader, however, the random permutation procedures are easier to understand than the other types of stochastic tests, and the permutation tests also have two major intellectual advantages. First, they provide a direct probability for the random likelihood of the observed distinction. Because the test statistic used in a random permutation test is the actual difference in the directly observed means or proportions, there is no need to calculate a separate indirect test statistic, such as t or X^2, and then to look up the associated P value in a special table.

Secondly, the distribution of the test statistic under the null hypothesis is obtained directly from permutations of the observed data. There is no need to invoke a hypothetical population, an estimated parameter, a theoretical repetitive sampling, a combination of pooled variances, or any other inferential assumptions that are used in the other stochastic strategies. With a random permutation test, what you get is what you see.

Furthermore, with modern computational devices, the calculational complexity of random permutation tests can be eliminated or sharply reduced. With a suitably programmed device, the P value of a random permutation test can be obtained with no more effort than it now takes to get an analogous value by other methods. As the intellectual superiority of the random permutation tests becomes accompanied by an increased computational simplicity, these tests will become the dominant procedures by which scientists determine stochastic distinctions.

9.4.1. *Random Permutation Tests*

The process described in Section 9.1 may have been easy to understand, but it was a computational disaster. We had to construct the 35 arrangements noted in Table 9–1 and then summarize them to get the P values noted in Table 9–2. If the values of 75% versus 33% came from numbers that were slightly larger but still as small as 6/8 versus 2/6, we would have had to examine 3003 rather than 35 arrangements. For numbers such as 15/20 versus 6/18, there would have been $33,578 \times 10^6$ arrangements. Fortunately, the process can be greatly simplified.

9.4.1.1. THE USE OF FACTORIALS

The numbers of the arrangements cited in the previous paragraph were determined with the formula, $n!/[(r!)(n-r)!]$, which indicates the number of combinatorial arrangements that can occur when a group of n members is divided into two groups, having r and $n-r$ members. The exclamation points in the symbols refer to an entity called a *factorial*. Thus, $n! = (n)(n-1)(n-2) \ldots 1$. For example, $7! = 7 \times 6 \times 5 \times 4 \times 3 \times 2 \times 1$. By convention, $0! = 1$. In Table 9–1, we had a group of seven people divided into two groups containing four and three members. The number of arrangements was $7!/[4! \times 3!] = (7 \times 6 \times 5 \times 4 \times 3 \times 2 \times 1)/[(4 \times 3 \times 2 \times 1)(3 \times 2 \times 1)] = 35$. The value of 3003 was obtained as $14!/[8! \times 6!]$. The value of $33{,}578 \times 10^6$ emerged from $38!/[20! \times 18!]$. Because many electronic hand calculators have a device that automates the calculation of factorials, the result of $n!$ can be achieved merely by pushing a button.

Although the calculation of these factorial quotients lets us know how many arrangements would need to be checked, the actual process of checking each arrangement is unfeasible for anything other than contrasts of tiny numbers such as 3/4 versus 1/3. The factorial calculations can be used, however, not only to simplify the process enormously but also to give us the p values for each of the summary arrangements noted in Table 9–2.

The strategy is as follows. Consider any fourfold table that has the following structure:

		VARIABLE 2		
		YES	NO	TOTAL
VARIABLE	YES	a	b	n_1
1	NO	c	d	n_2
	TOTAL	f_1	f_2	N

If we assume that variable 1 is the independent variable (such as treatment) and variable 2 is the dependent variable (such as success), the choice of treatment divided the N people into two groups of n_1 and n_2 members. The number of possible arrangements for those people is $N!/(n_1! \times n_2!)$. The remaining arrangements depend on what happened in variable 2. Because the marginal values for variable 2 are fixed, the number of arrangements for the YES group in variable 2 will be $f_1!/(a! \times c!)$. The number of arrangements for the NO group in variable 2 will be $f_2!/(b! \times d!)$. The total number of possibilities for arranging the interior of the table is therefore

$$\frac{f_1!}{(a! \times c!)} \times \frac{f_2!}{(b! \times d!)}$$

When this number is divided by the total number of all possibilities, we will have the random probability of obtaining the observed table. If we call this the i-th table, its random probability under the null hypothesis is

$$p_i = \frac{\dfrac{f_1!}{a! \times c!} \times \dfrac{f_2!}{b! \times d!}}{\dfrac{N!}{n_1! \times n_2!}}$$

With rearrangement of terms, we get a relatively simple formula for this probability. It is

$$p_i = \frac{f_1! \times f_2! \times n_1! \times n_2!}{a! \times b! \times c! \times d! \times N!} \qquad [9.1]$$

For example, consider the results we observed in Section 9.1. The contrast of 3/4 versus 1/3 can be expressed in a fourfold table as follows:

	Success	**Failure**	**Total**
Treatment A	3	1	4
Treatment B	1	2	3
Total	4	3	7

The probability of getting this particular distinction by random chance if the two treatments are equivalent is

$$p = \frac{4! \times 3! \times 4! \times 3!}{3! \times 1! \times 1! \times 2! \times 7!} = 0.343$$

Note that this is the same p value shown in Table 9–2 for the situation in which A was 42% better than B, i.e., the contrast of 3/4 versus 1/3.

For the contrast in which A was 100% better than B, the marginal totals of the fourfold table would remain the same, but the interior four cells would be $\begin{bmatrix} 4 & 0 \\ 0 & 3 \end{bmatrix}$. For this table, the chance probability is

$$p = \frac{4! \times 3! \times 4! \times 3!}{4! \times 0! \times 0! \times 3! \times 7!} = 0.029,$$

which is the same value noted in the first row of Table 9–2. For the third contrast shown in Table 9–2, the fourfold table would be $\begin{bmatrix} 2 & 2 \\ 2 & 1 \end{bmatrix}$ and the p value would be 0.514, calculated from $(4! \times 3! \times 2! \times 3!)/(2! \times 2! \times 2! \times 1! \times 7!)$. Finally, the contrast in which B is 75% better than A would come from $\begin{bmatrix} 1 & 3 \\ 3 & 0 \end{bmatrix}$, which would yield a p value of 0.114, calculated from $(4! \times 3! \times 2! \times 3!)/(1! \times 3! \times 3! \times 0! \times 7!)$.

Because all of these calculations involve the term $(f_1! \times f_2! \times n_1! \times n_2!)/N!$, it can be determined immediately and labeled as K. In this instance, $K = (4! \times 3! \times 2! \times 3!)/7! = 0.3428571$. This value can be stored as a constant in the calculator, and the p_i value for each individual table can then be found by dividing K by the values of $(a! \times b! \times c! \times d!)$ that appear in the interior cells of that table. According to the way P is to be interpreted, the p_i values for the individual tables are then added in either one direction or in both directions to yield the P value that is the exterior probability.

Note that the only tables whose p_i values are to be added are those with incremental differences that equal or exceed the observed difference in proportions. Note also that if two of the same marginal totals are equal in the observed results, i.e., if $n_1 = n_2$ or if $f_1 = f_2$, the "other" tail will have the same probability values as the first tail. In such situations, the two-tailed probability is simply twice the one-tailed probability. If this marginal equality does not occur, i.e., if $n_1 \neq n_2$ and if $f_1 \neq f_2$, then both tails must be determined separately, as in Tables 9–1 and 9–2.

Finally, before we leave this subject, please note that the total P value is calculated correctly only if it includes the p value for the observed table plus the sum of the p values for all tables with more extreme differences. Certain programs for hand-held calculators or even for digital computers may perform the test incorrectly because they include only the p_i value for the observed table, without adding in the p_i values for the more extreme tables.

9.4.1.2. **THE FISHER EXACT TEST FOR PROPORTIONS**

The process of obtaining a P value for a fourfold table in the manner just described can be called the *Fisher Exact Probability Test*,[1] but in the traditional curtailment of long eponyms, it is often truncated to the *Fisher Test* or the *Fisher Exact Test*.

To illustrate its calculation in a different example, suppose we wanted to perform a stochastic contrast of the 75% versus 33% noted when the numbers are 6/8 versus 2/6. The observed original table would be

	Success	Failure	Total
Treatment A	6	2	8
Treatment B	2	4	6
Total	8	6	14

The K factor would be $8! \times 6! \times 8! \times 6!/14! = 9667.1328$. The available tables and their associated percentages of increments in success rates for A − B are as follows:

$$\begin{vmatrix} 8 & 0 \\ 0 & 6 \end{vmatrix} \quad \begin{vmatrix} 7 & 1 \\ 1 & 5 \end{vmatrix} \quad \begin{vmatrix} 6 & 2 \\ 2 & 4 \end{vmatrix} \quad \begin{vmatrix} 5 & 3 \\ 3 & 3 \end{vmatrix} \quad \begin{vmatrix} 4 & 4 \\ 4 & 2 \end{vmatrix} \quad \begin{vmatrix} 3 & 5 \\ 5 & 1 \end{vmatrix} \quad \begin{vmatrix} 2 & 6 \\ 6 & 0 \end{vmatrix}$$

100%	71%	42%	13%	−17%	−46%	−75%
$p_1 = 0.0003$	$p_2 = 0.016$	$p_3 = 0.140$			$p_4 = 0.112$	$p_5 = 0.009$

The individual p_i values were calculated only for the three left-most tables, in which the increment was $\geq 42\%$, and for the two right-most tables, in which the negative increment was also at least 42%.

For a one-tailed interpretation, P would be $0.0003 + 0.016 + 0.140 = 0.159$. For a two-tailed interpretation, the values of 0.112 and 0.009 would be added to the one-tailed value of 0.159 to produce $P = 0.280$. If α is set at 0.05, we still cannot reject the null hypothesis for these results, although the P values are lower (as might be expected) with the 6/8 versus 2/6 comparison than with the previous comparison of 3/4 versus 1/3.

Although the arrangement and calculation of a p_i value for each possible table is somewhat of a nuisance, the Fisher test has the advantage of providing a direct probability value for the observed results and avoiding the need to look up a P value in a special table. Furthermore, for the relatively small sample sizes in which the Fisher test is best used, not too many tables need to be examined. Finally, with a programmable electronic hand-calculator, the performance of the Fisher test can be automated so that the only work needed by the user is to enter the values of the observed fourfold table and the one- or two-tailed direction of the P value. The only caveat is that the total group size must be ≤ 69, because contemporary hand-held calculators cannot handle numbers larger than 69!. If N is >69, the best way to do the Fisher test is with a program on a digital computer that has a larger capacity than contemporary hand-held calculators. (Alternatively, when N exceeds 69, certain handbooks will give the values of N! or of log N!. These values can then be used appropriately in a hand calculator.)

9.4.1.3. **THE PITMAN-WELCH TEST FOR MEANS**

The procedure just described for a stochastic contrast of two proportions can also be used when the data are dimensional, with the results expressed as a contrast of two means. Because the techniques were described independently and almost concurrently by Pitman[2] and by Welch,[3] the procedure can be called the *Pitman-Welch Test*.

With dimensional data, we cannot use factorial calculations as simplifying tactics when the individual values are permuted. Certain simplifications can be employed, however, particularly when the total numbers are small. The process is best illustrated with an example. Suppose the measured results in four patients who received treatment A were 8, 11, 13, and 21 units, so that the mean was 53/4 = 13.25. For four patients receiving treatment B, the results were 19, 25, 31, and 37, with a mean of 112/4 = 28.00. The incremental difference is 14.75 units and the ratio is 2.1, so the result seems quantitatively significant. Is it also stochastically significant?

To answer this question, we could consider all the ways of arranging the eight values— 8, 11, 13, 19, 21, 25, 31, and 37—into two groups, each containing four members. We could calculate the mean for each group in the arrangement, find the difference in means for each pair of groups, and determine how often the difference equals or exceeds 14.75. For the eight values divided into two groups of four each, there would be 8!/(4!)(4!) = 70 arrangements to consider.

Table 9–3 shows 35 of these arrangements. Because the two groups each contain the same number of members (four), the second set of 35 arrangements would simply be a mirror image of what is shown in Table 9–3, with all of the group A results appearing as group B and vice versa. This type of symmetry occurs for permutation tests of dimensional data whenever the two compared groups have the same number of members. If the numbers are unequal, the entire set of possible arrangements must be worked out.

The 35 arrangements in Table 9–3 can be summarized as follows:

Observed Difference in Means	Frequency
15.75	1
14.75	1
10 to 14	3
7 to <10	5
4 to < 7	7
0 to < 4	7
−4 to <0	7
−7 to <−4	2
−10 to <−7	2
Total	35

We now have the answer to the basic question. A difference of 14.75 units or more occurs twice in these 35 arrangements and would appear four times in the full total of 70 arrangements. The P value would be 0.029 (= 2/70) for a one-tailed and 0.057 (= 4/70) for a two-tailed test.

All of these arrangements and calculations can be avoided, however, if we think more carefully about the data in these small groups. Examining the actual results, we can note that the group receiving treatment A contains the three members with the lowest values (8, 11, 13) of the total array of values: 8, 11, 13, 19, 21, 25, 31, and 37. The fourth observed value in treatment A is 21, yielding the mean difference of 14.75 in the two groups. If we are looking for a difference in mean values that is more extreme, i.e., even larger than 14.75, the only way to obtain it is if the fourth member of group A were 19 rather than 21. For the group of values 8, 11, 13, and 19, the mean would be 12.75. The mean for 21, 25, 31, and 37 would be 28.50, and the difference in means would be 15.75. Thus, we would have only two ways of obtaining a mean difference that is at least as large as 14.75. Therefore, the one-tailed P value will be 2/70 or 0.03. Because there are four members in each treatment group, 35 (or half) of the possible 70 arrangements will be symmetric. Thus, there will be one arrangement in which the values 19, 25, 31, and 37 appear in group A, with 8, 11, 13, and 19 in group B. Consequently, the probabilities on the "other tail" will be distributed in a manner similar to those of the "first tail." The two-tailed P value will therefore be 0.03+0.03 = 0.06.

**Table 9–3. PERMUTATION ARRANGEMENTS TO COMPARE
MEANS OF TWO GROUPS**

Treatment A	Group A Mean	Treatment B	Group B Mean	Increment in Means: Group B-Group A
8,11,13,19	12.75	21,25,31,37	28.50	15.75
8,11,13,21	13.25	19,25,31,37	28.00	14.75
8,11,13,25	14.25	19,21,31,37	27.00	12.75
8,11,13,31	15.75	19,21,25,37	25.50	9.75
8,11,13,37	17.25	19,21,25,31	24.00	6.75
8,11,19,21	14.75	13,25,31,37	26.50	11.75
8,11,19,25	15.75	13,21,31,37	25.50	9.75
8,11,19,31	17.25	13,21,25,37	24.00	6.75
8,11,19,37	18.75	13,21,25,31	22.50	3.75
8,11,21,25	16.25	13,19,31,37	25.00	8.75
8,11,21,31	17.75	13,19,25,37	23.50	5.75
8,11,21,37	19.25	13,19,25,31	22.00	2.75
8,11,25,31	18.25	13,19,21,37	23.00	4.75
8,11,25,37	19.75	13,19,21,31	21.50	1.75
8,11,31,37	21.25	13,19,21,25	20.00	− 1.25
8,13,19,21	15.25	11,25,31,37	26.00	10.75
8,13,19,25	16.25	11,21,31,37	25.00	8.75
8,13,19,31	17.75	11,21,25,37	23.50	5.75
8,13,19,37	19.25	11,21,25,31	22.00	2.75
8,13,21,25	16.75	11,19,31,37	24.50	7.75
8,13,21,31	18.25	11,19,25,37	23.00	4.75
8,13,21,37	19.75	11,19,25,31	21.50	1.75
8,13,25,31	19.25	11,19,21,37	22.00	2.75
8,13,25,37	20.75	11,19,21,31	20.50	− 0.25
8,13,31,37	22.25	11,19,21,25	19.00	− 3.25
8,19,21,25	18.25	11,13,31,37	23.00	4.75
8,19,21,31	19.75	11,13,25,37	21.50	1.75
8,19,21,37	21.25	11,13,25,31	20.00	− 1.25
8,19,25,31	20.75	11,13,21,37	20.50	− 0.25
8,19,25,37	22.25	11,13,21,31	19.00	− 3.25
8,19,31,37	23.75	11,13,21,25	17.50	− 6.25
8,21,25,31	21.25	11,13,19,37	20.00	− 1.25
8,21,25,37	22.75	11,13,19,31	18.50	− 4.25
8,21,31,37	24.25	11,13,19,25	17.00	− 7.25
8,25,31,37	25.25	11,13,19,21	16.00	− 9.25

If $\alpha = 0.05$, the one-tailed probability will be stochastically significant, but the two-tailed probability will not be.

9.4.2. *Parametric Procedures*

A different basic strategy for performing stochastic contrasts is derived from the statistical inferences that were used at the end of Chapter 7 to estimate parameters in sample surveys. These parametric methods are the source of the Z test, t test, and chi-square tests that are the best-known and most commonly used procedures for determining statistical significance. As we shall see shortly, the Z test and t test correspond to the Pitman-Welch permutation procedure. The chi-square test corresponds to the Fisher permutation procedure.

For readers who may have forgotten (or avoided) the last part of Chapter 7, the method of parametric estimation will be briefly recapitulated here before we turn to its modification for stochastic contrasts.

9.4.2.1. **ESTIMATING A PARAMETER**

In the various subsections of Sections 7.5 and 7.6, we learned about the way that a population parameter can be estimated from the results of a random sample taken from the population. The population mean, μ, is estimated to be $\bar{X}$, the mean of the observed group. The population standard deviation, σ, is estimated to be s, the standard deviation of the observed group [calculated as $\sqrt{S_{xx}/(N-1)}$]. The standard error of the mean, $s_{\bar{x}}$, is calculated as $s/\sqrt{N}$, where N is the size of the group. A confidence interval is then placed around $\bar{X}$, using a value of Z_α that has been chosen for a $1-\alpha$ level of confidence. This confidence interval, which runs from $\bar{X}-Z_\alpha s_{\bar{x}}$ to $\bar{X}+Z_\alpha s_{\bar{x}}$, is then regarded as having a $1-\alpha$ chance of including the true parametric population mean, μ.

For a proportion, the same type of reasoning is used, except that the symbols are different. The observed proportion will be p, and the corresponding population parameter is π. The standard error of the proportion is usually calculated with n rather than $n-1$, and is expressed as $\sqrt{pq/n}$, where $q = 1-p$. A value of Z_α is chosen in an analogous manner, and the confidence interval used to estimate π runs from $p-Z_\alpha\sqrt{pq/n}$ to $p+Z_\alpha\sqrt{pq/n}$.

For example, suppose we have taken a random sample of 50 voters in Connecticut and have found that 27 (54%) intend to vote Republican in the next election. Can the Republican party leaders feel confident of victory? To answer this question we note that $p = 0.54$, $q = 1-p = 0.46$, and $n = 50$. We calculate $\sqrt{pq/n}$ as $\sqrt{(0.54)(0.46)/50} = 0.07048$. For a 95% confidence interval we choose $Z_{0.05} = 1.96$ and find the value of $0.54 \pm (1.96)(0.07048)$. Because this interval runs from 0.402 to 0.678, the Republican party leaders have no strong assurance that they will win the election. In fact, they might receive as little as 40.2% of the votes.

9.4.2.2. **THE Z TEST FOR A DIFFERENCE IN TWO MEANS**

The way we arrived at a confidence interval for a group mean was to pretend that we had repeatedly taken random samples from a population. When we formed a new group composed of the means found in those repeated samples, the *standard error* was the standard deviation found among the means.

To extend this tactic to study variations of a difference in the means of two groups, $\bar{X}_A$ and $\bar{X}_B$, we engage in another hypothetical act. We pretend that $\bar{X}_A$ is the mean of a random sample of size n_A, taken from a large population having μ_A and σ_A as its true mean and standard deviation. We pretend that $\bar{X}_B$ is the mean of a random sample of size n_B, taken from a large population having μ_B and σ_B as its true mean and standard deviation. We then calculate the value of X_C as the difference in the two sample means, $\bar{X}_A - \bar{X}_B$.

If we performed this sampling process over and over, each time taking samples of sizes n_A and n_B from the parent population and each time calculating X_{C_i} as the difference in the means of the two samples, $\bar{X}_{A_i}$ and $\bar{X}_{B_i}$, we would get a new sample (or group) consisting of the individual values of X_{C_i}. The new sample would contain: $X_{C_1} = \bar{X}_{A_1} - \bar{X}_{B_1}$; $X_{C_2} = \bar{X}_{A_2} - \bar{X}_{B_2}$; $X_{C_3} = \bar{X}_{A_3} - \bar{X}_{B_3}$; and so on. This new sample can be thought of as coming from a population whose true mean is μ_C and whose true variance is σ_C.

Because this hypothetical sample, consisting of differences in the means of two samples, will have a Gaussian distribution, we can construct a Z-score for our observed value, X_C, as

$$Z = \frac{X_C - \mu_C}{\sigma_C} \qquad [9.2]$$

From this value of Z, we could then find the associated P value for the exterior probability by which X_C differs from μ_C.

Under the null hypothesis, we assume that the two groups, A and B, come from populations having equal means. Because $\mu_C = \mu_A - \mu_B$, the assumption that $\mu_A = \mu_B$ will make $\mu_C = 0$. Equation 9.2 will be reduced to $Z = X_C/\sigma_C$. Because $X_C = \bar{X}_A - \bar{X}_B$, the equation becomes

$$Z = (\bar{X}_A - \bar{X}_B)/\sigma_C \qquad [9.3]$$

We now need to find or estimate a value for σ_C. It can be shown mathematically that the variance of a distribution consisting of the differences of means in two samples is

$$\sigma_C^2 = \frac{\sigma_A^2}{n_A} + \frac{\sigma_B^2}{n_B} \qquad [9.4]$$

If we estimate σ_A^2 and σ_B^2 respectively as s_A^2 and s_B^2 from the standard deviations found in groups A and B, we can then estimate σ_C^2 as

$$s_C^2 = \frac{s_A^2}{n_A} + \frac{s_B^2}{n_B} \qquad [9.5]$$

Substituting appropriately into equation 9.3, we can now construct the formula for the Z test of stochastic significance for a difference of the means in two groups (or samples). The formula is

$$Z = \frac{\bar{X}_A - \bar{X}_B}{\sqrt{\frac{s_A^2}{n_A} + \frac{s_B^2}{n_B}}} \qquad [9.6]$$

To illustrate the process, consider the two groups of people compared in Section 9.3.1.3. For treatment A, the results were 8, 11, 13, and 21, with a mean $\bar{X}_A = 13.25$ and a standard deviation $s_A = 5.56$. For treatment B, the results were 19, 25, 31, and 37, with mean $\bar{X}_B = 28.00$ and $s_B = 7.75$. To perform a stochastic contrast of these two means, we calculate $Z = (13.25 - 28.00)/\sqrt{(5.56^2/4) + (7.75^2/4)} = -14.75/\sqrt{7.728 + 15.016} = -14.75/\sqrt{22.744} = -14.75/4.77 = -3.09$. According to the values of Z shown in Table 7–2, the two-tailed exterior probability (or P value) of getting this result is somewhat less than 0.0027, and the one-tailed probability is 0.00135.

Although this process was performed correctly, it has produced a result different from what we found for the same data with the Pitman-Welch permutation test in Section 9.3.1.3. With the latter test, the two-tailed P was 0.06 and the one-tailed P was 0.03. The discrepancy should illustrate an important point for the reader: As with observations made by different clinicians, tests performed with different statistical procedures can yield results that do not always agree.

9.4.2.3. **THE t TEST FOR A DIFFERENCE IN TWO MEANS**

In Section 7.6.4.3, the *Central Limit Theorem* was cited as proof for the belief that a collection of repetitively drawn sample means will have a Gaussian distribution. This theorem holds true, however, only if the sample sizes are reasonably large. If the sample sizes are small, the spectrum of means will *not* be exactly Gaussian. Consequently, we were not completely correct when we turned to Table 9–2 to find a P value for the calculated value of Z in the illustration at the end of Section 9.3.2.2. The P and Z values of Table 9–2 can be properly associated only if the sample sizes are reasonably large.

The shape of the spectrum created by a collection of means of repetitive small samples was first noted by W. S. Gossett, who published his results pseudonymously as "Student."[4] He found that the means of repetitive small samples have a spectrum resembling a Gaussian curve, with slight differences that change according to the size of the samples. Figure 9–1 shows the shapes of two of these alternative curves, which are called *t distributions*. In general, the t curves are slightly shorter in the center and slightly taller at the tails than the Gaussian Z curve, but the differences begin to vanish as sample size increases.

Although the differences between the t and the Gaussian Z distribution are small, the statistical consequences have been extensive. Perhaps the main consequence is that the t test (or "Student's t test") has become the most popularly used statistical procedure for performing a stochastic contrast of the difference in two means. The other main consequences have been some additional complexity in performing the contrast.

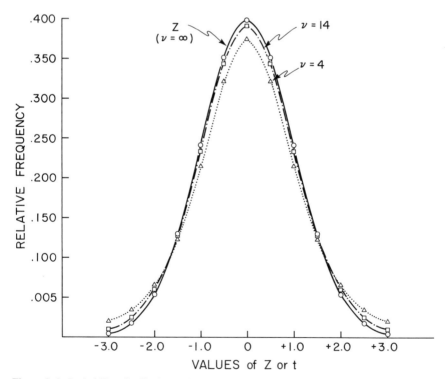

Figure 9–1. Probability distributions of Z and t. The relative frequencies show the probabilities of any single point of Z or t. The customary P values of statistics depend on the *area* under the curve, external to the point. The curves are shown for Z and for t values at 4 and 14 degrees of freedom (indicated by ν).

9.4.2.3.1. *The Pooled Variance*

In using the Z test, we made the null-hypothesis assumption that the two hypothetical populations, A and B, had equal means, i.e., $\mu_A = \mu_B$. We could have made the additional assumption, however, that the two populations also have equal variances, i.e., $\sigma_A = \sigma_B$. This assumption is not strictly necessary but can be used for the Z test. The assumption is desirable for the t test.

Because s_A may not always equal s_B, we need some way of estimating their common variance when we assume, with the null hypothesis, that $\sigma_A^2 = \sigma_B^2$. The tactic used for this estimation is analogous to what is done for obtaining an average of two proportions. If $p_1 = r_1/n_1$ and $p_2 = r_2/n_2$, we average the proportions as $(r_1 + r_2)/(n_1 + n_2)$. In this instance, because $s_A^2 = S_{xx_A}/(n_A - 1)$ and $s_B^2 = S_{xx_B}/(n_B - 1)$, we get the pooled variance as

$$s_p^2 = \frac{S_{xx_A} + S_{xx_B}}{n_A - 1 + n_B - 1} \qquad [9.7]$$

This can also be written as

$$s_p^2 = \frac{(n_A - 1)s_A^2 + (n_B - 1)s_B^2}{n_A + n_B - 2} \qquad [9.8]$$

When we substitute s_p^2 from equation 9.8 for both s_A^2 and s_B^2 in equation 9.5, we get

$$s_C^2 = \frac{s_p^2}{n_A} + \frac{s_p^2}{n_B} = \left(\frac{1}{n_A} + \frac{1}{n_B}\right)s_p^2 = \left(\frac{1}{n_A} + \frac{1}{n_B}\right)\left[\frac{(n_A - 1)s_A^2 + (n_B - 1)s_B^2}{n_A + n_B - 2}\right] \qquad [9.9]$$

This can be rearranged as

$$s_C^2 = \frac{(n_A - 1)s_A^2 + (n_B - 1)s_B^2}{n_A n_B} \times \frac{n_A + n_B}{n_A + n_B - 2} \qquad [9.10]$$

With this value of s_C substituted for s_A and s_B, the formula for calculating t (or Z) becomes

$$Z \text{ or } t = \frac{\overline{X}_A - \overline{X}_B}{\sqrt{(n_A - 1)s_A^2 + (n_B - 1)s_B^2}} \times \sqrt{n_A n_B} \times \sqrt{\frac{n_A + n_B - 2}{n_A + n_B}} \qquad [9.11]$$

For large values of n_A and n_B, the value of $\sqrt{(n_A + n_B - 2)/(n_A + n_B)}$ is essentially 1, and the values of $n_A - 1$ and $n_B - 1$ are close to n_A and n_B. The pooled-variance formula then reduces to

$$Z \text{ or } t \cong \frac{\overline{X}_A - \overline{X}_B}{\sqrt{\dfrac{s_A^2}{n_B} + \dfrac{s_B^2}{n_A}}} \qquad [9.12]$$

This formula is similar to that of equation 9.6, except for the reversal of n_B and n_A in the denominators.

For example, for the two groups noted in Section 9.3.2.2, the value of s_C^2, calculated without pooling the variance, was 22.744. To pool the variance we first calculate

$$s_p^2 = \frac{(3)(5.56)^2 + (3)(7.75)^2}{4 + 4 - 2} = \frac{92.74 + 180.19}{6} = 45.49$$

The value of s_C^2 is then $\dfrac{45.49}{4} + \dfrac{45.49}{4} = 22.744$.

In this instance, the unpooled and pooled variances are identical because $n_A = n_B$, and so $t = Z = -3.09$. In most instances $n_A \neq n_B$, and the values for the pooled and unpooled variances will differ. When $n_A = n_B = n$, the calculation of t or Z can be greatly simplified. It is merely

$$Z \text{ or } t = \frac{\bar{X}_A - \bar{X}_B}{\sqrt{s_A^2 + s_B^2}} \times \sqrt{n} \qquad [9.13]$$

9.4.2.3.2. *Interpretation of t*

To find P values, the t value is used like a value of Z, except that the corresponding values of P must be noted in a different table, and the associated t/P values must be examined for the appropriate degrees of freedom. In using Z, we added a subscript to let Z_α indicate the decision level at which we were working. With t, we add two subscripts to write the distinctions as $t_{\alpha,\nu}$, where α is the decision level and ν represents the degrees of freedom in the total sample. When two groups are under contrast, the degrees of freedom are $n_A + n_B - 2$.

Table 9–4 shows an excerpt of the corresponding t/P values at different degrees of freedom. If we apply this table to interpret the contrast for the two groups we have been considering, we note that our observed result, $t = 3.09$, is still stochastically significant. At 6 degrees of freedom, t would have to be at least 2.45 for P to be <0.05 (two-tailed), and our observed t value exceeds this demand.

Another important point to note is that for high degrees of freedom (usually 30 or greater), the values needed to achieve stochastic significance are almost identical for Z and t. The main distinction between the two is at small sample sizes, where the t test makes stricter demands (i.e., t must be higher than Z to yield a stochastically significant result).

9.4.2.4. **THE CHI-SQUARE TEST FOR TWO PROPORTIONS**

In the mathematical model used for the Z and t procedures, the test statistic was a special ratio, in which a difference in two means was divided by the standard deviation of their difference. This same model can be used, as shown later, for stochastically contrasting

Table 9–4. RELATION OF P VALUES TO VALUES OF t AND DEGREES OF FREEDOM*

Degrees of Freedom	Values of P (Two-Tailed)					
	0.5	*0.2*	*0.1*	*0.05*	*0.01*	*0.001*
3	0.77	1.64	2.35	3.18	5.84	12.94
6	0.72	1.44	1.94	2.45	3.71	5.96
9	0.70	1.38	1.83	2.26	3.25	4.78
20	0.69	1.33	1.73	2.09	2.85	3.85
40	0.68	1.30	1.68	2.02	2.70	3.55
100	0.68	1.29	1.66	1.98	2.63	3.39
∞ or Z	0.68	1.28	1.64	1.96	2.58	3.29

*Cells show value of t (sign ignored) that must be equalled or exceeded for the stated value of P

a difference in two proportions. A more popular mathematical model for this contrast, however, is the chi-square (pronounced to rhyme with eye-square) test.

Consider the contrast of 6/8 versus 2/6 that we evaluated in Section 9.4.1.2. The associated table was as follows:

	Success	Failure	Total
Treatment A	6	2	8
Treatment B	2	4	6
Total	8	6	14

In this table, $n_A = 8$, $n_B = 6$, and the contrasted rates of success are $p_A = 6/8$ and $p_B = 2/6$. The pooled rate of success for the two treatments is $P = 8/14$. (Note that the P here is a pooled proportion, not an exterior probability. I am sorry about the ambiguity, but it is part of traditional statistical symbols and nomenclature, and I dare not add neosymbolisms beyond the neologisms that already appear elsewhere in this book.)

Under the null hypothesis, we assume that groups A and B are random samples taken from the same population, whose true proportion of success is the parameter π. We estimate the value of π to be $P = 8/14$, and the value of $1 - \pi$ is estimated to be $1 - P = Q = 6/14$. We can now determine the successes and failures that would be expected for each treatment under the null hypothesis. For treatment A, the expected successes would be $n_A \times P = 8 \times (8/14) = 4.57$ and the expected failures are $n_A \times Q = 8 \times (6/14) = 3.43$. For treatment B, the corresponding expectations are $n_B \times P = 6 \times (8/14) = 3.43$ and $n_B \times Q = 6 \times (6/14) = 2.57$. The fractions of people encountered in these expectations may seem peculiar, but they must be preserved for the statistics to be correct.

We can now prepare a table showing the expected results. They are as follows:

	Success	Failure	Total
Treatment A	4.57	3.43	8
Treatment B	3.43	2.57	6
Total	8	6	14

Note that the marginal totals for these expectations remain the same as before.

The next step is to form a special test statistic, called X^2 (pronounced ex-square), which is calculated as the sum of the (observed-expected)^2/expected values in each cell. Thus

$$X^2 = \frac{(6-4.57)^2}{4.57} + \frac{(2-3.43)^2}{3.43} + \frac{(2-3.43)^2}{3.43} + \frac{(4-2.57)^2}{2.57}$$

$$= \frac{2.04}{4.57} + \frac{2.04}{3.43} + \frac{2.04}{3.43} + \frac{2.04}{2.57} = 2.43$$

This value of X^2 is interpreted using the statistical distribution of an entity called χ^2 (chi-square), which has different values of P associated with different values of χ^2 at different degrees of freedom. The number of degrees of freedom in a table with two variables is equal to $(r-1)(c-1)$, where r = number of rows and c = number of columns. Thus, in a fourfold table with two rows and two columns, there is $(2-1)(2-1) = 1$ degree of freedom.

The correspondence between χ^2 values and two-tailed P values at 1 degree of freedom is as follows:

Value of P	0.90	0.50	0.30	0.20	0.10	0.05	0.025	0.01
Value of χ^2	0.0158	0.455	1.074	1.642	2.706	3.841	5.024	6.635

Thus, for our observed value of $X^2 = 2.43$, we find that P lies between 0.20 and 0.10. This can be written symbolically as $0.10 < P < 0.20$. (You may recall that in Section 9.4.1.2, we found the exact two-tailed value for P to have the slightly higher result of 0.280.)

9.4.2.4.1. *Formula for Calculations*

To save all the labor of obtaining and calculating the values of the (observed-expected)^2/expected results, a relatively simple formula can be used for calculating X^2. If the table is expressed as

		VARIABLE 2		
		YES	NO	TOTAL
VARIABLE	YES	a	b	n_1
1	NO	c	d	n_2
	TOTAL	f_1	f_2	N

the formula is

$$X^2 = \frac{(ad-bc)^2 N}{f_1 f_2 n_1 n_2}$$
[9.14]

Thus, for our illustrative example

$$X^2 = \frac{[(6 \times 4) - (2 \times 2)]^2 \times 14}{8 \times 6 \times 8 \times 6} = 2.43$$

Another simple computing formula can be used if the data are presented in the form of $p_A = t_A/n_A$ and $p_B = t_B/n_B$ with $P = (t_A + t_B)/(n_A + n_B) = T/N$. In this situation,

$$X^2 = \left(\frac{t_A^2}{n_A} + \frac{t_B^2}{n_B} - \frac{T^2}{N} \right) \times \frac{N^2}{T(N-T)}$$
[9.15]

For our illustrative example, where $p_A = 6/8$, $p_B = 2/6$, $P = 8/14$

$$X^2 = \left(\frac{6^2}{8} + \frac{2^2}{6} - \frac{8^2}{14} \right) \left(\frac{14^2}{8 \times 6} \right) = 2.43$$

The labor of doing all of these calculations can be eliminated, of course, with a properly programmed hand-held calculator, but the formulas can be used to check that the calculator is working properly.

9.4.2.4.2. *The Yates Correction*

In 1934, arguing that the values of a fourfold table would always be discrete integers, whereas the distribution of χ^2 was continuous, Yates[5] introduced a continuity correction that was intended to make X^2 a more accurate approximation of χ^2. For practical calculations, the Yates correction converts equation 9.14 to

$$X_C^2 = \frac{[\,|\,ad - bc\,| - (N/2)]^2 \times N}{f_1 f_2 n_1 n_2}$$
[9.16]

For our illustrative example, the Yates-corrected value of X^2 would be

$$X^2 = \frac{[|(6\times4)-(2\times2)| - 7]^2 \times 14}{8\times6\times8\times6} = \frac{13^2 \times 14}{8\times6\times8\times6} = 1.03$$

The associated two-tailed P value for X_C^2 would lie between 0.3 and 0.5 and is still disparate from the result obtained with the exact probability test.

Although the Yates correction was popular for many years, it has now become controversial, with some statisticians arguing for and others against its usage. The argument is still unresolved, but its resolution may not be particularly important. For large values of N, the corrected and uncorrected values of X^2 are reasonably similar and yield P values that are reasonably close to the "gold standard" values obtained with the Fisher Exact Test. For small values of N, the Fisher Exact Test is easy to calculate and would be preferred over either type of X^2 calculation. With this principle, the main issue is to decide when the values of N are large enough to use X^2 rather than the Fisher test. Because statistical authorities also disagree about this decision, no general rule can be stated. My own preference, which is a conservative composite of the experts' recommendations, is to use the Fisher test whenever N<40 or if any of the expected values in the four cells is ≤5. Otherwise, X^2 (uncorrected) can be employed.

9.4.2.4.3. *Is Chi-Square a Parametric Procedure?*

In many statistical texts, the chi-square test is called *nonparametric* because it is used for categorical data, rather than for the dimensional data entered into a Z test or t test. If dimensional data are a prerequisite for parametric tests, chi-square is not parametric. On the other hand, the chi-square procedure uses the parametric strategy of making an estimate of π and obtaining P by referring to the hypothetical sampling distribution of a test statistic. Besides, as noted in the next section, the X^2 test (uncorrected) for a fourfold table yields the same results that would be obtained if a parametric Z test were applied to the binary data. For practical purposes, therefore, chi-square is a parametric test.

9.4.2.5. THE Z TEST FOR TWO PROPORTIONS

Because a binary proportion is analogous to a mean, the Z test can also be used for stochastic contrasts of the difference noted in two proportions. The formula is

$$Z = \frac{P_A - P_B}{\sqrt{\left(\frac{1}{n_A} + \frac{1}{n_B}\right)(PQ)}} \qquad [9.17]$$

When applied to the contrast of 6/8 versus 2/6, this formula would produce

$$Z = \frac{(6/8-2/6)}{\sqrt{\left(\frac{1}{8}+\frac{1}{6}\right)\left(\frac{8}{14}\times\frac{6}{14}\right)}} = \frac{0.4167}{\sqrt{(0.2917)(0.2449)}} = 1.56$$

This value of Z, as noted in Table 7–2, is associated with a two-tailed P value of slightly less than 0.134.

An interesting feature of Z = 1.56 is that if we square it, we get 2.43, which was the same value obtained earlier for X^2 in these data. In fact, it can be demonstrated algebraically that equation 9.17 yields a value of Z^2 that is identical to what is obtained with equations 9.14 or 9.15 for X^2. Thus, the stochastic tests of means and proportions are united by the common result that $Z = \sqrt{X^2}$.

9.4.2.6. **THE BINOMIAL TEST FOR TWO PROPORTIONS**

In addition to the three methods we have already learned—the Fisher test, chi-square test, and Z test—for doing a stochastic contrast of two proportions, a fourth method is also available. It relies on the binomial expansion as yet another strategy for determining probabilities. The procedure somewhat resembles what was done in the Fisher test.

You may recall from elementary school algebra that $(a+b)^2 = a^2 + 2ab + b^2$ and that $(a+b)^3 = a^3 + 3a^2b + 3ab^2 + b^3$. If we consider a sample of size n from a population whose parametric proportion is P, the probability expectations for that sample can be worked out from the expansion of $(P+Q)^n$.

Suppose we consider the chances of getting a six when a single die is tossed. The parametric value of P is $1/6 = 0.17$. With two tosses, we consider the expansion $(1/6)^2 + 2(1/6)(5/6) + (5/6)^2$. For getting a six in both tosses, the chance is $(1/6)^2 = 0.03$. For getting a six in one toss and something else in the other, the chance is $2(1/6)(5/6) = 0.28$. For getting a six in neither toss, the chance is $(5/6)^2 = 0.69$. For three tosses, we consider the expansion $(1/6)^3 + 3(1/6)^2(5/6) + 3(1/6)(5/6)^2 + (5/6)^3$. The results would yield the following probabilities: for three sixes, 0.005; for two sixes, 0.069; for one six, 0.347; and for no sixes, 0.549.

If you understand this principle, you can see how it might be readily adapted for parametric inferences. For example, suppose we want to perform a stochastic contrast of the two proportions, 6/8 versus 2/6. Estimating the population parameter to be $8/14 = 0.571$, we can then use the binomial expansion process to note the random likelihood for each set of observed results. Thus, for the group of six patients, we would inspect the binomial expansion of $(0.571 + 0.429)^6$. The expansion would have seven terms, with the binomial coefficients of 1, 6, 15, 20, 15, 6, and 1. The chances of finding two successes (or fewer) in those six patients would be the sum of relative frequencies for the last three terms. This would be $(15)(0.571)^2(0.429)^4 + 6(0.571)(0.429)^5 + (0.429)^6 = 0.167 + 0.050 + 0.006 = 0.223$. An analogous calculation could be done to find the random likelihood of achieving six successes in eight patients if the true probability of success is 0.571.

The binomial expansion technique is too cumbersome to be used for routine stochastic contrasts of two proportions, but it is particularly valuable for determining the confidence interval for a proportion or for a single increment in two proportions. These confidence intervals are usually calculated with Z or t procedures, which make the computations easy, but the results are really approximations of the definitive statement that is provided by a binomial expansion. The calculation of the binomial expansions can be avoided if appropriate tables are available. They can be found in sources such as Donald Mainland's excellent text.[6]

9.4.2.7. **ONE-SAMPLE TESTS**

The results of two groups sometimes become paired or matched in a way that allows them to be reduced to a single one-sample arrangement. This situation can happen for a before-and-after measurement of blood pressure, a comparison of two laboratories' measurements of serum cholesterol in the same specimens, or an appraisal of two radiologists' agreement in interpreting chest films as normal or abnormal.

Because variance among individuals is reduced, a paired reduction of two groups into one is more likely to achieve stochastic significance than a direct contrast of the two groups. The stochastic tests are done with special arrangements of the Z or t test for dimensional data or of the chi-square test for proportions.

9.4.2.7.1. *The One-Sample or Paired t (or Z) Test*

If X_i represents one of the paired dimensional measurements and Y_i represents the other dimensional measurement, each corresponding value of X_i and Y_i can be subtracted to form the incremental variable,

$$d_i = X_i - Y_i$$

Under the null hypothesis, d_i has a mean of 0 and a variance estimated from $S_{dd} = \Sigma d_i^2 - [(\Sigma d_i)^2/N]$, where N is the number of paired observations. The observed mean is $\bar{d} = \Sigma d_i/N$ and the standard error of this mean will be $\sqrt{S_{dd}/(N-1)}/\sqrt{N}$.

A t (or Z) test can then be done using the statistic

$$t = \frac{\bar{d}\sqrt{N}}{\sqrt{S_{dd}/(N-1)}} \qquad [9.18]$$

For example, suppose we want to evaluate an oral hypoglycemic agent. In eight normal volunteers who are maintaining a standard diet, we measure the morning fasting blood sugar on the day of the test, give one dose of the agent three times during the day, and measure fasting blood sugar again the next morning. The results are as follows:

Identity of Volunteer	FBS Before	FBS After	Increment
A	92	88	−4
B	89	85	−3
C	74	75	+1
D	75	75	0
E	87	81	−6
F	83	78	−5
G	71	69	−2
H	94	87	−7

For these data, $\Sigma d_i = -26$ and $\bar{d} = -3.25$. The standard deviation (s_d) = 2.816, and so we calculate $t = (-3.25)(\sqrt{8})/2.816 = 3.26$, which has P<0.05 at seven degrees of freedom. We can infer that a stochastically significant change occurred in the levels of blood glucose.

Because the total variance is reduced by the pairing, the denominator of the expression in [9.18] is smaller than it would be in the regular two-group t test. On the other hand, because the degrees of freedom are reduced from $2N-2$ to $N-1$, the criterion for obtaining a significant P value is somewhat tougher. Nevertheless, the reduction in paired variance is usually more important than the concomitantly tougher standard for P, and the one-sample or paired t test, when it is properly employed, is much more likely to achieve stochastic significance than the conventional two-group test.

9.4.2.7.2. *The McNemar Chi-Square Test*

Let us assume that two radiologists, A and B, have been asked to say Yes or No regarding the abnormality of a set of chest films. When the results are tabulated, we find the following values:

	Readings by		Number
Observer A		**Observer B**	**of Pairs**
Yes		Yes	a
Yes		No	b
No		Yes	c
No		No	d
		Total	N

These data can be organized into an arrangement called an *agreement matrix* as follows

		Observer B		
		Yes	**No**	**Total**
Observer	Yes	a	b	n_1
A	No	c	d	n_2
	Total	m_1	m_2	N

Despite a resemblance to the conventional fourfold table we have been considering, the table just cited is different, because it refers to agreement in two observations of the *same* variable. It does not refer to two different variables. If this table referred to two different variables, it would have to be formed as follows:

	Total Readings of		
	Yes	**No**	**Total**
Observer A	n_1	n_2	N
Observer B	m_1	m_2	N
Total	$n_1 + m_1$	$n_2 + m_2$	2N

For the latter table, we could calculate stochastic significance (if we wanted to do so) by using the conventional X^2 test on the difference in proportions of n_1/N versus m_1/N in the positive readings of observer A versus observer B.

To test the agreement or disagreement of the observers, however, the earlier table is more appropriate, because it shows the actual values of a, b, c, and d for each paired possibility of agreement or disagreement. For this type of stochastic contrast, McNemar[7] has demonstrated that the appropriate value of X^2 is calculated as

$$X_M^2 = \frac{(b-c)^2}{b+c} \qquad\qquad [9.19]$$

We shall see some examples of this procedure in Chapter 21, during a discussion of matched and unmatched data analyses for case-control studies.

9.4.3. *Nonparametric Procedures*

Although random permutation tests do not involve the use of parameters, the term *nonparametric* is customarily reserved for procedures that involve an analysis of the *ranks* of the observed data.

The strategies were first developed as an act of computational convenience by Frank Wilcoxon,[8] who, in the days before the numerical labors became eased by mechanical or electronic devices, wanted to simplify the calculational process by using the ranks rather than the actual magnitudes of the dimensional data. Instead of looking at the inferred null hypothesis distribution of a test statistic, such as t or Z, Wilcoxon developed a different test statistic based on sums of the rankings in the two groups. Under the null hypothesis, the possible number of these combinations was finite for groups of sizes n_A and n_B. All of the possibilities for sums of ranks could be determined, and the null hypothesis distribution of the sum-of-ranks test statistic could be examined. Tables could then be prepared to associate each sum of ranks with a P value.

Later on, when investigators began to use ordinal grades and ranked scales for expressing scientific results, the nonparametric procedure became an ideal mechanism for performing stochastic tests for ordinal data. When two or more items share the same ordinal grade, their rank is assigned using the tactic described in Section 7.2.3.3. The test statistic also receives an adjustment for the numbers of tied ranks. Consequently, for examining a stochastic contrast in two groups of ordinal data today, the appropriate nonparametric procedure is called the *Wilcoxon Rank Sum Test.* In recent years, a modification of this test has become more popular and is often used instead. The modification is called the *Mann-Whitney U Test.*

When a paired matching takes place so that two groups of ordinal data can be condensed to a single group, the nonparametric stochastic procedure is called the *Wilcoxon Signed Ranks Test.*

Details of these procedures can be found in good textbooks of statistics. For readers who like "cookbook demonstrations" and who are willing to risk the wrath of educators who rail against "cookbooks," the "Julia Child" set of demonstrations is contained in a little-known but clearly written text by Freeman.[9] Readers who want more formal mathematical discourse can find it in two other excellent texts.[10, 11]

9.5. PROBLEMS IN INTERPRETING QUANTITATIVE AND STOCHASTIC SIGNIFICANCE

For interpreting the results, the calculation of any stochastic test can be depicted as a general composite of the formula shown in equation 9.13. For the discussion that follows, the test statistic will be called Z, but the discussion pertains to any stochastic result examined in any of the permutation, parametric, or nonparametric procedures that have just been discussed.

The basic structure of the stochastic strategy involves starting with an observed distinction, which is then *multiplied* by the associated group size and *divided* by the associated variance. If we let d = observed distinction, N = group size, and v = variance, the basic structure for the calculation is

$$Z = \frac{dN}{v}$$

This composite formula will more nearly approximate the realities if we take the square root of the N/v term and cite the calculation as

$$Z = d \sqrt{\frac{N}{v}} \qquad [9.20]$$

After being calculated, this value of Z is compared with the value of Z_α that was previously chosen for the boundary of α. If $Z > Z_\alpha$, the value of P will be $< \alpha$, and we shall reject the null hypothesis, concluding that the observed distinction is significant. If $Z < Z_\alpha$, the value of P will be $> \alpha$, and we shall concede the null hypothesis. The observed distinction will be called *not significant.*

Because stochastic significance requires suitably large values of Z, equation 9.20 immediately lets us see why problems can often arise in the relationship between quantitative and stochastic importance. Quantitative significance depends primarily on d, the magnitude of the observed distinction. A large value of d, however, can fail to achieve stochastic significance if N is too small or v is too large. These are the stochastic penalties produced by small group sizes or by high variance in the groups.

Conversely, a value of d that is quantitatively small or unimportant can become stochastically significant if the sample size is large enough or if variance is small enough to make the calculated value of Z sufficiently big.

A large enough group can therefore make any distinction stochastically significant, no matter how trivial the distinction may be. To find the size of that group, all we need to do is choose a level of α at which we want to declare significance, find Z_α, find (or estimate) the variance, and then solve equation 9.20 for N. The required group size will be

$$N = \frac{vZ_\alpha^2}{d^2}$$

Note that the required magnitude of N will be increased by large variance, by large values of stochastic confidence (i.e., small value of α), and by small distinctions. Small distinctions are particularly important, because they appear in the denominator and they are squared. Thus, a difference of 0.10 in two groups becomes squared to 0.01 and it multiplies sample size by a factor of $1/0.01 = 100$, whereas a difference of 0.20 is squared to 0.04 and becomes a multiplicative factor of 25. Thus, if one distinction is half of another, the group size required for stochastic significance is four times larger.

9.5.1. *Contradictory Conclusions and Errors*

To draw conclusions from the statistical results of a completed study, standards must be set for several different decisions. The accuracy of the conclusions will depend on the way that those standards serve to either lead or mislead us when we seek to determine truth.

When the results are first appraised, they will show a particular distinction, d. This distinction will be expressed with one of the indexes of contrast we learned about in Chapter 8 (or with one of the indexes of association to be discussed in Chapter 10). By thinking about increments, ratios, or whatever other strategies we use in decisions about quantitative importance, we shall arbitrarily choose a value of δ to represent the magnitude of a quantitatively significant distinction for the relationship under consideration. In the true state of that relationship, the actual distinction is Δ, and the actual conclusion we want to draw refers to the state of Δ vs. δ. What we will have observed, however, is a distinction, d, which will or will not be called quantitatively significant according to whether $d \geq \delta$ or $d < \delta$.

In a second act of appraisal, which refers to the numerical fragility of the observed evidence, we establish a null hypothesis and then calculate Z as an index of stochastic significance. To make a decision about this calculated Z, we arbitrarily choose a value of Z_α to represent the magnitude required for stochastic significance. If $Z \geq Z_\alpha$, we reject the null hypothesis and declare significance. If $Z < Z_\alpha$, we concede the null hypothesis and declare that stochastic significance has not been achieved.

While all these appraisals, calculations, and decisions are taking place, there still remains the issue of truth. The conclusion we really want to reach is a decision about Δ, the true magnitude of the distinction in the relationship under consideration. We do not know this value, and none of our observed or calculated results will indicate what it really is. To do the stochastic calculation of Z, we make the *assumption* that $\Delta = 0$, but all we can say after we compare Z vs. Z_α is that the calculated results do or do not support the assumption. With respect to truth, we may be right or wrong when we decide to reject or concede the null hypothesis. Furthermore, the null hypothesis is itself incorrect if Δ does not equal zero and is actually $\geq\delta$.

In most of our final conclusions, the truth we want to know is whether $\Delta\geq\delta$—i.e., is there really a quantitatively significant distinction in the relationship? The assumption that $\Delta = 0$ is but one step in the chain of reasoning that precedes this conclusion; and the direct question (about whether $\Delta\geq\delta$) is not part of this reasoning. Even if we reject the assumption that $\Delta = 0$, we still do not know whether Δ is big enough to exceed δ.

As a result of all these phenomena, many different situations can be encountered in the statistical analysis. The situations arise as the different YES or NO possibilities for answers to the following three questions:

1. In the observed results, is $d\geq\delta$?
2. In the stochastic calculations, is $Z\geq Z_\alpha$?
3. In the true relationship, is $\Delta\geq\delta$?

The way we reach and use the decisions achieved in answering the first two questions will determine whether we are right or wrong in the concluding inference that represents our answer to the third.

In many statistical conclusions, the dominant decision depends on the answer to the stochastic question. The observed distinction is regarded as significant if $Z\geq Z_\alpha$. If $\Delta < \delta$, this decision will be wrong, and the false-positive conclusion is what statisticians call a *Type I error*. (Strictly speaking, of course, the stochastic conclusion is that $\Delta \neq 0$. This conclusion will almost always be correct, because Δ is seldom exactly zero. The idea we have in mind when we declare significance, however, is that $\Delta\geq\delta$.) When $Z<Z_\alpha$, the observed distinction is regarded as not significant. If $\Delta\geq\delta$, this decision will be wrong, and the false-negative conclusion is called a *Type II error*.

The interplay of the three pairs of magnitudes—for the observed d vs. the quantitatively significant δ, for the calculated Z vs. the stochastically significant Z_α, and for the reality of the true Δ vs. δ—can produce the eight different situations shown as sectors in the Venn diagram of Figure 9–2 and in Table 9–5. In four of these sectors (1, 3, 6, and 8), the stochastic conclusion is correct. In two sectors (5 and 7), the stochastic conclusion is falsely positive and produces a Type I error. In two other sectors (2 and 4), the stochastic conclusion is falsely negative and produces a Type II error. When the statistical decisions are made, however, we will not know the true value of Δ to tell us exactly where the observed results are located in Figure 9–2 and Table 9–5. We can readily compare the values of d vs. δ and Z vs. Z_α, but we cannot place them exactly without knowing the value of Δ vs. δ.

In trying to decide where we are, we can examine the concordance of our answers to the questions about the observed results for quantitative and stochastic significance. Because significance will be present quantitatively if $d\geq\delta$ and stochastically if $Z\geq Z_\alpha$, the two sets of values will be concordant in two ways as YES-YES and NO-NO, and discordant in two ways as YES-NO and NO-YES. The YES-YES concordance occurs in Sectors 1 and 5 of Figure 9–2 and Table 9–5. The NO-NO concordance is in Sectors 4 and 8. The YES-NO discordance is in Sectors 2 and 6; and the NO-YES discordance is in Sectors 3 and 7. The existence of concordant or discordant results for d and Z, however, will not solve our problem, since the stochastic conclusion will be wrong in one member of each of those pairs of sectors. Thus, the stochastic conclusion is correct in Sectors 1, 3, 6, and 8, and wrong in Sectors 2, 4, 5, and 7.

9.5.2. *Analysis of Problems*

Although the concordance of the observed quantitative and stochastic distinctions will not solve the problem, a careful analysis of the four situations may help us escape some of

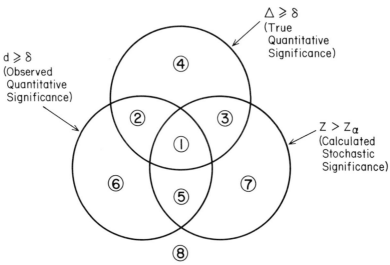

Figure 9–2. Truth, error, and interpretations in the eight types of possible results for statistical significance (see further details in text and Table 9–5).

the hazards or take additional mathematical steps to avoid them. The analysis will differ according to the four patterns of concordance.

9.5.2.1. **d⩾δ AND Z⩾Z_α**

When both types of significance seem present, in the YES-YES situation of Sectors 1 and 5, an erroneous conclusion cannot be prevented with any mathematical strategy. If the observed d is ⩾δ and is also stochastically significant, but if the true value of Δ is indeed smaller than δ, we have received a distorted set of results, either because of unkind fate or flawed research. Our only hope in avoiding error here is to perceive the distortion as a scientific rather than statistical phenomenon. By carefully evaluating the architecture of the research, our scientific appraisal may allow us to discern what may be wrong—or at least we may learn enough to be wary of the statistical conclusion that a significant distinction exists when it really may not.

9.5.2.2. **d<δ AND Z<Z_α**

When both types of significance seem absent, as in the NO-NO concordance of results in Sectors 4 and 8, the fear of error is that we may be missing a truly significant difference. If the error is caused by a flaw in research architecture, a careful scientific analysis may help detect it. The error, however, can also arise from "fragile" numbers, which can be discerned with the aid of a mathematical stretegy. The strategy depends on searching for the false-negative errors that may occur when a group (or sample) size is too small to show the true quantitative and stochastic distinctions.

This type of problem might arise, for example, if we have done a small clinical trial comparing treatment A, which has a true success rate of 80%, and treatment B, which has a true success rate of 40%. The quantitatively impressive difference in the two treatments

Table 9–5. TRUTH, ERROR, AND INTERPRETATIONS OF RESULTS SHOWN IN FIGURE 9–2

Sector in Venn Diagram	True Quantitative Significance	Observed Quantitative Significance	Calculated Stochastic Significance	Concordance of Observed and Calculated Significance	Concordance of Stochastic Conclusion and "Truth"
1	Yes	Yes	Yes	Yes	Yes
2			No	No	No (Type II error)
3		No	Yes	No	Yes
4			No	Yes	No (Type II error)
5	No	Yes	Yes	Yes	No (Type I error)
6			No	No	Yes
7		No	Yes	No	No (Type I error)
8			No	Yes	Yes

might be missed in small groups where the success rates turn out to be as low as 5/9 (59%) for A and as high as 4/8 (50%) for B. For these results, the increment of 6% and ratio of 1.1 may be dismissed as quantitatively unimportant, and the value of Z will not be stochastically significant. With a larger sample size, however, the results might have been more accurate, and the superiority of treatment A might have been manifested more convincingly.

The mathematical strategy used for detecting this numerical problem is to check the "power" of the stochastic calculations. The strategy involves the use of one or both of two tactics that receive detailed discussion in Sections 9.6 and 9.7. In one tactic, we examine the scope of the confidence interval for d. If this scope includes the value of δ, then a distinct possibility exists that the true value for Δ is indeed as large as δ. In the second tactic, we perform an additional test of stochastic significance, using the alternative null hypothesis that $\Delta = \delta$. If we are unable to reject this alternative hypothesis, then a distinct possibility exists that the original null hypothesis (i.e., $\Delta = 0$) is incorrect, and we may decide to accept the alternative hypothesis that $\Delta \geq \delta$.

9.5.2.3. $d \geq \delta$ AND $Z < Z_\alpha$

The mathematical strategy just described for checking the stochastic "power" of the data is particularly pertinent for the YES-NO discordance of Sectors 2 and 6. If the observed distinction is quantitatively significant but the stochastic calculation is not, the sample size may be too small.

For example, suppose two treatments actually have the extreme effects of a 100%

success rate for the first and 0% for the second. The observed distinction will be clearly shown in a trial of four people where the success results are 2/2 vs. 0/2. Because the actual numbers are so small, however, the quantitatively impressive distinction of 100% vs. 0% will not be stochastically significant. A Fisher test would show that the two-tailed P value is 0.33. (With one more person in each group, the quantitative significance would be the same, at 3/3 vs. 0/3, but the one-tailed Fisher P value would drop to 0.05. For a contrast of 4/4 vs. 0/4, the two-tailed Fisher P value would be significant at 0.028.)

Because a value of $d > \delta$ would make us particularly suspicious that significance really exists but was not detected stochastically, we would be especially eager in this situation to do the further mathematical analyses described in Section 9.5.2.2 and in Sections 9.6 and 9.7.

9.5.2.4. **$d < \delta$ AND $Z \geqslant Z_\alpha$**

This peculiar situation produces the NO-YES discordance of Sectors 3 and 7, where stochastic significance is achieved despite an unimpressive quantitative distinction in the observed results.

One obvious explanation for this type of discordance is a huge sample size, which can magnify trivial quantitative distinctions into being stochastically impressive. For example, treatment A may be regarded as significantly better than treatment B because a clinical trial showed $P < 0.05$ for the compared results. Quantitatively, however, the compared rates of success may have shown the unimpressive distinction of 56% vs. 52%. The stochastically significant value of Z that made $P < 0.05$ was achieved because 2400 patients were studied, with the observed numbers of success being 671/1198 for treatment A and 625/1202 for treatment B.

In this type of situation, the large sample size will give statistical stability to the results for each group, and we may be content to accept the observed distinctions as being numerically adequate. Giving priority to the absence of quantitative significance, we may want to overrule the results of the stochastic calculation. We would therefore decide that the distinction is *not* significant, despite an impressively large value of Z (or small value of P). Since this decision would carry the risk of a false-negative conclusion, we can again use mathematical prophylaxis to check the stochastic power of the data in sustaining a *negative* conclusion. If we do not get stochastic support for the possibility that $\Delta \geqslant \delta$, we may then be willing to maintain our negative conclusion that $\Delta < \delta$.

From the foregoing discussion of concordances and discordances, we see that in three of the four situations valuable mathematical help can be obtained from examining confidence intervals for d and from an additional test of stochastic significance, with the alternative null hypothesis that $\Delta = \delta$. This extra mathematical aid, which is discussed in Sections 9.6 and 9.7, will not save us from having to do careful scientific appraisals of the evidence, because mathematical tactics will seldom cure a scientifically flawed research architecture. Nevertheless, the additional statistical tactics can help prevent erroneous conclusions when the group sizes are too small or too big.

9.6. **FURTHER USES OF CONFIDENCE INTERVALS**

Regardless of what statistical methods are used to provide the P values of stochastic contrasts, the calculation and inspection of confidence intervals is a valuable procedure for data expressed in either means or proportions.

9.6.1. *The Precision of a Central Index*

As noted in Section 5.3.1, the scientific word *precision* refers to the amount of detail in a measurement. The same word is often used statistically, however, to describe the stability of a central index. If the observed values of data are closely bunched together, the central index is less fragile and more precise than if they are widely spread. Even if the data are widely spread, the central index will still be relatively stable if the group size is large. Both of these concepts were reflected in the $s_x/\overline{X}$ ratio that was cited in Section 7.6.4.5 for representing the fragility of a central index. The smaller this ratio, the less fragile is the index. Because $s_{\overline{x}}$ is calculated as $s/\sqrt{N}$, fragility increases as standard deviation increases but is reduced as the group (or sample) size gets larger.

An excellent way of determining the statistical precision of a central index is to examine its confidence interval. If the confidence interval is narrow or tight, the index is much more precise than if the interval is wide. If the sample sizes are large, the confidence interval is usually calculated as $\overline{X} \pm Z_\alpha s_{\overline{x}}$ for dimensional data and as $p \pm Z_\alpha(\sqrt{pq/n})$ for binary proportions. If the sample sizes are small, the Z_α in these formulas should be replaced by $t_{\alpha,\nu}$ where the ν represents degrees of freedom in the sample and α has the same connotation as before. (For proportions, the confidence interval is probably best calculated with the binomial technique mentioned in Section 9.4.2.6.)

For example, for the four people who received treatment A in Section 9.4.1.3, the results were 8, 11, 13, and 21. The mean was 13.25 and the standard deviation was 5.56. If we wanted to put a 95% confidence interval around this mean, the value of $t_{\alpha,\nu}$ would be $t_{0.05,3}$. In Table 9–4, this value is seen to be 3.18. The confidence interval would be $13.25 \pm 3.18(5.56/\sqrt{4})$, and would range from 4.4 to 22.1. The wide range around the value of 13.25 would indicate the imprecision and high fragility of this mean. An analogous example for binary data was presented in Section 7.6.4.5, where we found that the proportion of 55%, derived from 11/20, had a 95% confidence interval that went from 33.4% to 76.6%.

9.6.2. *Confidence Intervals as Substitutes for P Values*

In equation 9.6, we saw that Z was determined as the difference in two means divided by the standard error of the difference. The P value for this ratio will be stochastically significant at $\alpha = 0.05$ if Z exceeds 1.96.

Instead of calculating Z as shown in equation 9.6, we can choose a value for the desired confidence interval around the difference in means and then calculate the quantity

$$(Z_\alpha) \sqrt{\frac{s_A^2}{n_A} + \frac{s_B^2}{n_B}}$$

If the observed difference in means, $\overline{X}_A - \overline{X}_B$, is larger than this quantity, we will know that the difference is significant at $P < \alpha$. If the sample sizes are small, Z_α is replaced by the appropriate value of $t_{\alpha,\nu}$ for this calculation.

For example, in the two groups of treated people who were stochastically contrasted in Section 9.4.2.2, the value of

$$\sqrt{\frac{s_A^2}{n_A} + \frac{s_B^2}{n_B}}$$

was 4.77. At $N-2 = 6$ degrees of freedom, $t_{0.05,6} = 2.447$. The confidence interval on either size of the difference in means would be $4.77 \times 2.447 = 11.57$. Because the observed difference in means was $13.25 - 28.00 = -14.75$, it exceeds the confidence interval and would therefore be declared stochastically significant at $P < 0.05$.

An alternative way of making this same decision is to see whether the confidence interval around the difference in means excludes or includes the value of zero. If it includes the value of 0, the difference is *not* stochastically significant. Thus, the 95% confidence interval around the difference in means is -14.75 ± 11.67. This interval does not include zero and so the difference is stochastically significant.

9.6.3. *The "Shortcut" Crude Estimate of Significance*

Instead of using equations 9.5 or 9.10 to calculate the square root of the variance or pooled variance of the difference in means, we can get a crude estimate of this value by simply adding the two standard errors, $s_{\bar{X}_A}$ and $s_{\bar{X}_B}$. It can be shown[12] that the sum of the two standard errors is always larger than the standard deviation of their difference. Consequently, if $\bar{X}_A - \bar{X}_B$ exceeds the product $t_{\alpha,\nu}$ $(s_{\bar{X}_A} + s_{\bar{X}_B})$, the contrast will be stochastically significant.

An example of this distinction can be seen in the two groups we have been discussing, for which the standard errors of the mean are $s_{\bar{X}_A} = (5.56)/\sqrt{4} = 2.78$ and $s_{\bar{X}_B} = 7.75/\sqrt{4} = 3.875$. Their sum is $2.78 + 3.875 = 6.655$, which is larger than the 4.77 found previously as the standard deviation of their difference. When multiplied by $t_{0.05,6} = 2.447$, the result is $6.655 \times 2.447 = 16.28$. Because this number is larger than the observed mean difference of 14.75, we cannot reject the null hypothesis on this basis, and the regular t test procedure would be required.

In general, however, the addition of the standard errors for each group offers an excellent screening device for performing stochastic tests in one's head. If we assume that $\alpha < 0.05$ if $Z_{0.05} = 2$, the process is as follows: Add the two standard errors. Multiply their sum by 2. If the resulting product substantially exceeds the observed difference in central indexes, the contrast will not be stochastically significant at $\alpha < 0.05$. If the resulting product is substantially smaller than the observed difference, the contrast will be stochastically significant. If the resulting product is reasonably close to the observed difference (such as the 16.28 and 14.75 noted in the preceding paragraph), go ahead and do the formal mathematical procedure.

9.6.4. *Screening for Type II Errors*

In Sections 9.6.2 and 9.6.3, we used confidence intervals to screen for Type I errors. If one end of the confidence interval came close to 0, or if 0 was actually included in the interval, the results support the possibility that $\Delta = 0$ and that the observed difference is not significant.

The other end of the confidence interval can also be used to screen for Type II errors. If the other end of the interval approaches or exceeds the δ established as being quantitatively important, there is a good chance that the observed difference is indeed significant, despite the stochastic decision of nonsignificance.

For example, consider the situation in Section 9.5.2.2, when we contrasted the results of 5/9 for treatment A and 4/8 for treatment B. The observed increment was $56\% - 50\% = 6\%$, which was considerably smaller than what we might get in the long run as $80\% - 50\% = 30\%$. If we calculate a confidence interval for the 6%, however, we would find the following:

1. For the pooled estimate of P and Q, we get $P = (5+4)/(8+9) = 9/17 = 0.529$, and $Q = 0.471$. The standard error of the difference will be $\sqrt{[(1/9 + (1/8)][0.529][0.471]} = 0.243$. If we choose $1 - \alpha = 0.95$, Z_α will be 1.96, and the confidence interval will be calculated with $1.96 \times 0.243 = 0.48$. The actual interval will be 0.06 ± 0.48 and will run

from -42% to $+54\%$. Because the upper boundary of this interval exceeds 30%, we cannot reject the idea that the data came from a circumstance in which $\Delta = 30\%$.

2. If we do not pool the estimate for variance, the standard error of the difference is $\sqrt{(p_A q_A/n_A) + (p_B q_B/n_B)}$, which is $\sqrt{[(5/9)(4/9)]/9 + [(4/8)(4/8)]/8} = \sqrt{0.059} = 0.242$. Because $1.96 \times 0.242 = 0.47$, this interval would be 0.06 ± 0.47 and would also include both 0% and 30%.

9.7 STATISTICAL POWER AND THE ALTERNATIVE TYPE OF SIGNIFICANCE

All of the stochastic tactics discussed so far in this chapter began with the null hypothesis assumption that $\Delta = 0$, i.e., that there is essentially no distinction in the entities under contrast. The P values determined with this assumption tell us the stochastic likelihood of committing a false-positive or Type I error when we reject this hypothesis if it is true. In Section 9.5, however, we thought about an alternative possibility. The true value of Δ might be $\geq \delta$, so that a quantitatively significant difference really exists. If we concede the null hypothesis that $\Delta = 0$, we will fail to detect this distinction. The conclusion will be a false-negative or Type II error.

This hazard can arise in the two different ways noted in the previous discussion. The value of $d < \delta$ may have been produced by an unrepresentative sample, or the value of d may have correctly exceeded δ, but the sample size was too small to be stochastically significant.

We saw an example of the first problem in Section 9.5.2.2 where a confidence interval helped resolve the problem. Thus, although the observed value of d was only 6% for the contrast of 5/9 versus 4/8, the 95% confidence interval suggested that the value of Δ could range from -42% to 54%. This range would warn us to hesitate before conceding the idea that Δ was quite small and possibly $= 0$.

We saw an example of the second problem in Section 9.5.2.3, where stochastic significance was absent for a distinction in which the observed value of d was 100%. In this situation, we did not need a confidence interval to warn us that Δ might be substantially larger than 0. The warning was delivered by the observed value of d, which failed to be stochastically significant only because the sample size was so small.

Both of these problems could have been avoided with larger sample sizes. In the second instance, a contrast of 4/4 versus 0/4 rather than 2/2 versus 0/2 would have had group sizes big enough for Z to exceed Z_α. In the first instance, a larger sample size might have removed the fear that we had assembled unrepresentative groups. If the observed contrast of 56% versus 50% had came from success rates of 67/120 in treatment A and 59/118 in treatment B, the standard error of the difference would be $\sqrt{[(1/120) + (1/118)][0.2491]} = 0.065$. The 95% confidence interval around the observed difference would be $0.06 \pm (1.96)(0.065)$. It would run from -6.6% to 18.7%, and it would *not* include the increment of $\Delta = 30\%$. We might therefore be justified in concluding that the observed distinction was not significant or at least that the true difference in treatments was not as high as 30%.

9.7.1. *Sample Size and the Two Types of Erroneous Conclusion*

In equation 9.20 in Section 9.5, we noted the crucial role of sample size in stochastic contrasts. The formula was

$$Z = d \sqrt{\frac{N}{v}}$$

where d is the observed distinction in the two groups, v is the variance of that distinction under the null hypothesis, and N is the total sample size.

If the observed distinction, d, is larger than δ, which is the amount of a quantitatively significant distinction, we check for a false-positive result by seeing whether the associated value of Z exceeds Z_α, which is set at 1.96 for a two-tailed test at the 0.05 level. If Z fails to exceed Z_α, the sample size is too small (or the variance is too large).

If d is less than δ, however, we can check for a false-negative result by beginning with a different null hypothesis. We can start with the idea that the true distinction, Δ, is really as large as δ, rather than 0. The sampling variance of data under this alternative hypothesis can be determined as v_H. The Z value that corresponds to a value of $d = \delta$ would be

$$Z = \delta \sqrt{\frac{N}{v_H}}$$

Because d is less than δ, we are looking for the Z value at the negative point $d - \delta$, under the alternative hypothesis. This value will be

$$Z_H = (d - \delta) \sqrt{\frac{N}{v_H}} \qquad [9.21]$$

When converted to a P value, this value of Z_H will indicate the likelihood that the observed distinction comes from two groups having δ as their true difference. If this value of Z_H is large enough, we can reject the alternative hypothesis and conclude that the true difference is not as large as δ. If Z_H is too small, however, we must concede the alternative hypothesis. The conclusion would be that the two groups may indeed differ by a magnitude of δ.

To distinguish these two different activities, let us call Z_0 the value of Z that is calculated in equation 9.20 under the original null hypothesis, H_0. This value of Z_0 will give us a P value that can be called P_0. It is the conventional P value found in most stochastic tests. P_0 is compared and interpreted against the Z_α level determined by the choice of α and by one- or two-tailed decisions about probability.

In the other activity, shown in equation 9.21, we investigated the alternative hypothesis, H_H. (The alternative hypothesis is usually labeled as H_A in most statistics books. To avoid confusion with the Greek letter α, which pertains to H_0, I shall use H_H instead of H_A.) The Z_H value that emerges from the calculation in equation 9.21 corresponds to an alternative P value, P_H, which indicates the random likelihood of obtaining the observed distinction by chance under the alternative hypothesis. This value of P_H (or the corresponding Z_H) is compared and interpreted against a Z_β level, which is determined by an appropriate choice of β. Because the alternative hypothesis usually goes in only one direction, Z_β is usually chosen to be one-tailed. Because this level of β is used in testing for the possibility of Type II error, the procedure is sometimes called a check for *beta error*.

Equations 9.20 and 9.21 show the crucial role of sample size in obtaining stochastically significant decisions. If N is too small, its multiplication of a quantitatively significant value of d may still lead to a small value of Z_0 that is $<Z_\alpha$. The null hypothesis may then be mistakenly conceded, merely because of a small sample size.

On the other hand, if $d<\delta$, we need to consider the role of chance before we conclude that the true difference is really not significant. We therefore assume that $\Delta = \delta$, and we then establish an alternative hypothesis and calculate Z_H. If the value of P_H is $>\beta$, we cannot reject the idea that a true difference of Δ actually exists. If P_H is $<\beta$, we can reject the alternative hypothesis and then conclude stochastically that the observed difference is both quantitatively and stochastically insignificant. The sequence of the reasoning is shown in the flow chart of Figure 9–3.

The value of $1 - P_H$ is called the *power* of a stochastic contrast. Thus if $P_H = 0.10$, the power is 0.90 or 90%. This usage leads to such expressions as "the results had a 90% power of rejecting the null hypothesis at the 5% level for an incremental difference of 20%." In this expression the respective numerical values refer to $\beta = 0.10$, $\alpha = 0.05$, and $\Delta = 0.20$.

9.7.2. *Example of Calculations*

In a randomized trial, the results show success rates of 18/40 = 45% for new treatment A and 12/39 = 31% for old treatment B. The investigators, after performing the customary stochastic test, are disappointed to find that P>0.2 and that the null hypothesis (that $\Delta = 0$) cannot be rejected. The stochastic test could have been done with $X^2 = [(18 \times 27) - (12 \times 22)]^2 79/[(30)(49)(39)(40)] = 1.70$ or with $Z = [(18/40) - (12/39)]/\sqrt{([1/39] + [1/40])(30/79)(49/79)}} = 1.30$.

A statistical consultant, trying to assuage the investigators' sorrow, points out that an alternative hypothesis should be considered with these small sample sizes. Because the investigators believe that the new treatment A is proportionately at least 75% better than treatment B, the investigators examine the alternative hypothesis that the success rate

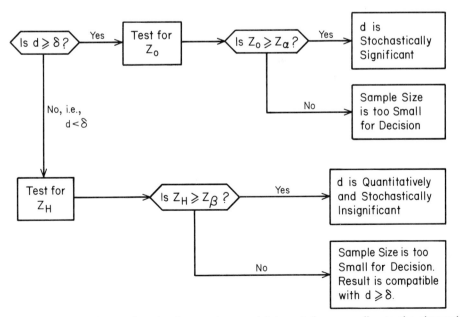

Figure 9–3. Sequence of stochastic procedures and interpretations according to the observed distinction (d), the quantitatively significant distinction (δ), and the calculated values of Z for the null hypothesis (Z_O) and the alternative hypothesis (Z_H). For further details, see text.

with treatment A is really $1.75 \times 31\% = 54.25\%$, so that the true value of Δ would be 23.25%. To use equation 9.21 here, the $\sqrt{N}/v_H$ term is calculated as $\sqrt{[(18/40)(22/40)/40] + [(12/39)(17/39)/39]} = 0.098$, and $d - \delta = 0.142 - 0.2325 = -0.0905$, so that $Z_H = -0.0905/0.098 = -0.923$. This value of Z_H is interpreted as a one-tailed test, because we expect treatment A to be better than treatment B. According to Table 7–2, the P_H value associated with a one-tailed Z_H of -0.923 lies between 0.3 and 0.16. We therefore cannot reject the alternative hypothesis that the true difference in treatments is really 23.25% and that the difference was not detected in this trial.

Freiman and associates[13] have pointed out the frequency with which this problem occurs in many clinical trials. When the observed results do not show stochastic significance, the authors often fail to examine the other side of the picture by noting the sizable distinction that might have been missed because the sample size was too small.

9.7.3. *The Doubly Significant Sample Size*

In most research hypotheses, the idea is to show a quantitatively significant distinction in which $d \geq \delta$. Sample size for this null hypothesis is calculated from equation 9.20 by specifying the level of α, by determining v_0, and by substituting δ for d. Because $Z_\alpha = \delta \sqrt{N}/v_0$, we solve for N by squaring and rearranging terms so that

$$N = Z_\alpha^2 v_0 / \delta^2 \qquad [9.22]$$

What we worry about, however, is that the observed value of d may be less than δ— a situation in which we will want to rule out the alternative hypothesis that $\Delta > \delta$. For this purpose, we would apply equation 9.21, using v_H for the variance and choosing a value of Z_β that would allow rejection of the alternative hypothesis. These substitutions would give us

$$Z_\beta = (d - \delta) \sqrt{\frac{N}{v_H}}$$

If we assume that v_0 and v_H are quite similar and can be replaced by one or the other as v, some algebra that the reader will be spared can then be used to show that the sample size needed for this achievement is

$$N = \frac{(Z_\alpha + Z_\beta)^2 v}{\delta^2}$$

Thus, because the $Z_\alpha + Z_\beta$ term is squared, the sample size needed for double significance may be about four times larger than what was needed for single significance. (The cited formula is a simplified version of the more elaborate procedure. Readers who want further details can find it in discussions elsewhere,[14, 15] with symbolism that differs from what is used here.)

9.8 THE PROBLEM OF MULTIPLE CONTRASTS

The last topic to be discussed before the reader is granted a parole from stochastic contrasts is the possibility that false-positive results may arise by chance when multiple stochastic contrasts are conducted. For example, if we stochastically contrast the mean *age* in two groups, the chance of obtaining a false-positive result is α. The chance of avoiding this result is $1 - \alpha$. If we now contrast the mean *weight* of the two groups, we have another α chance of obtaining a false-positive result and have an avoidance chance of $1-\alpha$. The chance of avoiding a false-positive result in the two contrasts will be $(1-\alpha)(1-\alpha)$.

If we also stochastically contrast the mean height, hematocrit, and serum cholesterol values of the two groups, the chance of avoiding a false-positive result in the five contrasts will be $(1-\alpha)^5$. Thus, for an α of 0.05, the chance of avoiding a false-positive conclusion in five contrasts will be $(0.95)^5 = 0.77$. The chance of obtaining a false-positive result will therefore be $1-0.77 = 0.23$. By performing five independent contrasts in the same set of data, our working false-positive level of $\alpha = 0.05$ has been functionally raised to a level of 0.23. In general, if α is the established false-positive level for an individual stochastic contrast, the functional false-positive level in a set of k contrasts is raised to

$$\alpha' = 1-(1-\alpha)^k$$

A variety of mathematical methods have been proposed for dealing with this problem,[16-18] which is further discussed in Section 22.6.3.2. Of those methods, the one that is statistically simplest is to lower the individual α level for each contrast to α/k. The value that emerges for α' will then approximate the originally desired overall level of α. Thus, if we want the overall level of α to be 0.05 and if we plan to perform five contrasts, the individual level of α would be set at $0.05/5 = 0.01$ for each contrast. Each contrast would then have a 0.99 chance of being correct. Because $(0.99)^5 = 0.95$, and $1-0.95 = 0.05$, the overall α would return to the 0.05 level.

9.9. SYNOPSIS

The term *stochastic contrasts* refers to mathematical tests of numerical fragility or chance probability for observed distinctions. Although the mathematical process is often called *hypothesis testing,* the latter term is best reserved for the complex issues involved in testing a scientific rather than a statistical hypothesis.

A stochastic contrast is conducted in six steps. In the first step, we choose a null hypothesis, which is contrary to the point we want to prove, and which will be rejected if the calculated results fulfill certain criteria. In the customary null hypothesis, the observed maneuvers are assumed to be equivalent or the observed groups are regarded as random samples from the same population. In the second step, we choose a particular test statistic, which can be the distinction noted in the central indexes of the observed groups or a special mathematical entity such as Z, t, or X^2. In the third step, we examine the distribution of the test statistic under the null hypothesis. With permutation or nonparametric tests, this distribution is obtained from all possible appropriate combinations of the observed data. With parametric tests, the distribution is provided by a mathematical model.

This distribution will show us, in the fourth step, the exterior probabilities of obtaining a result that is at least as large as the observed distinction in the data. The exterior probabilities can be examined in a unilateral (one-tail) or bilateral (two-tail) direction, according to the results expected from the scientific hypothesis. In permutation tests, such as the Fisher test for a contrast of proportions or the Pitman-Welch test for a contrast of means, the exterior probabilities are shown directly as P values. In parametric tests, the P value is found from the corresponding results contained in special tables that show the distribution of the test statistic. Among the currently popular parametric procedures are the chi-square test for contrasting proportions and the Z test for contrasting means. When sample sizes are small, the Z test is usually replaced by the t test. Proportions can also be stochastically contrasted with a Z or t test. The Mann-Whitney U test is commonly used for stochastic contrasts of two groups of ordinal data.

In the fifth step, we choose a boundary—called an α level—that is the criterion for rejecting the null hypothesis. The customary level of α is 0.05. In the sixth step, after comparing the calculated value of P with the selected level of α, we form a conclusion. If the exterior probability value for P is below α, the null hypothesis is rejected, and the observed distinction is called *stochastically* (or statistically) *significant*. If P exceeds α, we concede the null hypothesis and declare that the results are not stochastically significant.

The process just described can also be used for paired contrasts in which the results of two matched groups are reduced to a single group of incremental distinctions. These one-sample tests, which are usually more likely to achieve stochastic significance than the two-group tests, are identified with titles such as the paired t (or Z) test for dimensional data, the Wilcoxon Signed Ranks Tests for ordinal data, and the McNemar chi-square test for binary data expressed as proportions.

The interpretation of tests of stochastic significance is complicated by the interrelationship among the observed distinction in results, the true distinction in the biologic phenomenon, and the distinction regarded as quantitatively significant. In the general strategy of the stochastic procedure, the index of significance is obtained as a product in which the observed distinction is multiplied by group size and divided by group variance. A trivial distinction can thus become stochastically significant if group size is large enough (or group variance is small enough); conversely, an important quantitative distinction may fail to achieve stochastic significance if group size is too small (or variance is too large).

Although false-positive (Type I) errors can occur if a minor distinction is declared significant, false-negative (Type II) errors can occur if nonsignificance is declared when a major distinction exists. To avoid these problems requires careful attention to the magnitude of a quantitatively significant difference and to the paramount role of group (or sample) size in stochastic calculations. Confidence intervals can be used to estimate the possible extent of the observed distinction for considering both Type I and Type II errors. Before a distinction is declared stochastically nonsignificant, it can be tested for the statistical power with which the data allow exclusion of an alternative hypothesis regarding a major distinction. The alternative hypothesis can also be used for calculations of a doubly significant sample size in planning clinical trials.

When multiple tests of stochastic significance are performed on different variables in the same set of data, an unimportant difference can become significant (Type I error) merely by chance. This problem, which is further discussed in Chapter 22, is usually managed statistically by lowering the α level for the individual tests of the multiple contrasts.

EXERCISES

Exercise 9.1. In a particular randomized trial, the two-tailed P value for the observed distinction between active treatment and placebo was 0.001. Please comment on whether each of the following conclusions is right or wrong:

9.1.1. If the active treatment is inert, such a result could arise by chance once in 1000 such trials.

9.1.2. The active treatment is 1000 times more likely to be successful than the placebo.

9.1.3. If the active treatment is inert, the observed distinction or a larger one has a probability of 1/1000 of occurring by chance alone.

9.1.4. The odds are 1000 to 1 that the active treatment is effective.

9.1.5. Our chances of being wrong are 1 in 1000 if we conclude that the active treatment is efficacious.

9.1.6. The results have the statistical power of 0.999 for demonstrating efficacy.

Exercise 9.2. In a randomized trial of a new pharmaceutical agent, the rates of adverse reactions are determined for the active agent and for the placebo. Should the stochastic contrast of these rates be done with a one-tailed or two-tailed test? Please give the reason for your answer.

Exercise 9.3. An investigator has developed a new analgesic agent that allegedly costs less and has fewer adverse side effects than the standard agent. In a randomized trial of efficacy for two agents, the investigator finds that the mean pain relief scores were 1.7 ± 0.8 for six people receiving the new agent and 2.3 ± 0.9 for seven people receiving the standard agent. Although the standard agent's results are somewhat better, the investigator does a t test and finds that the difference is not stochastically significant. The investigator's conclusion is that the trial has shown the two agents to have similar efficacy. Please state why you agree or disagree with this conclusion.

Exercise 9.4. In a randomized double-blind trial, corticotrophin gel was compared with placebo gel for the ability to prevent pressure sores in patients undergoing surgery on the upper shaft of the femur or on the hip joint. The frequency of pressure sores postoperatively was 12/43 for the placebo group and 5/42 for the group receiving the corticotrophin gel. Please perform a test of stochastic significance for this contrast. What is your conclusion?

Exercise 9.5. In the trial described in Exercise 9.4, the authors stratified their patients into those who had fractured femurs and those who had hip replacements. The frequency rates of pressure sores for placebo versus actively treated patients were 7/27 versus 5/26 in the fractured femur group and 5/16 versus 0/16 in the hip replacement group, respectively. How do these stratified results affect the conclusion you formed in Exercise 9.4? Why?

CHAPTER REFERENCES

1. Fisher, 1934; 2. Pitman, 1937; 3. Welch, 1937; 4. "Student," 1908; 5. Yates, 1934; 6. Mainland, 1963; 7. McNemar, 1947; 8. Wilcoxon, 1964; 9. Freeman, 1965; 10. Siegel, 1956; 11. Bradley, 1968; 12. Feinstein, 1981; 13. Freiman, 1978; 14. Feinstein, 1975; 15. Fleiss, 1981; 16. Miller, 1966; 17. O'Neill, 1971; 18. Tukey, 1977.

Chapter 10

Statistical Indexes of
Association

All our comparisons so far have been a contrast of two things: one mean versus another mean; one success rate versus another success rate; or one risk versus another risk. We have not yet developed a way to compare more than two things at once, although we may often want to do so.

Having given a drug at different levels of dosage (such as 25 mg., 50 mg., 100 mg., and 200 mg.), we might want to see whether the response becomes progressively greater with increasing dosage. The goal would not be to contrast responses for the 25 mg. group versus the 50 mg. group, or the 50 mg. group versus the 100 mg. group, or the 25 mg. group versus the 200 mg. group. Instead, we want to examine the general trend of the dose-response curve. Does the response become progressively higher with increasing dosage; does it become flat; or does it decline?

In a different type of analysis, we might want to see if there is a relationship between patients' race and their use of one of four hospitals, **W, X, Y,** and **Z** in our community. For each hospital, we could determine the proportions of its patients who were **white, black,** or **other.** We could contrast those proportions for pairs of hospitals such as **W** versus

170

X, Y versus Z, etc., but the individual pairs of contrasts would not give us a single index of the relationship between race and site of hospitalization.

An analogous but different problem would arise if we asked two rheumatologists, A and B, to rate the degree of restricted motion in a series of knee joints, using a scale of **0**, **1+**, **2+**, **3+**, **4+**, in which **0** represents *no restriction* and **4+** represents *no mobility*. In this study of observer variability, we could see how often the rheumatologists disagree; we could calculate the incremental magnitudes of individual disagreements (e.g., by saying that a rating of **3+** by one rheumatologist and **1+** by the other is a **2+ disagreement**), and we could then calculate an average magnitude of disagreement; but this index would not describe whether the disagreements have an ordered relationship. Thus, if the average disagreement for 20 patients is **1+**, we would not know whether the observers tend to give close but disparate ratings for individual patients (with disagreements of **1+** versus **2+**, **3+** versus **4+**, and so on) or whether the observers agree completely on many patients but wildly disagree (with ratings of **0** versus **4+**) on others.

In each of the three situations just described, we wanted an index that would describe the relationship of data collected for two variables. In the first case, the two variables were *dosage* and *response*; in the second, *race* and *hospital site*; in the third, *ratings of rheumatologist A* and *ratings of rheumatologist B*. The statistical expressions that do this job are called *indexes of association*. Unlike the univariate indexes of spectrum and contrast, indexes of association are bivariate or sometimes multivariate. An index of spectrum describes the contents of a single variable; an index of contrast describes a comparison for the central indexes of a single variable in two groups; but an index of association describes what is found simultaneously in two or more variables. Those variables can contain dimensional data for an entity such as *age* or categorical data that describe groups and subgroups such as **old, middle,** and **young.**

The three cited clinical situations also illustrate some of the main differences in the kinds of associations for which indexes are desired. In the first two examples, we wanted to find the *trend* between two different variables: The first situation contained dimensional data (*response* versus *dosage*), and the second situation contained unranked nominal data (*race* versus *hospital site*). In the third example, we wanted to find the *concordance* (or agreement) for two different observations of the same variable. These three types of indexes—for trend in dimensional data, trend in unranked data, and concordance—are the basic expressions used for statistical associations.

10.1. MODELS AND STRATEGIES FOR INDEXES OF ASSOCIATION

In Chapters 3 to 5, we considered an intellectual model that could be used for evaluating the basic components of a research study. Intellectual models of strategy are also used in statistical activities. Without calling it a *model*, we used one such strategy in Chapters 7 to 9 when we decided to let a spectrum be represented by the mean that was "fitted" to the data. After determining a standard deviation, which depended on disparities between the individual items of data and their fitted mean, we calculated the coefficient of variation in Section 7.6.1. As a quotient of standard deviation divided by mean, the coefficient of variation indicates how well the model fits the data. The larger this coefficient, the worse is the fit.

To create indexes of association, we can use several strategies that employ this principle of fitting a model and examining departures from the fit. In all of the strategies, we develop an expectation for certain results, and we then determine the deviation between the observed and the expected values. For indexes of trend in dimensional data, the expected values are generated when the data are fitted by a model that is a straight line (or its multidimensional analog). For indexes of trend in nominal data, the expected values are obtained with a model that assumes the two variables are wholly unrelated. For indexes of concordance, the expected values depend on a model based on the agreement that might occur by chance alone.

10.2. INDEXES OF DIMENSIONAL TREND

Suppose we want to summarize the relationship of hematocrit to blood urea nitrogen (BUN) levels in the following set of data for a group of people with renal disease:

Person	Blood Urea Nitrogen	Hematocrit
A	80	29
B	32	40
C	138	18
D	36	31
E	70	27
F	23	43

The first (and best) thing to do with this information is to draw it in the scattergraph shown in Figure 10–1. By visual inspection of this graph, we can immediately determine that a distinct relationship exists, regardless of what emerges as a statistical index. If we want to obtain a quantitative summary for this relationship, however, we currently do not have a way to do so. If we let variable X represent BUN and variable Y represent

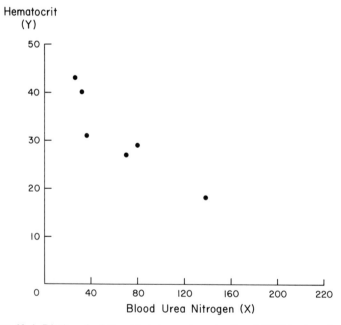

Figure 10–1. Display of relationship between hematocrit and BUN in six patients.

hematocrit, we can obtain a univariate summary for each variable. For blood urea nitrogen, we calculate $\Sigma X = 379$ and $S_{xx} = 9252.83$. The mean will be $\bar{X} = 63.17$, and the standard deviation (marked with an "x" subscript to show it pertains to variable X) will be $s_x = 43.02$. For hematocrit, we can calculate its univariate summary from $\Sigma Y = 188$, S_{yy} 413.33, $\bar{Y} = 31.33$, and $s_y = 9.09$. The univariate summaries, however, do not tell us how Y relates to X or vice versa.

Using what we have learned from univariate tactics, we could try to examine the changes in hematocrit that occur for each successive change in BUN. Thus, if we organize the data according to the rises in BUN, the sequence of BUN values is 23, 32, 36, 70, 80, and 138. The hematocrit values that correspond to each member of the BUN sequence are 43, 40, 31, 27, 29, and 18. For the first change, as BUN rises from 23 to 32, hematocrit falls from 43 to 40. Noting the subsequent changes, we can then arrange the following table of associated incremental responses:

	Change in Successive Values of BUN	Change in Corresponding Values of Hematocrit
	+ 9	− 3
	+ 4	− 9
	+ 34	− 4
	+ 10	+ 2
	+ 58	− 9
Mean of changes	+ 23	− 4.6

This table shows that if we take the ratio of the means of hematocrit and BUN changes, hematocrit tends to fall an average of $-4.6/23 = -0.2$ units for each unitary rise in BUN. This crude appraisal gives us the general idea that hematocrit goes down about 0.2 of a unit as BUN goes up, but the measurement is very coarse and has many imperfections. Fortunately, a much more elegant technique is available.

10.2.1. *The Regression Coefficient*

Still letting hematocrit be variable Y and BUN be variable X, we can draw a straight line, expressed as $Y = a + bX$, that best fits the points shown in Figure 10–1. The value of *a* will be the *intercept*, showing the point at which the line crosses the Y-axis when $X = 0$; and the value of *b* will be the slope, which shows the ratio of change in the Y values for unitary changes in the X values. This slope will correspond to the entity we were trying to measure in the preceding section.

For the actual data, this line is expressed as

$$\hat{Y}_i = a + bX_i.$$

The X_i values will be the individual values of 80, 32, 138, and so on that were observed for BUN. The $\hat{Y}_i$ values will be the corresponding values that are estimated by the model, i.e., the straight line equation, for Y_i at each point of X_i. (The "^" is placed over the $\hat{Y}_i$ to indicate that the value is estimated, rather than observed.) The difference, $Y_i - \hat{Y}_i$, between the observed and estimated values of hematocrit at each point of X_i will help indicate how well the line fits the data.

The values of *a* and *b* are calculated from the data using a strategy that produces the best-fitting line. The strategy is often called the *least squares method* because it depends on minimizing the sum of the squared deviations, $\Sigma(Y_i - \hat{Y}_i)^2$. With this strategy, whose mathematical proof is omitted here, the best fit occurs when

$$b = \frac{S_{xy}}{S_{xx}}$$

and when

$$a = \bar{Y} - b\bar{X}.$$

A new entity, S_{xy}, appears in the formula for b. It is called the *codeviance*, and it represents $\Sigma(X_i - \bar{X})(Y_i - \bar{Y})$, which is the sum of the codeviations calculated for each point of the data. A simple way of calculating S_{xy} is with the formula

$$S_{xy} = \Sigma(X_iY_i) - [(\Sigma X_i)(\Sigma Y_i)/N].$$

The construction of this formula for codeviance should not be strange, because it resembles

$$S_{xx} = \Sigma X_i^2 - [(\Sigma X_i)^2/N],$$

which we encountered earlier for calculating deviance in Section 7.4.2.3. When divided by N or by N−1, the codeviance yields an often mentioned entity called the *covariance*, which we shall not need for the calculations here. To calculate codeviance for the data in the cited table of BUN versus hematocrit, we have X_1Y_1 = 80×29 = 2320, X_2Y_2 = 32×40 = 1280, ... and X_6Y_6 = 23×43 = 989. The value of ΣX_iY_i will be $2320 + 1280 + 2484 + 1116 + 1890 + 989$ = 10,079. We can now insert our previously calculated values of ΣX and ΣY to find that the value of $(\Sigma X)(\Sigma Y)/N$ is $(379)(188)/6$ = 11,875.33. Therefore S_{xy} = $10,079 - 11,875.33$ = -1796.33. Placing our previously calculated value of S_{xx} into the formula b = S_{xy}/S_{xx}, we find that b = $-1796.33/9252.89$ = -0.194.

We now have a precise calculation of the desired index that expresses the statistical association. The index is b, the slope of the best-fitting line for the array of data. This line is regularly called the *regression of Y on X*, and the slope is therefore called the *regression coefficient*. (We can also take comfort in realizing that the precise calculation is quite similar to what we found in our previous crude estimation, i.e., that hematocrit goes down about 0.2 of a unit for each unitary rise in BUN.)

10.2.2. *Completing the Equation and Drawing the Line*

Having found the value of b, we can now obtain the value of a by substituting our previously calculated values of $\bar{X}$ and $\bar{Y}$ into the formula a = $\bar{Y} - b\bar{X}$. It produces a = $31.33 - (-0.194)(63.17)$ = $31.33 + 12.26$ = 43.59. We can now express the estimated line as: $\hat{Y}_i$ = $43.73 - 0.194X_i$.

Furthermore, because of two properties of the calculations, we can now immediately draw the line on the graph. We already know from the definition of a that the line goes through the point $(0,a)$. With some algebra not shown here, it can also be demonstrated that the line always passes through the point $(\bar{X}, \bar{Y})$. Thus if we mark the two points $(0, 43.73)$ and $(63.17, 31.33)$ on the graph, we can draw the line that connects them, as shown in Figure 10–2. As a further illustration of how things work, let us determine $\hat{Y}_i$ at the point where X_i = 36. The observed value of Y_i at this point was 31. The calculated $\hat{Y}_i$

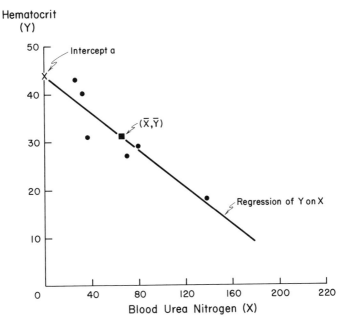

Figure 10–2. Best-fitting line if hematocrit depends on BUN.

is $43.73 - (0.194)(36) = 43.73 - 6.98 = 36.75$, which is the value shown on the line at that point in Figure 10–2.

10.2.3. *The Problems of Units and Two Regression Lines*

Our satisfaction with the preceding accomplishment is hampered by two problems with which we have not yet dealt. First, the value of the regression coefficient depends entirely on the units of measurement. It so happens that BUN here was expressed in units of mg./dl., but suppose it were expressed in millimoles rather than milligrams? If so, we would get a quite different value for the regression coefficient, even though the relationship between hematocrit and BUN would remain identical.

The second problem is that we were able to decide quite easily for these calculations to let Y = hematocrit and X = BUN because of our biologic realization that hematocrit should depend on BUN. However, we might conceivably have wanted to see what happens if we looked at things the other way around, determining the regression of BUN on hematocrit. If so, there would be a second regression line to consider. It would be expressed in the form

$$X_i = a' + b'Y_i.$$

Its slope would be

$$b' = \frac{S_{xy}}{S_{yy}},$$

and its intercept would be

$$a' = \bar{X} - b'\bar{Y}.$$

Substituting appropriately into these formulas, we would find $b' = -1796.33/413.33 = -4.35$; $a' = 63.17 - (-4.35)(31.33) = 63.17 + 136.16 = 199.33$; and so the "other" regression line would be

$$\hat{X}_i = 199.33 - 4.35Y_i.$$

When drawn on the same graph (in Figure 10–3) as the previous line, we see that this second line has a different location from the first one. The most shocking feature about the difference in the two lines, however, is that we now have a strikingly different alternative value, -4.35, for the regression coefficient. [It so happens in this instance that the reciprocal of -0.194 is $1/(-0.194) = -5.15$, which is reasonably close to -4.35. This reasonably close reciprocity will not necessarily occur, however, in other data sets.]

The availability of two lines and two regression coefficients is disconcerting. Which do we choose when a dependency relationship is not as clearly evident as for hematocrit and BUN? What do we do when we simply want to see how two variables are related interdependently, without one necessarily being biologically affected by the other? For example, in an appropriate group of patients, suppose we wanted to see how bilirubin and

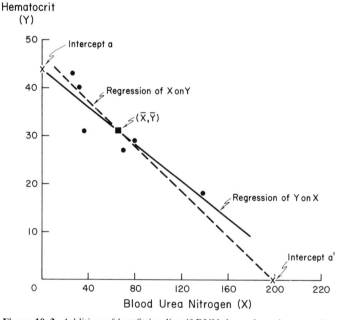

Figure 10–3. Addition of bestfitting line if BUN depends on hematocrit.

cholesterol values are related to one another, without making the assumption that bilirubin depends on cholesterol or vice versa? We would not know whether to regress bilirubin on cholesterol, or cholesterol on bilirubin.

Fortunately, a simple solution exists for both of these problems in units of measurement and in choice of regressions. As discussed in the next two sections, we can transform the data into dimension-free *Z-scores*, and we can then calculate a neutral entity called the *correlation coefficient*.

10.2.4. *The Use of Standardized Z-Scores*

A *standardized Z-score*, which we learned to use in Section 7.5.2.1, is calculated for each item in a univariate set of data when the deviation of that item from the mean is divided by the standard deviation. The formula is

$$Z_i = \frac{X_i - \bar{X}}{s_x}.$$

It transforms the original data into a new set of Z_i values that are dimension-free, because they are expressed in standard deviation units of the variable. For example, the Z-score for the first BUN value in the data of Section 10.2 is $Z_1 = (80 - 63.17)/43.02 = 0.39$. The Z-score for the fourth value is $Z_4 = (36 - 63.17)/43.02 = -0.63$. The corresponding Z-scores for the first and fourth hematocrit values are $(29 - 31.33)/9.09 = -0.26$ and $(31 - 31.33)/0.09 = 0.04$.

These standard deviation units make the data become commensurate and directly comparable regardless of the original units of measurement. For our current goal, the great value of Z-scores is that they provide an escape from the dilemma about which regression line to use. We do not have to calculate the Z-scores because they play a conceptual rather than empiric role in the new model, but they allow an intermediate line to be constructed for the equation.

10.2.5. *The Correlation Coefficient*

Suppose we expressed the Z-scores as $(X_i - \bar{X})/s_x$ for our BUN data and as $(Y_i - \bar{Y})/s_y$ for our hematocrit data. If we now went through all the algebra needed to calculate the regression of the standardized Z-scores for Y on the standardized Z-scores for X, we would form the following equation:

$$\left(\frac{Y_i - \bar{Y}}{s_y}\right) = r\left(\frac{X_i - \bar{X}}{s_x}\right).$$

The equation has a slope of r but would have no intercept, because the line passes through the origin of the graph. (Both of the Z variables have a mean of 0). If we decided, instead, to calculate the regression of the standardized Z-scores for X on the standardized Z-scores for Y, we would eventually form another equation:

$$\left(\frac{X_i - \bar{X}}{s_x}\right) = r\left(\frac{Y_i - \bar{Y}}{s_y}\right).$$

The great marvel of the standardized-score procedure is that the value of r would be the same in both of these equations.

Furthermore, if we worked out all the algebra that verifies the last assertion, we would find that r is a perfect blend of the two previous regression coefficients, b and b'. It is the square root of their product. Thus, $r = \sqrt{bb'}$. In a more usable and conventional form of expression, the value is

$$r = \frac{S_{xy}}{\sqrt{S_{xx}S_{yy}}}.$$

The most common name for r is the *correlation coefficient*. It is sometimes also called the *product-moment coefficient* (for reasons that are no longer pertinent) or *Pearson's correlation coefficient*, the eponym commemorating Karl Pearson, who first popularized the procedure.

For the data we have been considering we can substitute the appropriate values of S_{xy}, S_{xx}, and S_{yy} to calculate r as $-1796.33/\sqrt{9252.89 \times 413.33} = -1796.33/1955.63 = -0.92$. Because we already know the values of b and b', we can calculate r alternatively as $\sqrt{(-0.194)(-4.35)} = \sqrt{0.844} = -0.92$. [The latter calculation demonstrates the advantage of using the S_{xy} formula, which immediately tells us the sign of the result. With the $\sqrt{bb'}$ formula, we do not know whether to take the negative or positive value of the square root.]

We now have an excellent index for expressing the association of BUN and hematocrit. The index is r, the *correlation coefficient*, and its value is -0.92. It tells us that as one variable rises, the other falls, and furthermore (as we shall see in the next section), that this inverse correlation is quite strong.

10.2.6. *Interpretation of the Correlation Coefficient*

In any calculation of correlation for two variables, the value of r can range from -1 to $+1$. The peak values of $+1$ or -1 indicate a perfect correlation, and a value of 0 indicates no correlation at all, i.e., that the two variables are wholly unrelated. If r is positive, the two variables tend to go in the same direction. As one rises, the other rises; as one falls, the other falls. If r is negative, the two variables tend to go in opposite directions, with one falling as the other rises. The absolute (positive or negative) magnitude of r determines the *strength* of the correlation. To decide how strong a correlation may be is somewhat like answering the question, "How high is up?" An absolute r value of 0.92 obviously indicates a very strong correlation, and a value of 0.07 obviously indicates a very weak correlation (or essentially none). The interpretation of intermediate values depends on the interpreter. In general, considering the variability of medical data, r values of 0.5 or higher are regarded as quite good, but sometimes, particularly in certain types of epidemiologic or psychosocial data, the investigator may ecstatically report a "strong" correlation when the r value is only 0.13 or even lower.

One way for a reader to avoid being misled by an investigator's enthusiasm is to contemplate r^2, which is sometimes called the *coefficient of determination*. Because r lies between -1 and $+1$, the value of r^2 is always smaller than r, except when $r = 0, -1$, or $+1$. Thus, if $r = 0.5$, $r^2 = 0.25$; and if $r = 0.03$, $r^2 = 0.0009$. The importance of r^2 is that it indicates the proportion of the original variance or deviance in the system that has been reduced by applying the linear model. Thus, if we had only the results for Y_i, the hematocrit values, we would summarize them by fitting them with their mean, $\bar{Y}$. The residual deviance in the system would be S_{yy}, which in this instance is 413.33. By having available the associated values of X, however, and by estimating $\hat{Y}_i$ from the values fitted by the line, the residual deviance in the new system is $S_r = \Sigma(Y_i - \hat{Y}_i)^2$, which we have not yet calculated but which represents the sum of the squared deviations of the Y_i values around the values estimated by the regression line. Because S_r is almost always smaller than S_{yy}, the value of $(S_{yy} - S_r)/S_{yy}$ will represent the proportion of the original deviance that was reduced by applying the linear model. We do not have to calculate S_r to find this result because it turns out that

$$r^2 = \frac{S_{yy} - S_r}{S_{yy}}.$$

Because $r = -0.92$ for our data, $r^2 = 0.85$, and the linear model has reduced 85% of the original variance. A high value of r^2 thus also indicates that the straight line provides an excellent fit to the data.

The foregoing sentence should give the reader yet another warning. A low value of r or r^2 means only that the data are not well fitted by a straight line. It does not necessarily mean that the two variables are unrelated. For example, two variables may be closely associated in a U-shaped relationship that can be fitted perfectly with a parabolic curve such as $Y = X^2$, but the r value for this curve will emerge as zero because the variables cannot be well fitted with a straight line.

Finally, many investigators engage in the pernicious practice of reporting correlations not in the descriptive r values but in the associated P values of inferential statistics. The P value of the r (or b) coefficient is determined by calculating

$$t = \frac{r\sqrt{N-2}}{\sqrt{1-r^2}}$$

and by interpreting this value of t at $N-2$ degrees of freedom. Because $N-2$ appears in the numerator, the t values will enlarge with large group sizes. If the group size is big enough, t can easily exceed what is needed for a stochastically significant value of P. This achievement often leads to the claim of statistical significance being made for small correlations that achieve their significance only by virtue of being derived from large samples. Because statistical significance at $P<0.05$ can be obtained with a sample size only as large as 100 for an r value as low as 0.2 and with N of 2500 for an r of 0.04, a wary reader should always examine the actual value of r and should preferably inspect the scattergraph of the data, to determine whether a correlation is *really* significant for quantitative rather than probabilistic interpretations.

10.3. INDEXES OF TREND IN UNRANKED DATA

Suppose we have the following set of data for race and hospital utilization:

Race	Hospital A	Number of Patients Using Hospital B	Hospital C	Hospital D	Total
Black	78	85	10	26	199
White	658	340	262	287	1547
Other	20	6	17	7	50
Total	756	431	289	320	1796

We could try to make sense of this information in several ways. First, we could examine the proportions of black, white, or other people in the spectrum of each hospital. This examination would produce the following table:

Race	Hospital A	Proportion of Patients Using Hospital B	Hospital C	Hospital D	Total
Black	10%	20%	3%	8%	11%
White	87%	79%	91%	90%	86%
Other	3%	1%	6%	2%	3%
Total	100%	100%	100%	100%	100%

The results tell us that the percentage of black users was highest in hospital B and lowest in hospital C, that "other" users were highest in C and lowest in B, and a few other distinctions that may make us suspect that race has something to do with the patient's choice of hospitals. These percentages, however, will not provide a single overall index to distinguish a relationship, if any, between race and hospital site. Consequently, we need to develop some sort of model for expressing the relationship.

10.3.1. *The "Observed-Expected" Model*

The model we can use is similar to what was done for calculating X^2 in Section 9.4.2.4. Let us assume that race and hospital site are wholly unrelated. If so, the proportion of black, white, and other people can be expected to be the same at each institution. Our best approach for deciding what these proportions might be is to use the values found in the totals. Thus, the expected proportion of blacks at each institution would be 199/1796 = 11%; the expected proportion of whites would be 1547/1796 = 86%; and so forth. If we multiply the total number of people at each institution by these expected proportions, we get the expected numbers for each group. Thus, the expected numbers of blacks at hospital A would be $(199/1796) \times 756 = 83.77$. (For the accuracy of the ensuing calculations, we must maintain the decimal points and fractions of people in the expected values.) The expected number of *others* at hospital D is $(50/1796) \times 320 = 8.91$.

With this procedure we can determine the values entered in the following table:

Race	Hospital A	Expected Numbers of Patients Using Hospital B	Hospital C	Hospital D	Total
Black	83.77	47.75	32.02	35.46	199
White	651.19	371.25	248.93	275.63	1547
Other	21.05	12.00	8.05	8.91	50
Total	756	431	289	320	1796

Note that in this new table, the sums of the expected values (sometimes with minor differences due to rounding) have the same marginal totals as before for both rows and columns. Furthermore, note that the expected value in any cell of the table is obtained by multiplying the corresponding marginal totals and dividing by the grand total. Thus, the cell in the 2nd row, 3rd column of this table is 248.93. It was obtained by multiplying two numbers: the (horizontal) marginal total, 1547, for the 2nd row and the (vertical) marginal total, 289, for the 3rd column; the product was then divided by the total group size of 1796. Because of this principle, we would get exactly the same expected values if we made the assumption that the proportion of hospitals should be the same among the races instead of our previous assumption that the proportion of races should be the same among the hospitals.

10.3.2. *The Calculation of X^2*

From the observed and expected values, we now calculate X^2 as the sum of the (observed-expected)²/expected ratios in each of the cells in the table. Thus,

$$X^2 = \sum \frac{(o_i - e_i)^2}{e_i}$$

where o_i = observed value in the i-th cell, e_i = expected value in the i-th cell, and i ranges in this case from 1 to 12. If we went across each row and then downward for these calculations, we would get

$$X^2 = \frac{(78 - 83.77)^2}{83.77} + \frac{(85 - 47.75)^2}{47.75} + \ldots + \frac{(17 - 8.05)^2}{8.05} + \frac{(7 - 8.91)^2}{8.91}.$$

When this calculation is carried out, the result is $X^2 = 64.83$.

For a complicated calculation of this type, it is useful to have a simpler method of computing or check the result. An easier formula for this purpose is

$$X^2 = \sum \left(\frac{o_i^2}{e_i} \right) - N$$

This is calculated as

$$\frac{(78)^2}{83.77} + \frac{(85)^2}{47.75} + \ldots + \frac{(17)^2}{8.05} + \frac{(7)^2}{8.91} - 1796,$$

and this easier computation yields $1860.38 - 1796$, which is 64.38—the same result as before, except for variations due to rounding.

10.3.3. *Calculation and Interpretation of ϕ^2*

The X^2 entity can be used for statistical inference and interpreted with the mathematical distribution of *chi-square* for the appropriate degrees of freedom in the table. For descriptive purposes, however, we use X^2 to calculate

$$\phi^2 = \frac{X^2}{N}.$$

The value of ϕ^2 is the unranked-data analog of r^2, the coefficient of determination for dimensional data. The square root

$$\phi = \sqrt{\frac{X^2}{N}}$$

is analogous to the correlation coefficient, r, and is interpreted in the same way as r.

Thus, for the data we have been examining,

$$\phi^2 = 64.38/1796 = 0.03585$$

and

$$\phi = 0.189.$$

The result suggests that a distinct but low-level correlation exists between race and hospital site.

10.3.4. *Example of ϕ^2 for Dimensional Data*

An example of the way ϕ^2 can be used as a crude check on the results of r^2 is to convert dimensional data into nondimensional data. Thus, for the BUN and hematocrit data presented in Section 10.2, let us label each BUN reading *high* or *low* according to whether it is greater or less than the mean BUN of 63.17. Similarly, each hematocrit value will be labeled *high* or *low* in relation to the mean of 31.33. For the six people whose original data were shown at the onset of Section 10.2, the new set of data will be

Person	Hematocrit	Blood Urea Nitrogen
A	Low	High
B	High	Low
C	Low	High
D	Low	Low
E	Low	High
F	High	Low

These results can be used to form the following table:

BUN Value	Hematocrit Value Low	High	Total
Low	1	2	3
High	3	0	3
Total	4	2	6

Using the uncorrected calculational formula for this table,

$$X^2 = \frac{[(0 \times 1) - (3 \times 2)]^2 \times 6}{4 \times 2 \times 3 \times 3} = 3.00.$$

Accordingly, $\phi^2 = 3.00/6 = 0.5$ and so $\phi = \sqrt{0.5} = 0.71$, which is lower than the $r = 0.92$ found for the dimensional calculation, but is still a quite high correlation coefficient, particularly in view of the information lost when we transformed the data.

10.4. OTHER INDEXES OF TREND

The r index is pertinent when both variables are dimensional; and the ϕ index, when both variables are nominal or dichotomous. For other bivariate combinations, a large variety of other correlation coefficients have been created, adding eponymic wealth to statistical riches. For example, when both variables represent ordinal grades, an appropriate correlation coefficient is called *Kendall's tau*; when both variables represent unlimited ordinal ranks, the coefficient is *Spearman's rho*; and when one variable is dimensional and the other is nominal, the coefficient is called *Jaspen's multiserial M*. Other indexes of correlation are called *eta* (for dimensional versus nominal data) and the *biserial coefficient* (for dimensional versus dichotomous data).

When needed, the methods of preparing and calculating all of these indexes can be found in an appropriate statistical book, such as the texts by Bradley,[1] Fleiss,[2] Freeman,[3] and Siegel.[4] Simple illustrations of Kendall's tau and Spearman's rho are provided in a paper by Kramer and Feinstein.[5]

10.5. INDEXES OF CONCORDANCE

All of the cited indexes of association are satisfactory for the job they are asked to do in describing a trend between two different variables, but the indexes do not tell us about *agreement.* The trend will be perfect, with a correlation coefficient of 1, if the measurements made in one laboratory are exactly twofold higher or exactly 10 units higher than the corresponding measurement made in another laboratory. The close relationship would let us accurately predict one laboratory's results from the values found in the other laboratory, but the actual agreement in the two laboratories would be nonexistent.

If we want to describe concordance rather than trend alone, we need some additional indexes. To illustrate this situation, suppose we have done a study of observer variability, asking two ophthalmologists to check the members of the incoming freshman class at our university and to rate each retina as *normal* or *abnormal*. When the results are in, we find the following table:

Number of Students Rated by Ophthalmologist B as:	Number of Students Rated by Ophthalmologist A as:		
	Normal	*Abnormal*	**Total**
Normal	650	12	662
Abnormal	17	8	25
Total	667	20	687

We could summarize these results in the several ways noted in Sections 10.5.1 to 10.5.3.

10.5.1. *Indexes of Percentage Agreement and Bias*

Because the ophthalmologists agree on the rating for 650 normal and 8 abnormal students, we can use a simple index to express the *percentage of agreement*. In this instance, because the two raters agree on 650+8 = 658 occasions, the index is 658/687 = 96%, which suggests excellent agreement.

We could also note that ophthalmologist B has a somewhat greater tendency than A to call the retina abnormal. She reported it as abnormal in 25/687 = 4% of cases, whereas A said that 20/687 = 3% were abnormal. We might now want to know if these abnormal readings show a trend—that is, do B and A show a bias when they disagree? To answer this question, we can note that the two observers disagree in 17+12 = 29 cases. If the disagreements occur in an equitable manner, we would expect half of them to be in one direction (where A says *abnormal* and B says *normal*) and half in the other direction (where A says *normal* and B says *abnormal*). Consequently, if we found the numerical difference in the two types of disagreements and divided it by the total number of disagreements, we should get a result close to zero.

We can then obtain an index by expressing the difference in disagreements as a proportion of the total number of disagreements. This ratio is sometimes called *McNemar's Index of Bias*. In this case, it is $(17-12)/29 = 5/29 = .17$. Because the maximum value of the index is 1 (or -1)—a value that would occur if all 29 disagreements are found in an upper right or lower left corner of the four cells in the table—the observed value of .17 is elevated above 0 but not strikingly high.

10.5.2. *The Role of* ϕ

Although we used our new friend, ϕ, as an index of trend in Section 10.3.3, we can try applying ϕ to express concordance. Using the appropriate formula, we can calculate $X^2 = [(650\times8)-(12\times17)]^2 \times 687/[667\times20\times662\times25] = 77.67$, and so $\phi^2 = 77.67/687 = 0.11$, and $\phi = 0.34$. This result is somewhat dismaying because it suggests that the observed association is much weaker than the implications of the extremely high index for percentage of agreement.

If we start to think about why ϕ created this effect, we can recall that ϕ depends on the values that are expected in the data if there is no association between the two variables. In a study of observer variability, should we suspect that any agreement can occur by chance? The answer to this question is a resounding *yes*. In the study under discussion, the proportion of students rated as *normal* was 0.971 [= 667/687] by observer A and 0.964 [= 662/687] by observer B. If the two observers simply distributed these ratings at random, we would expect agreement on normal values to occur by chance alone in $0.971 \times 0.964 = 0.935$ of the readings. For ratings of abnormal, the corresponding total proportions were 0.029 by A and 0.036 by B, and so the chance agreement on abnormal readings would be $0.029 \times 0.036 = 0.001$. Thus, the total proportion of agreement that could be expected to occur in this study by chance alone is $0.936 + 0.001 = 0.937$, or about 94%. The observed percentage of agreement, which was 96%, is now no longer impressive.

It so happens that the study just described had a poor architectural design because of an inadequately challenging scope in the spectrum of input. A group of generally healthy young college students will have predominantly normal retinas and will not constitute a suitable test of variability in the ophthalmologists. Given that the poorly designed study has been conducted, however, what can be done to salvage the data and provide a suitable index for the results? A report of *96% agreement* would certainly be misleading and so ϕ would be a better index because it at least contains some provision for chance agreement.

The problem with ϕ, however, is that it makes provision for chance agreement but not for the magnitude and direction of disparities. For example, we would obtain exactly the same magnitude of ϕ as before from the following table of results:

Ratings by Ophthalmologist B	Ratings by Ophthalmologist A		Total
	Normal	Abnormal	
Normal	17	8	25
Abnormal	650	12	662
Total	667	20	687

This table would also yield a ϕ value of 0.34. The value would be negative rather than positive, and the negative value might tell us that something funny has happened, but it would not indicate that the percentage of agreement has dropped to $(17 + 12)/687 = 4\%$. [It would also not indicate that the McNemar Bias Index is now extremely high at 642/658 = 0.98.]

To avoid this problem in interpreting ϕ as an index of agreement, we can use the kappa index, described in the next section.

10.5.3. *The Kappa Index*

In Section 10.5.2, we found that the proportion of agreement expected by chance for the original table under discussion was 0.937. Because perfect agreement would have been a proportion of 1, the only real challenge offered to the observers was the difference between perfect agreement and what might occur by chance. Thus, the challenge was the increment of $1 - 0.937 = 0.063$. What the observers actually produced was an agreement proportion of 0.958 [= 658/687]. This performance differed from the chance expected agreement by an increment of $0.958 - 0.937 = 0.021$. The ratio of the actual increment and challenge increment forms *kappa*, the index of concordance. In this instance, kappa is $0.021/0.063 = 0.33$.

If we use the symbols p_o and p_c respectively to denote the proportions of agreement that were observed and those that could be expected by chance, then the formula for kappa is

$$k = \frac{p_o - p_c}{1 - p_c}.$$

If we express the conventional observer variability table (also called an *agreement matrix*) as

OBSERVER B	OBSERVER A		TOTALS
	Yes	No	
Yes	a	b	f_1
No	c	d	f_2
TOTALS	n_1	n_2	N

then kappa is calculated as

$$k = \frac{N(a+d) - (n_1f_1 + n_2f_2)}{N^2 - (n_1f_1 + n_2f_2)}.$$

In this instance

$$k = \frac{687(650+8) - [(667 \times 662) + (20 \times 25)]}{687^2 - [(667 \times 662) + (20 \times 25)]} = \frac{9992}{29915} = 0.33.$$

Another, perhaps simpler, calculational formula for kappa in these data is

$$k = \frac{2(ad - bc)}{n_1f_2 + n_2f_1}$$

which yields exactly the same results, calculated as $2[(650 \times 8) - (12 \times 17)]/[(667 \times 25) + (20 \times 662)]$.

The value of kappa, which is here slightly lower than that of ϕ, indicates that the excellent percentage in observed agreement of the ophthalmologists is substantially reduced when a correction is made for the agreement expected by chance. This correction for chance agreement is the main virtue of the kappa statistic and has made it the best currently available index for denoting concordance in dichotomous data. Despite its preferred status, however, kappa has an important disadvantage that will be discussed in Chapter 26.

Like the r coefficient of correlation, kappa varies from values of -1 to $+1$, but the interpretation is different. A value of 0 denotes agreement that is no better than chance, and negative values denote agreement that is worse than chance. For example, for the poor agreement noted in the table that just preceded Section 10.5.3, kappa would be $\{687(17+12) - [(25 \times 667) + (662 \times 20)]\}/687^2 - [(25 \times 667) + (662 \times 20)] = -9992/442,054 = -0.02$. To interpret the strength of the agreement when kappa is positive, Landis and Koch[6] have suggested the following guidelines:

Value of k	Strength of Agreement
<0	Poor
0– .20	Slight
.21– .40	Fair
.41– .60	Moderate
.61– .80	Substantial
.81–1.00	Almost perfect

10.5.4. *Other Indexes of Concordance*

In the method just described, kappa is an index of agreement for two observers reporting on binary data. For more than two observers, things get more complicated. We can compare each pair of observers separately and take an average of all the paired kappas; or we can use a more generalized form of kappa.[2] If the two observers used distinctly ordinal ratings (such as **normal, slightly abnormal,** and **substantially abnormal**), the index of concordance would be expressed in an adaptation[2] called *weighted kappa*. A simple example of its calculation was shown by Kramer and Feinstein.[7]

For evaluating diagnostic marker tests, as noted in Chapter 25, the index of concordance is expected to express accuracy rather than consistency alone. In this circumstance, kappa is seldom used and is generally replaced by other indexes, called *sensitivity* and *specificity*.

For studies of quality control in chemical measurements, the correlation coefficient, r, is often used as an index of agreement in the dimensional data obtained at two laboratories. Because r expresses trend rather than agreement, extremely high values of r can be obtained if the two laboratories have similar trends but different results. Thus, a perfect value of r can be obtained if laboratory A achieves results that are always twice as high or always 10 points higher than the results from laboratory B. To avoid the misleading index that may be produced when r is used for agreement rather than trend, the concordance of dimensional data should be expressed with R_I, the *intraclass correlation coefficient*.[2]

10.6. MULTIVARIATE TRENDS

In Section 10.2.1, we used $\hat{Y}_i = a + bX_i$ as the equation of a straight line showing the dependence of hematocrit on BUN. Suppose we had wanted an equation to show that hematocrit depended on BUN and also on serum ferritin level. If we let W represent ferritin level and c be its weighting coefficient, we could write

$$\hat{Y}_i = a + bX_i + cW_i.$$

This is the equation of a plane, which is a straight line in three-dimensional space. The coefficients a, b, and c could also be calculated using the method of least squares, and the residual deviance around the plane would be $S_r = \Sigma(Y_i - \hat{Y}_i)^2$. Each value of $\hat{Y}_i - Y_i$ would be calculated as the difference between the observed value, Y_i, and the expected value of $\hat{Y}_i$ on the plane at the observed point X_i, W_i. This value of S_r could be used to determine R^2, which is often called the *multiple correlation coefficient*. Like the squared simple correlation coefficient r^2, to which it is analogous, R^2 varies between 0 and 1 and indicates how well the mathematical model fits the data.

Each of the regression coefficients also has a distinctive role. In this instance, the coefficient b would indicate the amount by which Y changes for a single unitary change in X, with W held constant; and the coefficient c would indicate the corresponding change produced in Y by a unitary change in W, with X held constant. Because of these attributes, the coefficients in a multiple regression are called *partial regression coefficients*.

This technique can be extended to produce an equation in which Y depends on many more than two variables. The result is called a *regression surface,* because we do not have a better word to express a plane that occupies more than three dimensions. Because we would soon run out of alphabetical letters for expressing multiple variables, the symbols are changed so that the regression surface is cited as

$$Y = b_0 + b_1 X_1 + b_2 X_2 + b_3 X_3 + \cdots.$$

In these symbols, each of the X_i values represents a *variable,* rather than a single item of data. Thus, in the foregoing equation, if Y = hematocrit, X_1 might represent BUN; X_2 might represent serum ferritin level; X_3 might represent the patient's age; and so on. Each of the corresponding b_i values represents the analog of a regression coefficient for that variable, and b_0 is the intercept on the Y axis when all other variables are 0. To allow the importance of different variables to be compared without regard to the original units in which they are expressed, the b_i coefficients are regularly converted to *standardized regression coefficients*, which represent the values they would have if each of the corresponding variables were expressed in a standardized Z-score.

This technique, which is called *multiple linear regression,* is regularly used to analyze the predictive impact of different variables in prognosis of a particular ailment or as risk factors for a particular disease. The mathematical conceptualization of the model contains provisions for the misleading predictive results that might occur if certain correlated variables were considered only one at a time, as in simple regression. For example, in a simple regression for a particular ailment, suppose we noted that prognosis was poor for old people and good for young people. If most of the old people in the group were men and if most of the young people were women, a different simple regression analysis would suggest that gender was also an important prognostic feature. By performing the multiple regression analysis in which prognosis is examined simultaneously for both age and gender, we would discover that age is the key factor.

Like many other mathematical models, multiple linear regression is often more appealing in its concept than in its pragmatic accomplishments. The problems created in actual usage often lead to multiple linear regression being replaced by other mathematical models, such as *multiple logistic regression* or *discriminant function analysis.* Some clinical investigators, unhappy about the additive assumptions that are made in all of these models, prefer other analytic techniques called *multivariate stratification.*

10.7. SYNOPSIS

Statistical indexes of association are used to show the relationship between two (or more) variables. If the variables are different, the relationship is a trend. If the variables represent different observations of the same entity, the index is used to express concordance. The indexes are derived by fitting a model to the data and by noting the disparities between the observed values of data and the values expected or predicted by the model.

For two variables having dimensional data, the trend is shown with the correlation coefficient, r, that is calculated for the straight line of simple regression that best fits the data. The equation of the straight line is determined from calculations made with the variance (or deviance) of each variable and with their covariance (or codeviance). The correlation coefficient also represents the regression coefficient that would be obtained if the straight line were determined from the standardized Z-scores achieved when each variable is expressed in units of its own standard deviation. The value of r^2, which varies from 0 to 1, demonstrates how well the data are fitted by the straight line model. A low value of r^2 can indicate either no correlation or a poor model.

For unranked data, the trend in the two variables represents the closeness of their association. The trend can be construed as the accuracy with which one of the variables could be used to estimate the other. This trend is expressed with ϕ, the index of nominal or dichotomous association. It is interpreted in the same way as r, but it is calculated with a model in which the observed-expected deviations are formed on the assumption that the two variables are wholly unrelated. The descriptive value of ϕ is related to the X^2 often used for calculating stochastic significance. $\phi^2 = X^2/N$, where N = size of the group.

To express concordance in dichotomous data, the preferred index is kappa, which contains a correction for the agreement that can be expected to occur by chance among the observers. Other indexes, including *weighted kappa* and the *intraclass correlation coefficient,* are used when concordance is expressed for other types of data.

A *multiple linear regression* model of a mathematical surface is often used to express the relationship between a single outcome variable, such as prognosis or development of a disease, and multiple previous baseline variables, which can act as *prognostic factors* or *risk factors*. The *multiple correlation coefficient,* R^2, indicates how well the model fits the data, and the relative importance of each individual variable is indicated by its *standardized regression coefficient.* Because of various mathematical or scientific problems and appeals, many different models have been used to express multivariate relationships.

EXERCISES

The goal of these exercises is to get you to think about associations and to do a few simple calculations without having the calculations become too oppressive.

Exercise 10.1. After studying 11 patients with chronic bronchitis, a group of investigators[8] made two claims. They said that peak expiratory flow rate had a highly significant negative correlation with concomitant concentrations of histamine but not with concentrations of eosinophils in sputum. The conclusions were based on results found in multiple measurements during a 6-week period in each patient. The authors published a list of the lowest, highest, and mean values found in each patient's multiple measurements. The table below is excerpted from that list and shows each patient's mean value for the three variables. (The three parts of this assignment involve use of this table for checking the investigators' claims.)

	Y	X	W
		Mean Values per Patient	
Patient No.	***Peak Expiratory Flow Rate (% Predicted)***	***Sputum Histamine ($\mu g/g$)***	***Sputum Eosinophils (%)***
1	43.0	0.49	46.7
2	77.6	1.48	0.7
3	33.8	0.38	1.4
4	20.3	0.50	11.1
5	41.7	2.00	1.8
6	27.0	0.33	0.5
7	28.8	0.51	0.8
8	49.0	0.91	3.8
9	44.9	0.52	11.4
10	25.1	0.60	25.2
11	15.9	0.18	23.1

10.1.1. Without using a calculator and without doing any calculations (other than counting), how might you arrange this information to check the investigators' contention?

10.1.2. With a calculator available, what could you do to check the two claims?

10.1.3. Are you worried about any limitations for either of the two claims? If so, what is your concern and how might you check it?

Exercise 10.2. In a study of gender and handedness in 7688 school children, the investigators[9] found the following results:

Gender	Handedness *Right*	*Left*	**Total**
Male	3543	417	3960
Female	3404	324	3728
Total	6947	741	7688

How would you express this relationship statistically? What conclusion would you draw about its quantitative and stochastic significance?

Exercise 10.3. The registrar of your medical school has come to you with a problem. For various prizes at commencement or for internship recommendations, the registrar must prepare a class standing, ranking the members of the class for their total performance in five clinical clerkships. The problem is that each clinical group uses a different scheme for giving grades. The rating schemes are as follows:

Medicine: A, B, C, D, E (with A = highest and E = lowest)
Obstetrics & Gynecology: High honors, Honors, Pass, Fail
Pediatrics: Numerical examination grade ranging from 100 (= perfect) to 0
Psychiatry: Superior, Satisfactory, Fail

Because these rating schemes are all different, what kind of composite score would you suggest to provide a class standing?

Exercise 10.4. Here is a set of hypothetical data for a crossover study assessing the occurrence rate of substantial pain with treatment for 92 patients with chronic stable osteoarthritis of the knee. They were randomly assigned to receive either drug A or drug B first, followed by a washout period, followed by the other drug (B or A). The total results can be cited in two different ways:

		Drug A *No Pain*	*Pain*	**Total**
Drug B	No Pain	40	10	50
	Pain	2	40	42
	Total	42	50	92

	Drug A	**Drug B**	**Total**
No Pain	42	50	92
Pain	50	42	92
Total	92	92	184

10.4.1. What statistical indexes would you use for expressing the results of this study? Please give reasons for your choice.

10.4.2. What stochastic tests would you use for determining stochastic significance of the results? Please try at least two different tests. If they yield conflicting results, which set would you choose—and why?

Exercise 10.5. Assume that the first table in Exercise 10.4 represents the results of ratings given to each patient by two different observers. Thus, instead of "Drug A" and "Drug B," the tabular headings are "Observer A" and "Observer B." What indexes would you use for expressing the agreement of these two observers?

CHAPTER REFERENCES

1. Bradley, 1968; 2. Fleis, 1981; 3. Freeman, 1965; 4. Siegel, 1956; 5. Feinstein, 1980; 6. Landis, 1977; 7. Kramer, 1981; 8. Turnbull, 1978; 9. Hardyck, 1975.

PART THREE

ADDITIONAL PRINCIPLES OF CAUSE-EFFECT RESEARCH

We now have an outline of all the basic tools needed to prepare or evaluate a research project. Some of the tools are used for scientific architecture of the plans, and others are used for statistical analysis of the results.

One of the main reasons for understanding the statistical expressions is to keep them from causing confusions or fears that prevent a deeper look at the data. That deeper look is used to review the crucial architectural distinctions that determine scientific credibility and importance for the results. The architectural discussion thus far, however, has dealt with a broad overview, not with a deep look. Many other important details remain to be considered for both the external and internal architecture of a research project. The rest of this text is concerned with those details.

In the seven chapters of Part III, the focus is on additional principles of cause-effect research.

Chapter 11

The Role of the Maneuver in Cause-Effect Research

There are three reasons for devoting an entire chapter to the role of the *maneuver* in cause-effect research:

1. Many people may not recognize the diverse entities that can serve as maneuvers in cause-effect reasoning.

2. The selection of an appropriate comparative maneuver requires a clear identification of the principal maneuver.

3. The types of maneuvers being compared will determine both the actual structure of the research and the intellectual architecture used to evaluate the results.

11.1. IDENTIFICATION OF A MANEUVER

Many assertions in ordinary life contain the idea that event B followed event A and may have been caused by it. Consider the following statements: An apple a day keeps the doctor away; women are more home-oriented than men; people who eat raw clams are likely to get hepatitis; malaise is improved after treatment with chicken soup; the birth weight of a baby often triples in the first year of life.

Each of these statements can be diagrammed as a sequence of:

$$\text{BASELINE STATE} \xrightarrow{\text{MANEUVER}} \text{OUTCOME}$$

The arrangements for the preceding five statements are shown in the following table:

Baseline State	Maneuver	Outcome
Healthy person	Eating an apple a day	No doctor (or no illness)
Undifferentiated person	Female gender	Home orientation
Healthy person	Eating raw clams	Hepatitis
Malaise	Chicken soup	Improvement of malaise
Weight at birth	1st year of life	Increase in weight

When the sequence of events has a cause-effect implication, the *maneuver* is the entity regarded as the causal agent. The research is intended to demonstrate (or refute the idea) that the maneuver does indeed have the causal action attributed to it. The sequence of events can be planned in advance, with the maneuver deliberately imposed at a selected point in the pathway; or the maneuver can be suspected from observations made during or after the occurrence of events.

By using the word *maneuver* to refer to such diverse causal agents as causes of disease, therapeutic procedures, passage of time, and socioeconomic states, we can be liberated from some of the restrictions that have handicapped the analysis of scientific architecture in the traditional research of epidemiology, clinical medicine, and sociology. Epidemiologists have studied causes of disease; clinicians have studied treatment; and sociologists have studied socioeconomic agents—but the different investigators have often used different models for the analyses. With the concept of a maneuver, we can employ a single model that is applicable to research performed in all three of these domains and in many other domains as well. The model of BASELINE STATE/MANEUVER/OUTCOME seems perfectly obvious, but it has not been generally applied for studying the architecture of clinical, epidemiologic, or sociologic research.

11.2. THE PRINCIPAL MANEUVER

Whenever a set of results contains a cause-effect implication, we can begin our appraisal by identifying the principal maneuver. It is whatever is being proposed as the main agent responsible for the observed distinction. After reviewing the evidence, we may or may not agree with the proposal, but our first step in the review is to determine what is being "sold." We shall later decide whether we want to "buy" the proposal.

In many forms of investigation, the principal maneuver can be immediately identified from the expression of the research question. If the question is well stated, it will also identify a particular target event (or target variable) that is to be noted in the outcome, and the baseline state will also be implied or overtly expressed. Thus, in the first and third statements in the preceding section, the person exposed to such principal maneuvers as an apple a day or to raw clams could be assumed to be healthy at the time of exposure. For the implication that women are more home-oriented than men, we could assume that the persons under study had a genderless, undifferentiated baseline state. In the fourth and fifth statements, the baseline states were identified as malaise and newborn baby, respectively.

As the main agent whose impact is under consideration, the principal maneuver must be distinguished from other entities that can also affect the condition of the recipient. Among such entities are ancillary maneuvers, susceptibility factors, and identification processes.

11.2.1. *Ancillary Maneuvers*

Certain ancillary activities are regularly performed just before, during, or immediately after a principal maneuver is conducted. For example, blood transfusion may be used to prepare a patient for surgery; anesthesia is given while the surgery is in progress; and the monitoring functions of a recovery room occur afterward.

If surgery is the principal maneuver under study, all these other activities are ancillary to it. On the other hand, in a study of anesthetic agents, the anesthesia might be regarded as the principal maneuver, and the surgery would be ancillary. The distinctions are important for deciding what role each agent plays in the research architecture. An agent that is a principal maneuver in one study might be an ancillary maneuver in another.

11.2.2. *Susceptibility Factors*

The effect of an underlying maneuver of nature or disease can alter a person's susceptibility to an outcome event. When these distinctions are being investigated to establish their role as risk factors or prognostic predictors, they may be regarded as principal maneuvers. Thus, if we ask whether women tend to live longer than men, the female gender is regarded as the principal maneuver. On the other hand, if we want to investigate the effect of jogging on longevity, the principal maneuver is jogging. If gender is an important prognostic factor for longevity, we would divide the groups into men and women and examine the longevity of joggers and nonjoggers separately for each gender.

Thus, an agent that is a principal maneuver in one study might be a susceptibility factor in another.

11.2.3. *Information Processes*

Certain activities that are regularly used to acquire information about people may sometimes serve as principal maneuvers rather than merely as data-acquisition processes. For example, most physicians use history taking merely as a process that provides data about a patient's condition. For a psychiatrist, however, the communicative exchange that takes place during history taking may also serve as an agent of therapy and thus may, in certain studies, play the role of principal maneuver. If the research is intended to compare quality in a history taken by a person versus a history taken by a computer, the history-taking activities are compared as processes. If the research is intended to learn whether patients are more satisfied (as an outcome event) when histories are taken by a person rather than by a computer, the history-taking activities become compared as maneuvers.

During the initial investigations of the way in which people responded to an infused or ingested load of glucose, the glucose load was a principal maneuver. Today, however, the imposition of a glucose load has become a standard diagnostic procedure, used as an information process to provide the particular collection of data called a *glucose tolerance curve*.

In any individual study, therefore, an investigator will regularly encounter four sets of entities having the roles of principal maneuver, ancillary maneuver, susceptibility factor, or information process. The role played by each entity will be distinctive to that study and may vary substantially from one study to another.

11.2.4. *Problems of Attribution*

Although the principal maneuver may be clearly identified in the statement or conclusions of a research project, the observed impact may be caused by something else: an ancillary maneuver, susceptibility factor, or information process. These additional components can produce some of the biases and problems that were discussed in Chapter 4. An ancillary maneuver can produce performance bias. A susceptibility factor can produce susceptibility bias. An information process can produce detection bias or transfer bias. Because of these problems, the additional components must be considered before an observed impact is attributed to the selected principal maneuver.

For example, to test the validity of the aphorism offered as the first statement in Section 11.1, suppose we do an appropriate study and find that people who eat an apple a day are visited by doctors less often than people who do not eat a daily apple. The result confirms the original statement of the aphorism, but does it confirm the causal role attributed to apple eating? Several alternative causal explanations are possible. In susceptibility, people who choose to eat an apple a day may be initially healthier than those who do not. In ancillary maneuvers, the apple eaters may maintain occupations and life styles that are more conducive to health than the counterpart activities of non–apple eaters. In information processes, the home visits by doctors may occur less often because the apple eaters do not report their illnesses, solicit medical care for them, or have doctors who are willing to make house calls. If all these potential alternatives have not been considered and appropriately checked or adjusted, we might be quite wrong in concluding that eating an apple a day was indeed the cause of keeping the doctor away.

Similarly, to test the second statement in Section 11.1, we might assemble data showing that a group of randomly chosen women have higher scores than a group of randomly chosen men when completing a questionnaire that provides an index of home orientation. Does this result confirm the causal hypothesis that the biologic property of female gender is responsible for an increased degree of home orientation? We cannot reach this conclusion because we have not considered the biases in susceptibility factors and ancillary maneuvers that can be created by familial, educational, social, and occupational differences among women and men. As for the effect of information processes, we would need to check the sampling frame to see whether it was a suitable source for avoiding distorted assembly in the randomly chosen groups. We would also need to check the questionnaire to see whether it provided a suitable index of home orientation.

For these reasons, a cautious investigator and reviewer will always be concerned about the additional factors, rather than the selected principal maneuver alone, that may be responsible for the impact observed in a cause-effect study.

11.3. THE COMPARATIVE MANEUVER

The act of comparison is the *sine qua non* that allows conclusions to be drawn in a scientific manner. Without a comparative maneuver, the reasoning may simply produce the traditional *post hoc* fallacy described in Section 4.1. *Post hoc* reasoning was the source of many of the errors that occurred in the prescientific era of medicine, and the reasoning still occurs in many circumstances today. Because the use of comparative maneuvers is intended to eliminate the problem, the appropriate choice of one (or more) comparative maneuvers is a fundamental decision in a research project. Until this decision is made, the architectural plan cannot be established; and if the decision is inappropriate, the project may yield unsatisfactory results no matter how well the architectural plan is carried out.

In many research studies, the comparative maneuver may seem apparent from the expression of the research question. Thus, if we want to know whether eating an apple a day prevents illness or whether raw clams can cause hepatitis, the comparison would be with *not* eating an apple a day or raw clams. Even when the absence of the principal maneuver would seem obvious as the comparative choice, however, the selection may not be simple. For example, suppose the selected comparative maneuver for avoiding illness is eating two apples a day or eating an orange a day? What decisions could be drawn from these comparative maneuvers? Suppose raw oysters are chosen as the comparative maneuver for raw clams? In each of these instances, the comparative maneuver would be something other than the principal maneuver, but the choice would probably not be satisfactory for making the point that is intended as the conclusion of the research.

Because the choice of the comparative maneuver(s) is so vital to the success of a research project, the decision will be extensively discussed later on.

11.4. A CLASSIFICATION OF MANEUVERS

Because almost anything can be considered as a possible cause of something, the list of possible maneuvers is endless, and a taxonomy of maneuvers is difficult to establish. The taxonomy is worth developing, however, because most projects are identified according to the entity selected as the principal maneuver. One basic axis of classification depends on whether the maneuver is natural or imposed. Separate axes of classification can then be used for maneuvers that are demographic, social, medical, or other types of agents.

11.4.1. *Natural Maneuvers*

Most of the maneuvers studied in the cause-effect research of clinical epidemiology are etiologic or therapeutic agents that have been overtly imposed as interventions on a person's natural condition of health or disease. Not all maneuvers are overtly imposed, however. Some can occur as inherent features of nature. A person's inborn characteristics are natural in the sense that the person has no control over them. Such characteristics include age, biologic gender, and such genetic components as blood type and parental longevity. When compared to determine the different effects of age, gender, or blood type, these maneuvers are regarded as imposed on an underlying state of health or disease. Other natural maneuvers are constitutional entities arising from a combination of external environment and the body's metabolic capacity or internal milieu. Among these constitutional entities are levels of serum uric acid, cholesterol, and various lipid, protein, or lipoprotein components.

In certain studies, people may be followed over a period of time to observe the consequences of a phenomenon such as the natural processes of growth, development, homeostasis, or healing. In sick people, we can observe the clinical course that occurs after a disease has been established. In these circumstances, time is joined with the action of nature and disease to form the *natural maneuver* under consideration. For example, to determine the physiologic weight gain that occurs in infants during the first year of life (without considering the contributory roles of diet, family pattern, and so forth), we could descriptively note the weight status of a group of infants at birth and note their weight a year later. We could then regard the passage of time and physiologic growth as the natural maneuver for the increment in weight.

Similarly, to determine the subsequent development of retinopathy in a group of people with newly diagnosed diabetes mellitus, we could follow those people for the next 20 years, see how many of them develop retinopathy, and ascribe the change to a natural maneuver, which occurs as the effect of the disease during the passage of time.

In research architecture, the idea of a natural maneuver is useful because it allows a formal structure to be employed for many descriptive studies, and it also serves as an important background for comparative studies. For example, in a purely descriptive study, we could determine what proportion of newly discovered diabetic patients develop retinopathy during the next 20 years. In a cause-effect study, we might try to identify prognostic markers (or risk factors) that predict which patients are most or least likely to develop retinopathy. In a process study, we might appraise the accuracy of those predictions in a different group of diabetic patients.

11.4.2. *Imposed Maneuvers*

Most of the agents under study in medical research are imposed maneuvers, but not all of them are medical. The nonmedical entities that may be regarded as contributory causes of disease are: such demographic or public health features as socioeconomic status, education, religion, hobbies, and occupation; the behavioral features of smoking, diet, and exercise; and the environmental features of air and water. A series of noxious agents that are regularly suspected as causes of disease include chemicals and radiation as well as the classic microbes and toxins.

All of the pharmaceutical, surgical, physical, and other agents of modern medical therapy are imposed as maneuvers; and the array of medical maneuvers can also include the personnel (e.g., physician versus nurse practitioner), therapeutic milieu (e.g., special ward versus general inpatient care versus outpatient care), practice arrangements (e.g., group versus solo practice), and fiscal mechanisms (e.g., prepaid versus fee-for-service) that are used in health care delivery.

The background role of natural maneuvers is particularly important in evaluating prophylactic or remedial therapeutic interventions, because the treatment becomes a human maneuver imposed on a natural maneuver. The effects of the preceding natural maneuver must therefore be appraised both as a control and as a susceptibility factor for the outcome observed as a possible result of the intervention. Thus, the possible action of oral contraceptives in causing thromboembolism involves the imposition of a pharmaceutical maneuver upon the recipients' basic susceptibility, created by a natural maneuver. When a headache is treated with aspirin or when long-term hypoglycemic treatment is used to prevent vascular complications in diabetic patients, a pharmaceutical maneuver intervenes in the outcome that would be produced by nature, time, and disease as the natural maneuver.

The existence of this double-maneuver phenomenon makes clinical research much more complicated than the simple cause-effect models considered in many mathematical discussions of experimental design. The underlying actions of nature, disease, or both create differences in the baseline condition and outcome susceptibility of people who may otherwise seem similar because they share the same diagnosis of health or disease. Unless these distinctions of natural maneuvers are suitably recognized as risk factors (for healthy people) or prognostic factors (for diseased people), research projects concerned with prophylactic or remedial therapeutic maneuvers may yield misleading or distorted results.

11.4.3. *Other Types of Maneuvers*

Certain maneuvers are difficult to classify because they represent a mixture of natural and imposed components or they may be used to study effects other than health or disease.

The constitutional factors, such as serum cholesterol, that were mentioned in Section 11.4.1 represent a mixture of natural and imposed components. The term *risk factor* is often used for certain conditions, such as an elevated cholesterol or uric acid, that are not yet regarded as diseases and that can be evaluated as maneuvers leading to other diseases, such as atherosclerosis. A more striking example of a combination of nature and nurture is a person's psyche, which can greatly affect the results of many other maneuvers and which can also serve as a maneuver of its own in producing various psychosomatic problems.

Maneuvers such as a special educational program may be used to alter the behavior of clinicians in providing health care or to encourage patients to comply with prescribed medication or other instructions. In Exercise 2.2.9 at the end of Chapter 2, we encountered a maneuver that was intended to alter the diagnostic interpretations made by radiologists.

The key issue in these mixed-component or miscellaneous maneuvers is not what to call them, but to recognize their function in the investigation of cause-effect relationships.

11.5. **THE FUNCTION OF MANEUVERS**

The principal maneuver under investigation is usually expected to accomplish something. For example, if "absence makes the heart grow fonder," the imposed maneuver of *absence* is expected to augment the baseline magnitude of *cardiac fondness*. The expected accomplishment of a principal maneuver denotes its functional role. This accomplishment can be an effect that we anticipate from our knowledge of nature or that we deliberately seek to achieve as the purpose of the maneuver. Thus, we may believe that the natural event of exposure to measles will provoke the disease in a susceptible person. We may then deliberately vaccinate a susceptible person, as an act of medical intervention, for the purpose of preventing the disease.

In a taxonomy for the different functional roles of the many principal maneuvers studied in medical research, one major axis of classification depends on whether the effect of the maneuver is expected to be transient or persistent. Thus, when we determine a person's physiologic response to an infusion of potassium sulfate, we expect the effects to be brief and we expect the person to return afterward to exactly the same state that existed before the study. By contrast, a maneuver that involves growth and development over time, exposure to a noxious agent, a prophylactic intervention, effects of an established disease, or the action of active pharmaceutical therapy is expected to have an effect that will endure or persist for longer than a transient, ephemeral duration.

11.5.1. *Explication*

The transient-action maneuvers employed in medical research usually have an *explicatory* purpose. They are intended to provide a diagnostic label for a disease or an explanation of a pathologic, physiologic, or pharmacologic mechanism. They are not intended to change the basic condition of the person exposed to the maneuver, and, in fact, such maneuvers are usually abandoned or prohibited if they are noted to produce any persistent changes.

At least two types of explication can be distinguished. In one situation, which might be called *probative,* the imposed maneuver is really a stimulus. The response to this stimulus is intended to help identify an important antecedent maneuver, which may have led to a particular state of health or disease. Many laboratory tests and other diagnostic procedures were originally developed as probative stimuli and later became medical information processes, rather than research procedures. Examples of such activities are an electrocardiographic exercise stress test and a glucose tolerance test.

Many of the procedures used for gathering routine information in clinical medicine involve a transient, explicatory stimulus. Thus, all of the invasive diagnostic procedures that involve catheterization or intravascular injections as well as the less invasive procedures, such as the oral or anal receipt of radiographic contrast material or the performance of endoscopy, can be regarded as explicatory maneuvers or probative stimuli. The value of these diagnostic procedures was originally established (presumably) during research conducted as an explicatory investigation.

Later on, the procedures became used routinely so that they are no longer regarded as research, and they act merely as information processes. Because the signing of an informed consent for many of these procedures indicates that their effects are not always transient and reversible, another important point to be noted is that an ordinarily explicative stimulus may become regarded as a causal maneuver in certain types of research. For example, suppose we want to know whether cerebral arteriography is followed by more (or fewer) side effects than radionuclide scans of the brain. In this situation, the two procedures—although used explicatively for diagnosis—are regarded as maneuvers that can intervene to produce adverse consequences.

A different type of explication is concerned with probing the maneuver itself rather than the recipient's underlying state of health or disease. Such research is often intended to compare the effects of a series of graded doses of the principal maneuver. We might do this type of research as part of bioassay testing for a pharmacologic agent or for determining the level of exercise needed to evoke a suitable response in an exercise stress test for a healthy person. In these examples, we want to determine the dose or level at which the maneuver must be given to produce its action, and we are not specifically trying (in this part of the research) to discriminate between different states of health or disease. There is no good single name for this type of research. It might be called *pharmacologic* when the maneuver is a pharmaceutical substance and *maneuveral* when some other type of agent (such as an exercise test) is under investigation.

Because the effects are transient, most explicatory investigations are basically cross-sectional, not cohort studies. The outcome event is something that describes either the person's current state or an antecedent state, but not the future state that follows a therapeutic intervention.

11.5.2. *Natural Course*

The term *natural course* is usually reserved for natural, nontherapeutic maneuvers acting during a passage of time in which a distinct, persistent change is expected to occur between the baseline state and outcome.

To give names to these natural-course maneuvers, we need some new words and definitions. An *ontogenetic* maneuver produces normal growth and development. The natural effects produced by a disease can be considered for short-term and long-term passages of time. The short-term action, which can be called *pathodynamic,* produces effects that are often present when the disease is first diagnosed and that may disappear as the disease subsides or is brought under control. The long-term action, which can be called *pathogressive,* produces effects that are usually regarded as complications of an established chronic disease. For example, polyuria and polydipsia are pathodynamic effects of diabetes mellitus; retinopathy is a pathogressive effect. For viral hepatitis, jaundice is a pathodynamic effect and cirrhosis is pathogressive. For coronary artery disease, angina pectoris is pathodynamic and congestive heart failure is pathogressive.

Because of vagaries in the clinical behavior of disease, we may sometimes have trouble deciding whether a particular effect is short-term or long-term. The word *pathodynamic* can therefore be extended to apply to such effects. In fact, readers who dislike all of these neologistic distinctions can use *pathodynamic* for both the short-term and long-term actions of a disease. The key point is not the particular name, but the idea that disease plus time can act as a maneuver. Research intended to demonstrate such maneuvers often appears in medical literature, and is commonly arranged with the cross-sectional architecture discussed in Chapter 18.

11.5.3. *Intervention*

The classic agents explored in medical research are interventions. They consist of etiologic entities that can cause disease, and therapies that can prevent or alter disease.

11.5.3.1. **ETIOLOGY**

The terms *etiology* and *pathogenesis* are generally used for the instigation and development of an undesirable condition (or disease). Because the two terms are often used synonymously and because the pathways of instigation and development of disease are often difficult to distinguish, only one of the terms will be employed here. Because the *patho-* prefix already has important roles in reference to the *pathodynamic* and *pathogressive* outcomes of disease, we shall avoid a further and possibly ambiguous usage. The term *etiology* (or *etiologic*) will be employed for maneuvers that lead to the production of an undesirable condition, which, in clinical epidemiology, is commonly a disease.

Etiologic maneuvers can be either natural or imposed. For example, atherosclerosis is often regarded as having certain natural causes that arise as normal degenerative changes with aging, and certain contributory causes that are self-imposed by people who smoke, eat high-fat diets, or lead slothful lives. Sickle cell anemia can be regarded as having a natural maneuver, consisting of abnormal hemoglobin genes, or as having an imposed maneuver, consisting of the marital and procreational decisions of the gene carriers.

Etiologic maneuvers will thus be natural entities or imposed interventions, according to the context in which they are studied and the roles ascribed to them.

11.5.3.2. **THERAPY**

The term *therapy* will be used throughout this discussion to refer to medical interventions, regardless of whether the treatment is intended to prevent something that does not yet exist or to alter something that has already occurred. An imposed therapeutic intervention can be prophylactic, to prevent what might happen, or remedial, to change what has already occurred.

The idea of prophylactic therapy may initially seem odd, because the idea of prevention is often associated not with clinical medicine, but with such public health activities as disposal of sewage, purification of water, and elimination of atmospheric pollution.

Nevertheless, many interventions that clinicians impose on individual patients are intended to prevent something from happening. The use of vaccination is an obvious example, but other examples (described in Section 11.5.3.2.4) are more subtle. They occur when treatment is used to prevent the adverse effects, such as vascular complications or death, that are anticipated from an established disease.

Therapeutic interventions can have four different clinical goals, which can be described as contrapathic, salutary, remedial, and contratrophic.

11.5.3.2.1. *Contrapathic (Primary Prevention)*

The goal of a contrapathic intervention is to prevent the primary occurrence of an undesired outcome in a patient who is initially free of that outcome. In the usual situation, the person is healthy at baseline, and the undesired outcome to be prevented is a disease. A classic example of primary prevention with contrapathic therapy is vaccination of healthy children against poliomyelitis. The undesired outcome, however, might be pregnancy or an adverse drug reaction rather than a specific disease; and the person receiving the intervention need not be completely healthy at baseline. Thus, oral contraceptive pills might be used to prevent pregnancy in a woman with severe congenital heart disease; antacid therapy might be used to prevent gastric irritation in a patient receiving aspirin; and vaccines might be used to prevent influenza or pneumonia in patients with chronic pulmonary disease.

11.5.3.2.2. *Salutary (Health Maintenance)*

The goal of a salutary intervention is not specifically contrapathic, because a particular target disease is seldom cited as the outcome to be prevented. Examples of salutary maneuvers, intended to promote health maintenance, are eating a nutritious diet, exercising regularly, and getting adequate sleep. When the effects of a vaccine are evaluated by measuring antibodies rather than by noting the prevention of the disease, the vaccine is shown to be salutary, not contrapathic.

11.5.3.2.3. *Remedial*

A remedial maneuver is the classic therapeutic intervention of clinical medicine: an attempt to change or remove something that has already occurred. Examples of remedial therapy are aspirin for headache, antibiotics for gonorrhea, or chicken soup for malaise.

11.5.3.2.4. *Contratrophic (Secondary Prevention)*

With contratrophic interventions, a clinician engages in preventive medicine. The goal is to prevent the adverse progression (i.e., pathogression) of an established disease. The outcome event, which is not present in the baseline state, is something to be prevented or retarded. Examples are chemotherapy to prevent or delay death in patients with cancer, glucose regulation to avert vascular complications in diabetes mellitus, and antistreptococcal prophylaxis to prevent recurrences of rheumatic fever.

11.5.3.3. **PURVEYANCE**

We also need a name for various maneuvers that involve changing the delivery of health services, rather than altering states of health or disease. The maneuvers can be the educational tactics, personnel, institutions, administrative processes, or fiscal mechanisms that are involved in providing health care. Thus, we may want to compare the impact of an educational program on the way doctors order drugs, or the change in costs produced by different organizational arrangements, or the effect of nurse practitioners in improving satisfaction with care.

The word *purveyant,* which is offered as a general title for these maneuvers, is the best that Roget's Thesaurus and several excellent dictionaries seem to offer. Other available words have too many ambiguous meanings; and *delivery,* which is probably the clearest word, has become entangled with obstetric actions, religious salvations, and the United Parcel Service.

If the research deals with the outcome of a purveyant procedure, the investigation has a cause-effect structure. Thus, if the goal is to determine whether costs are reduced, doctors more cautious, or patients more satisfied with one of these procedures in comparison to another, the procedure is indeed a maneuver. On the other hand, if a specific outcome is not assessed and the focus of evaluation is the quality of the performed service, the activity is part of *process* research. Thus, if we assess whether bacteria disappear after treatment of a urinary tract infection, the research is oriented toward impact; if we check that the nurse practitioner ordered an appropriate antibiotic for the infection, the research is oriented toward process. If we conduct an educational program to alter the way in which antibiotics are ordered, the change in the ordering process becomes the outcome of the research.

11.6. ILLUSTRATION OF TYPES OF MANEUVERS

Table 11–1 contains illustrations of nomenclature, functional roles, baseline states, outcomes, and individual maneuvers for the diverse activities described in Section 11.5. Additional examples are provided in the exercises at the end of the chapter.

11.7. CONCEPTS AND AMBIGUITIES IN EVALUATION

In cause-effect research, the principal maneuver is evaluated by contrasting its outcome effects against those of the comparative maneuver. In process research, the quality or desirability of a particular procedure is evaluated by comparison with some selected standard of performance.

Because of different ideas about outcomes and comparisons, however, it may sometimes be difficult to decide whether a particular evaluation is process research or cause-effect research. For example, suppose we are asked to evaluate a medical school's elementary course in biochemistry. Our first step might be to determine the goal of the course. Is it supposed to help transform students into good doctors? If so, we need to be able to define a *good doctor* and arrange to determine the distinctive contribution made by biochemistry amid all the other interventions and susceptibility factors in medical education. Is the course supposed to convey certain cognitive information? If so, we need to devise an appropriate test for determining how much the students have learned. With either of these two goals—good doctor or biochemical connoisseur—we have defined an outcome for the course, but our evaluation may still be process research if we merely rate each student against a selected standard of performance or knowledge. To convert the evaluation into cause-effect research, we would have to compare the subsequent performance or knowledge of our students against that of a group of medical students who did not take this biochemistry course or who received some other form of instruction in biochemistry.

On the other hand, suppose we decided not to establish a goal for the course. Instead, we examine the pedagogic process itself. Were the lectures exciting and interesting? Were they organized in a logical sequence of development? Was the content of the lectures "relevant"? If we gave ratings to these individual components of the pedagogic activity

Table 11–1. ILLUSTRATIONS OF TYPES OF MANEUVERS

Functional Role of Maneuver	Baseline State	Maneuver	Outcome	Type of Maneuver
Explain physiology	Healthy	Exercise	Change in pulse	Probative
Explain pathophysiology	Coronary heart disease	Exercise	Change in ECG	Probative
Determine dosage	Healthy or diseased	Doses of beta blocker	Bradycardia	Pharmacologic
Normal growth	Healthy infant	Passage of time	Healthy child	Ontogenetic
Maintain health	Healthy	Daily jogging	Healthy	Salutary
Risk of disease	Healthy	Male gender	Coronary heart disease	Risk factor
Cause of disease	Healthy	Exposure to hepatitis	Hepatitis	Etiologic
Prevent disease	Healthy	Hepatitis vaccine	No hepatitis	Contrapathic
Short-term result of disease	Healthy	Hepatitis	Jaundice	Pathodynamic
Long-term result of disease	Healthy	Hepatitis	Cirrhosis	Pathogressive
Prognostic predictor	Hepatitis	Persistent jaundice	Cirrhosis	Prognostic factor
Improve manifestation of disease	Jaundice	Bed rest	Decrease in jaundice	Remedial
Prevent pathogression	Hepatitis	Steroids	No cirrhosis	Contratrophic
Alternative health care	Hepatitis	Nurse practitioner	Reduced psychic depression	Purveyant
Reduced costs	Hepatitis	Nurse practitioner	Reduction in cost of care	Purveyant
Education	Practicing physician	Postgraduate seminar	New knowledge about disease D	Purveyant

and then reached an overall conclusion about the course, the evaluation would clearly be process research.

The ambiguity here arose because of the different entities that can be the agents and subsequent states in comparative evaluations. If the subsequent state is an effect noted in a person exposed to the agent, the agent seems to have an impact, and the relationship would seem to be a cause-effect situation. Yet, if no comparative agent is investigated, a cause-effect conclusion cannot be established.

This distinction demonstrates that certain types of process evaluations are clearly concerned with procedure alone, whereas others, which focus on *output*, may resemble cause-effect research with a missing control group. The process evaluations are particularly likely to examine procedure alone when an output is difficult to define as a goal of the procedure, or when output data are difficult to collect. This situation commonly occurs in trying to evaluate certain services, such as teaching or medical care.

The uncontrolled cause-effect studies of process often occur when we try to evaluate new technologic agents, such as pulmonary artery (Swan-Ganz) catheterization, that can be used as both informational processes and therapeutic vehicles. Patients who have the appropriate clinical indications, such as certain types of congestive heart failure, will usually receive Swan-Ganz catheterization, so that few patients will be left to form an uncatheterized control group. Even if uncatheterized controls can be assembled, however, crucial data needed for the comparison will be missing because they can be collected only as measurements performed during the catheterization. Thus, certain evaluations of the impact of medical services or technologic agents may necessarily be conducted as process research, because the appropriate alternative comparison cannot be feasibly achieved to demonstrate cause-effect distinctions.

The idea of evaluation has now become so popular and fashionable among grant-giving agencies that the proponents of any research project are regularly asked to provide additional proposals indicating how the accomplishments will be evaluated. The granting agency's request for a special evaluation may seen particularly odd if the proposed project is itself an act of evaluation research. Thus, the proponent of a randomized trial of two therapeutic agents may be asked to prepare an additional proposal for the evaluation that appraises the research. In other circumstances, agencies infatuated with the idea that randomized trials are the only acceptable form of evaluation may turn down excellent proposals for appraising processes that cannot be subjected to randomized trials or even to comparison with a control group.

11.8. ACTUAL AND VIRTUAL MANEUVERS

For reasons of feasibility or convenience, the actual architecture of a research project may differ substantially from the intellectual architecture of the scientific reasoning.

For example, suppose we want to determine whether the development of diabetes mellitus tends to increase a patient's serum cholesterol level. The scientific reasoning here is that serum cholesterol in healthy people becomes higher if they develop diabetes mellitus than if they do not. The principal maneuver would be diabetes mellitus and the comparative maneuver would be the absence of diabetes mellitus. The architectural diagram would be

$$
\left. \begin{array}{l} \text{HEALTHY} \\ \text{PEOPLE} \end{array} \right\} \quad \begin{array}{c} \xrightarrow{\text{Diabetes Mellitus}} \\ \xrightarrow{\text{No Diabetes Mellitus}} \end{array} \quad \left\{ \begin{array}{l} \text{CHANGE IN} \\ \text{CHOLESTEROL} \end{array} \right.
$$

If the work is conducted as a *cohort study,* the research structure used for the investigation will directly correspond to the arrangement of the intellectual model. In a cohort study, the people under observation are followed forward in time after the imposition of the compared maneuvers. If the maneuvers are allocated by randomization, the research is called a *randomized trial* or *experiment*. If the maneuvers are allocated by nature or by the judgmental selection of a physician or of the recipient, the research is called an *observational cohort*.

Using a cohort structure to carry out this study according to the proposed model, we would assemble a large group of healthy people. We would then follow them forward in time to see what happens to serum cholesterol after one subgroup develops diabetes while the other subgroup remains free of diabetes. This cohort study could not possibly be conducted as a randomized trial. Even if we were ethically willing to try to make healthy persons diabetic, and even if we could get enough people to volunteer to take the risk of becoming diabetic, we do not know how to produce diabetes mellitus in a manner similar to its natural occurrence.

A more feasible approach, therefore, would be to perform the research as an observational cohort study. We would try to find a large group of healthy people who have been under careful medical surveillance for many years. If enough of these people have spontaneously developed diabetes while under observation, we might be able to use their data to indicate the diabetes-induced changes in cholesterol. These results could be compared against what was noted in the rest of the people, who did not develop diabetes. This project is reasonable but might be quite difficult to conduct. We might not easily be able to find a large enough group of people who were followed long enough for diabetes to develop, with cholesterol examinations performed at frequent enough intervals to provide the necessary data about changes. Thus, because of problems in assembling groups of adequate sizes, in duration of follow-up, or in details of data, an observational cohort study might be so difficult to do that it does not get done.

Consequently, if we wanted to answer the research question about whether diabetes mellitus raises serum cholesterol, we could not use the cohort structure that corresponds to the phrasing of the question. If we still wanted to obtain an answer, we would have to do some other type of research, using a different type of structure. The cross-sectional studies that were mentioned in Section 2.2.4 are commonly used for this purpose. Although their architecture will be discussed in greater detail in Chapter 18, cross-sectional studies are cited here to illustrate a research structure that does *not* follow the logical or temporal direction of the scientific architectural model.

In a cross-sectional approach, the investigator would assemble a group of diabetic patients and a control group of people who do not have diabetes. The cholesterol levels would be determined in the two groups, and if the levels are higher in the diabetics, the investigator might conclude that diabetes elevates cholesterol. With this design, the investigator would not observe the serial change in baseline state that was produced by the development of diabetes. The maneuver would have been imposed *before* the people were encountered in their outcome state. The only "maneuver" actually imposed in the research would be the information process of drawing blood to determine cholesterol levels in each patient.

To diagram the architecture of a cross-sectional study, we can use arrows that go downward rather than horizontally forward. The groups and investigative activities could be shown as:

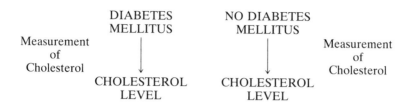

These two diagrams can be consolidated, in a manner analogous to what was done previously, into a single diagram that shows the research as:

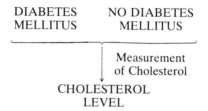

When these cross-sectional results are analyzed, however, the investigator will want to draw a cohort rather than a cross-sectional conclusion. The cross-sectional evidence might be that cholesterol is higher in diabetics than in nondiabetics, but the cohort conclusion would be that diabetes produces an elevation of cholesterol. For this cohort conclusion, diabetes mellitus is regarded as the maneuver, even though it was not investigated directly as a maneuver.

The term *virtual maneuver* can be used for a maneuver investigated with data that differ from cohort evidence of observed serial effects that followed the maneuver. In a cohort study, diabetes mellitus would be the maneuver that is actually observed. In the cross-sectional study, diabetes was a virtual maneuver. Its onset and subsequent consequences were not actually observed and followed in the research.

As another example, suppose we want to find the frequency with which hypertension produces vascular complications in patients who have had the disease for 20 years. In a direct cohort approach to this descriptive study, we would assemble a group of patients with newly diagnosed hypertension; we would follow them for 20 years; and we would see how many have vascular complications at the end of that time. In a cross-sectional approach, we would assemble a group of patients who have already had hypertension for 20 years and we would determine how many of them have vascular complications. In both approaches, we would examine the patients to detect vascular complications. In both approaches, we would regard the action of hypertension during a 20-year period as the principal maneuver responsible for the vascular complications. In the first approach, however, we would directly observe the serial changes that followed the principal maneuver, whereas in the second approach, we would not. In the first approach, the temporal effect of hypertension would be a *real* or actual principal maneuver, whereas in the second approach, the principal maneuver would be *virtual*. The two diagrams that follow indicate these distinctions:

Cohort: PATIENTS WITH NEWLY DIAGNOSED HYPERTENSION { Action of Hypertension for 20 Years } VASCULAR COMPLICATIONS

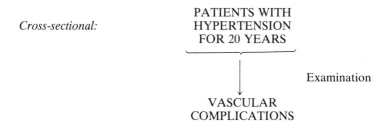

Cross-sectional: PATIENTS WITH
                                  HYPERTENSION
                                  FOR 20 YEARS

                                          | Examination
                                          ↓
                                      VASCULAR
                                  COMPLICATIONS

Cross-sectional (and heterodemic) data structures are regularly used for cause-effect investigations of virtual maneuvers. Because the results are interpreted serially (or longitudinally), the evidence must be evaluated with the same scientific criteria used for serial reasoning in a cohort study, but because the architecture of the noncohort research is so different, not all investigators (or readers) agree about the interpretations, criteria, and reasoning. Some of the controversies that arise from these disagreements will be discussed later.

11.9. PROFICIENCY OF A MANEUVER

Unless a maneuver has had an opportunity to do its job properly, the action of the maneuver cannot be fairly evaluated. The *proficiency* of the maneuver refers to the features that create this opportunity. They depend on an appropriate potency, intrinsic accompaniment, and extrinsic accompaniment for the maneuver.

11.9.1. *Potency*

The *potency* of a maneuver refers to its capacity to produce the intended target event in the outcome state. For pharmaceutical substances, this capacity depends on route of administration, dosage, frequency, and duration. For example, a drug that must be given parenterally will not be potent if taken orally. A drug that requires flexible dosage may be ineffective if given in fixed dosage, and a fixed-dosage drug may not work properly if the dose is too low or too high. A drug that should be taken four times daily for ten days may be inadequate if taken less frequently or for a shorter duration.

The decision about a schedule that will provide adequate potency is much easier when the maneuver is investigated for beneficial than for noxious effects. The exposure needed for a potent beneficial action is often investigated in animals, from which a suitable schedule can be estimated for people; and the beneficial effects in people can often be directly correlated with dosage if the effect is remedial. On the other hand, noxious effects in animals are often difficult to induce experimentally, or the required dosage may be so egregiously high that the results cannot be extrapolated to humans. Furthermore, the noxious effects in people may occur so infrequently that a suspected causal maneuver can seldom be directly related to an observed noxious effect.

For these reasons, the choice of a potent level of exposure is often difficult to determine when noxious maneuvers are under study. For example, how much conjugated estrogen taken for how long a period of time should be regarded as an exposure capable of inducing carcinoma in a postmenopausal woman? The issues become even trickier when the principal maneuver is a nonpharmaceutical etiologic entity, such as cigarette smoking or certain occupational toxins. How much smoking and for how many years should a person have smoked to be designated as a smoker? What is the strength of exposure needed for someone to be classified as exposed to vinyl chloride, lead, beryllium, asbestos, or the otopathogenicity of a discotheque? Because of the problems of choosing a single potent level of exposure, certain etiologic investigations may rely on the associations found in dose-response curves for multiple levels of exposure, rather than on a two-group contrast of results in exposed and nonexposed people.

If the maneuver depends on the personal performance of an operator, the skill of the operator is a primary determinant of the maneuver's potency, regardless of whether the maneuver itself consists of personal intercommunication, a physical procedure (such as manipulation of the spine, application of a cast, or insertion of an acupuncture needle), or a surgical operation (such as hysterectomy or cardiac transplantation). The personal performance of any of these procedures may differ when done by a neophyte, by an experienced expert, or by two different experts.

A different issue in the potency of a maneuver arises from the vulnerability of the person who receives it. This attribute is different from the baseline condition, discussed in Section 4.2.1, that reflects prognostic susceptibility to the outcome event. Prognostic susceptibility is determined exclusively by the underlying disease or clinical condition, and is estimated from what would presumably happen without any intervening maneuver. *Vulnerability* requires a distinctive combination of personal susceptibility plus the action of the maneuver.

For example, until someone develops hives as an idiosyncratic reaction that demonstrates vulnerability to a particular medication, we might have no evidence suggesting that this person was in any way susceptible to hives. Similarly, for a healthy woman who has previously had normal pregnancies and normal children, we would have no evidence to suggest an increased susceptibility to birth deformities. If this woman develops rubella at some point during the last two trimesters of her next pregnancy, we would not be particularly alarmed; but if the rubella occurs during the first trimester, when the fetus is vulnerable, the likelihood of a congenital anomaly would be sharply increased. The opportunity for rubella or any other agent to have a teratogenic impact in pregnancy depends not merely on the intensity of maternal exposure (or dosage regimen), but particularly on the vulnerability of the fetus. The question of appropriate vulnerability of the fetal recipient is particularly important although often ignored in etiologic studies of allegedly teratogenic agents.

A separate decision about potency comes from the hunch, suspicion, or rationale that leads to the selection and investigation of a particular agent as a possible potent maneuver. The initial idea that something may be an etiologic or therapeutic maneuver can be derived from experiments with animals, from logical deductions, from inspired hunches, or from flights of fancy. By recalling the many episodes in medical history in which accused causes of disease were later exonerated and in which allegedly efficacious treatments were later discarded, we can get an idea of the frequency with which physicians of every era have been able to engage in imaginative creativity or profound self-delusion, or both, about the potency of maneuvers.

Clinicians have always had an excellent physiologic rationale for almost every medical intervention, regardless of the era in which the intervention was used and regardless of its ultimate merits. Blood-letting would get rid of bad humors; complete dental extractions would remove foci of infection; high concentrations of oxygen would prevent premature babies from getting the respiratory distress syndrome; thalidomide would reduce a pregnant woman's nausea or anxiety. In more recent years, in treatment of angina pectoris, talc poudrage of the pericardium would stimulate new vasculature; internal mammary artery ligation would increase coronary blood flow; and arterial tunnel implants would bring more blood directly to the myocardium. Today, venous grafts provide detours around coronary blockages and transluminal angioplasty reams them out. Yesterday's Nobel prize for the physiologic triumphs of castration in prostatic cancer[1] is followed by tomorrow's controlled clinical trial,[2] showing no substantial survival value for either the operation or the use of estrogen therapy.

One way to avoid these difficulties is to perform the necessary clinical evaluation of a new treatment soon, rather than late, after it is introduced. Another way is to exercise more astute judgment in appraising the rationale and capacities of the intervention itself.

11.9.2. *Intrinsic Accompaniment*

Very few maneuvers can be administered in isolation. A pharmaceutical substance is customarily given in a vehicle, such as a tablet, capsule, or solution. A major surgical procedure is usually carried out with preoperative preparation, intraoperative anesthesia, and immediate postoperative care in a recovery room. A patient who is being monitored in a coronary care unit also interacts with other patients in the unit and with members of the professional staff. The term *intrinsic accompaniment* can be used to describe the entities that are an inherent part of a maneuver. The neglect of the intrinsic accompaniment is a frequent cause of defective comparisons or interpretations in appraising the action of maneuvers.

11.9.2.1. DIRECT INTRINSIC ACCOMPANIMENT

The direct intrinsic accompaniment of a maneuver consists of features that are a necessary constituent of its administration. Such features include the vehicle in which a pharmaceutical agent is prepared or conveyed, the anesthesia associated with surgery, the paper in which cigarette tobacco is wrapped for smoking, and the personal manner with which a psychiatrist conducts a particular therapeutic method (such as Freudian analysis).

These accompanying constituents must be considered when comparative maneuvers are selected, because the constituents may often be the best choice of a comparative maneuver. Thus, according to the relative situation under consideration, the comparison for an injected treatment may be an injected placebo; the comparison for cutaneous cortisone in base lotion may be base lotion, not just any placebo lotion; the comparison for a surgical operation may be a sham surgical operation (anesthesia, incision, and manipulation of principal structures, but no alteration of those structures).

11.9.2.2. INDIRECT INTRINSIC ACCOMPANIMENT

The indirect accompaniment of a maneuver consists of the environment in which the maneuver is carried out. The effects attributed to the principal maneuver may sometimes arise from these indirect accompaniments.

The indirect accompaniment includes such *associated maneuvers* as the use of a recovery room after surgical operations; dietary therapy during pharmaceutical treatment of diabetes mellitus or peptic ulcer; and chair rest, early ambulation, or elastic stockings during pharmaceutical treatment of myocardial infarction. The *site of the maneuver* may also play an important role. Examples of the effect of the hospital site are its function as a form of "environment-ectomy" during the treatment of peptic ulcer, "parent-ectomy" during treatment of childhood asthma, and "incarceration" during treatment of obesity.

Another indirect accompaniment is the impact of *associated personnel*. Examples are the psychic or other forms of support given by nurses, social workers, and doctors. A different effect of this indirect accompaniment can be created by the psychic resolution needed to maintain an unappealing diet. The need to develop this resolution may selectively alter the population of people who comply with the program. (Because this effect occurs after rather than before the treatment begins, the bias that may be produced differs from the type of pure susceptibility bias discussed in Section 4.2.1.)

11.9.3. *Extrinsic Accompaniment*

The extrinsic accompaniment of a maneuver consists of other agents, not regarded as an inherent part of the maneuver, that are given essentially at the same time and that can affect the action of the maneuver or the outcome events. These external agents can be given *conjugately,* as part of a deliberate plan for producing a combined action of two or more maneuvers; *conditionally,* when the second agent is given in response to an effect that follows the first maneuver under study; or *incidentally,* for some other reason unrelated to the prime maneuver. For example, a woman with breast cancer may receive a modified radical mastectomy as the principal therapeutic maneuver. Adjuvant chemotherapy may have been given as a conjugate maneuver just before the surgery. In the postoperative period, when a metastasis is noted in the lung, she may receive radiotherapy as a conditional maneuver. While all this was taking place, her diabetes mellitus may have been treated with insulin as an incidental maneuver. These external maneuvers, which are sometimes called *co-maneuvers* or *co-interventions,* must be carefully appraised, because all three types of co-maneuver can "contaminate" or otherwise alter the results of the maneuver under study.

11.9.3.1. CONJUGATE MANEUVERS

A *conjugate maneuver* is juxtaposed concomitantly just before, during, or just after the main maneuver. An example of concomitant juxtaposition is the simultaneous use of two antibiotics (such as penicillin and gentamicin) or two antihypertensive agents. An example of sequential juxtaposition is the use of adjuvant chemotherapy just before surgery for cancer or the preplanned use of radiotherapy just after the surgery. The direct and indirect internal accompaniments of a maneuver are really conjugate maneuvers that are commonly overlooked because they may not have been regarded as maneuvers.

The term *conjugate,* however, is usually reserved for a specified agent that is deliberately regarded as a maneuver and that was *chosen with the same decision* used to select the main maneuver. Thus, postoperative radiotherapy is a conjugate maneuver if it will be given regardless of what is found at surgery, but is a *conditional* maneuver if given only when surgery reveals positive lymph nodes or other evidence that the tumor has spread.

The obvious (or nonobvious) use of conjugate maneuvers creates many problems in evaluating single maneuvers, particularly when conjugate maneuvers that were unauthorized can either act in the same way as the principal maneuver, or have a direct impact on the outcome event. For example, in studies of pain-relieving agents, the patients assigned to an active nonsalicylate preparation or to placebo may supplement their treatment with aspirin, thereby confusing the evaluation of changes in pain.

An important type of unauthorized conjugate maneuver is called *contamination of the control group.* In this circumstance, persons assigned to the comparative passive maneuver learn about the special intervention being used as the active maneuver and begin to apply that intervention themselves. An example of this problem occurred in the Multiple Risk Factor Intervention Trial,[3] in which many members of the control group apparently changed their diets, lost excess weight, and lowered elevated blood pressures without being specifically encouraged to do so. When the outcomes were relatively similar for the people assigned to active or passive treatment in that trial, the absence of a major distinction was attributed to contamination of the control group. A similar type of problem occurs in trials of medical versus surgical therapy for coronary artery disease, when members of the medically treated group decide to have surgery.

11.9.3.2. **CONDITIONAL MANEUVERS**

A conjugate maneuver, which is prescribed as the result of a single decision made for what is known about a patient's condition at a particular point in time, must be distinguished from a *conditional maneuver,* which is added because of a change in the patient's condition. The change may occur because of an apparent success or failure of the main maneuver or it may be purely intellectual, arising from the acquisition of new information that was not available when the main maneuver was chosen.

For example, in the treatment of depression, the decision to treat with verbal and chemical psychotherapy followed by electroshock would be a conjugate maneuver if the electroshock is given no matter what happens during the verbal and chemical psychotherapy. The electroshock is a conditional maneuver if it is reserved only for circumstances in which the verbal and chemical psychotherapy are ineffectual. As noted earlier, a conjugate maneuver in the treatment of cancer arises from the single plan to perform surgery immediately followed by postoperative radiotherapy, regardless of what is found at the time of the operation. If ordered only when the tumor is found to have spread to lymph nodes or beyond, the postoperative radiotherapy is a conditional, not a conjugate maneuver.

The distinction between conjugate and conditional additions must be borne in mind when combinations of maneuvers are evaluated. A conditional maneuver will usually have been given to people whose pretherapeutic condition was different from the corresponding state of people treated with a conjugate maneuver. For example, the groups of patients treated with the sequence of surgery followed by chemotherapy for breast cancer will be different if the chemotherapy is given conjugately, regardless of what is found at surgery, or if chemotherapy is ordered conditionally for patients found to have lymph node metastases.

Conjugate and conditional maneuvers should also be distinguished from susceptibility factors that can influence the outcome event. In most analyses of etiology or therapy, the conjugate and conditional maneuvers are specific interventions—such as diets, smoking, or therapeutic agents—that have been imposed on the natural state of the recipients. The susceptibility factors will be demographic and pathologic conditions of health or disease that exist in those recipients when the maneuvers are imposed. For example, a patient who discovers a familial history of coronary disease as a susceptibility factor may decide to stop smoking and may, on discovering hypercholesterolemia as another susceptibility factor, later change to a low-fat diet as a conditional maneuver. Another patient, in response to the initial discovery of the familial history alone, may stop smoking and adopt a low-fat diet simultaneously as conjugate maneuvers. Similarly, surgery and chemotherapy may be given as conjugate maneuvers for a patient with the susceptibility factor of Stage I cancer; or the surgery may be given alone, with chemotherapy added later when prognostic susceptibility has changed to Stage III.

11.9.3.3. **INCIDENTAL MANEUVERS**

Unlike a conjugate or conditional maneuver, which is usually aimed at the same target as the main maneuver, an incidental maneuver is aimed at a different target. For example, patients with cancer may receive chemotherapy as a principal maneuver for its cytotoxic effect on the tumor and may receive such incidental maneuvers as blood products, antibiotics, or steroids that are supportive therapy for various clinical problems that may occur concomitantly. Because these incidental maneuvers can affect survival, which is the customary outcome event used in appraising the treatment of cancer, their contribution must be considered when two chemotherapeutic regimens are compared. Unless the incidental supportive therapy was reasonably similar for both regimens, performance bias (as discussed later) may create a major distortion in the comparison.

When causes are sought for the adverse effects of a particular maneuver, the list of candidate suspects may include the interaction produced by an incidental maneuver. In such circumstances, the concomitance of the incidental maneuver creates a vulnerability that would not otherwise occur for the person exposed only to the main maneuver. Although the complex phenomena of drug/drug interactions are usually analyzed exclusively according to the metabolic interplay of the drugs, the vulnerability of the recipient also requires suitable evaluation.

11.10. SYNOPSIS

Although any phenomenon can be investigated as a possible cause of some other phenomenon, the entity regarded as *the* cause is the principal maneuver. It must be clearly identified so that a suitable comparative maneuver can be chosen, and its role must be separated from the contributions and possible biases that can arise from ancillary maneuvers, susceptibility factors, and the information processes used to assemble the individual data or the compared groups.

Maneuvers can be divided into the natural actions of growth, development, healing, and progression of a disease, and the imposed agents of etiology, therapy, and other activities. The imposition of an additional maneuver upon an underlying natural maneuver creates complicated distinctions that are often oversimplified in experimental designs concerned with only a single maneuver.

Maneuvers can be used to provide explications, create natural courses, or produce interventions. The effects of explicatory maneuvers—which are employed in physiologic, pathophysiologic, or pharmacologic research—are usually transient or ephemeral, and the recipient returns to the status that existed before the research. Natural-course maneuvers lead to ontogenetic growth and development, or to a disease's short-term pathodynamic or long-term pathogressive consequences. Interventional maneuvers can be the imposed agents and constitutional risk factors involved in the etiology (or pathogenesis) of disease, and the therapeutic agents used for contrapathic, salutary, remedial, or contratrophic effects. Additional sets of purveyant maneuvers, usually relating to delivery of health services, are performed by educational tactics, personnel, and administrative facilities.

Although evaluations can be conducted to appraise the quality of processes or the impact of cause-effect maneuvers, certain processes may be examined for procedure alone, without a defined output. In other circumstances, a maneuver having a definite impact is evaluated by process methods because a control group, receiving a comparative maneuver, cannot be feasibly assembled.

When the cohort structures used in the intellectual architectural model of cause-effect reasoning cannot be readily applied, the research may be conducted with a cross-sectional or other structure that uses different architectural arrangements. The maneuvers compared in the intellectual analysis of these alternative structures are applied in a *virtual* manner rather than under the *actual* observations given to the consequences of the maneuvers in cohort research.

For an effective evaluation, each of the compared maneuvers in a cause-effect study should be checked for proficiency in the potency with which the maneuver itself is administered, in the direct and indirect features that constitute the intrinsic accompaniment of the maneuver, and in the additional occurrence of conjugate, conditional, or incidental maneuvers that constitute the extrinsic accompaniment. Neglect of these issues in proficiency can lead to selection of an unsuitable comparative maneuver or to a comparison whose results are distorted by various forms of performance bias.

EXERCISES

Exercise 11.1. In Exercises 2.2.1 to 2.2.11 at the end of Chapter 2, you were asked to classify various features of a set of research projects. Eliminating Exercises 2.2.1, 2.2.6, and 2.2.10 from consideration and analyzing the remaining eight projects, please do the following for each project: Name the principal maneuver under investigation, classify its function (according to the taxonomy of Sections 11.5. and 11.6), and indicate whether the maneuver was actual or virtual.

Exercise 11.2. What are some of the most important problems you would anticipate from ancillary maneuvers, susceptibility factors, or information processes in causal statements that have the following conclusions:

11.2.1. Health maintenance organizations reduce the costs of hospitalization associated with ordinary forms of clinical practice.

11.2.2. Passing a voluntary recertification board examination helps prevent incompetent specialists from being foisted on the public.

11.2.3. Breast-feeding improves the bonding between mother and child.

11.2.4. The results are usually very good when chicken soup is used to treat the malaise of acute viral infections.

11.2.5. Ivy League education is desirable because graduates of Ivy League colleges achieve a higher socioeconomic status than graduates of other colleges.

Exercise 11.3. In Exercise 3.1 at the end of Chapter 3, you were asked to obtain further specifications for the objectives of 13 research projects. Please eliminate projects 3.1.3, 3.1.6, 3.1.7, 3.1.9, and 3.1.10. For the remaining eight projects, indicate the pertinent baseline state of the people who might be studied in the research and the most cogent target you would observe in the outcome state. Then characterize the function of the principal maneuvers under study as ontogenetic, etiologic, and so forth. (Note that the role of the maneuver may vary according to what you choose as the outcome.)

Exercise 11.4. We are planning to study the cause-effect impact of the following principal maneuvers, and we want to be sure that each maneuver has been imposed with suitable proficiency. For each of the following maneuvers, name the one or two most important aspects of proficiency that would be your main concern in determining the maneuver's suitability. You may assume that each pharmaceutical agent has been given in proper daily dosage.

11.4.1. Adjuvant chemotherapy for treatment of breast cancer.

11.4.2. Aspirin treatment as a cause of Reye's syndrome.

11.4.3. Hormonal treatment during pregnancy as a cause of birth defects.

11.4.4. Hormonal treatment during pregnancy as prophylaxis against premature delivery.

11.4.5. A newly proposed surgical operation in prevention of future bleeding in patients with esophageal varices.

11.4.6. A newly proposed grapefruit and cornflakes diet in treatment of obesity.

11.4.7. The role of a grapefruit and cornflakes diet in childhood as a possible cause of anorexia nervosa in later life.

11.4.8. Beta blocker therapy to prevent recurrent myocardial infarction.

CHAPTER REFERENCES

1. Huggins, 1966; 2. Veterans Administration Cooperative Urological Research Group, 1967; 3. MRFIT, 1982.

Chapter 12

Strategy of Comparison in Cause-Effect Research

When the basic objective is formulated for a cause-effect research project, the principal maneuver is usually obvious or easily chosen. It is the particular agent whose effects the research is intended to demonstrate or document. Thus, each of the principal maneuvers is readily evident in research intended to answer such questions as whether bypass surgical grafting is beneficial for patients with coronary disease, cigarette smoking causes cancer of the bladder, women can be successful urologic surgeons, or Health Maintenance Organizations reduce the costs of medical care.

After the principal maneuver has been identified, the next main step in cause-effect research is to choose the comparative maneuver and then to arrange to observe what happens when the maneuvers are imposed and compared. The choice of the comparative maneuver is a particularly crucial decision, because no amount of subsequent design or analysis can salvage a project in which the fundamental maneuvers were inappropriately compared.

The selection of a suitable comparative maneuver involves issues of judgment, feasibility, and science. The *judgment* arises from the basic goals of the research. What does the investigator want to prove? What will be needed to make the proof convincing? Who is to be convinced? The answers to these three questions will determine the manner in which the principal maneuver is to be given (or defined), the choice and manner of administration of the comparative maneuver, and the mechanism used for allocating the maneuvers and collecting data. Thus, if we want to prove that Excellitol is an effective agent, we can compare it against nothing or placebo; if we want to prove that Excellitol is more effective than any other available agent, the comparison should be against all other agents or against whatever is regarded as the most effective of those other agents. If we want the proof to be as convincing as possible, we might have to arrange an experimental trial of Excellitol versus the comparative agent. If we think we can obtain convincing proof without a formal experimental trial, or if such a trial is unfeasible, we might use an observational structure for the research.

The issue of *feasibility* arises because the ideal experimental plan for comparing the two maneuvers may be impossible or unfeasible to carry out. We may not be able to solicit or randomly assign people to receive a maneuver that is suspected of being harmful rather than beneficial. We may be forbidden from using sham surgery as a comparative maneuver for real surgery. We may not be able to acquire enough people to participate in the study, or follow them long enough, or obtain all the special data we might like to have. In all of these (and other) circumstances, the choice of a comparative maneuver and even the selection of the basic research structure—as an experimental trial, observational cohort, or case-control study —may represent a compromise between what is ideal, what is convincing, and what is possible.

The issues of *science* arise in various aspects of individual suitability for the principal maneuver and for the comparative manner. Has each one been planned in a way that makes it suitably administered? Has the comparative maneuver been chosen to cope appropriately with various problems that can create an unsuitable comparison? The distinctions between an unsuitable and a biased comparison are important. In an *unsuitable* comparison of maneuvers, we are contrasting the wrong things. In a *biased* comparison, we might contrast the right things, but the contrast is not carried out properly. Thus, if we want to know whether Excellitol is the *best* available inexpensive agent to relieve pain in rheumatoid arthritis, a comparison against placebo is unsuitable. A comparison against aspirin might be suitable, but would be biased (against aspirin) if the aspirin were given in fixed dosage rather than in the flexible dosage needed to titrate each patient's threshold of response.

Because so many different issues are involved, this chapter is divided into two main parts. The first part, Section 12.1, deals with issues of proficiency and contrast in choosing a comparative maneuver or maneuvers. The remainder of the chapter, Sections 12.2 and 12.3, deals with the chronology of comparison and allocation of maneuvers.

12.1. SELECTION OF COMPARATIVE MANEUVERS

Any comparative maneuver must have two different types of suitability. First, it must be suitable in its individual proficiency, according to the features discussed at the end of the previous chapter. Second, it must be suitable for the comparison it is intended to provide. This section deals with decisions about necessity and relativity that determine a maneuver's suitability for its role in comparison. Other important decisions, discussed in subsequent sections of this chapter, arise from the reversibility, multiplicity, and concurrency of the compared maneuvers.

12.1.1. *Necessity for Comparison*

Although comparison or control groups are regarded as a necessity of science, a comparison group may sometimes be reasonably omitted from research that otherwise fulfills scientific requirements. In other circumstances, the comparison group may be chosen in an unusual way that creates major problems in appraising fulfillment of the requirements.

12.1.1.1. **NO CONTROL NECESSARY**

In a descriptive survey, no comparative maneuver is needed or desired, because the goal of the study is to describe, not to compare. Examples of descriptive questions are the following: What is the cost of a routine pregnancy? What is the death rate for coronary disease in British Columbia? Are elderly people interested in moving from private individual housing to an old-age home?

Obtaining descriptive data is a crucial prelude to many other forms of research, and the importance of descriptive surveys should not be minimized because of any statistical or scientific belief that control groups are an absolute necessity of research. For many important issues in health care (such as the accomplishments and true costs of clinical services), the appropriate descriptive data do not yet exist, and their acquisition by suitable surveys is the all-important first step in the investigation (or evaluation) of the services.

12.1.1.2. **VIRTUAL USE OF HISTORICAL CONTROLS**

When the conventional treatment for a particular condition has been strikingly and consistently unsuccessful (or successful), the background historical experience with this treatment can sometimes serve as a virtual control group when a new treatment is evaluated. For example, the effect of the first usage of insulin in patients with diabetic acidosis or of penicillin in patients with bacterial endocarditis was so dramatic in comparison with historical experience that no direct control groups were needed, and conclusions could be drawn from the results in a single patient. Similar examples occurred with the demonstration that renal dialysis could alter uremia and that adrenocorticosteroids could remove adrenal insufficiency. The frequency of infants with phocomelia, compared with the historical incidence of phocomelia after conventional pregnancies, was prime evidence in the indictment of thalidomide as a noxious agent for pregnant women.[1]

The reports of the initial therapeutic triumphs (or disasters) with the agents just cited contained no overt control groups because the historical controls were an obvious, well-known reference group for clinical readers. In other circumstances, in which the therapeutic effects are less dramatic, a control group is necessary—and the use of nonconcurrent historical controls arouses considerable controversy. The subject is discussed in a later section on the concurrent features of control groups.

Another point to be noted about uncontrolled studies is their occasional use to demonstrate the technical ability to carry out an extraordinary new maneuver, such as cardiac or hepatic transplantation. The results of such reports, however, merely indicate that the maneuver can be technically accomplished. They do not indicate when it should be done or what its overall value may be. For the latter decisions, control groups are necessary.

12.1.1.3. **CONTRIVED CONTROLS**

In certain types of epidemiologic research, the results of a maneuver may be compared against a control group that is not directly observed or followed. The group is contrived from various forms of general vital statistics data. For example, a gynecologist who has treated a large number of postmenopausal women with replacement estrogens and who has noted the subsequent occurrence of breast cancer in those women may create his control group by using what has been reported to the National Center for Health Statistics as the occurrence rate for breast cancer in a general population of women of the same age group.[2]

This type of comparison contains many problems that will be discussed later in greater detail. One immediate problem is that the control group contains a mixture of people, exposed and not exposed to the main maneuver under study. A second problem is that the baseline condition of the control group is completely undefined, whereas the actively treated group had to fulfill deliberate clinical criteria before being exposed to the treatment. A third problem is that the outcome event (in this instance, breast cancer) may have been sought and diagnosed with different degrees of intensity in the actively treated group and in the general population. The contrived comparisons are thus easy prey for all three major forms of bias in proficiency, susceptibility, and detection.

12.1.1.4. **NO PERFECT CONTROL POSSIBLE**

In many circumstances of evaluation for modern technology, a perfect control group may be impossible to achieve, and the investigator must settle for a less-than-perfect comparison. For example, although sham surgery was performed in clinical trials[3, 4] many years ago to test the value of internal mammary artery ligation for coronary disease, such sham operative procedures are generally unacceptable today. To test the efficacy of a surgical procedure, the comparative "no-operation" procedure would usually have to be medical therapy.

A different type of problem arises when a suitably chosen injected active medication is compared against a suitably chosen oral active medication. In this circumstance, double-blinding could be achieved only by arranging for each treatment group to receive two medications: An oral placebo would also be given to the injected group, and an injected placebo would also be given to the oral group. Because the arrangement would require that patients receiving the oral active treatment undergo the nuisance of a placebo injection, the research plan may be rejected either by the institutional review board or by the patients to whom the plan is proposed. If the clinical trial is conducted without the accompanying placebos, the two compared agents will still have been properly selected, but the subsequent results may be difficult to evaluate because the identity of the treatments was not suitably masked.

Yet a different type of problem arises if two active oral agents are being compared in a test of *compliance-mediated efficacy* rather than *intrinsic efficacy*. If one of the agents must be taken four times daily and the other agent is taken once daily, a double-blind trial intended to compare their intrinsic efficacy would require that the once-a-day agent be supplemented by three daily placebos. Such a design, however, would be unsatisfactory if the once-a-day agent is expected to be more effective because it leads to better compliance than the agent that must be taken four times daily. In the latter circumstance, the trial would have to be conducted with the two treatments taken in their natural dosage pattern. Although the compared agents would be suitably selected, the absence of suitable masking might create problems in evaluating the results.

The cited imperfections, which occur as a necessity in formulating a suitable comparison, should be distinguished from the contrived comparison discussed in Section 12.1.1.3. A contrived comparison is created mainly for the convenience of the investigator. For example, an investigator who is prepared to exercise suitable imagination and effort should be able to find and obtain follow-up data for a group of postmenopausal women who did not receive estrogen replacement therapy. The group need not be contrived, in "arm-chair research," from statistical data for a general population.

12.1.1.5. NO CONTROL POSSIBLE

Finally, in certain circumstances of modern technology, a suitable control group may be impossible to obtain. For example, when the heart-lung pump was first developed, its physiologic advantages were so immediately apparent that surgeons would have been ethically reluctant to conduct clinical trials in which a control group received open-heart surgery without the use of the pump.

A different kind of example occurs with efforts to evaluate the use of the Swan-Ganz (pulmonary artery) catheter that is now often employed in the management of certain types of congestive heart failure and other problems in fluid retention. The accomplishments achieved with the catheterization are often best documented with paraclinical data obtained through the catheter. Such data cannot be obtained from an uncatheterized control group because a similar catheter would not have been inserted to allow acquisition of the necessary information.

In circumstances of the types just cited, the comparison of a new maneuver may have to be conducted against an unsatisfactory historical control group. Alternatively, the focus of the evaluation can be altered so that its main objective is not to compare the new maneuver against an old maneuver. Instead, the research may be aimed at identifying the particular kinds of patients who are most likely to be benefited or harmed by the new maneuver. With this change in the objective, the maneuvers under study become the patients' clinical conditions rather than the technologic agent.

12.1.2. *Relativity of Comparison*

The relativity of a comparison refers to the kind of conclusion to be drawn from the research regarding the superiority of a maneuver and its distinctiveness.

12.1.2.1. TYPE OF SUPERIORITY

The first issue in comparison is to decide what a maneuver is to be compared against. Is it supposed to be superior (or inferior) to nothing, to an inert maneuver, or to some other active maneuver?

Cochrane[5] has introduced a somewhat confusing but useful group of terms for these distinctions. He refers to *efficacy* as the decision that a maneuver actually does something—that it "works." The appropriate comparison is against nothing or against a presumably inert maneuver, such as placebo. *Efficiency* refers to the decision that a maneuver works better (or worse) than some other active maneuver. The appropriate comparison is with a standard maneuver whose efficacy is well demonstrated or at least generally accepted.

Cochrane has also used a third term, *effectiveness,* which refers not to a comparison, but to the impact of a therapeutic agent in the community. For example, although shown to be both efficacious and efficient in clinical trials, a new treatment may be ineffective when introduced into community practice because the agent is so inconvenient, uncomfortable, or expensive that patients refuse to take it. The agent may also be ineffective because people are not motivated to maintain treatment. An example of efforts to deal with the latter problem is shown by current campaigns to improve the community usage of antihypertensive agents.

The choice of a comparative agent is crucial for making decisions about the action of a principal maneuver, and the choice involves scientific, clinical, and ethical problems that are particularly prominent in the testing of new therapeutic agents. For most clinical purposes, a new agent should be compared for efficiency against a standard active agent. Such a comparison would allow a practicing clinician to decide whether the old treatment warrants replacement by the new one. If many standard active agents are available, however, a major problem arises about which one to choose. A comparison of new agent X against old agent A will not be convincing to clinicians who regularly use agents B, C, D, or E. On the other hand, if X is to be compared against each of the existing agents, the cost of the clinical trials—to say nothing of feasibility—may be prohibitive.

A second problem in comparison with standard active agents is that the active agent may not be unequivocally efficacious or the comparison may not be conducted under suitably challenging circumstances. For example, suppose a prophylactic daily regimen of drug X is compared against a similar regimen of oral penicillin for the ability to prevent group A streptococcal infections in patients who have had rheumatic fever. If no or few infections occur in either the drug X group or the oral penicillin group, the conclusion might be that drug X has been just as efficacious as oral penicillin. On the other hand, it is possible that very few streptococcal infections took place in the community during the period in which the trial was conducted. The compared agents may have seemed equally efficacious because neither one was adequately challenged.

To eliminate both of these problems—the choice of one among many active agents and the possibility of inadequate challenges—new agents are commonly tested against placebo. In fact, the FDA in the United States usually demands placebo-controlled trials for any new therapeutic agent. The placebo acts as a standard of both comparison and efficacy. The scientific advantages of this arrangement are obvious, but it also creates clinical and ethical problems. Clinically, the practitioner who reads the published results may want to know how the new drug compares with standard treatment, not with placebo. Ethically, a great many objections (which are beyond the scope of discussion here) can be raised about the use of placebos.

12.1.2.2. INTERPRETATION OF PLACEBO RESPONSE

Although frequently discussed in both medical and nonmedical literature, the placebo response is seldom divided into its distinctively different passive, active, and psychic components. The passive component arises from the natural course of the disease under investigation. For example, in a self-limited ailment such as the common cold, most patients will be placebo responders because they will improve spontaneously after a brief period of time regardless of how they are treated and sometimes despite treatment. To refer to natural healing as a *placebo response* seems peculiar, yet the term is often used in this manner.

An active component of the placebo response is often produced by an unrecognized accompaniment of the principal maneuver. In this situation, for example, a skin lesion may be healed more by the cream in which the steroid is delivered than by the steroid itself; and a patient's diabetes mellitus may be controlled more with the dietary therapy than with the concomitant hypoglycemic agent. Other types of accompaniment that can produce the placebo response were discussed in Sections 11.9.2 and 11.9.3. These features of the accompaniment of the principal maneuver need thoughtful consideration for suitable choice of any comparative maneuver, including placebo.

The psychic component is what most people have in mind when they refer to *placebo response.* The patient may experience a sense of well-being merely by anticipating therapeutic benefit from whatever treatment is taken. This sensation can occur whether the treatment is chosen by the patient (as with over-the-counter, nonprescription medication) or by a clinician, who may also deliver it. An additional source of benefit for the patient is the iatrotherapy provided by a doctor's communication, concern, and bedside manner while the overt agent of treatment is being given. Although an important and often invaluable accompaniment of any form of clinical treatment, the role of iatrotherapy is often overlooked when therapeutic agents are evaluated. Furthermore, a suitable appraisal of iatrotherapy often requires an open acknowledgment that clinicians, like patients, can be placebo reactors.

This problem arises because the strains of a busy practice may drain or substantially reduce the enthusiasm with which a clinician is willing to make the effort needed to provide iatrotherapy. A clinician who believes the therapeutic agent is effective will often make this effort, even if the agent eventually turns out to be as worthless as some of the many later-discredited treatments that have been enthusiastically used throughout medical history. On the other hand, if the agent is regarded merely as an ineffective placebo, the clinician may not develop the self-motivation needed to evoke the accompanying iatrotherapy. Thus, as long as the agent has not been demonstrated to be ineffectual, the clinician's placebo response may produce iatrotherapy that is beneficial for the patient.

This contributory component in the total impact of clinical care is often overlooked when therapeutic agents are evaluated. A major purpose of double-blind placebo treatment is to ensure that the accompanying maneuver of iatrotherapy occurs equally in all the groups under comparison, but the full impact of clinical care may be obscured unless a "no-treatment" group is also tested.

For example, consider the following results in a hypothetical randomized clinical trial containing ample numbers of patients:

Treatment X:	68% Improvement
Placebo:	67% Improvement
No treatment:	5% Improvement

In this situation, the active treatment appeared no better than placebo, but either type of intervention (treatment X or placebo) was substantially better than no treatment at all. The results suggest that iatrotherapy produced a major improvement that failed to occur in the untreated patients. If treatment X is rejected because it is no better than placebo, and if no other treatment is available for this clinical condition, the decision will be scientifically proper, because it identifies treatment X as an apparently worthless therapeutic agent. Clinically, however, the patients who are deprived of treatment X (or its placebo) will also be deprived of the iatrotherapy that can be highly beneficial. The ethical problems associated with this decision and with other aspects of placebo therapy will be further discussed in Chapter 29.

12.1.2.3. FORMATS FOR COMPARATIVE AGENTS

The exact format of the placebo or comparative agent(s) is important for double-blind or double-masked studies, in which an attempt is made to hide the identity of the maneuver from both the patient who receives it and the person who observes and records its outcome.

If the principal maneuver is an oral medication, the comparative agent can easily be prepared in a similar oral format. For other types of maneuvers, however, the appropriate format of the contrast may be difficult or unfeasible to achieve. Some of these problems were discussed in Section 12.1.1.4. For example, if the principal maneuver is a surgical operation, can sham surgery be used as a placebo? If the principal maneuver consists of daily injections of a substance such as insulin, should the control group receive daily injections of an inert substance? If the principal maneuver is acupuncture, is a suitable placebo constructed by arranging for acupuncture needles to be inserted in the wrong sites?

A different type of problem arises if the principal maneuver must be given in an adjusted dosage, which is raised or lowered according to certain clinical or laboratory measurements of the patient's response. For example, the dose of anticoagulants is customarily regulated according to the patient's prothrombin time, and insulin is changed according to levels of blood sugar. Because the adjustment requires a knowledge of the response variable, e.g., prothrombin time, blood sugar, etc., the person who performs the adjustment cannot be kept unaware of the results or of the identity of the maneuver. To deal with this problem, the maneuvers are often given in a double-observer rather than double-blind format. One observer, who is aware of the treatments and responses, adjusts the dosage for both the active and the placebo agents. The second observer, who is kept singly blind by being unaware of the treatment, examines the patient and records the responses.

In circumstances in which the response to treatment is an overt clinical phenomenon, such as relief of pain, a double-blind mechanism for regulating the treatment regimen can be attempted by giving both the active agent and the placebo in an escalating pattern of dosage. The escalation is usually allowed to continue until some upper boundary of dosage is reached. If pain (or some other target symptom) has not been relieved at the highest dosage, the agent is regarded as a failure and other arrangements are made for the patient's treatment.

12.1.3. *Distinctions of Alternative Vs. Additive Maneuvers*

A further decision in choosing the comparative maneuver depends on whether it is to be used in an alternative or additive manner.

Two compared maneuvers are *alternative* if one can readily be substituted for the other. Thus, antacid X and antacid Y are alternative if the "winner" of their comparison would be preferred and used alone thereafter as a substitute for the "loser." Similarly, a mechanical contraceptive device and oral contraceptive pills are usually regarded as alternatives.

The compared maneuvers are *additive* if they consist of different tactics or mechanisms that do not act as alternatives for one another, and that might act together for a combined effect that is more cogent than the effect of either maneuver alone. Thus, digestive distress can be treated with an antacid, with an antispasmodic, with a histamine-receptor antagonist, with dietary regulation, or with combinations of two, three, or all of these procedures. An extraordinarily cautious person might use both mechanical and oral agents of contraception.

The choice of an additive or alternative comparison depends on the question that the research is intended to answer. If we want to know whether agent X is efficacious in treating digestive distress, the appropriate comparative maneuver would be an alternative procedure such as placebo or a known efficacious agent. If we want to know whether agent X offers the best way to treat digestive distress, the appropriate comparative maneuver might be an additive combination of agent X and some other maneuver.

The contrast of additive maneuvers creates considerable complexity in the design of the research because of the problems of assessing conjugate combinations of maneuvers as well as the individual maneuvers alone. The complexity includes the choice of appropriate combinations as well as the appropriate placebos. Suppose we want to compare an oral drug, Excellitol, against whiskey in the relief of severe headache. Because each agent presumably works in a different manner, we might also want to assess the effects of a combination of Excellitol and whiskey. To check all possible arrangements of treatment, we might have to examine many different maneuvers: Excellitol alone; whiskey alone; Excellitol and whiskey; Excellitol and whiskey placebo; Excellitol placebo and whiskey; Excellitol placebo and whiskey placebo; Excellitol placebo only; whiskey placebo only; no treatment. Because a test of many maneuvers is too complicated for practical realities and because all these maneuvers need not be tested to reach clinical conclusions, the experiment would be designed to compare only the most cogent maneuvers of the nine that have just been cited. The reduction of the nine maneuvers to a smaller but more manageable number is discussed in Exercise 12.8 at the end of this chapter.

12.1.4. *Reversibility of Maneuvers*

The reversibility of a maneuver refers to its ability to be "washed out" so that the patient can return to the baseline state at some reasonably short time after the maneuver is discontinued. For example, all of the maneuvers used in explicatory investigations of pathophysiologic phenomena are intended to be reversible. Most oral pharmaceutical agents and injections are reversible. Most surgical maneuvers and psychotherapy are *not* reversible.

The concept of reversibility becomes important in Section 12.2 when we consider the chronology of comparison. A desirable way of comparing two maneuvers (when possible) is to do a cross-over study, in which the same persons receive each maneuver. In a parallel study, the two maneuvers are compared in two different groups. In a cross-over study, there are two groups of data—one for each maneuver—but only one group of patients.

For the underlying structure of a cross-over study to be effective, two conditions must be met:

1. Each of the compared maneuvers must be reversible, so that its immediate action is gone when the next maneuver begins.

2. The underlying clinical condition must be relatively stable so that the recipient is in the same baseline state on both occasions. For example, although aspirin and chicken soup are both reversible maneuvers, they could not be used in a cross-over study of treatment for the common cold because the patient's evolving baseline condition would not necessarily be similar when each agent is begun.

12.1.5. *Simultaneous Comparison of Multiple Maneuvers*

In many well-designed scientific projects, a single principal maneuver is contrasted with a single comparative maneuver, but in certain circumstances more than two maneuvers are contrasted simultaneously. The simultaneous multiple contrast of more than two maneuvers can have major advantages and disadvantages

12.1.5.1. ADVANTAGES OF MULTIPLE MANEUVERS

The contrast of multiple maneuvers has a major advantage when the research is intended to find a "best" agent among a set of contenders, none of which appears better than any other for the intended purpose. The entire set of contenders may be tested simultaneously to determine which agents are most effective. A second advantage occurs in pharmacologic research for such activities as bioassay, in which the principal maneuver is given at different levels of dosage. A third advantage for multiple maneuvers occurs in certain probative activities. For example, suppose a maneuver such as ergometric exercise with a bicycle has been noted to produce certain responses. The objective now is to determine which aspect of the exercise is most cogent for eliciting the response: the duration of the exercise, the amount of resistance, the placement of the foot pedals, and so on. These different components can be tested separately but simultaneously as multiple maneuvers.

In *large-scale therapeutic trials,* multiple maneuvers are commonly investigated for pragmatic rather than scientific advantages. Because of the complex logistics involved in planning and carrying out a large-scale therapeutic trial, the project is not easy to repeat. The investigators may therefore try to test several different therapeutic procedures in order to gain as much information as possible. For example, in the celebrated UGDP trial[6] of hypoglycemic therapy for adult-onset diabetes mellitus, five different therapeutic regimens were contrasted simultaneously: placebo, tolbutamide, phenformin, a flexible dose of insulin, and a fixed dose of insulin.

12.1.5.2. **DISADVANTAGES OF MULTIPLE MANEUVERS**

In exchange for these advantages, the contrast of multiple maneuvers has some major drawbacks. The first arises from the problem of *similarity in baseline state.* If the maneuvers can be applied to standardized animals, to identical human twins, or repetitively to the same people, the problems of attaining a similar baseline state in the contrasted groups are minimized. Thus, in using animals to screen pharmaceutical agents, or in using the same people repetitively for pharmacologic or probative maneuvers, the investigator can often be reassured that each maneuver is applied to individuals who are similar in the baseline state. In many studies of remedial or prophylactic therapy, however, this assurance is seldom possible because the same people cannot be tested repetitively, and parallel groups must be created for each treatment. The greater the dispersion of the population into different therapeutic groups, the greater is the likelihood of major disparities in the baseline states of the groups.

The second problem, which is often more difficult than the first, is the *evaluation of multiple targets in the outcome state.* If only a single target variable (or event) is under appraisal, its response to multiple maneuvers can readily be appraised. For example, we can readily determine whether serum cholesterol level, as the main focus of the outcome, was most reduced by drug U, V, W, X, Y, or Z. If more than one outcome variable is under appraisal, however, certain value judgments must be applied to give weights to the different responses, and each maneuver may rank differently for these different responses. Thus, drug X may rank 1st in relieving symptoms, 3rd in reducing cholesterol, 1st in high number of adverse side effects, 4th in ease of maintenance, and 1st in high cost. If only two maneuvers are under study—such as deciding whether drug X is better than drug Y—the comparison of multiple target variables is not too difficult. We can arrive at an overall judgment by considering the importance of each of the different responses and ascribing different weights or trade-off values to them. Thus, although drug Y may not relieve symptoms quite as well as drug X, drug Y may be preferred because it has fewer side effects, is easier to take, and is cheaper.

If multiple maneuvers are contrasted for multiple outcomes, however, the creation of these judgmental weights can be formidable. For example, is relief of symptoms more important than cost? Is avoidance of side effects more important than relief of symptoms? To answer such questions, we have to consider not just two sets of multiple ranks in the responses, but three, four, or more such sets. The common sense judgments that can be used in contrasting multiple ranks for two maneuvers become obscured by the complexity of data encountered when multiple maneuvers have diverse ranks for multiple targets.

A separate problem in multiple comparisons occurs when tests of statistical significance are applied to the results. Assuming that significance is proclaimed when the P value found in the test is below a standard α level of 0.05, we have 1 chance in 20 of getting a falsely positive significant difference in a contrast of two treatments, X and Y, that are really equivalent. If the comparison contains four treatments—W, X, Y, and Z—there are six possible pairs of contrasts: W versus X, W versus Y, W versus Z, X versus Y, and so on. If each of those six contrasts is also conducted at an α level of 0.05, our chance of getting a false positive result among the tests, if all four treatments are equivalent, becomes elevated to about 1 in 3. [This is calculated as $\{1-(1-0.05)^6\} = 1-0.74 = 0.36$.] To avoid this problem, special statistical strategies are used to adjust the α level downward when multiple comparisons are conducted. These strategies increase the complexity of the statistical activities and usually reduce the comprehensibility of the results.

The need for examining only a single target variable is a major scientific advantage of laboratory research. In clinical epidemiology, and particularly in health care research, an array of different outcome variables must often be evaluated. To simplify the problems, many research projects are designed (when possible and feasible) so that a single principal maneuver is contrasted with a single control maneuver.

12.2. CHRONOLOGY OF COMPARISON

Concepts of time can be used in at least five different ways in the architecture of research. The first and most obvious usage refers to the time elapsed since each person's birth. This is occasionally called *life time* or *generation time,* although the simplest word is *age.* The second usage, which was discussed in Section 2.2.4, refers to a *temporal direction.* The people under investigation may have been examined cross-sectionally at a single point in time or followed forward in time longitudinally. The other three usages of time are discussed in the rest of this section. They refer to the timing of data collection, the calendar dates of events, and the serial landmarks in a person's clinical course.

12.2.1. *Retrolective and Prolective Studies*

Arrangements for collecting the data used in research may be made before or after the actual occurrence of the events described by the data. If the research is planned before the maneuvers are imposed, the investigator can develop special techniques, formats, or other procedures that are deliberately aimed at collecting high quality data for the investigation. Experimental research, such as a randomized clinical trial, is always conducted in this manner (although the investigators may sometimes have to go back later to assemble information that was originally overlooked).

In many other research circumstances, however, the investigation is not planned until after the main events have occurred. The data used in the research are obtained from information that was routinely entered in such archives as medical records, college health records, state health departments, tumor registries, etc. For example, patients' medical records are the customary starting point for most published cohort surveys of treatment and for most case-control studies of the etiology of disease.

We need some new terms to describe this third type of temporal distinction, which occurs in the time relationship between the imposition of maneuvers and the collection of research data. The words *prospective* and *retrospective* are often used to distinguish the difference between advance plans for obtaining the data and plans that are developed afterward, but the usage is ambiguous because the same words are also often applied for a different type of temporal distinction, in direction of observations. Thus, *prospective* may also refer to the forward, longitudinal direction in which people are followed in a cohort study; and *retrospective* may also refer to the backward direction in which the "follow-up" occurs in an etiologic case-control study. Because scientific language should avoid rather than create ambiguity, the use of *prospective* and *retrospective* for two different sets of ideas is particularly unattractive. To eliminate the ambiguity, the straightforward terms *prolective* and *retrolective* can be used to distinguish the timing of collection for the research data.

To illustrate the problem, suppose we want to compare the subsequent four years of growth and development for bottle-fed versus breast-fed babies who were born at Yale–New Haven Hospital during 1979. The study is obviously *prospective* in direction, because a cohort of children will be followed forward in time from birth. On the other hand, the study can be conducted in at least two different ways. In one way, the plans for the study are made before 1979. Starting in 1979, we arrange to monitor each birth and to observe each child thereafter, using special arrangements to follow the children and to collect data about their subsequent feeding patterns and their outcome state four years later in 1983. In the second approach, we decide to do the study in 1984. Using medical records and other compendia of information, we identify each child born during 1979, we determine whether each child was breast-fed or bottle-fed, and we try to learn the status of each child in 1983.

With both of these approaches, we would be performing a prospectively directed cohort study, following the same group of children and collecting data about the same kinds of phenomena. The collection of data, however, would be prospective in the first approach and retrospective in the second. To avoid having two different meanings for *prospective* and to eliminate such jarring phrases as *prospective prospective study* and *retrospective prospective study*, a different set of terms is necessary. The word *prospective* can be eliminated entirely and replaced by *cohort* to refer to a forward-directed longitudinal study. The terms *prolective* and *retrolective* can then be used in reference to the plans made for assembling the groups under study and collecting the data. Thus, the two studies of newborn children described in the previous paragraph could be described with the terms *prolective cohort* and *retrolective cohort*. (In the alternative phrases used by other writers, the word *prospective* is often reserved for a study that is doubly prospective in both direction and data, i.e., a prolective cohort. Such writers will then use *historical prospective, historical cohort,* or *retrospective cohort* for what is here called a *retrolective cohort.*)

12.2.2. *Secular Time and Serial Time*

The fourth type of temporal distinction, *secular time,* would be more rapidly understood and would not contain any religious connotations if it were called *calendar time.* It refers to the actual dates, noted on the calendar, when the research was being performed or when the maneuvers under observation were imposed. When changes in the annual occurrence or mortality rates of disease are noted over a long period of calendar time, the observed results are often called *secular trends.*

Serial Time, which is the fifth type of temporal distinction, refers to the time elapsed in a particular person's clinical course before or after the zero-time imposition of the maneuver under investigation. The point at which the maneuver is imposed is usually chosen to be *zero time,* but other points in serial time may sometimes be chosen because of various distinctions in the research. For example, if the maneuver under study is the pathodynamic or pathogressive effect of a particular disease, the exact time of onset of the disease can seldom be determined, and so zero time may be chosen to be the date of first diagnosis.

In a randomized trial, zero time can be either the moment at which the maneuver was randomly assigned or the moment at which it was imposed. The distinction is important for subsequent analysis of the data. For example, in a randomized trial of medical versus surgical therapy, the medical treatment is usually begun immediately as soon as the randomized assignment is noted. The assigned surgical operation, however, may not be scheduled to occur until several days later, during which time the patient may die or may change his mind about accepting the surgery, so that the operation is not actually performed. A major problem may then arise, as discussed in Chapter 29, about whether to include or exclude the latter patients when results of the surgical group are analyzed.

A different type of problem occurs in a randomized trial of treatment for a clinical condition whose exact identity cannot be determined until after treatment has begun. For example, if we want to test a particular antimicrobial agent in the treatment of an acute staphylococcal pneumonia, we would not want to delay the treatment until bacterial cultures have confirmed the identity of the infecting organism. In this circumstance, the candidate patients can be admitted to the trial, randomization can be conducted, and the compared maneuvers can be administered at zero time, but the patients who do not qualify because their bacterial cultures fail to demonstrate staphylococci would later be "de-admitted" from the trial.

Another type of problem occurs in studies of etiologic maneuvers that were self-selected by the recipients. The exact date of onset can seldom be determined for such maneuvers as cigarette smoking or high-fat diets, and furthermore, the people included in a cohort study of such maneuvers are usually assembled long after each maneuver was first imposed. In addition to these difficulties in choosing an appropriate zero time for members of the group exposed to the principal maneuver, the investigator must choose a zero time for the comparative unexposed group. This decision involves answering such questions as: When did a nonsmoker begin not to smoke? The problems created by these distinctions will be discussed in Chapter 17.

Regardless of how zero time is chosen, the baseline state, or zero state, will be the person's clinical condition at that moment. The events that preceded zero state will have occurred in the *prezero interval* and the subsequent events in the *postzero interval*. Thus, if zero time is the date at which treatment was imposed, we can measure the pretreatment duration of certain manifestations, such as abdominal pain or an abnormal chest x-ray. We can also measure the post-treatment interval at which certain events, such as success or death, occurred.

All of these different kinds of time can enter into the architecture of a research project. The following statement contains an example of an investigative structure that makes use of all five chronologic concepts: "In a retrolective cohort study, performed from 1973 to 1975, we found that the 5-year survival rate of elderly people with disease D had sharply increased during the two decades from 1949 to 1969." In this statement, the "elderly" refers to the timing of age; the "cohort" denotes temporal direction; the "retrolective" indicates the time of research data collection; the "5-year survival rate" is an entity of serial time; and the calendar dates of 1973 to 1975 and 1949 to 1969 refer to secular time.

When two maneuvers are being compared in an experiment, certain chronologic problems need not be considered. By virtue of the architecture used in an experiment, the maneuvers are almost always tested under similar circumstances for both secular and serial time. In a survey, however, this aspect of equality in the comparison cannot be taken for granted. The maneuvers may have been concomitant in neither serial time nor secular time.

12.2.3. *Concurrent Maneuvers and Inception Cohorts*

Two maneuvers are compared concurrently if they are tested during the same secular interval and imposed at the same point in serial time for the treated condition. This concurrency is readily attained in experiments in which a *parallel* comparison is arranged for the groups who receive the maneuvers. Concurrency of maneuvers is not always achieved, however, in surveys. For example, a "dys-serial" comparison occurs if patients who are receiving chemotherapy as a second or third course of treatment for a cancer are contrasted against patients whose radiotherapy was a first course.

A "dys-secular" comparison occurs if the results of a new therapeutic agent for condition C are contrasted with the results obtained several years earlier with an older agent. This type of "dys-secularity" is an inevitable feature of the use of historical control groups. Such comparisons have two main hazards. The first hazard is that secular changes may have occurred in diagnosis, so that the most recent treatment is given to patients with milder or earlier diagnosed diseases than before. The second hazard arises from ancillary accompaniments to the main therapy. Thus, secular improvements in the postsurgical survival of patients with a variety of diseases may be due to better anesthesia, availability of better antibiotics, and use of improved postoperative recovery-room monitoring, rather than better techniques of surgery itself.

Another aspect of concurrency refers to place rather than time. Even though two maneuvers, A and B, are compared with similar features of secular and serial time, the rest of the comparison may be unfair if maneuver A is given exclusively to persons in institution A or region A, and if maneuver B is given exclusively to persons in institution B or region B. Because of differences in the institutions or regions, the persons assembled for the comparison may be different in their baseline states and in subsequent features of the comparison. To avoid all these problems in nonconcurrency, the maneuvers in an observational cohort study should be investigated in an *inception cohort* of people who are similar in serial time, in secular time, and in place where the compared maneuvers were imposed.

12.2.4. *Successive Alternative (Cross-over) Maneuvers*

In certain experimental situations, often called *cross-over trials,* each or most of the compared maneuvers are tested successively and alternatively in each participating subject. The great appeal of such designs is that the members of the compared groups are essentially identical, thus eliminating the vicissitudes of the different people who are compared when the maneuvers are contrasted in parallel. (An additional appeal is the opportunity to plan the cross-overs with the Latin, Greco-Latin, Youden, and other squares that are often the focus of attention in statistical approaches to experimental design.)

The main problem with cross-over studies is that they allow us to compare the same people, but we really want to compare the same baseline states. If a person receives treatment X for two weeks and is then crossed over to treatment Y, we must be assured that he has the same baseline state at the inception of both treatments. Otherwise the comparison of results may be improper. Two different types of hazard—serial changes and carry-over effects—can create changes in the initial states that are successively compared.

12.2.4.1. **SERIAL CHANGE IN BASIC CONDITION**

During the course of treatment X, the patient's clinical condition may have changed so that he is in a substantially different state when treatment Y begins. For example, if we want to give drug A for 10 days, followed by drug B for 10 days, to compare relief of symptoms of a cold in a cross-over trial, we may find that the patient no longer has any symptoms after the first 10 days.

For this reason, cross-over trials have an extremely limited set of pertinent clinical applications. The trials can generally be used only in testing the short-term effects of pharmaceutical agents in healthy people, in situations in which a chronic disease has a stable level of activity, and in conditions in which a recurrent manifestation appears consistently. Examples of such conditions are menstrual cramps, uncomplicated angina pectoris, and pain or disability in osteoarthritis. Even in these conditions, however, the relief or prevention of pain by one therapeutic agent may have an important psychic effect that may carry over into the action of the next therapeutic agent. Thus, a patient who has become intensely depressed by chronic pain may become so exhilarated by its relief that the exhilaration may transiently mask the subsequent return of the painful stimulus.

12.2.4.2. CARRY-OVER EFFECTS

The cited type of carry-over effect is the second major problem that can impair the propriety of a cross-over design from one agent to another. The carry-over effect may be pharmacologic, occurring because the first agent has not yet been excreted, or psychologic, occurring because of a sustained psychic effect lasting longer than the period of direct pharmacologic action. For these reasons, a wash-out period, in which the patient receives a placebo or no treatment, is often used between the successive maneuvers administered in a cross-over trial.

12.2.5. *Zero-time Choices in Retrolective Cohort Studies*

The choice of zero time is a particularly important feature in retrolective cohort studies. In an experimental trial, zero time is established by the investigator and is usually the date of randomization or the onset of the randomized therapy. In most prolective studies, zero time is also easily determined as the date when an eligible person begins the maneuver under observation. In a retrolective study, however, the investigator begins with archival data—often a patient's complete medical record—that may contain an account of the patient's entire medical lifetime. From the many events noted in that record, the investigator must choose a zero-time date that serves two major purposes. The choice is used first to convert the recorded secular time, which is the calendar date at which events actually occurred, into a serial time that denotes a suitable chronology for the prezero and postzero occurrences in the patients' clinical course. The choice of zero time also demarcates the *zero-state* condition, which will be the baseline state for which the patient is admitted, classified, and analyzed in the research.

To help keep bias out of the research and to allow the results to approximate what would have been found in an experimental trial, the zero-state condition should be catalogued only according to the information that was actually clinically available at zero time. For example, a patient's medical record will often contain reports of evidence that was clinically discovered after zero time and that would alter the designation or interpretation of the zero-state phenomena. Because such evidence would not have been available when the patient was admitted to a randomized trial at zero time, the evidence should *not* be used in classifying the patient's zero state. If the evidence would require de-admission of the patient or other special analytic procedures, the procedures should be employed in the same way as they might have been used in a randomized trial.

Some of the subtle decisions involved in choosing a suitable zero time are presented in Exercise 12.6 at the end of the chapter.

12.3. ALLOCATION OF MANEUVERS

The main groups under comparison in a cohort study are usually designated by the names of the maneuvers they received. Thus, we can refer to the surgical and medical groups in a trial of treatment for coronary disease, or to the takers and nontakers in a survey of the adverse effects attributed to oral contraceptive pills. Because membership in these groups is created when the maneuvers are imposed, the allocation of maneuvers is so fundamental a constituent of research architecture that the research is called an *experiment* or *survey* according to the method used for allocation.

The allocation usually takes place when the maneuvers are assigned (by a clinician) or self-selected by the recipient (as in a person's decision to smoke cigarettes or in a patient's decision to refuse treatment). In an experiment, the investigator can establish a specific research plan for allocating the compared maneuvers. In a survey, the allocation occurs in an *ad hoc* manner, and the investigator must identify the maneuvers that were employed.

The groups whose maneuvers are compared in a longitudinal research project are seldom assembled directly as groups. Instead, the maneuvers are successively assigned to, or determined for, different individual people. At some point during or after the sequence of assignments or determinations, we assemble the people who received each maneuver and call them a *group*. Thus, the "treatment A group" would be created as the array of people who, during a particular secular interval, successively received treatment A.

Because of the judgmental decisions that are involved, the selection of the maneuver is a prime source of distortion (or bias) in the comparison of postmaneuveral results. The allocations may have been conducted in a manner that assigned the good-risk people to one maneuver and the poor risks to another. Having major differences in baseline susceptibility, the two groups cannot be fairly compared thereafter, because differences in their outcomes may be due to baseline inequalities, not to effects of the maneuvers.

One of the main virtues of an experiment is that randomization can be used to prevent this source of bias. Within the limits of chance and the luck of the draw, a randomized allocation of maneuvers allows each eligible recipient an equal opportunity to be assigned to each of the maneuvers under investigation. (Randomization is also usually lauded for having the virtue of allowing the quantitative results to be tested for stochastic contrasts that rely on an unbiased allocation of maneuvers. This virtue does not appear to be a statistical necessity, however, because the same stochastic tests are regularly and uninhibitedly applied to survey data in which the maneuvers were allocated selectively without randomization.)

12.3.1. *Allocation in Surveys*

In a survey, the maneuver must be ascertained for each person under investigation. This activity may be difficult if the maneuver was started or completed before the survey began. In retrolective research, the ascertainment depends on the previously recorded data regarding such maneuvers as therapy, smoking history, dietary patterns, and so on. In prolective research, the ascertainment often depends on the reliability of the patient, but may also require the use of previously recorded data.

In addition to all the other forms of criteria (discussed later) that are necessary to define baseline states and outcomes, a separate set of criteria is usually necessary to define what is to be regarded as a maneuver. For example, how many cigarettes per day and what duration of usage are necessary to call someone a *cigarette smoker*? What kind of nutritional intake pattern is required, and for how long, to be cited as a *high-fat diet*? Does the designation of *simple surgical resection* apply to a patient who received no other therapy after his cancer of the rectum was removed as an excisional biopsy?

A tricky problem in retrolective surveys of prognosis and treatment for a particular disease is the decision about what to call the principal maneuver. The archival data that describe the patient's entire clinical course may describe many available candidates from which to choose. For example, in a patient with lung cancer who initially refuses thoracotomy and then begins to receive radiotherapy two years later, what should be called the principal maneuver: the refused surgical resection or the accepted radiotherapy? If, after initially refusing the thoracotomy, the patient accepts a surgical resection that is carried out two years later, which date should be called zero time: the refusal or acceptance of the surgical resection? These and other difficult decisions are usually resolved by reviewing the basic objective of the research, by clearly specifying the questions to be answered in the research, and by choosing the option that provides the best answer. Thus, in a study of prognostic features for the clinical course and outcome of lung cancer, the date of the patient's refusal of thoracotomy might be chosen as zero time. In a study of the specific consequences that follow different treatments, the principal maneuvers would be the treatments that were actually administered.

In noncohort investigations, such as the case-control studies discussed in Chapter 23, the maneuvers must be ascertained as "outcome data" in the people initially selected as cases or controls. The ascertainment process creates many problems, reserved for discussion later, that are not present in cohort studies.

12.3.2. *Allocation in Experiments*

The great appeal of an experiment is that it permits the investigator to assign the maneuvers. With this opportunity, the investigator can arrange for such strategies as randomization, balancing, proportional assignments, and stratification.

The detailed techniques used for these activities will be described in Chapter 16. For the moment, we can note that *randomization* consists of assigning treatment by a chance mechanism that allows all potential recipients an equal opportunity of being selected. Although randomization can be conducted by tossing a coin or by drawing from an appropriately arranged deck of playing cards, the standard procedure is to have a randomization schedule generated from an appropriate computer program or table of random numbers.

The randomization is *balanced* when the schedule is constrained to assign equal numbers of people to each of the maneuvers under comparison. (If the assignment is conducted without this constraint, the luck of the draw might assign seven of the first 10 people to treatment A and three to treatment B. In the long run, if many people are admitted to the study, the numbers assigned to each treatment should become similar, but in a relatively small study, they may be substantially unbalanced.) The balancing is obtained with use of a *balancing interval*. Thus, in a comparison of two treatments, if six is chosen to be the balancing interval, three of every six successive patients will randomly be assigned treatment A and three will be assigned treatment B. In certain circumstances, the balancing interval may be as small as two. To avoid bias, the investigator should be kept unaware of the size of the selected balancing interval.

Proportional assignments can be used to create a deliberately unbalanced assignment of the compared maneuvers. For this purpose, the randomization schedule may be arranged to let half the patients receive placebo, with the other half being divided between two active treatments—A and B. In some other study, one third of the patients might be given placebo, with the other two thirds assigned to active treatment C.

In a *complete randomization,* the treatments are assigned without regard to the clinical location or condition of the patients. In a *stratified randomization* (which statisticians often call a *block randomization*), the patients are first divided into groups, called *strata,* and a separate randomization schedule is prepared for each stratum. The purpose of the stratified randomization is to ensure that the treatments are equally divided within each stratum.

The strata may be demarcated according to the good or poor prognostic expectations of the patients under study, the accompanying maneuvers, the sites of the research, or combinations of these features. In a cooperative clinical trial, in which several different institutions collaborate and pool their results, the randomization is usually stratified at least for each institution.

An example of hazards in the luck of the draw is a complete randomization of 32 patients that produced a balanced assignment of 16 patients to each of treatments A and B, but the 16 patients in treatment A included 10 people with good prognosis and six with poor prognosis, whereas the group assigned to treatment B comprised five with good prognosis and 11 with poor prognosis. This type of undesirable prognostic imbalance can be avoided with a stratified randomization. Because a stratified randomization may be cumbersome to do, or because the appropriate prognostic characteristics may not be well identified before the trial begins, the treatments may be assigned with complete randomization, but the subsequent results may be "post-stratified" for analysis within groups whose characteristics are demarcated after the trial is completed.

Randomization, although the most popular and generally accepted procedure today, is not the only method of experimentally assigning the maneuvers in a clinical trial. They can be allocated according to various other strategies—labeled with such names as *minimization, play-the-winner,* and so on—that are further discussed in Chapters 16 and 29.

12.3.3. *Diagrams for Allocation of Maneuvers*

As shown in Section 4.1, the standard diagram for contrasting maneuver A with a comparative maneuver B would be as follows:

$$\text{BASELINE} \quad \left\{ \begin{array}{c} \xrightarrow{\ \ A\ \ } \\ \xrightarrow{\ \ B\ \ } \end{array} \right\} \quad \text{OUTCOME}$$
$$\text{STATE}$$

A special symbol, (R), can be introduced to show randomization so that the diagram becomes

$$\text{BASELINE} \underline{\quad} (R) \overset{A}{\underset{B}{\Big\langle}} \left. \begin{array}{c} \longrightarrow \\ \longrightarrow \end{array} \right\} \quad \text{OUTCOME}$$
$$\text{STATE}$$

This diagram shows a parallel randomized comparison for the two maneuvers, A and B. The maneuvers under parallel contrast are sometimes called the *arms* of the trial.

In a cross-over study, randomization determines the sequence of which maneuver, A or B, is received first. The cross-over can be depicted as follows:

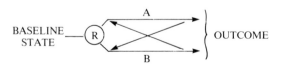

A stratified parallel randomized trial containing three maneuvers and two prognostic strata could be shown as follows:

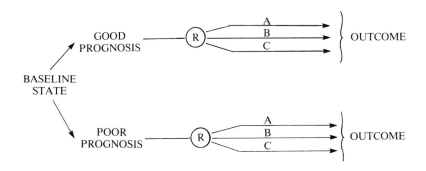

12.4. SYNOPSIS

When decisions are made about choosing a comparison maneuver, the investigator should be aware of circumstances in which the comparison is unnecessary, necessarily imperfect, or impossible. The investigator should also beware of the scientific hazards associated with the appealing convenience of using historical or contrived control groups.

The actual choice of the comparative maneuver depends on whether the comparison is intended to show the principal maneuver's efficacy in being better than nothing or its efficiency in being superior to other active maneuvers. When a placebo is used for studies of efficacy, the placebo response should be divided into its active, passive, and psychic components, and the psychic components should be separated according to their source in the responding patient or clinician. The compared maneuvers are alternative if one would customarily be substituted for the other, and additive if they might both be used for a combined action. Additive combinations must be considered when the investigator searches for a best treatment rather than for an efficacious or efficient treatment. The simultaneous comparison of multiple maneuvers can be logistically advantageous in a large-scale complex clinical trial, but has many scientific (and statistical) disadvantages when multiple outcome events must be appraised for each maneuver.

The chronology of comparison contains five major temporal distinctions: the age of the investigated persons; the longitudinal or cross-sectional directions in which the people are followed; the prolective or retrolective arrangements used for collecting the research data; the secular timing of calendar dates of events; and the serial time that can precede or follow the zero-time imposition of the maneuver in each person's clinical course. The choice of zero time can be difficult if the maneuver is an etiologic or pathodynamic rather than a therapeutic agent, or if a therapeutic maneuver is to be chosen retrolectively from all the candidates available in the archival data that describe a person's complete clinical course. To avoid bias, maneuvers should be compared concurrently in an inception cohort of people who are similar in serial time, secular time, and place where the maneuvers were imposed. Therapeutic maneuvers can be employed in successive alternative (or cross-over) patterns if the patients do not undergo a serial change in their basic condition and if each maneuver has reversible effects that can be washed out before the next maneuver begins.

The groups of people who are associated with each maneuver under investigation in a survey were created as the maneuvers were allocated successively during the individual decisions made by clinicians or by recipients of the maneuvers. To avoid the biases that can be produced by these decisions, maneuvers (when possible) can be allocated experimentally with a randomization schedule that allows each potential recipient an equal opportunity to receive the maneuvers under comparison. The randomization may be constrained to yield a balanced assignment of equal numbers for each treatment or a deliberately unbalanced assignment for the proportions of patients receiving the different treatments. The randomization is often stratified so that treatments can be balanced according to institutional locations, prognostic features of the patients, or other important clinical attributes that may not be equitably assigned if a complete randomization is done without attention to the pertinent strata.

EXERCISES

Exercise 12.1. Indicate the comparative maneuver(s), if any, that you would want to use for research projects intended to reach the following conclusions.

12.1.1. Treatment with Excellitol is the best way to prevent weekend hangovers.

12.1.2. With appropriate surgical techniques, a traumatically severed limb can be successfully rejoined.

12.1.3. People who stop smoking live longer and develop fewer smoking-related diseases than people who continue to do so.

12.1.4. Lung cancer can be caused by pumping cigarette smoke into the trachea of beagle dogs.

12.1.5. The respiratory distress syndrome is particularly likely to develop in premature children delivered by cesarean section.

12.1.6. People who eat a high-fat diet are particularly prone to develop coronary artery disease.

12.1.7. Gargling with Xanadine shortens the duration of symptoms in people with sore throats.

12.1.8. It is very expensive to provide medical care for elderly people living in an old-age home.

12.1.9. It is beneficial to perform Pap smears for early detection of cancer of the cervix or uterus.

12.1.10. People with congestive heart failure who are treated with digitalis and diuretics have an excessively long duration of hospitalization.

12.1.11. Replacement of the hip joint with a prosthesis is an effective treatment for patients whose fractured hip has been shattered or failed to heal after an injury.

Exercise 12.2. Which of the 11 projects cited in Exercise 12.1 can be well performed with a cross-over design for the maneuvers? In which project(s) is there a substantial risk of distortion due to performance of a conditional maneuver?

Exercise 12.3. A randomized clinical trial has been conducted to determine the value of daily oral penicillin prophylaxis in preventing recurrences of group A streptococcal infections in children and adolescents who have had rheumatic fever. The control group received a daily regimen of oral sulfadiazine, because the long-term use of a placebo was regarded as ethically improper in such patients. At the end of the study, the attack rates of streptococcal infections are found to be similar in both groups of patients, and the investigators are worried about the virulence of the streptococci that challenged the two regimens. Without starting a new study, what can the investigators do to help convince themselves that either agent or both was indeed efficacious?

Exercise 12.4. For a six-month period in 1970, the manufacturers of Bayer aspirin advertised on television that "Bayer is better" than other aspirins. The advertising was then discontinued by the marketing executives, replaced by some other campaign, and has not been resumed. The original claim was based on pharmacokinetic data showing that Bayer aspirin had fewer disintegration-chemical impurities, was more soluble, and produced higher blood levels than the 223 competing brands of aspirin. Although Bayer was first among the 223 competitors in the ranking of each of these three features, the quantitative magnitude of the differences was quite small. The Federal Trade Commission, trying to preserve truth in advertising, later contended that Bayer was not justified in claiming it was "better," because the evidence was pharmacologic rather than therapeutic. The FTC wanted Bayer to conduct therapeutic trials to demonstrate its superiority. In the absence of such trials, the FTC wanted Bayer (in 1980) to present retrospective corrective advertising to warn the public of the previous deception. Because Bayer refused to do so, the matter became legally disputed and adjudicated. *Briefly* outline the arguments you would offer if you were testifying on behalf of Bayer or on behalf of the FTC. What decision would you make as the judge?

Exercise 12.5. An investigator suspects that workers in steel mills are harmed by their exposure to the furnaces, fumes, and heat of their occupation. From records kept at a large mill, he assembles a retrolective cohort of exposed workers and determines their survival rate 10 years later. For comparison, using records of the state health department, he notes the 10-year survival rate of people for the same secular era and having similar age and gender in the same region where the steel mill was located. At the end of the study, the investigator is shocked to discover that the exposed workers had a *higher* survival rate than the comparison group. What do you think may have been wrong with the study?

Exercise 12.6. You are going to use hospital medical records and other archival data to perform each of the following retrolective cohort studies. For each study, indicate the date that you would choose as zero time in the clinical course of each pertinent person admitted to the study. If you chose this date against a cogent alternative candidate, briefly give the reasons.

   12.6.1. Development of a new predictive staging system to determine the likelihood that major problems, requiring care of the child in a newborn special care unit, will occur at the time of delivery.
   12.6.2. Development of a new staging system to classify infants in a newborn special care unit for their prognostic risks for (a) survival beyond first year of life and (b) survival with high-quality life.
   12.6.3. A staging system to help in comparing the merits of radical versus simple surgery versus nonsurgical treatment in patients with lung cancer.
   12.6.4. Comparison of medical versus surgical therapy in patients with angina pectoris.
   12.6.5. A study of the impact of baseline co-morbidity (previous heart failure, stroke, etc.) on the long-term outcome of hospitalized adults with recently diagnosed diabetes mellitus.
   12.6.6. Impact of good versus nongood regulation of blood glucose in adults with recently diagnosed diabetes mellitus.

12.6.7. Impact of serum pepsinogen level, noted during a screening test on entrance to college, in predisposing freshman college students to subsequent development of peptic ulcer.

12.6.8. Effect of sickle cell trait (versus its absence) on growth and development of black children.

12.6.9. Outcome of care in patients with sore throats when care is given by nurse practitioner versus M.D.

12.6.10. Development of a staging system for evaluating the effect of psychotropic agents in allowing schizophrenic patients to leave state hospitals for satisfactory activities in the community.

Exercise 12.7. A particular disease is so rare that only about two or three cases are seen each year at major medical centers. Several such centers have arranged to do a cooperative randomized trial, testing new treatment X against the standard old treatment. Patients with the disease can be well demarcated into fair and poor prognostic categories. The collaborating investigators have asked your help in preparing a randomization schedule for the trial. What type of randomization would you recommend?

Exercise 12.8. In Section 12.1.3, we noted nine different formats for the regimens that might be used in comparing Excellitol against whiskey in relieving severe headaches. An investigator to whom you suggested this design complains that it contained too many regimens, and refuses to divide the patients into nine groups. What would you offer instead as a format that would have fewer regimens while still giving a suitable answer to the basic question?

Exercise 12.9. Find any longitudinal study in any subject in which you are interested. The study, which should contain a comparison of at least two maneuvers, can be a survey or an experimental trial. After indicating the basic outline of the study, note whether you detect any flaws in the potency, accompaniment, relativity, or chronology of the maneuvers under comparison. The study you choose should preferably deal with a complex clinical condition rather than a relatively simple problem (such as relief of toothache); and you are more likely to encounter "juicy" flaws if you choose a survey rather than a trial, although you may find appropriate defects if you choose a trial whose results are known to be controversial.

CHAPTER REFERENCES

1. McBride, 1961; 2. Hoover, 1976; 3. Dimond, 1960; 4. Cobb, 1959; 5. Cochrane, 1972; 6. University Group Diabetes Program, 1970.

Suitability of Variables

At this point in the model of reasoning used for a cause-effect research study, we have finished thinking about most of the major points in the basic architecture. We have outlined the objective of the research by citing the baseline state, principal maneuver, and outcome. We have determined the comparative maneuver and method of allocating maneuvers; and we have carefully considered the suitability, i.e., proficiency, of each of the compared maneuvers.

Having noted these basic conceptual elements, the reviewer of a completed project can proceed to examine what actually occurred and can begin a judgmental evaluation of the results. If the project is still being planned, however, an important step remains to be considered. The baseline state and outcome event(s) have been identified as basic components in the research, but the identification was quite coarse. The baseline state may have been cited as *coronary disease, schizophrenia,* or *severely ill*; and the outcome may have been cited as *success, fall in serum cholesterol,* or *relief of pain*—but we do not yet know what is meant by these entities.

We may have a good idea of what *coronary disease* is, but we have not yet indicated what particular kind of coronary disease is to be included in the research. The general concept of *success* is readily understood and always pleasing, but the attributes that will create success for people admitted to this project are still unidentified. At this stage in the research design, therefore, we need additional specifications for the entities selected as the baseline state and outcome(s) in the research. The concern at this point is still with conceptual strategy rather than implemental tactics. Thus, if we learn that *success* will be defined as a disappearance of symptoms, we know what the investigator basically has in mind as the focus of the outcome event, but we do not yet know the exact tactics that will be used for examining patients and determining that symptoms have disappeared. We shall consider those tactics later, when we contemplate the implementation of the research strategy, but at least we now know the selected outcome event.

The additional specifications for the baseline state and outcome events have three important roles. First, they identify the particular phenomena on which the observations will focus. The selection of a focus is always valuable for letting an investigator or reviewer know where intellectual energy is to be concentrated. Second, the focal observations will be expressed in variables. The measurement of these variables will be a prime topic of attention later when the tactical methods of the research are selected, implemented, and appraised. Third, the focal phenomena and variables can be promptly evaluated to determine the suitability of the baseline state and outcome.

For example, if the investigator decides to identify coronary disease via the routine performance of coronary arteriography in *all* patients under study, this decision may make the selected form of coronary disease quite suitable as a baseline state for a clinical trial of medical versus surgical therapy, but quite unsuitable as an outcome event in a prophylactic trial of multiple risk factor intervention for large numbers of relatively healthy people. As another example, if success is defined as a disappearance of symptoms, the selected outcome may be quite suitable for a study of remedial therapy with analgesic agents, but not for a study of oncologic agents intended to eliminate morphologic manifestations of cancer.

The rest of this chapter is concerned with the choice of entities and variables that are used to specify the focus of the baseline state and outcome events. An additional set of variables, describing the performance of the maneuvers, must also be considered, because the desired proficiency of the maneuvers cannot be assessed unless we examine the actual way in which they were conducted. This attention to the suitability of variables is needed to ensure that the stated components of the objective will indeed emerge as the achieved goals of the research. The specific methods used to measure those variables will be discussed later, as part of the implementation of the research. Our main concern now is with certain general ideas and principles that can encourage, impede, or divert the pursuit of the desired goals.

13.1. **PROBLEMS OF MENSURATION**

In Chapter 6, we learned about the challenges of measuring clinical phenomena and expressing the results in suitable scales. The main discussion now is for problems that arise when an available system of mensuration does not seem satisfactory.

If attractive methods do not exist for collecting information about certain desired variables, what should the investigator do? Should those variables be omitted? Should some other variables be chosen instead? Should the research be delayed until attractive methods are developed? Should the main research be started anyhow, with additional research undertaken to develop attractive methods concomitantly? Should data about the desired entities be collected and stored with the hope that suitable scales and analytic systems will be developed later?

For example, suppose an investigator wants to know the impact of a particular intervention on the patient's quality of life and family relationships. If no standardized rating scale exists for recording a single state or transitional changes in these two outcome variables, the investigator must decide what to do about them. This decision, which occurs at the level of architectural implementation, has consequences that may extend back to the earlier outline of the basic objective. Thus, suppose the investigator decides these two variables are too difficult to measure. If they are replaced with patient's income and medical costs as easily measured variables, the originally desired outcome events will have been altered from a human quality to a fiscal quantity.

Because the decision to replace quality of life by a fiscal outcome was made while the research was being planned, the fiscal outcome may be presented as though it were part of the original objective, and the change of goals may not be apparent. A reviewer of the results, however, will often want to contemplate not just what *was* done in the research but also what *might* have been done. Some of the dissatisfactions and controversies that have occurred after carefully planned clinical studies can be attributed to this problem. The objections arise not from what the investigators actually did but from the omissions or changes that made the research depart from a presumably more desirable mission.

These departures are often caused by insurmountable problems of logistics or feasibility in assembling groups and performing maneuvers, but other departures are due mainly to problems in mensuration. As the investigator decides which variables will be included or omitted in the research, an important point to bear in mind is that mensurational difficulties can alter the original basic objective of the study. To preserve that objective, the investigator may have to resolve the mensurational difficulties by developing suitable new indexes of expression. If those indexes are not developed, and if their absence leads to a change of the basic objective, the investigator may have to re-appraise the desirability of the research and decide whether to go ahead with it. The investigator should also be prepared to receive relatively negative appraisals from reviewers who do not admire the altered objective.

The list that follows contains examples of the way that surrogate variables have often been substituted for desired variables in modern research.

Desired Variable	Surrogate Variable
Number of people living in New Haven in 1984	Census data for New Haven in 1980, adjusted to 1984
Number of people with coronary artery disease	Numbers of deaths attributed to coronary artery disease
Quality of a nation's health care	Infant mortality rate for that nation
Quality of an individual clinician's care	Performance of throat culture before prescribing antibiotics for sore throat; duration of patients' hospitalizations
Improvement of a patient's alcoholism	Patient's fidelity in keeping clinic appointments
Severity of patient's clinical illness	Anatomic dissemination of cancer; height of blood glucose; level of blood urea nitrogen
Palliation of patient with cancer	Survival time; size of tumor
Anxiety	Size of pupils; level of catecholamine
Intelligence	Score on multiple-choice psychometric test

13.2. GENERAL SELECTION OF VARIABLES

Of the many phenomena that can be noted before and after administration of a maneuver, only certain ones will be specifically observed and recorded; and of those that are recorded, not all will be analyzed.

For example, the recorded data will usually include certain administrative information, such as the patient's name, residence, and an identification number (such as hospital or Social Security number), but these data are used almost exclusively for personal identification and seldom receive any formal analyses. Other administrative information that may be collected but unanalyzed includes name of employer, place of employment, name of referring physician, name and relationship of next of kin, and religion.

The type and amount of administrative information needed for each project can usually be easily determined without creating any major difficulties. The tricky problems arise in decisions about what and how much data to collect for the key variables that describe each person's baseline state, outcome event, and performance of maneuvers.

13.2.1. *Scope of Variables*

The larger the research study in effort, costs, duration, and size of the group under observation, the more likely is the investigator to try to obtain as much information as possible. Because no one can be completely sure in advance about what data may or may not be valuable, the investigator usually prefers to collect too much rather than too little. If more information is acquired than seems needed, there is always the chance that someone may later come up with interesting ideas for analyzing the extra material. On the other hand, if something cogent is later found to be left out, the investigator may be chagrined or embarrassed (or both) to discover a possibly irremediable omission of important data.

To avoid this hazard, the investigator may use an observe-everything approach that creates an alternative hazard: the collection of too much data. Occupied with assembling a vast array of information, the investigator may not have time to give adequate attention to obtaining high-quality data for certain important phenomena. The data may be omitted entirely or they may not be observed or recorded adequately.

Although important variables may be omitted because they are crowded out by all the other information, a separate problem occurs when the data are deliberately omitted as being too "soft," subjective, or unworthy of scientific attention. For example, in many therapeutic trials and surveys, the main endpoints chosen as outcome events are "hard," objective, and scientifically cogent for documenting the pharmacologic, pathophysiologic, or therapeutic effects of treatment. The result of such studies may be satisfactory for pharmacology or therapy of *disease* but unsuitable for making clinical decisions about the treatment of patients, because the data contain no information about disability, comfort, convenience, and other human effects on the patient and the patient's family.

Although "hard" data may be highly desirable for certain statistical goals, the "soft" data that describe clinical human phenomena are often crucial for decisions in patient care. The omission of such data may create a major restriction in the scope of variables and may keep the results of a clinical trial from being enthusiastically accepted by practicing clinicians and patients. A special nomenclature has been suggested[1] to describe this distinction in data. The term *therapeutic trial* was proposed for clinical trials having a restricted target, such as death or relief of symptoms, as the outcome variable; and *patient care trial* was proposed for studies in which the outcome variables were expanded to include additional pertinent issues in patient care. The restricted-scope-of-variables problem has often occurred in many randomized clinical trials, and the problem is particularly striking in studies of therapy for the palliation of patients with advanced cancer.[2] The outcome events may refer to survival, size of tumor, impact on enzymes, and many other dimensional measurements, but the palliation of patients is seldom described for relief of symptoms, changes in functional capacity, or general quality of life.

13.2.2. *Displacement of Targets*

As noted in Section 13.1, when an important phenomenon under study is not easily measured, the target variable may be shifted to a different phenomenon. During this displacement (which Yerushalmy[3] has called "the substitution game"), the main purpose of the research may be lost or irrevocably diverted. For example, the relief of angina pectoris may be studied by reporting changes in the electrocardiogram rather than changes in chest pain or functional capacity. The improvement of exercise capacity is often studied by noting performance on a treadmill ergometer rather than performance in activities of daily living. The consequence of the substitutions is that a clinical reader of the results does not discover what has happened in the relief of angina pectoris.

13.2.3. *The "Hardening" of Soft Data*

Many important outcome variables must be expressed in transition categories that reflect judgments about magnitude (e.g., *larger, shorter, costlier*) or desirability (e.g., *good, better, improved, more convenient, less anxiety*). These judgments are often difficult to validate in an objective manner. How do we prove that a weight loss of 4 lbs. is trivial in a patient who weighs 300 lbs.? How do we prove that oral therapy is more convenient than injections of a similar agent? How do we prove that going back to work is a good outcome for the patient?

Because the decisions represent subjective judgments by patients and doctors, such phenomena may be dismissed as "soft" and either omitted from the research or deliberately replaced by "hard" entities, such as survival time, white blood count, or electrocardiographic evidence. The best way to preserve important soft data is to "harden" them. The hardening process consists of establishing specific indexes for describing the phenomena, specific scales for summarizing the descriptions contained in each index, and specific criteria for denoting or demarcating each element in the scale.

The creation of hardened indexes is an important clinimetric challenge in clinical research.[4] Many indexes still remain to be developed for important entities. Many of the ones that have already been developed are satisfactory for identifying a single state but not transitions in states. (For example, is a change in Apgar score a good way of identifying the progress of a sick newborn child?) Many indexes that may seem satisfactory for their role in identifying either single states or transitions are used inconsistently because rigorous criteria have not been stipulated for the elements and scales contained in the index.

13.2.4. *Consensuality and Creativity*

One of the best ways to establish a new index is by consensual authorization. For this process, a selected group of authorities is chosen. The members get together, discuss the issues, dissect the judgmental elements, and recombine them into the scale of the index that emerges. After the authorities reach agreement on the procedure, their approval constitutes a type of validation for the results. This technique has been responsible for all of the hard data that now exist in scientific research. Conventions of experts were responsible for such standards as the length of a meter, the weight of a kilogram, and the nomenclature (and identification) of anatomic structures, microbiologic organisms, and chemical elements.

One of the prime problems of contemporary clinical research is that either the analogous meetings have not been conducted or the meetings have been ineffectual. The experts may agree on nomenclature but may not supply operational criteria for identifying the categories in the scale. (An outstanding example of this difficulty is demonstrated in the nosologic taxonomy that is called the *ICDA classification of disease.*[5] The names and organizational categories of diseases have been carefully selected by an international panel of authorities, and the taxonomy is periodically revised to keep it up to date, but no criteria have ever been issued for making the diagnoses.)

Alternatively, the experts may not have been well chosen. Thus, a group of academic clinicians may not be the appropriate authorities for establishing standards of outpatient clinical practice; a group of clinicians may not be suitable for establishing standards of patient satisfaction; and a group of ethicists may be too academically distant from reality to make decisions about patients' desires in medical ethics.

Because of the difficulties in obtaining consensual validation, an individual investigator may decide that the required effort is too arduous and may therefore abandon the consensual validation but not the data. The investigator will then use his or her own creativity to establish the necessary indexes, scales, and criteria. If the work is worthwhile, it may then become generally accepted and can receive its consensual validation in that manner. Imperfections that are later recognized in the index can also be modified in subsequent activities. A classic example of such a procedure is the Jones Diagnostic Criteria for rheumatic fever. First established as a solitary act by T. Duckett Jones[6] in 1944, the criteria have now received three successive sets of modifications[7-9] by formal committees of the American Heart Association. The criteria have also become worldwide in their application, and the major-minor decision logic introduced by Jones has been emulated in approaches for creating diagnostic criteria for other diseases.

13.3. LEVELS OF DISAGREEMENT ABOUT SUITABILITY

Because decisions about suitability will vary from one project to another and also from one evaluator to another, disagreements can regularly be expected to occur. A committee of experts who managed to smooth out minor individual differences and to achieve unanimous belief that their research plan was eminently suitable may be shocked or angered to discover that the results are regarded as highly unsuitable by other evaluators and even by other experts. Such disagreements are inevitable, given the diversity of human opinions and values, but certain procedures can be used to reduce the frequency of the disputes and even occasionally to resolve them.

The most important step is to determine the level of the research plan at which disagreement is produced. Proceeding from high order to low order inspection, these levels can occur in the basic objective of the research, in the structure used to conduct the research, in the entities selected as foci of observation, in the variables that identify those entities, and in the criteria used to demarcate the variables. For example, suppose an investigator proposes a large observational cohort study to determine whether the treatment of hypertension prevents death from coronary artery disease.

13.3.1. *Disagreement About Objectives*

At the level of basic objective, someone may believe that such research is not worth doing and that the expended energy and funds would be better used for more fundamental investigation of the etiologic and pathophysiologic mechanisms that lead to hypertension or to coronary disease. A person who regards the basic objective of the research as unsuitable will often find flaws in everything else thereafter.

13.3.2. *Disagreement About Research Structure*

At the level of research structure, someone else, while accepting the value of the basic objective, may believe that the only way it can be properly investigated is with a randomized controlled trial. No matter how well the rest of the research proposal is developed, this person may find the work unsuitable if not conducted as an experimental trial. Alternatively, another person, who is willing to let the work be done as an observational cohort study, may dislike the research plan because it calls for a retrolective rather than prolective assembly of the cohort's data. This second person may believe that medical records and other archival information cannot be used as a suitable source of evidence for the observational research.

13.3.3. *Disagreement About Foci of Observation*

At the level of foci, someone who accepts the basic objective and structure of the research may be unhappy because the investigators plan to examine only the relationships of hypertension, treatment, and death from coronary disease, without including such additional phenomena as baseline co-morbidity, adverse psychic effects of antihypertensive treatment, and outcome events other than coronary disease.

13.3.4. *Disagreement About Variables*

If these additional foci have been included in the research plan, disagreements may be evoked at the level of variables, because baseline co-morbidity has been defined as "treatment for any disease other than hypertension," because adverse psychic effects of antihypertensive treatment will be measured only as "number of days lost from work," and because "noncoronary deaths" will constitute the only outcome event other than coronary mortality.

13.3.5. *Disagreement About Demarcations*

Finally, someone who agrees with everything else that has thus far been proposed may dissent at the level of demarcations, disputing the criteria used for decisions within the scale of each variable. Such a person, for example, may believe that hypertension itself, as an admission criterion for the study, should be demarcated with a diastolic pressure of 85 rather than the proposed 90 mm. Hg. This person may accept the idea of using *days lost from work* as a surrogate variable for *adverse psychic effects* but may insist that a specific illness be documented for each lost day or that no days be counted as lost unless they exceed more than five each year. The use of *nonantihypertensive therapy* may also be accepted as a substitute for measuring *co-morbidity,* but additional demands may be placed on the types and duration of treatment that can be regarded as *nonantihypertensive therapy.*

This dissenter may also agree that *coronary artery disease* is the main outcome event in the research but may argue that it should not be demarcated only as *death attributable to coronary artery disease* and that the outcome event should also be counted for survivors who develop angina pectoris or myocardial infarction. An additional argument might be offered that nonfatal strokes and impaired renal function should also be counted as outcome events.

13.3.6. *Resolution of Disagreements*

Because any or all of these different types of disagreement can lead to decisions that the research has unsuitable components, the sources of the disagreement must be identified if the investigator is to make any useful efforts to repair the perceived flaws and to try to evoke better agreement. The ease with which the flaws can be repaired will usually be directly proportional to the level at which the disagreement occurs. Thus, at the level of demarcating variables, which is the lowest order of the levels cited here, compromise solutions can often be readily achieved in criteria for delineating selected attributes. At the next higher level, the selected variables can often be improved with greater efforts in clinimetric mensuration. At the preceding level, which deals with foci, the investigator must usually be persuaded to expand the scope of variables to include those that have been omitted, but the persuasion may not be hard to accomplish.

The disagreements that are most difficult to resolve are at the first two levels of dissent, because disputes about high order issues in the basic objective or structure of the research usually involve matters of policy rather than methods of scientific investigation. Someone who devoutly believes that the basic objective is not worth pursuing or who will accept results from only one particular type of research structure (such as a randomized trial) is not likely to be persuaded by any repairs or alternative arrangements except a proposal that the research be abandoned or totally transformed into another structure. An investigator whose proposal is given this type of reception and who does not want to change the basic objective or structure of the proposal can do little to help his cause. He can only hope that somewhere in a pluralistic society he will find other evaluators (and sources of support) whose concepts of scientific policy are more sympathetic to his own.

13.4. DIFFERENTIATION OF VARIABLES

After the variables to be observed have been selected, they can be divided according to their different functional roles in administration, zero state, outcome, and performance of maneuvers. The reason for this division is to be sure that the role of each variable has been suitably identified and that adequate procedures become developed (later, during implementation) for acquiring the necessary data.

13.4.1. *Administrative Variables*

The *administrative* variables, such as patient's name, address, and identification number, refer to the administrative aspects of conducting the study and coordinating the research personnel, investigated people, and data. The administrative variables usually have no scientific function in the research, although sometimes they may be applied in a subsequent investigation concerned with demographic or socioeconomic attributes that happen to be described and available in the administrative data.

13.4.2. *Zero-State Variables*

These are the variables that identify each person's baseline condition at zero time. Some of these variables are noted only for their role in the prezero interval and at zero time, and they do not recur for measurement thereafter in the postzero interval. Among such variables are items of family history, past medical history, demographic features, and certain clinical and paraclinical manifestations that are not followed and repeatedly observed after the imposition of the maneuver at zero time.

Other zero-state variables are recorded for their values at zero time but are then retained for additional observations in the postzero interval. For example, in a study of therapy for hypertension, the patient's history of an antecedent myocardial infarction would be used to characterize zero state only. The patient's blood pressure, retinal appearance, and manifestations of cardiomegaly would be used to characterize zero state but would also be followed thereafter for changes that would help identify outcome events.

13.4.3. *Outcome Variables*

The variables used to record the outcome events can be divided according to their roles as primary, ancillary, and incidental targets. A *primary target* is the main outcome that is expected to be prevented, altered, or otherwise changed by the maneuvers under study. For the research that was proposed in Section 13.3, the primary target variable was the development of coronary disease (or death due to coronary disease).

The *ancillary targets* consist of important additional phenomena (noted as potential changes, benefits, side effects, or adverse reactions) that can be anticipated with the investigated maneuvers. In the research proposal of Section 13.3, the potential ancillary-target variables were described with such titles as *days lost from work* and *adverse psychic effects.* (The variables for *noncoronary death, stroke,* and *impaired renal function* would be either target or ancillary variables according to the way in which the investigator and the critics resolved their dispute.)

An *incidental target* is a variable that is observed just in case something happens. This function is commonly performed by a large array of paraclinical tests and by check lists of questions about various clinical manifestations. No incidental targets were mentioned in the research proposed in Section 13.3. If such research were conducted, measurements of serum cholesterol and potassium would probably be included as incidental-target variables.

In the UGDP clinical trial of treatment of diabetes mellitus,[10] the primary-target variable in the published analysis was *cardiovascular death* rather than the *cardiovascular complications* that were specified as primary targets in the original research design. Cardiovascular complications in living patients were analyzed as an ancillary variable. The investigators also reported changes in serum lipids as an incidental variable. Part of the ongoing, unresolved dispute about that trial arose from the change in stated targets and also from the absence of any data for such additional ancillary variables in diabetic therapy as *infections, hypoglycemic reactions,* and patient's *convenience in using the regimens.*

13.4.4. *Performance Variables*

The performance variables refer to the proficiency with which the maneuvers are conducted. These variables are used to record information about each patient's compliance with a prescribed regimen, the quality of regulation or control for certain intermediate target variables (such as blood pressure or blood glucose) that may be directly affected by the main maneuvers, and the usage of additional therapy (or other activities) that can act as co-maneuvers.

The performance variables can also be used to record data about a patient's mainte-nance of the research protocol (e.g., keeping appointments, bringing in specimens, and so on) and about the surveillance methods (e.g., frequency of routine tests, criteria for ordering *ad hoc* tests, etc.) that are used to detect the entities noted as outcome events.

In earlier writing,[11] I referred to the performance variables as *synchronous,* because they refer to events occurring while the maneuver is in progress. This aspect of timing distinguishes them from the *prochronous* zero-state variables, which occur beforehand, and the *postchronous* outcome variables, which occur afterward. Because *zero state, performance,* and *outcome* are simpler titles and are already well-established words, I trust they will be received with reasonable joy by neologophobes, who hate new words.

13.4.5. *Value of Differential Classification of Variables*

There are several important reasons for engaging in a differential classification of variables. The most obvious reason, as noted earlier, is to be sure that adequate procedures become developed for acquiring the necessary data. A second reason is that this organized classification of variables can be used as a "review of systems" by both an investigator and an evaluator of either the proposed or completed research. From this classification, the reviewer can promptly determine which variables are regarded as most important in the research and can readily identify any important variables that have been overlooked.

Two other valuable reasons will become apparent later, when we consider the analysis of data for a completed project. First, when a prognostic analysis is performed—using stratification or other combinations of data—the choice of cogent variables for the analysis will depend on their role in affecting the susceptibility to the primary target event(s). A clear, unambiguous identification of the primary target(s) is therefore essential for prognostic analysis. Secondly, if certain outcome variables are to be used as transition indexes, indicating a change between the baseline and subsequent state, arrangements must be made for collecting suitable data. If the data are expressed in dimensional scales, transitions can readily be measured from one state to another. If the data are expressed in nondimensional scales, however, a single-state scale may contain too few categories to permit discernment of distinct but subtle transitions. To record these distinctions, the investigator may need to create separate *transition variables* for describing the outcome events.

13.5. **SUITABILITY VS. SIMILARITY**

The discussion thus far in Chapters 12 and 13 has dealt with suitability for the four main components of a cause-effect study. We want to make suitable choices for the particular entities that will be selected as baseline state, outcome, principal maneuver, and comparative maneuver(s) and also for the variables that will be used to identify those entities. If these choices, which establish the fundamental design of the research, are later regarded as unsuitable, the results will usually be unacceptable, regardless of the excellence with which the study is carried out or the fervor with which the statistical results are analyzed.

A quite different source of unacceptable results arises from the problem of similarity in the compared components. Unless we can be assured that each set of components was fairly compared, the subsequent results may be unacceptable because they have been distorted by bias. These two different problems produce two different reasons for rejecting the results of a research study. For problems in suitability, we think the wrong things were done. For problems in similarity, we do not believe what was found in the comparison.

Problems of suitability are usually created by inappropriate choices in the basic plans for baseline state, outcome, and maneuvers; but problems in similarity are usually created as or after the maneuvers are imposed. Dissimilar comparisons are generally produced by unanticipated disparities in the action of nature or people when maneuvers are selected and carried out, and when the results are analyzed. These differences between suitability and similarity create major differences in some of the main scientific challenges of experimental and observational research. In an experimental trial, the investigator can easily make plans to avoid the disparities produced by natural events, but must worry about whether the research plan contains a suitable simulation of nature's realities. In observational research, a suitable set of research components can easily be chosen for the natural events that transpire, but the investigator must worry about the dissimilar comparisons that may arise because the maneuvers were not allocated experimentally and because the research often begins after the maneuvers have already occurred.

Because the problems of dissimilar comparisons usually arise during implementation of the maneuvers, a discussion of these problems will be reserved for Chapters 15 to 17. At this point in the rational architecture of a research study, we have finished formulating a suitable set of basic plans. Before they are carried out, we shall pause for a brief appraisal—discussed in the next chapter—that may help prevent a great deal of wasted effort.

13.6. SYNOPSIS

In a cause-effect study, the variables chosen to identify the baseline state, outcome, and performance of maneuvers should be suitably selected to denote the scope of desired information. If an adequate system of mensuration does not exist for important phenomena, the investigator can often develop one, using individual creativity or consensual authorization. The development of a suitable new variable is usually preferable to the substitution of an alternative variable that is more easily measured but unsuitable.

Disagreements about the suitability of a particular project can arise at different levels of appraisal for the basic objective of the study, for the structure used to conduct the research, for the entities selected for observation, for the variables that identify the entities, or for the criteria that demarcate the variables. Disputes about the basic objective or research structure can seldom be resolved without drastic changes in the research, but reasonable alterations can often be made to achieve a satisfactory suitability of foci, variables, and demarcations.

The selected variables should be differentially classified for their roles in the administration of the project and in identifying the zero-state (baseline) condition, performance of maneuvers, and primary, ancillary, or incidental targets noted as outcome events. The differential classification is useful for reviewing the selection of variables and for subsequent activities, when the research plan is implemented, in arranging for suitable methods of observation, prognostic analysis, and identification of transitions.

EXERCISES

The assignment here is to find three published reports of cause-effect comparative studies and to comment on the suitability of the variables used in the research. You may use any source you want to obtain appropriate literature for review. For Exercise 13.1, the study should be a randomized controlled trial of a therapeutic agent. For the next two exercises, the study should have been performed observationally, without experimental allocation of the compared maneuvers. In Exercise 13.2, the research should be a cohort (retrolective or prolective) study of therapy. In Exercise 13.3, the maneuver should be an etiologic agent that allegedly causes a disease. The actual structure (cohort, case-control, etc.) used in the etiologic research is unimportant as long as you can distinguish the basic conceptual model.

For each of these three projects, prepare a diagram and *brief* verbal description of the basic objective and structure of the research. Then list and classify the main variables that were actually analyzed (in statistical summaries, tables, or graphs) to describe the baseline state and type of outcomes associated with the maneuvers under investigation. Do any of these variables seem to be substitutes for the real targets that the investigators had in mind? Reading these reports as a practicing clinician who wants to use the information in patient care, are you content with the variables that were analyzed? If not, what additional variables would you like to know about? Finally, note and comment about whether any variables were used (or efforts made) to determine the proficiency with which the maneuvers were carried out.

Exercise 13.1. Randomized trial of a therapeutic agent.

Exercise 13.2. Observational cohort study of a therapeutic agent.

Exercise 13.3. Observational study of an etiologic agent.

CHAPTER REFERENCES

1. Spitzer, 1975; 2. Rudnick, 1980; 3. Yerushalmy, 1966; 4. Feinstein, 1983; 5. International Classification of Diseases, 1980; 6. Jones, 1944; 7. American Heart Association, 1955; 8. American Heart Association, 1965; 9. American Heart Association, 1984; 10. University Group Diabetes Program, 1970; 11. Feinstein, 1972.

Preliminary Appraisal of the Outline

For an experimental trial or prolective cohort study, the plans developed in Chapters 11 to 13 are now ready to be implemented. During the implementation, the investigator converts the general architectural outline into a specific set of procedures and instructions for carrying out the research. These activities require arrangements to provide operational identifications for all the selected variables and states, assemble suitable numbers of people for the study, allocate the maneuvers or determine which ones were received, and obtain the necessary follow-up data.

Suppose the general architectural outline shows the following diagram:

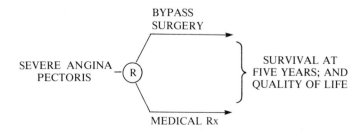

The implementation of this randomized trial would require some of the following proce-dures: operational criteria to define severe angina pectoris; methods of assembling such patients; tactics for persuading them to enter the trial; arrangements for suitable perform-ance of the surgery or medical therapy; preservation of the medical group from contami-nation by unassigned surgery; selection or creation of a scale for measuring quality of life; and mechanisms for following both groups for at least five years to determine quality of life, causes of death, or other outcome events.

The problems encountered (or created) during the plans for implementation or during the actual research may sometimes alter, distort, or badly compromise the objective of the research. The compromises may make the results difficult to compare, to interpret, or to apply in subsequent clinical activities. Even without such added problems, however, the basic outline of the research may be flawed with fundamental defects that cannot be improved no matter how elegantly they are implemented. Before all the work of the implementation begins, therefore, the basic outline of the research should be evaluated.

The goal of this evaluation is to determine whether the research project is (or was) worth doing. By doing this evaluation immediately after the basic architecture is outlined, the investigator may discover the need for major modifications of the objective, including the possibility that the project should be drastically altered or abandoned. The evaluation of a research project should take place at all phases of its planning, but a particularly good time for the appraisal is early in the work, just after the basic outline has been completed. Many research proposals that were accompanied by a carefully detailed implementation have been unaccepted or disapproved not because the implementation was unsatisfactory but because the subsequent evaluators rejected the basic outline.

The subsequent evaluators can be members of a committee from an agency that provides grants to support the research, the reviewers or referees who determine whether the report of the completed research warrants publication, the practicing clinicians and other persons who read the published report to help in decisions of patient care, or policy makers who use the results to establish regulations, legislation, guidelines, or other acts of public policy. When these people evaluate the research, it will be either a fully developed proposal or a report of the completed project. Their evaluation will usually begin with a preliminary appraisal of the basic plans and will then be extended to cover what was done or proposed during the implementation. For the investigator, the main purpose of a preliminary appraisal is prophylactic: to avoid making elaborate arrangements for carrying out an unsatisfactory basic plan. Many projects that have been meticulously implemented have been rejected or badly flawed because they were performed without benefit of such an appraisal. This same appraisal can also be conducted, of course, after the research has been completed. At that time, however, the appraisal becomes a postmortem examination rather than a potentially beneficial act of prophylaxis.

The preliminary appraisal of the basic outline can be conducted in four steps. The first two steps, which involve attention to the fundamental questions and stipulations, are used to determine what the investigator wants to do. The next two steps are devoted to value judgments about whether the work is worth doing and to the feasibility with which it can be carried out.

14.1. THE FUNDAMENTAL QUESTIONS

Before any other decisions can be made about a research project, the evaluator, consultant, and investigator must all have their heads clear about the basic outline of the research. The fundamental activities here are to find out what the investigator wants to do and to be sure that the proposed research outline is aimed at the main question it is supposed to answer.

14.1.1. *What Is the Question?*

The investigator's first step is to state the question to be answered in the research and to indicate the basic outline of the baseline state, compared maneuvers, and outcome events used in the architectural reasoning. The actual architectural structure proposed for the research need not coincide with this reasoning, but the basic outline of the reasoning should coincide with the question to be answered.

This coincidence may not always occur. The investigator may say he wants to determine whether food preservatives are dangerous, but the research outline may indicate a study in which cancer of the stomach is the only outcome event. The proposed question may emphasize an attempt to palliate patients with a particular condition, but the proposed outline may be concerned solely with duration of survival.

The disparity between basic question and basic outline can have several sources. To produce a feasible proposal, the investigator may have truncated the basic goal of the research. Thus, because every possible danger of food preservatives cannot be investigated in one study, cancer of the stomach might have been chosen as a starting point. In such a situation, the investigator might reconsider whether the outcome should be restricted to just one disease, and if so, whether cancer of the stomach is the best candidate. Another possibility is that the basic goal of the research may have been displaced rather than merely truncated because the investigator, seeking hard data, decided to measure survival rather than palliation. In this circumstance, the investigator might be reminded of creative opportunities for developing new indexes to measure the original goal while simultaneously pursuing the quest of hard data.

A more difficult and delicate problem occurs when the investigator does not readily state the basic question that the research is intended to answer. Not all investigators are equally experienced, articulate, or concise in expressing their ideas. Just as clinicians may sometimes be asked to help patients who do not clearly state a chief complaint, research consultants may have clients who do not succinctly specify the corresponding attribute of a research project. When asked to indicate the basic question or basic outline, the investigator, like a garrulous patient, may ramble on about diverse concepts and hypotheses, describe the findings of previous research activities, emphasize the importance of the proposed project, and discuss the kinds of assistance and collaboration that may be needed—all without a clear statement that outlines the basic goal of the research. The research consultant, like a good clinician faced with an analogous problem in obtaining a patient's history, may then have to exercise suitable forms of ingenuity in deciding when to interrupt, how to probe, and where to direct the flow of information.

A strategy that I have found particularly helpful as a research consultant is to ask the investigator to "begin at the end." This strategy is useful regardless of how well the basic outline is presented and is particularly effective in clearing heads for both investigator and consultant. For this process, the investigator is invited to engage in an act of scientific divination. Pretending that the research project has been finished and that the results have confirmed what was anticipated, the investigator is asked to give a summary of the two, three, or four most important points that were found.

By preparing such a summary in advance, the investigator is often forced to engage in acts of intellectual clarification that might otherwise take much longer to occur. By reading the summary, the research consultant (or other critics and evaluators) can get a prompt, reasonably good idea of what is sought and expected in the project. The investigator and consultant can then work backward from this summary to be sure that the research is constructed in a way that can potentially provide the evidence needed for the summary. This *begin-at-the-end* strategy has been so effective throughout the years that I now use it routinely in consultative work, even when the investigator can clearly outline the basic questions and objective of the proposed research.

14.1.2. *What Will Be Done with the Answer?*

The answer to this question often reveals the *latent objective* of the research. It indicates either the investigator's immediate next step, after the work is done, or a hitherto unstated major purpose (or hidden agenda) for the research. Table 14–1 contains some examples of the questions (or answers) that would indicate the overtly stated objective and the unstated latent objective for each of a series of research proposals.

Learning the latent objective of a research project is an invaluable activity, mainly because it often allows the stated objective of the research to be corrected or expanded so that the *latent* objective becomes directly included as part of the *stated* objective. For example, after we learn the latent objective of project 1 in Table 14–1, we might arrange to compare Excellitol against an active drug, whereas previously we might have compared it only against placebo. In project 2, we might recognize that a convincing answer to the latent objective can be obtained only with a study in which the performance of nurse

Table 14–1. EXAMPLES OF STATED AND UNSTATED LATENT OBJECTIVES FOR RESEARCH PROJECTS

Project Number	Stated Objective	Latent Objective
1.	Is Excellitol treatment good for rheumatoid arthritis?	Can we use Excellitol instead of aspirin or nonsteroidal anti-inflammatory drugs?
2.	Are nurse practitioners safe and effective?	Can we rely on them instead of physicians?
3.	Can we develop a better staging system for cancer?	Can we get rid of the various barbarities produced by radical therapy?
4.	What are the costs of health care?	Do we need a system of national health insurance?
5.	What is the mechanism of DNA transfer across the bladder of a ferret?	I have already worked out the mechanism in toad bladders, but I need additional funds to keep my lab going.
6.	What is the attitude of the suburban community toward neighborhood health centers?	Our epidemiologic large-scale survey team is finishing its current project and we are looking for something new and big to do.
7.	We want to evaluate the accomplishments of the medical school's new curriculum.	The president of the university has become infatuated with the idea that everything must have a formal evaluation. We must do this in order to get him off our back.

practitioners is directly compared against that of physicians. In project 3, we might ask the investigator to specify what is to be classified with the better staging system. Is it the baseline condition of the patients before treatment or the barbarities that occur after treatment or both?

By learning the latent objective, we may also be able to suggest other strategies that either provide an easier way of achieving the desired goal or that revise it into a more desirable goal. In project 4, for example, the investigator might be cautioned that merely learning the costs of health care may not answer the question about national health insurance. In projects 5 and 6 we might ask the investigator whether the pursuit of a different, more exciting question might not evoke the same salubrious fiscal blessings as those sought originally. In project 7; we might contemplate a simpler and more efficient mechanism for placating the university president.

The latent objective thus has two crucial roles: It may indicate targets, hitherto omitted from the outline of the research, that should be directly incorporated as part of the activities; and it may at times suggest that the planned research be replaced by a quite different approach for attaining the investigator's main goal.

14.2. **THE FUNDAMENTAL STIPULATIONS**

After the basic research question has been clarified, its effective implementation will demand that the investigator stipulate specific answers to a series of additional questions about elements of structure and function in the research architecture.

14.2.1. *Are All Major Elements of the Architecture Clearly Indicated?*

For example, we can readily contemplate implementation of the basic objective if it is expressed as "Does cigarette smoking cause coronary disease?" We would not be sure of what to do next if the question is asked as "What happens when people smoke?" or as "Is smoking harmful?"

14.2.2. *Are the Specifications Sufficiently Specific?*

Even when the main architectural elements are clearly indicated, they may not have been specified in enough detail to indicate the things that need to be implemented. For example, in the previous question about cigarette smoking and coronary disease, the goals seem reasonably clear, although we shall later have to know how many cigarettes and how many years of smoking are to be regarded as cigarette smoking and what kinds of clinical ailments are to be called coronary disease (e.g., angina pectoris, overt myocardial infarction, silent electrocardiographic evidence, etc.). On the other hand, if the objective were expressed as "Does smoking cause heart disease?" we do not really know what the investigator has in mind. For example, would we want to check whether a father's cigar smoking can cause congenital heart disease in a child?

The requirement for specificity at this phase of planning, therefore, is to be sure that the basic intentions are clear.

14.2.3. *Will the Results Answer the Question?*

Our concern here is with potential major problems in suitability of the research. In order to achieve a specific research model, has the basic question been asked in an inappropriate manner? Would some other question be better? For example, the proficiency of the principal maneuver may be greatly impaired if the investigator plans to test a fixed dosage of a drug that requires flexible dosage. The outcome event may be displaced if it is measured with an inadequate item of hard data instead of with the soft data that actually describe the outcome under study. The credibility of the research may be destroyed if it is performed with a research structure that is convenient for the investigator but inappropriate for getting a convincing answer to the main question.

14.2.4. *To What Population Will the Results Apply?*

The group of people admitted to most research projects in clinical epidemiology represents a convenient sample, obtained because the people were readily available to the investigator. They may not truly represent the outside world population for which the research is intended and to which the results will be extrapolated. If not, is the study worth doing anyhow?

The answer to this question, which is further discussed in Chapter 15, depends on the particular level at which the investigated people have been constrained and on the consequences of the constraints. Certain distortions can be produced by the mechanisms that make people available for the research, and other distortions are created by the investigator's decisions about whom to choose from the available people. Thus, if the research is performed at a Veterans Administration hospital, the available patients may include relatively few women and may omit men with ailments that excluded them from military service in young adult life. On the other hand, the relatively unselected population available at a general community hospital may be sharply constrained by the investigator's choice of criteria for eligibility. For example, to eliminate the impurities caused by diverse ages, races, genders, and co-morbidity in the spectrum of patients with coronary artery disease, the investigator may plan a randomized trial of medical versus surgical therapy for white men, ages 35 to 50, who have only coronary disease and no major co-morbid ailments such as hypertension, diabetes mellitus, or gout. When obtained in this pure group of patients, will the results of the trial be pertinent for the many impurities treated in clinical practice? Will they be useful when a clinician decides whether to choose surgery for the coronary disease of a 68-year-old black woman with diabetes mellitus and hypertension?

14.2.5. *Has the Principal Maneuver Received an Adequate "Pilot Test"?*

When the principal maneuver is a new pharmaceutical substance or surgical procedure, the maneuver will almost always have been tried out in animals before it is proposed for application to people. The purveyant maneuvers that consist of human interventions, however, can seldom be tested in animals. For example, suppose we want to determine whether a special educational program will be better than the existing pattern of medical communication in helping patients manage their clinical problems. Because this maneuver cannot be evaluated in animals, the only way to determine its possible efficacy is to try it directly in people.

Because randomized trials have become a generally desired procedure for evaluating interventional maneuvers, the investigator may propose that the new educational program be immediately tested with a randomized trial. This approach may be reasonable if the program itself has already been developed and has received a few "pilot trials" to show that it can work. The expense and efforts of a randomized trial may not yet be warranted, however, if no evidence exists to demonstrate that the program can indeed be created and applied.

The controversies discussed in Chapter 29 about when to start a randomized trial all refer to maneuvers that are pharmaceutical or surgical interventions; and the focus of the dispute is whether observational pilot studies should first be performed in people before the results of animal experiments are converted into the human experiments of randomized trials. When animal experiments cannot be used for previous demonstration of the possible efficacy of purveyant maneuvers, however, some sort of pilot testing will usually be desirable—if only to show that the maneuver itself can be developed—before randomized trials are undertaken.

14.3. THE FUNDAMENTAL VALUE JUDGMENTS

Decisions about values depend on neither science nor method. They rest on issues of policy, fashions, or ideology that reflect the way in which a particular research project fits into the smaller and larger world in which it takes place.

Someone who believes that basic biologic mechanisms are the only topic worth studying and that clinical therapy is merely "halfway technology" may have great difficulty developing enthusiasm for research concerned with patient care. Someone else who regards basic biologic research as "irrelevant enzyme grinding" may not be persuaded to support anything that deviates from a direct therapeutic objective. A third person who believes that basic biology and clinical therapy are both important scientific goals may have little or no intellectual tolerance for investigations concerned with the personnel, administrative, and fiscal mechanisms involved in health services research. A fourth person may feel that all the other activities are minor and perhaps wasteful, unless the achievements of basic biology and clinical therapy are converted into effective delivery of health care.

Agreement about the basic goals of research may be followed by major dissent about the values of different architectural structures used for materials and methods. In basic biologic investigation, the disputes may focus on the value of different technologic approaches and on the systemic, histologic, cytologic, or molecular level of investigation that determines whether the research is sufficiently basic. In studies of therapy, randomized trials may be regarded as a religious shrine, which is worshiped by devout believers who refuse to accept the results of nonrandomized studies. The shrine may be shunned, however, by heretics who attack the high costs of the trials and the occasional misdirected efforts and confusion they produce. In epidemiologic studies of etiology, scientists accustomed to cohort directions in research may be baffled or repulsed by the backward logic of case-control studies and by the statistical machinations of heterodemic analyses.

As noted in Section 13.3, there is very little an investigator can do if the basic goals of the research are rejected. Perhaps the only solution is to find a different agency, committee, journal, or atmosphere that will be more hospitable to the goals and more likely to share a common set of values. If the basic architectural structure is rejected, the investigator can re-evaluate the proposed materials and methods, and can attempt either to change them accordingly or to present a more persuasive defense of their value.

Because a pluralistic society needs good research directed at each of the cited goals and because a pluralistic medical science needs each of the cited research structures, the main hazard for both society and science is that value judgments about research will depend on ideology rather than quality. Certain projects that are excellently conceived, planned, and implemented may be rejected only because they deviate from popular fashions and paradigms.[1] Conversely, other projects that are neither well planned nor well implemented may contain sufficiently fashionable concepts to receive enthusiastic support from a peer group review conducted by experts who establish and maintain the popular paradigms. In this way massive funds may be expended for pedestrian basic research in molecular biology; for dehumanized, overly statisticated clinical trials in therapeutics; for ineffectual sentimentality in health services research; or for grandiose apparitions in computerized management information systems.

The basic value judgments about research occur as answers to the following two questions:

14.3.1. *Is the Question Worth Asking?*

What is the importance or significance of the research? Assuming that the answer has been obtained, will its subsequent usage (the latent objective) be worthwhile? Almost every research proposal or published report has a section in which the investigator explains the significance of the work. The composition of this discussion is particularly cogent, because it lets the reader know *why* the work is desirable.

Different people will obviously have different criteria for making the decision about what is worthwhile or important. Among the principles that can affect these criteria are the following:

14.3.1.1. HOW COMMON IS THE PROBLEM UNDER STUDY?

A common condition, such as dementia in elderly people or schizophrenia in younger people, will often be regarded as more important than an uncommon disease, such as scleroderma.

14.3.1.2. HOW SERIOUS IS THE PROBLEM?

Although less common than tension headaches, dementia or schizophrenia may be deemed more important because their impact is much more serious. (Criteria for deciding what is serious will also vary, of course; and members of the public often wish that "nonserious" phenomena such as tension headaches, dysmenorrhea, impotence, or the common cold would receive as much scientific attention as lupus erythematosus and thalassemia.)

14.3.1.3. HOW CREATIVE IS THE PROPOSAL?

Even though the problem may be uncommon or not particularly serious, its study may be warranted because of exciting creativity in the proposal. What the investigator achieves may be seminal in developing a new field of research. For example, relatively few clinicians may have expected that a new way of producing insulin would emerge from basic investigations in the molecular biology of DNA. Alternatively, even though a new field of research is not developed, the proposal may have fundamental value in clarifying an existing activity. An example of such research would be the attempts to develop a taxonomy for important clinical phenomena, such as severity of illness, that currently lack suitable systems of classification.

14.3.2. *Is the Answer Worth Getting?*

Although the question may be worth asking, it may not rank high in the priority of other contenders to which human effort and financial support can be given. The latent objective may be so distant from the direct objective that the connection is too remote to be appealing. For example, an investigator proposing any form of basic biologic research can always claim that the results may eventually help eliminate cancer or contribute to its cure. Because this same claim could also be made by someone who wants to study the botanic flora of Nepal, ichthyologic variation in Madagascar, or meteorologic vicissitudes in Antarctica, the evaluators may seek a stronger oncologic link before deciding that the research should be supported mainly because its latent objective is important. Conversely, the latent objective, although immediate and worthwhile, may not be attainable. For example, suppose we find that an intensive program of psychotherapy can be highly beneficial for elderly people living in nursing homes. Would we decide to institute such programs throughout the nation?

When the value of the answered question is appraised, the evaluators may also wonder whether the latent objective could be better achieved in some other way. For example, several years ago a randomized experimental trial was conducted to show that emergency-room patients were more likely to keep their subsequent clinic appointment if a clerk telephoned to remind them of the appointment than if no reminders were given. The latent objective of the research was to convince a hospital administrator that funds should be allocated to hire such a clerk. An evaluator of the research might comment that if the administrator required randomized-trial data to convince him of the value of such a clerk, the clinical investigators could have made better use of their time by trying to get a new administrator. There might be many reasons for not wanting to hire such a clerk in contrast to other types of desired personnel, but an administrator who refused to recognize the value of such a clerk, without obtaining randomized-trial evidence, would be too rigid in too many other decisions to be more than a bureaucratic nuisance.

14.4. ISSUES IN FEASIBILITY

Finally, or perhaps concomitantly with all the other questions, there is the matter of feasibility. Even if the basic objective is worthwhile and well designed, the project may be impossible to carry out because of difficulties in ethics, numbers, or other aspects of human life. These difficulties, which usually arise from the particular structure used in the research, become especially prominent when the investigator proposes an experimental or observational cohort study. Because of problems of feasibility in trying to conduct experiments or observational cohort studies, they are often replaced by the case-control, heterodemic, or other noncohort observational structures that are discussed later in the text.

14.4.1. *What Barriers Prevent an Experimental Allocation of Maneuvers?*

If the investigators are proposing an experiment or if a reviewer would prefer an experimental rather than observational structure for the research, the first point to be considered is the ethical or human barriers that would prevent the maneuvers from being allocated experimentally. For example, in comparative evaluations of contraceptive agents, we might be able to contrast one presumably active agent against another, but ethical constraints would forbid the assignment of women to be left unprotected as a placebo group. Because of human behavior, we could not conduct clinical trials in which cigarette smoking or breast feeding was randomly assigned.

It is possible, of course, to obtain data for women who do not use contraceptive agents; for smokers, nonsmokers, and ex-smokers; and for breast-feeding mothers and those who use bottles—but the research would have to be done as an observational survey, not as an experiment. The maneuvers will have been self-selected by the recipients.

14.4.2. *Can Enough People Be Obtained for the Study?*

The problem here is to obtain large enough numbers for the results to be quantitatively convincing and stochastically significant. The condition under study may be so uncommon that enough cases cannot be obtained at a single institution. Alternatively, the occurrence of the investigated condition may have been artifactually rarefied by restrictions imposed in the criteria established for admitting people to the study. Finally, even if enough potential candidates are available, many of them may refuse to volunteer for randomization or for whatever else is proposed in the research.

One of the main virtues of cooperative (or multi-institutional) research studies is that results can be pooled for people with conditions that cannot be obtained in sufficient numbers at a single medical setting. In exchange for the important statistical advantages, however, cooperative studies contain some major disadvantages. The multi-institutional collaboration creates a cumbersome set of logistics in carrying out the study and some difficult scientific hazards in arranging standardized procedures for materials and methods. Although cooperative studies can be used for observational research, they have become particularly common for the experiments of randomized trials and will be further discussed, together with other special aspects of randomized trials, in Chapter 29.

14.4.3. *Can the Outcome Events Be Observed and Suitably Analyzed?*

The prime issue here is whether the people investigated in an experimental or observational cohort study can be observed long enough and well enough to determine the performance of maneuvers and occurrence of the main outcome events. For example, could the research actually be conducted if the plan was to assemble a large cohort of 20-year-old men and see what happens to their serum cholesterol levels during the next 40 years? In a free-living and reasonably mobile society, how many of those men would report for annual, biennial, or other interval measurements of cholesterol, and how many would still be available for appraisal of their status 40 years later? How many of the investigators would still be available to do the appraisals? If we wanted to determine, in another long-term prolective cohort study, whether the nuances of ongoing familial interaction lead to schizophrenia, would we be able to obtain all the necessary details of the nuances of familial interaction?

A separate problem in long-term outcome events is the difficulty of separating the effects of the maneuver under scrutiny from all the other co-maneuvers that can occur as an external accompaniment during the follow-up interval. For example, suppose we decide to follow a cohort of 30- to 35-year-old people to determine whether the use of artificial sweeteners during the next 20 years leads to an increased incidence of certain cancers. How will we disentangle the effects of the artificial sweeteners from all the other potential carcinogens to which the people may be exposed during that interval?

14.5. SUBSEQUENT RE-APPRAISAL

For an investigator, the type of appraisal just described should occur at least twice. The first appraisal begins just after the outline of the research has been formulated. When the appraised outline has been fully implemented, by methods discussed in Chapters 15 to 17, the proposed research should be re-appraised.

The purpose of the second appraisal is to discover certain problems that were not apparent in the broad outline and that may have become evident only after the further implementation was developed. For example, in establishing procedures to gather data, is the investigator seeking too many details or not enough? During collection of data for a large array of different variables, has the investigator lost track of the main objective so that satisfactory information is not being acquired for the principal variables? Conversely, could additional data, collected without impairing the basic goals, yield answers to further questions of major importance in the research?

14.6. **SYNOPSIS**

The baseline state, outcome event(s), and compared maneuvers in a cause-effect research project constitute a basic architectural outline that should be appraised before additional plans are made to implement the research. The purpose of the appraisal is to avoid extensive efforts in arranging to carry out a defective fundamental plan.

The first two steps of this appraisal involve clarifying and stipulating the goals of the research and the main entities to be observed. A *begin-at-the-end* strategy, in which the investigator summarizes the main findings that are anticipated in the research, is often helpful in determining the particular entities that must receive major attention. Establishing the *latent objective* of the research is also helpful in deciding whether the proposed investigation can meet its goals or should be substantially altered. The entities noted in the basic outline should be checked to ensure that they have been specified without ambiguity, that they are suitable for the objectives of the research, that the groups under study appropriately represent the people to whom the results will be applied, and that the proposed maneuvers have previously been appropriately tested with animal or human pilot studies.

The next step in the appraisal is concerned with judgments about the value of doing the research. These decisions often depend on issues of public policy or on paradigmatic fashions in scientific ideology, rather than on the creativity or quality of the research itself. To overcome the prejudice of evaluators who are unsympathetic to the basic goals or structure of the research, the investigator needs to justify why the main question of the research is worth asking and the answer is worth obtaining. The justification often involves citing the importance of the problem under study, the necessities and innovations contained in the proposed methods, and the direct relationship of the results to a desirable subsequent objective.

The last step in the appraisal is devoted to problems of feasibility. Cooperative studies, in which multiple investigators and institutions collaborate to pool their data, may be needed to acquire sufficient numbers of people who have conditions that occur uncommonly or that have been rarefied by the admission criteria or other procedures used in the research. Prolective cohort studies may be unfeasible because enough people cannot be obtained for certain investigations or because the people cannot be followed long enough or well enough to obtain satisfactory data about the outcome events, the intervening maneuvers, and the differential impact of intervening maneuvers. In addition to the problem in long-term follow-up, certain experimental trials may be unfeasible because the proposed maneuvers would be either unethical if allocated by randomization or unacceptable to the people invited to volunteer as participants in the trial.

EXERCISES

Exercise 14.1. Comment *briefly* on the value and feasibility of each of the proposed projects that follow. For *value,* the main point is whether you regard the study as important or unimportant. If you think it is unimportant, please cite your reasons. For feasibility, the main point is whether you think the study can be successfully accomplished with the proposed research structure. If not, why not? Please also comment *briefly* on the stipulations of each project. The idea at this stage in the research outline is simply to be sure you have a good idea of what the investigator is talking about. Please do not pick nits about intensive details or criteria. For example, if the investigator proposes surgery for coronary artery disease, you need to know whether the intended maneuver is a bypass graft or cardiac transplantation, but if bypass grafting is proposed, you need not ask about how many grafts or from what site they will be taken.

14.1.1. In a prolective cohort study, does the mother's nutrition during pregnancy affect the subsequent intellectual capacity of the child?

14.1.2. In a randomized clinical trial, will ambulatory patients be more satisfied with their care if the clinical setting is refurbished with comfortable chairs, attractive walls and draperies, and up-to-date magazines than in the current unattractive facility used at our hospital?

14.1.3. In a prolective cohort study, what are the types and frequencies of adverse side effects that occur during a five-year period after initiation of contraception with pharmaceutical agents, as compared with mechanical forms of contraception?

14.1.4. In a randomized clinical trial, can nurse practitioners function just as effectively as physicians in providing primary health care?

14.1.5. In a randomized clinical trial, we want to determine whether hard-core unemployed people who are trained to act as communicators, counselors, and other sources of psychic support can improve preoperative anxiety and postoperative quality of life for elderly people undergoing major surgery.

14.1.6. In a randomized clinical trial, does radical surgery produce longer survival than simple surgery (or lumpectomy) for women with breast cancer?

14.1.7. In a randomized clinical trial, are blinded veterans more likely to respond to a notice of an appointment to a special rehabilitation clinic if the notice is sent as a mailed written letter or as a tape-recorded announcement?

14.1.8. In a prolective cohort study, can disturbed patients be helped just as well by concerned, empathic, reasonably skilled personnel (such as nurses, social workers, clergymen, appropriately selected grandparents) as by formally trained psychotherapists?

14.1.9. In a prolective cohort study, does a high-fiber diet reduce the risk of getting gastrointestinal cancer or other chronic GI diseases?

Exercise 14.2. Choose any *observational cohort* study of a cause-effect relationship in which you are (or might be) interested. State its basic objective and draw the schematic model for the architectural outline. Indicate the major advantages that might occur if this project were performed as an experiment rather than as an observational survey. State why the project is not being done as an experiment.

Exercise 14.3. Choose any two cause-effect research projects in which you are (or might be) interested. For each project, state the basic objective; draw a schematic architectural model for the reasoning used in the comparison; and state at least one latent objective for the study. Indicate how the project might be (or has been) a failure if the latent objective was not suitably considered when the project was designed. Can you find and briefly describe a published project that was a failure because of this problem?

CHAPTER REFERENCE

1. Kuhn, 1970.

Implementation of the Outline:
Baseline State

The cause-effect study that was outlined in Chapters 11 to 13 and possibly revised in Chapter 14 is now ready to be implemented. Having decided what is to be observed, the investigator must now arrange to observe it and determine what happened.

15.1. THE CHALLENGES OF INNATE BIAS

The things that happen "naturally" in the ordinary circumstances of human life and medical practice are not planned or intended to be scientific activities. Arrangements are not always made to obtain and record data of high scientific quality; the maneuvers to which people become exposed are selected and changed with personal judgments; and the outcomes are also observed and interpreted judgmentally.

Experiments are used to avoid the "innate" biases produced by these personal decisions, which can lead to distorted assembly of the group of people receiving maneuvers, susceptibility bias in the choice of compared maneuvers, performance bias in the way the maneuvers are carried out, detection bias in the way the outcomes are observed, and transfer bias in the information available for the research. With suitably designed and conducted experiments, all these biases can be eliminated or reduced. This desideratum is often provided by randomized controlled trials and makes them so scientifically attractive in clinical epidemiologic research.

For many cause-effect investigations, however, randomized trials are either impossible or unfeasible. Instead of being able to make comparisons with the scientific rigor of an experiment, the investigator must analyze comparisons that occurred under natural circumstances. The investigator can sometimes arrange to get high-quality data for these nonexperimental comparisons but must often work with data, of uncertain scientific quality, that were obtained and recorded by someone else.

These distinctions create major differences in the scientific challenges that occur when the plan of a research study is implemented. In an experiment, the innate biases can be eliminated in the planned design, and the investigator's job in implementation is to carry out the plans. In a nonexperimental research structure, some or all of the innate biases will be contained in the assembled information, and the investigator's job, as part of the research implementation, is to make suitable plans for discerning the biases and for removing or adjusting them. While making plans to deal with the innate biases received in the data, the investigator is also challenged to avoid methods of analysis that will introduce additional problems beyond those that may already be present.

15.2. **DISTINCTIONS AND CONSEQUENCES OF ARCHITECTURAL STRUCTURES**

The activities in implementing the plan of a cause-effect outline will differ not only for experimental and nonexperimental research but also for different nonexperimental structures. Some of the main distinctions of these structures are shown in Figure 15–1.

In a cohort study, the main groups under investigation are selected according to their baseline state before the maneuvers were imposed. In a case-control or other non-cohort study, the basic groups are chosen according to their outcomes or other postmaneuver states. Furthermore, in the noncohort structures, all of the investigator's information about baseline state, maneuvers, and outcomes is assembled after these events have already transpired.

In a prolective study of an inception cohort, the investigator enters the research scene

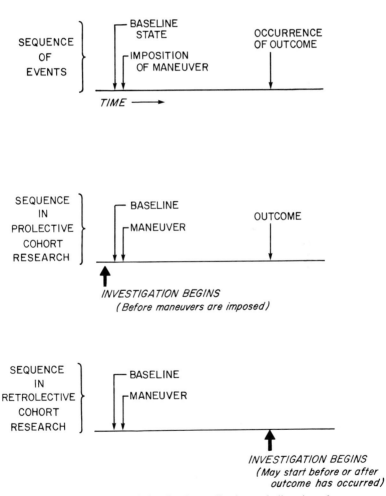

Figure 15–1. Distinctions of timing for data collection and allocation of maneuvers.

before the maneuvers are imposed. The investigator can then arrange beforehand to collect suitable data for identifying the baseline state and subsequent events. In a retrolective cohort study, the investigator begins collecting the research data after imposition of the maneuvers. To identify the maneuvers and baseline states, the investigator must depend on recorded archival data or other "retrospective" sources of information.

A prolective cohort study becomes an experimental trial if the maneuvers are allocated according to a specific investigative plan, such as randomization. In all other research structures, the maneuvers are chosen by practicing clinicians or are self-selected by the exposed people, without a specific plan for investigative assignment.

For example, suppose we want to know whether tea drinking causes gallstones. In an experimental trial, we would arrange for a group of healthy young adults to volunteer to receive and maintain a randomized assignment to drink or not drink tea. We would follow the people long enough thereafter to observe the subsequent development (or nondevelopment) of gallstones.

In a prolective cohort study, we would find healthy young adults just before they have made their own decision to begin drinking or not drinking tea. We would let them carry out the decision and follow them thereafter. In a retrolective cohort study, we would start the research after the tea drinking decisions have already been carried out. One way of assembling the people might be to do a household survey. We could then ask each interviewed person to tell us what has been going on since young adulthood, determine their current status, and follow them thereafter. Alternatively, if suitable records were available somewhere, we might be able to find groups of people who were noted long ago in young adult life to be tea drinkers or non–tea drinkers. We would then try to locate those people and identify their subsequent development of gallstones.

In a case-control study, we would start with a group of people who are already known to have gallstones, and we would choose a "control" group of people who do not have gallstones. We would then ask the members of each group about their antecedent drinking of tea. In a heterodemic study, we would not have to examine any people directly. We could get data about the annual occurrence rates of gallstones in a particular region and see whether changes in those rates are related to changes in the annual sales of tea in that region.

The type and amount of implementation done by the investigator will therefore depend on the architectural structure used in the research. In all structures, the investigator must assemble data for the groups of compared people, but the groups are chosen differently for cohort and non-cohort research. In all structures, the investigator must contemplate data to identify each person's baseline state, imposed maneuvers, and subsequent outcomes, but in prolective studies, advance plans can be made to acquire information that is complete and reliable. In the retrolective cohort (or non-cohort) structures, the investigator must work with whatever has been recorded in various archives or recalled by individual people. In an experimental trial, the investigator has the additional job of arranging the allocation of maneuvers, but in nonexperimental studies, the investigator must find out which maneuvers were received and what biases may have occurred because of the selectivity with which the maneuvers were chosen and carried out.

In this chapter and the two that follow it, the discussion will be concerned with the events that occur during and after the imposition of maneuvers. The basic viewpoint will be that of a cohort study in which the maneuvers are observed prolectively, with or without an experimental allocation. Because this type of research structure coincides with the basic architectural reasoning used to interpret the results of cause-effect research, the challenges of forming groups, getting data, and analyzing results for the imposed maneuvers will be relatively straightforward. The imposition of the maneuver and the implementation of the investigator's research plan will occur at the same time.

In a retrolective cohort study, the intellectual and actual architecture of the research will still coincide, because the cohort is followed in a longitudinal forward direction, but the investigator may have many additional problems in forming groups and obtaining satisfactory data after the events have already occurred. In case-control, heterodemic, and other non-cohort research structures, the actual procedures used in the research form a structural model that is drastically different from the scientific model with which the results are interpreted. The investigator must not only find out what happened but must analyze the non-cohort results in a manner satisfactory for scientific reasoning.

Because the scientific principles of cause-effect reasoning remain the same regardless of what structure is used to perform the research, the discussion here will focus on the challenges produced when maneuvers are imposed. The challenges are readily perceived and discussed for research conducted with cohort structures. The same challenges also occur and must be considered for noncohort investigative structures, but the disparities between the components of the research and the architecture of scientific reasoning produce special additional problems that will be discussed separately in Chapters 18 to 22 of Part IV.

15.3. **ADDITIONAL CHRONOLOGIC DISTINCTIONS**

In addition to the cohort or non-cohort direction of the research and the prolective or retrolective timing of data collection, the information can be obtained and analyzed with several other chronologic distinctions. In certain retrolective studies, part of the data can be obtained "prolectively," i.e., with advance planning for direct observation, and in certain prolective studies, phenomena that received little or no attention in the original research plan can be analyzed "retrospectively."

A retrolective cohort study acquires a "prolective" or direct-data component when the outcome of the cohort is observed directly. In this type of study, the investigator assembles the cohort retrolectively, using special surveys or archival data to find the members and to identify the baseline states and initiation of maneuvers. The members of the cohort are then located in their subsequent state, and the investigator directly observes their outcome condition. This type of activity was demonstrated during the examples of Section 15.2 when the investigator used a household survey to assemble a cohort of people who may have started tea drinking many years earlier but whose subsequent gallstones would be determined directly. The research described in Exercise 12.6.7 at the end of Chapter 12 is another example of a retrolective cohort study with direct data outcomes. The cohort was assembled retrolectively from data for measurements of serum pepsinogen obtained many years previously in members of a college's entering freshmen class. Using alumni records to determine the current location of members of the cohort, the investigators then tried to reach each member to get prolective data about the outcome events.[1]

A more clinical example of a *retrolective-prolective cohort* design was used for a study of growth and development in children with sickle cell trait.[2] The groups of investigated infants and their newborn baseline states, with and without sickle cell trait, were identified retrolectively from existing medical data assembled several years earlier in a perinatal cord-blood screening project. The outcome state, which represented a serial time 4 to 5 years later, was identified when each invited child appeared for a special examination conducted by the investigators.

A reversal of the prolective direction of planning occurs when the results of a clinical trial are analyzed in a "retrospective" manner. For example, data from several randomized trials may be combined many years after the trials were completed for a retrospective analysis of the pooled information.[3] A more common example of retrospective analysis is the type of stratification, described briefly in Section 12.3.2, that is used for further analysis of results obtained with a "complete" (or "unstratified") randomization in a single trial. If the originally assembled information is adequate, the data used in the retrospective analyses will have been obtained prolectively. If the original information is inadequate, the investigators may make retrolective efforts, after the trial is completed, to obtain what is missing or to fix the defects.

Retrolectively acquired data can be used to improve the description of any necessary feature of the baseline states, performance of maneuvers, or outcomes in a prolective study. For example, in the UGDP randomized trial of therapy for diabetes mellitus,[4] the investigators were initially concerned with vascular complications rather than death as the principal outcome event in the research. When a substantial number of deaths occurred during the trial, the prolectively assembled death certificate information was scientifically inadequate for identifying causes of death. The investigators then made retrolective efforts to assemble better data about each patient's moribund phenomena.[4, 5]

The outcome observed in the cohorts of a randomized clinical trial can also be extended retrospectively to encompass phenomena occurring long after the original trial was completed. For example, when diethylstilbestrol (DES) became suspected of causing abnormalities in the children whose mothers received it during pregnancy, the hypothesis was investigated by obtaining additional follow-up data,[6] many years later, from a randomized trial in which DES had been originally tested only for its immediate effects on the gestation.[7]

The main point to be noted before we leave this section is that research data can be collected and analyzed with both "prospective" and "retrospective" methods, regardless of the structure used in the research. Furthermore, regardless of the research structure or the timing of data collection, each component of the states and maneuvers used in scientific reasoning about a cause-effect relationship should be suitable for the question framed in the research and should be compared in a similar, unbiased manner.

To avoid an excessively long batch of reading, this chapter is concerned only with problems of suitability and similarity for the baseline state of the people in whom the investigated maneuvers are imposed. Chapter 16 is devoted to analogous problems in performance of the maneuvers themselves, and Chapter 17 to the states that occur as outcome events.

15.4. ACQUISITION OF BASELINE DATA

In addition to providing a suitable identification of the baseline states that are compared during cause-effect reasoning, the premaneuver data have several other important roles that must be considered when the data are acquired. The information can be used to "screen" candidates for admission to the study, to determine their prognostic susceptibility to outcome events, and to appraise transitions between baseline and outcome states. The rest of this section is devoted to the role of the baseline information in issues of suitability, admission to the study, prognostic analysis, and transitions.

15.4.1. *Suitability of Variables in Prolective and Retrolective Studies*

From the discussion in Chapter 13 we might conclude that suitable variables can be chosen much more easily in prolective than in retrolective research. After all, the prolective investigator can decide what information to collect, whereas retrolective research depends on what someone else has recorded. The conclusion is correct, but things do not always work out that way.

When choosing the variables in a prolective study, the investigator may be affected by fashionable paradigms that constrain or alter the focus of the research. The investigator may then emphasize the collection of "hard data" as a substitute for "soft data" that may be more important and suitable but more difficult to measure. Because the information assembled prolectively depends entirely on previous decisions about which variables to measure, the investigator may find after the project is finished that certain important or crucial information was omitted.

This type of problem can also arise when unexpected outcome events occur in a randomized trial. To determine the patients' prognostic susceptibility to these outcome events requires a suitable analysis of data describing the patients' baseline conditions—but the most cogent descriptive data may not have been collected. For example, in a randomized trial of sulfinpyrazone therapy to prevent recurrent myocardial infarction,[8] the investigators found unexpected benefits for active treatment in preventing sudden death. Because many of the sudden deaths were presumably due to arrhythmias, a prognostic analysis was needed to show that the compared groups were similar in their baseline susceptibility to developing arrhythmias. Such an analysis, however, would require information from a 24-hour period of monitoring cardiac rhythm in ambulatory patients. Because arrhythmias had not been suspected as outcome events, the prognostic monitoring had not been performed in the patients' baseline states.

In a retrolective study, the data inscribed in medical records may not have the high quality that is possible in prolective research, but the retrolective information may often have the advantage of having been recorded without any prejudicial judgments about scientific importance. The archival sources may thus contain valuable soft data that have been deliberately excluded, because of the "hard-data" zeitgeist, from prolective studies of the same topic. By developing appropriate systems of taxonomy for dealing with the soft information, the retrolective investigator may be able to demonstrate its importance, use it to improve the analysis of results, and establish its value for future research. For example, the importance of performance status as a cogent prognostic factor in patients with cancer was demonstrated by retrospective analysis of data originally assembled as an incidental variable in randomized trials of chemotherapy.[9] Other soft but cogent prognostic variables have been demonstrated from retrolective surveys of medical records of patients with cancer. Among such variables are the cluster of symptoms, severity of symptoms, chronometry and auxometry (rate of growth) of manifestations, and impact of co-morbid ailments.[10–13]

The data recorded in archival sources (as well as in prolective studies) will often omit many important items of information. In most studies of nonpsychiatric therapy, the patient's psychic status is usually described poorly or not at all. No reasons may be mentioned for various decisions in the patient's medical itinerary of transfers from one clinician or institution to another. A precise stipulation may not be entered for the reasons why one particular treatment was preferred to another or why certain treatments were started or stopped. Trying to determine whether prominent clinical symptoms have been relieved, the investigator may find that the medical progress notes contain only the results of paraclinical tests and that changes in the patient's clinical condition are recorded only in the increasingly infrequent entries of nurse's notes.

Nevertheless, because the archival information was inscribed spontaneously without the specifications or limitations of a research protocol, the existing records sometimes contain important data that were omitted from a prolective research plan prepared without adequate attention to suitability of variables. An alert investigator who is uninhibited by the mensurational fashions, and who is willing to accept a slight reduction in quality of data in exchange for a major increase in the cogency of variables, can often take advantage of this scientific opportunity.

15.4.2. *Disparities Between Desired and Admitted Groups*

No one appears spontaneously in a research study. To be counted in the results, the investigated people had to be invited or selected to contribute their data. The acceptances and rejections that occur during this solicitation can lead to substantial distortions in the results of the research.

Although the investigator cannot prevent disparities between the groups who are desired and admitted to a research project, several precautions can be taken to reduce the magnitude of the disparities, to analyze their effect, and to arrive at appropriate adjustments and interpretations. The precautions all require a suitable identification of the people who were considered or solicited but not included in the study. Many details of the baseline state of these people may be unknown because they were not examined, but other details—such as place of residence and basic demographic and diagnostic status—will have been acquired as part of the information that led to each person's consideration as a possible candidate for the study. This pre-admission information about the baseline state can then be used to compare the characteristics of the people who were or were not actually included in the study.

15.4.3. *Appraisal of Transition Variables*

When a change occurs between outcome and baseline state for a dimensional variable, such as blood pressure or serum cholesterol, the measured distinction can readily be expressed as an increment, ratio, or proportionate increment. If the measurement is expressed in nominal, dichotomous, or ordinal categories, however, the scales of expression may be too coarse to permit the identification of distinct, important changes that can occur while a patient remains in the same category.

For example, according to the New York Heart Association criteria for functional capacity,[14] a patient who is bedridden is cited in Class IV of the disability scale. After receiving treatment, the patient may become continent, oriented, and able to feed himself while still remaining bedridden and therefore still in Class IV. The substantial functional improvement would go unrecognized because the four categories available for classifying functional disability do not provide a method for denoting an improved transition in a bedridden patient.

To avoid this type of problem, the investigator should review the proposed list of baseline variables and note whether outcome transitions are to be determined from the subsequent state of those same variables. If a particular baseline variable is not suitable for identifying transitions, the investigator should consider expressing the corresponding phenomenon in a separate, distinctive *transition variable*,[15] which is used directly to identify changes rather than a single state.

15.4.4. *Preparation for Prognostic Analysis*

Despite common fulfillment of the admission criteria, the people admitted to a study may be distinctly different in their susceptibility to the outcome events. Thus, in an investigation of treatment for breast cancer, the persons with localized tumors have better survival expectations than those with involvement of regional lymph nodes. In a general population, older people have a much shorter additional life expectancy than younger people.

To ensure that the maneuver is evaluated appropriately, the members of a cohort are regularly classified according to their baseline prognostic status—before the maneuver is imposed—for susceptibility to the outcome event. The prognostic classifications have at least three different purposes: to identify the prognostic composition of compared cohorts; to determine whether the compared maneuvers have disparate effects in people with different prognostic susceptibility; and to allow precise extrapolation of the results.

In the next three subsections, which illustrate the roles of prognostic classification, we shall assume that the prognostic distinctions are cited in partitioned composite categories, called *strata*. The strata are often identified with titles such as **good risk, fair risk,** or **poor risk.** A well-known example of a prognostic stratification is the system of stages, designated as **I, II,** or **III,** that is commonly used in the TNM classification of patients with cancer.[16]

15.4.4.1. COMPOSITION OF COHORTS

Prognostic categories are regularly used to show the *spectral partition* or *spectral proportions* of the baseline states contained in the cohort exposed to each maneuver. The purpose is to check the similarity (or disparity) of the cohorts produced by either randomization or whatever mechanism was used to allocate the maneuvers. For example, the baseline state of 150 persons receiving treatment A might be summarized with a spectral partition showing that 40 *(27%)* were in the **good** prognostic stratum, 80 *(53%)* were in the **fair** stratum, and 30 *(20%)* were in the **poor** group. If the corresponding spectral proportions for 154 persons receiving treatment B were 43 *(28%)* **good,** 79 *(51%)* **fair,** and 32 *(21%)* **poor,** we would conclude that cohorts A and B had similar prognostic compositions (at least for what was included in the categories designated as **good, fair,** and **poor**).

15.4.4.2. STRATIFICATION FOR EFFECTS OF MANEUVERS

The results of the spectral partition in Section 15.4.4.1 will tell us about the baseline states of the compared cohorts but not what happened after the maneuvers were imposed. For the latter purpose, the results would be presented as a stratification that shows the outcome of each maneuver in each of the prognostic strata. Thus, in the foregoing cohorts, treatment A, with a *50%* success rate, might seem to have had results quite similar to treatment B, with a *52%* success rate. A baseline stratification for the results of each treatment, however, might show the following distinctions in rates of success:

Prognostic Category	Treatment A	Treatment B
Good	26/40 *(65%)*	37/43 *(86%)*
Fair	39/80 *(49%)*	40/79 *(51%)*
Poor	10/30 *(33%)*	3/32 *(9%)*
TOTAL	75/150 *(50%)*	80/154 *(52%)*

We now see that the two treatments had some dramatically different effects. Although both treatments had similar rates of success in the **fair** prognostic group, treatment B was substantially better than treatment A in the **good** group and substantially worse in the **poor** group. This distinction would have been completely missed if we had inspected only the total results for each treatment.

The tactic of prognostic stratification is constantly used in public health epidemiology, as discussed in Chapter 20, to compare mortality or morbidity rates in general populations for whom the compared maneuvers are different geographic regions (such as the U.S. and the U.K.) or different secular eras (such as 1969 to 1974 and 1979 to 1984). For this purpose, the populations can be stratified according to different baseline categories of age, race, and gender, and the outcomes can be cited in such stratum-specific phrases as *mortality rate for white men, ages 40 to 54.* To avoid having to compare rates across different strata, the stratum-specific results for a single region or single secular era are often adjusted or standardized to a single value. In the customary standardization, which is further described in Chapter 20, the stratum-specific outcome rates are multiplied by the proportions that each stratum would occupy in a standard population. The products of these multiplications are then added to form a single *standardized rate* or *age-gender-race adjusted rate* for each population, and these adjusted rates are then used for comparisons of public health maneuvers.

15.4.4.3. EXTRAPOLATION OF RESULTS

Although the standardization process just described could be used to adjust baseline prognostic disparities when treatments are compared in clinical epidemiology, a clinical evaluator seldom wants to obtain a single adjusted value for the results of different treatments. Instead, the clinician wants to know what happened for each treatment in the different prognostic strata. Besides, the adjustment process is useful only for dealing with disparities in the spectral partition of the baseline states. The adjustment would not show the disparate interplay between baseline state and treatment that produced the post-therapeutic distinctions noted in Section 15.4.4.2. For this reason, a clinician usually wants to see the results of treatment A versus treatment B compared separately in each of the **good, fair,** and **poor** prognostic strata.

Beyond the cited role in avoiding misleading post-therapeutic results, a stratified analysis has three important functions when the results of the research are extrapolated for application afterward. First, in clinical activities, a clinician choosing treatment for an individual patient wants to know what each potential treatment has previously accomplished in similar patients. This similarity can be more easily determined if previous results are prognostically stratified than if everything is lumped together as a total for each treatment. Second, when statistical estimates are made to determine the possible distortions produced by the absence of appropriate candidates who were *not* included in the study, the estimates will depend on results found for people who were in strata similar to those of the absentees. Third, by examining the spectral partitions for different strata, we can determine how well the investigated group represents the population to which the total results might be extrapolated. Thus, if the spectral partition shows ample numbers and proportions of *old men, young women,* and *old women* but very few *young men,* we might conclude that young men have been substantially underrepresented in the cohort. The results found in the first three strata might be quite suitable for extrapolation to other members of those strata, but the results in the total cohort should not be generalized.

15.4.4.4. CHOICE OF COGENT PROGNOSTIC VARIABLES

For all these reasons, the investigator will want to be sure that data have been collected, whenever possible, to identify cogent prognostic variables in the baseline state of the cohorts under study. Because prognostic susceptibility depends on the particular event that is chosen as the outcome, different choices of this outcome will make different baseline variables become prognostically cogent or relatively unimportant.

For example, in a patient with acute myocardial infarction, the cogent prognostic variables may differ strikingly according to whether the selected outcome event is *prompt disappearance of chest pain, survival at 30 days,* or *return to former occupation.* The baseline variables that predict the likelihood of prompt disappearance of pain may depend mainly on characteristics of the pain; short-term survival may depend mainly on physiologic derangements in cardiac function; and return to former occupation may depend mainly on the person's job, psychic status, and life style.

Because a prognostic analysis is only as good as the baseline variables it includes, and because the analysis will be inadequate if cogent variables are omitted, the choice of these variables is a particularly important but difficult scientific judgment. What makes the judgment so difficult is that some variables are important for one prognostic goal but unimportant for another, and that other variables, although clinically well recognized as important, are either omitted from analysis because they lack a taxonomic classification or are inadequately analyzed because the classification is unsatisfactory.

As an example of changes in prognostic importance for different variables, *age* and *gender** would be much more cogent than *serum cholesterol* and *familial history* in predicting susceptibility to pregnancy but might be substantially less cogent in predicting susceptibility to coronary artery disease. None of these four variables would be particularly cogent in predicting the immediate outcome of an acute myocardial infarction. For the latter prediction, the cogent variables would be such features as shock, congestive heart failure, arrhythmias, and co-morbidity. Among the many clinically recognized cogent variables that are usually omitted from prognostic analyses of therapy are the symptomatic, chronometric, and co-morbid patterns mentioned earlier (in Section 15.4.1). When patients' performance status is considered, the investigators seldom distinguish pathophysiologic from psychologic causes of impairment. In epidemiologic analyses of risk factors for development of disease, familial ailments and longevity are regularly omitted; and the complexity of the human psyche, when considered at all, is usually designated only with the crude binary categories of *type A* and *type B*.

Because of the vital importance of choosing cogent prognostic variables, they warrant careful scientific attention, regardless of the particular architectural structure used in the research.

15.5. ADMISSION CRITERIA

Despite the large amount of statistical literature devoted to sampling and particularly to random samples, the research projects of clinical science are almost never performed upon a sample. The groups of people whose data are collected and analyzed did not get there by haphazard chance or by random selection. A great many human decisions were involved in the process by which the people were transferred from their state of scientific anonymity at home to their statistical exaltation as members of a group of analyzed data. The people had to decide to seek medical attention, to accept what clinicians offered, and to participate in the research. The personal clinicians had to make decisions about diagnosis, prognosis, and therapy; and the investigators had to decide whom to include in the research.

---

*Because sex is an important human activity as well as an inborn biologic attribute, I have throughout this book reserved *sex* for the activity and *gender* for the attribute. In many epidemiologic analyses, people have the chance to be "broken down by sex," but here the breakdown is by gender.

All of these human decisions create abundant opportunities for the subsequent groups of data to receive distortions that can produce improper statistics and defective research.

The sequence and components of these different decisions warrant detailed attention for the same reason that biochemists try to decompose a metabolic pathway into its constituent events: If we want a scientific understanding of what is happening, we need to know precisely how it happens. This section is concerned with the decisions, made by practicing clinicians and mainly by investigators, that determine who will be admitted to a research project. Section 15.6, which follows, describes the decisions made by the people under investigation.

The admission criteria chosen for a cohort study determine the baseline state of the persons who will enter the investigation as having received the compared maneuvers. The baseline state—which is also sometimes called the *initial state, baseline condition, pretreatment condition, starting point, zero state,* or *focal state*—becomes specified with two decisions. One decision involves a stipulation of the set of conditions that would make a person diagnostically eligible to be a candidate for the study. The other decision contains boundaries that may exclude a person from admission, even though diagnostically eligible. These two decisions produce the combination of *eligibility criteria* and *exclusion criteria* that constitute the *admission criteria.*

For example, in a study designed to test the remedial effects of Excellitol on ordinary headaches, the eligible people would be those who fulfill criteria for the diagnosis of "ordinary headache," but not all such people would be admitted to the study. We might exclude pregnant women, persons who are taking chronic salicylate therapy for arthritic disorders, or persons known to be allergic to any of the ingredients of Excellitol.

15.5.1. *Eligibility Criteria*

The main requirements of eligibility criteria are suitability and consistency. The criteria should obviously be suitable for choosing appropriate people for admission. To be consistent, the criteria should be described in a manner that is clear enough to allow them to be understood by the reader and to be used reproducibly, if desired, by another investigator. Thus, if the investigator says the study is concerned with acute myocardial infarction, we would not know exactly what is required for a patient to be admitted. If the investigator says he admitted patients according to the WHO criteria for acute myocardial infarction,[17] we would have a much better idea, although we might still have problems deciding what is meant by "shock" or "abnormal enzymes" in the WHO criteria.

15.5.2. *Exclusion Criteria*

Although the investigator's results are aimed at the population of eligible people, this population is always constrained by a series of exclusions that produce the groups actually studied in the research. Some of these exclusions are inevitable, occurring because many of the potentially eligible participants are either geographically unavailable for the study or unwilling to participate in it. Many other exclusions, however, are deliberately imposed by clinical practitioners or investigators for reasons of therapeutic exigency, prognostic susceptibility, therapeutic vulnerability, contamination of maneuvers, spectral homogeneity, investigative efficiency, or biased referral. These decisions, which are discussed in the next few sections, are made with data obtained for the candidate person's baseline diagnosis, co-morbidity, co-medication, demography, patterns of behavior, and medical itinerary. As noted later, the decisions can have profound effects on the similarity of comparisons conducted in the research and on the suitability of the results.

15.5.2.1. THERAPEUTIC EXIGENCY

The patients admitted to a randomized trial or other comparison of therapeutic agents should be suitable for receiving any of the compared agents. For a particular patient, if one or more of the compared agents has the therapeutic exigency of being mandatorily indicated or contraindicated because of the severity, co-morbidity, or other features of the patient's baseline state, the patient would be excluded from the proposed comparison.

For example, because patients with insulin-dependent diabetes mellitus cannot be left without insulin treatment, they would not be admitted to a trial in which they might be assigned to receive only oral hypoglycemic agents or placebo. In a trial in which anticoagulants will be compared against placebo in the treatment of acute myocardial infarction, the patients to be excluded because of therapeutic exigency might include those with concomitant deep venous thrombosis, for whom anticoagulant therapy might be mandated, or those with gastrointestinal bleeding, for whom anticoagulants would be contraindicated. A highly neurotic patient with inflammatory bowel disease, who might become psychotic if subjected to a total colonic resection with permanent colostomy, could be excluded from a trial containing this surgical procedure as one of the therapeutic possibilities.

15.5.2.2. PROGNOSTIC SUSCEPTIBILITY

Patients at the extremely good or poor ends of the spectrum of prognostic susceptibility to the outcome event may be deliberately excluded from a trial because of the belief that their anticipated outcome cannot be adequately affected by the proposed maneuvers. For example, patients with a shortened life expectancy because of advanced cancer would not be admitted to a trial assessing the long-term outcome of surgery for coronary disease. Alternatively, patients with mild conditions might be excluded from a trial intended to pose a suitable challenge to the tested treatments. For example, in a randomized trial of surgery versus medical therapy for children with tonsillitis, the admitted patients were restricted to those with a documented history of repeated, clinically severe episodes.[18]

In studies of oral contraceptive agents, the people to be admitted would be those susceptible to becoming pregnant. The excluded patients would therefore be men (unless the contraceptive agent is intended to act on men) and nonfecundable women, who are premenarchal or postmenstrual, who have had hysterectomy or bilateral ovariectomy, or who do not have suitable sexual exposure.

15.5.2.3. THERAPEUTIC VULNERABILITY

The idea of *vulnerability*, which was briefly mentioned in Section 11.9.1, refers to a specific interaction between human host and maneuver rather than to the prognostic susceptibility that is an attribute of the baseline condition alone. Without having any of the foregoing therapeutic exigencies or distinctive prognostic susceptibilities, patients would be excluded from a comparative trial of therapy if they seem particularly vulnerable or invulnerable to any of the maneuvers under study.

A patient is invulnerable if the treatment seems to offer no potential benefit. For example, to receive surgical bypass for coronary artery disease, a patient must have an anatomically remediable lesion. If the coronary arteriogram shows insufficient or no evidence of occlusion, or if too many vessels are occluded, the patient would be denied admission to a cohort receiving surgical bypass. When non-narcotic analgesic agents are to be tested, patients with very severe pain, which might respond only to treatment with narcotics, are often excluded from admission. If we wanted to investigate the adverse effect of sexual hormones on a gestating fetus, pregnant women would be excluded from the study if they have passed a suitable stage of fetal vulnerability, which is usually the first trimester of pregnancy.

A patient is also vulnerable to a treatment if it is known to bear the threat of immediate harm. This potential threat from a presumably beneficial maneuver is the reason for excluding actually or potentially pregnant women from many therapeutic trials, and also for excluding people who have previously had allergic reactions to any of the proposed pharmaceutical agents. The potential for adverse reaction, rather than a previously demonstrated sensitivity, can be another reason for exclusion. Thus, because of the bronchospastic potential of many beta-blocking drugs, people with asthma or chronic pulmonary disease are often omitted from trials of such agents. Patients would be denied an operation if they are so ill that they might not be able to tolerate the anesthesia or the performance of surgery. Patients who can survive the operation itself might be excluded if its anatomic consequences are hazardous. Thus, a patient with severely impaired pulmonary function might not be able to spare the non-neoplastic tissue removed in a proposed pneumonectomy for localized cancer of the lung.

15.5.2.4. CONTAMINATION OF MANEUVERS

A different clinical reason for excluding people from a study of therapy is that they are receiving a concomitant medication that may contaminate the action or the appraisal of one of the main maneuvers under investigation. For example, a person receiving anticoagulant therapy might not be admitted to a study testing the effects of aspirin on platelet function. A person being treated with doses of aspirin for arthritis might be excluded from a study of analgesic agents for headache or postepisiotomy pain.

15.5.2.5. SPECTRAL HOMOGENEITY

The four previous types of exclusion were necessitated by clinical aspects of the baseline state, the treatments, or their interactions. Two other types of exclusion may be created for the convenience of the investigator in analyzing the results or conducting the research.

If the group under study contains a heterogeneous spectrum of different types of people and clinical conditions, the results of the research may be difficult to analyze. To avoid this problem, the investigator may try to make the spectrum more homogeneous (or "clean") by constraining its boundaries to exclude patients who have certain co-morbid ailments or who might be demographic outliers in the cohort under investigation. For example, although a man with gout might have no clinical or pharmaceutical reasons for being denied appropriate treatment for coronary artery disease, such a patient might be excluded to purify the group tested in a trial of medical versus surgical therapy. Because of demographic infrequency in the cohort, women might be excluded from a study conducted at a Veterans Administration hospital. Black people might be excluded from a study conducted in an environment where most of the patients are white (or vice versa).

15.5.2.6. INVESTIGATIVE EFFICIENCY

To save potentially wasted effort, the investigators may exclude patients who might move away from the site of the investigation while the trial is in progress, who appear unwilling to cooperate with the examination procedures needed for the research protocol, who might not suitably comply with the prescribed maneuvers, or who might not be able to give a suitably informed consent for admission to a trial.

Among the clinical and demographic features that might lead to such exclusions are alcoholism, dementia, psychiatric disorders, or the geographic mobility produced by an occupation such as military service.

15.5.2.7. BIASED REFERRAL OR MIGRATION

By clinical referral or self-selection (as discussed further in Section 15.6), many patients come to specialized medical centers from zones outside the usual catchment areas of those centers. Because the migrating extrazonal group may have substantial prognostic differences from the intrazonal group, the subsequent results of the mixed group at the immigrant location cannot be fairly compared with an unmixed set of intrazonal results.

Agrez and coworkers[19] demonstrated this type of bias in clinical studies by showing that surgical therapy was needed less often for Crohn's disease in groups of patients demarcated from defined populations than in groups collected at medical referral centers. In epidemiologic public health studies, such biases can be produced by the geographic migrations noted in Section 15.6.1.2.

In a randomized trial, the problem is often irrelevant, because the prognostic distinctions would presumably be equally distributed among the compared therapeutic maneuvers; but in observational studies in which the institutions or geographic zones become regarded as the compared maneuvers, the comparisons may be biased. For observational clinical research, the investigators can therefore review each patient's medical itinerary and confine the inception cohort to people who have been acquired from the appropriate populational zone. In public health studies, the adjustment is usually impossible because the necessary information is unavailable.

15.5.3. *Qualification Period*

To ensure that the admission criteria are fulfilled, investigators may sometimes test patients during a qualification period before admitting them to a randomized trial. The qualification period can be used to check the persistent maintenance of certain eligibility criteria, such as an elevated blood pressure or arthritic pain when untreated. Qualification periods can also be used to wash out the potential contamination produced by carry-over effects from previous treatment, and to establish the absence of conditions—such as metastatic cancer or poor compliance—that might otherwise lead to the patient's exclusion from the study.

15.5.4. *Substitutes for Inaccessible Candidates*

As noted in Section 15.6, the people who fulfill admission criteria for a particular study may not all be admitted to it. Although the effect of their absence must always be appraised, our concern in this section is with the substitutes chosen for inaccessible candidates.

In prolective studies in which the cohort is obtained by accrual of successive patients in a clinical setting, the substitutes for candidates who refuse to participate are usually the next patients who appear at the site of the research and who fulfill the admission criteria. In surveys that assemble the cohort from responses to a mailed questionnaire or a telephone call, the substitutes will usually come from the next names on the list. If the list has been exhausted, the investigators may enlarge the scope of the geographic region or other sources of the list. If the desired person is not at home when the interviewer appears in a household survey, data about that person may be obtained from a relative or friend, or the interviewer may go to an adjacent home.

Retrolective cohort studies contain some special problems. The investigator may not be able to find the archival data to describe the baseline state of each person on the list of potential candidates. In a retrolective-prolective cohort, whose candidates enter the study only if their outcome data are acquired by direct communication, the investigator will lose those members with whom communication could not be established. If the size of the cohort is fixed (as in the study of pepsinogen measurements for a single group of college freshmen), there is no way to replace the losses. Many other retrolective cohorts, however, are demarcated by a secular boundary, e.g., children born at a particular hospital during 1973 to 1976, or patients treated for omphalosis during 1979 to 1981. If enough members of the candidate cohort are inaccessible, the secular boundary can be extended to cover a larger period of time, thereby allowing more patients to become eligible.

15.5.5. *Postmaneuver Withdrawals*

After having been admitted to a randomized trial or other cohort study, certain persons may later withdraw from it and be unavailable for examination of their outcome state. They may have died, for reasons related or unrelated to the investigated maneuvers, before the end of the planned duration of observation. They may have decided to drop out of the study for clinical reasons, such as a major improvement or worsening of symptoms, or for personal reasons, such as moving away or losing interest. Alternatively, the decision to withdraw the patient may have been made by the attending clinician because of an adverse drug reaction, or by the investigator because the patient was later deemed ineligible for admission or was cooperating poorly with the research protocol.

In a prolective cohort study, the investigator, knowing which members of the cohort have withdrawn after onset of the maneuvers, can decide how best to include or exclude the withdrawals when denominators are counted for expressing the results of different outcome phenomena. The reasons for the withdrawals and the way they are counted in the subsequent analysis of data can substantially alter what is found for members of the cohort who persisted in the study.

These problems, which can be managed (and disputed) in prolective studies by using methods discussed in Chapter 29, become much more thorny in nonprolective research. In a retrolective cohort study, the investigator who cannot reach members of the cohort to determine their status after admission has no idea whether they are dead or alive. If the missing members occupy a large proportion of the total cohort, the results of the entire study may be unreliable. In non-cohort research, the problem is potentially even worse, because an actual cohort was not assembled. The investigator therefore has no way of knowing what proportion of the cohort was withdrawn, and how and why the withdrawals occurred. During the scientific reasoning with which the non-cohort results are interpreted for the cohort of people who received the original maneuvers, there is no way of assuring the investigator (or the reviewer) that the original cohort is accurately represented by the remnants collected in a case-control or other non-cohort study.

15.6. OTHER RELATED DECISIONS

While these decisions were being made by the investigator, the investigated persons were making their own decisions, and some other people may also have contributed to the activities.

15.6.1. *Decisions by the Investigated Persons*

If the maneuver is self-selected—as with cigarette smoking, "prudent" diets, and a "healthy life style"—the main phenomenon under investigation will have been chosen by the investigated persons. The other main decisions by the investigated people consist of seeking (or accepting) contact with the medical establishment, choosing where the contact will occur, and accepting what is subsequently offered.

15.6.1.1. **SELECTION OF MANEUVERS**

For prescribed medications, surgical procedures, and all other maneuvers that are recommended by clinicians, the maneuver is imposed on someone who may play a relatively passive role in its selection. The recipient can become more active by refusing a proposed treatment and by choosing (or agreeing) to do something else; but aside from this circumstance, the patients who are studied in clinical epidemiologic research participate as the subjects of the research, not as its designers.

For studies of the adverse effects of nonprescription (or over-the-counter) drugs, however, and for investigations of most of the smoking, eating, exercising, and other self-selected maneuvers that receive epidemiologic attention as risk factors for disease, the people who receive the maneuvers also plan the main phenomenon studied in the research. They allocate the maneuvers.

The baseline factors that made people choose or reject a self-selected maneuver seldom receive adequate attention as a source of susceptibility bias when the effects of the maneuvers are later analyzed. The recipients are often classified for demographic similarity in age, race, or gender but not for similarity of antecedent clinical, psychic, or genetic attributes that can affect both the choice of the maneuver and the subsequent outcome events. For example, suppose the option to engage in vigorous jogging is rejected by middle-aged men who have a mild angina pectoris that they have not told anyone about. Such men, who are also likely to have reduced longevity because of their coronary disease, will be absent from the group of healthy middle-aged men whose longevity will then appear fallaciously prolonged by the jogging. Conversely, if the "silent angina" men decide to begin jogging in the hope of helping their angina, some of their subsequent sudden unexpected deaths while jogging may be offered as an example of its adverse effects.

Although this type of bias in the self-selection of maneuvers is seldom documented, a striking example of its effect was provided in a classic study by the late Elizabeth Stern.[20] In women who were choosing a method of contraception, she found no differences in the conventional demographic data (age, religion, ethnic group, age at first intercourse, age at first pregnancy, number of children) in women choosing oral contraceptive pills versus mechanical methods of contraception. The women who chose the pill, however, were different clinically. They had a substantially higher rate of cervical dysplasia. The results cast major doubt on previous assumptions, based on the customary epidemiologic use of demographic data alone, that susceptibility to cervical cancer did not affect the choice of contraceptive methods.

A different problem in susceptibility bias occurs when people migrate from one geographic region to another and when rates of mortality are later compared for the two regions. If health status was exactly similar for the migrators and for the people who remained behind, the rates of mortality should be unaffected. If the migration involved certain factors of good (or poor) health, however, or if the migration was provoked by psychic states that can also affect longevity, the migrating group will be different prognostically from the nonmigrators. The migration bias will produce susceptibility bias when mortality results are later compared for the people or pathologic impact of selected environmental factors at the two geographic regions.

Another way in which the recipients of maneuvers can distort the baseline state of the investigated cohorts is with decisions to volunteer for participation in a study in which the cohort is chosen by a mailed questionnaire or direct interview. This type of decision is considered as part of the stimuli discussed in the next section.

15.6.1.2. **IATROTROPIC STIMULUS**

The iatrotropic stimulus[21] is the particular reason why a person decided to seek medical attention at a particular time. This stimulus is often different from the chief complaint, almost always stated in a medical record, which consists of the main symptoms reported by the patient. The chief complaint may be "chest pain, 9 mos.," but the iatrotropic stimulus may be anxiety produced by the recent death of a relative, the concern of a worried spouse, the publicity of a recent campaign regarding some aspect of health, some other symptom that is the patient's "latent objective," an examination previously scheduled for follow-up of some other disease, a pre-employment physical examination, and so on. For a practicing clinician, the iatrotropic stimulus is particularly important as a guide to various decisions in communication. For an investigator, the iatrotropic stimulus helps indicate where the patient should be placed in the complainant or noncomplainant spectrum of whatever disease is under study.[21]

If the person is solicited by mailed questionnaire, telephone call, or other invitation to participate in a survey, the counterpart of the iatrotropic stimulus is the reason for accepting or rejecting the invitation. It may be rejected because of fears of disease or because the activity seems to be a nuisance. It may be accepted because of altruism, neurosis, or the associated monetary reward. It may also be accepted or rejected because of outcome events that followed the imposition of the maneuvers. These different reasons for volunteering to participate can strikingly affect the composition of the acquired cohort. By determining the outcomes for nonresponders as well as responders to a mailed questionnaire, Axelsson and Rylander[22] provided an excellent example of the major distortions that can occur if investigative conclusions are based only on the results of a responder cohort. Some additional problems in volunteer cohorts are discussed in Section 15.8.3.

15.6.1.3. **IATRIC ATTRACTIONS**

This term refers to the reputation, costs, ethnicity, location, or other reasons why a person chose to seek care at one medical setting in preference to another. For example, the men who are treated at a Veterans Administration hospital may have substantial differences (in employment patterns, familial relations, alcoholism, etc.) from men treated elsewhere who are otherwise similar in age, race, and diagnosis.

Iatric attractions can produce migratory phenomena, analogous to those cited in Section 15.6.1.1, that also lead to susceptibility bias when results are compared for different medical institutions. For example, the people who decide to seek care at a specialized center that is quite far from their homes must be able to travel to that center. To undertake the journey, the people usually must be in better average health (and more affluent) than other people with apparently similar clinical conditions who receive treatment at their local medical institutions. The better health (and affluence) that allowed the migration may produce susceptibility bias when post-therapeutic results are compared for the specialized center and for local institutions.

In responding to solicitations, people may be affected by the prestige of the solicitor. Thus, someone who regularly refuses to complete questionnaires sent by an advertising agency may be willing to return information for a listing in *Who's Who*. An invitation is more likely to be accepted if it comes from the person's own physician than from a distant unknown investigator.

15.6.1.4. **ACCEPTANCE OF PROPOSALS**

These decisions occur when a person refuses or goes along with proposals regarding referrals to other medical settings, diagnostic work-ups, therapeutic procedures, admission to a randomized trial, maintenance of assigned treatment, or return for subsequent examinations. The decisions can be an important source of bias in clinical epidemiologic data.

15.6.2. *Decisions by Incidental Medical Personnel*

In studying a clinical phenomenon, the investigator may neglect the effect of incidental personnel whose activities come between the desired population and the people available for research.

15.6.2.1. INTER-IATRIC REFERRALS

These decisions affect the likelihood that patients will appear at the particular medical setting in which research is being conducted. The decisions determine a patient's referral from a family physician to a specialist, from one specialist to another, from ambulatory status to hospitalization, from one hospital to another, from one service within a hospital to another, or from private care to release for admission to a randomized trial.

15.6.2.2. RETRIEVAL OF MEDICAL RECORDS

Investigators who do retrolective research quickly discover the enormous importance and contributions of the personnel who maintain an institution's medical records. The investigated cohort is often identified according to the diagnostic listings prepared by these persons; and the medical records of the members of the cohort must be retrieved, reviewed, and excerpted to provide the research data. A major problem can arise if certain records cannot be retrieved. Do the unlocated records refer to patients who are missing for random reasons, or are they the ones who have died? Has some other investigator, doing some other study, sequestered the records of people with a special phenomenon whose absence from the cohort will distort the results?

15.6.2.3. SCOPE OF SOURCES FOR MEDICAL RECORDS

Another important point in retrolective cohort studies is whether the investigator has included a wide enough scope of sources in seeking medical records of patients with a particular clinical condition. At many medical centers, the medical record library maintains diagnostic listings and filing systems for patients who have been admitted to the institution, but not for those who were treated only on an ambulatory basis. Consequently, an investigator who wants to find all patients with the cited condition may need to check the separate files (if they exist) of records for emergency rooms, radiotherapy departments, chemotherapy clinics, and other outpatient settings.

15.7. INTAKE OF THE COHORT: THE FILTRATION PROCESS

The diverse decisions discussed in Sections 15.5 and 15.6 should demonstrate the scientific futility of assuming that the groups studied in medical research were random samples for which a "sampling error" can be calculated and applied in statistical inferences. Such calculations can be used stochastically to determine whether certain differences might arise by chance because of small numbers in the groups under study, but the customary sources of "sampling error" in clinical epidemiologic research arise from intake, not from sampling. These nonsampling errors, which can seldom be assessed by quantitative calculations, are produced by distortions that occur as people are transferred and filtered from existence at home to appearance as counted units in an investigated group.

For subsequent discussions of bias, the filtration process can be cited according to eight different populations, containing four main sets of transfers through which the people migrate en route to the final statistics. If the process is viewed with the architectural model of a randomized trial, the first two transfers bring the people to the attention of an investigator. The next three transfers allow the investigator to make an offer that he hopes will not be refused. In the next two transfers, the offer is negotiated and acted upon. In the last transfer, the research subject or the researcher has second thoughts and may alter the previous decision.

15.7.1. *Intended Population*

This group, which is sometimes also called the *target population,* consists of the external population of people who have the particular condition under study as the baseline state. These are the people to whom the results of the study will presumably apply when extrapolated. Because of what occurs during the filtration process, however, the intended population is seldom the same as the actual group of people studied in the research.

15.7.2. *Available Group*

Except for the intended population, who reside in the outside world beyond the cloistered scene of an investigator's office, all the other people under consideration can be regarded as groups, rather than populations. The available group contains the people who have left their anonymous location in the outside world and who have appeared in a milieu in which a research project is being conducted. Thus, if we work at hospital H and want to study condition C, the available group consists of people with condition C who appear at hospital H.

15.7.3. *Candidate Group*

The candidate group consists of members of the available group who come to the attention of the investigators. For example, if we consider only the people who are seen on the medical service with condition C, we will not include the patients with condition C who were treated on the surgical, obstetric, radiologic, psychiatric, or other services of hospital H.

15.7.4. *Eligible Group*

These are the members of the candidate group who fulfill diagnostic or other criteria for basic eligibility for the study. Thus, we may have decided to study only elderly men who have had condition C for less than six months or only the patients who fulfill some other set of diagnostic criteria.

15.7.5. *Qualified Group = Nonexcluded Group*

The qualified group contains the members of the eligible group who are not excluded for any of the various reasons cited in Section 15.6.2. Thus, an elderly man who satisfies eligibility criteria requiring that he have had condition C for less than six months may be excluded because he also has far-advanced cancer; or he takes a drug that might alter the outcome of the principal maneuver; or he is deemed too unreliable or noncooperative to be a worthwhile participant in the study.

15.7.6. *Receptive Group*

The receptive group consists of the qualified people who are willing to participate in the proposed research. Refusals can occur because the people either do not like the general idea or are repelled by certain features of the particular project. The two most common reasons for refusal are unwillingness to participate in the follow-up process or in randomization.

In any prolective cohort study, the investigator must arrange to follow the people who receive the maneuvers. The follow-up process may contain special tests, frequent examinations, or other activities that, if adequately explained, may make many persons unwilling to participate in the research study, although willing to receive the maneuver. In a randomized trial, the most common reason for a person's refusal to participate is not the follow-up process but the randomized allocation itself. Many patients do not want their treatment to be chosen by the equivalent of the "toss of a coin," particularly if the contrast is something as dramatic as medical versus surgical therapy. The problems of obtaining informed consent and other ethical difficulties in soliciting patients for randomized trials are further discussed in Chapter 29.

15.7.7. *Admitted Group*

After all of these transfers have been completed, the members of the receptive group are admitted to the study. They are then randomized or otherwise associated with the maneuvers under investigation.

15.7.8. *Counted Group*

Although the filtration process would seem to be completed after the people have been randomized or admitted, it is still not finished. Just before or after imposition of the maneuvers, certain events may occur to make the investigator eliminate members of the admitted group from being included in the people whose data are analyzed and counted as the final results.

Some patients may die during the interval that elapses between randomized assignment and actual onset of treatment. Other people may die so soon after a treatment begins that the death cannot reasonably be associated with the treatment. Some of the people who were randomized may change their minds after the randomization is completed but before the maneuver is imposed. They may drop out of the study without knowing the maneuver, or they may refuse to accept a known treatment (such as medical versus surgical therapy) to which they were randomly assigned. After treatment has begun, the investigator may discover that certain patients were ineligible and should not have been admitted. A variety of other postmaneuver phenomena mentioned in Section 15.5.5, as well as other events discussed in Chapters 16 and 17, may also make the investigator want to remove certain people from being counted in the results.

An unresolved controversy has developed about the policy to be used for deciding which patients to include in counting the results of a randomized trial.[23] The crux of the debate is a choice between two reasonable and justifiable but opposing policies. One policy is oriented to a fastidious avoidance of bias, even if the clinical pertinence of the results becomes compromised. The other policy is oriented to clinical pragmatism, even if the results become "messy." Although the controversy is further discussed in Chapter 29, its implications extend to all aspects of cause-effect research, not just to randomized trials. The proponents of strictly unbiased research may sometimes accept, in a nonrandomized study, major sources of bias that would instantly be rejected if encountered in a randomized trial.

15.7.9. *Illustrations*

To illustrate the distinctions of the filtration process, its seven component groups (excluding the counted group) are shown in Table 15–1 for the diverse cohorts that would be under investigation in: (A) an etiologic study; (B) a study of contratrophic therapy; (C) a probative study of healthy people; and (D) a probative study of laboratory animals.

A separate diagram in Figure 15–2 shows the sequence of acceptances and rejections that convert the intended population for a study of clinical therapy into the group that is actually admitted. If this diagram were suitably rotated (so that the *admitted group* were at the top rather than the bottom), it might demonstrate even more strikingly the way that the people studied in clinical research often represent merely the "tip of the iceberg" for the phenomenon under consideration.

15.8. SCIENTIFIC PROBLEMS IN DISTORTION AND BIAS

A reader who has not been exhausted by the preceding discussion is now ready to consider the scientific consequences of all the foregoing decisions and transfers. (Exhausted

Table 15–1. THE FILTRATION PROCESS FROM INTENDED POPULATION TO THE ADMITTED GROUP (OR "SAMPLE") IN FOUR RESEARCH PROJECTS

	A. Etiologic Study	B. Study of Contratrophic Therapy	C. Probative Study in People	D. Probative Study in Animals
Type of study	Cigarette smoking as cause of disease	Treatment of maturity-onset diabetes mellitus to prevent vascular complications	Reactions to psychologic stress test	Physiology of ACTH
Intended population	Healthy people	People with maturity-onset diabetes mellitus	Healthy people	Healthy dogs
Available group	British physicians cited in registry of physicians	People admitted to 12 medical centers participating in a cooperative clinical trial	College students	Dogs in city pound
Candidate group	Those who responded to questionnaires	People diagnosed as having diabetes and referred to the research clinic	Those who answered the ad for volunteers for a new test	Dogs sent by pound to research center
Eligible group	Those whose responses were legible	Those who fulfilled the glucose tolerance criteria	The volunteers who were deemed suitable by investigator	Dogs selected from cages and who survived adrenalectomy
Qualified group	Those whose responses had adequate information re smoking	Those who had no anticipated major problems in co-morbidity or compliance		
Admitted group	Those who were classified as smokers or nonsmokers	Those who accepted the randomly assigned treatments	Those who took the test	Survivors given ACTH or saline infusions

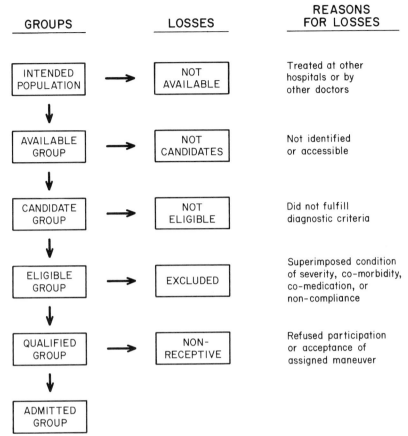

Figure 15–2. Diagram showing successive transfers from the intended population to the group admitted to a study of therapy.

or nonreceptive readers should pause for revival of spirit before admitting themselves to the next group of sections in the text.)

As a result of the cited events, enormous opportunities arise for the research data to be distorted or biased. Although the term *selection bias* is sometimes used for these problems, they can take two different forms, which have two different sets of consequences. In the first type of problem, called *distorted assembly,* the investigated group does not properly represent the intended population. In the second type of problem, called *susceptibility bias,* the groups receiving the contrasted maneuvers were unfairly compared. With distorted assembly, we have difficulty in generalizing the results externally, beyond the groups who were studied. With susceptibility bias, the results contain the internal difficulty of a distorted comparison.

15.8.1. *Distorted Assembly*

If a random sample can be obtained from the intended population, the likelihood of distorted assembly is substantially reduced, although we would still have to worry about differential distinctions in the people who accept the invitation to participate. Random samples of an intended population, however, have never been used in epidemiologic and clinical investigations of the etiology or treatment of disease. (A rare exception to the "never" in the preceding sentence might be claimed for certain descriptive surveys, performed under the auspices of the U.S. National Center for Health Statistics,[24] in which random samples were chosen from community populations. These surveys, however, have not been aimed at specific etiologic or therapeutic goals. The data obtained during household interviews by the nonclinical personnel have been demographically splendid, but the medical information is seldom sophisticated enough for scientific studies of disease.)

Because the groups under investigation have been collected by filtered intake rather than by random sampling, distorted assembly can be suspected in *every* clinical and epidemiologic research project. The main questions about distorted assembly are not whether it exists, but how to reduce its effects and evaluate its consequences.

15.8.1.1. THE SCREENING LOG

In research emanating from a medical setting, the investigator usually has no way of knowing how the intended population was altered during the transfer to the available group. After a group becomes available at the medical setting, however, the investigator can usually identify and quantify the characteristics of the people who were checked at each subsequent step of the transfer process.

This activity, when properly performed, is usually noted in a screening log, which cites each candidate considered for a study, regardless of whether the candidate was admitted. By keeping track of all the available people, the investigator can determine their cogent characteristics, note why the available people did not become candidates, why candidates were not eligible, and why eligible people were disqualified or otherwise not admitted. When these data are tabulated, the quantitative and qualitative results will denote what has been omitted from the cohort. The results can then be evaluated to determine how well the people included in the cohort represent the intended population.

15.8.1.2. EVALUATION OF DISTORTED ASSEMBLY

If the research requires that the intended population be suitably represented by the cohort, the occurrence of distorted assembly can be a fatal flaw. For example, if we wanted to know the characteristics of people who develop group A streptococcal infections, the results found in patients hospitalized with group A streptococcal infections would be grossly misleading. If we wanted to determine the merits of maintaining rigorous control of blood glucose in diabetic patients who require insulin, the question would not be answered with a randomized clinical trial of hypoglycemic agents in patients who are not insulin-dependent.

On the other hand, most cause-effect research is directed at determining whether a principal maneuver exerts a particular impact; and the investigator (and reviewer) may not want to know whether this impact is universal. For example, if we suspect that hearing is impaired by prolonged exposure to the noises of a discotheque, an appropriate study of the young people who attend discotheques might suffice to prove the point. The absence of elderly people from the research would not alter the basic conclusion.

For most cause-effect studies, therefore, distorted assembly will not affect the internal comparison conducted *within* the assembled groups. The main consequence of distorted assembly will be externally, in the extrapolation of results. We may be uncertain about how extensively the results can be extrapolated, or we may be unable to extrapolate them to people who are substantially different from those included in the study. For example, the efficacy of antibiotic prophylaxis in preventing recurrences of rheumatic fever was demonstrated in randomized clinical trials in which the investigators made vigorous efforts to encourage the patients to maintain faithful compliance with the assigned regimens. Because this vigorous encouragement and faithful compliance might not occur outside the setting of a randomized trial, the effectiveness (rather than the efficacy) of antibiotic prophylaxis might be lowered when applied to the intended population in the outside world. If surgical therapy is shown to be better than medical therapy in a randomized trial of white men, ages 35 to 55, with stable angina pectoris and no major co-morbidity, the results may be impossible to apply when a clinician later encounters the previously mentioned 65-year-old black woman who has unstable angina, diabetes mellitus, and hypertension.

15.8.2. *Susceptibility Bias*

Susceptibility bias occurs in cause-effect research when the baseline states of the compared groups have substantially different prognostic susceptibilities to the outcome event. In experimental research, the bias can usually be prevented by using randomization to assign the compared maneuvers. In a randomized trial, all of the transfers that excluded various types of people from receiving a particular maneuver took place before the maneuvers were allocated. The subsequent comparison of maneuvers may be difficult to extrapolate, but it will be conducted without distortion.

In nonrandomized comparisons, however, people who were excluded from receiving a particular maneuver may be compared against those who satisfied the pretherapeutic admission criteria for receiving it. Such comparisons may be grossly distorted by susceptibility bias, because the excluded people may have been destined to have substantially worse (or better) outcomes than those who were admitted.

For example, suppose we want to do a randomized trial comparing the relative efficacy of two narcotic agents in relieving pain. During the screening procedures, we exclude people with mild pain. They are given non-narcotic analgesic agents, but we keep track of those people to determine the promptness with which their pain is relieved. After the randomized trial of the two narcotic agents is completed in the patients with severe pain, we note that the patients excluded from the trial had better results than either group treated with narcotics. If we tried to conclude that non-narcotic analgesics are better than the two narcotic agents, the silliness of the conclusion would be immediately apparent.

Nevertheless, an analogous type of susceptibility bias has been overlooked in many clinical and epidemiologic studies of cause-effect relationships in which the maneuvers were not allocated with randomization. Without considering the allocation decisions that led to certain maneuvers being received or not received, and without considering the prognostic impact of the particular characteristics that led to the allocation decisions, the investigators simply compare results in people in whom the maneuvers were or were not imposed.

The problem of susceptibility bias was dramatically demonstrated during the early era of randomized trials when randomization was used to study the merits of medical versus surgical therapy for bleeding esophageal varices.[22] After excluding patients who were unsuitable candidates for surgery, the investigators conducted the trial and found that the group actively treated with surgery did *not* have substantially better results than the control group treated medically. In the excluded patients, however, who had been maintained as a separate control group receiving medical therapy, the investigators were surprised to discover that the medical treatment was followed by substantially worse results in the excluded controls than in the admitted controls.

One possible conclusion from the data is that patients who will receive nonsurgical treatment for bleeding esophageal varices should be admitted to randomized trials, because results are so much better for patients who participate in the trials. The correct conclusion, of course, is that the admission criteria for surgical therapy will demarcate people with particularly good prognoses. With this susceptibility bias, such patients will usually have better outcomes—even if surgery is not performed—than patients who did not fulfill the admission criteria.

The problem of susceptibility bias has now generally become well recognized in clinical studies of the benefits of therapeutic agents, but the problem is still rampant and generally ignored in epidemiologic studies of the adverse effects of therapy. The problem can be eliminated or substantially reduced in observational (nonrandomized) studies by a relatively simple change in current investigative procedures. The people admitted to the cohort, case-control, or other groups assembled for such studies should be restricted to those who would fulfill the admission criteria for a randomized trial of the maneuvers under study. Unless such admission criteria are applied equally in randomized and nonrandomized research, the results of the nonrandomized studies will continue to contain the major distortions of susceptibility bias.

Some of these issues are elaborated in the exercises at the end of this chapter. Others are further discussed in later chapters.

15.8.3. *Nonspecific Selection Bias*

In prolective cohort research, with or without randomization, the investigator works with a group of available candidates whose subsequent exclusions can usually be clearly documented for evaluating their impact on distorted assembly and susceptibility bias. In certain types of retrolective cohort research, however, the people under study may not become available until they have responded to the investigator's request to make themselves available. Because this request occurs after the maneuvers have been imposed, and because the investigator may not have access to the people who fail to respond to the request, there is no good way to determine how the responders and nonresponders differ in diverse features that would create distorted assembly, in premaneuveral features that would create susceptibility bias, or in outcome events that may have occurred after imposition of the maneuvers. In such circumstances, when the format of the research blurs the possibility of distinguishing the different types of bias, the problems are often given the nonspecific title of *selection bias*.

For example, in Section 15.3, we considered a retrolective-prolective cohort study of the outcome of pepsinogen levels in college freshmen. Suppose people with a very high pepsinogen level were particularly likely to develop peptic ulcers but also had a personality that made them unwilling to respond to mailed solicitations to submit information about their current health. In data assembled from the responders, the investigator might notice that information is absent for many of the people who originally had very high pepsinogen levels, but—without access to the nonresponders—the investigator might not be able to arrive at a correct conclusion in the research.

The problem is even trickier when the investigator must rely on the responders to supply not only the cohort under study but also the data about the imposed maneuvers. For example, in the classic Doll-Hill study[26] of the subsequent development of lung cancer in relation to the smoking habits of British doctors, the group under study was acquired by sending out questionnaires to the physicians listed on the roster of the British Medical Association. The physicians who returned the questionnaires became the assembled cohort. Their response to the question about smoking indicated the allocated maneuver. The data on their subsequent death certificates indicated the occurrence or nonoccurrence of lung cancer as the outcome event. Because the self-allocated maneuvers as well as other outcome events might affect the likelihood that the initial questionnaires would be returned, the possibilities and consequences of different forms of selection bias are difficult to evaluate in this study. A major potential problem cited by a prominent biostatistician is discussed in Exercise 15.4 at the end of the chapter.

The cited problems in a biased selection of compared cohorts are really issues in *transfer bias*. The problems arise when the members of a cohort are recruited not just after the maneuvers were imposed but after many of the outcome events have already occurred. The sources and effects of transfer bias will be discussed more extensively in Chapter 17.

15.9. SYNOPSIS

The cause-effect relationships evaluated with scientific reasoning can be studied with various research structures that are arranged quite differently from the format of the conceptual architecture. The people studied in the research can be assembled according to their conditions before or after the maneuvers were imposed; and the research data can be collected before or after occurrence of the events described by the data. For the scientific reasoning to arrive at correct conclusions, the assembled groups and data must allow a satisfactory analysis of why the investigated maneuvers were selected and what happened before and afterward.

The collected data must be suitable for identifying the baseline states of the investigated people before the maneuvers were imposed. This baseline state information will be used to compare the composition of the cohorts, to prepare the transition variables, to allow a cogent prognostic stratification of the outcome events for each maneuver, and to facilitate the extrapolation of results.

The cohorts of people receiving the maneuvers under investigation are demarcated by sets of eligibility criteria and exclusion criteria that constitute the admission criteria. The eligibility criteria indicate the basic condition under investigation; and the exclusion criteria indicate the otherwise eligible people who are excluded for reasons of therapeutic exigency, prognostic susceptibility, therapeutic vulnerability, contamination of maneuvers, spectral homogeneity, investigative efficiency, or referral bias. A qualification period may be used before the maneuvers are imposed to demonstrate that the admission criteria are fulfilled. The contents of the admitted cohort can also be affected by substitutes for inaccessible candidates and by people who are eliminated from the cohort because of withdrawals occurring after the maneuvers were imposed.

These decisions, made by investigators and practicing clinicians, will be accompanied by other decisions that can affect the cohorts under comparison. The people under investigation may have selected the maneuvers, volunteered to participate in cohorts recruited by solicitation, decided when and where to seek medical attention, and agreed to accept the proposed clinical procedures. The compared cohorts will also be affected by patterns of inter-iatric referral and by the effectiveness and scope of the sources used for retrieving archival data, such as medical records. Because of all these decisions, the actual cohorts under study may greatly differ from the population for which the results of the research are intended. The differences arise during the decisions with which members of the intended population are sequentially transferred and filtered to the groups who are available, recognized as candidates, eligible, qualified, receptive, admitted, and counted in the results of the cohort for each maneuver.

The consequences of these transfers may create a distorted assembly that makes the results misleading or useless for application to the intended population. Such problems can be substantially reduced if a screening log is maintained and suitably analyzed, or if the study is concerned mainly with internal comparison of maneuvers rather than external extrapolation of results. The internal comparison of maneuvers can be greatly distorted by the susceptibility bias that can arise if the compared cohorts are chosen without suitable admission criteria. In cohorts recruited by solicitation after the maneuvers have been imposed, several types of bias can be combined into a selection bias that arises because of diverse phenomena associated with the solicitation process, the imposition of maneuvers, or the subsequent outcomes.

EXERCISES

Exercise 15.1. Please review the particular cause-effect studies that were previously described in Exercises 2.2.3, 2.2.5, 2.2.7, and 2.2.8 for Chapter 2, and in Exercises 3.1.2, 4.1.2, 4.1.4, and 4.1.5 that followed Chapters 3 and 4, respectively. Without regard to the actual structures used in the research, cite the particular variables that you would regard as most cogent for the prognostic analysis of results. (You are limited to no more than two variables in each study, and preferably you should choose one.)

Exercise 15.2. You are planning to do randomized therapeutic trials of one form of treatment versus another for the baseline states and events listed in the table that follows. Two different sets of criteria—cited as I and II in the table—can be demanded for admitting patients to the study and allocating treatment randomly. How might your ability to perform the trial and to generalize the results be affected if you use criteria I or II? (Please bear in mind that the criteria must be satisfied before patients can be admitted and randomized.)

	Baseline State	Outcome Event	Admission Criteria I	Admission Criteria II
15.2.1.	Cancer of lung	1-year survival	Must have histologic evidence of cancer	May have histologic or cytologic evidence of cancer
15.2.2.	Acute myocardial infarction	30-day survival	Must have electrocardiographic evidence of infarct	May have clinical and/or laboratory evidence if ECG is negative
15.2.3.	Acute sore throat	Relief of symptoms	Laboratory evidence of β-hemolytic streptococcus	Clinical evidence of pharyngeal inflammation
15.2.4.	Acute sore throat	Prevention of rheumatic fever or glomerulonephritis	Laboratory evidence of β-hemolytic streptococcus	Clinical evidence of pharyngeal inflammation
15.2.5.	Low back pain (in primary care medical practice)	Relief of symptoms	Appropriate clinical evidence plus negative x-ray of spine	Clinical evidence of pain and/or muscular spasm
15.2.6.	Psychiatric depression	Relief of symptoms	Must have suitable score on a selected self-rating scale for depression	Clinical diagnosis of depression

Exercise 15.3. One of the most famous randomized clinical trials in modern medicine is a cooperative study of antihypertensive therapy in men at U.S. veterans' hospitals.[27] In that trial, the investigators deliberately chose to perform the research on a compliance cohort. Before admission, each potential patient was tested for several weeks to determine whether he would take the medication faithfully and be prompt in keeping return appointments to the clinic. Patients who did not properly comply in either medication-taking or appointment-keeping were excluded from admission

to the trial. According to the screening log of the study, about 50% of the eligible patients were thereby excluded from the trial. The results of the trial showed distinct superiority for the antihypertensive drugs versus placebo in preventing subsequent cardiovascular complications. How might the pretrial exclusion procedures have created a problem in the results? How might this problem affect our ability to extrapolate the results to the intended population?

Exercise 15.4. Perhaps the most famous epidemiologic investigation in modern medicine is the Doll-Hill study[26] of cigarette smoking in physicians, mentioned in Section 15.8.3. After assembling the original cohort from physicians who responded to a mailed questionnaire about their smoking habits, the investigators later made additional efforts to discover the characteristics of the nonresponders. The additional data showed that doctors who smoked were much less likely than nonsmokers to return the questionnaires and become members of the cohort.

Making the assumption that smokers and nonsmokers had similar rates of illness at the time they received the questionnaires, and making the further assumption that smokers and nonsmokers actually had similar rates of subsequent death, a biostatistical heretic[28] created a scenario in which he claimed that the differential rate of returning questionnaires had produced a selection bias that falsely elevated the death rates subsequently calculated for the smoking and nonsmoking cohorts. What do you think this scenario was? (Hint: Try making up some numbers or using some algebra to show what might happen.)

Exercise 15.5. Here are a series of proposed conclusions in cause-effect relationships that have been (or might be) studied epidemiologically with research structures in which the maneuvers were *not* allocated with randomization. Without regard to the particular structure used in the research, and without regard to any controversy that may exist about the conclusion, which of these relationships might be made falsely positive because of a neglected aspect of *susceptibility bias?* (Another way to approach this issue is to answer the following question: If you were investigating these phenomena in a prolective cohort study, what would be the admission criteria you would use for the compared cohorts, and what cogent feature of those criteria, if neglected, might produce a major susceptibility bias in the results of the study?) For each relationship in which you think such a bias could arise, please list the way in which it could occur.

   15.5.1. Suitable exposure to asbestos may cause mesothelioma.
   15.5.2. Cigarette smoking may cause coronary artery disease.
   15.5.3. Cigarette smoking may cause cancer of the bladder.
   15.5.4. Use of saccharin may cause cancer of the bladder.
   15.5.5. Using sexual hormone tests to diagnose early pregnancy may cause deformities in the fetus.
   15.5.6. Using diethylstilbestrol (DES) to help avoid threatened abortion in early pregnancy may cause clear cell vaginal carcinoma in the female children.
   15.5.7. Coffee drinking may cause cancer of the pancreas.
   15.5.8. Use of tampons during menstruation may cause toxic shock syndrome.
   15.5.9. Use of reserpine (or rauwolfia products) may cause cancer of the breast.
   15.5.10. Drinking tea may cause gallstones.

Exercise 15.6. Choose any two longitudinal cohort studies with which you are familiar or that you can learn about. Both studies should be concerned with the comparison of maneuvers, but one should be a study of therapy and the other should be a study of etiology or pathogenesis. Neither study should have been previously cited as an example in the text. After briefly outlining the objective of each study, note the procedures that were used for assembly of the cohorts and indicate whether these procedures have produced any difficulties in the extrapolation of results. If you do note any difficulties, please be specific in citing where they arise and what effect they would have on the extrapolation. For example, it is not sufficient to say that a study of 7-year-old girls could not be extrapolated to apply to 6-year-old girls. What aspect of the age distinction would create the distortion that prevents the extrapolation? (Cohort studies of therapy are readily available in medical literature, but cohort studies of pathogenesis are harder to find. If you have difficulty, please look at some of the references cited in Kessler and Levin's anthology of public health epidemiologic cohort studies.[29])

CHAPTER REFERENCES

1. Chuong, 1981; 2. Kramer, 1978; 3. Chalmers, 1977; 4. University Group Diabetes Program, 1970; 5. Feinstein, 1976; 6. Bibbo, 1978; 7. Dieckmann, 1953; 8. Anturane Reinfarction Trial Research Group, 1978; 9. Peto, 1976–1977; 10. Feinstein, 1968; 11. Charlson, 1974; 12. Wells, 1977; 13. Feinstein, 1982; 14. New York Heart Association, 1964; 15. Feinstein, 1977; 16. American Joint Committee, 1978; 17. World Health Organization, 1962; 18. Paradise, 1984; 19. Agrez, 1982; 20. Stern, 1971; 21. Feinstein, 1974; 22. Axelsson, 1982; 23. Sackett, 1979; 24. National Center for Health Statistics, 1973; 25. Garceau, 1964; 26. Doll, 1964; 27. Veterans Administration Cooperative Study Group, 1970; 28. Berkson, 1955. 29. Kessler, 1970.

Chapter 16

Implementation of the Outline: Maneuvers

Many cause-effect studies get into trouble before they begin because of decisions made when the maneuvers were chosen in the basic outline of the research. If subsequent reviewers disagree with the suitability of individual maneuvers, with the choice of comparative maneuvers, or with the plan used for comparing them, the rest of the work may be regarded as misdirected. No amount of elaborate statistical analysis will be able to salvage it.

For example, if a reviewer believes that Excellitol was given in the wrong dosage or that the omphalorrhexis was performed with the wrong surgical technique, the evaluation of these principal maneuvers would be unsatisfactory regardless of what they are compared against. Even if each maneuver was individually suitable, the reviewer may still have wanted Excellitol to be compared against an active agent rather than placebo (or vice versa) or to be compared against active agent B rather than active agent C. Even if all the maneuvers were suitably chosen and compared, a reviewer may still reject the research because its architectural structure is deemed unsuitable: the results came from an observational cohort or case-control study, not from a randomized trial.

If these complaints are anticipated, the investigator can try to avoid them by changing the basic outline of the research. If problems of feasibility prevent the necessary changes from being made, the investigator can proceed with the original plan but may then have to persuade a skeptical critic by explaining or justifying why the unsuitable choices were really suitable. The investigator's main hope here is that the reviewers will be rational and reasonable—a hope that is not always fulfilled, particularly if the investigator's ideas and approaches differ from the fashionable paradigms[1] of the era.

Assuming that the basic outline is satisfactory, the investigator's next step is to determine the maneuvers. In this step, the investigator arranges either to allocate the maneuvers in an experiment or to ascertain which ones were imposed nonexperimentally. The investigator also decides whether any special problems occurred while the maneuvers were being carried out.

16.1. DETERMINATION OF THE MANEUVERS

In an experimental trial, the investigator must develop a plan to allocate the maneuvers, impose them, and find out how proficiently they were performed. In all other research structures, the maneuvers are allocated by someone else, and the investigator must afterward learn what happened.

16.1.1. *Experimental Allocation of Maneuvers*

The opportunity to allocate the maneuvers permits an investigator to achieve four things that are seldom possible in ordinary observational circumstances: assignment within strata, proportional assignment per treatment, balanced allocation, and randomization.

16.1.1.1. ALLOCATION WITHIN STRATA

The purpose of a stratified randomization, in which maneuvers are allocated within specified subgroups of a cohort, is to have the compared maneuvers suitably distributed among those subgroups. Without such precautions, the luck of the draw during randomization might produce some of the imbalances noted in Section 12.3.2. For example, although equal numbers of patients might be allocated to treatments A and B, the group assigned to A might contain a substantially higher proportion of patients with good prognoses.

The strata chosen for the allocation may be demarcated according to prognosis, ancillary maneuvers, the site of the research, or combinations of these (or other pertinent) factors. For example, suppose we have three hospitals participating in a therapeutic trial of treatments A and B for good-risk and poor-risk patients who may or may not receive special instructions about compliance. The assignment schedule could be prepared for 12 strata: 3 hospitals × 2 risk groups × 2 instruction groups. Within each of those 12 strata, a separate schedule would be prepared for the sequence of assignments to treatment A or treatment B.

In a randomized trial in which I collaborated many years ago, the work was done at a single institution, but eight strata were used to assign treatment.[2] The strata, labeled A through H, were demarcated by dichotomous boundaries for three variables: presence or absence of rheumatic heart disease, age above or below 10 years, and time elapsed (above or below 15 months) since previously active rheumatic fever. After fulfilling the basic criteria for admission, each patient who entered the trial was first diagnosed as being in one of those eight strata. For the three treatments under comparison in the trial, a separate randomization schedule had been previously prepared for each stratum, and the allocations were enclosed in a series of opaque envelopes numbered A-1, A-2, A-3, . . . , B-1, B-2, . . . , C-1, and so on. The envelopes were opened as patients were sequentially admitted to each stratum. Thus, the fifth patient admitted to stratum G would receive the treatment identified in envelope G-5. The next patient admitted in stratum G would receive the treatment marked in envelope G-6.

In most cooperative clinical trials, the randomization is usually stratified for the collaborating institutions, so that a separate allocation schedule is prepared for the patients of each institution (or investigator). The institutional stratification has two main goals. If patients are later found to differ substantially at the different institutions, the results can easily be analyzed separately for each source of patients in the total study. By allowing a balanced allocation of treatment within each institution, such a stratification also helps keep the individual investigators happy about participating in the trial. For example, if an institution will ultimately contribute 15 patients to a trial of medical versus surgical therapy, the participating surgeons may be quite distressed if randomized fate happens to assign 11 of those patients to medical therapy and only four to surgery.

From time to time, particularly if the treated condition is rare, the randomization is deliberately arranged to be central rather than institutional. The purpose is to ensure a balanced allocation of treatment for all patients entered in the study or for patients within selected prognostic strata. An example of this situation was provided in Exercise 12.7 at the end of Chapter 12.

Institutional stratifications are usually easy to arrange, but things can become difficult if a stratification depends on specific clinical features of the patients. The clinical features that are most cogent for the stratification may not be known or agreed upon before the trial begins; or the patients may sometimes be classified in the wrong stratum, so that the assigned treatment is taken from an incorrect location in the randomization schedule. To avoid these problems, many randomizations are not stratified for any attributes other than the institutional sources of the patients.

Randomizations that do not depend on individual characteristics of the patients are called *complete,* in contrast to *block* or *stratified* randomizations, in which the patients are first divided into distinctive institutional, clinical, or other groups. (The word *block* arises because modern randomized trials were first developed in an agricultural setting in which the land could be divided into different blocks or lots within which different treatments would be tested.[3]) With complete randomizations, any prognostic or other pertinent clinical analyses are performed according to retrospective stratifications.

16.1.1.2. **PROPORTIONAL ASSIGNMENT PER TREATMENT**

In most clinical circumstances, the investigators want the treatments to be distributed in a proportionally equal manner among the patients. For two compared treatments, half the patients in the total cohort would get each treatment. For three treatments, the total cohort is divided into thirds. For N patients receiving k treatments, each treatment group would contain N/k patients. Aside from the appealing rational esthetics, the results of an equiproportional arrangement are more likely to be statistically significant than when the treatments are assigned disproportionately.

A disproportionate arrangement can be deliberately sought, however, in four different situations. In one of these situations, someone has qualms about using placebo. It may be needed to provide a convincing comparison, but the investigators want to give placebo to as few people as possible. The proportions may therefore be arranged so that 75% of the admitted patients get the active treatment and only 25% receive placebo.

In an opposite situation, when a single placebo group will be used for multiple comparisons against several other active agents in the same trial, the investigators may want the placebo group to be larger and therefore more statistically stable than the others. Thus, if five active treatments and a placebo are all to be compared in the same study, each regimen would ordinarily be given to 1/6 of the patients. To increase the size of the placebo group, it may be proportionally assigned to receive 2/7 of the patients, with each of the five active treatments getting 1/7 of the patients.

In a third circumstance, the disproportions are intended to allow a single drug to be studied in different dose regimens that can later be combined for the total results. For example, if N people enter a trial, N/2 may be assigned to placebo, N/4 may be given a low dose of drug X, and N/4 may receive a high dose of drug X. These three regimens can later be compared individually, but placebo can also be compared against the combined results of drug X in a contrast that will contain an equiproportioned N/2 versus N/2 people.

The fourth reason for disproportionate allocations arises when an additional new treatment is brought in for evaluation after the trial has been in progress. To let the new treatment "catch up," so that each treatment has equal numbers by the end of the trial, the new randomization schedule may give a disproportionately large number of patients to the new treatment. For example, suppose we begin a randomized trial intended to compare treatments A, B, C, and D in each of four groups containing 200 patients. The original allocation schedule would call for each treatment to receive 1/4 of the patients, assigned in a ratio of 1:1:1:1. After 600 patients have been accrued, so that each treatment group contains 150 patients, we decide to add a fifth treatment, E, to the total comparison; and we want treatment E as well as the other treatment groups each to contain 200 people when the trial is finished. We would therefore want to add 400 more patients, with 50 being randomized to each of treatments A, B, C, and D, and 200 going to treatment E.

The latter strategy can equalize the statistical numbers but might be scientifically dangerous. The 400 patients in the second randomization will be accrued at a later secular date than the first 600 patients; and major hazards can arise if the new group of 400 comes from a set of institutions different from the sources used to recruit the first 600. Although the patients in treatments A, B, C, and D could continue to be compared as an inception cohort, the patients receiving treatment E would be nonconcurrent in both time and place. Nevertheless, if the statistical or other merits of the strategy seem compelling, we could carry it out with a 1:1:1:1:4 allocation ratio in the new randomization schedule. (This type of double randomization—with a proportionate schedule of allocation in the first six institutions and a disproportionate schedule in the second set of six institutions—was used when phenformin was later added, as a fifth treatment, to four other regimens under previous investigation in the UGDP randomized trial of therapy for diabetes mellitus.[4])

16.1.1.3. **BALANCED ALLOCATION OF TREATMENT**

If we wanted the allocation to be equally divided between two treatments, we could do so by tossing a coin or using some other appropriate mechanism. We could feel sure that in the long run this mechanism would allocate the two treatments quite equally.

Anyone who has visited Las Vegas, Atlantic City, Monte Carlo, or other centers of stochastic activity, however, knows that strange things can happen in the short run. The roulette wheel may produce the color *red* on five consecutive rotations—an event whose probability is $(18/38)^5 = 0.024$. The shooter at dice may roll four consecutive passes, an event whose probability is $(6/36)^4 = 0.0008$. Despite the fiscal joy of bettors who correctly anticipated these improbable short-term events, things become evened out in the long run, thus allowing the proprietors of the coordinating statistical centers to maintain profitable operations.

In a randomized clinical trial, an investigator will generally prefer not to trust the long run of fate to provide the desired equalization—particularly if the sample size is small enough to make the distribution a short-run event. To guard against the inequities of randomized fate, arrangements are made for the numbers of assigned treatments to be balanced at regular intervals. If k treatments are being studied, the balancing interval is usually 2k, 3k, or some other multiple of k. For example, if fate alone creates the schedule for a comparison of treatment A versus treatment B, the randomization might assign the first 10 patients as follows: A, B, A, A, A, B, A, B, A, A. Although this 7-3 split might later be equalized, it would persist as a major problem in the analysis if only 10 patients were admitted to the trial. To prevent this problem, the randomization could be constrained, without losing its basically random attribute, so that the treatments are equally allocated after every 2, 4, 6, 8, or 10 patients.

The tactics of disproportionate assignment and balancing were well illustrated in the Coronary Drug Project,[5] a mammoth randomized trial in which six treatment groups were studied simultaneously. Five treatments were active drugs—daily doses of estrogen 2.5 mg., estrogen 5.0 mg., dextrothyroxine 6 mg., nicotinic acid 3.0 g., and clofibrate 1.8 g. The sixth was a lactose placebo, 3.8 g. daily. The treatments were assigned in a ratio of 5:2:2:2:2:2, so that five patients received placebo for every two patients assigned to active drugs. With this disproportionate distribution of drugs, separate randomization schedules were prepared, within two strata of risk, for each of the 53 participating institutions. The schedules were balanced after every 15 allocations of treatment within each of the 106 strata.

16.1.1.4. **MECHANISM OF ALLOCATION**

The main goal in the *scientific* allocation of treatment is to remove human judgment from the decision. These judgments by either patients or clinicians or both can lead to the biased allocations described previously, in which different maneuvers are selectively chosen for people with different prognostic distinctions. The resulting susceptibility bias may then destroy or vitiate the similarity of comparison when results of the maneuvers are later contrasted.

Although many mechanisms can be used to eliminate judgmental decisions when maneuvers are allocated, the most popular mechanism is randomization because it also has a modest statistical advantage. The other mechanisms will be considered after randomization is discussed.

16.1.1.4.1. *Methods of Randomization*

Although sometimes misused to refer to any mechanism for allocating maneuvers, the word *randomization* is strictly applicable only when the allocation is done with a formal procedure for which the probabilities of different assignments can be calculated.

This procedure can be achieved by tossing a coin, which is suitable for assigning two treatments; by using the suit noted on a card picked from a deck of ordinary playing cards, which (when reshuffled after each choice) is suitable for four treatments; or by rolling a die, which is suitable for assigning one of six treatments. A die could be used, in fact, for assigning anywhere from two to six treatments. Thus, for two treatments, A could be assigned if the die toss yields a *1, 3,* or *5*; and B if the toss is a *2, 4,* or *6*. For three treatments, assign A for tosses of *1* or *2*, B for *3* or *4*, and C for *5* or *6*. Six treatments can be assigned in exact correspondence to each of the six possible numbers. For four treatments, assign A for a toss of *1*, B for *2*, C for *3*, and D for *4*; toss again if the die yields *5* or *6*. For five treatments, assign E for *5* and toss again for *6*.

Although quite satisfactory for a small study, these manual procedures may become cumbersome for a large randomization schedule or for various forms of balancing. Accordingly, the preferred mechanism of randomization is to use one of three statistical techniques. The first technique employs a *table of random numbers,* which were generated in batches of digits by some appropriate mechanism. Table 16–1 contains an array of random numbers, spanning the interval from 0 to 99. For a particular randomization, this table would be entered at some randomly chosen (i.e., close your eyes and point) location. The chosen number and those that follow it determine the sequence of randomized assignments. For an unconstrained randomization of two treatments, even numbers might be assigned to treatment A and odd numbers to treatment B.

The rank of the random numbers can be used to preserve randomness while allowing a randomization to be constrained. For example, suppose we wanted a balanced randomization after six allocations of treatments A and B. We can take six consecutive random numbers and assign the first three to A and the next three to B. We then arrange the *sequence* of allocation to occur according to the *rank* of the random numbers. Thus, suppose we start with the number 42 in the 31st row of digits in Table 16–1. We assign the first three numbers (42, 56, and 54) to treatment A; we assign the next three numbers (45, 54, and 20) to treatment B. Because 54 has occurred twice, we give treatment B the very next number (51) instead of 54. We now arrange the six random numbers, in order of rank, as 20, 42, 45, 51, 54, and 56. The sequence of random allocation will be B, A, B, B, A, A.

A more convenient modern mechanism for preparing randomized schedules is to let a computer do the work and to use *computer-generated random numbers.* To produce each successive random number, the computer relies on a special algorithm, which generates a decimal that lies randomly somewhere on the unit interval between 0 and 1. The generated number is multiplied by an integer whose size depends on the number of treatments to be considered. Thus, suppose we want to randomize four treatments A, B, C, and D. We would multiply the generated number by four and then truncate the result to integer level. In this arrangement, digits that are randomly generated from 0.0000 to 0.2499 will become *0*; 0.2500 to 0.4999 become *1*; 0.5000 to 0.7499 become *2*; and 0.7500 to 0.9999 become *3*. A truncated *0* is then assigned to treatment A, *1* to B, *2* to C, and *3* to D. The table that follows shows how this process would work.

Sequence of Generated Number	Generated Random Number	Multiplied by 4 Becomes:	Truncated to	Treatment Assignment
1	0.1465	0.5860	0	A
2	0.7041	2.8164	2	C
3	0.7781	3.1124	3	D
4	0.3249	1.2996	1	B

A particularly convenient mechanism for achieving balanced randomizations for two or more treatments is to use a *table of random permutations.*[6] In such tables, an array of integers, ranging from 1 to 8, 1 to 16, or 1 to 100 (or more) is arranged in a random sequence. Treatments can then be assigned according to the even or odd (or other appropriate features) of the digits encountered in the balanced interval demarcated by the sequence. For example, the following array of digits shows a random permutation of the integers from 1 to 16:

9	6	10	11
13	7	1	2
15	5	8	4
12	3	14	16

Table 16–1. RANDOMLY GENERATED NUMBERS FROM 1 TO 100*

75	59	24	33	65	67	35	89	71	4	14	22	58
16	23	47	7	23	32	7	47	57	23	1	5	10
26	26	69	64	41	79	88	73	91	2	81	13	89
34	43	5	78	9	69	94	95	99	11	75	79	10
43	60	27	50	68	46	62	73	32	53	19	27	73
40	18	75	67	87	90	31	35	19	73	79	51	94
24	95	86	98	17	80	55	2	69	59	13	36	5
47	78	30	30	42	17	82	69	38	71	88	67	25
72	1	42	31	25	41	87	81	72	65	77	32	49
40	4	65	6	52	56	22	88	7	93	99	12	4
70	45	0	28	42	78	62	75	87	11	46	9	20
69	6	16	18	27	0	98	62	16	27	86	56	0
70	44	73	21	7	67	22	0	42	14	17	35	56
12	86	62	88	82	88	0	27	57	61	86	50	50
38	18	84	44	66	84	60	18	57	9	43	45	73
97	67	3	60	62	6	32	55	65	6	12	2	74
79	55	46	62	4	7	4	39	45	46	50	48	92
81	83	48	16	27	18	11	88	48	27	22	72	92
85	93	12	90	94	74	30	20	6	57	81	80	21
93	16	8	78	10	24	8	38	11	65	49	24	66
0	49	82	2	24	98	22	2	78	23	41	2	81
38	54	11	75	64	18	32	22	95	41	4	78	84
92	94	58	59	21	57	36	74	53	22	45	60	67
74	81	64	70	8	42	76	34	41	37	64	79	87
21	80	23	60	37	72	87	95	34	8	36	18	24
78	67	52	32	83	27	43	40	85	22	64	60	61
91	60	48	27	96	85	19	67	27	98	83	82	33
13	54	10	36	35	94	49	70	13	33	96	81	3
64	75	1	42	81	44	61	94	49	6	31	18	92
97	25	57	88	31	23	37	15	66	83	32	49	74
42	56	54	45	54	20	51	17	45	22	97	84	78
8	43	30	50	25	57	91	0	25	88	91	80	50
83	26	67	5	2	53	22	57	0	53	98	88	79
21	42	6	70	93	46	85	28	86	6	47	18	85
56	37	47	78	82	50	27	63	33	38	97	81	80
91	70	41	82	30	4	60	82	25	61	98	80	0
12	31	61	68	61	48	96	89	57	52	58	97	99
4	60	36	85	41	76	52	70	84	63	22	24	4
66	63	92	92	46	47	19	4	1	8	95	58	51
95	19	33	73	34	99	91	0	76	81	1	18	72
66	77	33	78	74	30	25	56	76	67	4	54	34
60	28	62	14	16	48	57	84	28	91	62	11	76
54	62	95	94	64	85	70	90	66	80	59	5	17
65	34	57	58	20	46	40	35	73	49	14	82	98
87	88	22	26	16	39	92	50	50	59	74	28	33

*This table was generated on an IBM 370/158 computer system, using software of the Statistical Analysis System (SAS). The uniform function program of SAS was instructed to generate random numbers ranging from 1 to 100. The number *100* appears as *0* in the table.

If we let odd numbers receive treatment A and even numbers receive treatment B, and if we work across the rows from left to right and then from top to bottom, this permutation would provide a balanced randomization, with eight patients for each treatment, in the following sequence: A, B, B, A, A, A, A, B, A, A, B, B, B, A, B, B.

16.1.1.4.2. *Advantages of Randomization*

In addition to removing human judgment from the allocation of maneuvers, randomization has an attractive statistical virtue. Because statistical tests of significance are based on the idea of random probabilities, the application of such tests is particularly appropriate when the maneuvers are assigned according to random probabilities. This statistical virtue is relatively unimportant, however, because tests of significance refer to the numerical size rather than the scientific quality of the data; and the tests are constantly performed for data obtained without randomization. In fact, if randomization were a prerequisite for doing tests of statistical significance, the medical literature would have to be expunged of all the P values, confidence intervals, and other inferential statistical indexes that have been calculated for epidemiologic and clinical studies in which nothing was randomized.

The major virtue of randomization is its unpredictability rather than its probabilistic attributes. This unpredictability may be lost when nonrandomized approaches are used by investigators trying to avoid the complexity of having to prepare and use a formal randomization schedule. One simple approach is to assign the compared agents in alternating sequence, i.e., the first patient gets treatment A, the second gets B, the third gets A, and so on. Other schemes may use even or odd digits in the patient's date of birth, hospital unit number, or date of hospitalization.

Unless the treatments are given under totally double-blind conditions, however, all of these procedures would allow a conniving investigator (or clinician) to anticipate the treatment scheduled for a particular patient and to manipulate the circumstances so that the patient receives a desired treatment. A famous example of this type of manipulation occurred early in the days of large-scale controlled trials when anticoagulant therapy was being tested against placebo in the management of patients with acute myocardial infarction.[7] Because the treatments were openly assigned alternatingly on even- or odd-numbered days, a clinician who wanted his patient to receive anticoagulants could delay the hospital admission by 24 hours if the infarction occurred on the wrong day. Because patients are at greatest risk of death in the first day of a myocardial infarction, those who survived to be admitted to receive anticoagulants on the second day were in a better prognostic state than those who were admitted immediately.

When anticoagulants emerged as unequivocally superior to placebo in this trial, the results set off a controversy that has still not been fully resolved more than 30 years later. In subsequent trials in which randomization was used, anticoagulants were slightly but not statistically significantly better than placebo. Subsequent analysts[8] then claimed that the randomized trials were undersized, containing too few patients for the superiority of anticoagulants to be demonstrated stochastically. In more recent nonrandomized research,[9] the conclusion was that anticoagulants are efficacious for poor-risk patients with myocardial infarction, but not for the good-risk group.

16.1.1.4.3. *Alternatives to Randomization*

As long as the attending clinician and patient cannot anticipate the impending assignment, various mechanisms can be used instead of randomization to allocate treatment. The purpose of the alternative methods is either to eliminate problems of prognostic disparity or to avoid some of the ethical difficulties in using placebo or an inferior treatment. A tactic called *minimization*[10] tries to reduce prognostic disparity in the treated groups by having the investigator keep an ongoing tally of important clinical attributes of the admitted patients. Successive treatments are then assigned in such a way as to minimize the differences among those attributes in the treated groups. If the results of each treatment can be promptly determined after its imposition, a variety of techniques—among them a method called "play-the-winner"[11]—has been used to reduce the likelihood of assigning patients to an inferior treatment.

A different approach deals with the problem of ethics. The treatments are still assigned by randomization, but the patients' consent is sought after the randomization rather than before, and consent is solicited only from those patients assigned to a previously untested agent.[12, 13]

16.1.2. *Ascertainment of the Maneuvers*

When cause-effect research is not conducted as an experimental trial, the investigator must find out what maneuvers were imposed. The ascertainment process is relatively easy in prolective studies, because the investigator can determine what agents people received while they were receiving them. When the research is conducted afterward, however, the recipients may have problems in recalling what happened a long time ago, or the investigator (and the recipients) may be biased by the outcomes that followed the maneuvers. Although double-blinding is often used in experimental trials to prevent a knowledge of the maneuvers from biasing the detection of the outcome events, investigators in nonexperimental studies often neglect the parallel scientific importance of preventing a knowledge of the outcome events from biasing the ascertainment of the maneuvers.

16.1.2.1. **INTERVIEWER BIAS**

The term *interviewer* is used here to refer to the person who tries to ascertain the maneuver. The ascertainment is often conducted by interview with the potential recipient but can also be attempted from review of medical or other appropriate records. The main problem in ascertainment is that when the interview (or review of old records) is conducted after the outcome events have taken place, the procedure may be biased by a knowledge of the outcome and of the research hypothesis. For example, an interviewer who believes that tea drinking causes gallstones may readily take "no" for an answer when checking for the antecedent drinking of tea in a person without gallstones, but may inquire much more carefully and intensively to find evidence of previous tea drinking if the person is known to have gallstones.

One way of avoiding this problem is to keep the interviewer (or data reviewer) ignorant of either the research hypothesis or of the outcome events. Another approach, when data come from a direct interview, is to use a rigid, formal structure of questions for the interview and to be sure that exactly the same structure is applied to each person who is interviewed. A good scientific principle to apply in these situations is that the investigator who has established the research hypothesis should *not* be the person who acquires the data that will later be used to prove or disprove the hypothesis.

16.1.2.2. **RECALL (ANAMNESTIC) BIAS**

Even if the person acquiring the data is objective and unbiased, the person who provides the data may not be. This problem is particularly likely to arise in case-control studies, in which exposure to previous maneuvers is ascertained after the outcome event has occurred. For example, compared with the mother of a normal baby, a woman who has just given birth to a deformed child is much more likely to search her memory to recall every medication and any other events that may have occurred during pregnancy. Because an unfortunate outcome is almost always likely to be followed by rumination about antecedent events that may have led to that outcome, and because this rumination is much less likely to occur in people who did not have the unfortunate outcome, the possibility of recall bias is substantial and must be suitably considered.

Aside from the possibility of biased results, the data may simply be inaccurate. For example, when a group of women were asked *after* pregnancy was completed to cite the medications they had taken during the pregnancy, the responses often disagreed with information obtained from those same women while the pregnancy was in progress.[14]

16.1.3. *Size of Groups*

At least three different tactics can be used to determine the number of people needed for statistical significance in a comparison of maneuvers. In the most common method, the sample size is calculated to be just large enough for significance in the anticipated distinctions of the groups. Patients are then admitted to the study consecutively until this predetermined sample size is reached.

The second method depends on a technique called *sequential analysis*. When this technique is used to compare two treatments, patients are paired on admission and randomly allocated to the two treatments. The results of each pair are then appraised as a tie, or as a win or loss for one of the two treatments. The wins and losses are then plotted sequentially on a special graph, marked with precalculated boundary lines. When the plotted line passes outside the boundaries, statistical significance is reached, and the trial is terminated.

Despite the attraction of getting the minimum sample size needed for significance, the sequential analysis method has many impracticalities that reduce its successful application. It cannot be used in long-term studies, because the outcome event must occur soon after treatment to allow prompt determination of a winner for each new pair of compared patients. Furthermore, because the sample size depends on this single outcome event, the trial may be concluded with groups that are too small to yield stochastically significant differences for other outcomes that are also of interest in the research.

The third method, although often disdained mathematically, is particularly common in pragmatic reality. A fixed-size sample is calculated at the beginning of the trial, but because the calculation requires many guesses about the outcome events, the investigators rely on checking what actually happens in the trial. After the study begins, the investigators try to admit all the patients they can get, but someone regularly "peeks" at the accruing results. If clinically impressive and stochastically significant differences have begun to appear, the trial may be ended prematurely before the planned duration of follow-up or before the initially calculated sample size has been assembled. Conversely, at the end of the planned trial period for the planned sample size, if the differences are found to be impressive but not stochastically significant, the investigators may arrange a "postmature" extension, in which the trial period is prolonged or more patients are admitted.

Despite considerable discussion[15, 16] (to which the reader is referred), no statistical agreement has been reached about how best to manage the stochastic consequences of multiple "peeks" at the accruing data, and how best to make other decisions about premature termination or postmature extension of a trial with a predetermined sample size.

16.2 PERFORMANCE OF THE MANEUVERS

Regardless of how suitably the maneuvers were chosen, they cannot act until they have been imposed on the recipients. While the maneuvers are being performed, their action can be substantially altered by features that affect proficiency. The features can be general aspects of timing or potency, or factors involving compliance, regulation of intermediate targets, or superimposition of additional maneuvers.

16.2.1. *Timing of Maneuvers*

To be regarded as a possible cause of a subsequent effect, a maneuver should be imposed before the effect has occurred and at a time when the effect can be influenced. These two criteria seem so obvious that their statement may seem superfluous. Nevertheless, both criteria are sometimes given inadequate attention, and the ensuing problems can bias the results compared in the research.

Although randomized allocation of maneuvers can distribute the problems equitably, they can become prominent sources of distortion in nonrandomized research. One of the problems can be called *protopathic bias*. It occurs when the outcome event has already taken place but is not adequately recognized before the maneuver is allocated. The maneuver, which is evoked by an early manifestation of the outcome event, is then fallaciously held responsible for causing it. For example, although given to a child who is ill with fever that is a prodromal manifestation of Reye's syndrome, aspirin may later be accused of causing the Reye's syndrome. A second problem, which can produce *vulnerability bias*, occurs when subsequent events are attributed to a maneuver that was given too soon, too late, or too inappropriately to be held responsible for any beneficial or adverse effects that may follow it. Both of these problems, although produced by the timing of maneuvers, really depend on the baseline state of the people receiving the maneuvers; and the problems lead to susceptibility bias of the compared groups. The problems will be discussed later during further considerations of susceptibility bias.

16.2.2. *General Proficiency*

The plans made for an experimental trial are not always carried out exactly as intended, particularly in studies in which the participation of multiple institutions allows ample opportunity for individual variability. The management of protocol violations in an experimental trial is discussed further in Chapter 29. The rest of the discussion now is concerned with the problems created by nonproficient maneuvers in either experimental or nonexperimental research.

For individual psychotherapy, surgical operations, and other maneuvers that depend on personal skill, the proficiency of the maneuver is seldom ascertained because the skill of the performance is difficult to measure. In the absence of methods for assessing these skills, major problems can arise and controversies can flourish. For example, although many controlled trials have been conducted for psychotropic pharmaceutical agents, which are standardized by the manufacturer, no such trials have been attempted to compare the efficacy of psychotherapeutic doctrines, such as Freudian analysis and Jungian analysis, which are not standardized for their performance by individual psychotherapists.

As noted in Exercise 4.4.2 at the end of Chapter 4, the rate of postoperative deaths or complications can sometimes be used as a surrogate index of surgical skill. In the controversy about the merits of surgical bypass versus medical therapy for coronary disease, the relatively high rate of postoperative deaths in the VA cooperative clinical trial[17] was used as an argument that the surgery had not been proficiently performed.[18] The counterargument was that the postoperative mortality rate at VA hospitals, although higher than at certain specialized centers, was the same as the national average for the operation.[19]

For pharmaceutical agents, smoking, diet, or other substances that are appraised as maneuvers, decisions must be made about the particular amount of exposure that will be regarded as proficient. In what quantity and for how long must a woman have taken estrogen replacement treatment to be classified as *exposed*? What is the amount and duration of cigarette smoking that is required to label someone as a *smoker*? In a randomized trial of pharmaceutical agents, what is done about patients who took their assigned drug faithfully but who used the wrong dosage or the wrong schedule of administration?

Although these questions have no definitive answers, variations in the answers can substantially alter the results of the research. For example, the odds ratio for the relationship of endometrial carcinoma and postmenopausal estrogen replacement therapy ranged from 5.1 to 0.9 in the same study, according to the definition used by the investigators for *exposure to estrogens*.[20]

16.2.3. *Problems in Regimen Compliance*

The word *compliance* refers to a person's maintenance of a prescribed program. *Regimen compliance* refers to maintenance of a therapeutic regimen, in contrast to *protocol compliance,* which deals with schedules for clinical examinations, blood tests, or other plans of a clinical trial. (Some readers may not like the term *compliance,* because it can connote servility by the patient or paternalism by the clinician; but alternative words, such as *adherence* and *fidelity,* seem to have even greater disadvantages.)

In circumstances of free daily life, the maintenance of a prescribed diet or exercise, the ingestion of a prescribed oral medication, and sometimes the daily injection of a medication depend completely on the patient's decision to comply with the prescribed regimen. In nonexperimental research, the investigator determines what the patient actually did, and the patient is classified accordingly. In experimental trials, however, the assessment of compliance is particularly important because the prescribed regimen may differ from the received regimen.

Two regimens (or maneuvers) that would produce the same results if well maintained would not be fairly compared if one of the maneuvers receives excellent compliance and the other does not. To assess this possibility requires methods of ascertaining how faithfully each patient maintained the maneuver, development of criteria for classifying fidelity, and analysis of outcome data according to categories of fidelity. The analysis of maneuveral compliance is particularly important for oral medication, dietary therapy, and exposure to noxious substances, such as cigarettes, alcohol, or industrial toxins. In each instance, the investigator will have to decide how much compliance or exposure is required to regard the maneuver as having been proficiently administered.

The mechanisms used for assessing (and encouraging) compliance have been well discussed elsewhere[21] and are too extensive for recapitulation here. The main issues to be considered now are certain problems, biases, and opportunities related to distinctions in compliance.

16.2.3.1. NEGLIGENT NONCOMPLIANCE AND PROBLEMS IN APPRAISAL

If someone merely forgets to take a particular medication, and if the negligence is not related to a particular feature of the baseline state, maneuver, or outcome, the main consequence of the negligence is that an efficacious medication may appear ineffective. Thus, unless a clinician discovers that a patient has failed to take a prescribed antihypertensive drug, the persistently elevated blood pressure may be incorrectly regarded as a failure of treatment, and some other medication may be prescribed.

This type of negligent noncompliance can sometimes be valuable for demonstrating therapeutic efficacy in an experimental trial in which placebo was not employed. Thus, as noted in Exercise 12.3 at the end of Chapter 12, when similar results were found for two regimens of antibiotic prophylaxis against recurrent streptococcal infections, the investigators were able to convince themselves that both regimens were efficacious because the results were substantially better in compliant than in noncompliant patients.

If noncompliance is produced by reasons other than mere negligence, however, the possible causes should be carefully explored and analyzed. For example, a particular medication may receive poor compliance because of its inconvenience. It may taste terrible, be hard to swallow, or have to be taken eight times daily. Since these features do not involve pharmacologic efficacy, a rearrangement of the vehicle or dosage schedule for the medication may allow it to be more effective in general usage.

If poor compliance is produced by an unrecognized outcome event, the results of the regimen may be erroneously interpreted. For example, if a patient stops taking a remedial medication because all symptoms have been relieved, the successful outcome will be undetected if the patient is merely cited as a noncompliant drop-out. Conversely, if the medication receives poor compliance because symptoms have become worse or an adverse effect has appeared, the unsuccessful outcome may also be missed if the noncompliance is ascribed merely to negligence.

16.2.3.2. COMPLIANCE-DETERMINED SUSCEPTIBILITY BIAS

A particularly tricky problem occurs if compliance depends on certain personality traits that may also be associated with the outcome event, or if maintenance of the regimen creates stresses that also have relationships to both personality and outcome. For example, if coronary disease and cigarette smoking are both directly related to psychic tension, the people with lesser degrees of tension will be destined to develop lesser amounts of coronary disease, but will also be more able to comply with a regimen that calls for them to stop smoking. Such a circumstance can create a *compliance-determined susceptibility bias*. The exsmokers will appear to have lower rates of coronary disease than the persistent smokers, but the lowered rate may occur because compliance with the nonsmoking maneuver served to demarcate a group with lowered susceptibility to the outcome event.

Compliance-determined susceptibility bias was dramatically demonstrated in the randomized trial called the *Coronary Drug Project*.[22] The patients who complied well with the clofibrate regimen that was aimed at reducing blood lipids were shown to have significantly lower fatality rates than patients who complied poorly. This evidence might have been interpreted as showing the efficacy of clofibrate were it not for a simultaneous analysis of data in the patients allocated to placebo. The patients who complied well with the placebo regimen were also found to have significantly lower fatality rates than those who complied poorly.

In addition to indicating the important role of personality factors in coronary disease, this evidence helps sustain the controversial argument—discussed in Chapter 29—that the results of a randomized regimen should be analyzed only in the total group of people assigned to it, without separate analyses for differences in compliance.

16.2.4. *Regulation of Intermediate Targets*

In many therapeutic circumstances, the achievement of a long-term goal is attempted through the regulation of an intermediate target. For example, we may try to keep blood glucose or blood pressure at normal levels to prevent the vascular complications that can occur in patients with diabetes mellitus or hypertension. The degree of regulation is sometimes cited as the *control* of the intermediate target. Examples of such regulation are shown in Table 16–2.

To achieve the appropriate intermediate regulation, the dosage of treatment for each patient is usually "titrated" according to the results noted in the regulated entity. The achievement of such regulation creates major problems and challenges.

16.2.4.1. COMPLIANCE VS. REGULATION

If a particular treatment must be applied in a regulatory dosage, a measurement of compliance alone is unsatisfactory. A patient may comply perfectly with the prescribed regimen, but the prescribed dosage may not be adequate to achieve the desired regulation. Conversely, certain patients may be excellently regulated despite poor compliance. Because the goal of therapy is usually to normalize the levels of such things as an elevated blood pressure, glucose, or lipids, a clinician appraising the results wants to know not whether the patients took the prescribed medication faithfully but whether the desired normal levels were actually attained. Consequently, when a regulatory maneuver is evaluated, one of the variables under consideration must be a direct indication of the degree of achieved regulation.

This distinction has not always been appreciated in the statistical analysis of randomized trials of regulatory agents. The results have often been presented for the total cohort receiving the agent or for subgroups with different degrees of *compliance* but not for subgroups with different degrees of *regulation*.

16.2.4.2. DOUBLE-BLIND ADJUSTMENTS

To adjust the dosage of a particular regulatory treatment, the clinician must know both its current dosage and the level of the regulated target. In a trial conducted under double-blind conditions, this requirement creates a problem that might be called "the bind of the blind." The clinician must regulate the treatment but cannot do so without becoming unmasked and learning its identity.

The problem can be dealt with in two ways. The first is to maintain the conventional double-blind arrangement while allowing all the compared agents to be given in an escalating or "de-scalating" pattern of dosage. The observer can raise or lower the dosage

Table 16–2. LONG-TERM GOALS AND INTERMEDIATE REGULATION FOR SIX THERAPEUTIC AGENTS

Treatment	Long-Term Goal	Intermediate Regulation
Hypotensive agents	Prevention of vascular complications	Reduction of blood pressure
Anticoagulants	Prevention of thromboembolic phenomena	Alteration of clotting mechanisms
Digitalis	Maintenance of cardiac compensation	Cardiac rate or blood level of digitalis
Hypoglycemic agents	Prevention of vascular complications	Reduction of blood sugar
Antibiotic agents	Eradication of microbial organisms	Blood level of antibiotic
Hypolipidemic agents	Prevention of vascular complications	Reduction of blood lipids

of the agents in accordance with the desired regulation. The hazard of this arrangement, of course, is that the observer may break the double-blind code by noting the response achieved after each change of dosage. Thus, if no regulatory action occurs despite many escalating increments that have reached presumably high dosage, the agent is probably placebo.

To avoid this hazard, dosage adjustments may be performed with a double-observer technique. One clinical observer, aware of therapy, regulates the dosage; the second observer, kept double-blinded, makes the pertinent observations of the outcome events. Although cumbersome, the double-observer technique is often the best way to maintain double-blinding when dosage of treatment must be adjusted in accordance with measurements of its regulatory action.

The regulating and examining observers must be sure not to communicate with one another; and the regulating observer must be careful that the patient does not discover what treatment is being used. To avoid such discoveries, the regulating observer may sometimes arrange to change dosages of placebo. If the patient does become aware of treatment, plans should be made, if possible, to keep this knowledge from the examining observer, although the knowledge can obviously affect subjective features of the responses reported by the patient.

16.2.4.3. REGULATION-DETERMINED SUSCEPTIBILITY BIAS

A difficult problem in evaluation occurs if the ability to maintain good regulation is also related to susceptibility to the outcome event. This circumstance can produce a *regulation-determined susceptibility bias*. For example, patients with brittle diabetes mellitus, which is difficult to regulate at normoglycemic levels without frequent episodes of hypoglycemic shock, may also be particularly likely to develop vascular complications. In the era before the insulin pump, such patients often had poorly regulated blood glucose levels and also had high rates of vascular complications. The lower rate of complications noted in patients who could be easily regulated was then attributed to the regulation.

If satisfactory trials can be designed to test the insulin pump, the results may finally resolve the long-standing controversy about whether the low rates of vascular complications in well-regulated diabetic patients are due to regulation-determined susceptibility bias or to the regulation itself. The controversy might have been resolved much sooner if satisfactory studies had been conducted to achieve improved prognostic analyses of diabetic patients, using brittleness and other cogent variables that are not discerned merely by categorizing *maturity-onset, insulin-dependent,* or other clinical features used in conventional analyses.

16.2.5. *Contamination of Maneuvers*

Among the things to which people are exposed in daily life, so many substances can act as co-maneuvers that we may be either heroic or foolhardy in trying to isolate a single maneuver as responsible for a particular outcome. Dietary components, life style, psychic factors, occupational exposures, and atmospheric pollutants, as well as unprescribed and prescribed medications can all play roles in contaminating the specific maneuvers that are under investigation. The contamination can facilitate, distort, or disguise the effects of the investigated maneuver. For investigative analysis, the contamination can be classified according to the contrast, similarity, or interaction of the co-maneuvers.

16.2.5.1. CONTRASTING MANEUVERS

The most striking form of contamination occurs when people assigned to a particular treatment in a randomized trial receive one of the contrasted treatments. One aspect of this phenomenon is called *contamination of the control group*. For example, in studies of aspirin versus placebo for prevention of myocardial infarction, members of the placebo group may become contaminated by taking aspirin for various other purposes, including the incentive produced by publicity about the alleged benefits of aspirin. In a randomized trial of medical versus surgical therapy for coronary disease, some or many of the patients assigned to medical treatment may decide to have surgery. When vigorous multiple risk–factor intervention did not produce better results in the treated than untreated group of the MRFIT randomized trial,[23] the investigators contended that the control group had been contaminated by unauthorized, self-imposed attempts to reduce risk factors.

16.2.5.2. **SIMILAR MANEUVERS**

In the circumstance just cited, the comparative efficacy of an active principal maneuver will have been falsely reduced by its concomitant application in the inactive group. In the reverse situation, a maneuver's efficacy is falsely elevated by the concomitant use of other maneuvers having a similar action. For example, in clinical trials of continuous daily antibiotic prophylaxis to prevent recurrent streptococcal infections in patients who have had rheumatic fever, the patients may receive additional antibiotics from their family physicians to treat intercurrent infections in respiratory, urinary, or gastrointestinal tracts. Unless the role of this additional treatment is suitably analyzed, a falsely high efficacy may be ascribed to the prophylactic agent.

16.2.5.3. **INTERACTING MANEUVERS**

Certain maneuvers may accomplish their good or evil effects only when combined in an interaction with other maneuvers. This situation has been well recognized pharmacologically as drug-drug or drug-food interactions. In epidemiologic studies, which can seldom be as precise or decisive as pharmacologic experiments, the concept of interaction has been expressed in such phrases as *tumor promoters* and *tumor initiators*. The search for such interactions is often used as the rationale for some of the epidemiologic "data dredging" described in the next section and in Chapter 22.

16.3. **RETROACTIVE HYPOTHESES ABOUT MANEUVERS**

In experimental or nonexperimental cohort studies, the research structure is determined by the maneuvers under investigation. The investigator's hypothesis about the maneuvers must be formulated before the research begins, because the basic groups under study are established by the maneuvers they received. In such research, a large number of different outcomes can be examined, but the maneuvers under study are limited to those chosen at the outset of the investigation.

For non-cohort research, however, the basic groups are determined by something other than the maneuvers. In one classic type of cross-sectional survey, as noted in Chapter 18, the basic group consists of members of a geographically defined community. The investigator can then inquire about many possible exposures to maneuvers and many possible outcome events. In a classic etiologic case-control study, discussed in Chapter 23, the basic groups are chosen as cases or controls according to a selected outcome event, such as a particular disease. From each diseased case or nondiseased control, the investigator can then obtain data about antecedent exposure to a large number of possible etiologic maneuvers. In the heterodemic studies of Chapter 24, no basic groups are assembled. The investigator can take information about the ecologic or secular occurrence rates of a particular disease and correlate it with the corresponding rates of usage (or sales) for various substances that can then be suspected as etiologic maneuvers.

In all these non-cohort types of research, the investigator may begin with a hypothesis about a particular maneuver, but data about many other possible maneuvers are readily available. In an era of computers, the additional data can easily be analyzed for the possible role of alternative maneuvers about which no etiologic hypotheses were formulated or even suspected before the data dredging activities took place. The additional analyses seem reasonable, because we might as well check everything when we do not know what causes a disease, but the activity creates some major scientific hazards.

The main hazard of data dredging, which is often given the more genteel name of "hypothesis-generating research," is that positive results may be interpreted as demonstrating a causal relationship, although they merely show a statistical association between the indicted maneuver and the outcome event. Such an association is not necessarily causal and not even necessarily accurate. It may be highly biased by factors that have been overlooked during the data dredging; and it may even be an accidental event of stochastic chance. As noted earlier, at an α level of 0.05 for statistical significance, one of every 20 examined associations can be expected to be positive by chance alone, even though a true association does not exist.

For this reason, investigators and reviewers of non-cohort research must always recall the old scientific maxim that hypotheses cannot be proved by the data with which they were generated. A hypothesis that has been retroactively created in a data-dredging study cannot receive serious scientific attention until it has been deliberately tested in a separate study, conceived and designed for the purpose of performing the test. If this scientific principle were carefully observed, the public would be spared various problems that resemble the process of shouting "fire" when a match is lit in a crowded theater. One notable recent example was the highly publicized but now discredited[24-26] association that was found between coffee drinking and pancreatic cancer in a data-dredging case-control study.[27]

16.4 SYNOPSIS

The maneuvers under investigation are determined in an experimental trial by the investigator's mechanism of allocation and in nonexperimental research by ascertainment of what was imposed on the recipients.

In an experimental trial, the investigator can arrange to allocate the maneuvers within strata defined by the institutions or clinical features of the patients. Plans can also be made to divide and balance numbers of patients according to the proportions desired for each maneuver and to schedule the sequence of allocation by using randomization or some other mechanism that removes personal judgment from the assignments. When maneuvers are retrospectively ascertained in nonexperimental research, suitable precautions are needed to avoid recall bias in the people who supply the information and interviewer bias in the people who acquire it. The size of the groups needed for statistical significance in a comparison of maneuvers can be fixed with advance calculations, determined by sequential analysis, or adjusted by a "calculate-then-peek" technique.

The performance of maneuvers should be checked for appropriate timing of onset in relation to outcome events and particularly for skill, dosage, or other factors that will allow each maneuver to have been proficient. The maneuvers will not be fairly evaluated if they lack suitable proficiency because of inappropriate timing, inadequate skill in performance, or inadequate schedules for dosage and/or duration of medication. For allegedly etiologic maneuvers, a definition should be established for the amount and duration of a suitably proficient exposure.

Compliance must be monitored and analyzed to assure a fair comparison of maneuvers;

but compliance-determined susceptibility bias can arise if personality factors simultaneously affect both compliance and the outcome event. When an intermediate target, such as elevated blood pressure, is regulated to prevent a long-term adverse outcome, such as vascular complications, the degree of regulation should be monitored and analyzed to provide clinically cogent results. In a double-blind study, suitable regulation can be achieved with techniques of escalating dosage or using double observers. A regulation-determined susceptibility bias can arise if people who have the greatest difficulty (or ease) in achieving good regulation are also prognostically most (or least) likely to develop the adverse outcome events.

The appraisal of maneuvers can be distorted or confused by the contamination that occurs when members of the control group receive the principal maneuver, when individual maneuvers are supplemented by other maneuvers having similar action, or when additional maneuvers interact with the main maneuvers under study.

Because multiple maneuvers can readily be investigated without preceding hypotheses in non-cohort research, data dredging analyses can often yield positive statistical associations that occur by chance alone. The etiologic hypotheses generated in such statistical expeditions cannot be eligible for serious scientific attention until checked in subsequent research that is suitably designed to test the hypotheses.

EXERCISES

Exercise 16.1. These three exercises will give you a chance to do some randomizations yourself.

    16.1.1. Using the random numbers provided in Table 16–1, prepare a complete randomization schedule for the first 30 patients entering a parallel trial of three therapeutic agents, A, B, and C. Briefly note the strategy you used in working out the schedule.

    16.1.2. Perform the same task you did in 16.1.1, except arrange for the randomization to be balanced after every six admissions to the trial.

    16.1.3. Two agents, A and B, are to be tested in a randomized cross-over trial in which each agent is taken for two weeks, followed by a two-week wash-out period, followed by administration of the other agent. Prepare a randomization schedule for the 10 patients who will enter this study. Briefly outline your procedures in preparing this schedule.

Exercise 16.2. In a recent clinical trial comparing treatment alternatives in women with advanced breast cancer,[28] the investigators used a randomized consent design to allocate patients to the compared treatments. Eligible patients were recruited for the study if they satisfied the admission criteria. Patients were then randomized either to group A (do not seek consent) or group B (seek consent). Patients randomized to group A were not approached for entry into the study and received the best standard therapy available. For patients assigned to group B, informed consent was requested: The patients were asked to participate in a clinical trial and to accept the experimental therapy. If the patient agreed, she received the experimental treatment; if she refused, the best standard treatment was given instead. Please diagram both the randomized consent design and a more conventional design for this randomized trial. Describe the advantages of the new design. Discuss what you perceive as the major limitations of the randomized consent design.

Exercise 16.3. A group of investigators planning to conduct an experimental double-blind trial of two agents, A and B, do not wish to go through the complexities of using a randomization schedule. They plan to assign treatment A to all patients with odd hospital admission numbers and treatment B to all patients with even numbers. They state that because the double-blinding is effective—i.e., the two treatments cannot be distinguished—personal judgments will not enter the assignment and therefore randomization can be avoided. Do you see any pitfalls in this plan? If so, what are they?

Exercise 16.4. A psychiatrist wants to test the merits of classic Freudian analysis versus modern behavioral therapy. He has found a group of psychiatrists who are adept at using both types of therapy and who are willing to participate in a randomized trial of the two forms of treatment. The psychiatrists say they can find a large enough number of patients who would consent to participate in such a study, who would comply with whatever treatment is assigned, and who would remain in the study long enough for the outcome events to be observed. Having read Section 16.2.2, the principal investigator is worried about the personal variability and possible prejudices of the participating psychiatrists in using the two forms of treatment. What sort of design would you suggest for a randomized trial that can deal with this problem?

Exercise 16.5. When fatality rates with anticoagulants failed to show superiority over placebo in randomized trials of treatment for patients with acute myocardial infarction, the pro-anticoagulant clinicians claimed that the dosage of anticoagulants had not been suitably regulated. Would it have been fair for the investigators to review the intra-trial results of the prothrombin times (or other suitable indexes of anticoagulation), classify the patients as well-regulated or not well-regulated, and separately compare the fatality rates in well-regulated patients versus the rates in placebo?

Exercise 16.6. For treating patients with obesity, a practicing clinician has developed a new dietary regimen consisting of 900 calories per day of bread, wine, and cheese supplemented by a daily vitamin-mineral pill. He says that patients who have maintained this regimen have lost an average of 40 pounds. Do you believe him? If not, why not?

Exercise 16.7. A group of investigators has come to you for help in deciding whether the basic comparison of maneuvers has been properly planned in their proposed research. The consultees want help not in arranging the allocation of maneuvers (i.e., randomization versus clinical judgment), but in choosing an appropriate comparison. What criticism or advice would you offer for each of the following proposals:

    16.7.1. We want to determine the best way of rehabilitating people who have developed paraplegia after a traumatic accident. One group of people will receive especially careful attention to training in the use of mechanical aids, such as braces, crutches, and wheelchairs. The other group will receive routine mechanical therapy but intensive attention to psychologic, social, and occupational adjustments.

    16.7.2. We want to determine whether a new nonsteroidal anti-inflammatory drug, Inflamex, is better than aspirin in relieving the chronic pain of people with rheumatoid arthritis. Previous tests have shown that the optimal dosage of Inflamex is 500 mg., 4 times daily. One group of patients will receive Inflamex in this manner. The other group will receive aspirin in the same dosage schedule as the Inflamex.

    16.7.3. We want to test a new therapeutic regimen that can allegedly save lives in patients with acute myocardial infarction. To avoid the logistic problems of performing a randomized clinical trial in the hospital, we decide to test the new regimen in the following way. All patients treated during January 1, 1983 to December 31, 1984 (before the new regimen was instituted) will be the control group. After the new regimen is started, on January 1, 1985, it will be given to all patients thereafter until December 31, 1986. The results for the two forms of treatment will then be compared.

16.7.4. A gynecologist has performed 100 routine abortions using a vacuum extractor device that seems to have been safe, effective, convenient, and relatively inexpensive. We want to acquire such a device for use at our hospital. A member of the hospital's evaluation committee claims that the gynecologist's results are not valid because a control group was not tested. Do you agree?

16.7.5. Radiotherapists have claimed that the survival results after cancer surgery are improved by preoperative radiation of the cancer. We plan a randomized therapeutic-trial to perform the following comparison in operable patients. One group of patients will receive surgery immediately. The other group will receive a course of intensive radiotherapy for a month, followed by a month of recovery. At the end of the second month, surgery will be performed in those patients who are still operable. The results will be compared in those patients who received surgery alone versus those who received radiotherapy plus surgery.

16.7.6. We want to determine whether the use of a special low-fat diet can prevent the development of coronary artery disease. The large number of people accepted into the trial will be randomly assigned to receive diet or no diet. The no-diet group will be allowed to continue their customary patterns of eating. The diet group will be assigned the special diet. After 10 years, the rate of occurrence of coronary disease will be noted in the control group and in those who maintained the special diet.

16.7.7. We want to determine whether diethylstilbestrol (DES) given during pregnancy causes cancer in the subsequent offspring. We have available the medical records of a large institution in which DES was often used many years ago. Excellent follow-up information is available for all patients and offspring. From the old medical records, we shall assemble a retrolective cohort of women who were treated during pregnancy with DES. We shall then obtain outcome data for the current status of each child. For a control group, we shall match each DES-treated mother with the next pregnant woman, seen at the same institution in the same era, who did not receive DES. We shall do a similar follow-up for the children of these women.

16.7.8. A gynecologist wants to prove his belief that postmenopausal estrogen replacement therapy keeps women looking young and beautiful. Using a random sampling household survey technique, he will assemble a group of women who have been using such therapy and an age-matched control group of women who have not. Each woman will then be rated for her youthful looks and beauty by a panel of judges who are kept ignorant of the therapy. The "pulchritude indexes" will be compared in the groups who do or do not receive estrogen therapy.

CHAPTER REFERENCES

1. Kuhn, 1970; 2. Wood, 1957; 3. Fisher, 1935; 4. University Group Diabetes Program, 1970; 5. Coronary Drug Project, 1973; 6. Moses, 1963; 7. Wright, 1948; 8. Chalmers, 1977; 9. Horwitz, 1981; 10. Taves, 1971; 11. Zelen, 1969; 12. Zelen, 1979; 13. Horwitz, 1980; 14. Klemetti, 1967; 15. Pocock, 1978; 16. McPherson, 1982; 17. Murphy, 1977; 18. Proudfit, 1978; 19. Chalmers, 1978; 20. McDonald, 1977; 21. Haynes, 1979; 22. Coronary Drug Research Group, 1980; 23. MRFIT, 1982; 24. Lin, 1981; 25. Feinstein, 1981; 26. Whittemore, 1983; 27. MacMahon, 1981; 28. Santen, 1981.

Chapter 17

Implementation of the Outline: Outcome Events

For suitable analysis in a cause-effect research project, the outcome events must be properly characterized; the people under investigation must be observed long enough and well enough for their outcomes to be noted; the outcome events must be properly timed and detected; and appropriate mechanisms must be used to deal with the problems arising from diverse transfers that can occur between the onset of maneuvers and the collection of research data.

17.1. CHARACTERIZATION OF OUTCOME EVENTS

Everything that happens after the imposition of a maneuver can be regarded as an outcome event. Some of these events will have been anticipated and chosen as specific foci in the research. Other events will be expected but regarded as incidental. Yet other events will occur as pleasant or unpleasant surprises.

The challenge of choosing suitable variables to describe both baseline and outcome events was outlined in Chapter 13. The rest of this section is concerned with certain distinctive phenomena that receive attention as outcome rather than baseline variables.

17.1.1. *Temporal Components of Variables*

Three different locations in serial time affect the types of variables observed after the imposition of maneuvers. Some of the variables refer to new single-state events; others refer to transitions; and yet others deal with the maneuvers themselves.

17.1.1.1. SINGLE-STATE EVENTS

Many phenomena noted in the postmaneuver outcome are new individual events that were not present or defined when the baseline-state variables were established. For example, if the effects of prenatal care are being evaluated, the outcome includes many features of late-stage pregnancy, labor, delivery, child, and neonatal period that were not noted in the patient's baseline state. The criteria used to characterize these features should therefore be included when the outcome variables are chosen. If healthy people are receiving special diets or other maneuvers for the primary prevention of atherosclerosis, the definition of atherosclerosis, which may not have been considered in the baseline state, becomes an important challenge in the outcome variables. The development of an adverse reaction such as a skin rash, diarrhea, or oculomucocutaneous syndrome is obviously a new event that was not part of the baseline state variables.

17.1.1.2. TRANSITIONS

Many outcome events are characterized as transitions rather than as single-estate occurrences. The transition may be described in a specifically comparative term, such as *rise, fall, same, larger,* or *smaller,* or in a phrase that describes the postmaneuver response as *excellent, poor, improved, deteriorated, success,* or *failure.*

New sets of indexes, scales, and criteria are usually required to demarcate the transition phenomena, and individual transition variables may need to be developed separately (as noted in Section 13.4.3) for circumstances in which the baseline variable has too crude a scale to show subtle but important changes.

17.1.1.3. CHARACTERIZATION OF MANEUVERS

With attention centered on characterizing the baseline state and outcome events, investigators may sometimes neglect what comes between them: the performance of the maneuvers. As noted in Chapter 16, these performances must be characterized for the features that indicate the proficiency of each maneuver, the co-maneuvers, and, when pertinent, the patient's compliance with therapy and regulation of intermediate targets.

17.1.2. *Differentiation of Events*

In Section 13.4.3, the outcome events were divided according to their anticipated roles as primary, ancillary, and incidental targets in the research. Our main concern now is with undesirable events that are unanticipated.

Any event that occurs after the imposition of a maneuver can be designated as desirable, undesirable, or neutral. The desirable events are usually regarded as the benefits of the maneuver; and the undesirable events are usually regarded as the risks. The undesirable events are often given such names as *complications, untoward events, side effects,* or *adverse drug reactions.* These events can range from a transient skin rash or brief pain at the site of an injection to the occurrence of a deformed child or death. An essential step in characterizing undesirable events is to decide what kinds of events are sufficiently undesirable to warrant attention. For example, brief pain at the site of an injection might be ignored, but pain that persists for several days or that causes problems in using the injected limb might be regarded more seriously.

17.1.2.1. **THE RISK/BENEFIT RATIO**

The characterization of both desirable and undesirable events is important for developing the risk/benefit ratio that is often thought about when different maneuvers are appraised. (Because the risks and benefits are seldom quantified in commensurate units, and because a numerical ratio is almost never actually calculated, the term *risk/benefit ratio* is incorrect. Nevertheless, it is preserved here to avoid afflicting the reader with another neologism, such as *risk/benefit comparison.*)

During this appraisal, maneuvers that can be highly beneficial may be rejected because their risk/benefit ratio is too high. For example, thalidomide was a very effective agent in treating the nausea of early pregnancy, but its phocomelic deformities in the fetus were unacceptable. Conversely, phenothiazine frequently produces tardive dyskinesia as an undesirable side effect, but the drug remains acceptable and popular because of its benefits in treating uncontrolled schizophrenia.

Despite the intellectual appeal of the name, risk/benefit ratios are often evaluated inadequately because many of the benefits are not specifically cited or quantified, sought with the same zeal used in the quest for risks, or publicized with the same fervor as the risks. The problem is well illustrated with the furor that occurred several years ago when replacement estrogen therapy was accused of being a cause of endometrial cancer in postmenopausal women. Regardless of the scientific merits of the accusation, the idea of cancer is well established as a detrimental risk, but evaluators of the risk/benefit ratio for estrogen therapy could find no data to indicate the happiness of women whose hot flashes and other distressing manifestations of the postmenopausal syndrome had been relieved by estrogens; and no attention had been given to the subjective value of the benefits in those women who regarded the cosmetic effects of estrogens as highly desirable and who might be quite willing to accept those benefits in exchange for the slight risk (if true) of a cancer that almost always had an excellent prognosis.[1, 2]

Furthermore, when several colleagues and I undertook case-control research to evaluate the potential benefits of estrogen in preventing postmenopausal osteoporosis, we discovered that we were pioneers in using an epidemiologic case-control study in deliberate search of a benefit.[3] The many previous case-control studies reported in medical literature had all been aimed at finding adverse effects or had been conducted as data-dredging exercises, without a preestablished hypothesis. Finally, when the results of our case-control study and of several subsequent ones all suggested that estrogens helped prevent hip fractures and other osteoporotic hazards, the findings were generally ignored by the same media that had so heavily publicized the possible risk of endometrial cancer.

If risk/benefit ratios are to be used in enlightened public policy decisions about the value of a particular treatment or other maneuver, the appraisals cannot be satisfactory if the predominant emphasis is given to risk. A major expansion will be needed in the current methods used to define, discover, and acknowledge benefit.

17.1.2.2. PROBLEMS IN ADVERSE DRUG REACTIONS

An undesirable (or desirable) event is not necessarily attributable to the antecedent maneuver. The event can be due to a co-maneuver, to the natural evolution of the baseline condition, to a newly imposed co-morbid disease, or to something else, such as a complication from a diagnostic test procedure. Certain events can be psychogenic, such as fatigue and depression. In patients with cancer, the anticipated side effects of nausea and vomiting can occur psychogenically *before* chemotherapy has had the opportunity to produce them.

In an era in which new drugs are constantly being developed and marketed, a reasonable concern has developed for identifying their adverse side effects. In a careful scientific approach, the first step would be to develop standardized operational criteria, as described in Section 6.4.1, for differentiating the various causes of an undesirable event to decide that it is an adverse drug reaction in that patient. If the undesirable event occurs long after the maneuver was stopped, its relationship to the maneuver will be difficult to discern and will require special investigation. If the event occurs, however, while the maneuver is in progress or soon afterward, clinical judgment can be employed to decide whether the event can reasonably be related to the maneuver. For example, if a patient develops a skin rash soon after receiving an antibiotic, a relationship between the two events can readily be suspected. If the skin rash develops several years later, without any intervening antibiotic therapy, the relationship is hardly tenable.

This type of clinical judgment has been the traditional method for deciding that undesirable events were adverse drug reactions, and for preparing case reports that have been either published in medical literature or submitted to agencies concerned with public policy regarding drugs and health. An interesting irony in the current state of medical science is that clinical judgment has been rejected for cause-effect decisions about benefit but is often accepted for analogous decisions about risk. To claim that a patient was helped by a particular drug, a clinician would have to submit data fulfilling rigorous scientific criteria for every aspect of the information and reasoning. The nebulous vagaries of an unspecified clinical judgment would be unacceptable. On the other hand, to claim that a patient was harmed by a particular drug, the clinician need merely submit a case report to an appropriate agency. The report may then be accepted and included in the agency's dossier without further questions.

Casually prepared case reports have been solicited and analyzed for many years by agencies in various countries, but no standardized requirements or criteria have been established to denote the types of evidence and judgment needed for the operational identification of an adverse drug reaction. A few individual investigators[4-6] have suggested criteria for the process, but the agencies that conduct the process as a formal responsibility have not issued their own operational specifications. In the absence of such criteria, various mathematical strategies can be proposed for statistically analyzing the assembled case reports to make decisions about a drug's production of adverse reactions,[7-10] but the information used in the analysis is often of lamentably low quality. For example, in an appraisal of 26 case reports in an agency's collection of adverse reactions to a particular drug, 20 of the reports were found either to describe events that were incompatible with an adverse drug reaction or to contain such poor data that no justifiable decision could be formed.[11]

In the randomized controlled trials that are conducted before new drugs are marketed, adverse reactions are usually identified not by specific operational criteria but by a comparison of the incidence of undesirable events in the actively treated and placebo groups. This tactic is useful when direct control groups are available, but it has many scientific deficiencies. It does not distinguish events that are drug-related from those that are not. Thus, if a clinical trial happens to be conducted while an epidemic of influenza or viral gastroenteritis passes through the community, manifestations attributable to these co-morbid diseases will be included among the tabulation of undesirable events. Furthermore, if a study is conducted with statistical precision but without clinical judgment, silly results may sometimes emerge, as in the suggestion several decades ago that gonorrhea was an adverse side effect of oral contraceptive pills.

Clinical epidemiologists are confronted by an intricate scientific challenge in creating adequate surveillance mechanisms to protect the public against adverse drug reactions. Although the details of this challenge[10] are beyond the scope of the discussion here, a crucial first step is to develop a standardized, scientific mechanism for deciding that an individual event occurring in an individual patient is an adverse drug reaction.

17.2. MAINTENANCE OF THE COHORT

In non-cohort research and in retrolective cohort studies, the investigator need not make any prospective plans for following a group of people forward in time. In prolective cohort research, however, with or without randomization, suitable methods must be developed to observe the cohorts long enough and well enough to discern what happens in the outcome state.

In ordinary laboratory experiments, this maintenance procedure does not create a major problem. Laboratory experiments are generally short, so that a protracted serial time does not elapse between the imposition of the compared maneuvers and the occurrence of the outcome. The laboratory groups of animals (or chemicals) are a totally captive population, with no freedom to migrate elsewhere, to drop out of the project if they are discontent with it, to appear at the wrong times for examination, to refuse the examination procedures, etc. The laboratory investigator governs the timing and distribution of all subsequent examinations and can be sure they are performed with equal intensity and frequency in the compared cohorts. The laboratory investigator usually works in his own laboratory and seldom has problems with collaborators and data from multiple other institutions. All these scientific luxuries of the experiments conducted in laboratory cohorts are, alas, seldom available in the longitudinal surveys or experimental interventional trials performed for the prolective cohort studies of clinical epidemiology.

17.2.1. "Fail-Safe" Procedures

The establishment of fail-safe procedures, which consist of the mechanisms used for dealing with undesirable events, is vital both for the ethical conduct of a randomized trial and for making it attractive to potential participants. The mechanisms may contain provisions to unmask the identity of a medication given blindly, to discontinue or alter medication, and to institute additional treatment as needed.

The fail-safe mechanisms may also include the monitoring of certain variables—such as blood counts or chemical measurements—to detect early evidence of undesirable phenomena before they have progressed to overt clinical manifestations. Thus, if an agent is suspected of having the potential to produce leukopenia or cataracts, the patient's white blood count or ocular status would be checked at regular intervals for evidence indicating that the agent should be stopped or changed.

17.2.2. *Preservation of Participants*

In persuading the observed persons to remain under observation, to comply with prescribed medication, and to return for the examination procedures, the investigators may need extensive efforts to make the process attractive and convenient. This activity, which is often crucial to the success of a long-term project, is seldom adequately documented in research publications. An unusually complete account, which is recommended for your reading, was presented[12] for a randomized trial in which the investigators had to maintain an outpatient cohort of about 600 children and adolescents for six years, during which the patients were asked to return to the research clinic for monthly examinations and bimonthly blood tests. The investigators made special arrangements for a clinic schedule that kept groups of patients together as a type of "club," for transportation of patients who were unable to use public facilities, and for home visits by nursing staff to patients who were ill or delinquent in keeping appointments. The investigators also provided certain services, ordinarily relegated to social workers, that helped maintain a personal liaison between the clinical researchers and the patients.

Regardless of whether the cohort is assembled prolectively or retrolectively, skills must be developed for tracing and ascertaining the outcome status of patients who may have become lost to follow-up. The investigators may need considerable ingenuity in checking with neighbors, clergymen, insurance companies, and other sources of suitable information. (The name *tolper*, derived from an old radio program called "Mr. Keen, Tracer Of Lost Per*sons*," has been proposed for the people who develop this skill in locating and obtaining data about patients who would otherwise have to be classified as missing.) Boice[13] has reviewed some of the literature on this subject and has presented a quantitative account of yields for different methods of tracing former patients in a retrolective cohort study.

17.2.3. *Preservation of Protocol*

When several different investigators are collaborating in a cooperative study, arrangements must be made (and checked) for the investigators to be consistent in performing the various examinations and interpretations that are planned in the protocol.[14] In many instances, a central laboratory may be used to receive specimens (such as serum and electrocardiograms) from all the collaborating institutions and to report the results of the examination of those specimens.

17.2.4. *Preservation of Investigators*

In any long-term ongoing study, a hazard exists (particularly at academic medical centers) that the investigative personnel may leave their association with the study before it is completed. Losses of investigative personnel can occur because of new jobs, transfers, or (occasionally) loss of interest in the study. An important challenge for the principal or coordinating investigators in a cooperative study is to find suitable substitutes for any departing personnel and to arrange for an orderly transfer of responsibility.

17.3. PATTERNS AND PROBLEMS IN CHRONOMETRY

An intricate pattern of chronometry can be created by relationships in the timing of four different sets of phenomena: the baseline state at zero time, the onset and performance of the maneuvers, the tests and procedures used to detect the outcome event, and the occurrence of the outcome event. In the usual model of scientific reasoning, this pattern is simple: The maneuver is imposed on the baseline state at zero time and is followed by the occurrence of the outcome. In medical reality, however, this simplicity often vanishes. The maneuver may not start at the chosen date of zero time and may not begin to act promptly. The maneuver may be administered not as a single deed but repetitively over a long interval of time. The outcome may not be an overtly recognized event, and it can escape detection unless suitable tests are performed at suitable intervals.

17.3.1. *Onset of Maneuvers*

Section 12.1 described the choice of a zero time at which the maneuver is regarded as imposed on the clinical course of whatever condition is under study. In an experimental trial, the act of randomization is intended to reduce any bias that may arise because members of the compared cohorts have different durations in their prezero clinical course before the intervention begins.

17.3.1.1. POSTRANDOMIZATION DELAY

Randomization may not be successful in equalizing the prezero clinical course of the compared patients if one of the assigned treatments is delayed or given conditionally. For example, if patients assigned to surgery in a randomized trial must first receive a period of preoperative preparation, the surgery will not occur until later than the compared medical therapy, which often begins immediately. If measured from the onset of treatment rather than from the date of randomization, the postzero interval will be relatively shorter in the surgical than in the medical group. If the assigned surgery is not carried out because of something (such as death) that happens during the preparation interval, the results of the maneuver will be unfairly compared if the pretherapeutic deaths are omitted from the surgical cohort but deaths occurring in the corresponding interval of time are counted in the medical cohort.

17.3.1.2. LEAD-TIME PROBLEMS

An interesting set of lead-time problems occurs when a disease is classified according to either diagnosis alone or nonclinical manifestations (such as anatomic morphology), without provision for the clinical manner in which the disease was detected. In many patients, a disease becomes identified after it has produced symptoms or other manifestations that evoke medical attention and the ordering of suitable diagnostic tests. In other patients, however, the tests may have been ordered for screening purposes while the disease was in a lanthanic stage, without any symptoms or clinical complaints to call attention to itself. If the disease is an outcome event, these different modes of diagnostic discovery can lead to substantial problems in detection bias, as noted in Section 17.4. If the disease is a baseline state, and if zero time is the point of first diagnosis, the postzero interval will have different durations for patients discovered because of either clinical manifestations or screening procedures.

An example of the difficulty is shown in Figure 17–1, which demonstrates how the screening detection of a disease can raise the duration of survival without affecting the patients' clinical course. The problem could be avoided and the zero state distinction could

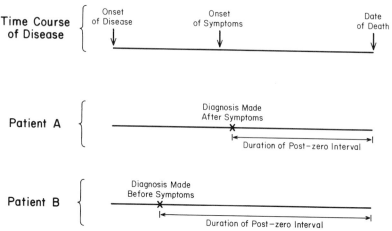

Figure 17-1. Illustration of lead-time bias. Because of presymptomatic detection of disease during screening, the post-zero interval of survival appears to be longer in Patient B than in Patient A, although no change has occurred in the total clinical course.

be properly analyzed if the diseased patients were suitably classified according to their iatrotropic stimulus and mode of clinical detection. Because these classifications are generally neglected, an enormous amount of erroneous data can be assembled about the virtues of screening in improving disease survival; and major problems in bias can be created when durations of survival are used as outcome data in groups whose different treatments are compared without regard to major differences in diagnostic mode of detection.

17.3.1.3. OTHER PROBLEMS IN CHOOSING ZERO TIME

In nonrandomized research concerned with etiology of disease, the compared cohorts may consist of people who received a particular maneuver, such as cigarette smoking, and those who did not. For the outcome intervals of the latter group to be compared, a zero time must be chosen for the date on which a maneuver was *not* imposed. This issue is often resolved by defining zero time as the date when the maneuver might have been imposed at a time when the potential recipient was qualified to receive it.

Regardless of whether the maneuvers are studied in an experiment or a survey, the choice of zero time will greatly affect the ability to generalize the results. Thus, if treatments A and B are tested in a chronic disease and if no distinction is made about whether patients are in their first, second, or later courses of treatment, the results will be difficult to generalize for future applications.

17.3.2. *The Potency Interval for Maneuvers*

Many maneuvers do not become effective immediately after they begin, and their action does not cease as soon as they are stopped. Most pharmacologic agents, for example, require a lapse of time before an administered dose has produced an effective blood level; and the agent may remain in the blood long after the last dose. The relative timing of the onset, duration, and ending of this potency interval can create many difficult problems in cause-effect research.

Two of those problems have already been discussed (Sections 11.9.1 and 15.5.2.3) for decisions in defining a potent maneuver and relating it to a baseline state. To decide that someone has been exposed to the maneuvers of smoking, high-fat diet, vigorous physical activities, or estrogen replacement therapy, we would need to choose not only an effective dosage for each exposure but also an effective duration. For example, it would not seem reasonable to ascribe the occurrence of coronary disease at age 65 to a few rich meals or heavy cigarette smoking in early adulthood, followed thereafter by a life of abstinence. To allow the maneuver an opportunity to be potent, its onset must occur at a suitable point of vulnerability in the recipient's baseline state. If given only in the last trimester of pregnancy, thalidomide would not affect a fetus; and if not begun until several days after the acute manifestations of myocardial infarction, lidocaine prophylaxis would have little or no value in preventing arrhythmias.

The potency interval creates a different set of chronometric problems when decisions must be made about relating an outcome event to the preceding maneuver. For example, if a patient has a pulmonary embolism shortly after the first dose of an oral anticoagulant and before the anticoagulant has had a chance to act on the blood, should the embolism be associated with the treatment and regarded as a failure of anticoagulation? To avoid this problem, the investigators may demarcate a post-therapeutic interval, sometimes called a *window*, during which the treatment is allowed to build up its potency. Any undesirable events occurring during this window are not ascribed to the treatment, and the zero time date for onset of treatment is essentially moved to the end of the interval. The policy seems clinically reasonable, but because it occurs after randomization and therefore carries the hazard of bias, its application is frowned upon by many statisticians. The use of such a window was an important source of controversy about the efficacy of sulfinpyrazone in preventing recurrent myocardial infarction.[15-17]

The temporary persistence of short-term potency after a maneuver has been stopped is sometimes called its *carry-over effects*. The duration of this carry-over period is important in designing a cross-over trial, because we would not want a second maneuver to begin while the preceding one is still active. To avoid this problem, patients often receive a wash-out period between successive maneuvers in a cross-over study. Because the complexity and expense of the trial may be greatly increased by these wash-out periods, they are sometimes eliminated with the hope that sophisticated statistical analyses will be able to adjust and compensate for the unwashed carry-over effects. The scientific justification for this hope is that the same interval of time will allow potency to be lost by the first maneuver and gained by the second. Because a true baseline state is not established before onset of the second maneuver, its baseline state is either determined from statistical calculations, or extrapolated from the baseline that existed before onset of the first maneuver.

A trickier problem in dating the effective termination of a maneuver arises when an undesirable event occurs relatively long after the maneuver has been stopped. For example, as a counterpart of the situation described earlier, suppose a patient has a pulmonary embolism one week after cessation of potent anticoagulant therapy. Should the embolic event be associated with the treatment and regarded as a failure of anticoagulant therapy? Questions of this type are difficult to answer, and the answers may evoke disagreements in both clinical judgment and scientific policy. The clinical disputes will arise from different beliefs about how long a maneuver must act to be potent and how much potency it retains after being stopped. For example, if we are unwilling to regard a thromboembolic event as a failure of anticoagulant therapy that stopped three years previously, should a lung cancer be ascribed to cigarette smoking that stopped 33 years previously?

The disagreement in scientific policy will arise from different beliefs about how to count and attribute events in a randomized trial. For example, no sensible clinician would regard the foregoing thromboembolic event as a failure of long-discontinued anticoagulant therapy. Nevertheless, according to the intention-to-treat policy[18] that is discussed further in Chapter 29, the thromboembolism would be counted as a postanticoagulant event if the patient had been assigned long-term anticoagulants in a randomized trial.

17.3.3. *Duration of Follow-Up Period*

The follow-up period should be long enough to allow an appropriate time for the target event(s) to occur and to be evaluated, but short enough to avoid creating major logistic obstacles in carrying out the research. For example, three months is probably too short a time for useful assessments of the impact of therapy on the survival of patients with a chronic disease such as cancer, diabetes mellitus, or coronary heart disease. On the other hand, a duration of 30 years might be too long a time for the investigators to be able to maintain attentive surveillance of the cohort. As another example, consider the famous Canadian randomized trial of the work of nurse practitioners in primary care.[19] The comparison of the nurse practitioners and family physicians was conducted with superb research methods, but the period of follow-up observation for patients occupied one year. Was this a satisfactory duration of time to allow the compared groups to be subjected to an adequate scope of challenges in family practice?

Analogous problems arise in choosing an optimum duration for the follow-up period in investigations designed to determine whether cigarette smoking causes lung cancer or coronary disease, whether hypotensive therapy prevents vascular complications in patients with hypertension, and whether the procedures of Health Maintenance Organizations improve the quality and costs of medical care.

17.3.4. *Frequency of Examinations*

Follow-up examinations serve at least three purposes: they provide the necessary follow-up data; they allow treatment to be modified, if necessary, for more effective regulation or to reduce the potential for adverse phenomena; and they help preserve interest, communication, and liaison between investigators and the people under investigation.

The interval between successive follow-up examinations should obviously be short enough to allow detection of the phenomena under surveillance. On the other hand, the examinations should not occur so frequently that they become a nuisance for the patients, leading either to drop-outs or to the patients' appearing at inadequate or irregular intervals for the examinations. Thus, to assess the occurrence of rises in antibody titers for detecting a group A streptococcal infection, sera need not be obtained more often than every two months; but to assess the development of anicteric hepatitis after a blood transfusion may require performance of liver function tests every two weeks.

If the outcome event—as in the two foregoing examples of streptococcal infection and anicteric hepatitis—must be discerned from transitions in the results of consecutive diagnostic tests, an inadequate timing of those tests can produce an important problem. Even in a randomized, double-blind study, the type of detection bias noted in the next section can arise if the diagnostic tests for a particular cohort are not or cannot be performed at suitable intervals.

17.4. **DETECTION OF OUTCOME EVENTS**

Three distinctive activities must take place to detect an outcome event that requires a medical diagnosis. The patient must receive medical attention; the appropriate diagnostic procedures must be done; and the evidence obtained during those procedures must be interpreted.

The medical attention is part of the surveillance mechanism for people followed in a cohort study. The surveillance may occur in a routine periodic manner, with clinical examinations performed at annual, biweekly, or other intervals. The routine surveillance may be supplemented (or occur exclusively) during *ad hoc* examinations solicited by members of the cohort because of specific symptoms or other problems.

In response to what is noted during the surveillance, different diagnostic procedures will be ordered by different clinicians. For example, when a postmenopausal woman reports she has had vaginal bleeding, one clinician may be content to look no further if the pelvic examination and cervical Pap smear are negative. Another clinician may order a dilation and curettage of the endometrium.

The evidence obtained during the diagnostic procedures is interpreted with different judgments by different observers. The same pelvic examination or Pap smear may be deemed negative by one observer and positive by another. The same specimen of endometrium may be interpreted as hyperplasia by one pathologist and as carcinoma by another.

A plethora of opportunities exists for one or more forms of detection bias to arise during these three activities.

17.4.1. *Detection Bias and The Role of Double-Blinding*

The use of double-blind procedures has become so thoroughly accepted as a component of modern randomized trials that the individual roles of randomization and double-blinding are sometimes confused. A critic who dislikes the idea of allocating treatment without clinical judgment may attack double-blinding, whereas a critic who opposes the objective evaluation of outcome events may attack randomization.

The main role of double-blinding is to prevent the observers and decision makers from being biased when surveillance is applied, diagnostic tests ordered, and evidence interpreted in the diagnostic detection of outcome events. In a secondary role, double-blinding also can help prevent bias or contamination in the clinician's (or patient's) management of maneuvers and co-maneuvers. For example, a patient who knows she is getting placebo or something other than the active treatment may seek and receive the active agent. A clinician may use ancillary treatment in a different manner if aware of the main treatment being given to the patient.

Like many other terms in clinical epidemiology, *double-blind* has become thoroughly accepted despite its linguistic disadvantages. The idea of double-blinding is that both the patient and the clinician are kept unaware of the specific treatment being received by that patient. The word *blind* seems odd, however, when applied to the observers who perform a specifically visual examination, such as the interpretation of a roentgenogram or histopathologic specimen; and it is frightening when applied to therapeutic trials in ophthalmology. (How many patients would want to enter a "double-blind study" of treatment for cataracts or glaucoma?) The term *double-blind* is also used inappropriately when the process is applied in a manner that is really *single-blind*. For example, when reviewing certain diagnostic material, radiologists or pathologists may be desirably kept blind to the patients' treatment, but the patients may have been fully aware of what treatment they were getting.

An alternative phrase, *double-masking*, seems less harsh than *double-blinding*, but has its own disadvantages in the caparisoned imagery it conveys. Another alternative term, *objective*, indicates the desired elimination of subjective prejudice but is often too nonspecific to denote the distinctive method that is used. Because no better alternatives seem available, and because readers may be delighted that I have no neologistic substitutes to offer, *double-blind* and *double-blinding* will be preserved here.

The main problem in double-blinding is that it is often impossible, inconvenient, or delusionary. It is impossible in research that has a nonexperimental structure or in experimental trials of medical versus surgical treatment in which a sham operation would today be usually regarded as unethical. (The ethics of a sham surgical procedure are open for discussion in Exercise 17.5 at the end of the chapter.)

Double-blinding is inconvenient if the compared agents have a distinctively different appearance or are delivered by different routes of administration. For example, if treatment A is given in liquid form and treatment B as a capsule, double-blinding would require that the recipients of A also take a capsule placebo and that the recipients of B also take a liquid placebo. If A is injected and B is taken orally, the recipients of B would have to receive a placebo injection that is necessitated by scientific rather than clinical considerations. These problems may create ethical difficulties (as cited in Exercise 17.6) but may also cause scientific hazards in evaluating the maneuvers. Compliance may be reduced if the patient's regimen schedule is complicated by the demands of double-blinding, and the intermediate regulation needed for a treatment's optimal potency may be compromised, as noted in Section 16.2.3.2, unless the double-blinding is conducted with a double-observer technique.

The most common unrecognized problem in double-blinding is that it is often a delusion. It provides the "window dressing" needed to satisfy evaluators who insist that the results of a trial are unacceptable unless double-blind procedures were used, but the double-blind masks are frequently perforated by unavoidable differences in the compared treatments. The construction of a perfectly mimetic placebo is often impossible, and even if the two agents are made to look the same, patients or clinicians can often smell or taste the compared agents to try to discern their distinctions. As a nonclinical example, suppose we wanted to conduct a double-blind trial of the culinary efficacy of mustard. What placebo could be used that looks like mustard, smells like mustard, and tastes like mustard? (The challenge of conducting such a trial is presented in Exercise 17.4.5.) In other circumstances, treatments that otherwise seem similar may often be distinguished by their physiologic side effects, such as the bradycardia that accompanies beta-blocking pharmaceutical agents.

An interesting by-product of double-blinding is its occasional adverse effect on the clinicians who provide care for the patients. I know several clinicians who, after participating in a long-term double-blind study, have refused to engage in any others. The clinicians' main complaint was the frustration of caring for patients without learning anything from the experience, because the post-therapeutic results could not be immediately correlated with the treatment. By the time the double-blind code was broken several years later to identify the treatments, the results would have to be studied retrospectively; and the clinician's learning experience would have to be acquired as a literary and statistical rather than directly pragmatic exercise.

For all these reasons, double-blind procedures can be used for their intellectual appeal, but unless the double-blind arrangements are impeccable, the goal of objectivity can sometimes be better achieved by improving the measurement process than by blinding the observers. Rigorous, consistent methods and criteria can be established for observations and interpretations that can provide hardened data, as discussed earlier. When double-blind methods *are* used, their efficacy should be checked in suitable circumstances to assure the investigators and reviewers that the masking was successful.[20]

Even if double-blinding was not used in the original performance of maneuvers, an appropriate form of single-blinding can still be applied when outcome data are reviewed. For example, when evidence is examined to make crucial decisions about causes of death in a randomized trial or any other research structure, the people who prepare an excerpt of the evidence can be kept blind to the research hypothesis, and the people who make decisions from the excerpts should be kept blind to the antecedent treatment. In the current technologic era, this process is readily achieved with a tactic sometimes called *differential xeroxing*. Replicate copies are made of the medical record or other information needed to decide the cause of death, but any data about therapy are removed from the material supplied to the decision maker.

17.4.2. *Outcome-Interpretation Bias*

Perhaps the most common (or most commonly known) form of detection bias occurs when outcome phenomena are interpreted subjectively. A patient who knows what drug he is getting may readily be influenced by that knowledge as he decides whether he feels better or worse after treatment. A clinician who knows the identity of the treatment may affect the patient's own perception and responses, or may subconsciously distort what the patient reports.

The clinical information submitted to a consultant may be regarded as desirable for ordinary patient care but can often be a major source of bias if the consultant's diagnoses are to be used in research. A radiologist interpreting a chest film may be prejudiced by a knowledge of the patient's occupation and smoking habits. A pathologist who knows whether a patient received estrogen therapy may be influenced by that knowledge when interpreting the histology of an endometrium. Some of the controversy about the efficacy of BCG vaccine in preventing tuberculosis arose from controlled trials in which the positive skin test produced by the vaccination was incorporated among the evidence used to diagnose tuberculosis.[21]

17.4.3. *Surveillance and Test-Ordering Bias*

Although the importance of blinding is easily recognized and acknowledged when diagnostic evidence is interpreted for an outcome event, the role of blinding or of equality in detection procedures is just as important, although not as well recognized, for activities in surveillance of the compared maneuvers and in the ordering of diagnostic tests.

In a controlled experimental study, the protocol would call for the compared groups to be similar in frequency and intensity of surveillance, and in diagnostic procedures for finding the target event(s). This type of equality is seldom assured, however, if the research is being performed as an observational survey. When maneuvers are imposed under natural, nonexperimental conditions, the general medical surveillance and ordering of diagnostic tests can regularly be expected to differ for exposed and nonexposed people. The differences can be due to disparities in the baseline state of the people who receive the maneuver, in their pattern of medical care, or in ancillary phenomena associated with the maneuver.

17.4.3.1. SURVEILLANCE BIAS

Surveillance bias is particularly likely to occur whenever a new treatment is under study. To be sure that no adverse effects occur, the patients will be monitored much more closely than people who are not receiving that treatment. For example, when minor pain develops in a calf muscle, the event may be ignored if the pain disappears in two days. If the woman is receiving a new oral contraceptive agent or is a nurse, however, the increased medical surveillance may evoke diagnostic attention to the pain. It may then be recorded as an episode of thrombophlebitis, which would have been undetected in some other person. Surveillance bias is also likely to occur in patients receiving regular medical checkups for treating or monitoring the status of a chronic disease, such as diabetes, hypertension, asthma, or epilepsy. During these check-ups, the clinician may find and work up diverse unrelated phenomena that would escape detection in a person who did not have the co-morbid chronic ailment. Whatever treatment is being used for the co-morbid ailment may then be falsely associated with the unrelated phenomena.

17.4.3.2. **TEST-ORDERING BIAS**

Test-ordering bias can occur if a particular maneuver produces a manifestation that is worked up to determine its diagnostic source. The diagnostic procedures may then reveal silent instances of an unrelated disease that may otherwise have been undetected. For example, suppose a laxative given to treat constipation frequently produces the side effect of gastritis, and suppose the gastritis frequently leads to a small hematemesis. The imaging or endoscopic procedures used to diagnose the hematemesis may reveal a silent gastric ulcer or gastric cancer that might otherwise be undetected (or not detected until a much later date). The ulcer or cancer, however, may then be fallaciously associated with the laxative. (The detection problems produced by co-morbidity bias and co-manifestation bias will be further discussed in Chapter 21.)

17.4.4. *Consequences of Detection Bias*

For all the reasons just cited, a substantial detection bias may occur in nonexperimental research if the members of cohort A, exposed to maneuver A, have had a greater (or smaller) opportunity to have the target event detected than the members of cohort B, exposed to maneuver B. When exposure to the compared maneuvers occurs in different regions or secular eras, the outcome events may be detected disparately because of differences in nosologic principles of diagnosis or in the availability and usage of diagnostic test procedures.

The tilted targets that can occur as a consequence of inequalities in surveillance, in test ordering, and in test interpretation are one of the major sources of error in classical epidemiologic research as well as in more modern forms of clinical epidemiology. For example, does disease D really occur more frequently in region A than in region B, or is the disease more likely to be detected in region A? Does the sharply rising secular rate of occurrence of disease E mean that it has begun to appear as an epidemic or has there been an epidemic of tests for it? Does thrombophlebitis really appear more often, or is it more likely to be detected when it occurs, in women who use oral contraceptive pills than in those who use mechanical forms of contraception? When workers in a particular industry receive intensive screening tests for cancer and are then found to have a higher rate of cancer than the general population, is the increase in cancer due to the occupational exposure or to the diagnoses revealed by the screening procedures? When disease F is found more often in people with disease G than in people who do not have disease G, is the higher rate of disease F due to a pathodynamic effect of disease G or to the diagnostic work-ups and discoveries that occur when patients with disease G receive their medical examinations?

Aside from nosologic caprices (discussed in Chapter 24) in the methods used for choosing a single diagnosis as the cause of death when death certificates are tabulated to produce the data of vital statistics, the neglect of detection bias has been perhaps the single greatest source of scientifically unreliable information in modern epidemiology. When dropsy was eliminated as one of the great killer diseases of the 19th century, no one claimed that the disease had been reduced by improvements in sanitation, life style, nutrition, or industrial pollutants. Dropsy was generally recognized to have been conquered by a change in nosology. It was given another name, with its patients distributed among such "new" diseases as congestive heart failure, hepatic decompensation, venous insufficiency, and nephrosis. The role of nosologic changes and technologic diagnosis does not yet seem to have been suitably analyzed, however, during 20th-century rises and falls in the occurrence of gastric cancer, pancreatic cancer, coronary artery disease, thromboembolic disease, lung cancer, systemic lupus erythematosus, and many other ailments for which diverse maneuvers have been either credited or blamed.

An interesting unpublished example of this problem occurred about two decades ago. A graduate student seeking a doctoral degree in a distinguished department of epidemiology had prepared a case-control study intended to determine the cause of an epidemic of streptococcal infections that had begun in a particular state in 1961. According to the state health department's tabulations, the annual occurrence of streptococcal infections had remained fairly constant in that state for many years, but in 1961 the occurrence rate suddenly rose to a new high level at which it had remained thereafter. The student's case-control study had been reasonably well designed and the interviews were aimed at rounding up the usual suspects (in nutrition, environmental exposures, and so on) that might be producing the epidemic. After all the plans for the research had been completed and after the first interviews had begun, the student discovered that the state health department, in late 1960, had introduced a new service for physicians practicing in that state. Each practitioner had been mailed a set of plastic Petri dishes, containing suitable culture media for streptococci. The dishes were to be used, without charge to physicians or patients, for throat cultures that would be sent to the state health department for incubation and diagnosis.

The role of diagnostic testing was promptly recognized as the cause of the streptococcal "epidemic," but analogous or more subtle distinctions in the availability and usage of diagnostic technology have seldom received adequate attention in epidemiologic surveys of etiology. Even in a randomized, experimental comparison, however, differences in maneuvers may play unsuspected roles in producing an unequal detection of outcome events. An example of this situation was cited in Section 4.2.3. As another example, consider a non–double-blind randomized study in which anticoagulants are being administered on a long-term basis. When the anticoagulant recipients report for the tests used to regulate dosage, other clinical phenomena can also be reported or noted. These other phenomena may then be detected in the anticoagulant group at a higher rate than in people not receiving anticoagulants. A different type of example occurs if a treatment produces a side effect, such as belching, that may evoke diagnostic tests such as cholecystography and ultrasonography. The silent and otherwise undetected gallstones that are revealed during these tests may then be attributed to the treatment.

17.5. THE CHRONOLOGIC ROLE OF THE VIRGULE IN SUMMARIZING OUTCOME EVENTS

When quotients are constructed to calculate the averages, proportions, or rates that summarize data for a group of people, each quotient has three components: a numerator, a denominator, and a virgule. The virgule is the diagonal slash mark (/) that separates the numerator and denominator. In the days before computer printouts made the division sign ($\div$) difficult to distinguish from the plus sign ($+$) used for addition, the quotients were often written as $a \div b$ or $\Sigma X \div N$. Today, quotients are almost always written as a/b or as $\Sigma X/N$.

In ordinary arithmetic, the virgule merely denotes the act of division. When we calculate the mean weight and the proportion of women in a group of 14 people respectively as $1015/14 = 72.5$ kg. and as $5/14 = 36\%$, the virgule plays no special role other than its mathematical symbolism. When we calculate the group's mean weight loss as $72.8/14 = 5.2$ kg. and the group's fatality rate as $3/14 = 21\%$, however, the virgule has an additional scientific function. It denotes the passage of time in the cohort. For weight loss and survival to be properly interpreted as outcome events in this cohort of 14 people, we need to know the particular period of postzero serial time that is under consideration. Was the mean of 5.2 kg. lost in 4 weeks, 4 months, or 4 years? Is 21% the fatality rate at 6 months or at 6 years?

The passage of time itself can be used to summarize cohort outcomes in such expressions as a mean or median survival time of 8.7 years. In almost all other expressions of cohort outcomes, however, the time interval of serial follow-up disappears in the virgule and must be cited separately for the results to be clearly expressed. This requirement is responsible for the chronometric component that appears in such cohort expressions as *3-year survival rate, mean weight loss per week,* or *annual mortality rate.*

The virgule also creates two additional scientific demands beyond its demarcation of the postmaneuver interval. A zero time must be chosen to indicate the chronologic point at which the serial follow-up interval began; and any rates or proportions that are calculated thereafter for subsequent points in serial time (such as 6 months or 3 years) will imply that everyone in the calculation has been followed for the stipulated length of time. We would have no idea of what is really meant by a *3-year survival rate* if we did not know when the 3 years began for each person, and the rate would be misleading if only a few people in the cohort had actually been under observation for as long as 3 years.

Thus, although a cross-sectional proportion, such as *36% women,* can be expressed without any special chronologic or mathematical accoutrements, a cohort proportion, such as *17% fatality rate,* is accompanied by three additional requirements: the zero-time point or event from which the serial time interval begins; the duration of the serial interval; and the number of people followed for that duration. An expression such as *17% fatality rate* for a cohort of 14 persons will be mathematically unclear and scientifically inaccurate unless we know that the interval began with the onset of a particular treatment, that it refers to the status of people 3 years after treatment, and that only 12 of the 14 treated people have been followed for as long as 3 years. Because two of the 12 people had died during that interval, the 17% fatality rate in this instance was calculated as 2/12.

These chronologic issues create major scientific problems in using statistics to summarize the outcomes of a cohort. What do we do about people who were followed for a while and then lost? What should be done with people whose outcome event cannot be observed because they have not been followed long enough or because they died of an unrelated cause? What happens if the cohort is assembled after zero time and does not include all of the people who were exposed to the maneuver? What is the effect of including people whose follow-up in the cohort began at various serial times after onset of the maneuver under investigation?

The basic problems cited in these questions can be divided into two types: denominator losses and numerator losses. In the denominator-loss problems, which are discussed in the next section, people who should be included in the cohort have been omitted. The cohort under study is a residue of what should have been investigated. In the numerator-loss problems, which are discussed in Section 17.7, the cohort contains all its appropriate members, but the outcome events for some of the members are unknown or uncertain. A series of statistical adjustments, often called *life-table analyses,* can be used to deal with the purely mathematical challenges of numerator losses, but the main issues, of course, are scientific. Serious distortions and biased results can be produced either by a residue cohort or by unrecognized disproportions in numerator losses.

17.6 **TRANSFER BIAS IN RESIDUE COHORTS**

Transfer bias is produced, after the imposition of maneuvers and occurrence of outcome events, by phenomena that distort the relative proportions of the maneuver-outcome relationships in the groups collected for comparison of results. The bias can arise in many different ways. The most common mechanism in cohort research is a disproportionate loss of members from the compared groups. These losses can be produced by death or migration of the cohort members, by the investigator's decisions in collecting data, or by decisions made when living cohort members accept or decline invitations to participate in the research.

In the architectural model with which we usually think about a cause-effect relationship, the research begins with the assembly of a clearly demarcated cohort whose members each had a baseline state that qualified them for admission to the cohort. When the maneuvers were allocated, by either experimental assignment or judgmental selection, the total cohort became divided into the smaller cohorts exposed to each maneuver. The members of the cohort receiving each maneuver were then followed to observe what occurred as the outcome events.

Although this scientific model seems quite obvious and straightforward, it is not always used and sometimes cannot be used in epidemiologic studies. For diverse reasons of ethics, feasibility, convenience, or prejudices that may be conscious or subconscious, the cohort under study may be assembled *after* rather than *before* the maneuvers were imposed; or a prolectively assembled cohort may be altered when its results are analyzed. A simple example of the latter problem is the common surgical practice of reporting the results of an operation only for people who survive the postoperative period. Thus, if 90 people receive a particular operation, with 12 postoperative deaths and with 40 successes in the 78 postoperative survivors, the success rates are commonly cited as $40/78 = 51\%$, rather than $40/90 = 44\%$. In a medical example of this statistical malfeasance, the results of various treatments for obesity are regularly reported for the people who continued the dietary regimen, omitting all the unsuccessful drop-outs.

The flaws of this tactic are quite evident when it is used in cohorts receiving clinical therapy; and most clinical readers—being intuitively familiar with the ideas that a cohort is created whenever people receive a particular treatment and that the results of the treatment should be cited for all of the people who received it—can promptly recognize the truncated cohort and the potentially inaccurate data that are produced by the truncation. The same sort of problem can occur, but the consequences can be much more difficult to recognize and interpret, when a cohort is not assembled as a prospective clinical series and when the method of assembly allows the collected group to be the residue of the actual cohort to which the results will be applied.

The rest of this section is concerned with the various forms of transfer bias that can arise when residue cohorts are assembled or created by truncation, multiserial collection, augmentation, or contrived simulation. Although the different forms of transfer bias can be readily anticipated and are frequently discussed, they are seldom actually measured. An excellent quantitative demonstration of the problem in population surveys was recently reported by Bergstrand and coworkers.[22]

17.6.1. *The Truncated Cohort*

A cohort that is appropriately uni-serial, because all members are followed from the same point in serial time after imposition of the maneuvers, can be truncated by the deliberate elimination of certain members or by the absence of members who are not available for study.

The deliberate elimination of members was illustrated in the foregoing examples of the truncated cohorts formed to report the results of surgical and anti-obesity therapy. An example of truncation due to unavailability was cited in Section 15.6.2.2, when the investigator was unable to obtain medical records for all of the people cited as members of the cohort. A more subtle issue in unavailability occurs when the cohort is assembled, after the outcome events have already appeared, as the group of people who volunteered to respond when asked to submit information about their current status. This type of volunteer-cohort situation was described in Section 15.3, when the investigator attempted to determine which members of a college freshman class had developed a peptic ulcer in later life.

When people have been deliberately eliminated from an inception cohort, the rates calculated for subsequent events may be inaccurately high or low. If these rates are compared against those of an untruncated cohort, the comparison may be distorted by transfer bias. An unbiased comparison can presumably be obtained if the eliminated people are restored to the truncated cohort and if the correct rates are then calculated. Sackett and Gent[18] have cited an example in which a randomized trial of medical versus surgical therapy would yield results that are either unfavorable or favorable to the surgery, according to whether an inception or residue cohort is used for calculating the rates of success.

When some of the members of an inception cohort are unavailable, the potential problem of transfer bias is more difficult to evaluate because we do not know whether the available people suitably represent the maneuver and its outcomes. Thus, if the absentees occur in a random manner, they may not affect the rates of events calculated for the residue of the cohort. If people are missing because of phenomena that involve maneuver-related outcomes, however, their absence will produce inaccurate rates and subsequent biases in comparison. For example, when a cohort is assembled from archival records, a falsely high survival rate will be calculated for the surgical group if records are missing for most of the people who had postoperative deaths and if the investigator does not know why those records are missing.

If data are available to describe the baseline state of the original inception cohort, the likelihood of bias can be checked by comparing cogent attributes of the original and residual cohorts. Thus in the situation described in Section 15.3, the investigator could determine whether the same proportions of people with high, medium, or low pepsinogen levels were contained in the missing group and in the truncated cohort collected from the responding original members. If these proportions are similar in the two groups, the residual cohort is less likely to be biased than if the proportions are disparate.

If the baseline state and maneuvers are unknown for the absentees—as in the medical record problem just described—there is no way to do the proposed checking. The main hope for an unbiased result is that the proportion of missing people will be too small to have a substantial effect on the results. An analogous problem, occurring in epidemiologic rather than medical record studies, can produce the attritions that lead to the type of transfer bias described by Neyman.[23] In this situation, the contents of the original cohort are unknown, so that the proportion of losses cannot be determined. If assembled long after the original maneuvers were imposed, the residue cohort will fail to contain the people who died in the interim. The absence of these people from the denominator of the residue cohort will inevitably alter the accuracy of any survival rates calculated for outcome events. These problems are further discussed in Section 20.5.

17.6.2. *The Multi-Serial Cohort*

A multiserial cohort is assembled when the investigator, at a single cross-section in secular time, collects a group of people whose exposure to the maneuver began at diverse serial times *before* they entered the cohort.

This type of problem commonly occurs in clinical studies of the course of a chronic disease. For example, to obtain data about the future vascular complications of diabetes mellitus, the investigator may assemble the group of patients who were treated in a diabetes clinic during 1966 to 1968. After following the patients thereafter for the next 15 years and determining each patient's outcome state during 1981 to 1983, the investigator can prepare statistics about the long-term rates of survival and vascular complications in diabetes. He may even divide those rates according to the good or poor ways in which the glucose was regulated during the follow-up interval.

In the reported results, however, a fundamental problem is created by the way in which the cohort was assembled as a multi-serial cross-section of patients who appeared in the clinic during 1966 to 1968. Some of those patients may have had newly diagnosed diabetes, but others may have had their diabetes diagnosed 1, 2, 10, or 20 years previously. The subsequent events can be reported as the 15-year outcome rates of diabetes mellitus in the assembled group, but the information will be chronometrically uninterpretable, because many members of the multi-serial cohort will have had diabetes for much longer than 15 years.

An even greater hazard is produced if the investigator decides to partition the multi-serial cohort according to the previous duration of diabetes and to report results for the total interval elapsed since each patient's zero time. Thus, after following the clinic group for 15 years, the investigator might cite 20-year outcome rates for those patients whose diabetes had been first diagnosed 5 years before they entered the study, and 25-year outcome rates for people with a 10-year antecedent duration of diabetes. The hazard of this tactic is that we have no way of knowing the true fate of the inception cohorts whose residues were acquired in the multi-serial group. Among patients whose diabetes was first diagnosed 10 years earlier, in 1956 to 1958, those who are found in the clinic in 1966 to 1968 may completely misrepresent the original group. Many members of the inception cohort may be dead; some may have transferred to other sources of care because of difficulties in maintaining whatever regimen was being advocated in the clinic; some may have stopped coming because their diabetes disappeared; and others may be attending other clinics because of additional medical problems that are related or unrelated to the diabetes. If the residue members encountered in the clinic are followed for the next 15 years, we surely cannot conclude that the results found in this subgroup accurately represent what happens to people 25 years after their diabetes mellitus is first detected.

In addition to the inaccuracies or distortions of any rates of outcome events that are calculated for the multi-serial cohort, the results may be strongly biased if the rates are compared among patients receiving different treatments, because responses to previous treatment may have altered the composition of the assembled cohort.

The problems of multi-seriality are less obvious when the cohort is assembled epidemiologically to study the subsequent occurrence of a particular disease rather than its clinical course. The customary epidemiologic procedure is to collect a group of presumably healthy people who have volunteered for the study by responding to a mailed questionnaire, allowing a household interview, or accepting an invitation delivered in some other way by an investigator or by a participating friend or neighbor. The admission status of individual members of the cohort is determined from information obtained after they have volunteered to enter the cohort and to be followed thereafter for observation of subsequent events. This type of healthy volunteer cohort has been assembled for studying the effects of cigarette smoking, various nutritional patterns, or other risk factors on the subsequent occurrence of cancer or cardiovascular or other diseases.

The procedure seems quite reasonable and is probably the only feasible way to perform long-term cohort studies of the many phenomena that become suspected as etiologic risk factors in modern life. Nevertheless, such studies are fraught with many scientific hazards.

One immediate hazard is that of multi-seriality. The habits of smoking, eating, drinking, or exercising that are regarded as the maneuvers in such cohorts have been imposed for different durations of serial time before the people enter the cohort. Another problem, noted in Section 17.3.1, is the difficulty of establishing a zero time for the nonimposition of a maneuver in someone who does *not* smoke, drink alcohol, or exercise regularly. To deal with these two problems, the data are usually stratified according to the age of the people included in the cohort, and the outcome results may be reported as survival rates at specified intervals for people who entered the cohort at ages 30 to 34, 35 to 39, 40 to 44, and so on. This type of demographic adjustment is probably the best thing that can be done under the circumstances, but it does not deal with the multi-seriality problem created if one person has been smoking for 2 years and another for 20 years before the two people each enter the same stratum of the cohort at age 35 to 39.

The results noted in the residues assembled in the cohort can also have more serious hazards. One hazard is bias from the attrition described by Neyman.[23] Suppose a particular maneuver has the action of killing many people relatively soon after they are exposed, but "immunizing" the survivors who continue receiving it. A cohort consisting of people who have been receiving the maneuver for several years will omit all the exposed people who died early, and the residual cohort will have a particularly long survival. The early dangers of the maneuver will not only be completely missed, but the maneuver will appear to produce unusually good longevity.

When a multi-serial cohort is acquired from volunteers, a relationship between the maneuver and an intermediate outcome status that followed its onset may affect (and distort) the composition of the people who volunteer or who are invited to enroll. An example of one potential problem was cited in Section 15.8.3 and Exercise 15.4. Such a transfer bias, if it occurs, could falsely lower the survival rates of smokers in comparison with nonsmokers. A somewhat analogous problem might occur if participants in a study of high-fat versus low-fat diets are recruited by neighbors who believe that low-fat diets are particularly healthful. In soliciting people to enter the study, the neighbors might selectively invite their healthy-looking friends who take low-fat diets and their non–healthy-looking friends who take high-fat diets, while ignoring those friends who do not conform to the desired pattern.

Some of these postulated problems may seem far-fetched, but all of them represent the kinds of alternative hypotheses that must be considered and ruled out as part of the basic principles of scientific reasoning in cause-effect explanations. Unfortunately, very few of these alternative hypotheses can be thoroughly checked without studying the inception cohort whose unfeasibility necessitated the substitution of a multi-serial cohort.

17.6.3. *The Augmented Cohort*

In Section 12.2.3, we considered the scientific advantages of an inception cohort that is not only uni-serial but also uni-secular and uni-zonal. The uni-seriality is desired to avoid the multi-serial problems that have just been described. A uni-secular cohort, whose members' zero times all occurred during a well-demarcated and relatively small secular interval of several calendar years, is desirable to avoid the problems of change due to different technologic methods in diagnosis and treatment during a prolonged secular interval.

For example, suppose we decide to compare the outcomes of radiotherapy versus surgical therapy for all patients whose lung cancer was first treated at our institution between January 1, 1950, and December 31, 1983. The cohort is uni-serial, because we would include only people receiving radiotherapy or surgery as a first treatment. The cohort is also uni-zonal, because it includes only people who were treated at our institution. The 33-year span of secular time, however, would make the total results (if they were so combined) very difficult to interpret. The changes in diagnosis during that interval would have been substantial; and the earlier secular results would contain no provision for the later diagnostic impact of flexible bronchoscopy, improvements in sputum cytology, mediastinoscopy, or new methods of thoracic and extrathoracic imaging. The changes in ancillary therapy, as well as in surgery and radiotherapy, would also have been so substantial that a comparison of the two treatments might be uninterpretable unless the mega-secular interval were demarcated into smaller secular periods.

The scientific advantages of a uni-zonal cohort are less obviously apparent. A cohort is uni-zonal if it contains all the appropriate members whose zero times occurred in the particular zone to which the cohort refers. In most clinical studies of prognosis or therapy, this zone is usually a particular clinician's practice, a medical institution, or a consortium of collaborating clinicians and institutions. In the epidemiologic studies devoted to risk factors or etiology of disease in presumably healthy people, the zone may be a demarcated geographic region, an industrial or commercial setting, or such special locations as a retirement community or a housing project.

If members are lost by ex-migration from a uni-zonal cohort, the consequences are straightforward: they are the hazards of a truncated cohort, as discussed in Section 17.6.1. A more difficult type of problem is created when a uni-zonal cohort is augmented by the in-migration of members whose zero time occurred elsewhere. For example, suppose we compare the case-fatality rate for low-birth-weight babies treated in the newborn special care units at two different institutions. The results that may emerge are shocking. They show substantially better survival rates at the small institution, A, which has relatively primitive facilities, than at the large institution, B, which has the full panoply of modern technologic splendor. The shock disappears, however, when we examine the sources of the compared cohorts. At institution A, the cohort consists entirely of infants born at that institution. Institution B, however, is a regional referral center. In addition to low-birth-weight children born at institution B, its special care unit receives the sickest babies born at other institutions. Because the actual inception cohort born at institution B is augmented by the in-migration of poor prognostic residues from cohorts born elsewhere, the total fatality rate becomes increased at institution B.

The transfer bias produced by an augmented cohort is readily apparent in the clinical situation just described. The bias is less overtly evident but can be even more dramatic, however, when the cohort is assembled as a registry of information sent from diverse sources to an agency soliciting reports or other referrals of cases with a particular clinical condition. When assembled exclusively from such volunteer reports, the cohort has no identifiable zonal source and no specifically demarcated populational denominator to which its data can be referred. Although often suspected in these circumstances, transfer bias is difficult to demonstrate because the necessary data are absent.

In one striking recent example, however, the transfer bias of an augmented cohort could be clearly documented. To study the long-term effects on children whose mothers had received diethylstilbestrol (DES) during pregnancy, the investigators assembled and planned to follow a uni-serial, uni-secular, uni-zonal inception cohort assembled retrolectively from the medical records of pregnancies managed at several collaborating institutions.[24] An additional noninception cohort was formed by people who had volunteered or who had been referred to join the group under surveillance. When the adverse outcome events were noted and tabulated, the rates were essentially similar for the groups exposed or not exposed to DES in the inception cohort. In the augmented group of volunteers, however, the rates were substantially higher than in the members of the inception cohort.

17.6.4. *The Simulated Cohort*

A popular tactic in "armchair research" allows the investigator the convenience of avoiding the effort needed in "shoe-leather research" to assemble, follow, and study a cohort. Instead, the investigator contrives or simulates a cohort from sources of data that are readily available, having been assembled by various governmental or commercial agencies.

These simulations are often necessary because they are the only feasible way for the research to be conducted. For example, if we really wanted to know the exact annual mortality rate for people living in a particular region during a particular year, we would have to arrange to count all those people on a single day and to obtain follow-up information for everyone's status a year later. This research might be feasible if the region and its number of inhabitants were small, but for larger regions and numbers of people, the investigation is usually impossible. Instead, we can simulate a cohort study by using census bureau data to estimate the number of inhabitants and by using another source of data, perhaps the regional health department, to determine the number of deaths in that region during the year.

These simulated cohorts, created from the data of agencies concerned with vital statistics, are the source of all the mortality rates used in regional, national, and international comparisons. In fact, an interesting irony about the current use of *cohort* for a longitudinally followed group of people is that the word was originally proposed and applied for the simulations performed with vital statistics data.[25] People born in the same year were called a *cohort*, or an *age cohort*; and the cohort's life expectancy was (and still is) determined by calculating the survival proportions that remain as the cohort passes through the mortality rates noted for people of correspondingly increasing age at annual secular intervals.

The cohorts simulated from vital statistics data have certain scientific imperfections, such as not accounting for people who have migrated into or out of the original inception cohort, but the results have been a valuable index of total mortality rates in demographic groups of a particular region and era. Things become scientifically much more difficult and much less credible when the outcome data are differentiated for causes of death rather than for total mortality alone. The main problem here is not the simulation of a cohort but the problems of detection bias noted earlier in Section 17.4.3.

A much greater hazard arises when a cohort contrived from vital statistics data is used as a control group for patients receiving a particular clinical treatment. For example, the hazards of postmenopausal estrogens in possibly causing breast cancer were studied in a retrolective cohort of postmenopausal women assembled from the medical records of a gynecologist who often prescribed estrogen replacement therapy.[26] The women identified as estrogen recipients were then checked for the subsequent occurrence or nonoccurrence of breast cancer. Although a comparison group of nonestrogen users might have been assembled as a retrolective cohort from the medical records of an estrogenophobic gynecologist in the same region, the investigators decided to simulate a control group by using vital statistics data. From the annual rates of breast cancer reported in that region, the investigators contrived a control group of women having the same age-race composition as the actual observed cohort. The carcinogenic risk of estrogen therapy was then determined as a ratio of the directly observed rate of breast cancer in the estrogen-exposed women and the rates expected from the contrived control group.

The scientific flaws of such a comparison are manifold. First, the control group is contaminated, because it comes from the general population as a mixture of women who did and did not receive estrogens. Second, the exposed women in the control group are a multi-serial cohort with heterogeneous durations of previous exposure to estrogen. Third, aside from demographic similarity in age, gender, and race, the baseline state of the contrived control group is completely unknown and cannot be suitably compared with the clinically studied pretherapeutic conditions of the group receiving the principal maneuver. Fourth—and perhaps most important for an outcome event such as breast-cancer, whose detection depends entirely on appropriate examination procedures—the surveillance and diagnostic processes were almost surely conducted differently in the groups under comparison.

The use of simulated cohorts as comparison groups for specific maneuvers has been a fertile source of error in epidemiologic research. The best known of these errors has even received a specific name, the "healthy worker effect,"[27] which was discussed in Section 4.2.1.

17.6.5. *Problems in Non-Cohort Research*

The ultimate form of a residue cohort is assembled when the research is conducted as a cross-sectional survey or case-control study, in which the scientific model of cohort reasoning is applied to groups who were not collected or followed as a cohort. The multiple scientific problems of these alternative but often necessary research structures will be considered when they are discussed in Chapters 18 to 22 of Part Four.

[*Because the remaining sections of this chapter deal mainly with issues in descriptive statistics, an intermission can now be declared to divide the chapter into two parts. The exercises at the end of the chapter are arranged accordingly.*]

17.7 STATISTICAL MANAGEMENT OF NUMERATOR LOSSES

To be related to the preceding maneuver and baseline state, the outcome events must be observed in all members of the assembled cohort. If not all members have been accounted for, the results in the remaining group may misrepresent what actually happened. For example, suppose we have follow-up data for 70 members of an original group of 100 people exposed to maneuver X. We do not know what has happened to the 30 lost people, but for the remaining 70, we know that 45 are alive and 25 are dead. Accordingly, we decide to express the survival rate for maneuver X as 45/70 = 64%.

This expression seems to be the best we can do under the circumstances, but it has some major risks. If the missing 30 people are all alive, we have substantially underestimated the cohort's survival: It should be (45 + 30)/100, or 75%. If the missing 30 people are all dead, we have grossly overestimated the survival rate: It should be 45/100, or 45%. Thus, according to the fate of the missing people, the true value of the survival rate can range from 45% to an almost twice higher value of 75%. (Note also that 45%, the lower value of this range, is substantially below what we would get from the statistical tactic of putting a 95% confidence interval around the observed value of 64%. Using the formula $\sqrt{pq/N}$ for the standard error of a proportion and multiplying by 1.96 to get a Gaussian estimate of 95% confidence, we would calculate the lower boundary of the confidence interval as $0.64 - 1.96 [\sqrt{(45/70)(25/70)} \div 70] = 0.64 - 0.11 = 53\%$.)

The foregoing example shows but one of several major problems that can occur when real-world people undergo real-world transfers between the imposed maneuver and the data that are analyzed for a cohort in cause-effect research. Because the members of a cohort must be assembled, exposed to the compared maneuvers, followed over time, and accounted for at the end, diverse difficulties can arise at each step in the process. The rest of this section contains a discussion of the statistical methods that can be used to deal with the problem of expressing results in cohorts that have had numerator losses. In this situation the denominator of the cohort was well defined and enumerated, but certain people cannot be accounted for in the numerator because their outcome is uncertain or unknown.

17.7.1. *Sources of Numerator Losses*

A person's postmaneuver outcome may be difficult to determine if the person has disappeared or not been followed long enough, or if events have been altered by a competing risk.

17.7.1.1. **LOST TO FOLLOW-UP**

The ultimate act of noncompliance is for a patient to drop out of a study and become lost to follow-up. In this circumstance, the investigators know that the patient was alive and in some particular clinical condition at the last time of examination, but nothing further is known about why the patient has dropped out or what happened thereafter.

With careful investigative methods, these losses can be kept to a minimum. In a suitably organized study with appropriate techniques of the "tolpery" described earlier, the researchers should usually be able to discern at least the life or death status of each cohort member. A high rate of losses to follow-up suggests that the investigators have not been particularly thorough in their work. If the outcome event is life or death, the number of losses to follow-up should ordinarily be quite small, perhaps below 1% or 2%.

17.7.1.2. **INSUFFICIENT DURATION**

When the outcome data are collected for analysis, certain members of the cohort are still being followed, and their current status is known, but their postzero serial time does not yet have a long enough duration for the occurrence of the outcome event. For example, suppose we want to determine each patient's survival status as alive or dead 3 years after a particular treatment, and suppose we start assembling this cohort in 1979, intending to admit all patients who received that treatment at our institution during 1979 to 1982. When we write our first research report, at the end of 1983, the patients who entered the cohort during 1981 and 1982 will not yet have had the opportunity to survive 3 years.

17.7.1.3. **COMPETING RISKS**

In the statistics assembled for a cohort's results, each member's outcome events will be directly related to the antecedent maneuver and baseline state. The possibility of forming this relationship may be impeded, however, by unwanted events that can intervene between the imposition of the maneuver and the outcome.

One such unwanted event is death, but death need not have a statistical sting if due to an appropriate cause. Thus, if a patient is being treated for cancer and dies because of the cancer, the outcome is sad but can be readily associated with both the maneuver and the baseline state. Suppose, however, that a patient who is apparently free of cancer and in excellent health 2 years after treatment is killed in an automobile accident or has a sudden fatal myocardial infarction. How should this patient's death be managed statistically when 3-year survival rates are calculated for the cancer cohort? Conversely, suppose we are studying long-term survival rates after medical treatment of myocardial infarction. What should be done about a patient who develops and dies of an intervening cancer?

The competing risks that create these problems need not be due to an unrelated death. The long-term treatment that is under investigation may have been stopped after a brief duration because of a minor adverse drug reaction or because the patient acquired a co-morbid ailment for which the main treatment is contraindicated. More strikingly, the patient—for clinical or personal reasons—may have transferred to the opposite treatment under comparison. Thus, after 2 years of medical therapy in a randomized trial of medical versus surgical treatment, the patient may have sought and received the surgical procedure that was denied by the randomization.

In all of these instances, a competing event, which affects either the maneuver or the outcome, will thwart the possibility of easily associating the investigated maneuver and the anticipated outcome.

17.7.2. *Scientific Policies in Statistical Summaries of Cohort Results*

Several different statistical methods have been devised to deal with the problems just cited and with other difficulties in creating quantitative expressions for the outcome of a cohort. The statistical methods, however, are merely mathematical devices for carrying out the policies chosen in at least four major scientific decisions. Because perfect solutions do not exist for the problems, and because each scientific policy can receive different justifications, a variety of statistical methods can be used to implement the scientific decisions, which are described in the four sections that follow. The scientific policies involve choices of the numerators and denominators to be entered into each of the quotients used for the subsequent statistical expressions.

17.7.2.1. MANAGEMENT OF CENSORED PATIENTS

Statisticians have introduced the useful but somewhat disquieting word *censored* to refer to patients who have become lost or who have an insufficient duration of follow-up. Such patients can be dealt with in one of two ways. They can be either completely eliminated from the original denominator, being regarded as though they never entered into the cohort, or they can be maintained in the denominator for partial intervals until a point in time when they become decrementally censored. In the decremental reduction process, if one of 50 patients becomes lost after the first year, the first-year denominator would contain 50 patients, but denominators thereafter would contain 49. A second patient in this group, who has been followed for only a little more than 2 years, would be counted in the 2-year denominator, but the group size would drop to 48 for subsequent annual calculations. In the complete elimination process, neither one of those two censored patients would be counted in calculations for the cohort; and both the first and second year denominators would be based on 48 people.

Because the complete elimination of censored patients might lead to substantial losses of data and potential distortions in results, the decremental reduction process seems preferable and is used in almost all modern statistical methods. An important point to bear in mind for residue cohorts (or non-cohort groups) assembled *after* the outcome events have occurred is that the statistical calculations depend exclusively on the patients acquired by the investigator. Not only are none of the censored patients accounted for, but many of the people who died may also be missing from the data.

17.7.2.2. MANAGEMENT OF COMPETING RISKS

Because competing risks can occur as either inappropriate outcomes or contaminating maneuvers, two different sets of policies must be considered.

17.7.2.2.1. *Inappropriate Outcomes*

If the patient has an appropriate outcome event, such as a death that is easily associated with the baseline state and maneuver under study, things are quite simple statistically. The death can be counted as an event related to the maneuver, and the patient's follow-up status will be known, no matter how long the cohort is followed thereafter.

If observation of the anticipated outcome event has been precluded, however, by the competing risk of an alternative outcome event such as death due to an unrelated cause, the statistical situation becomes difficult, and the data can be managed in several different ways. In one approach, the unrelatedness of the death is ignored, and all deaths are associated with the maneuver, regardless of their cause. The advantage of this policy is that it eliminates the difficulties of establishing differential diagnoses for causes of death. The disadvantage is that appropriate and inappropriate deaths are all associated with the main maneuver and may thereby obscure its actions and effects. The appraisal of all deaths rather than appropriate deaths, however, may also have substantial advantages in evaluating the total impact of a maneuver. For example, in a randomized trial conducted to show the benefits of screening for breast cancer,[28] the fatality rates for breast cancer were lower in the screened women than in the unscreened group. On the other hand, the total fatality rates for all causes were not significantly different in the two groups.

In a second policy, after the deaths are classified as related or unrelated, patients with an *unrelated* death are regarded as lost (or "withdrawn alive") when they die, and their data are managed as though they had been censored at that time. The censoring process is then carried out according to the policies described in Section 17.7.2.1. The patients may be decrementally removed from the denominators as the unrelated deaths occur, or they may be totally eliminated from consideration. When patients are decrementally removed, separate quotients can be constructed, if desired, to report the occurrence of the unrelated events. For example, in an evaluation of prognosis for patients with cancer of the larynx,[29] rates of death were calculated separately for causes ascribed to the cancer and to co-morbid diseases.

The policy of totally eliminating co-morbid deaths has often been used in cohort statistics in which the survival rates after treatment of a cancer are cited only for the *evaluable* patients who died of oncogenic causes. Despite the intellectual appeal of the policy, it can sometimes lead to major distortions in evaluating the total impact of a maneuver, particularly when the patients are elderly and may have many co-morbid ailments besides the particular condition under investigation. For example, when the outcomes were confined to evaluable patients, who were either still alive or whose deaths were ascribed to cancer, the use of castration and/or estrogen therapy was initially regarded as highly beneficial for men with cancer of the prostate. At about the time that the inventor of this treatment was receiving a Nobel prize, however, a randomized trial was completed showing that the *total* fatality rate was actually higher in the estrogen-treated patients than in the placebo group.[30] The hormone therapy may have reduced deaths from cancer while promoting deaths from other causes.

17.7.2.2.2. *Inappropriate or Contaminating Maneuvers*

A separate and particularly controversial problem in competing risks deals with the management of inappropriate or contaminating maneuvers. If a patient maintains the assigned maneuver with a poor compliance or poor intermediate regulation, the outcome events can at least be associated with that maneuver; and any dispute about the policy can rest on the fairness of evaluating maneuvers that were not given in a suitably proficient manner. Suppose, however, that the patient has completely stopped taking an assigned medication or, even worse, has transferred to the opposing competitor that is under investigation in the same trial.

This problem can be approached in at least three different ways. One policy (which happens to be my own preference in randomized trials) is to regard an appropriately contaminating event—when treatment was stopped or transferred—as a phenomenon that produces censoring. The patient would be dropped from the study at that point and the existing data would be managed according to whatever policy has been adopted for censored data. A second policy is used constantly and sometimes inadvertently in all studies conducted without experimental randomization. Patients are classified according to whatever pattern of treatment they actually received. In nonexperimental studies, a patient who refuses the offer of surgery for cancer and who instead receives radiotherapy is counted as part of the radiotherapy cohort. If a patient with peptic ulcer received antacid therapy and was later transferred to histamine-suppression therapy, he would be counted, according to the choice of zero time and outcome duration, as having had either antacid-then-histamine-suppressor treatment, antacid treatment that failed, or histamine-suppressor treatment.

Because decisions about starting and stopping treatment can produce the susceptibility bias described previously, and because randomization is intended to prevent this bias in an experimental trial, a reasonable argument can be offered that any postrandomization changes in maneuvers can be a source of bias. This anti-bias argument is the basis for the third policy, which is particularly encouraged by many modern statisticians, that is often called the *intention-to-treat* approach.[18] According to this policy, anything that happens to a patient after a treatment has been randomly assigned in a trial is thereafter included in the events ascribed to that treatment, regardless of why and how the events occurred.

Despite its statistical appeal, the intention-to-treat policy may sometimes reduce bias at the cost of removing clinical sensibility from the results. For example, using the intention-to-treat policy in a trial of medical versus surgical therapy, a patient randomized to medical therapy who refuses the treatment, seeks surgery elsewhere, and dies postoperatively would have his death associated and counted with the results of medical treatment. Conversely, a patient who suddenly dies before the randomized surgery can be carried out or who refuses the offered surgical procedure would have his death or survival associated with an operation he never received.

Because there are no unequivocally right or wrong answers to questions about what scientific policies to maintain in the analysis of outcome data and contaminating maneuvers in randomized trials, the justifications that can be offered for diametrically opposed viewpoints have helped produce some of the major controversies discussed in Chapter 29. An interesting irony during these disputes has been the double standard of evaluation sometimes maintained by advocates of the intention-to-treat policy. Although the sanctity of randomization can reasonably be advocated as a prime method for reducing bias after imposition of maneuvers, the importance of the policy is often disregarded in cause-effect studies in which the maneuvers were not assigned with randomization. The possibility of premaneuveral or postmaneuveral susceptibility bias seldom receives adequate attention when data are evaluated from studies conducted without randomization.

17.7.2.3. POINTS VS. CURVES FOR STATISTICAL EXPRESSIONS

Regardless of the policies adopted for managing data for censored patients and competing risks, separate decisions are needed for policies about citing a series of phenomena that can occur at various serial times after imposition of the maneuvers. Should events be cited for their cumulative occurrence at individual points in time, such as 1 year or 5 years after onset of the maneuvers, or should the expression depend on the entire curve of the pattern formed by those points? For example, if 120 members of a cohort of 200 people are noted to be dead when the cohort is checked after 5 years of postzero serial time, the cohort's 5-year survival rate is $80/200 = 40\%$. If 100 of those members had been dead at the 3-year point, the 3-year survival rate would have been $100/200 = 50\%$. The pattern of the curve would show the drop from 50% survival at 3 years to 40% at 5 years.

The rates of survival at individually specified time points are particularly valuable for clinicians estimating prognosis for individual patients. The rates noted at different points in serial time are what a clinician uses to answer questions raised by a patient who wants to know his "chances." The time-point rates are also useful when reviewers try to compare the results of different maneuvers. The comparison is conceptually clear and straightforward if the reader can compare survival rates of treatment A versus treatment B at specified intervals such as 1, 3, or 5 years after treatment. On the other hand, despite their value in prognostication and in direct comparisons of treatment, the rates at single points in time may not indicate the total pattern of what has happened. Figure 17–2 shows strikingly different survival curves for two cohorts, each having survival rates of about 50% at 3 years and 40% at 5 years. In cohort A, survival was excellent for the first 2 years, with no deaths occurring until the third year, and with no deaths occurring after the fourth year. In cohort B, most of the deaths occurred in the first year, with a slowly declining survival rate thereafter. This distinction in the two cohorts would have been completely missed if we had compared only their survival rates at 3 years and 5 years.

To avoid the latter problem, the results of cohort outcomes have increasingly been depicted visually in graphs, with curves (or polygonal lines) that show the entire pattern of rates for the postmaneuver events. The curves have the major statistical advantage just described, but also have some substantial scientific and clinical disadvantages. One obvious but minor problem is that the curve cannot be summarized into a single expression that will tell a patient his chances. He can be shown the curve, if appropriate, but a prognostic estimate of chances usually requires the use of individual time-point rates as probabilities.

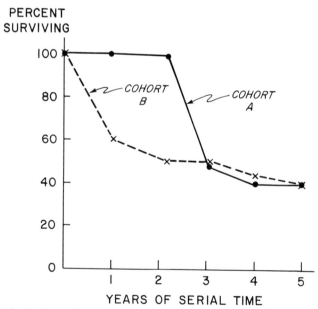

Figure 17–2. Survival curve in two cohorts having survival rates of 50% at three years and 40% at five years.

A second problem, which is more cogent intellectually, is the difficulty of comparing two treatments whose results are expressed in curves rather than single measurements. When survival rates at 3 years for two contrasted treatments are expressed as 34% (29/85) versus 46% (40/87) or as median survival times of 1.6 years versus 2.8 years, we can readily determine what happened; we can form a quantitative index of contrast (by methods described in Chapter 8), and we can then easily form an opinion about the statistical comparison.

This intellectual task is much more difficult if the results are cited in curves. The only single expression that might be used to summarize each treatment is the area under the curve, but such an expression is strange and unfamiliar for most scientists and is almost never cited. Without quantitative indexes to describe the results, the evaluator can make the comparison with qualitative visual judgments, which seem unsatisfactory for decisions about a contrast whose individual components have been so carefully quantified. Alternatively, the evaluator can do a test of statistical significance on the two curves, using the log-rank test or other fashionable tactics in statistical inference,[31] but the result indicates only the stochastic aspects of probability, not the quantitative importance of the difference. Like all tests of statistical significance, the results are strongly affected by the size of the groups under study. Important clinical differences can fail to achieve statistical significance if the groups are small, and trivial clinical distinctions can become statistically significant if the groups are large enough.

A separate problem is not inherent in the use of curves, but commonly occurs in published literature because of the laxity of investigators and of editorial standards. With decremental reduction of denominators in managing data for censored patients, the points at the far end of a curve may show rates obtained from only a few patients. Thus, although a cohort began with 95 patients, the point shown for the 5-year survival rate may depend on only six people who were followed that long. Although such distinctions should clearly be marked to let the reader beware of the fragile numerical stability of the rate, the points on the curve are often presented without any indication of their associated denominators. For this reason, a curve of rates should always be accompanied by information denoting the denominators included at each point—and preferably, by a standard error or confidence interval for the rate shown at that point.

From the foregoing discussion, it should be apparent that a useful statistical reporting of cohort rates requires both types of expression for the results. The time-point rates should be cited for individual prognostic appraisals and clear scientific comparisons; the curves should be cited to show the entire pattern of the rates and to avoid misleading comparisons.

17.7.2.4. **MEANS, MEDIANS, AND AVERAGE INTERVALS**

In the preceding section, the results were expressed as rates of occurrence for the selected outcome events. Because the events occur at specific time intervals after the onset of maneuvers, the average duration of those intervals can be used instead of rates to provide a single summary expression for the occurrence of outcome events. Rather than saying that a particular cohort had a 3-year survival rate of 40%, we could say that the mean survival time was 2.9 years (if that was the value). The most obvious advantage of the average time is that it provides a single quantitative index, which eliminates the problems of either choosing a single value from the individual rates at multiple time points or having to evaluate the total scope of a curve.

The main disadvantage of using a mean or median is that unlike the rates at time points, these two methods of expressing an average cannot be adjusted to include contributions from patients who have been lost to follow-up. The mean, furthermore, has the additional disadvantage that was noted in Section 7.4.1.2. A mean cannot be calculated for patients with an insufficient duration of follow-up. Thus, the people who have not yet died cannot be included in a calculation of mean survival time. In the rankings used to obtain a median, such people will be at the upper end of the rankings, and someone who has already died will be near the middle. Because a median can almost always be determined, and because of its other virtues in citing central tendency, the median has become the preferred statistical index of expression for summarizing the events of a cohort according to the average serial time of their occurrence. In fact, if you are looking for a simple, single index that summarizes the total array of events, *and* if relatively few people in the cohort have been lost to follow-up, *and* if you will be content with so simplified an expression, the median serial time for events is probably the best of all the available expressions. Because this degree of simplicity alone is seldom satisfactory, however, the curve of rate points should also be inspected and analyzed.

17.7.2.5. METHODS BASED ON PERSON-DURATIONS

A fifth issue in scientific policy refers to an analytic method that is seldom used or approved today. It is mentioned here because it is often encountered in older literature and because it is still sometimes worthwhile.

In the preceding four sections, when we tried to avoid the loss of data that might be contributed by censored patients, the main strategy was to decrement the denominators progressively as the patients became censored. This strategy allowed the outcomes to be expressed in the customary units of events per patient at risk, such as a survival rate of 40%. An alternative strategy that can preserve data from censored patients, while also yielding a single summary expression for the entire set of observations, is to convert the denominators from counted persons into added person-durations. With this strategy, the denominator is attained by adding the duration of follow-up for each member of the cohort, regardless of how long the individual members have been followed. The total number of events observed in the cohort is then used as the numerator, and the result is expressed as a rate of events per person-durations.

For example, suppose a cohort contains 100 people who have each been followed for 1 year, 50 people each for 2 years, and 25 people each for 3 years. The cohort has accumulated 275 person-years $[= (1 \times 100) + (2 \times 50) + (3 \times 25)]$ of follow-up. If nine myocardial infarctions have been observed in this cohort during that time, we could refer to the myocardial infarction attack rate as 9/275 person-years or as 3.3 per 100 person-years.

The person-duration technique of expression has its main advantages when relatively few people have been lost to follow-up, when everyone has been followed for relatively similar lengths of time, *and* when the outcome event is something that can occur repetitively (such as an infarction) in the same person. For example, in studies of prophylaxis against recurrent streptococcal infections in a closely followed cohort of children and adolescents who had had rheumatic fever,[32] the incidence of new streptococcal infections was quite usefully expressed as an attack rate per 100 patient-years.

The main disadvantage of the person-duration method occurs when different members of the cohort have striking differences in the lengths of follow-up. For example, 200 person-years can be accumulated in the denominator if 200 people are each followed for 1 year or if 20 people are each followed for 10 years. A separate disadvantage of the person-duration method is that it makes no provision for risks that change with time. If the risk of an adverse outcome in the first year is different from the risk in the second year of serial time, the distinction will not be discerned with the person-duration method.

When the outcomes are individually repetitive events, a problem arises in distinguishing between the occurrence of events and the susceptibility of "eventful" people. For example, suppose the streptococcal infection attack rate is 10 per 100 patient-years. This numerator can be attained if 10 patients each had one infection, or if two people each had five infections.

There is no easy way to manage this type of numerator difficulty, even if everyone has been followed in the denominator for an identical length of time. To avoid ambiguity, two rates can be cited, one for the occurrence of infections and the other for the occurrence of infected patients. Thus, if patient-years appears in the denominator, we could express the results as attack rates of 10 streptococcal infections per 100 patient-years and 2 streptococcally infected patients per 100 patient-years. If the denominator is expressed in patients, the same results might be cited as an attack rate (among 50 patients) of 10/50 (20%) for infections and 2/50 (4%) for infected patients.

For all these reasons, when the outcome event is a nonrepetitive entity (such as death) that removes the person from further follow-up, or when any of the other disadvantages become important, the statistical situation is probably better managed with the progressive decrementation of denominators than with the person-duration technique.

17.7.3. *Statistical Methods for Decrementing Denominators*

At least three different statistical methods can be used to decrement denominators for an appropriate calculation of the rates of events associated with censored numerators. The first method is quite direct and simple, requiring no intricate procedures. The second method is adapted from the strategy used by the actuaries of life insurance companies to compute expected life spans for establishing the premiums paid on insurance policies. Because of this intellectual ancestry, the method is properly called *actuarial analysis,* but because of the tabular arrangements of data and the frequent application to study survival, the method is often called *life-table analysis* (even when the adverse outcome event is something other than death). The third method, which is the most recent and currently most popular of the three techniques, is often cited eponymically as the *Kaplan-Meier method.* It depends on rates calculated at the variable intervals produced by the occurrence of individual events.

The principles of the three techniques are merely outlined here. Details of their application can be found in suitable publications.[33, 34]

17.7.3.1. **THE DIRECT METHOD**

With this technique, event rates are calculated at clinically meaningful fixed intervals, such as 1 year, 2 years, and so on. The censored patients are removed from the denominator after the last interval for which their follow-up was complete. Thus, if one of 50 patients drops out after 1 year, if another has been followed for slightly more than 2 years, and if all other patients have been followed for more than 3 years, the denominators for calculating the rate of events would be 50 at 1 year, 49 at 2 years, and 48 at 3 years.

For example, in the cohort just cited, suppose one person died in the first year, two more in the second, and three more in the third. The cumulative mortality rates for the cohort would be calculated as 1/50 at the end of the first year, 3/49 at the end of the second year, and 6/48 at the end of the third. The corresponding survival rates, each calculated as 1 minus the mortality rate, would be 0.980, 0.939, and 0.875.

Although the process is easy enough to be accomplished without formal tabulations, a set of data for the direct method would be arranged as shown in Table 17–1 for the 50 patients under consideration.

The direct method has the major advantage of simplicity and overtness. The results are easy to calculate and understand, and the numerator and denominator can be overtly demonstrated as the actual patients included in each rate. The main disadvantage of the direct method is that it contains no contributions from censored people for the interval in

Table 17–1. DIRECT ARRANGEMENT OF SURVIVAL DATA FOR 50 PATIENTS

Interval	Censored During Interval	Cumulatively Followed from Onset Throughout This Interval	Died During Interval	Cumulative Deaths	Cumulative Mortality Rate	Cumulative Survival Rate
0–1 yr.	0	50	1	1	0.020	0.980
1–2 yr.	1	49	2	3	0.061	0.939
2–3 yr.	1	48	3	6	0.125	0.875

which they were censored. Thus, a person who was censored after 11 months in the second year would be contained in the denominator for the first year, but his 11/12 of a year's follow-up would be omitted from the denominators for the second year.

The simplicity of the direct method is thus achieved by a slight deflation in the true size of the denominators. The result is a slight overestimation of mortality rates and a corresponding slight underestimation of survival rates. The actuarial method described in the next section makes an attempt to correct this defect, but the complexity of the effort makes the results more difficult for clinicians to understand and interpret.

17.7.3.2. **THE ACTUARIAL METHOD**

In the actuarial method, the rates of events are also calculated at fixed intervals of time, but the denominators are adjusted to include interval contributions of the censored people. To allow this contribution, a separate individual mortality rate is calculated for each interval rather than for the cumulative mortality determined with the direct method. Each of the interval mortality rates is converted to a survival rate for that interval; and the cumulative survival rate at the end of an interval is the product achieved by multiplying all the preceding survival rates.

One way of adjusting the denominator for people censored in each interval would be simply to add the fractions of years in which the censored people were followed. Thus, in the example used in Section 17.7.3.1, after one person died in the first year, 49 people were at risk at the beginning of the second year. Of those people, 48 (including the two who died) had complete follow-up for the second year, and one person was followed for $11/12(= 0.92)$ of that year. The adjusted interval denominator for that year would be 48.92, and the adjusted interval mortality during that year would be $2/(48.92) = 0.0409$.

Because this approach can become cumbersome if many people have been censored, the tactic used in the actuarial method is to assume that the censored people were all followed for half of the interval in which they were censored. The strategy is carried out by subtracting half the number of censored people from the total number of people who began the interval. Thus, in the actuality of the actuarial method, the adjusted denominator for the second year would be $49 - 0.5 = 48.5$; and the interval mortality would be calculated as $2/(48.5) = 0.0412$.

Because of the adjusted denominators, interval mortality rates, interval survival rates, and cumulative survival rates, a special table must be constructed to keep track of what is going on in an actuarial analysis. The cohort we have been discussing would be actuarially displayed as shown in Table 17.2. In these results, the cumulative survival rates are obtained as the product of the interval survival rates. Thus, the cumulative rate for the second year

Table 17–2. ACTUARIAL ARRANGEMENT OF SURVIVAL DATA FOR 50 PATIENTS

Interval	At Risk at Beginning of Interval	Censored During Interval	Adjusted Denominator for Interval	Died During Interval	Mortality Rate for Interval	Survival Rate for Interval	Cumulative Survival Rate
0–1 yr.	50	0	50	1	0.020	0.980	0.980
1–2 yr.	49	1	48.5	2	0.041	0.959	0.940
2–3 yr.	46	1	45.5	3	0.066	0.934	0.878

is $0.980 \times 0.959 = 0.940$; and the cumulative rate for the third year is $0.980 \times 0.959 \times 0.934 = 0.878$. These cumulative survival rates would then be plotted on a graph as the rate points showing the annual survival for this cohort. (It so happens in this instance that the direct and the actuarial methods produced quite similar cumulative annual survival rates. As shown at the end of the chapter in Exercise 17.12, this similarity does not always occur.)

In the two methods just demonstrated, no provision was made to differentiate the results for competing risks of death or for the problems of contaminated maneuvers. If such patients are managed as though they were censored (while being "withdrawn alive"), their data can be handled with the same approach used for adjusting denominators in either the direct or the actuarial method. Chiang[35] has developed and demonstrated a modification of the actuarial method for dealing with deaths due to competing risks.

A quite different approach to the competing-death problem has been proposed by Cutler and Ederer.[36] They first calculate cumulative survival rates in a conventional actuarial analysis with all deaths included, regardless of cause. Mortality data from the general population, supplied by an appropriate national agency dealing with vital statistics, are then used to calculate the annual cumulative survival rates that would be expected for a cohort composed of people having the same individual ages and genders as the cohort under analysis. These expected survival rates are assumed to represent the effects of deaths due to unrelated causes. The *relative survival rates,* which are calculated as the rates of the observed to the expected rates, would then represent the impact of the related mortality in the observed cohort. Despite the statistical ingenuity that provided a brief period of popularity, the relative survival rates are seldom used today. The expected survival rates are cumbersome to calculate; an undifferentiated general population is seldom a good source of comparative data; and the relative annual ratios of observed to expected rates can sometimes produce values exceeding 1, which have peculiar implications.

17.7.3.3. **THE VARIABLE-INTERVAL (KAPLAN-MEIER) METHOD**

In the variable-interval method, the main focus is on the entire curve of mortality rather than on the traditional clinical concern with rates at fixed periodic intervals. To make this curve as accurate as possible, the intervals are defined by the events occurring in the observed cohort; and a new rate is calculated whenever a death (or other appropriate event) occurs. The patients who were censored during one of these death-defined intervals are simply eliminated from the denominator of that interval, as in the direct method, without any adjustments for their contributions to that interval.

Because the exact timing of events is so important, the individual serial durations must be carefully examined to use this method. For the cohort of 50 people we have been discussing, let us assume that the cited six deaths and two censorings occurred at the following points in serial time:

Deaths occurred at: 0.5, 1.4, 1.8, 2.1, 2.3, and 2.9 years.
Censorings occurred at: 1.9 and 2.3 years.

To avoid ambiguity in the Kaplan-Meier calculations, deaths and censorings cannot occupy the same time boundary. The reasonable assumption is therefore made that deaths actually occurred just before their reported point in time and that withdrawals due to censoring occurred somewhat afterward. Accordingly, when a death and censoring are reported for the same time point, as for the 2.3 years point in the foregoing data, the death is assumed to define the interval that ends at 2.3, and the censoring occurs in the subsequent interval.

Because each death in the Kaplan-Meier method creates a boundary for a preceding and subsequent interval, the tabular process is easier to follow if shown with the seven intervals created by the six deaths in our cohort of 50 people (Table 17–3).

The first interval in Table 17–3 begins with a cumulative survival rate of 1.000 and ends with the death at 0.5 year. Since the interval survival rate is 49/50 = 0.980, the second interval begins with a cumulative survival rate of 1.000 × 0.980 = 0.980. After the death in the second interval, the third interval begins with a cumulative survival rate of 0.980 × 0.980 = 0.960; and the interval survival rate is 47/48 = 0.979. During the fourth interval, the person censored at 1.9 years is removed from the number alive before the fourth death at 2.1 years. The fourth interval survival rate is 45/46 = 0.978, and cumulative survival before the fifth-interval death becomes 0.940 × 0.987 = 0.920. The fifth interval ends with the death at 2.3 years; and the person who was censored at 2.3 years is removed from the denominator of people alive in the sixth interval. The sixth interval survival rate is 42/43 = 0.977. The seventh interval begins with a cumulative survival of 0.900 × 0.977 = 0.879, and with 42 people who are alive and being followed. Since no further deaths have occurred, the table ends here. If you can visualize the numbers that are cancelled as the operations proceed, you will note that this final cumulative survival rate is actually calculated as (47/50) × (44/46) × (42/43) = 0.878. (The value of 0.879 in the table is due to intermediate rounding.)

The graphic results of the variable-interval method of analyzing a cohort's outcome are shown in Figure 17–3. Because the rates are calculated for inconsistently varying durations, the resultant curve looks like a staircase with uneven steps. The results of the fixed-interval methods of analysis for this same cohort are also shown in Figure 17–3. In this instance, the fixed- and variable-interval methods have yielded almost identical results at the same time points. Because the three methods are all doing essentially the same thing, the agreement among them can be expected to be quite good, although disparities may occur in different sets of data.

Table 17–3. VARIABLE-INTERVAL (KAPLAN-MEIER) ARRANGEMENT OF SURVIVAL DATA FOR 50 PATIENTS

Number of Interval	Cumulative Survival Rate Before Death(s)	Time of Death(s) That End(s) Interval	Number Alive Before Death(s)	Number of Deaths	Number of Survivors	Interval Survival Rate	Censored Before Next Death
1	1.000	0.5	50	1	49	0.980	0
2	0.980	1.4	49	1	48	0.980	0
3	0.960	1.8	48	1	47	0.979	1
4	0.940	2.1	46	1	45	0.978	0
5	0.920	2.3	45	1	44	0.978	1
6	0.900	2.9	43	1	42	0.977	0
7	0.879	—	(42)	—	—	—	—

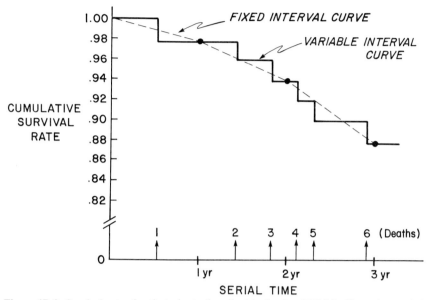

Figure 17–3. Survival rates for the cohorts described in Section 17.7.3.3. The points and dotted lines show the results obtained with the fixed-interval techniques of the direct and actuarial methods of analysis. The solid line "staircase" shows the results obtained with the Kaplan-Meier method. The vertical arrows on the abscissa show the timing of the six deaths used to demarcate the Kaplan-Meier intervals. In this instance, the fixed-interval and variable-interval methods give almost identical results for the fixed-interval points at 1, 2, and 3 years.

The main advantage of the variable-interval method is its attention to the true shape of the survival curve, thus allowing the discernment of subtleties that might be missed with the fixed-interval techniques, and avoiding the possible distortions created by the lines drawn to connect the locations of rates noted only at the fixed-interval points. The chance of missing such subtleties or creating distortions can always be minimized, of course, if small boundaries are selected for the fixed intervals. To avoid any possible misinterpretations at the transition points of a Kaplan-Meier curve, the vertical lines should be omitted in the graph and the rates drawn merely as a set of unconnected horizontal lines. Because a reader who will misinterpret the regular staircase will probably also misinterpret the ghostly staircase that occurs when the vertical lines are omitted, they were included to enhance the visual esthetics of Figure 17–3. The Kaplan-Meier method also has the purely statistical advantage of being readily amenable to the log-rank test or other procedures[31] that can be used for calculating statistical significance when two survival curves are stochastically contrasted.

Like the direct method described in Section 17.7.3.1, the variable-interval method does not allow the censored patients to contribute to the denominators of the interval in which they are censored; and the survival rates are therefore likely to be slightly underestimated. Perhaps the main disadvantage of the variable-interval method is its unfamiliarity to clinicians who are accustomed to thinking about single summary indexes (such as a median) or about the summaries provided by survival rates at fixed points in time. When desired, the rates at fixed points can readily be discerned from the variable-interval curves, but the discernment may be difficult when the curve is published in a reduced image, and the component numerators and denominators may be impossible to distinguish unless a separate chart has been published to accompany the graph. Because such a chart, as demonstrated by Table 17–3, occupies much more space for a variable-interval analysis than when the intervals are fixed, the charts are seldom published for the readers' edification.

17.7.3.4. **CHOICE OF THE THREE METHODS**

As in many other issues in the communication of statistical information, the decision about which of these three methods to choose depends on the viewpoint of the investigator and reader. Because the denominators are reasonably well decremented for censored patients in all three methods, any one of the three offers a reasonably satisfactory approach for expressing the results of a cohort. If the purpose is to provide a readily understandable descriptive communication, the fixed-interval methods seem preferable, and the direct method is particularly desirable. If the purpose is to achieve statistical approbation, the Kaplan-Meier variable-interval method is currently most popular, despite its abrupt truncation of intervals for censored patients.

Perhaps the greatest communicative advantage of the direct method is that it displays the actual numbers of patients who comprise the numerators and denominators for any of the cumulative rates; and the cumulative rates are determined directly from those numbers. The constituent numbers are often omitted from the curves shown for data reported with actuarial and Kaplan-Meier methods. The denominators are sometimes displayed for patients who were actually followed to the time points at various intervals, but these numbers cannot be directly converted to rates and interpreted without recourse to the concatenated multiplications that produce the cumulative rates calculated in the nondirect methods.

When the actual numbers are available in the direct method, a reader can even evaluate things for himself by performing a chi-square test or some other simple procedure for checking statistical significance. This tactic will often be disdained as statistically wicked, because it uses data only for one time point rather than for the whole curve or because it fails to use more elegant methods of stochastic inference. Nevertheless, it offers an excellent screening test for investigators or readers who like to check results for themselves and who do not want to be completely dependent on statistical procedures whose principles and ramifications they may not understand. Besides, as other statisticians have pointed out,[37] even the log-rank test is not immune from imperfection.

Regardless of their relative merits, none of the three main methods deals with the problem of *why* the censored patients were lost to follow-up and whether bias was produced by differential losses in different prognostic subgroups of people exposed to the maneuvers under comparison. The question of bias can be approached, if suitably cogent prognostic variables were cited in the data, with a new statistical technique, sometimes called the *proportional hazards model,* or *Cox's regression.*[38] It consists of a procedure that (in essence) combines multiple regression with decrementation of censored patients.

17.8. **SYNOPSIS**

The outcome events of a cohort must be suitably identified. The different variables must account for single-state phenomena that were not described at baseline, for transitions, and for the performance of maneuvers. Although the outcome events can be categorized for their anticipated roles as primary, ancillary, and incidental targets in the research, unanticipated events will often occur and require decisions about their desirability, causes, and consequences. These decisions are often impeded by inadequate data for the benefits used in risk/benefit appraisals, and by the absence of specific operational criteria for diagnostically identifying adverse drug reactions.

The performance of prospective follow-up studies in people is much more difficult than in the customary environment of laboratory science. The persons under study must be protected with fail-safe procedures while being encouraged to maintain participation and compliance. A central laboratory technique may be needed for consistency in certain measurements, and a special coordinating center may be required to maintain the data. In long-term studies, the investigators themselves may sometimes need replacement.

Chronometric problems occur in several situations. The maneuvers under comparison may be imposed at different times in the serial course of the clinical conditions; and individual maneuvers may have a dosage, duration, or timing that does not let them achieve potent action. To allow outcome events to be ascribed to the preceding maneuvers, conflicting policies have been applied regarding therapeutic windows, potency intervals, wash-out periods, and carry-over effects. Additional difficulties arise if the follow-up period is too short to allow ample opportunity for the outcome events to occur and if the examinations needed to discern important transitions are not performed frequently enough.

The outcome events are detected during the three-stage process of medical surveillance, ordering diagnostic procedures, and interpreting the evidence. Detection bias, a prime source of error and distortion in clinical and public health epidemiologic data, can occur when any of the three stages of this process has substantially differed in the compared cohorts. Although double-blind techniques can be used to reduce detection bias in randomized trials, the techniques are often not feasible or they may not be effective.

The statistical expression of outcome events for a cohort is complicated by the interval of time that elapses between the onset of the maneuver and the occurrence of the outcomes. The statistical results may be substantially distorted by the transfer biases that can occur in residue cohorts. A residue cohort is formed when an inception cohort is truncated by the absence of members who had received the maneuvers, when a heterogeneous multi-serial group of people is collected for a follow-up that begins at diverse times *after* onset of the maneuvers, or when an inception cohort is augmented by people referred because of postmaneuver events. Other major problems can arise when a contrived-control cohort is simulated from the easily available but often scientifically dubious data of vital statistics.

A separate set of statistical challenges involves problems in managing data for censored patients who are lost to follow-up or followed for an insufficient duration, and for competing-risk patients whose outcomes cannot be suitably observed because of alternative-outcome events or contamination of maneuvers. The customary scientific policy is to regard the censored and competing-outcome patients (and perhaps those with contaminated maneuvers) as "withdrawn alive" during the postzero interval in which the withdrawing events occur. The cohort's denominators are then progressively decremented at these intervals. The life-table analyses used for the decrementation can be conducted at variable intervals or at fixed intervals, with either direct or actuarial adjustments. Alternatively, outcome events can be cited for the median duration at which they occur or for denominators determined by the sum of durations for which each member was followed.

EXERCISES

[Exercises 17.1–17.8 refer to Sections 17.1 through 17.6 in the text. Exercises 17.9–17.12 refer to Section 17.7.]

Exercise 17.1. The transitional outcomes of a cohort are often expressed as an average transition rather than as a rate of transition events. Thus, the results of antihypertensive treatment may be reported with the statement that "the mean fall in blood pressure was 8.2 mm. Hg" rather than with statements such as "20% of patients achieved normal blood pressure." What do you perceive as the strengths and weaknesses of this policy for characterizing outcomes?

Exercise 17.2. A patient develops nausea and vomiting soon after receiving a particular medication. What questions would you ask to decide whether the event is an adverse drug reaction? If you were allowed only one additional procedure to obtain data for this decision, what procedure would you choose?

Exercise 17.3. A randomized trial is being conducted to compare medical versus surgical treatment for a particular condition in which surgery is substantially delayed after randomization until certain preparations have occurred. The surgeons are willing to accept the intention-to-treat policy in ascribing all pretreatment deaths to surgery, but they insist on measuring the average survival of all other patients from the date of the actual surgery, not from the date of randomization. They want you to adjust the results of the medically treated group to reflect this distinction. What adjustment would you use?

Exercise 17.4. A federal agency has asked you to consult in the design of randomized trials to evaluate the efficacy of over-the-counter (nonprescription) pharmaceutical agents and other analogous substances for which cause-effect claims are made. A prime concern in the research is the construction of suitable double-blind arrangements when the evaluated agents have such distinctive appearances, tastes, smells, or other attributes that an appropriate placebo comparison may be difficult to create. What proposals would you offer for a comparison maneuver (or strategy) that would provide a suitably objective evaluation of the maneuver/outcome relationships in the following claims:

17.4.1. Heartburn gets fast relief with Rolaids.
17.4.2. Gargling with Listerine makes a sore throat feel better.
17.4.3. Clogged nasal passages are opened when Vicks Vapo-Rub is applied to an infant's chest.
17.4.4. Adolescent pimples are reduced by the use of Acnorrhexis Lotion.
17.4.5. The taste of sautéed chicken is improved if mustard is added to the gravy.
17.4.6. Lux soap makes skin lovelier

Exercise 17.5. The ligation of the mammary artery is one of several surgical procedures that have been proposed in the past few decades to increase coronary blood supply in the treatment of coronary artery disease. In 1959, when this operation had received widespread acceptance and was being frequently performed, it was subjected to two randomized trials.[39, 40] In each trial, after patients were suitably prepared and anesthetized in the operating room, a ligature was passed around the mammary artery. At this point, the surgeon opened an opaque, sealed, appropriately sterilized envelope containing the randomized instruction: TIE IT or DON'T TIE IT. The surgeon who carried out this assignment was the only clinical person who knew what had been done and did not participate in the subsequent management or evaluation of patients. The subsequent results, which showed that angina pectoris had improved in about 70% of each of the two treated groups, led to the abandonment of the operation not long afterward.

Because the trial was conducted before modern concerns with ethics, a thoroughly informed consent was not obtained from the patients who participated in the study. The use of the sham surgery can either be criticized as highly unethical, because its recipients did not consent to the possibility, or lauded as an appropriate and desirable response of clinicians to the alternative societal obligation to demonstrate the value of treatment and eliminate useless therapies. What are the reasons for your position in this dispute? If you believe the research is not ethical, what mechanism would you propose for getting an answer to the societal question?

Exercise 17.6. Suppose we wanted to do a double-blind comparison of two active agents, one of which is injected once a day and the other taken orally three times a day. Both agents are to be maintained for a period of 5 years. To make this study double-blind, each group would require an unnecessary extra pattern of treatment: The injected group would have to take an additional oral placebo three times daily; and the oral group would require an additional daily injection of placebo. An argument can be offered that such a trial is scientifically and clinically improper (and perhaps unethical), even if the patients give a suitably informed consent before entering the trial. An unnecessary placebo injection daily for 5 years is certainly undesirable; the complex pattern of treatment used in the trial would differ from what would occur in clinical practice; and the observed efficacy of the regimens might be affected by the patients' difficulties in complying with the complexity. What are your reasons for agreeing or disagreeing with this argument? If you agree, what would you propose as an alternative approach in designing the trial?

Exercise 17.7. Each of the statements in the following exercises contains a causal claim that might be or has been made at the end of an investigation. Without regard to any other aspect of the research design, what side effect or other feature associated with each maneuver would you suspect as a possible cause of detection bias for the outcome event? (Please confine your speculation to detection bias, not to any issues in the susceptibility bias of the people who receive the maneuvers.)

17.7.1. Although no studies have been conducted recently, observational research performed several years after the introduction of oral contraceptive agents showed a higher rate of thrombophlebitis in women using these agents than in those using the alternative existing barrier methods, which (at that time) consisted of either male condoms or the *ad hoc* insertion of diaphragms. Consequently, oral contraceptive agents have been regarded as a possible cause of thromboembolic phenomena.

17.7.2. In studies conducted at about the same time as those cited in 17.7.1, oral contraceptive agents were also implicated as a possible cause of gonorrhea. The conclusion was that gonorrhea occurs more commonly in women using oral contraceptives than in those using diaphragms or other *ad hoc* barrier methods.

17.7.3. Air pollution is a contributing cause of lung cancer because the rate of lung cancer is much higher in urban than in rural regions.

17.7.4. Estrogen replacement therapy causes endometrial cancer in postmenopausal women.

17.7.5. Postmenopausal women using estrogen replacement therapy have a less satisfactory sex life than those who do not use the hormone.

17.7.6. Jogging prevents sudden death due to coronary artery disease.

17.7.7. Fluoride treatment of municipal water supplies to prevent dental caries may raise the rate of cancer in those municipalities.

17.7.8. Appendectomy can be a cause of colon cancer.

17.7.9. Gastric cancer may be caused by treating gastric ulcer with cimetidine or other histamine-suppressor agents.

Exercise 17.8. Indicate the potential sources of any type of important bias you can think of that should be considered as a source of false conclusions drawn from the following statements:

17.8.1. Among elderly people who had children and who were interviewed in an old age home, most said they would rather live there than with their children.

17.8.2. People of Irish descent living in the United States have higher death rates than their counterparts living in Ireland.

17.8.3. Cardiac damage occurs in all patients with rheumatic fever, because it is invariably found at autopsy of those who die during an acute attack.

17.8.4. The contention that the Welby University Medical Center delivers poor primary medical care has been refuted by the high degrees of satisfaction reported in a survey of patients attending Welby's General Medical Clinic.

Exercise 17.9. Here is a set of data for the subsequent survival of a group of patients with a particular disease.

Table 17–4. SKELETON TABLE TO BE COMPLETED FOR EXERCISE 17.9.1

(1)	(2)	(3)	(4)	(5)	(6)	(7)	(8)	(9)
Years After Diag-nosis	Alive at Begin-ning of Interval	Died During Interval	Lost to Follow-up During Interval	Withdrawn Alive During This Interval, i.e., Insufficient Follow-up	Adjusted Denomi-nator for the Interval	Mortality Rate for the Interval	Survival Rate for the Interval	Cumu-lative Survival Rate
0–1	126	47	4	15				
1–2		5	6	11				
2–3		2	0	15				
3–4		2	2	7				
4–5		0	0	6				

17.9.1. Using an actuarial method of analysis, and calculating all rates to at least three decimal places (to avoid errors due to rounding), please complete Table 17–4.

17.9.2. Using the direct method of decrementing denominators, calculate the cumulative survival rates at each of the cited intervals in Table 17–4.

17.9.3. Comment on the different results obtained for 5-year cumulative survival rates with the two methods of calculation. Which method would you prefer to use as a clinician evaluating treatment and making decisions in patient care?

Exercise 17.10. For the data shown in Exercise 17.9, assume that the investigators checked each patient's status every 6 months. The deaths and censored events listed in the data were noted at the following times:

	During Interval		Deaths at
	Lost to Follow-up	"Withdrawn Alive"	end of interval
0–6 mos.	3	5	32
6–12 mos.	1	10	15
12–18 mos.	3	7	3
18–24 mos.	3	4	2
24–30 mos.	0	8	2
30–36 mos.	0	7	0
36–42 mos.	1	3	0
42–48 mos.	1	4	2
48–54 mos.	0	5	0
54–60 mos.	0	1	0

From this additional information, prepare a variable-interval (Kaplan-Meier) analysis of the survival proportions of the cohort.

Exercise 17.11. Prepare a graph showing the results of the actuarial and Kaplan-Meier analyses of these data. (You need not recalculate the previous data of Exercise 17.9.)

Exercise 17.12. Like the direct method, the variable-interval method does not augment the interval denominators to include contributions from people censored during an interval. In Exercises 17.9 and 17.10, are the results of the variable-interval method more like those of the direct method or those of the interval-augmenting actuarial method? What is your explanation for the observed distinction?

Exercise 17.13. Here is an interesting exercise that may appeal to you if you would enjoy some mathemedical algebra. In the actuarial method of decrementing denominators for a cohort of N people, let d_i represent the deaths occurring during any interval and let l_i represent the adjusted denominator for that interval. The mortality rate for the interval is calculated as $q_i = d_i/l_i$ and the interval survival rate is $p_i = 1 - q_i$. Thus, for five deaths and an adjusted denominator of 75, the interval survival rate would be $1 - (5/75) = 0.933$. The cumulative survival rate, P_i, at any interval is the product of that interval survival rate and all the preceding interval survival rates. Thus, $P_4 = p_1 \times p_2 \times p_3 \times p_4$. Your assignment here is to prove that when no losses occur due to censoring or competing risks, the direct method, the actuarial method, and the Kaplan-Meier method all yield exactly the same cumulative rates at the end of the follow-up period for the cohort.

CHAPTER REFERENCES

1. Chu, 1982; 2. Wells, 1981; 3. Hutchinson, 1979; 4. Irey, 1966; 5. Karch, 1975; 6. Kramer, 1979; 7. Finney, 1974; 8. Levine, 1977; 9. Moussa, 1978; 10. Feinstein, 1974; 11. Kramer, 1980; 12. Gavrin, 1964; 13. Boice, 1978; 14. Ramshaw, 1973; 15. Anturane Reinfarction Trial Research Group, 1980; 16. Temple, 1980; 17. Anturane Reinfarction Trial Policy Committee, 1982; 18. Sackett, 1979; 19. Spitzer, 1974; 20. Howard, 1982; 21. Clemens, 1983; 22. Bergstrand, 1983; 23. Neyman, 1955; 24. Robboy, 1981; 25. Frost, 1939; 26. Hoover, 1976; 27. McMichael, 1975; 28. Shapiro, 1982; 29. Feinstein, 1977; 30. Veterans Administration Urological Research Group, 1964; 31. Peto, 1976–1977; 32. Wood, 1964; 33. Lee, 1980; 34. Miller, 1981; 35. Chiang, 1964; 36. Cutler, 1958; 37. Haybittle, 1979; 38. Cox, 1972; 39. Cobb, 1959; 40. Dimond, 1960.

PART FOUR

STRUCTURE, SCIENCE, AND STATISTICS IN CROSS-SECTIONAL RESEARCH

Regardless of a reader's scientific background in physical, biologic, or social sciences, the architectural model of scientific cause-effect reasoning is not hard to understand and interpret. Observing the outcome of a maneuver imposed on a baseline state, we engage in the conventional scientific act of noting a "before," doing a "something," and seeing an "after." To decide that the maneuver has caused the observed effect, we use the conventional scientific act of comparing what happens when some other maneuver is imposed. To allow the results to answer the question we asked, we make suitable choices of the baseline states, the outcomes, and the particular maneuvers that are compared. To be sure that the results are not distorted by bias, we add a further scientific requirement that the compared groups be similar in prognostic susceptibility of the baseline states, in performance of the maneuvers, in detection of the outcome events, and in transfer of people from baseline state to analyzed data.

When the research is conducted as a cohort study, and particularly when the maneuvers are imposed and followed experimentally, the architectural structure used in the research coincides with the architectural model of the scientific reasoning. Reading the reports of such research, we can easily apply and check the principles that will make the results scientifically acceptable, because we can easily (or reasonably easily) find what we need to know. When we examine the reported methods and results, everything is (or should be) presented for its occurrence in a direct, straightforward sequence of events. That sequence of events will be quite similar to the scientific sequence we learned in studying the experiments of elementary chemistry, elementary physics, or other examples of scientific activity.

In many clinical and epidemiologic activities, however, the scientific sequence of a cohort structure is not or cannot be applied. The use of an experiment may be unethical or unfeasible for studying the etiologic impact of an alleged cause in producing a human disease. We may be forbidden, by ethics or law, from deliberately exposing people to noxious agents; even if not forbidden, we may not know which agents to test or how to produce the disease consistently; and even if we knew what to do and were allowed to try it, we might not be able to convince enough people to participate willingly as experimental subjects. When the research questions are therapeutic rather than etiologic, we may still be unable to do all the experiments we might like. Randomized trials may be unethical, unfeasible, or too costly to be used for studying the prophylactic and remedial actions of *all* the therapeutic agents that must be evaluated for *all* the clinical conditions that receive attention in modern medical science.

Although an observational cohort study would seem to be the best substitute for an experiment, the cohort approach is either inappropriate or unfeasible for many research projects. The approach is inappropriate for studies in which the research is not intended to answer questions about the cause-effect outcome of a maneuver. A cohort study is usually not required for many kinds of descriptive data or for process research concerned with observer variability, diagnostic markers, or clinical competence. When cause-effect questions are being asked, the cohort approach is often unfeasible for studies, particularly in etiology of disease, in which the suspected agent must act for a long duration and has a low attack rate for the outcome event. Such studies would require investigation of a huge cohort followed for protracted periods of time. Even if we could develop suitable facilities to collect, maintain, and follow a cohort of 50,000 people for 20 years, very few investigators could be found to do the work.

A clinical investigator who wants to avoid these difficulties cannot escape them in epidemiologic research. The only complete escape is to abandon the topics pursued in the research and to ask a different set of investigative questions, while working in a laboratory setting where the models, methods, and materials are more amenable to experimentation and to other principles of scientific research. For etiologic and therapeutic challenges that cannot be explored in a laboratory setting, however, clinical investigators will have to cope with the difficult realities of assembling and studying the groups of people who can provide answers to the research questions. When the questions cannot be answered with the cohort structures that follow a conventional scientific sequence of events, the investigators will have to use different structures.

The non-cohort structures of epidemiologic research create enormous scientific problems for both investigators and readers. For investigators, the main problems are to satisfy the principles of scientific reasoning in the architectural model of cause-effect research while analyzing information collected with methods in which the groups, data, and statistical expressions have an entirely different structure from those of conventional science. For readers, the main problems are to understand what the investigators have done amid the alien models, structures, and statistics.

Chapter 18

An Outline of Cross-Sectional
Research Studies

Cross-sectional studies are the most versatile and probably the most common type of research that appears in medical literature. A reader may not always recognize the activity because it does not receive the fancy title of *cross-sectional study*. Nevertheless, such studies are routinely performed to provide the descriptive data used for diverse decisions in health policy, to investigate normal growth and development, to explore the pathophysiology of diverse diseases, to evaluate such processes as observer variability and diagnostic marker tests, and to apply cause-effect reasoning for appraising the impact of diverse etiologic agents, risk factors, and clinical therapies.

The defining characteristic of a cross-sectional study is that the basic state of each person in the research is examined essentially once. When quotients are calculated to summarize the results as means, proportions, or rates, the conditions that are entered in the numerator and denominator for each person are both determined at the time of that single-state examination. By contrast, in a cohort study, each person must be examined on at least two distinctly different occasions: the first time, to delineate the denominator condition; and the second time, to identify the subsequent outcome that appears in the numerator.

Although cross-sectional data refer to a single state for each person, the information about the numerator and denominator conditions need not have been obtained simultaneously at a single examination session. For example, the data assembled in the massive decennial surveys conducted by the census bureau are regarded as cross-sectional for each person and for each nation, even though the census takers may sometimes have to make several visits to obtain all the information for a particular household, and even though many months may be needed to survey all the households of a nation. In categorizing a person's cross-sectional status for level of blood pressure or for diagnosis of diabetes mellitus, we may list a single-state value obtained as an average of several previous measurements or as the pattern of different temporal values in a glucose tolerance test. To quantify the cross-sectional prevalence of retinopathy in patients attending a clinic devoted to hypertension or to diabetes, the denominator may consist of the number of different people attending the clinic for single visits and examinations during an interval of several months; the numerator would consist of the number of those people who were found to have retinopathy. In a diagnostic marker study, the carcinoembryonic antigen (CEA) test used to make a positive or negative diagnosis of colon cancer may have been performed on one day, and the surgery that shows the definitive status of the colon may have been performed several days later.

In all of the circumstances just cited, the individual items of the associated cross-sectional information were not noted simultaneously. Nevertheless, when the information is presented and analyzed, the underlying idea is that the numerator and denominator data were obtained concomitantly at a single state in time. Data arranged in this manner have a cross-sectional *structure*, regardless of the particular type of *study* in which the data were obtained. For example, the baseline state of people in a cohort study could be summarized with such cross-sectional data structures as statements that the 408 people had a mean age of 43.2 years, a mean weight of 68.5 kg., and a 73% proportion of women. Similarly, if we said that 92% of 37 survivors in this cohort were satisfied with their care, the expression would be a cross-sectional data structure, because it refers to the single-state concomitance of two conditions: the outcome (survival) and degree of satisfaction at the time of the outcome.

The example just cited can provide an additional way of indicating some of the flaws previously noted in research conducted with residue cohorts: The results of a residue are often expressed with a cross-sectional rather than a cohort data structure. Thus, the satisfaction rate of 92% in the 37 survivors is a cross-sectional structure in which the denominator is a residue of the cohort, not the original cohort. To determine the results of the original cohort, we would need to know about satisfaction in the inception group of 408 people, not just in the 37 survivors.

Although data from *cohort* studies can be reported in cross-sectional structures for a single state of the cohort, data from *cross-sectional* studies can be used—as noted later—to simulate the results of cohort research. This simulation gives cross-sectional studies their great versatility, power, and investigative appeal. With suitable arrangements of data, the results of cross-sectional studies can make the research seem to be directed forward, concurrently, or backward in time. In exchange for these advantages, however, the cross-sectional results may contain many ambiguities, inaccuracies, and biases that make the work difficult to understand or impossible to interpret.

The rest of this chapter is concerned with outlining the diverse uses of cross-sectional studies in medical research. The chapter is long because it contains three main components: an overview of the basic axes of classification for research goals and methods; a demonstration of symbols for the research structures and formats for the results; and an annotated inventory of the different types of cross-sectional studies. Some of the topics (such as explicatory experiments and pharmacologic research) receive a relatively detailed discussion, because they are not described elsewhere in the text, whereas other topics are outlined briefly, with further details reserved for later chapters. Thus, the additional application of cross-sectional studies will be discussed for cause-effect research in Chapter 23, for process research in Chapters 25 to 27, and for descriptive research in Chapter 28.

Because the results of cross-sectional *studies* always yield cross-sectional data *structures,* the latter term will often be used throughout the discussion. The methods and results can then be contrasted, as desired, with the cohort structures that have already been discussed and with the heterodemic structures described in Chapter 24.

18.1. AXES OF CLASSIFICATION FOR CROSS-SECTIONAL RESEARCH

The five main axes used in Section 2.2 to classify the general goals and methods of medical research are also pertinent for classifying specific distinctions in cross-sectional research.

18.1.1. *Purpose, Agents, and Sources of Data*

In general purpose, cross-sectional studies can be used for descriptive or comparative goals. In types of agents, the comparisons can be aimed at evaluating the procedures of a process or the cause-effect impact of a maneuver. In sources of group data, the information can be obtained homodemically from groups observed directly or heterodemically from groups that have been studied or contrived indirectly.

The other two axes of classification—which refer to experimental or nonexperimental allocation of agents and to the temporal direction in which the research is oriented—involve some special distinctions that require additional attention.

18.1.2. *Experimental Planning in Cross-Sectional Studies*

The word *experiment* can be used in at least two different ways. In one usage, an experiment occurs when an investigator carries out research in which careful plans have been made for assembling groups and collecting data. In a different usage, as defined in Section 2.2.3, an experiment occurs when the investigator allocates the agents under investigation. The first meaning of *experiment* is regularly employed to describe the design of studies in the social sciences and in other forms of research in which the main experimental design refers to the prolective collection of groups and data, not to the planned allocation of agents. The second meaning of *experiment* is the one we have been considering thus far. It requires prolective plans not only for collecting groups and data but particularly for allocating agents. In fact, as noted in Section 2.2.3, the investigator's opportunity to allocate the agents under investigation was defined as the main feature that distinguishes an experiment from a survey. The most obvious example of a clinical epidemiologic experiment occurs in a randomized trial when treatments are allocated experimentally to compare their therapeutic action.

In this classic example, the compared agents are cause-effect maneuvers, and the data are obtained with prolective plans established before the agents are imposed. The role of prolective planning is so much a fundamental part of experimental design in randomized trials that its identity is not always recognized as a separate constituent of the research methods. For example, the ability to use double-blind procedures is sometimes erroneously attributed to the randomization rather than to the prolective planning made possible by an experiment. Double-blind procedures can be used regardless of the mechanism that allocates maneuvers; and furthermore, as noted earlier, the data can be planned and collected prolectively in cohort studies that are not experiments. It is even possible to use experimental randomized trials for research in which important features of the data are obtained in retrospect. Thus, the mothers and children exposed to DES in a randomized trial[1] conducted in the 1950s were later checked in the 1970s in search of long-term adverse effects.[2, 3]

These experimental distinctions in allocation of agents and in prolective planning are noteworthy in cross-sectional research, because certain cross-sectional studies can be designed experimentally, using prolective planning and even randomization to investigate agents that are *not* cause-effect maneuvers. Conversely, certain experiments that seem to have the classic cause-effect experimental structure of cohort research are not concerned with cohorts and must be analyzed as cross-sectional studies.

18.1.2.1. EXPERIMENTAL DESIGN IN PROCESS RESEARCH

Because the prevention of bias is just as important in process research as in cause-effect research, such experimental strategies as randomization and double-blinding (or their appropriate counterparts) can be used to provide the necessary precautions in cross-sectional research evaluating such processes as observer variability, quality control, marker tests, and clinical competence. For example, in a study of interobserver variability among histopathologists, we would certainly want each pathologist to interpret each slide of tissue "blindly" without knowing what anyone else has said about it. To study intraobserver variability by having each pathologist later reinterpret the same set of slides, we could keep the pathologists unaware of their own previous statements, and we would send the same slides back with different numbers in a sequence that has been randomly rearranged.

The precautions needed to avoid bias are readily apparent and are usually instituted in special investigations, such as studies of observer variability, in which data for the process research can be obtained only if a specific study has been deliberately planned. The problems of bias may be less apparent and less likely to receive suitable attention in marker studies or in clinical audits in which the data used for the investigation are taken retrolectively from the records of routine medical practice. The problems of these nonexperimental process studies will be further discussed in Part Six.

18.1.2.2. EXPERIMENTAL DESIGN IN DESCRIPTIVE RESEARCH

Because comparative analyses are not performed in purely descriptive studies, no precautions are needed for arranging an unbiased allocation and observation of the compared procedures or maneuvers. The main experimental challenge in descriptive research is the prolective planning needed to be sure that the groups accurately represent the populations and that the acquired data accurately represent the groups.

The acquisition of accurate data (as discussed earlier) is always a fundamental scientific challenge, regardless of whether the work is observational or experimental, and regardless of what topic is being investigated. The acquisition of "accurate" groups of people, however, is often pursued quite differently in medical research and in the social sciences. For sociologists, economists, political poll-takers, market analysts, and other students of public opinion, a prime investigative activity is the descriptive research conducted to determine the attitudes and attributes of large populations by noting the results found in smaller samples of those populations. Consequently, an enormous amount of vigorous intellectual and mathematical attention has been given to the experimental design of randomized sampling methods that will allow the surveyed groups to be accurate representatives of the larger populations. Readers who are interested in the intricate strategies of survey sampling can find further details in appropriate publications.[4-6]

In clinical and epidemiologic research, however, we use randomization for allocating, not for sampling. The main medical concern is to avoid bias in assigning agents to the groups under study, and we seldom worry about how well those groups—which are almost never obtained as samples—represent the intended population. Besides, the realities of medical research and clinical practice would keep us from regularly acquiring our groups as random samples, even if we wanted to. In medical descriptive studies, we are therefore usually satisfied with obtaining the descriptive information to use for whatever purpose it may be applied; and in comparative studies, the intellectual energy is usually centered on the comparison of agents, not on the extrapolation of results to an outside population. The consequences of this *laissez faire* approach are the frequent occurrences of the distorted assemblies discussed earlier (in Sections 4.3.2 and 15.8.1) and the common complaint by practitioners that the results of many clinical investigations, including vastly expensive randomized trials, are not pertinent for the problems of clinical practice.

This distinction in the investigative approaches of the medical and social sciences can also sometimes produce major misunderstandings when the two types of investigators jointly discuss research methods and experimental design. For medical investigators, who are most often concerned with exploring cause-effect relationships, an *experiment* refers to the planned comparison of interventions; randomization is used to reduce bias in allocating the interventions; and extrapolation is deemed relatively unimportant. For social scientists, who seldom engage in the direct, personal imposition of the prophylactic and remedial interventions that create the cohorts studied in clinical care, the evaluation of treated cohorts is seldom a major challenge. Consequently, many social scientists regard an experiment as the planned acquisition of descriptive data that can be accurately extrapolated; randomization is used to reduce bias in sampling the groups under study; and the comparison of imposed agents is relatively unimportant. The two fundamentally different approaches may lead to considerable confusion when investigators from the medical and social domains use the same words to refer to disparate ideas and techniques.

18.1.2.3. CROSS-SECTIONAL EXPLICATORY EXPERIMENTS

A unique type of cross-sectional experiment in clinical epidemiology is almost never regarded as an activity in epidemiology. Just as Molière's *bourgeois gentilhomme* was astounded to discover that he spoke in prose, many modern clinical investigators may be astonished to learn that their explicatory experiments are cross-sectional studies in clinical epidemiology.

In all of the experiments discussed in Part Three, the principal maneuver was an intervention intended to produce a distinctive change in the baseline state of the recipient. Because a change may not always occur, the way we determine a maneuver's efficacy is to contrast the observed changes against those achieved with an inert maneuver, such as placebo treatment or the absence of exposure. The experiments are longitudinal, because the subsequent changes—whether temporary or permanent—are the main outcome at which the maneuver is aimed in its etiologic, prophylactic, remedial, or other interventional action.

In a different type of human experiment, however, the maneuver is used as a probe, not as an intervention. The goal is not to change the basic state of the recipient but to jostle it transiently for an explicatory purpose. The jostling is intended to reveal or explain something about physiology, pharmacology, or pathophysiology, not to produce any lasting changes; and the recipient of the maneuver is expected to return to the baseline state after the experiment is completed. In fact, if the experimental maneuver has more than a transient action, the investigator (as well as the subject) will be dismayed.

These explicatory experiments, which were briefly discussed in Section 11.5.1, are frequently performed in the special laboratory environments or clinical research centers of modern medical institutions. Although sometimes reported in traditional medical journals, the results commonly appear in publications that are specifically devoted to clinical research and that usually emphasize the explicatory studies conducted as clinical investigation in people or animals.

Explicatory experiments in people can be quite complicated to design and analyze because different types of maneuvers can be used as stimuli for preparatory, provocative, or informative purposes. A preparatory stimulus may consist of a special diet given for several days before imposition of the provocative stimulus, which is an injection or ingestion of a substance such as glucose or norepinephrine. The informative stimulus might be the injection of small amounts of a radioactively labeled substance, whose uptake or turnover is measured as the response to the preceding stimuli. The active stimuli used for preparation and provocation can be compared with control stimuli, such as a regular diet or the injection of saline. The informative stimulus, which indicates the response, can sometimes be administered not to the person who receives the preceding stimuli but to specially prepared animals or media, such as cell cultures. The response is noted after these external recipients are exposed to the stimulus of cells, fluid, or tissue derived from the investigated persons.

As an example of a relatively simple explicatory experiment, we might measure the before-and-after responses of serum corticosteroids to infusions of ACTH and saline given to patients with Addison's disease and to healthy volunteers. When the corticosteroid levels after stimulation by ACTH show a substantial rise in the healthy group but not in the diseased group, we will have demonstrated an important point about the pathophysiology of Addison's disease. Another example of a relatively simple explicatory experiment was presented in Exercise 2.4 at the end of Chapter 2, in which the pathophysiology of the kidney in patients with omphalosis was examined by noting the responses of renal blood flow to infusions of sodium sulfate and sodium chloride.

As an example of a more complex experiment, we might want to explore the physiologic metabolism of lipoproteins. As preparation for the provocative stimuli, the volunteers might receive a special high-fat or special low-fat diet for several days. As comparative preparation, a regular diet may be given to the same volunteers in a previous or subsequent cross-over arrangement or to a different group of volunteers studied in parallel. For each of the compared preparatory stimuli, the provocative stimuli may consist of repeated infusions of glucose or propranolol and comparative infusions of saline. The responses may be measured as the turnover, in each subject, of low-density lipoprotein that has previously received radioactive labeling in that subject's plasma. (I have made up this experiment, as an illustrative example, from a composite of several reports recently published in the *Journal of Clinical Investigation*. I hope the design does not get me expelled from the society that publishes the journal.)

For readers who are not intimately involved in studying the particular topics of biomedical research projects, the explicatory studies can be extremely difficult to understand and interpret. The reader usually needs a highly sophisticated knowledge of the state of the art not only for the complex technology used to create stimuli and measure responses, but also for contemporary concepts of the physiologic, pharmacologic, or pathophysiologic mechanisms under investigation. To determine the design of the experiments, the reader must often perform an intellectual dissection of the diverse activities described in a long account of methods for the cross-over or parallel plans in which an array of different stimuli and people have been arranged with potentially four different types of controls for informative, preparatory, provocative, and pathodynamic comparisons. The informative stimuli may be compared with a control that provides background data for such phenomena as the uptake of radioactivity. The preparatory and provocative stimuli may each be compared against controls that are used to differentiate the action of the main or active stimulus. And people with a particular disease state may be compared against controls who are healthy or in some other state of disease.

Nevertheless, after all the complexity has been sorted out, the investigator and reader emerge with a particular index that represents the main response to something that is regarded as a principal maneuver. The various other tactics that seemed like experimental maneuvers were actually being used as stimuli to probe the effect of the underlying causal agent that is under investigation. This causal agent, which plays the role of the principal maneuver in the ultimate scientific reasoning, is usually a state of health or disease, or the action of a drug. After all the elaborate experimental stimuli have been administered, the principal maneuver may turn out to be a physiologic mechanism of the human body, the pharmacologic mechanism of a drug, or the pathophysiologic derangement produced by a disease. When the relationships of maneuvers and responses are extrapolated beyond the people studied in the research setting, the activity becomes an exercise in clinical epidemiology, requiring a set of scientific principles quite different from those used in planning and conducting the research itself.

The research is cross-sectional because the responses and the maneuvers are categorized for clinical conditions that are noted at a single state in time. In studies of physiology and pathophysiology, the clinical conditions are the healthy or diseased states that serve intellectually as the principal maneuvers. In studies of pharmacologic mechanisms, the healthy or diseased conditions also serve as single-state maneuvers that can affect the action of the drug.

The clinical epidemiology of the investigated cross-sectional states becomes important when they are used to represent the condition that is the maneuver. If the research is aimed at a physiologic or pharmacologic response of healthy volunteers, can we assume that the investigated group, which often consists of college or medical students, suitably represents the analogous responses that might occur in healthy people who are much older or younger? If the volunteers consist only of men, would the responses be the same in women?

Although we usually need not worry too much about the representativeness of the healthy people investigated during studies of normal physiology or pharmacology, things can become quite troublesome if the research is concerned with the pathophysiologic impact of a particular disease. In this circumstance, the suitability of the disease state and the suitability of the compared control(s) become crucially important for cause-effect interpretations of the results. Because the experiments are difficult to conduct, only a few subjects may be assembled to represent each disease under investigation. For example, a study of the pathophysiology of renal disease might involve three healthy volunteers as well as four patients with obstructive uropathy, one with renal artery stenosis, and two with acute glomerulonephritis. Although statistical significance can usually be obtained with diverse analyses of the multiple variables studied at multiple time points in these small groups, the epidemiologic problem is whether the "universe" of obstructive uropathy, renal artery stenosis, or acute glomerulonephritis is suitably represented by the handful of patients who were studied for each state of disease.

A more substantial problem is in the cause-effect reasoning that occurs when the disease state becomes regarded as the maneuver responsible for the observed responses. Thus, if the index of response for a group of patients in an advanced stage of cancer differs from the corresponding index in healthy volunteers, is the difference due to the cancer itself or to the associated malnutrition, antecedent therapy, or co-morbid ailments? Would the same difference be found if we had investigated a group of patients with the same cancer but in a localized, newly detected stage? Would the results differ if the control group had contained patients with some other cancer, with advanced congestive heart failure, or with hepatic decompensation, rather than healthy volunteers?

The clinical epidemiologic problems of comparing results in different cross-sectional groups will be extensively discussed later in this chapter and particularly in Chapters 21, 23, and 25. The main point to be noted now is simply that the explicatory experiments conducted in clinical investigation often contain the major scientific difficulties of other cross-sectional studies in clinical epidemiology. The epidemiologic hazards of the groups selected for comparison do not vanish merely because the stimuli are given experimentally, and, in fact, the hazards are particularly likely to be overlooked because the critical reviewers tend to concentrate on the ingenuity with which the stimuli and responses were created by the experimental methods. When explicatory experiments produce interpretations that are later refuted, the basic source of the difficulty may often be not in the experimental design itself but in an unrecognized case-control problem of cross-sectional clinical epidemiology.

The epidemiologic problem is important not only for its consequences in cause-effect reasoning about pathophysiology, but also because the main stimulus used in the explicatory experiments is sometimes later converted from a purely investigative function to an expensive new technologic role as a marker test in clinical practice. Most of the current diagnostic procedures that involve the stimulus-response effects of ingestions, infusions, and contrast media—including the glucose tolerance test, lactose tolerance test, and dexamethasone suppression test, as well as radioisotopic imaging procedures—were all originally investigated with cross-sectional explicatory experiments.

If suitably evaluated during the experimental investigations, the explicatory stimuli can function quite effectively as diagnostic procedures. Unfortunately, however, because most of the experimental research is aimed at pathophysiologic explication, not diagnostic differentiation, the case and control groups selected for the explicatory experiments may be suitable for demonstrating pathophysiologic distinctions but not for demarcating diagnoses. The inadequacy of the technologic procedure as a diagnostic marker in clinical practice may not become apparent until many years of confusion, expense, and wasted effort. To avoid inaccurate or distorted results, the cases and controls used to evaluate the *diagnostic* efficacy of these technologic procedures should be chosen with the same scientific standards (discussed in Chapter 25) that are needed in the clinical epidemiology of other forms of diagnostic-marker research.

18.1.3. *Temporal Directions of Orientation*

When the temporal direction of a research study's orientation was discussed in Section 2.2.4, we thought about the way in which we look at, or follow, a group of people. We can follow them forward, to see what happens later; or concurrently, to see what is going on right now; or backward, to see what occurred previously. Thus, if we collect a group of adults and determine each person's blood pressure, the direction is concurrent. If we ask about childhood illnesses, the direction is backward. If we check later to see how many of those people have developed fractured hips during the next 5 years, the direction is forward.

An unusually distinctive attribute of cross-sectional studies is that data collected at a single cross-sectional examination can be oriented or interpreted as though the research contained a backward, concurrent, or forward direction; and sometimes exactly the same set of data can be interpreted in all three directions, according to the whims or goals of the interpreter. For example, suppose we cross-sectionally examine a group of patients with adult-onset diabetes mellitus and a control group of people without diabetes. For each person we obtain the following data: the values for hematocrit and serum cholesterol; an estimate of approximate magnitude for the intake of candy, sugar, and other sweet substances during adolescence; the duration of serial time since diabetes was diagnosed; and the presence or absence of diabetic retinopathy. All of this information is cross-sectional, having been obtained for each patient at a single state in time.

In analyzing this information, we may compare data from the diabetic and the control groups to look *backward* or retrospectively at the prevalence of an elevated adolescent intake of sweets, which is being suspected as a possible etiologic cause of diabetes. In expressing the central tendency and spread of hematocrit values in the diabetic group, our direction is *concurrent*. We simply want to know the group's condition now, possibly to alert the clinic personnel that some of the patients may be anemic. If we divide the group of diabetic patients according to their postdiagnostic diabetic durations of 0 to 5 years, 6 to 10 years, 11 to 20 years, and >20 years, and if we report the prevalence of retinopathy for the subgroups contained in each interval, the direction is *forward*. The implication is that the diabetes mellitus has been a pathodynamic maneuver and that the occurrence of retinopathy has been affected by the amount of time elapsed since onset of the diabetes.

The opportunity for directional versatility is much greater if we demarcate the serum cholesterol values as elevated or normal and if we then determine the prevalence of elevated values in the diabetic and control groups. Suppose we find that the rate (or proportion) of hypercholesterolemia is substantially higher in the diabetic group than in the control group. The interpretation of this result is a matter of "dealer's choice." We can think etiologically in a backward direction, viewing the hypercholesterolemia as a possible antecedent cause of the diabetes. We can think pathodynamically in a forward direction, interpreting the hypercholesterolemia as a subsequent effect (or complication) produced by the diabetes. Alternatively, we might conclude that a causal relationship almost surely exists, but we do not know which way it goes: whether hypercholesterolemia causes diabetes or diabetes causes hypercholesterolemia. In yet another option, we can regard the results as showing not a causal relationship, but a noncausal association in which the diabetes and cholesterol are either unrelated to one another or both produced by some undetermined cause. If the concurrent association is striking enough, we might suggest that hypercholesterolemia can be used as a diagnostic marker for diabetes, or vice versa. Amid all the available options, the only thing we can say for sure is the classical concluding statement: "This interesting finding warrants further research."

Each of these four different conclusions—containing backward, forward, bi-directional, or concurrent interpretations of the observed relationship—can be offered for the same set of results obtained in the same case and control groups of the same cross-sectional study. A calculation of statistical significance will not solve the problem of how to think about the data, because the same statistical test could be used for any of the four possible directions of interpretation. (In this instance, the statistical test would probably be chi square, although other tactics are available, particularly if the relationship is being offered as a possible diagnostic marker.)

This versatility of temporal interpretation is one of the greatest powers of cross-sectional studies. It allows them to be applied for many types of both cause-effect and process research and allows the research to be relatively quick, easy, and inexpensive. The real costs of this "free lunch," however, are in the associated scientific hazards and statistical obstacles that will be discussed later.

18.2. SYMBOLS FOR STATISTICAL ARCHITECTURE

In chemistry, physics, and other sciences, symbols and diagrams have been developed to serve as a type of shorthand for indicating the entities or ideas under discussion. In statistics, such symbols as Σ, Π, $\overline{X}$, and S_{xx} are used respectively to indicate a summation, multiplication of products, mean, and deviance. The diagrams in Sections 3.2.2 and 12.4.3 represent an attempt to show the *conceptual* architecture of cause-effect reasoning in medical research. In cohort studies, the conceptual and actual structures are similar. In non-cohort studies, their structure of the research is different and requires different diagrammatic patterns.

Because statistical expressions are the ultimate outcome of both cohort and non-cohort studies, the results may become particularly easy to understand if a set of symbols is available to show the simultaneous relationship between the statistical, conceptual, and actual structures of the research. Such a set of symbols can easily be created if we begin by considering the structures used in the main statistical expressions of results. Those statistical structures occur either as quotients, when a numerator is divided by a denominator, or as associations between variables. If we use appropriate alphabetical letters to represent such conceptual ideas as baseline states, maneuvers, and outcomes, the alphabetical letters can then be placed in numerators, denominators, or symbols for associations that will help represent the actual structure of the research.

These symbolic expressions, which represent a combination of ideas that can be called *statistical architecture,* are seldom needed for cohort studies, because statistical expressions for the outcome of a cohort usually provide a straightforward citation for the conceptual and actual structures of the research. When studied in a cohort, a cause-effect relationship is investigated and is statistically expressed in the customary scientific direction of going from cause toward effect. The symbols of statistical architecture can be particularly valuable, however, for the difficult task of getting one's head clear about what is going on when the statistical expressions emerge from research that may have been structured in a confusing jumble of different temporal directions for potential causes and potential effects.

18.2.1. *Descriptive Statistical Symbols*

No matter how the research is conducted, the results for each group in the study are usually cited with one of two types of expression that were discussed in Chapters 7 and 10: an index of spectral distribution or an index of association. The index of spectral distribution provides a summary for the distribution of data found in the spectrum of a single variable in the group. If the variable is dimensional, such as *age,* this index might be a mean and standard deviation or a median and inner 95-percentile range. If the variable, such as occupation or degree of severity of congestive heart failure, contains the nondimensional categories of a nominal or ordinal scale, the index might be a set of proportions for the subgroups in each category. If the variable contains the two binary categories used to describe the presence or absence of an event, such as acute myocardial infarction, the index is also a proportion and is often called a *rate*.

Indexes of association are used to show the simultaneous relationship of two or more variables. When these relationships are the trends noted as correlations or regressions, they are generally shown for two or more variables in the same group. For the checks of agreement that are expressed as concordances, the indexes refer to the same variable, as noted by two different methods, observers, or judges.

18.2.1.1. SYMBOLS FOR SPECTRAL DISTRIBUTIONS

To arrive at a simple way of showing a spectral distribution, we need to recall that quotients are used to cite the main indexes of central tendency, such as a mean, and all the proportions or rates that represent categorical groups. In the numerator of a mean, the symbol "$\Sigma(\ )$" is used to indicate the act of adding the amounts observed for the data of each person in the group. We can use the counterpart symbol "$N(\ )$" to indicate the act of counting the frequencies observed in each category of the data. The symbol "V" will represent a variable. With this convention, in a group containing N members, the symbol $\Sigma(V)/N$ would represent the mean of a dimensional variable; and $N(V)/N$ would represent the proportions (or rates) for categorical variables.

We can now extend this convention in three ways. First, because of the way proportions are reported, the citations for $N(V)/N$ indicate the full spectrum of the variable because they show the equivalent of both an index of central tendency and an index of dispersion. Thus, when we cite a group's occupation as 52% **blue collar**, 27% **white collar**, and 21% **other**, the proportions show the full spectrum of data for *occupation*. The citation of $\Sigma(V)/N$, however, gives only the index of central tendency, as a mean. Let us therefore agree that $\Sigma(V)/N$ will symbolize both an index of central tendency and an index of dispersion. Thus, if the index of dispersion is a standard deviation, $\Sigma(V)/N$ for age in a particular group might be expressed as 46 ± 13.

Secondly, let us also agree that $\Sigma(V)/N$ will be cited in whatever indexes of central tendency and dispersion are most appropriate for the dimensional variable that is under consideration. If central tendency is best expressed as a median or geometric mean rather than as a customary arithmetic mean, and if dispersion is best expressed with a range or inner percentile range, these will be the expressions denoted by $\Sigma(V)/N$.

Once we have agreed that $N(V)/N$ and $\Sigma(V)/N$ represent the preferred methods of citing the proportions for a categorical variable or the indexes of central tendency and dispersion for a dimensional variable, the third step is easy. Both pairs of symbols now summarize the same thing: the spectrum of distribution for a variable. We can therefore eliminate the "$N(\ )$" and "$\Sigma(\ )$" components of the symbols. Either one can now be shown quite simply as V/N.

With this convention, V/N represents an appropriate set of indexes that summarizes the spectrum of distribution for a single variable in a group of N people. If we actually wanted a portrait of this spectrum, it would be shown for dimensional data with a histogram or frequency polygon. For categorical data, the proportions of the individual categories V_1, V_2, and so on would be calculated as V_1/N, V_2/N, and so on. The results would be displayed in a bar graph or pie graph.

18.2.1.2. SYMBOLS FOR ASSOCIATIONS

In an association of trend for two different variables, such as a correlation or regression of hematocrit and blood urea nitrogen, the variables can be shown with different symbols, such as V and W.

If the association has a definite directional orientation, with one of the variables regarded as independent and the other as targeted or dependent, the *vs.* symbol can be used to show this orientation. A regression of V on W would be cited as V vs. W. If V is hematocrit and W is blood urea nitrogen, the V vs. W expression would summarize the data we examined earlier in Section 10.2, as the regression of blood urea nitrogen on hematocrit. If the directional association involves more than two variables, the symbol "{ }" can be used to represent the variables examined in a multivariate manner. Thus a multiple regression in which survival time is expressed as dependent on age, weight, and stage of disease could be cited as V vs. {W}, where V represents survival time and {W} represents the multivariate matrix of variables for age, weight, and stage of disease. In a more general sense, if we do not want to use the curly brackets, the W of V vs. W can represent the single or multiple variables that are independent in the regression.

In many instances, the associated trend is a correlation for which the relationship is regarded as interdependent or bi-directional. We do not believe that V depends on W or that W depends on V; or we may not want to commit ourselves to a uni-directional decision about which way the interrelated dependency goes. In this situation, the correlated trend can be shown as V × W (or W × V).

18.2.2. *Symbols for Cohort Studies*

With the statistical symbols of V/N to show the distribution of a spectrum, and V × W (or other arrangements) to show an association, we can now use alphabetical letters in those symbols to denote the architecture of the scientific reasoning and investigative structures. The easiest way to begin this procedure is to show it for a cause-effect cohort study. The ideas can then be expanded to include cross-sectional research.

In choosing symbols for the conceptual architecture of cause-effect research, we can use M for maneuvers, S for baseline states, and F for outcome fates (to avoid confusing the letter O and the number zero). With these symbols, the contrast of maneuvers A and B in the customary diagram of a cohort study would be

$$S\left\{\begin{array}{c} M_A \longrightarrow \\ \\ M_B \longrightarrow \end{array}\right\} F$$

When the study is completed, we want to compare the outcome rates for the two maneuvers. To do this, we need to enumerate the people who are in the groups S_A, F_A, S_B, and F_B. Using R for rate and "N( )" to show the act of counting, we would compare

$$R_A = \frac{N(F_A)}{N(S_A)} \quad \text{vs.} \quad R_B = \frac{N(F_B)}{N(S_B)}$$

Thus, we might compare the rates of 5-year survival as the outcome fate in patients with the baseline state of angina pectoris treated with medical or surgical therapy.

The statistical comparisons for the outcome of cohorts are almost always presented and labeled according to the maneuvers; and the baseline states are implicit although omitted in the expressions. Thus, the usual statistical contrast would be cited as 5-year survival rates for medical versus surgical therapy. Accordingly, the rates could be cited as

$$\frac{N(F_A)}{N(M_A)} \text{ vs. } \frac{N(F_B)}{N(M_B)}$$

Because the same outcome fate is being examined in both numerators, and because the numerator groups are always a subset of the denominator groups that are studied homodemically in cohort or cross-sectional research, the subscripts can be omitted from the numerator groups, and the rate can be written as

$$\frac{N(F)}{N(M_A)} \text{ vs. } \frac{N(F)}{N(M_B)}$$

Next, we can eliminate the cumbersome symbol of "N( )" if we agree to let the capital letters denote both the attribute and the number of people having that attribute. With this convention, the compared rates would be expressed as

$$\frac{F}{M_A} \text{ vs. } \frac{F}{M_B}$$

Finally, to make things more generally applicable, we can use M to represent the principal maneuver and $\overline{M}$ to represent the comparative maneuver. The foregoing rates would now be compared as

$$\frac{F}{M} \text{ vs. } \frac{F}{\overline{M}}$$

and (even more simply) as F/M vs. $F/\overline{M}$.

These symbols indicate the statistical structure of the comparison while simultaneously denoting the conceptual and research architecture. In this instance, F/M is the rate of the outcome in people receiving maneuver M; and $F/\overline{M}$ is the corresponding rate for people receiving the comparative maneuver.

To allow the same symbols to be applied when the outcome is something other than a single event, we can agree that the numerator symbol will represent an appropriate aggregation and expression for the spectrum of distribution in whatever type of variable is being used to describe the outcome event. Thus, if F represents survival at a particular time point after maneuver M, the expression F/M represents the incidence rate calculated as $N(F)/N(M)$. If F is a variable that denotes the individual survival durations of each patient, and if we were citing the mean survival and standard deviation of the group, the expression F/M would indicate both the mean value, $\Sigma(F)/N(M)$, and the appropriate standard deviation. In other circumstances F/M might denote the median and range of survival times for the group or a set of proportions for the patients whose outcome has been designated as *excellent, good, fair,* or *poor*. Thus, regardless of whether the outcome is expressed in a dimensional or categorical variable, F/M would represent an appropriate summary expression for the spectral distribution of F in the group of people who were exposed to M.

In certain circumstances, the variables used for the outcomes and also for the maneuvers are expressed in ranked (ordinal or dimensional) scales, and the relationship is cited as an association rather than as a contrast of two or more groups. For example, we might determine the rapidity with which pain is relieved after four different dosages of an analgesic agent. Such results could be cited as F/M_1 vs. F/M_2 vs. F/M_3 vs. F/M_4 for each of the four dosage groups. Alternatively, the association of relief time and dosage might be depicted conceptually as a line on a graph and expressed as F vs. M. The absence of the virgule sign (/) would indicate that the expression is an association, and the sequence of F vs. M would indicate that M is the independent variable in the association.

If the baseline state has been partitioned into strata having such distinctions as good, fair, or poor prognoses, the strata can be denoted with subscripts such as S_1, S_2, and S_3. The architectural diagram for the cohort study would be

$$S \longrightarrow \begin{matrix} S_1 \\ S_2 \\ S_3 \end{matrix} \bigg\} \;\; \begin{matrix} \xrightarrow{\;M\;} \\ \\ \xrightarrow{\;\overline{M}\;} \end{matrix} \bigg\} \; F$$

The results of the maneuvers compared in each stratum would be expressed as

$$S_1: \text{ F/M vs. F/}\overline{\text{M}}$$
$$S_2: \text{ F/M vs. F/}\overline{\text{M}}$$
$$S_3: \text{ F/M vs. F/}\overline{\text{M}}$$

Because the separate comparison of maneuvers is clearly shown in each stratum, this type of expression is probably better than trying to represent the strata with subscripts on the maneuvers. Thus, the stratified comparison could be shown as F/M_1 vs. $F/\overline{M}_1$, F/M_2 vs. $F/\overline{M}_2$, and so on, but the use of superscript bars and subscript numbers might be cumbersome. Besides, if we wanted to depict the compared maneuvers as M_A and M_B rather than M and $\overline{M}$, the result would require a doubly subscripted notation, such as F/M_{A_1} vs. F/M_{B_1}. Because the alphanumeric mixture is unappealing, we would probably relabel the maneuvers as M_1 and M_2 and then write the stratified comparisons as F/M_{11} vs. F/M_{21}, F/M_{12} vs. F/M_{22}, and so on. This type of doubly subscripted numerical notation is regularly used by statisticians, who are accustomed to working with it and can easily avoid the confusion of mixing up the numbers for maneuvers and strata. For readers who are not statisticians, the arrangement will be easier to understand if the strata are identified with colons, as in the original expression of S_1: F/M vs. F/$\overline{M}$, etc. If the maneuvers are identified with letters (or numbers), the symbols could be illustrated as S_1: F/M_A vs. F/M_B.

The maneuvers and the strata happen to coincide in certain epidemiologic studies in which an element of time, i.e., age, is the main maneuver and in which the different age strata become the denominators of the contrasted stratum-specific rates of the outcome event. Thus, the mortality rate of 40- to 49-year-old people (stratum 1) might be compared with the mortality rate of 50- to 59-year-old people (stratum 2) as F/S_1 vs. F/S_2. Because age is the main maneuver under contrast, these rates could also be shown as F/M_1 vs. F/M_2, in which M_1 represents age 40 to 49 and M_2 represents age 50 to 59.

18.2.3. *Symbols for Cross-Sectional Studies*

For cross-sectional research studies, the basic symbols that have been developed can be expanded to cover the array of phenomena that may be under scrutiny. In using the symbols, we need to remember the difference between a study and a data structure; and we need to recognize that the alphabetical symbols will indicate the scientific intent of the study and the way the data are arranged, but may not necessarily indicate the structure used in the research.

For example, the symbol V/N is a data structure that indicates the spectral distribution of a variable, such as the mean weight of a group of people. The data structure does not show, however, whether it is a cross-sectional or longitudinal expression. It might come from a cross-sectional study, indicating the weights measured at a single point in time; or it might come from a cohort study. If emanating from a cohort, the data structure could represent the mean weight of people in the baseline state or at the outcome. If desired, we could use alphabetical letters to show these distinctions. Letting E represent a variable observed in a cross-sectional study, the distinctions could be shown as E/N for mean weight in the cross-sectional study, S/N for mean weight in the baseline state of the cohort, and F/N for mean weight in the outcome of the cohort.

In general, however, this degree of distinction is seldom needed, and the alternative symbols of V and W are easier to use for variables in most situations unless we need E, F, M, and S (or a few other letters that will be introduced shortly) to show important distinctions in the architectural concepts of the research. The main additional symbols we will need for cross-sectional studies are the letters D (for diagnosis, disease, or clinical condition) and T (for the results of a test). In the cross-sectional studies concerned with certain diagnostic tests or procedures that are done to identify or mark the presence of a particular disease state, the results of positive tests can be shown as T and negative tests as $\bar{T}$. The groups of diseased and nondiseased people receiving the tests can be shown as D and $\bar{D}$. Thus, as discussed in Chapter 25, T/D would represent the nosologic sensitivity of a marker test, which is its proportion of positive results in diseased people. $\bar{T}/\bar{D}$ would represent the marker's nosologic specificity, which is the proportion of negative results in nondiseased people.

The alphabetical symbolism becomes particularly valuable when we are trying to understand what happens in cross-sectional studies that are used for cause-effect relationships. Although cross-sectional results become interpreted with the scientific model of cause-effect reasoning, the research itself uses a quite different architectural structure. For example, suppose we want to determine the subsequent occurrence of gallstones as the outcome (F) in healthy people (S), who do or do not drink large quantities of tea (M). In a cohort study, the rates of the outcome event would be compared directly as F/M vs. F/$\bar{M}$. In the cross-sectional research structure that is often called a *retrospective case-control study*, however, we would begin by assembling a case group of people who have already developed the outcome event of gallstones and a control group of people who have not. These two groups can be symbolized as F and $\bar{F}$. The members of each group would then be checked to ascertain their antecedent exposure to the principal maneuver, which in this instance is tea drinking. The actual research would be diagrammed as

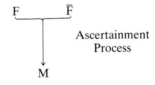

The rates that would be compared are the prevalences of tea drinking in the groups with and without gallstones. These rates would be shown symbolically as M/F vs. M/$\bar{F}$. These symbols immediately demonstrate some of the scientific and statistical difficulties, discussed later in greater detail, that are created by the architectural structure of a retrospective case-control study. In the architectural *model* of scientific reasoning and in the *cohort structures* of cause-effect research, the rates that we compare are F/M vs. F/$\bar{M}$. When a *case-control structure* is used to answer the same research question, however, the comparison contains a quite different set of entities—M/F vs. M/$\bar{F}$.

This catalog of symbols will suffice for most of the phenomena encountered in cross-sectional data studies. A few additional details will be introduced later as needed to describe the different types of cross-sectional research contained in the inventory of Section 18.4.

18.3. DISPLAY OF STATISTICAL RESULTS

Most statistical portraits of data appear as graphs or tables showing the relationship of two variables. For each variable, a graph usually shows the location of concomitant points; and a table usually shows the frequency counts for concomitant categories. The word *association* is often applied to these relationships, even though tabular data are frequently summarized with indexes of contrast rather than indexes of association.

Because each graph or table has a distinctive orientation, one of the variables must be shown in a position suggesting that it is the target or dependent variable. The position of the other variable (or variables) then suggests a role as the independent features that presumably affect the associated trend. In the usual algebra for two variables, y symbolizes the dependent variable and x the independent variable. The relationship is usually expressed as y vs. x. For statistical architecture the symbols can be V vs. W, if V is used as the outcome, target, or dependent variable. If the variables are definitely identified as maneuvers and outcomes, the relationship can be expressed as F vs. M.

In graphs, y is displayed as the ordinate variable and x as the abscissa. In tables, this horizontal-vertical orientation is often reversed to follow the usual direction of time as the reader's eye moves from left to right. The outcomes shown in the columns on the right side of the tables appear after the maneuvers listed on the far left, in the rows.

For example, the dependency of hematocrit and blood urea nitrogen was shown in Figure 10–1, with the independent BUN values moving horizontally and the dependent hematocrit values vertically. If this same information were categorized into low, medium, and high values for each variable, the table would usually be presented with BUN vertically in the rows and hematocrit horizontally in the columns. The skeleton table would look like this:

BUN Values	Hematocrit Values			
	Low	*Medium*	*High*	**Total**
Low				
Medium				
High				
Total				

This reversal of orientation for graphs and tables can generate considerable confusion when the axes are chosen for displaying a table. The results can be consistently displayed if the outcome (or output) variables are always placed in the columns and if the maneuver (or input) variables are placed in the rows.

18.4. AN ANNOTATED INVENTORY OF CROSS-SECTIONAL RESEARCH

The different types of cross-sectional studies can be catalogued mainly according to their roles in descriptive, process, and cause-effect research. The statistical architecture will be cited with the symbols discussed in Section 18.2.

18.4.1. *Descriptive Studies*

These studies are used to provide complete or abridged details of a set of observed phenomena in one or more groups. The abridged results may be expressed statistically with any of the univariate, bivariate, or multivariate indexes discussed in Chapters 7, 8, and 10. If comparisons occur, they are not intended to evaluate the quality of processes or the cause-effect impact of maneuvers.

Because the basic statistical expressions show the spectrum of results found in a single group of data, the term *spectral* has been used for the corresponding studies or data structures.

18.4.1.1. SPECTRAL REDUCTIONS

This title encompasses both the summaries shown with univariate indexes and the associations shown with indexes of trend. In either instance, the result provides an abridged expression or statistical reduction of the full spectrum of data. Spectral reductions can be presented as the deliberate product of a descriptive study or they can be used as data structures to express descriptive results in other studies.

18.4.1.1.1. *Spectral Distributions*

This name describes a set of old acquaintances: the means, proportions, ranges, standard deviations, and other univariate summary indexes that are the most common type of statistical data structure: V/N. If the variable is dimensional, the distribution of data is commonly summarized with indexes of central tendency and spread; and the spectrum is displayed with a histogram. If the variable is categorical, the distribution is summarized with the proportions of the subgroups formed by such categories as V_1/N, V_2/N, and so on; and the spectrum is displayed with a bar graph or pie graph.

To avoid confusion between V_1 and V_2 as symbols of different variables or as categories of a single variable, we can substitute other letters appropriately. Thus, for a group of diseased patients containing 18% in stage I, 39% in stage II, and 43% in stage III, the spectrum could be cited as D_1/D, D_2/D, and D_3/D. Note that the proportions expressed in a spectral distribution all have the same denominator. Recalling this distinction may save you from the frequent error—noted in Exercise 8.5 at the end of Chapter 8—of confusing the difference between a spectral proportion, D_1/D, for the prevalence of middle-aged people in the group with a particular disease, and the occurrence rate, D/N_1, for the relative frequency of that disease in the middle-aged people of a community.

18.4.1.1.2. *Spectral Associations*

In this type of study or data structure, a relationship of correlated trend is shown between two (or more) variables, without arriving at a decision about biologic dependency or causal impact. Thus, a descriptive index, table, or graph might be prepared to show the correlation between hematocrit and cholesterol or between the religion of patients and the types of nursing homes in which they are located. The most common correlations are bivariate, having the statistical structure of $V \times W$.

A correlation and reduction of multiple variables is sometimes used in an effort to create a new mensurational index. For example, the statistical procedures of factor analysis, principal component analysis, or cluster analysis might be applied to a set of data with seven variables, trying to reduce them to the three or four main factors, components, or clusters that provide a presumably better description of the interrelationships. Because no dependent variables are involved as targets for these activities, the multivariate interdependent relationships can be shown simply as {W}.

The data structures in this section have been listed as *associations,* which is the traditional, familiar title. The word *association* is quite ambiguous, however, because it refers to both concordances and trends and because *trends* can refer to both interdependent correlations and dependent regressions. A better name for the cited data structures is *spectral correlations.* To specify that the correlation involves two or more variables within the spectrum of a single group rather than a comparison across the spectra of different groups, the best term would be the cumbersome *intraspectral correlations.* I trust that readers who hate neologisms will give me credit for avoiding this one.

18.4.1.2. SPECTRAL RESEMBLANCES

Two different spectral distributions or associations are sometimes compared to see whether they are similar or different. The goal is to check for resemblance, not to perform the contrasts needed in evaluating a process or appraising a cause-effect impact. A spectral resemblance comparison might be used to determine whether the demographic characteristics are similar for the people who responded or did not respond to a mailed questionnaire.

Cross-sectional resemblances are commonly checked in cohort studies to see whether the contrasted groups were similar at baseline before the maneuvers were imposed. For example, in a randomized (or nonrandomized) comparison of the actions of treatments A and B, the baseline states of groups A and B might be compared for their similarity before treatment began. For this comparison, the spectral distributions in groups A and B might be checked for such individual features as age, gender, weight, stage of disease, or other cogent variables. For each variable, the comparison can be shown as V/N_A vs. V/N_B or as S/M_A vs. S/M_B if we want to indicate specifically that the variables are baseline states for maneuvers. A comparison of baseline state is sometimes conducted by combining several individual variables into a single multivariate score or into the clustered partitions of categories in a staging system. Groups A and B would then be checked for spectral distributions of the multivariate scores or categories.

18.4.1.3. SPECTRAL DEMARCATIONS

A special subset of spectral distributions is a *spectral demarcation,* in which certain boundaries are placed on a spectral distribution to establish a range of normal for the variable under consideration. The demarcation can be established directly from the statistical data or with other considerations to be discussed in Chapter 28.

18.4.2. *Process Studies*

Details of the architecture of these studies will be discussed in Chapters 25 to 27. They are listed here mainly to indicate that they are part of the inventory of cross-sectional studies. In all process studies, the quality of a procedure is evaluated by noting its performance with different approaches, one of which is often regarded as the reference or definitive standard.

18.4.2.1. CONCORDANCE STUDIES

In concordance studies, the same *procedure* is compared for its performance by different observers, methods, or judges. The procedures can be the observer variability noted among clinicians, radiologists, or histopathologists, the quality control determined in laboratory measurements, the audits conducted for clinical practice, or the examinations administered to check clinical competence for licensure or specialty certification.

The basic structure of the statistical comparisons is $V_1 \leftrightarrow V_2$, but the results may often be expressed with an elaborate set of statistical indexes, particularly in psychometric appraisals of examinations used to test clinical competence. Many studies of concordance receive inadequate statistical expressions because they are cited with indexes of correlated trend, as $V_1 \times V_2$, rather than with indexes of concordant agreement as $V_1 \leftrightarrow V_2$.

18.4.2.2. MARKER STUDIES

In marker studies, the same *entity* is designated or marked by two different procedures, one of which is the definitive standard. The usual purpose of the studies is to see how well the tested procedure can be used as a substitute for the definitive procedure.

18.4.2.2.1. *Diagnostic Markers*

In this situation, the marker procedure—which is commonly called a *diagnostic test*—is evaluated for its ability to discriminate a particular disease, D, among the spectrum of all other diseases and states of health. The positive (T) and negative ($\overline{T}$) results of the marker procedure are noted in people who have the disease and in a control group of people, $\overline{D}$, who do not have the disease. Thus, we might evaluate the proportionate frequency with which an elevated alkaline phosphatase test is found in patients with and without cancer. If the study is well conducted, we would recognize that the test has poor diagnostic discrimination, and we would not want to use it clinically for this purpose.

The results of these diagnostic studies are usually expressed as the sensitivity (T/D) and specificity ($\overline{T}/\overline{D}$) attained by the marker test in its nosologic identification of people with or without the disease. In clinical usage of the marker, however, a clinician wants to know the predictive diagnostic capacities of positive results as D/T and negative results as $\overline{D}/\overline{T}$. The clinician must therefore convert the statistical expressions from nosologic indexes based on disease to diagnostic indexes based on test results. The strategies used for these conversions, or for reaching the desired goals without them, are discussed in Chapters 20 and 25.

18.4.2.2.2. *Spectral Markers*

In a spectral marker study, a particular variable is evaluated for its ability to distinguish different subgroups in the spectrum of a single disease or clinical condition. The results are often expressed by citing the prevalence of a particular positive result, U, in the subgroups as U/D_1, U/D_2, and so on. For example, we might find that an elevated alkaline phosphatase occurs in 1% of patients with stage I of a particular cancer, in 10% of patients with stage II, and in 35% of patients with stage III. The results might also be expressed—still in a format such as U/D_1 and U/D_2—by citing the mean or other indexes of distribution for alkaline phosphatase in each stage.

These citations, with the spectral subgroup placed in the denominator, also create subsequent problems in clinical usage, because the clinician, appraising the result of a marker test as U_i and wanting to apply it to a particular patient, needs to know the values of D_1/U_i, D_2/U_i, D_3/U_i, and so on rather than the inverted statistical citations of U/D_i.

Diagnostic and spectral marker studies can become difficult when the results of the marker test are expressed in a ranked ordinal or dimensional variable. In these situations, a boundary must often be chosen somewhere on the scale of the variable to separate the regions of *positive* or *negative* results for the test. As discussed in Chapter 25, this decision can be made with specifically clinical judgments or with various mathematical procedures, such as the analysis of *receiver operating curves*.

18.4.2.2.3. *Prognostic Markers*

Although the word *predictive* is commonly applied to the work done when clinicians use the results of marker procedures to diagnose diseases or to identify subgroups within the spectrum of a disease, the activity is really cross-sectional and concurrent. The patient's true clinical condition coexists at a single point in time with the result obtained in the marker test.

A marker is really predictive when it is used prognostically to estimate the occurrence of future events. In these predictions, the same test whose results are used as a marker for diagnosis or for identifying spectral subgroups can also be applied as a prognostic marker. Thus, we might assemble data showing that patients with an elevated alkaline phosphatase have a 76% chance of surviving 3 years.

The data needed for such forecasts require cohort rather than cross-sectional studies, but investigators may sometimes approach this challenge by substituting conveniently available cross-sectional information. Thus, the baseline (pretherapeutic) phosphatase values may be available for a group of people who survived 3 years and for another group of people who did not. The distribution of alkaline phosphatase in the cross-sectional groups of survivors and fatalities may then be compared for some sort of conclusion about the prognostic role of the test.

18.4.3. *Cause-Effect Studies*

We now come, at long last, to the main topic for discussion in the rest of this chapter: the use of cross-sectional studies in research that has cause-effect implications. The previously mentioned temporal versatility of the studies is particularly evident in the different arrangements that follow.

18.4.3.1. SPECTRAL DEPENDENCIES

The studies and data structures used for spectral dependencies are similar to those discussed in Section 18.4.1.1.2, except that the trend is investigated with a definite direction of orientation. Because one of the variables is chosen to be the target or dependent variable that is affected by the independent variable(s), the graphs and tables of a spectral-dependency data structure usually convey a cause-effect implication; and a dose-response relationship in such structures is often used as evidence of a causal impact. These dependency structures contain two main hazards in nonexperimental data. The relationship between dose and response may be produced by bias; and the format of the data presentation may be produced by the investigator's prejudice. Because data for an interdependent noncausal correlation between two variables cannot be displayed in a graph or table without choosing one of the variables to be shown in a horizontal (or vertical) direction, readers (and investigators) must beware of interpreting the display of a correlation as indicating a dependency.

An additional hazard for both readers and investigators occurs when the research involves the "massage" of data from a collection whose total spectrum contains multiple variables. In an era in which computers can easily do the statistical processing, each of the individual variables can be examined separately as the dependent variable, while all the others can be analyzed simultaneously as independent variables to see if something significant emerges from the computer's work in number crunching. If enough variables are available for the multiple massagings of data, something positive may easily emerge by chance alone. The scientific problems created by such data-dredging activities are discussed in Section 22.6.

18.4.3.2. BIODYNAMIC STUDIES

The term *biodynamic* is used here to refer to the cross-sectional explicatory experiments, described in Section 18.1.2.3, in which the main maneuver under investigation is either the physiologic function of the body or the inherently pharmacologic actions of a drug. (If these experiments are labeled as *physiologic and/or pharmacologic,* the *biodynamic* neologism can be avoided, but it provides a useful contrast for the *pathodynamic* research described in Section 18.4.3.3.1.)

In biodynamic research, the clinical condition of the people under investigation is not intended to affect the main stimulus or maneuver under study. The subjects selected for the research are usually healthy, but diseased people may be chosen for certain pharmacologic studies that are best justified if the drug is pertinent for the particular disease. Extremely ill or moribund people may sometimes altruistically volunteer for studies in which the stimuli seem too dangerous to be given to patients with a long life expectancy, or in which the responses will be discerned from postmortem examination of tissue or cells.

18.4.3.2.1. *Types of Stimuli*

The stimuli used in biodynamic research may be ingested, inhaled, injected, inserted, or applied in some other way, such as exercise, and the responses consist of changes noted either clinically, in such variables as heart rate and temperature, or paraclinically, in such variables as electrolytes, lipids, or the metabolic products of a drug. In certain psychologic experiments, the stimuli may expose the subject to a particular vignette or scenario, and the response may be determined from the reactions reported in an interview or questionnaire. The diverse purposes of pharmaceutical stimuli are so numerous that they warrant a section of their own.

18.4.3.2.2. *Pharmacologic Research*

Pharmacologic explicatory experiments are usually divided into three main types, with further subdivisions that create a special taxonomy for the research. When the response is concerned with the distribution, degradation, or turnover of a drug, the investigations are usually called *pharmacokinetic;* when concerned with the drug's effect on electrolytes, lipids, or other conventional biochemical functions of the body, the research is called *pharmacodynamic;* and when the main goal is to find the amount (or dosage) of the pharmacologic stimulus that will evoke a particular response, the research is called *bioassay.*

The term *bioavailability* is applied when these activities are combined to study the temporal pattern of distribution, degradation, or metabolic responses for a drug at different dosages; and *bioequivalence* is used when bioavailability is compared for two or more different formulations of the same drug. (Because the goal of bioequivalence is to compare the agreement of two agents performing the same process, these studies can also be classified as a type of the concordance research described in Section 18.4.2.1. The particular variables used to measure bioavailability for each drug may be quite complicated, because they can involve areas under a curve of multiple responses at different times, but the basic statistical structure of the comparison is $V_1 \leftrightarrow V_2$.)

Beyond the categories just cited, the different goals in pharmacologic investigation have led to an additional taxonomy of phases for the research. When a new pharmaceutical substance is tried for the first time in human beings, the main goal is a bioassay to determine suitable dosage, but certain features of pharmacokinetics and pharmacodynamics may also be measured. These studies are usually called *Phase I,* and they are usually conducted in healthy volunteers.

After the drug's dosage and initial safety have been demonstrated, *Phase II* studies are done to test the drug in a few patients with the disease. These studies are usually both interventional and explicatory. The drug is examined for its therapeutic role as a maneuver that can change a distinctive feature of the disease, but at the same time, additional information is collected to help explicate the drug's pharmacologic action. A control or comparison stimulus is sometimes applied, with either a cross-over design or to a different parallel group, to help delineate either therapeutic or pharmacologic responses. The components of Phase I and Phase II studies are sometimes intermingled because diseased people may be the initial human recipients of the drug and because the pharmacologic attributes of the drug can be studied during both phases.

When the results of these early studies seem promising, the next step is *Phase III*, which involves larger studies of the drug's therapeutic efficacy. These studies contain a direct controlled comparison of the new drug versus placebo or alternative active drugs. To be approved according to the current policy of national regulatory agencies, these comparisons are almost always conducted as randomized trials. After the new drug is marketed, *Phase IV* studies may be used to determine its effects when given to a broader clinical spectrum of people and for longer durations of time than could be examined in the Phase III clinical trials. These additional studies of therapeutic impact may or may not be designed with specific control groups.

To expedite the marketing of new agents that seem strikingly valuable, or to reduce the enormous costs of the randomized Phase III trials, a drug may be approved with the proviso that additional studies, called *postmarketing surveillance,* be conducted afterward. The postmarketing observations are not limited to formal studies, however, and practicing clinicians may regularly find important new therapeutic uses (or indications) for a drug beyond the particular clinical conditions studied in the formal research of Phases I to IV. The practitioners may also be the main source of important observations about adverse effects. The term *Phase V* has sometimes been applied to these informal clinical observations and to the subsequent research that may follow them in efforts to substantiate either the new spectrum of efficacy or the suspicions of toxicity.

The activities conducted during Phases III to V are obviously cause-effect studies, with results that must be appraised according to the scientific architecture of cause-effect reasoning. The therapeutic impact studied in Phase II is also a part of cause-effect research. The pharmacologic responses studied in Phases I and II are cross-sectional explicatory experiments.

18.4.3.3. PSEUDOCOHORT STUDIES

A pseudocohort study yields results that have the appearance of a cohort investigation, but the data are obtained cross-sectionally. The principal maneuver under investigation can be the pathophysiologic effect of a disease or the long-term effect of normal physiologic growth and development. The data are presented in the statistical architecture of a cohort study. The arrangement may be F/M vs. F/$\overline{\text{M}}$ (or F/D vs. F/$\overline{\text{D}}$) when effects are compared for the presence or absence of a disease; and F/M_1 vs. F/M_2 when the maneuvers represent durations of serial time for a disease or for normal growth. The results for the outcome and the maneuvers are obtained cross-sectionally, however, from groups of people in whom the maneuvers and outcomes have already occurred when the people are chosen for the research.

Pseudocohort studies have two common formats. In a *pathodynamic study,* phenomena attributed to a disease (or other suitable maneuver) are investigated without specific regard to the serial timing of their occurrence. In a *longitudinal prevalence study,* the serial time elapsed after imposition of the maneuvers determines the groups under investigation.

18.4.3.3.1. *Pathodynamic Studies*

In pathodynamic studies, a particular disease is usually the maneuver that is held responsible for the outcome event. The outcome event is observed or inferred from an entity whose distribution is compared in a group of *cases,* who have the disease, and in a group of *controls,* who do not. This particular type of case-control study was the source of the pathodynamic relationship we examined in Section 18.1.3 when diabetes mellitus was regarded as a possible cause of the associated hypercholesterolemia.

Although relatively uncommon in traditional epidemiologic research, pathodynamic case-control studies are frequently performed in modern clinical investigation. Many of the explicatory experiments discussed in Section 18.1.2.3 are examples of such research; and many other clinical investigations, conducted without a direct experimental stimulus, are also done to illustrate or explicate the pathophysiologic actions of a particular disease. Some of the pathophysiologic investigations have an elaborate research design for experimentally imposing stimuli and measuring responses in cells, fluids, or tissues of the diseased and control patients, but eventually a main index of response is compared in the cases and controls. The comparison is sometimes arranged to contrast groups within the spectrum of the same disease rather than compare diseased versus healthy patients. Thus, the uptake of a radioactive substance may be compared in diabetic patients with and without vascular complications or in patients with localized or metastatic cancer. To provide better discrimination in the research, the cases may contain groups of patients from different parts of the spectrum of the same disease; and the controls may contain groups of people in different states of health or other diseases.

Because diseases are not or cannot be produced at the convenience of the investigator, the cause-effect maneuvers that are the main focus of comparison in pathodynamic research are imposed without an experimental plan, despite the elaborate stimuli-response experiments that may be devised to elicit data for the outcome events attributed to the maneuvers. Because cause-effect decisions in the research depend on the observation of effects ascribed to maneuvers that were not imposed experimentally, the scientific evaluation contains all the customary hazards of cross-sectional studies. The people in the selected groups may not suitably represent the clinical condition under study; the responses ascribed to a particular state of health or disease may really be due to an unrecognized co-maneuver in the associated co-morbidity or antecedent therapy; and other problems may arise as discussed in Chapter 21.

One problem relatively distinctive to pathodynamic research is the difficulty of disentangling the temporal sequence of cause and effect when two phenomena are observed simultaneously. We encountered this problem in Section 18.1.3, when we were trying to decide whether diabetes causes hypercholesterolemia or vice versa. We might want to say that diabetes is the causal agent, because it precedes hypercholesterolemia in the clinical sequence observed in most patients; but someone else, arguing for the etiologic role of cholesterol in diabetic patients who have no overt derangement in lipids, might claim that the hypercholesterolemia is latent or that existing methods are inadequate to detect the real cholesterol abnormality.

A cause-effect sequence of pathophysiologic explication may sometimes be reversed from one medical era to the next. For example, the general belief for many decades was that the occlusion of coronary arteries precedes and then leads to myocardial infarction. Today, after the advances of modern technology have demonstrated myocardial infarctions in occasional patients with apparently normal unoccluded coronary vasculature, the pathogenetic proposal has been offered that a myocardium infarcted or rendered ischemic by reduced blood flow (perhaps due to spasm) sets in motion a chain of events that later leads to vascular occlusion.

In other alternatives of pathophysiologic mechanisms, the two concomitantly observed phenomena are regarded as caused not by one another but by an underlying separate cause that is common to both. For example, when mild, symptomless diabetes mellitus is first discovered in an elderly patient hospitalized for treatment of a peripheral ulcer of the foot, many clinicians are reluctant to make the diagnosis of diabetic ulcer, and will, instead, ascribe both the diabetes and the ulcer to a common atherosclerotic pathogenesis. According to some investigators[7] (including the eminent statistician, Sir Ronald Fisher[8]), both cancer of the lung and cigarette smoking may be caused by an underlying constitutional predilection or diathesis.

In circumstances in which the causal sequence is not clear or in which an underlying mutual cause may be responsible for two phenomena that clearly seem intertwined in a cause-effect relationship, the investigator may decline to choose a single temporal direction for the sequence of events. This type of conclusion produces the bi-directional *pathoconsortive studies* described in Section 18.4.3.4.

18.4.3.3.2. *Longitudinal Prevalence Studies*

In a longitudinal prevalence study, the prevalence of an outcome event is compared in a set of groups who have different serial intervals after onset of the principal maneuver. The maneuver can be physiologic or pathodynamic, and the groups are often called *longitudinal cross-sections*. This was the type of research described in Section 18.1.3, when we noted the prevalence of retinopathy in cross-sectional groups of patients who had diabetes mellitus for durations of 0 to 5 years, 6 to 10 years, 11 to 20 years, and >20 years.

Longitudinal prevalence studies are sometimes the only feasible way to investigate certain types of normal growth and development. For example, suppose we wanted to study the changes that occur in serum cholesterol as healthy people grow older from age 20 to age 60. In a cohort study, we would assemble a group of 20-year-old people, determine each person's serum cholesterol, and repeat the determinations at regular intervals (such as every 5 years) until the cohort becomes 60 years old. The concept is splendid, but the research would be extremely difficult to carry out. Even if the people could be maintained for 40 years, and even if they were willing to re-appear periodically for the tests, we might not be able to find an investigator who would sustain interest in the research over so protracted a time.

To get around this problem, we can quickly answer the basic question by conducting the research as a longitudinal cross-section. For this activity, we would assemble nine groups of people—ages 20, 25, 30, 35, 40, 45, 50, 55, and 60—and determine the average cholesterol values in each group. The change in cholesterol with aging would then be deduced from the pattern of the successive values in each age group.

Longitudinal cross-sections are commonly used in pediatrics to show the growth and development of normal children. The various growth curves that are demarcated into percentiles for height, weight, or other features related to age have the appearance of cohort data but are obtained by cross-sectional studies of the prevalence of these features in different age groups. Because the features under study are not likely to be associated with early deaths whose absence might distort the data for the residual survivors of the inception cohort, the pediatric results are probably trustworthy, although unconfirmed by specific cohort studies. When the longitudinal prevalence studies are concerned with the effects of a disease, or with the prevalence of an entity, such as cholesterol, whose high or low values may be associated with early deaths in an aging cohort of adults, the results can contain some of the serious distortions described in Chapter 21.

18.4.3.4. **PATHOCONSORTIVE STUDIES**

These studies have the ambiguous temporal interpretation mentioned at the end of Section 18.4.3.3.1. The investigator has assembled a group of cases who have a particular disease or several groups who represent different parts of the spectrum of the disease. A control group has also been assembled, consisting of healthy people or people representing other diseases. In these groups of cases and controls, the investigator compares the prevalence or distribution of a focal entity, E. The basic statistical architecture of the comparison is E/D vs. E/$\overline{\text{D}}$. For example, the investigator may find that the average levels of immunoglobulin zeta are distinctly elevated in patients with multiple sclerosis but not in healthy people or in patients with other neurologic diseases.

After pondering the results, the investigator may feel sure that a causal relationship exists between immunoglobulin zeta and multiple sclerosis, but the investigator cannot decide which came first. Did the multiple sclerosis produce the elevated levels of immunoglobulin zeta? If so, the research is structured pathodynamically, in a forward direction, as F/M vs. F/$\overline{\text{M}}$. Did the elevation in immunoglobulin zeta act as a provocative or contributory cause of multiple sclerosis? If so, the research is structured etiologically, in a backward direction, as M/F vs. M/$\overline{\text{F}}$.

When the investigator refrains from making this temporal decision (or when the report is written in a way that makes the decision difficult to determine), the uncertainties of a two-way temporal direction can be used to label the study as *pathoconsortive*. The performance of such bi-directional studies has been enhanced in modern clinical investigation by the availability of new technology for discerning metabolic products, cellular constituents, radionuclide images, and other entities that could not be measured formerly. (Readers who dislike the neologisms created to describe ideas in clinical epidemiology are paradoxically often quite satisfied with the new words that are coined to describe all the novel substances or concepts produced by the new technology.[9])

In other types of cross-sectional cause-effect studies, the temporal direction is (or seems to be) relatively easy to decide, because its plausibility is supported by a well-established background of laboratory experiments and clinical observations. Thus, when certain entities are noted in strong association with cases of disease, there is usually relatively little argument about forward decisions that the entity of retinopathy came after the onset of diabetes mellitus, that rheumatic fever followed a streptococcal infection, or that uremia was a consequence of glomerulonephritis. There is also relatively little argument about backward decisions that cigarette smoking preceded lung cancer, that maternal use of estrogens came before vaginal cancer in daughters, and that a high-fat diet had been consumed before an acute myocardial infarction. When abnormal entities are revealed by new technology, however, no previous measurements may exist to hint at their time of onset for patients studied in only a single state, and no background of documentary evidence may be available to suggest the most plausible single direction for the observed two-way relationship. The investigator is always free to speculate about the direction, but many researchers will often prefer the cautious, accurate conclusion that the direction is uncertain and that the observed relationship is pathoconsortive.

Because the statistical architecture of the research usually takes the form of E/D vs. E/$\overline{\text{D}}$ and the entity E is usually expressed in a dimensional measurement, the existence of a relationship is demonstrated statistically in results analyzed as a contrast of means (or medians), no matter whether the cause-effect direction is assumed to go one way, the other way, or both.

18.4.3.5. RETROSPECTIVE CASE-CONTROL (TROHOC) STUDIES

In three previous types of cross-sectional studies that use a case-control structure, the prevalence of an entity was interpreted in three different temporal directions: concurrently, the entity was evaluated for its role as a marker; forward, for its occurrence as a consequence of the clinical condition or disease noted in the cases; and bi-directionally, for its distinctive but temporally uncertain relationship as a cause or effect. These three types of studies are commonly done by clinical investigators concerned with questions about diagnosis and pathophysiology of disease. Yet a fourth type of cross-sectional case-control structure, with a fourth type of temporal direction, has been commonly used for epidemiologic research. Before this additional type of case-control research is discussed, we need to consider the problem of what to call it.

18.4.3.5.1. *The Scientific Problems of Nomenclature*

When a single cross-sectional research structure—the case-control study—can be used for the three different temporal directions and three different interpretations that have already been discussed, the ambiguity of the *case-control* nomenclature can create major scientific and intellectual obstacles for people trying to understand the results. The obstacles are both demonstrated and further increased when the term *case-control* is misunderstood and is misapplied as a label for yet another type of research study, having a quite different type of architectural structure.

The mislabeling may occur in circumstances in which the investigator has assembled a group of people from medical records and has followed them forward in serial time to note the outcomes that occur after exposure or nonexposure to a particular maneuver, which is usually a therapeutic agent. Such a study is constructed as cohort rather than cross-sectional research, because the observed group is followed forward from maneuvers to outcome. The retrospective feature of the data collection in such a medical record cohort study has been designated as *retrolective* in this text and as *historical* by other writers.

Nevertheless, the retrospective approach, which here refers to the collection of data rather than the temporal direction of the groups under study, may create a confusion that mixes up maneuvers and outcomes. The members of the exposed cohort may then become called *cases*, the nonexposed cohort become regarded as *controls*, and the *retrolective* (or *historical*) *cohort study* becomes mislabeled as a *case-control study.* This type of error regularly appears even in prestigious medical journals; and in one recent instance, when chastised about their incorrect nomenclature, the investigators were able to blame the editors for altering the original text to create the linguistic misdemeanor.[10] In some circumstances, the investigators may become so confused that the title *case-control* is applied to a retrolective study[11] in which the cross-sectional spectrums and subsequent outcomes of ankylosing spondylitis were compared in groups of women and men.

These four types of scientific ambiguity in the *case-control* label can be avoided by using the terms *marker, pathodynamic, pathoconsortive,* and *retrolective cohort* for the four types of studies and research structures that are under consideration. What still remains, however, is the confusion and potential intellectual bewilderment produced by a fifth type of case-control study, which is perhaps the most common of all the five types, and which is usually labeled merely as a *case-control study* or as a *retrospective case-control study.* In this type of research, which has been a basic staple of epidemiology for several decades, the prevalence of the investigated entity in the cases and controls is interpreted in a backward direction for its role as a possible cause of the clinical condition noted in the cases.

The term *etiologic case-control study* might be used to distinguish this type of research structure, but the structure is not reserved for studying etiology of disease and has often been employed to investigate the adverse or sometimes beneficial effects of therapy. The phrase *retrospective case-control study,* which is often used as another label, creates the problem described earlier in which *case-control* becomes misapplied to describe a retrolective *cohort* study. Besides, all case-control studies that investigate the cause-effect outcome of a maneuver are conducted in retrospect, after the maneuver has already been imposed.

Because the word *control* is sometimes misunderstood by readers who think it refers to a comparison maneuver rather than a comparison outcome, substitutes have sometimes been proposed for the word *control.* In the proposed substitutions, the research structures are called *case-compeer* or *case-referent* studies. Unfortunately, because a comparative maneuver is not clearly represented by any of the controls studied in marker, pathodynamic, or pathoconsortive case-control research, each of those studies also has a case-compeer or case-referent structure.

More than a decade ago, after my consultants in Greek and Latin were unable to offer a better substitute, I suggested that the word *cohort* be inverted to describe these backwardly directed case-control studies and that they be called *trohoc* research. The word obviously lacks a good linguistic pedigree, but it clearly denotes the structure and orientation of the research; it removes the scientific confusion of using *case-control* alone or *retrospective case-control*; and it probably has at least as much claim to etymologic legitimacy as the acronymically created *vipoma* and *radar,* the wholly imaginary *quark,* the hybridized bilingual *antibody,* and several other neologisms that have become generally acceptable. Nevertheless, for reasons cited in the smaller print that follows, the backward directed case-control studies will often be labeled as *retrospective case-control* or as *case-control* rather than *trohoc* in this text.

The main problem with the word *trohoc* is that it evokes outrage or hostility in many of my epidemiologic colleagues. Some of them regard the word as strongly unpleasant if not overtly offensive, and a few have never forgiven me for being its evil progenitor. At the time I introduced the word,[12] my scientific respect for retrospective case-control studies was low. I believed they were a grossly inferior substitute for cohort studies and—because all of my own previous cause-effect epidemiologic research had contained cohort structures that were used to investigate prognosis and therapy—I did not fully appreciate the logistic problems of trying to obtain cohorts with which to study etiology of disease. During the ensuing years, however, I have participated in retrospective case-control studies that were aimed at either etiology of disease or therapeutic relationships for which cohort research was unfeasible. I now realize that my main objections to backward-directed case-control studies were provoked by their relatively low level of scientific standards rather than by their backward temporal orientation. As noted in Chapter 23, I now believe that the studies are valuable, important, and indispensable for certain research questions. If conducted with suitable improvements in scientific quality, trohoc studies can often deserve and receive serious scientific attention and credibility.

The foregoing personal "confession" is intended to reassure my epidemiologic colleagues that I respect the importance of trohoc research. In fact, I respect it so much that I believe major efforts are warranted to develop scientific methods, standards, and criteria for its performance. Because one of the first steps in any form of scientific research is to try to remove imprecision and impurity, the persistence of the heterogeneous *case-control* or the misleading *retrospective case-control* names as a title for these studies is scientifically unsatisfactory. Because I proposed *trohoc* during the long-ago essay in which I was disdainful of the scientific value of retrospective case-control studies, however, some of my colleagues persist in believing that *trohoc* was also itself intended to reflect that disdain, and they hate it as a pejorative or denigrating term.

I did not intend *trohoc,* however, to be disdainful, pejorative, or denigrating. I wanted it to be a legitimate, reasonable word; and I spent many hours with diverse dictionaries and appropriate literary colleagues seeking a satisfactory substitute, before concluding that *trohoc* was better than *retrohort* (the other contender). Having subsequently become a convert, who believes that trohoc studies can be extremely valuable, I still feel the name is satisfactory. It clearly communicates what is happening in the research, and it clearly separates this type of case-control study from all the others. If my epidemiologic colleagues still do not like *trohoc* but still want to advance the scientific stature of epidemiology, they should propose a better name.

About a century ago when our clinical epidemiologic ancestor, Ignaz Semmelweis, was trying to get his medical colleagues to sanitize their clinical practice by washing their hands, he encountered vehement opposition from people who did not want to change their entrenched patterns of operation. I suspect that this type of inertia, not the repulsiveness of *trohoc,* is the main problem today when many of my epidemiologic colleagues are urged to sanitize their scientific taxonomy. Because the younger generation will not have this problem, and because I am much more concerned with improving the science than with christening the improvements, I have no reluctance to de-emphasize or even abandon *trohoc* if the greater scientific goals can be achieved.

To help in achieving those goals and to avoid giving needless agony to older colleagues (or compeers) whose teeth gnash, eyes bulge, and minds snarl whenever they see *trohoc,* I shall use the term sparingly in this text. The younger generation may accuse me of "copping out," and my friends may think this outbreak of diplomacy is definitive evidence of senescence, but I shall generally go along with "the establishment" and often refer to this type of research not as a *trohoc study* but as a *case-control study,* with *retrospective* or *backward-directed* sometimes added as adjectives. Because none of the other forms of case-control studies described in this text are called *case-control,* the term should be reasonably unambiguous, at least within the confines of this book.

18.4.3.5.2. *The Structure of Retrospective Case-Control Studies*

In a backward-directed case-control study, the goal is to obtain supporting evidence for a cause-effect relationship between an antecedent agent and the clinical condition (or disease) assembled in the cases. The activities were illustrated earlier in Section 18.2.3, when we investigated the cause-effect relationship of tea drinking and gallstones by comparing the prevalence of antecedent tea drinking in a group of cases with gallstones and in a group of controls without gallstones. After the prevalence of previous exposure to the suspected causal agent is ascertained in the case group and in the controls, the statistical architecture of the research has the structure of M/F vs. M/$\overline{F}$. The comparison of M/F vs. M/$\overline{F}$ is the most unusual statistical structure in all of clinical epidemiology. It is the only statistical structure in which the *outcome* appears in the *denominator* and the antecedent *maneuver* in the *numerator*.

The uniqueness of this statistical structure is a direct reflection of the uniqueness of the research itself. These studies are the only type of epidemiologic research in which the group under investigation is followed in an overtly backward direction. Furthermore, because of the types of agents investigated as possible etiologic maneuvers, the studies have four other important or unique distinctions:

1. Unlike the three other forms of cross-sectional, cause-effect, case-control studies that were previously described, trohoc studies of etiologic maneuvers rely on information obtained mainly from interviews of patients. The interviews may have been performed in a special manner for the research; or they may have occurred many years previously, with their results inscribed in medical records.

2. While evidence is being sought to ascertain previous exposure to the suspected principal maneuver, the patients and their medical records can also be checked for many other previous activities: occupation, smoking, drinking alcoholic and nonalcoholic beverages, education, physical activities, marital status, medications, nutritional intake, food supplements, and so on. Because each of these exposures can also be analyzed as a possible maneuver in the M/F vs. M/$\overline{F}$ format, no other form of cause-effect research has the same cornucopia of opportunities to check a plethora of etiologic suspects in a single investigation.

3. Because the agents suspected as antecedent maneuvers are often defined as events, such as cigarette smoking or usage of oral contraceptive agents, the M/F vs M/$\overline{F}$ data are often reported as prevalence proportions (or rates), rather than as the means, medians, or other average values cited in other forms of cause-effect case-control studies.

4. Because these prevalence rates allow certain additional special statistical calculations that cannot be performed with means or medians, the results of case-control studies, almost unique among all other forms of clinical epidemiologic research, are cited in an unusual statistical expression called the *odds ratio.*

These unique or distinctive attributes have allowed case-control studies to be generally quick, easy, and convenient for studying cause-effect relationships; and the case-control technique has become an ascendant[13] and often pre-eminent method for studying the etiology of disease. Because the maneuvers studied as etiologic suspects have often been events or factors that are imposed on the healthy people of a community, the investigators have often been epidemiologists based in departments of public health or community medicine. Unaccustomed to hearing the research presented at clinical meetings or clinical conferences, and being taught about it only during frequently unpopular public health courses in medical school, most clinicians are unfamiliar with the research methods and structures. Clinicians then tend to think of the studies as distant activities in epidemiology rather than as clinical research.

In recent years, however, the retrospective case-control technique has been applied beyond the etiology of disease to investigate topics that are a distinctive part of clinical investigation: the evaluation of the cause-effect impact of therapeutic agents. Most of the impacts investigated with case-control studies have been risks rather than benefits, but the techniques have been applied to investigate both types of outcome. The methods and results of this new type of clinical epidemiologic investigation pose a new set of challenges and problems for the non–clinically-oriented epidemiologist and the non–epidemiologically-oriented clinician. The epidemiologist must deal with a series of phenomena that are not found in the customary studies of etiology of disease in healthy people. These phenomena, although pertinent in any cause-effect relationship, are particularly striking when the relationship involves the outcome of therapy. The phenomena include the complexity of prognostic distinctions in pretherapeutic baseline states and the potential biases created when treatments are allocated without randomization and when outcomes are detected without standardized objectivity. The clinician must deal with a series of phenomena that are not met in the customary studies of clinical therapy for patients. These phenomena, although sometimes difficult to evaluate when presented in reports of randomized or nonrandomized cohort studies, may become inscrutable when the research architecture and statistical expressions are unfamiliar or alien to the customary processes of scientific thought.

Some of these challenges and problems will be discussed further in Chapters 20 and 21. Others will appear in Chapter 23, which is devoted exclusively to retrospective case-control studies.

18.5. SOURCES OF GROUPS

The people admitted to cross-sectional (and cohort) studies can come from so many locations and be chosen in so many ways that an entire chapter will later be devoted to the "sampling" procedure. In thinking about the bias that might be present in those samples, the main point of emphasis is what was known about each person's critical status for the two major variables (maneuver and outcome) *before* that person became selected for the study.

In certain circumstances, such as a community survey, none of this critical information is obtained until after the person is admitted to the study. In other situations, such as a hospital-based selection of cases and controls, information about the person's status for one of the two main variables is known before the person is admitted to the study; and the information can affect the likelihood of the person's selection. In yet other circumstances, such as a case-control study based at a special registry, information about the patient's status for both main variables was known before the patient's case was reported to the registry and may have affected the likelihood that a report would be submitted.

These different degrees of critical knowledge—before the person (or the person's data) was sent to the site of the research and before the investigator decided to include that person in the research—can produce the diverse problems cited in Chapter 21.

18.6. HYBRID STRUCTURES IN CAUSE-EFFECT RESEARCH

All of the cause-effect research structures discussed so far have been homodemic: information about the two critical variables of maneuver and outcome was determined individually for each person in the research. All of the structures discussed so far have also had groups that came from a single format, which was either a pure cohort or a pure cross-sectional arrangement.

In two types of research structure, however, a hybrid is created. One of the hybrids contains homodemic data for one of the critical variables and heterodemic data for the other. The second hybrid contains one group selected in trohoc fashion and another group selected like a cohort.

18.6.1. *Semi-Homodemic Ecologic Cross-Sections*

In this type of hybrid structure, a pathodynamic study is conducted by public health epidemiologists examining the inhabitants of small communities, rather than by clinical investigators examining patients. The variable that represents the outcome is observed homodemically, from direct examination of a cross-section of people in the region under investigation. The variable that represents the maneuver, however, is observed heterodemically, not as something that has been imposed or not imposed on each person but as something happening in the ecologic region in which the examined people live or work. The recipient of the imposed maneuver is the region rather than the individual persons.

One example of this type of *semi-homodemic ecologic cross-section* was a study[14] in which the investigators clinically examined 736 people in 17 villages in Nepal. The prevalence of goiter found in the people of each village was then correlated with the corresponding values for iodine content, fluoride content, and hardness of water in each village. In an analogous study,[15] diverse cultural, physical, and chemical variables were noted during the direct examination of 510 adults in three regions of the South Pacific territory of Palau. The results were then correlated with the modernization that each region had undergone.

The research conducted in these studies can be classified as having pseudo-cohort intentions, because the denominators are formed by maneuvers and the outcomes are numerators. Because goiter is a disease, the first study in the previous paragraph is clearly etiologic. The investigated groups were chosen according to the regions whose ecologic exposures formed the variables that defined the maneuvers. In that study, the maneuvers received by each region were the chemical attributes of the water. The statistical structure can be cited as either F/M_1 vs. F/M_2 vs. F/M_3 . . ., or F vs. M. Because the maneuvers are not imposed on individual people, the association examined as F vs. M in this research structure differs from the customary data arranged to relate one variable versus another in individual people. Each of the variables associated here is a spectral distribution of data for the region. Thus, an array of prevalance rates for goiters in each region is associated with an array of means (or other summary expressions) for the corresponding chemical values of the water in that region.

In the second study, the cultural, physical, and chemical outcomes can be regarded as salutary or etiologic, according to whether the investigators thought the observed cultural and other changes were either developmental growth or bad things, equivalent to disease. The three groups under study were defined by the three villages, which had differences in degree of modernization as their compared maneuvers. The outcome in each village was the spectral distribution of data for the examined cultural, physical, and chemical variables. The statistical structure is also F vs. M or F/M_1 vs. F/M_2 vs. F/M_3.

18.6.2. *Trohoc-Cohort Studies*

In this type of hybrid format, a group of cases is selected in the classic retrospective case-control manner from people who already have the effect (or disease) that is under etiologic investigation. The control group, however, is chosen from a group of people located in the same catchment region as the cases, but assembled at a serial time that *preceded* the development of the outcome event in the cases. The structure of the architecture is shown in the numbered sequence of Figure 18–1. (Because the architecture has elements of both cohort and trohoc structures, the impulse must be resisted to call these structures *cohocs* or to claim *trohoc-cohort* as a pioneering palindrome in the neologistic taxonomy of epidemiologic methods.)

The trohoc-cohort approach was illustrated in a study in which the investigators began with 3700 patients who had a definite or probable acute myocardial infarction during 1964 to 1970.[16] Among that group of potential cases, the investigators found 464 persons who had *previously* received a complete Multiphasic Health Check-up (MHC) in the Kaiser-Permanente health care system. These 464 people became the cases of the case-control study. Using the files of the MHC system as a catchment population, the investigators then chose, for each case, a control who fit certain demographic and other matching criteria and who had had an MHC examination on a date close to that when the case was originally examined. The properties found at the earlier MHC cohort examination were then compared as risk factors in the cases and controls.

A somewhat different example of this approach occurred in research in which the investigators[17] began with information for a catchment study population of more than 700,000 children born in 37 large maternity hospials during 1947 to 1954. Among this group, 556 children were noted to have subsequently died of cancer. They were chosen to be the cases, and their medical records were then reviewed to determine antecedent exposure to intrauterine x-rays. A control group, selected as 1% sample of the remaining 700,000 births, was similarly reviewed. The prevalence rates of intrauterine radiation exposure were 15.3% in the cases and 10.6% in the controls, leading the authors to conclude that an excess cancer mortality was associated with the intrauterine radiation.

Although the hybrid structure initially seems peculiar, it gives the research some of the major scientific advantages discussed in Chapter 20 for *population-based* or *closed-cohort* case-control studies. The investigation depends on a delineated cohort, thus avoiding many of the potential transfer biases occurring in the residues of cohorts that usually become selected as cases and controls in conventional studies. By using the hybrid arrangement, the investigator can achieve the basic virtues of a cohort study without having

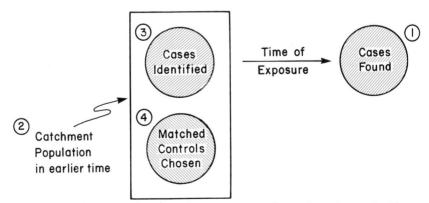

Figure 18–1. Timing of events and architectural sequence in a trohoc-cohort study. The cases are found in step 1; their earlier catchment population is the source found in step 2; the cases are identified in the source group in step 3; and a matching control group is chosen in step 4.

to examine and follow huge numbers of people to find a relatively sparse group of cases who develop the outcome event. The data structures have the statistical economy of a trohoc comparison of M/F vs. M/F̄, but the underlying arrangement is that of a cohort.

18.7. BENEFITS AND RISKS OF CROSS-SECTIONAL RESEARCH

Everything in life has benefits and risks, whether the entities under appraisal are technologic products, personal behavior, or investigative procedures. In the world of medical research, the versatility of cross-sectional studies as investigative procedures offers the striking benefits that have just been outlined. The studies allow us to examine a great many relationships and phenomena that cannot be investigated with the controlled, carefully planned experiments that would be scientifically ideal.

We may be able to persuade small numbers of volunteers to participate in experiments in which the potential harm is small and transient, but many of the other experiments that might be desired for ideal scientific evidence cannot be conducted. We either do not know how to create the disease to be studied or we cannot deliberately expose large numbers of human beings to the threat of harm.

We cannot take healthy people and deliberately expose them to suspected noxious agents in order to see whether those agents are etiologically capable of producing a disease. We cannot take healthy people and deliberately give them that disease in order to study the pathophysiologic phenomena, diagnostic markers, spectral markers, prognostic predictors, and long-term complications that occur as the disease begins, develops, and evolves. To study the pharmacologic action of drugs, we cannot maintain large colonies of human beings who would be exposed to huge doses for checking toxicity and who could be sacrificed to determine the drug's distribution and pharmacokinetics. If we suspect that an otherwise beneficial therapeutic agent has major adverse effects, we cannot deliberately give that agent to large numbers of people in order to study the frequency and consequences of the effects.

Even when the proposed investigation contains no threat of induced harm, we may still be unable to conduct the research according to a carefully designed plan that lets us arrange and observe everything from start to finish. We cannot follow large groups of people during an entire lifetime from birth to death in order to study all the physiologic changes that occur with normal growth, development, and aging. We cannot govern all the inherited genetic and metabolic factors, educational activities, marital choices, psychosocial interchanges, occupational selections, and other features of human life that can have profound effects on health and disease. Even if an experimental trial of therapy contains no risks, being intended to determine which of several beneficial agents is most effective, we do not have the time or resources to do all the randomized trials that would be needed for an experimental evaluation of each of the diverse therapeutic regimens made possible by modern technology.

Consequently, if we still want to study people to obtain answers to important medical questions about the physiology of human health, the pharmacology of drugs, and the etiology, pathophysiology, diagnosis, prognosis, and therapy of human disease, we cannot apply the tactics that are customarily regarded as the experimental method in science. In using resourcefulness and ingenuity to choose substitute tactics, medical investigators are challenged to preserve the scientific principles of the experimental method while evaluating the results of the natural or haphazard experiments designed by nature, by practicing clinicians, and by people themselves.

Cross-sectional studies have the virtue of being a prime substitute tactic with which to exercise that resourcefulness and ingenuity. Cross-sectional research can be used to investigate every one of the foregoing list of phenomena that cannot be studied with deliberate experimental plans.

The scientific risk we take in exchange for the investigative benefits of these substitutes is high. We may be able to do the research, but the results may be misleading, worthless, or wrong. We know that erroneous data and distorted comparisons may occur when experimental planning is impossible, but we may have great difficulty discerning the defects, minimizing their occurrence, and avoiding their deceptions. The ease with which cross-sectional studies allow us to do the research is more than compensated by the obstacles they produce in choosing suitable plans for the investigations, in understanding what emerges, and in preventing deluded conclusions.

The prevention of deluded conclusions is particularly important in medicine today because modern technology has produced so many risk/benefit ratios that require suitable evaluations and because physicians have such a long tradition of making wrong evaluations. The history of medicine demonstrates the humanitarian motives, personal dedication, and altruistic compassion that physicians have brought to their Samaritan function[18] in patient care, but also contains an unending sequential account of all the deluded conclusions that were reached in every era of medicine, from antiquity onward, during the investigation of every aspect of human health ranging from normal anatomy and physiology to the etiology and therapy of disease.

There is no reason to believe that modern medical intellects are immune from analogous errors when evaluating the risks and benefits of modern technology in causing, preventing, or curing disease. In fact, the opportunity for error is now much greater than ever before, because the scope of the challenges has been so enlarged. There are many more agents to be evaluated, many more conditions to be considered in the spectrum of health and disease, many more intricate complexities that can mask or distort the true phenomena, and many more investigations being conducted to yield results that may obscure rather than illuminate.

In clinical epidemiology, the process of evaluating risks and benefits involves an intricate interplay of scientific and statistical methods. Although the methods of science and of statistics are often discussed as separate topics, relatively little attention has been given to the way these two sets of methods are combined in medical research. Because the combination creates a distinctive pathway of reasoning when any type of research is conceived or evaluated, and because the opportunity for error is particularly high in cross-sectional studies, the sequential symbiosis of science and statistics will be discussed in the next chapter before we return afterward to the particular opportunities and hazards of cross-sectional research.

18.8. SYNOPSIS

In contrast to a cohort study, which obtains data for the outcomes that follow an initial state, a cross-sectional study contains information describing each person's condition at a single state in time. Cross-sectional research can be used to evaluate cause-effect relationships, to study processes, or to provide purely descriptive data; and the research can be designed with experimental scientific principles that can enhance accuracy and reduce bias in the data and groups under investigation. Special forms of cross-sectional explicatory experiments are regularly conducted in the pathophysiologically oriented research of contemporary clinical investigation.

Although only a single main state is investigated for each person, cross-sectional research structures can be arranged with an extraordinary versatility that can give the investigated relationships an apparently backward, forward, concurrent, or bi-directional orientation in the temporal sequence of events. This versatility allows cross-sectional research to be used for a large variety of investigations, whose structure can be displayed with symbols that denote both the architecture of the research and the basic statistical expressions.

Cross-sectional studies can have a forward orientation in biodynamic investigations of physiology or pharmacology, and in pseudo-cohort investigations that are used to discern pathodynamic effects of disease or other effects in longitudinal prevalence groups. The studies have an ambiguous temporal orientation in pathoconsortive relationships in which the cause-effect sequence is unclear. The orientation is backward in retrospective case-control studies of the effects attributed to etiologic or therapeutic agents.

The cross-sectional format often allows critical information about outcomes or maneuvers (or both) to be known before the investigated groups are chosen; and the format also can be used for hybrid arrangements of groups or variables.

This flexibility has made cross-sectional studies popular, inexpensive, and applicable to every type of question in descriptive or comparative research. In exchange for these investigative benefits, cross-sectional studies increase the risks of obtaining biased groups, erroneous data, and deluded conclusions in the research.

EXERCISES

Exercise 18.1. At the end of Chapter 2, Exercises 2.2.1, 2.2.2, 2.2.4, 2.2.6, 2.2.9, 2.2.10, and 2.2.11 all contained summaries of results of cross-sectional studies. Please classify each of these seven studies according to designations available in the inventory listed in Section 18.4. For each study, cite the two main variables being compared, choose appropriate symbols for those variables, and prepare a symbolic expression (as shown in Section 18.2) to indicate the comparison conducted in the research. (Because this is a difficult assignment, please do not worry if your responses do not coincide with the "official" answers. The goal is to get you to think about the contents and structure of these studies. Your ability to dissect and identify the components of the research will improve as you learn more about the studies in subsequent chapters.)

Exercise 18.2. Using any source of literature at your disposal, find the following types of research study:

      18.2.1. Cross-sectional explicatory experiment
      18.2.2. Spectral marker study
      18.2.3. Longitudinal prevalence study
      18.2.4. Pathodynamic study
      18.2.5. Pathoconsortive study

For each study, *briefly* outline (in no more than one or two sentences) what was done in this research. Prepare and provide a suitable explanation for a symbolic expression showing the comparison conducted in the research.

CHAPTER REFERENCES

1. Dieckmann, 1953; 2. Bibbo, 1978; 3. Bibbo, 1977; 4. Yates, 1980; 5. Kish, 1965; 6. Schaeffer, 1979; 7. Burch, 1980; 8. Fisher, 1959; 9. Feinstein, 1981; 10. Stuart, 1983; 11. Marks, 1983; 12. Feinstein, 1973; 13. Cole, 1979; 14. Day 1972; 15. Labarthe, 1973; 16. Friedman, 1974; 17. MacMahon, 1962; 18. McDermott, 1983.

Chapter 19

The Symbiosis of Science and Statistics in the Interpretation of Evidence

The evidence obtained in any type of research consists of raw data, usually cited in statistical expressions, for the groups arranged in an architectural structure chosen by the investigator. The evidence is then evaluated to draw conclusions and extrapolations. In cross-sectional studies, this evaluation is complicated by the diverse ways in which the actual structures of the research have been substituted for the desired structure of an experimental investigation.

The act of drawing conclusions and extrapolations is often called *inference*. In statistical inference, the evidence found in a substitute, called a *sample*, is extrapolated to the desired goal, called the *parent population*. The procedures of *statistical inference* are therefore concerned with standards for evaluating the accuracy and potential error of the sampled substitute. In cross-sectional studies, we often use an alternative research structure as a substitute for the architectural arrangement that we had in mind but could not construct. The procedures of *scientific inference* must therefore be concerned with standards for evaluating the accuracy and potential error of the architectural substitute.

Although the procedures and standards of statistical inference are frequently described, discussed, taught, and practiced, scientific inference is a generally unspecified activity. Unaccustomed to regarding the evaluation of evidence as an inferential procedure, some readers may even be surprised to see the noun *inference* preceded by the adjective *scientific* rather than by the usual prefix *statistical*. The inferences formed from ideas of scientific method and scientific experimentation often appear in published literature and in classroom discussions, but the ideas are usually presented as general concepts, and they are seldom accompanied by a citation of specific constituents in a specific sequence of inferential reasoning.

Because so many well-known scientific errors have occurred when conclusions were drawn from acquired evidence, the process of scientific inference warrants deliberate attention. This chapter, which provides that attention, could be placed anywhere in this text. It is put here because cross-sectional studies, to which we shall return when the chapter is finished, create a special challenge in scientific inference. In all the research discussed in preceding chapters, we were thinking about conclusions drawn from observed data and groups that were substitutes for the desired data and groups. In cross-sectional studies, the scientific inference contains a new and different challenge: we draw conclusions from research structures that were substitutes for the desired architecture.

The discussion in this chapter will outline the way that statistics and science are joined to form the data, groups, and structures that constitute the evidence of scientific research. This evidence becomes the "news" that is then subjected to the "editorial" processes called *inference* and *interpretation*.

19.1. PROBLEMS AND STANDARDS IN SCIENTIFIC INFERENCE

The main sources of error in drawing scientific conclusions from evidence can usually be attributed to flaws in the data, in the comparisons, or in the interpretations. The data that serve as basic information may be wrong or inappropriate; the comparisons may have been nonexistent or unsuitable; and even if the evidence is correctly obtained and compared, the observed distinctions may be ascribed to actions of the wrong agent.

The major intellectual advances of scientific method in the 19th and 20th centuries have been the establishment of standards for the scientific acceptability of comparisons and interpretations. In comparison, investigators are now obligated to provide a control for the proposed active agent, and, in interpretation, the investigators must rule out alternative hypotheses that might also explain the observed phenomena.

Because these two methodologic standards have been developed mainly in laboratories, where the investigators can readily arrange the studied groups of animals or inanimate substances, and where powerful technologic instruments can readily be used to get reliable measurements, the problems of flawed data have not received the same intensive attention that has been given to flawed comparisons and interpretations. When a laboratory investigator looks for alternative hypotheses to be ruled out, the focus is usually on other agents and actions. The investigator need seldom give serious attention to a different alternative explanation: defects in the basic evidence.

In clinical epidemiology, however, the data often come from observations that were not made under laboratory conditions, and the groups that produced the data are often formed arbitrarily by diverse human decisions and selections. The problems of flawed evidence therefore become a fundamental source of alternative explanations that must be considered. Before proceeding to "editorial" thoughts about alternative mechanisms of action for the distinction noted in the observed evidence, we first need to think about alternative mechanisms for the "news" itself. Before we formulate alternative hypotheses for the action of a principal agent, we must first formulate alternative hypotheses about biased data or a biased comparison that can distort the results of the structural mechanism from which the evidence has come.

The need for an additional set of alternative hypotheses greatly increases the opportunity for wrong conclusions in scientific inferences about the action of the agents studied in clinical epidemiology. A laboratory investigator, relatively free of problems in groups and data, can concentrate intellectual energy and imagination on thinking about alternative agents that may have been overlooked. A clinical epidemiologist must worry not only about alternative agents but particularly about the basic groups and data.

19.2. SCIENTIFIC METHOD AND THE PATHWAY OF "INTELLECTUAL METABOLISM"

The act of dissecting structures has been fundamental to scientific progress. The beginnings of modern medical science are often traced to Vesalius, who decided to study people rather than the writings of authorities, and who dissected the anatomic structures of the human body. Modern pathology began when Morgagni started systematic efforts to observe and dissect the morbid anatomy that lay beneath the exterior of a diseased body, and when Virchow later used a microscope to "dissect" the gross anatomic structures into tissues and cells.

In biochemistry, a pathway of biologic metabolism is constantly dissected into the sequential constitutents that occur at each stage. One of the earliest and best known of these pathways was Krebs' demonstration of constituent elements in the cycle with which carbohydrate was converted into carbon dioxide and water. The achievements of modern molecular biology depend on the awesome dissections made possible by electron microscopy and newer forms of biomedical technology.

The process of dissection is sometimes denounced as a reductionism that threatens the integrity of organismal biology and the dignity of human life. Because the pains and discomforts, sorrows and joys that occur only in living people cannot be observed in the dissected structures of biology, the reductionist techniques of scientific research sometimes become mistaken for scientific method itself and become attacked with the argument that science creates a diversion from many of the most important human phenomena that require creative intellectual attention. According to this argument, science can be used for investigating the reductionist phenomena of human biology and disease, but not for the organismal (or holistic) phenomena of human behavior and illness (or dis-ease).

The argument is particularly important for clinical epidemiology, because the basic phenomena of the research occur in individual persons or groups of people, and cannot be studied with the techniques of reductionist biomedical experimentation. If the distinctively human phenomena that have both humanistic and scientific interest cannot be investigated with scientific methods, the argument implies that the thought of doing scientific research in clinical epidemiology is itself a delusion and should be abandoned.

The argument, however, contains a fundamental error in reasoning. It is based on the assumption that scientific methods are carried out only with the *physical* (or chemical) dissections performed in reductionist biology. The human and humanistic phenomena of clinical epidemiology are all amenable to investigation with scientific methods, but the techniques are necessarily different from those of reductionist biomedical research. In particular, the dissections to be carried out in clinical epidemiology involve *intellectual* rather than physical structures and functions. The planning and evaluation of clinical epidemiologic research involve an intellectual pathway of *rational* "metabolism," during which a research plan is converted into a scientific conclusion. The pathway contains scientific reasoning that provides the "converting enzymes" for a sequential series of statistical structures that form the substrate of the metabolism.

This chapter contains a dissection of form and function for the symbiosis of statistical and scientific elements in that intellectual pathway. Our extraordinary ability to prevent or remedy disease in modern medical science has arisen mainly because we have learned to dissect the constituent elements of biochemical and physiologic pathways, to identify the different sites at which derangements can occur, and to develop appropriate focal interventions that can thwart or alter the derangements at those sites. Analogously, to prevent or remedy deluded conclusions in the interpretation of research evidence, we need appropriate dissections, identifications, and focal interventions for the intellectual pathways of analytic reasoning.

19.3. STRUCTURES AND FUNCTIONS IN THE INTELLECTUAL PATHWAY OF ANALYSIS

When an investigator conducts a research project in clinical epidemiology, the sequence of activities contains eight major constituents: (1) selection of a research hypothesis; (2) selection of a research structure; (3) acquisition and transformation of raw data; (4) organization of data into statistical structures; (5) scientific decisions about quantitative significance; (6) statistical inferences about stochastic significance; (7) scientific inference about the observed and desired architectural structure of evidence; and (8) research conclusions about confirmatory decisions, explicatory hypotheses, and policy decisions.

When a reader of the completed work decides to take a hard look at the evidence, the main outward evidence consists of statistical expressions that summarize the raw data of groups arranged according to the structure used in the research. The look usually begins superficially with a check that the two types of significance are indeed significant, i.e., that the observed distinctions are large enough to fulfill stochastic standards of probabilistic distinctiveness and scientific standards of quantitative importance. The look becomes hard when it penetrates beneath the exterior of the statistical expressions to evaluate the scientific quality of the raw data and to perform the scientific inference.

During that scientific inferential process, the evaluator decides whether the architectural structure that was planned or produced during the actual conduct of the research can be used as a satisfactory substitute for the architecture implied by the research hypothesis, which now appears as a stated conclusion of the research. If this inference confirms the substitution, the evidence can be accepted as supporting the hypothesis.

After accepting the evidence as "news" during these editorial appraisals, we can then advance to the more complicated editorial interpretations and judgments. They involve decisions about whether the hypothesis is confirmed rather than supported, whether alternative explanations are available for the observed phenomena and relationships, and whether the results should be followed by changes in scientific or public policy.

The sequence of these eight steps is listed in Table 19–1. The first three steps contain the plans and work that produce the news in the fourth step. The fifth, sixth, and seventh steps contain editorial appraisals of the distinctions and credibility of the news. The eighth step contains the main editorial judgments about the consequences in confirming and explaining the hypothesis and reaching policy decisions.

An investigator and a reader of the completed work go through the same constituent elements of the same intellectual pathway but use a different sequence. The rest of this chapter is concerned with the sequence in which investigators and readers use those constituents. (The next two chapters will be devoted to the reader's problems in evaluating the investigator's products.) Several of the constituent elements, which have already been

Table 19–1. SEQUENCE OF ACTIVITIES IN THE INTELLECTUAL PATHWAY OF CAUSE-EFFECT OR PROCESS RESEARCH

The Plans and Work	1. Choose a research hypothesis 2. Choose a research structure 3. Obtain the data
The News	4. Organize the data into statistical structures
Editorial Appraisal of Distinctions and Credibility of the News	5. Decide about quantitative significance 6. Decide about stochastic significance 7. Check the scientific inference from research structure to desired architecture
Editorial Judgments Re Consequences	8. Form conclusions about confirmatory decisions, explicatory hypotheses, and policy decisions

discussed, will be briefly recapitulated here. Others will be outlined in preparation for more detailed discussion later.

19.3.1. *Selection of a Research Hypothesis*

The research hypothesis consists of the question or questions that the research is designed to answer. In the comparisons used to answer questions about processes or cause-effect relationships, the hypothesis is expressed with the investigator's outline of the initial state, the principal agent, the comparative agent(s), and the subsequent state. To avoid the research equivalent of shooting arrows aimlessly into the air, the investigator can augment this four-component outline by stating the distinction that is expected in the compared results. In this statement, the investigator can indicate how big the distinction must be for the results to be regarded as similar or different; and if a difference is expected, the investigator can indicate which of the compared agents is expected to show it.

In a completely precise statement of the research hypothesis, the investigator might say something like, "I want to see whether the occurrence of an outcome event is increased to a value of w_A when people with a particular initial state are exposed to agent A, in comparison to the value of w_B that is expected when similar people are exposed to agent B." Because the exact magnitudes of w_A and w_B are often difficult or impossible to anticipate, the investigator may often omit their precise stipulation. The well-stated but quantitatively imprecise research hypothesis then becomes something like, "I want to see whether the occurrence of an outcome event is significantly raised (or lowered or similar) in people with a particular initial state who are exposed to agent A, in comparison with similar people exposed to agent B."

As noted earlier, the main flaws of many research projects occur at this very first step in choosing and stating the research hypothesis. The desired conclusions may not be sustained by the results of the research if the investigator has made unsuitable choices of the individual components of initial state and outcome event(s), or unsuitable choices of the compared agents. The subsequent quantitative and mathematical decisions about what constitutes a scientifically important and stochastically acceptable distinction may also be impaired if the magnitude and direction of the distinction were initially ignored. The reader and investigator may even have difficulty, as noted later, in deciding whether the conclusions of the research have come from a tested hypothesis or have merely been adapted to fit the unanticipated findings noted in the results.

19.3.2. *Selection of a Research Structure*

Having stated the distinction of the research hypothesis, the investigator next chooses the research structure with which to test it. At this point, the scientific architecture of the hypothesis and the actual structure of the research may become dissociated. Although a prolective experimental plan is implicit in the hypothesis, the realities of nature, people, and research may not permit the plan to be carried out.

The investigator may therefore have to substitute a retrolective rather than prolective plan for collecting data and for observing what happens after the compared agents are imposed. The agents may be imposed without an experimental allocation; the groups receiving the agents may consist of conveniently available cross-sections rather than inception cohorts; and the people receiving the agents may be studied heterodemically as groups rather than homodemically as individuals.

These alterations in the intellectual architecture of the research hypothesis are usually necessary to provide the substitute structures with which the research can actually be carried out, but the substitutions can create formidable barriers during subsequent intellectual efforts to understand the results of the research and to perform the penetrating analyses needed for sound conclusions in scientific inference.

19.3.3. *Acquisition and Transformation of Data*

If the research structure contains retrolective data, the investigator is at the mercy of whatever foci and quality were used when the archival information was observed, noted, and recorded. If the research structure is prolective, the investigator can establish methods to collect basic raw data that are suitable in both focus and quality. As noted earlier, these methods may be inadequate because a quest for high quality may omit a focus on important soft data, or because an appropriate focus on soft phenomena may not be accompanied by an adequate quality in the descriptive information.

Regardless of whether the basic data come from prolective or retrolective sources, the investigator must make many subsequent decisions that transform the raw information into the categories and scales of the simple or composite variables that become the basic elements of the descriptive statistics. These transformations may be carried out without suitable justification for the decisions, without documentation of the efficacy of the transformations, and without stipulated criteria that would allow the transformations to be performed with consistent reproducibility.

19.3.4. *Organization of Data into Statistical Structures*

Regardless of the quality of the data and the variables chosen to express the results, the overt evidence of the research is produced as the lists of numbers, rectangular tables, linear graphs, bar and pie graphs, and other displays that show the messages called *descriptive statistics*.

19.3.4.1. **PROBLEMS IN DESCRIPTIVE MESSAGES**

The format of the descriptive messages, which are usually the first item encountered by a reader taking a hard look at the evidence, may be a substantial impediment to their communication and to the subsequent efforts needed for the reader (and investigator) to get below the surface of the numerical information. The statistical structures may be strange and unfamiliar objects. The medical reader may comprehend a rate, but not an age-standardized rate or an actuarially-adjusted rate; a mean, but not a geometric mean; a risk, but not a relative risk or an attributable risk; an ordinary ratio, but not an odds ratio; a simple coefficient of correlation, but not a standardized coefficient of multivariate association; regression of a tumor, but not regression of one variable on another; an index of percentage agreement, but not a kappa coefficient of chance-adjusted agreement.

The communication of the descriptive message, which is the "news," may also be obscured by the intrusion of mathematical vocabulary from the "editorials" produced as stochastic inference. The medical reader may comprehend an error, but not a standard error; an interval of time, but not an interval of confidence; a normal state of health, but not a normal distribution of data; an asymptomatic patient, but not an asymptotic curve; a tea or tee, but not a t-test; a T-square, but not a chi square.

19.3.4.2. DIFFICULTIES IN CROSS-DISCIPLINARY COMMUNICATION

Because statistical expressions and statistical analyses have become so integral and essential in medical research, the interdisciplinary domain of biostatistics has been entered separately by statisticians and clinical biologists. Sometimes aided but usually encumbered by their previous background and education, the clinical biologists and statisticians may then have considerable difficulty in crossing disciplines to achieve a suitable understanding of the other domain's ethos: its motivating purposes, fundamental attitudes, underlying assumptions, and strategy of reasoning. In achieving this cross-disciplinary understanding, the statistician usually has a harder time than the medical person, although medical people are usually less successful.

The statistician may be as confused by the language and concepts of medical biology as the medical person is by the corresponding aspects of statistics. Familiar with the ideas associated with such statistical eponyms as Fisher, Pearson, "Student," Gauss, Wilcoxon, Mann-Whitney, Kaplan-Meier, and Cox, the statistician may be overwhelmed by the much larger series of eponyms used in clinical biology. Accustomed to thinking rather than memorizing or classifying, the statistician may give up the struggle to master the enormous taxonomic catalogs of terms acquired during medical instruction in anatomy, microbiology, physiology, pathology, pharmacology, and diverse clinical specialties, as well as the additional taxonomic catalogs containing concepts of ever-changing explicatory mechanisms for the biologic functions of the body in health and disease. The statistician may then apply his analytic talents to process the research information, but may not really understand what it means or implies.

The statistician may also not fully perceive the investigator's goals in doing a "statistical analysis" and the research difficulties in getting data. Having been educated in a mathematical setting where statistical analysis always begins *after* the data became available, the statistician may be unfamiliar with fundamental, primordial scientific challenges manifested in the acts of observation and description that convert existing phenomena into the human artefacts called *data*. Having learned to perform stochastic inference in an imaginary world of hypothetical populations from which samples could be chosen randomly, repetitively, and infinitely to achieve asymptotic estimates of the populational parameters, the statistician may not fully appreciate the dilemma of an investigator whose scientific inference depends on the results found in a single collection of data, obtained from assembled groups rather than from random samples, in a single project that may never be repeated.

The medical person, on the other hand, is often *innumerate* (the quantitative counterpart of *illiterate*) and is unaccustomed to the precise specifications, rigorous thinking, and consistent logical mechanisms of statistical methods. Medical investigators and readers who can overcome this intellectual barrier should have a much easier time learning the basic ethos of statistics than statisticians have in feeling comfortable with the immense diversity of biologic phenomena in medicine. As shown in Chapters 7, 8, and 10, the main descriptive techniques of statistics can be understood by any intelligent person who has made the effort to learn about indexes of central tendency, spread, trend, and concordance for one or two variables. When these indexes are extended to multivariate descriptions, the details become complicated and may often seem inscrutable, but the basic principles of the ideas are not too difficult to grasp. The basic principles of statistical inference can also be understood by any intelligent person who has made the effort to learn about estimating a parameter and to discover the strategies of doing a stochastic contrast with parametric methods, such as the t-test and chi square, or with nonparametric methods, such as the Fisher test and the Wilcoxon or Mann-Whitney U test.

Nevertheless, because medical people are so unaccustomed to numerate thinking and because their statistical instruction in medical school was often either nonexistent or unsuccessful, the medical people usually have much greater difficulty than statisticians in crossing the interdisciplinary boundary. Having a well-developed intellectual mechanism for rigorous analytic reasoning, statisticians can always get definitions for unfamiliar medical words; but medical people—whose education may emphasize prudence and judgment but not specifications for prudence and judgment—may be unable to shift their intellectual gears into unfamiliar patterns of thought.

The difficulties of cross-disciplinary communication are made worse by the many individual words that are used in substantially different ways by members of the two disciplines. The statistician and medical person may thus think they understand one another when they use the same word, but they may be thinking quite different thoughts. As noted earlier, the words *normal, error, regression,* and *interval* have different meanings in the two disciplines. *Variable* is usually an adjective to clinicians but always a noun to statisticians. *Variance* and *deviance* represent calculated quantities for statisticians but may be used by clinicians to describe abnormal patterns of behavior or a defective prosthesis (e.g., ball-valve variance[1]). Clinicians use the word *reliable* to denote something that is trustworthy; statisticians, to denote a process that is consistent or reproducible.

Clinicians use the word *precise* for a measuring instrument that produces a high degree of descriptive detail, i.e., one that can measure π as 3.14159 rather than 3.1. Statisticians, who are usually concerned with rounding, reducing, or summarizing data to eliminate excessive detail, have no word for a high degree of descriptive detail and instead use *precise* to refer to the spread of a set of measurements around the mean—a property that clinicians might label as *compactness* or *consistency*.

19.3.4.3. THE INTELLECTUAL PATHOGENICITY OF "SIGNIFICANCE"

And then there is *significance*—a word that is probably the single greatest intellectual pathogen in both biologic and statistical domains today. The word *significance* is an editorial, not a descriptive message of news, and it refers to two different things: a quantitative distinction in the results, which denotes their importance; and a mathematical attribute of the numbers, which denotes the probability that the observed distinction might arise stochastically, by chance alone, if there was no real difference in the compared agents. If the rates of success are 60% for treatment A and 40% for treatment B, the distinction is quantitatively significant. If the actual numbers that produce those rates are 3/5 vs. 2/5, the distinction is not stochastically significant. If the rates of success are 50% for treatment A and 49% for treatment B, the distinction is quantitatively not significant. If the actual numbers that produce those rates are 11,976/23,952 vs. 11,766/24,013, the distinction is stochastically significant.

Both types of significance require an editorial judgment that establishes a boundary. For quantitative significance, this boundary is δ, the size of the incremental difference that will be regarded as important. If the observed increment, d, exceeds δ, the observed distinction will be called *quantitatively significant*. In the two foregoing examples, the designation of *significant* was applied when d was 20% but not when it was 1%.

For stochastic significance, the judgmental boundary is called α. If the value of a calculated probability, P, is at or below α, we decide that the observed distinction is *stochastically significant*, i.e., it did not arise by numerical chance alone from agents that may actually have identical effects. Because α is commonly set at 0.05, the first distinction (3/5 vs. 2/5) was not stochastically significant because P exceeded 0.05; the second distinction (11,976/23,952 vs. 11,766/24,013) was stochastically significant because $P < 0.05$.

The two types of significance have a direct relationship to one another, as discussed in Section 9.5. The most important feature in this relationship is N, the size of the groups. If N is too small, as in the comparison of 3/5 vs. 2/5, a quantitatively important difference may not get its P value under the 0.05 stochastic boundary. If N is huge, as in the comparison of 11,976/23,952 vs. 11,766/24,013, the large value of N will multiply a quantitatively unimportant difference, such as 1%, and will make P stochastically significant. Thus, for the stochastic aspects of significance, nothing will be significant if the group size is too small, and anything can be significant if the group is big enough. Archimedes is said to have claimed that using a lever long enough and strong enough, he could move the earth. In the contrasts performed for statistical inferences about probability, the most infinitesimal difference can become stochastically significant if the group size is large enough.

The need for an adequate size of groups was often overlooked in older medical literature. Investigators would claim significance for the observed distinctions and would draw conclusions from groups whose sizes were so small that the distinctions could easily arise by chance alone. Whatever their importance, eminence, or implications, the results were stochastically nondistinctive. A laboratory investigator might make sweeping claims with results based on three animals. A clinician might hail a new treatment based on striking successes in two patients.

If the investigators were sufficiently insightful (or lucky), the claims of significance might be quite correct. In fact, a group size of $N = 1$ has been strikingly satisfactory in medical research in a single patient to show that insulin could promptly reverse diabetic acidosis, that penicillin could cure bacterial endocarditis, that a traumatically amputated arm could be re-attached, that an osteoarthritic hip could be replaced, and that a living heart could be successfully opened or even transplanted. Nevertheless, because few acts of medical research have such dramatic results and so convincing a set of historical controls available for comparison, critical reviewers and editors began to insist that statistical evidence be accompanied by a demonstration of its stochastic distinctiveness.

This decision inaugurated and encouraged the publication of the P values and other tests of "statistical significance" that now pervade the literature of medicine and public health. As prophylactic and remedial therapy for the stochastic maladies of statistics in medical research, the demand for stochastic distinctiveness has been splendidly efficacious, but like many other beneficial treatments, it has had major adverse side effects, including counterproductive abuse and addiction.

If the critical demand had been that the research have both types of statistical significance—that the statistical distinctions be significant in their stochastic as well as in their quantitative attributes—the current intellectual ailments might not have occurred. Unfortunately, however, the word *significance* was reserved for a purely stochastic connotation and the word *statistical*, which can refer to either the quantitative description or the stochastic inference, was attached to create statistical significance as a stochastic decision that has become a primary standard of quality, importance, and analytic evaluations in medical research.

At one of the world's leading medical journals, "statistical significance" became not only demanded as a prerequisite for publication, but the word *significance* was removed from general circulation and restricted to an exclusively stochastic usage.[2] "Significance" was allowed to appear in a manuscript only if accompanied by an appropriate P value or confidence interval. At a prestigious journal in psychology, the editor[3] decided to elevate the quality of the research by changing the stochastic boundary of α from 0.05 to 0.01. Papers would be accepted for publication only if the stochastic calculations showed P<0.01. Implemented also by other journals and by granting and regulatory agencies, the new policy announced that significance was now to be determined by mathematical calculations of stochastic probability, not by clinical or biologic judgments about substantive importance.

Although decisions about either quantitative or stochastic significance require judgmental answers to questions such as "How large is big?" and "How tiny is small?," the policy was easy to implement. Neither medical nor statistical people had given much attention to the judgmental boundaries needed for using δ as a standard of quantitative significance; but because quantitative significance was to be ignored, no boundaries had to be considered. To have a standard of stochastic significance, however, a judgmental boundary for α was already available. It had been set at 0.05 many years earlier, as an arbitrary, convenient custom used by Sir Ronald Fisher in making stochastic judgments and statistical inferences; and the boundary had been widely accepted by many investigators and statisticians thereafter. The difficult judgments involved in making quantitative and stochastic decisions and in choosing demarcations for δ and α could thus be neatly eliminated. The ultimate appraisal of significance for a research project could be reduced to determining whether its P value was above or below a single number that was precise, consistent, reproducible, and unequivocal: 0.05.

The policy has had a major adverse impact on the descriptive communication of research data, because investigators may be encouraged, or at least permitted, to publish results in which citations of significance have replaced the presentation of evidence. Instead of reporting the news that shows what was actually found in the research, investigators may present only the editorials that were determined as P values. A type of Guide-Michelin rating system has been developed to eliminate the need for reporting even the P values. Using *, **, and *** as respective symbols for P<0.05, <0.01, or <0.001, the investigator may present celestial tables in which the data have been replaced by stars.

The absence of the basic evidence makes it impossible for a reader to take a hard look at the evidence; but even when the basic data are reported, the current policy for determining significance has been a fundamental intellectual impediment to the reasoning and judgments needed during the next three steps in the pathway of scientific analysis.

19.3.5. *Scientific Decisions About Quantitative Significance*

Because the importance of a distinction inevitably depends on the particular subject that is being evaluated, decisions about quantitative significance are, like beauty, in the eye of the beholder. Because these decisions often are appropriately relegated to connoisseurs of the subject matter, statistical textbooks contain no discussion of the role of indexes of contrast in making the decisions. The increments, ratios, and proportionate increments that were discussed in Chapter 8 all appear in statistical literature, but they are presented either as purely descriptive indexes or as information inserted into the formulas used for calculating t, Z, X^2, or other test statistics used in stochastic contrasts. There is little or no discussion of the role of the descriptive indexes in performing quantitative contrasts and no attention to the need for examining two indexes: an increment and a ratio (or a proportionate increment).

Because clinicians have a long tradition of avoiding any specifications for quantitative judgments, and because no clinical biologist has had the towering influence, like Ronald Fisher in statistics, to have his convenient customs accepted as sacrosanct dogma, there are no medical standards for quantitative significance. As noted in Chapter 8, probably no one would dispute a fall in failure proportions from 0.60 to 0.40 as being quantitatively important and a fall from 0.05 to 0.49 as being unimportant. There might be considerable dispute, however, about a fall from 0.10 to 0.075 and even more dispute about the importance of a fall from 0.005 to 0.001. For the values of 0.005 and 0.001, however, the ratio of 5 is higher than the three preceding ratios, which are, respectively, 1.50, 1.02, and 1.33.

The absence of standards of quantitative significance for contrasted increments and ratios has been a boon for investigators, pharmaceutical companies, editors, and regulatory agencies. It has enabled the accomplishments of pharmaceutical substances or other maneuvers to be appraised exclusively according to standards of stochastic significance, while allowing editors and regulatory agencies to be consistent in approving (or disapproving) the results. If P is <0.05, the investigator is granted approval for the claim that the observed distinction is significant or that the tested drug is efficacious. Because the desideratum of $P<0.05$ can always be obtained, no matter how trivial the quantitative importance of the observed distinction, investigators who were wise enough (or fiscally supported enough) to study large groups have been able to achieve significance and to gain editorial or regulatory approval for claiming a significant action for agents that had minor importance in science or in clinical therapy. Conversely, however, an investigator who has found an agent of major quantitative importance may have his paper rejected for publication or his drug disapproved for marketing because one or two patients dropped out of the study, thereby raising the P value above 0.05 to the disastrous height of 0.06.

This policy continues to be generally applied during editorial and regulatory decisions about significance in medical research, even though the policy has been disclaimed or condemned by Fisher himself and by other prominent leaders in the world of statistics. Fisher[4] said that a rigid demarcation of a α level is "absurdly academic, for in fact, no scientific worker has a fixed level of significance at which from year to year, and in all circumstances, he rejects hypotheses; he rather gives his mind to each particular case in the light of his evidence and his ideas." Frank Yates,[5] known to medical investigators as the eponym for a correction in the calculation of X^2, used his presidential address several years ago to the Royal Statistical Society to complain about the "misuse of mathematical reasoning" that produces "irrelevant and misguided" decisions about significance. In the contemporary "bible" of statistics, an encyclopedic trio of four volumes called "The Advanced Theory of Statistics," Maurice Kendall and Alan Stuart[6] refuse to use the term *significance* because it "can be misleading." In an R.A. Fisher Memorial Lecture to the American Statistical Association, George E. P. Box[7] lamented the impact on investigators "overawed by what they do not understand," who "mistakenly distrust their own common sense and adopt inappropriate (mathematical) procedures."

Because the history of medical research also shows a long tradition of maintaining protracted loyalty to established doctrines long after the doctrines have been discredited or shown to be valueless, we cannot expect a sudden change in this medical policy merely because it has been denounced by leading connoisseurs of statistics. On the other hand, readers of the literature and investigators who have no incentive to (in Box's words) "mistakenly distrust their own common sense" can try to establish their own standards of quantitative significance, even if no one else wants to do so.

Such standards are almost always employed informally when individual investigators take their own first hard look at the research results. If the results did not come from a computer print-out that automatically produces P values along with the descriptive statistics, the investigators will first inspect the indexes of contrast to see whether a quantitatively significant distinction has been demonstrated. If so, the next step is to do the particular statistical tests that will denote whether the distinction is also stochastically significant.

The informal standards have a paramount value in appraising quantitative significance for the distinction observed in any set of comparative data. Although the standards are constantly applied in an informal unspecified manner, a formal decision is now required for two of the contrasts that were discussed in Chapter 8. In the first decision, when etiologic risk is evaluated for agents suspected of causing disease, the rates of individual risk are usually quite small. If the compared attack rates are as small as 0.0005 and 0.0001, clinicians, patients, and other members of society will have to use their own standards of importance for deciding what kinds of changes are warranted in personal life style and in national policy. If the decision depends on the total societal impact of the incremental risk, a society of 10,000,000 people exposed to an agent with an incremental risk of 0.0004 will have an additional 4000 cases of the disease. If the decision depends on individual human beings, however, an incremental risk of 0.0004 may not be persuasive enough to evoke major changes in personal life style.

The second decision requiring a formal standard of quantitative significance occurs when plans are made for large-scale clinical trials and other studies in which the investigators want to be sure to avoid the problems of type II statistical errors.[8] For this purpose, as discussed in Chapter 9, a level of δ is chosen as the quantitatively significant difference. The sample size of the study is calculated to be big enough to produce stochastic significance regardless of whether the observed distinction, d, turns out to be negative (i.e., $<\delta$) or positive ($\geq\delta$).

The actual process used to choose this crucial value of δ is seldom reported, but in a few available accounts, the investigators seem to have relied exclusively on θ, the proportionate increment in the two sets of occurrence rates expected as p_1 in the actively treated group and p_2 in the control group. Because $\theta = (p_1 - p_2)/p_2$ and $\delta = p_1 - p_2$, the value of δ can be promptly calculated as $\theta \times p_2$ after θ is selected. The usual choice of θ has been 0.5 or 0.25, which seems quite reasonable. Unfortunately, because a separate decision is not made about an important incremental value for δ, its size can be substantially altered by the choice of p_2 or its complementary value, q_2, for multiplication by θ.

An example of the problem was given in Section 8.5.1, and the difficulty will arise whenever separate decisions are not made for the levels of *both* θ and δ. The choice of complementary rates for success/failure or survival/mortality will befuddle not only the investigators but also the readers who evaluate the results of a completed trial. Suppose the investigators have shown that the mortality rate was 7.5% in the treated group and 10% in the control group and that the value of $d = 0.075 - 0.10 = -0.025$ is stochastically significant. Using the formula $\theta = (p_1 - p_2)/p_2$, the observed proportionate reduction in mortality is 25% $[= (0.075 - 0.10)/0.10]$, a value that may be regarded as quantitatively significant despite the relatively unimpressive incremental value of 0.025. A reader who decides to view the results as a proportionate improvement in survival rate rather than in mortality rate would calculate $\theta = (0.925 - 0.90)/0.90$ and would get a much less impressive θ (about 3%) for exactly the same set of data.

19.3.6. *Statistical Decisions About Stochastic Significance*

We can now resume the analytic sequence of reasoning at a point where the investigator (or reader) has observed a distinction, d, which has been deemed quantitatively significant enough to warrant being checked for stochastic significance. The quantitative distinction may be either large enough to suggest the conclusion that the results in the contrasted groups are different or small enough to suggest that they are not different.

The diverse stochastic tests that can be used to check either a difference or a similarity were outlined in Chapter 9 and are further discussed in appropriate textbooks of statistics. The main discussion now is confined to two important points that clinical epidemiologists should bear in mind when using the stochastic tests. The first point deals with the strategic principle used to determine stochastic significance, and the second, with the scope of the stochastic inference.

19.3.6.1. PRINCIPLES OF STOCHASTIC STRATEGY

The people who practice a particular craft—whether the craft be delivering health care or performing stochastic contrasts—usually operate under certain basic principles of strategy. In health care, these principles refer to a system of belief or school of thought about the mechanisms of human physiology, pathophysiology, pharmacology, or nonpharmacologic therapy. The practitioners of health care today include believers in such different systems as osteopathy, homeopathy, and naturopathy as well as the allopaths who hold M.D. degrees. In current Western society, the allopathic M.D.'s are the most prevalent, influential, and respected of these different types of practitioners, but the distinction does not hold true throughout the world.

Among practitioners of the particular forms of statistical inference used for stochastic contrasts, there are also at least three different schools of thought. All three are reasonably well respected, but the *relative frequentist* school is currently the most prevalent and influential. The relative frequentists work with the P values and confidence intervals that most medical readers are accustomed to seeing.

Although medical people usually assume that the frequentist approach is the only form of stochastic strategy, there are two other schools of stochastic thought. They are often labeled with the names *likelihood* and *Bayesian*. Members of the *likelihood* school (sometimes called the "likelihood brotherhood") work with various arrangements of "relative betting odds." Thus, a relative frequency of 0.05 might become a relative betting odds of 19 to 1. Members of the *Bayesian* school of inference work with subjectively anticipated probabilities, which are then compared with the actually observed rates of probability for outcome events. (The procedures used in Bayesian inference should not be confused with Bayes theorem, which is discussed in Chapter 20. Bayesian inference is a highly complex scheme of reasoning; Bayes theorem is a simple algebraic truism.)

Just as practitioners holding different systems of beliefs about health care may offer different treatments for the same ailment, practitioners of different systems of statistical inference may sometimes reach different conclusions about the stochastic significance of the same set of contrasted results. In one particularly interesting recent paper,[9] a clinical group of Bayesian analysts appraised results from several well-known randomized trials. The conclusions about stochastic significance were strikingly different in some instances from those previously obtained with the conventional relative frequentist approach. This demonstration of observer variability when different strategies are used for statistical inference is worth remembering, particularly by readers whose stochastic faith is devoutly placed in the frequentist icon of $P = 0.05$.

19.3.6.2. THE SCOPE OF STOCHASTIC INFERENCE

Regardless of which inferential strategy was used for the stochastic contrast, the investigator (and reader) must now contemplate the scope of the subsequent inference. To what decision do we project or extrapolate the results?

The principles of statistical inference were originally developed for the purpose of substitution. When a small sample substitutes for a larger parent population, the results found in that single sample are projected or extrapolated to the larger population. The concept of random sampling was developed to allow the sample to be an accurate, unbiased representative of the parent population.

The statistical inference that extrapolates results from a random sample to the larger population constantly occurs when political poll-takers, market analysts, social scientists, and other investigators conduct sample surveys to estimate the parameters of the population. When the results of two or more medical groups are contrasted for stochastic distinctiveness, however, neither group is chosen as a random sample from a larger population; and the investigator usually has no interest in estimating the parameters of a larger population. The investigator wants to know whether the group sizes are large enough to provide stochastic sustenance for the observed distinctions. Even when randomization was used to allocate the treatments that formed the groups, the groups themselves simply divide the total cohort admitted to the trial. The total cohort was not itself *randomly* selected from a larger population.

In addition to this scientific distinction in the two or more groups being contrasted, the statistical methods for performing a stochastic contrast are different from those used to estimate a parameter for a single group. To indicate this difference, statisticians usually refer to the inferential procedure of a stochastic contrast as *hypothesis testing*. The key distinctions of the frequentist, likelihood, and Bayesian schools of statistical inference are not in the way they estimate parameters, but in their methods of hypothesis testing for stochastic contrasts.

In the traditional frequentist technique, the basic method of parametric estimation from a single sample to a population is modified to form the two-group stochastic contrasts described in Section 9.4.2. The observed central indexes (as means or proportions) are assumed to be the results of random samples from two hypothetical populations. In the customary *null hypothesis*, the parameters for the central indexes are assumed to be equal in the two populations. The ensuing mathematical calculations then produce the P values or confidence intervals from which the data analyst decides to reject or concede the null hypothesis.

This statistical decision is very different from the inferential projection in which a substitute is used for estimating the real thing. In statistical hypothesis testing, the conclusion is a decision to reject or concede a hypothesis, not an inferential estimate that extrapolates a sample to a population. This distinction is recognized in the statistical vocabulary, which refers to a stochastic contrast as *hypothesis testing,* not as *differential inference, contrasted inference,* or some other name that might indicate an extrapolated conclusion beyond the observed data.

Regardless of what name is used for the statistical reasoning, a data analyst will choose a frequentist, likelihood, Bayesian, or other method for performing the stochastic contrast and will choose a standard (such as $\alpha = 0.05$) for demarcating the significance that occurs after decisions to reject or concede the null hypothesis. After completing the choices and the calculations, the investigator (or reader) makes the decision about stochastic significance.

If the observed distinction is regarded as stochastically nonsignificant, the pathway of intellectual metabolism may stop. The proposed conclusions of the research may be regarded as unacceptable because the numerical evidence is not stochastically adequate. The observed distinction may arise from numerical chance rather than from a definite biologic relationship. If the distinction is stochastically significant, however, the special nomenclature and concepts of the statistical reasoning can be crucial impediments to the next step in the scientific reasoning. During the scientific inference, the evidence obtained in a substitute research structure is to be inferentially extrapolated to the real thing. This scientific inference may be impaired or even ignored if the investigator fallaciously assumes that it was already accomplished during the statistical inference.

19.3.7. *Scientific Inference About Architectural Evidence*

Several assumptions or requirements are needed before extrapolations and other statistical decisions can emerge from stochastic reasoning about parameters and hypotheses. To estimate a parameter, we must assume that the sample was obtained randomly and that the test statistic has a particular type of distribution. (These distributions are often named eponymically after such people as Gauss, Poisson, and Bernoulli, but some have generic names, such as *hypergeometric* and *negative binomial*.) To test a statistical hypothesis, we need many more assumptions and/or requirements beyond random samples and distributions for test statistics.

For certain types of statistical tests, the samples must be *homoscedastic*, i.e., the observed variances in the groups must not be too disparate. To check this requirement, cautious analysts will perform special tests for heteroscedasticity before proceeding with a t-test or Z-test. For other types of tests, the samples must be *large enough* to sustain the basic assumptions about the distribution of the test statistic. Requirements of this type have led to the use of the t-test for small samples and the Z-test for large ones. (The requirement has also led to the current controversy about when and whether the standard chi-square test should receive the Yates correction or be replaced by the Fisher test.)

In making a scientific inference from the observed evidence to the concluded relationship, a scientific reader also makes a set of assumptions. They involve three important points that must be checked carefully, particularly if the observed evidence came from an architectural structure that substituted for the desired structure. According to these assumptions, (1) the observed raw data must reasonably represent the things they were supposed to measure; (2) the observed groups must be suitable surrogates for the larger groups they were supposed to represent; and (3) the research structures (as experiments or observational studies, cohorts or cross-sections, homodemic or heterodemic) must suitably represent the architectural structure that is intended or implied by the observed relationship.

These assumptions about data, groups, and architecture constitute the fundamental background for scientific inference. If the data are too inaccurate, if the compared groups are too unsuitable or biased, and if the structures used in the research do not contain adequate compensation for the potential distortion produced by their substitution for the "real thing," the observed relationship cannot be scientifically accepted and extrapolated.

After all the foregoing six steps of analysis have been completed, therefore, someone who is taking a hard look at the evidence that justifies a scientific inference is really looking for three things: hard data, hard groups, and hard structures. The reason for the scientific popularity of randomized trials is that they can, if suitably designed, provide hardness in all three attributes. The reason for the frequent controversies about randomized trials is that the data and compared groups, although hard in the sense of being accurate and unbiased, may be regarded as unsuitable for answering the focal clinical questions to which they were addressed.

The reason for the difficulties in forming scientific inferences from nonrandomized studies of maneuvers is that the nonexperimental structure may provide a suitable focus in data and groups, but the quality of the data may be low and the results in compared groups may be distorted. When a cohort structure is used for this nonrandomized comparison of maneuvers, however, the research has a reasonably familiar architectural format; and the investigator and reader usually have no difficulty discerning the potential flaws in data and groups.

The most formidable set of difficulties in scientific inference occurs for research done without a cohort structure. The difficulties are created by disparities between the ideal and actual structure of the research, by intervening events that can distort the collected evidence for the outcome of baseline states, and by the unfamiliar statistical expressions that are often used to communicate the results. Because of all these problems, the reader may have difficulty not only in analyzing the effects of the structural substitution but also in understanding what transpired to create the basic data and the compared groups.

These challenges in scientific inference often require a great deal of hard thinking for a reader who is trying to evaluate the evidence. Because this type of cerebral activity is not a popular indoor sport, many readers will avoid it if they can. One simple form of avoidance has been abetted by the vocabulary of the terms used in the preceding statistical reasoning. The words *inference* and *hypothesis testing* are regularly applied to the statistical activities, although these terms are particularly pertinent for the quite different scientific reasoning in which the reader is now engaged. In statistical reasoning, the inference is from a substitute sample to an extrapolated population; in scientific reasoning, the inference is from substituted evidence in data, groups, and structures to an extrapolated conclusion about the true state of an architectural relationship. In statistical reasoning, hypothesis testing is expressed in a simple symbolic expression about numbers, such as $H_o: \mu_1 = \mu_2$. In scientific reasoning, hypothesis testing refers to a relationship between initial states, compared agents, and subsequent states. A simple symbolism might be $F/M > F/\bar{M}$. Because of the massive confusion created by the ambiguity of using similar names for different ideas, neither the statistician nor the nonstatistician may be suitably prepared for the intellectual challenges of scientific inference and scientific hypothesis testing.

The statistician's background may provide little or no attention to quality in data, to the major problems that can occur when groups are not randomly sampled, and to the even greater problems of research in which the observed evidence does not arise from an experimental design. As noted by the biostatistician Marvin Zelen,[10] "The statistical design of experiments . . . as taught in most schools seems so far removed from reality, that a heavy dose may be too toxic with regard to future applications." Statisticians may even have been taught that there is no difference between the statistical and scientific testing of a hypothesis. As stated by G.W. Snedecor,[11] a prominent leader and teacher in modern statistics, "The purpose of an experiment is to produce a sample of observations which will furnish estimates of the parameters of the population together with measures of the uncertainty of these estimates." A statistician's excellence as a biostatistician depends largely on the ability to overcome the intellectual barriers of this type of misconception about scientific research.

For medical readers, the educational barriers that must be overcome are often formidable. Many people entered the world of medicine and public health because they were attracted by the soft, non-numerate phenomena of human clinical biology. Such readers neither desire nor welcome the irony of fate that later forces them to make decisions about those phenomena by having to take hard, numerate looks at statistical expressions of evidence.

The educational preparation for those hard, numerate looks was often either non-existent or grossly inadequate. The clinician's exposure to "scientific method" was usually confined exclusively to the type of research that can be done in an investigator's laboratory. Such research requires little or no attention to the wholly different strategies and tactics that are needed for using the scientific method to study groups of people under experimental or nonexperimental circumstances. The student may emerge having learned about scientific method in laboratory research, but the instruction may be as useless as extensive training in soccer might be for someone whose main athletic challenge in later life will be to play tennis.

If any instruction at all was given for the investigation of human groups, the curriculum did not focus on research methods, research architecture, or scientific reasoning. Instead, the instruction was usually devoted to elementary principles of statistical description and statistical inference. Because of problems in the way these principles are taught, however, students usually stay away in droves and fail to learn even the components of the statistical-scientific symbiosis needed to take hard scientific looks at the statistical evidence presented in medical literature.

For most medical readers, therefore, the job of taking these hard looks is a doubly onerous task. The reader did not originally anticipate or want to do such work; and now that it has been thrust forward as an inescapable professional obligation, the unprepared or confused reader feels incompetent and uncomfortable.

The vocabulary and concepts of statistics can then become particularly seductive in relieving this discomfort. If statistical inference is accepted as a substitute for scientific inference, the reader can fashion an escape. By regarding *statistical significance* as a merit badge that denotes both stochastic and substantive importance, the reader can avoid all of the hard reasoning needed to make decisions about quantitative significance in step 5 of the analytic pathway. By accepting the statistical consultant as an authority who knows how to do stochastic testing, by realizing that investigators and editors will usually pick competent statistical consultants, and by recognizing that editors will seldom publish work that fails to fulfill stochastic standards, the reader need not learn or know the tests and standards used in step 6 of the reasoning.

By regarding statistical hypothesis testing as tantamount to scientific hypothesis testing, the reader can also escape the arduous reasoning needed for step 7. The scientific hypothesis must be correct because it has already been tested. It need not be further examined because it has already been confirmed by the statistical act of hypothesis testing. The confirmation was delivered by the statement that the conclusion was *statistically significant.*

All of these blessings can be obtained by letting the two words *statistically significant* verify and replace three different major acts of scientific reasoning: that the observed distinction is important, that the distinction is numerically stable, and that the evidence was obtained with methods suitable for confirming the scientific hypothesis.

A reader who accepts this substitution can even extend its blessings beyond the radical medical resection it performs to amputate stages 5, 6, and 7 from the analysis. Because the reader is not going to examine the descriptive statistics to discern the importance of the observed distinction, the statistical structure of the organized evidence need not be checked, and step 4 can be eliminated. If the evidence deals with the evaluation of efficacy for a therapeutic agent, a reader who also accepts occasional advice[12] to disregard any evidence from structures other than randomized trials can eliminate many of the issues involved in step 2. A reader who gets no intellectual workouts during step 2 may then be in no condition to do the analyses needed when nonrandomized research structures are used to evaluate therapeutic agents for adverse reactions and safety, and when nonrandom-ized structures are used to evaluate hypotheses about physiology, pharmacology, etiology, pathophysiology, diagnostic procedures, prognosis, and many other aspects of medical care—but step 2 can be eliminated for issues in therapeutic efficacy. Because therapeutic efficacy is often the main interest of practicing clinicians, the removal of step 2 also helps ease the analytic burden.

Finally, if the reader accepts the principle that the investigators must have known how to obtain the basic information, because their work would not have been approved and published if they did not, step 3 can also be eliminated. The reader can thereby avoid worrying about the methods used to make observations, convert the observations into raw data, transform the raw data into statistical variables, and transmit the statistical variables into the coded information that is processed by the computer.

With all of these intervening steps having been accomplished by the investigator and either accomplished or eliminated by the reader, both the investigator and the reader are now ready for the grand finale.

19.3.8. *Subsequent Conclusions*

At this point in the intellectual pathway, the investigator and reader have each decided that the evidence is significant (both ways), that the scientific inference is justified, and that the results appraised in step 7 are regarded as consistent with the hypothesis stated in step 1. We can now conclude that the research hypothesis is supported by the observed results, but the reasoning is not yet finished. Before a final conclusion is reached, there are usually three more things to be done: the confirmatory decision, the explicatory hypothesis, and the policy decision.

For the confirmatory decision, we determine whether the results merely support the hypothesized relationship or actually prove it. Are we certain that the relationship indeed exists? If so, we can go on to the explicatory hypothesis, which provides an explanation for the particular action or mechanism that produces the relationship. Is the principal agent indeed responsible for the observed relationship, or might some other agent be doing the real work? If the principal agent does indeed do it, how does it do it? Regardless of what the explicatory hypothesis may be, the policy decision involves a consideration of what to do next. What beliefs should we change or what actions should we take as a consequence of what has just been demonstrated in the research? To answer these questions, we leave the arena of evidence—the methods, materials, results, and analyses that produced the "news" of a scientific report—and we move to a new enclave, usually called *discussion*, that produces the main "editorials."

19.4. **ADDITIONAL DECISIONS AND HYPOTHESES**

After the judgmental inferences that make the news acceptable, the subsequent editorial reasoning is usually concerned with two additional decisions and an additional act of hypothesis formulation. Because at this point in the intellectual pathway we have already accepted the evidence, the reasoning that produces the subsequent decisions and hypotheses can be uninhibited. It can proceed without any attention to flawed data or flawed comparisons as the source of an alternative explicatory hypothesis or as a restraint to conclusive decisions. We have already accepted the news; and we can now focus exclusively on the editorial conclusions.

Thus, we need not worry that surgery seems better than medical therapy because the medical treatment was reserved for sicker patients. We need not be concerned that people who choose to smoke may be prognostically more likely to get coronary disease than non-smokers. If antihypertensive agent A seems more efficacious than B, we can attribute the superiority to pharmaceutical reasons rather than poor compliance by patients or biased measurements of blood pressure. If people with well-regulated diabetes mellitus have fewer complications than those with poorly-regulated disease, we need not contemplate the likelihood that diabetics destined to have more complications are also more likely to have difficulty in regulation. If oral contraceptives are associated with an increased incidence of thromboembolism, we need not consider the possibility that thromboembolism has been defined and detected differently in women who do or do not use oral contraceptive agents.

All of these potential alternative hypotheses or decisional inhibitions —arising from flaws in data or from susceptibility bias, performance bias, detection bias, or transfer bias—can be disregarded now because they were all presumably considered during step 7, when the data and comparisons were evaluated during the act of scientific inference. If these alternative possibilities were not suitably considered and ruled out during step 7, they will remain as major sources of intellectual delusion and conceptual blunder when the reasoning, in step 8, focuses on the subsequent conclusions.

19.4.1. *Confirmatory Decisions*

The confirmatory decision involves the conclusion that the relationship demonstrated in the research is indeed demonstrated. This is the point where we check to see whether the research hypothesis was actually tested and confirmed in the research, or generated to fit the observed data. If the hypothesis was generated, it cannot be used as confirmation and must be tested in subsequent studies.

For confirmation, we usually require evidence from several studies, not just one, and the studies should preferably be done by different investigators working in different locations. This principle of demanding consistency or reproducibility for the observed relationship is a standard requirement in conclusions about confirmation, but the principle refers to editorial decisions rather than scientific news. As Harold Dorn[13] has pointed out, "Reproducibility does not necessarily establish validity, since the same mistake can be made repeatedly."

A lunatic in a mental hospital who repeatedly says he is Napoleon is consistent but not accurate. The consistently successful results that often followed the use of blood-letting in ancient medical therapy did not confirm its therapeutic efficacy. In much more recent times, a relationship between reserpine and breast cancer was subsequently discredited[14] despite the concomitant appearance, in the same issue of the same prestigious medical journal, of three different investigations[15–17] that were all consistent in supporting the relationship.

19.4.2. *Explicatory Hypotheses*

Regardless of whether the observed relationship deals with a process or a cause-effect impact, scientific investigators will usually try to develop an idea about the mechanism that explains the relationship. In process research, if two laboratories produce different measurements of a substance or if two practitioners make different decisions in patient care, what is the reason for the disagreement? In therapeutic research, what is the mechanism by which a particular agent creates its benefits or harm? In etiologic research or in other research concerned with mechanisms of health or disease, the investigator's data may support one mechanism, but other possible mechanisms always have to be considered.

Thus, for the research demonstrations that were contemplated just before Section 19.4.1, we might need to answer questions about the following alternative explicatory hypotheses: Is the surgery itself really superior to medical therapy, or does the beneficial effect arise from the associated anesthesia? Is cigarette tobacco the real etiologic culprit, or is it the paper in which the cigarettes are wrapped? In the pathophysiologic mechanism of hypertension, where does agent A act to produce its superiority over agent B? In diabetic patients, how does a well-regulated blood glucose level prevent or retard the development of atherosclerosis? What action of oral contraceptive agents produces an adverse effect on the physiologic mechanism of bleeding and clotting?

19.4.3. *Policy Decisions*

Finally, assuming that the suspected relationship is confirmed or that the explicatory hypothesis seems correct, what do we do about it? Do we change our belief about a fundamental scientific paradigm, concluding perhaps that the earth revolves around the sun, rather than vice versa? Do we institute new activities in health policy regarding sanitation and vaccination? Do we allow certain drugs to be marketed, removed from the market, or sold only with special warning labels? Do we allow health insurance plans or other agencies to pay for certain therapeutic procedures and to deny payment for others?

19.4.4. *The Seductiveness of the Confirmed Belief*

In all of the conclusions just cited, the investigator and reader become confronted by yet another hazard in scientific reasoning. Because no one approaches these conclusions without having some previous ideas, a person always holds some basic beliefs about the relationships, explicatory hypotheses, or policies that are being considered as conclusions. A characteristic feature of human nature in any act of reasoning is the ready acceptance of conclusions that confirm basic beliefs and a vigorous resistance to conclusions that contradict those beliefs.

The seductiveness of having a previous belief confirmed during the editorial process of interpretation may create a retrograde impact on the evaluation of the antecedent news. If the conclusions are agreeable, the reviewer may not conduct a careful search for flaws in the evidence and may then accept erroneous evidence; conversely, if the conclusions are disagreeable, a reviewer intent on discrediting the evidence may refuse to evaluate it rationally or may magnify trivial blemishes into major imperfections.

This type of intellectual seduction has been another fundamental barrier to rational scientific thought throughout the centuries. When the conclusion suggested by the research is compared with the belief held by the reader or by the scientific community, all further aspects of rational analysis may vanish. If the results confirm what we believe, the customary human tendency is to assume that they must be right. The research methods need not be examined closely because there is no need to do so. Having produced the right answer, the methods must also be correct. Conversely, if the results are contrary to what we believe, the research methods must be wrong, no matter how good they seem. According to the magnitude of the conceptual icon that is threatened by the research, the investigator who has produced the results may even be regarded as evil, dangerous, or deranged. The greater or more entrenched the paradigm that is threatened, the more likely is the reader to resist accepting the results and the more likely is the investigator to be assailed not merely for flawed research but also for flawed intellect or character.

19.4.5. *Examples of "Editorial" Triumphs and Blunders in Plausibility*

The history of science is replete with these "editorial" irrationalities, of which the assaults on Galileo and Darwin are two of the most prominent examples. The assaults occur when the observed results or proposed conclusions differ from the *doctrine of plausibility*. This doctrine usually represents the conceptual paradigms of the era: the basic beliefs whose statements often begin with "Everybody knows that . . . ."

In scientific activities, we think of plausibility as a type of educated common sense, formed by combining ordinary common sense with the additional wisdom acquired during instruction and experience in practicing a particular type of science; and we depend on this educated common sense to save us from deluded conclusions. Like other imperfect prophylactic agents, however, the doctrine of plausibility has many risks that accompany its benefits. The main risk is the *doctrine of entrenched resistance to implausibility*. The way we work out this risk/benefit ratio usually determines the triumphs or blunders that occur when scientific results are interpreted.

It is entirely plausible to demand that a cause be demonstrated to have preceded the effect. If a person was dead before the bullet was fired, the gunshot cannot be regarded as lethal. It is not plausible to believe (at least today) that storks bring babies, even though changes in the birth rate in Copenhagen once showed a positive correlation with the number of storks sighted flying over the city. In the days of ancient medicine, when plausible concepts of pathophysiology depended on an imbalance of four humors in the body, the medical therapy of the era was entirely plausible and "rational": the blood-letting, blistering, purging, and puking changed the balance of those humors. In more modern medicine, it was entirely plausible to use high concentrations of oxygen as prophylaxis for the respiratory distress syndrome that commonly occurs in premature infants. When many of the babies were blinded by retrolental fibroplasia, it was not plausible (at least initially) to regard the oxygen as the etiologic agent.

Using the doctrine of plausibility, a reader may be reluctant to accept conclusions or proposals that differ from what we already rationally believe or suspect. If the proponent of the irrational conclusions persists in pursuing the irrationality, the authorities who establish and maintain the plausibility of the attacked paradigm may then defend it by resorting to the doctrine of entrenched resistance. To avoid any invidious citations, my medical illustrations of this process are restricted to the work of people who are no longer alive.

In medical science, almost every plausible concept that has been held throughout the centuries about the causes, mechanisms, and treatment of disease has been either wholly wrong or so deficient that it was later overthrown and supplanted by other concepts. Furthermore, the people who proposed the conceptual corrections or improvements usually received substantial opposition and vilification. In fact, as we today recall the difficulties encountered by Vesalius, Sydenham, Morgagni, Hunter, Laennec, Virchow, Bernard, and Pasteur in trying to rectify errors in medical thinking, we may fall into yet another trap. Knowing the obstructions and calumny that were imposed upon these giants of anatomy, physiology, pathology, and microbiology, we may become hesitant to use our critical faculties lest we, too, become as recalcitrant and irrational as some of our professional ancestors. With this fear, whatever capacities a modern reader may have for rational analysis of plausibility may be suspended; and the reader may accept wildly implausible conclusions, such as the idea that storks bring babies, because the results are statistically significant.

In epidemiologic "editorial" reasoning, which has a much shorter history than the rest of medical science, there is a smaller number of outstanding episodes to demonstrate the two extremes. Nevertheless, examples can be cited for conclusions that were triumphantly correct despite overtly flawed methods, entrenched conceptual resistance, and colossal blunders that occurred after plausible interpretations of research conducted with what seemed to be the best methods of the era.

James Lind,[18] in 1753, performed a clinical trial of the treatment of scurvy, using non-randomized allocation of maneuvers, non-blinded observation of subjective endpoints, and an inadequate sample size—but he correctly demonstrated an accurate hypothesis about the use of citrus fruits in both treating and preventing scurvy. John Snow,[19] in the seminal act of modern public health epidemiology, performed an intervention that was non-randomized, that was appraised with historical controls, and that had major ambiguities in the equivocal time relationship between his removal of the handle of the Broad Street pump and the end of the associated epidemic of cholera—but he correctly demonstrated that the disease was transmitted through water, not air.

On the other hand, William Farr, still revered today for his pioneering role as the founder of modern vital statistics, performed a well-designed analysis[20] of carefully collected vital statistical data and noted that the occurrence rate of cholera was smaller in mountainous or other regions of low atmospheric pressure than in sea level regions, where atmospheric pressures were higher. Convinced of the plausibility of the miasma theory of transmission of epidemics, Farr interpreted his data as showing that cholera was produced by high atmospheric pressure; and for most of the rest of his life he vigorously fought the alternative hypothesis proposed by Snow.[21]

In one of the first public health epidemiologic investigations that actively obtained homodemic data from an ecologic cross-section, the Siler-McFadden commission[22] found pellagra occurring mainly in families and in neighboring households. Interpreting the results according to the prevailing concepts of etiologic plausibility, the investigators concluded that pellagra was an infectious disease with familial elements of vulnerability. When Joseph Goldberger,[23] in an ingenious set of epidemiologic investigations, later demonstrated correctly that pellagra was due to a dietary deficiency, his findings were initially vigorously opposed or outrightly dismissed.

In clinical epidemiologic studies of therapy for hospitalized patients, two of the pioneering investigators were Pierre Ch.A. Louis and Ignaz Semmelweis. Louis, developing the numerical method that made him probably the first clinical investigator to express statistical results in means rather than proportions, did a retrolective cohort study of bloodletting.[24] Because blood-letting had been used for centuries as the principal technique of non-surgical therapy, Louis was unable to find an untreated control group. He therefore compared the average duration of illness in patients who had received early versus late blood-letting. The study was non-randomized, retrolective, did not account for other therapeutic co-interventions (such as blistering, purging, and puking), and had a group size too small to avoid a significant type II error in its negative conclusion. Nevertheless, as the first quantitative evidence that blood-letting was generally ineffective, the work of Louis helped put an end to a treatment that had produced more harm than good. His work also brought him denunciation and opprobrium from leading members of the medical establishment at home and abroad.[25]

Semmelweis, after forming a hypothesis by studying retrolective data on the comparative occurrence of puerperal sepsis in two hospital wards, conducted a non-randomized prolective trial with historical controls. When the medical personnel of both hospital wards carefully washed their hands, the occurrence of puerperal sepsis was found to be much lower than in previous years, when the customary unsanitary practices were maintained. Semmelweis then indicted medical personnel themselves as agents in transmitting postpartum disease.[26] For many physicians of the era, who had already been unhappy about the use of statistical evidence to attack blood-letting, the statistical accusation that they themselves were causing disease was intolerable.

After Louis received the counter-attack on his work in blood-letting, he left the world of active clinical investigation, but his departure may have been prompted by depression developing after the death, at age 18, of his only child.[25] Semmelweis, although spirited enough to carry out and defend his pioneering research, did not promptly write up and publish its results. The prominent professors who had initially defended him against attack by obstetricians were angered by Semmelweis' failure to get his evidence into print. In an early demonstration of the "publish-or-perish" principle, the professors stopped giving him public support and Semmelweis was left to endure the calumny alone. Whether due to unrecognized Alzheimer's disease or to paranoid psychosis, he became unable to function, and his investigative career ended.[27]

The non-rational aspects of human behavior in interpreting and reacting to evidence were not unusual in that era, and are not unusual today. The occurrence of non-rational responses can readily be expected in scientists, because they are human, and particularly because the scientific method itself does not deal with human responses. The scientific method provides a rational procedure for getting evidence, not for making decisions about it afterward. The first seven steps in the intellectual pathway of scientific method determine whether the "news" is accurate and credible. The eighth step involves the "editorials" with which the news is interpreted and acted upon.

The enormous hazard of the editorial function—in any aspect of human life as well as in science—is its retrograde intrusion to distort or ignore the news. When determined to maintain a particular belief, the editorial writer or reader may misconstrue or neglect a suitable evaluation of the evidence that constitutes the news. Good news, although false, may be credulously accepted; and bad news, although true, may be tenaciously rejected.

This distinction is particularly important for the editorial judgments made when several studies are appraised to make decisions about causality.[28] For deciding about the benefits of modern therapy, the experimental clinical trial has been an important advance in scientific method, because it sets a standard for the quality of the evidence that will be accepted as "news." For deciding about the risks of therapy and of suspected etiologic agents that cannot be tested with experimental trials, however, no analogous scientific standards have been established for quality of evidence. The principles that have been developed for deciding about causality in non-experimental research are devoted to the editorials, not the news.

The scientific method used to evaluate quality of evidence is therefore particularly important in clinical epidemiology, because a well-established set of standards does not currently exist. As we return to the cross-sectional studies that are the most frequently used research structure in clinical epidemiology, the need for such standards and the problems of creating them will become particularly prominent.[28, 29]

19.5. SYNOPSIS

In studying mechanisms of biology and disease, scientific methods involve a physical "dissection" that reduces larger entities to smaller constituents. In studying the phenomena of clinical epidemiology, scientific methods involve an intellectual "dissection" of constituent elements in a pathway of reasoning. The pathway of intellectual "metabolism" in clinical epidemiologic research contains eight constituent steps.

In the initial step, the investigator forms the research hypothesis to be examined. In the second step, a research structure is chosen for the examination. In the third step, the investigator collects the basic data. In the fourth step, the data are organized into the descriptive statistical structures used for presenting the results. These four steps produce the descriptive evidence that becomes reported as the "news."

The collaborating clinicians and statisticians may often have difficulty in communicating and understanding the descriptive statistical messages. Statisticians, concentrating on the stochastic activities that come later on, may not fully appreciate the investigator's goals in the research or the basic difficulties in obtaining suitable groups and data. Clinicians, flustered by the unaccustomed demands of numerate reasoning, may be unfamiliar with the statistical expressions and may mistakenly assume that the news has been properly reported when it receives the stochastic rating of "statistically significant."

These problems in communication and understanding may impair the critical appraisals, occurring during the next three steps of the intellectual pathway, which determine the credibility of the news. The observed distinctions are evaluated for quantitative significance in step five and for stochastic significance in step six. Although principles of *statistical inference* are used in step six, the seventh step contains crucial issues in *scientific inference*. The scientific inference determines whether the observed data, groups, and research structure are suitable substitutes for the data, groups, and architecture of the relationship proposed in the research hypothesis.

At the end of these seven steps, if the evidence has been deemed distinct and credible, the intellectual pathway advances from accepted news to editorial interpretations. The editorial interpretations of the eighth step can contain three types of conclusions. One conclusion involves decisions about whether the hypothesized relationship has been confirmed or merely supported. The data used to generate a hypothesis cannot be used to confirm it; and consistently supporting data in several studies are not always confirmatory, because the same error can occur repeatedly.

A second interpretive conclusion involves formation of an explicatory hypothesis for the mechanism of the action noted in the main hypothesis. The third type of conclusion involves decisions about scientific and public policy. Which scientific beliefs should be changed and which public policies should be established or altered in response to the preceding conclusions?

These editorial interpretations often have a retrograde effect on the appraisal of the news. The news may often be accepted (or rejected) not because of its scientific quality as evidence, but because of its conformity (or non-conformity) to preexisting beliefs. The long history of medical science contains many examples of blunders produced by the plausible reasoning of an erroneous doctrine and of triumphs achieved despite an implausible contradiction of existing beliefs.

EXERCISES

Exercise 19.1. In several preceding exercises (13.1, 13.2, 13.3, 14.2, 14.3, and 15.6), you found examples of interesting research projects. Your assignment now is to retrieve some of those projects (or new ones, if you prefer) on the following topics:

    19.1.1. Randomized trial of a therapeutic agent.

    19.1.2. Observational cohort study containing a controlled comparison of a therapeutic agent.

    19.1.3. Observational study (cohort or non-cohort) containing a controlled comparison of an etiologic agent.

For each of the three studies you choose, briefly outline the research structure and tactics, and please give *brief* answers to the following questions:

    a. Did the published report contain specific attention to the quantitative (rather than stochastic) significance of the results? What are your reasons for believing that the results are (or are not) quantitatively significant?

    b. Did the published report contain specific attention to the issue of scientific inference for data, groups, and research structures? Do you agree that the reported evidence is scientifically acceptable? If not, *briefly* state the main reason for your disagreement.

c. Does anything about the published report suggest that the basic appraisal of the evidence was affected by preexisting beliefs about explanatory mechanisms or scientific policies? If so, briefly describe what happened.

Exercise 19.2. Section 19.3.4.3 contained several examples of research in which an important medical principle was demonstrated with the investigation of a single patient. Can you cite some examples of other principles that have been (or might be) convincingly shown by research conducted in a single patient, i.e., where N = 1?

Exercise 19.3. This exercise is intended to give you (and your colleagues) a brief review of your scientific ancestry and historical heritage. Different members of the class can be assigned to read the "old classics" cited in the list that follows and to present brief summary reports in class. The summaries should outline what was done, found, and concluded in the research. The reporter should indicate (if possible) which obstacles produced the blunder or had to be overcome in the triumph. The topics are as follows:

19.3.1. James Lind's study[18] of therapy for scurvy.
19.3.2. Pierre Louis' study[24] of therapeutic effects of blood-letting.
19.3.3. Ignaz Semmelweis' study [26, 27] of prophylaxis against puerperal sepsis.
19.3.4. William Farr's study [20] of the etiology of cholera.
19.3.5. John Snow's study[19] of public health prophylaxis against cholera.
19.3.6. The Siler-McFadden Commission's study[22] of the etiology of pellagra.
19.3.7. Joseph Goldberger's study[23] of the etiology of pellagra.

The reference numbers attached to each study in the foregoing list indicate a good starting place for your research on each topic.

CHAPTER REFERENCES

1. Hylen, 1968; 2. Ingelfinger, 1968; 3. Melton, 1962; 4. Fisher, 1959; 5. Yates, 1968; 6. Kendall, 1977–1983; 7. Box, 1976; 8. Freiman, 1978; 9. Diamond, 1983; 10. Zelen, 1969; 11. Snedecor, 1950; 12. Department of Clinical Epidemiology and Biostatistics, McMaster University, 1981; 13. Dorn, 1955; 14. Labarthe, 1979; 15. Boston Collaborative Drug Surveillance Program, 1974; 16. Armstrong, 1974; 17. Heinonen, 1974; 18. Lind, 1753; 19. Snow, 1855; 20. Farr, 1852; 21. Eyler, 1973; 22. Siler, 1914; 23. Terris, 1964; 24. Louis, 1836; 25. Feinstein, 1974; 26. Semmelweis, 1861; 27. Nuland, 1979; 28. Feinstein, 1979; 29. Feinstein, 1982.

Chapter 20

Statistical Communication of Cross-Sectional Evidence

Anyone who understands a national rate of unemployment, an index of average stock market prices, or a graph showing how inflation has changed with time should have no mathematical difficulty with the proportions, means, and associations that usually appear as descriptive statistical expressions in medical research. A person who knows what is involved in getting data and formulating statistical expressions for the cited economic indexes can readily look beneath the outer statistics to discern potential flaws when the economic evidence is used inferentially for cause-effect claims about political, social, or commercial interventions. The observed effects may be caused by the interventions but may also be artefacts of the statistical formulations. The rate of unemployment can rise or fall according to what is defined as *unemployed* and who is counted in the denominator. The stock market index can change drastically according to which group of stocks is used for the calculation. The movement of inflation can seem slow or rapid, ascending or descending, according to the points chosen as intervals of time on the graph.

In the foregoing economic examples, it was relatively easy to appraise the underlying structure rather than the external presentation of the evidence. We knew what was meant by the statistical expressions for the economic indicators, and we knew how the data got there. In clinical epidemiologic research, however, the outer statistical expressions can be a formidable impediment to communication of the interior news. The statistical expressions may be strange or unfamiliar items, such as an actuarial analysis, a relative risk, an odds ratio, a sensitivity index, a likelihood ratio, or an index of multivariate association. Beyond the problem of understanding what is being said by these "foreign" statistical terms, the reader may also be confused by scientifically unfamiliar methods of assembling groups and data.

These two sources of confusion in comprehending the news may then impair the reader's subsequent ability to perform editorial judgments. The reader may never get beyond the news to use the same common sense and intelligent thought that would be applied for judgmental appraisals of the statistical descriptions communicated in other aspects of daily life. The consequence is an intriguing paradox for people whose professional careers are concerned with medicine or public health. Despite no problems understanding the statistical evidence used in weather forecasts, sporting events, commercial activities, and the "political arithmetic" that gave rise to the word *statistics,* medical readers may have great difficulty comprehending the statistical evidence that appears in their own professional literature.

A capacity for penetrating beneath the outer layer of statistical expressions, for identifying the substantive interior distinctions, and for evaluating those distinctions is one of the main prophylactic agents needed to avoid intellectual blunders in scientific reasoning. After the interior distinctions have been identified for evaluating evidence in clinical epidemiology, we can use the architectural principles of scientific reasoning that were discussed in Chapters 11 to 17. We may never reach those inner distinctions, however, if we do not go beyond the external statistical expressions. A major block at this early stage of intellectual metabolism can completely thwart the sequential process of penetration, identification, and evaluation that constitutes an editorial appraisal of the news.

20.1. IMPEDIMENTS IN COMMUNICATION

The problem of obscure statistical communication is particularly likely to occur in cross-sectional epidemiologic research, because so many expressions have a format and orientation that differ substantially from what is used in other scientific structures. The obscurity can then produce three types of pre-empting block in the sequential process of editorial appraisal for the news. In the first situation, the editorial appraisal is never initiated. A reader who does not understand the superficial inferences conveyed by P values and by other stochastic indexes may be content to accept their proclamations of significance and to pay no further attention to the descriptive statistical results.

The second type of pre-emptive block often occurs when the reader falls victim to the confirmed-belief syndrome discussed earlier. If a cherished belief is contradicted, the reader will usually try to scrutinize the evidence closely. If a large ratio, a substantial increment, or the right direction for an inclining curve provides support for a cherished belief, however, the reader may decide that the evidence does not require checking.

A third type of pre-emptive block occurs when a reader who is ready and willing to take a hard look at the evidence actually tries to do so but has difficulty understanding it. Because the evidence consists of basic data, organized groups, and statistical expressions, each of these three components must be considered separately as well as collectively. The problems of obtaining and evaluating raw data for individual people were discussed in earlier chapters. The problems of organizing groups for cross-sectional studies will be considered further in Chapter 21. The rest of this chapter is devoted to the statistical difficulties of expressing and understanding results for cross-sectional studies.

Many epidemiologic studies, particularly in cross-sectional research, contain statistical expressions and arrangements of data that are distinctively different from the descriptive results presented in other types of scientific research. Although these descriptive distinctions can occur in the results of cohort as well as cross-sectional studies, the cross-sectional structure is particularly likely to create the five problems discussed in this chapter. Four of these problems are caused by a reversed orientation of data, by unfamiliar expressions, by the absence of reference denominators, and by an unknown attrition of denominators. A fifth problem is that the descriptive statistics may not even be available for inspection and evaluation.

20.2. **ORIENTATION OF DATA**

The diverse temporal orientations of cross-sectional studies can produce major ambiguities in the statistical data used to express the results.

Scientific thinking always goes in a forward direction: from cause to effect, from existence of a risk factor to occurrence of the actual hazardous event, from result of a laboratory test to the subsequently established diagnosis, from prognostic prediction to later outcome, from imposed treatment to ensuing response. In ordinary human logic, the statistical evidence used in this thinking might be expected to follow a similar orientation. The statistical data would be cited as effect per cause, hazard per risk factor, diagnosis per test result, outcome per prediction, or response per therapy.

In many cross-sectional studies, however, the structure of the research often produces statistical expressions having a reversed orientation. The data are collected and cited in such terms as cause per effect, risk factor per hazard, or test result per diagnosis. This reversed direction in the statistical expressions creates two main difficulties for the reader: the first problem (which is discussed throughout this chapter) is to retain mental clarity and orientation amid the disoriented statistics. The second obstacle (discussed in the rest of Section 20.2) is to understand the names and effects of the unfamiliar statistical activities.

20.2.1. *Ambiguity in Cause-Effect Case-Control Studies*

In a cohort study of a cause-effect relationship, the maneuvers determine the denominator groups who become the exposed or nonexposed cohorts. When an outcome numerator is divided by the corresponding cohort denominator to form an occurrence rate, we know that the quotient represents the incidence of an outcome per maneuver. In a cause-effect case-control study, however, the denominators can be formed by either the maneuvers or the outcomes—and either tactic can be confusing.

To make the statistical issue more concrete, let us consider the data that might have been obtained in the cross-sectional case-control study described in Section 18.1.3. Suppose we had assembled 80 patients with diabetes mellitus and the same number of control

Table 20–1. FOURFOLD TABLE SHOWING HYPOTHETICAL RESULTS IN A CROSS-SECTIONAL CASE-CONTROL STUDY

Presence of Hypercholesterolemia	Diabetes Group	Control Group	Total
Yes	21	6	27
No	59	74	133
Total	80	80	160

patients without diabetes. Let us also suppose that impeccable methods were used to measure each patient's serum cholesterol and to define hypercholesterolemia, which was found to be present in 21 of the diabetic patients and in six of the controls. These data would be arranged in the customary fourfold (or 2 × 2) statistical structure shown in Table 20–1.

For readers who approach the analysis of tabular results by first asking about stochastic significance, the answer can immediately be offered that it is indeed present in Table 20–1. The value of X^2 is 10.0 and P is <0.005. With this stochastic issue out of the way, we can turn to the descriptive analysis.

In thinking about the meaning of what is shown in Table 20–1, we can calculate several different proportions that would represent a statistical occurrence rate for the observed phenomena. The decision about which rates to calculate, however, would depend on what we think the phenomena represent. If we begin by considering diabetes as a possible pathodynamic cause of hypercholesterolemia, we would use the maneuvers as denominators. The occurrence rates of hypercholesterolemia would be calculated as 26% (= 21/80) in the diabetic group and 8% (= 6/80) in the controls. Although the comparison is structured as F/M vs. F/M̄, these occurrence rates are certainly not incidence rates, because a cohort was not assembled and followed. What has been calculated for each group is a cross-sectional prevalence rate that has a cohort connotation. Although we have not used serial time durations in the manner described in Section 18.3.3.3.2 for longitudinal prevalence studies, the occurrence rate obtained in this type of pathodynamic study can be called a *longitudinal prevalence rate*.

Now suppose we decide to regard hypercholesterolemia as a maneuver that may cause diabetes. With this hypothesis, we would again put the maneuvers in the denominators and use an F/M vs. F/M̄ comparison if we calculated the longitudinal prevalence rates of diabetes as 78% (= 21/27) in the hypercholesterolemia group and as 44% (= 59/133) in the people with normal cholesterol values. These calculations, however, are scientifically unacceptable for two different reasons. The rates are statistically illegitimate because the groups were originally assembled according to their attributes as diabetic or nondiabetic, not according to their cholesterol values. The use of cholesterol status to demarcate the denominators would not properly denote the way the samples were chosen. Unless the groups were selected according to their elevated or normal values of cholesterol, the denominators used for the occurence rates of 78% and 44% are statistically unsatisfactory. A second scientific flaw, even if we were willing to condone the proposed structure of the statistical rates, is that the results are clinically bizarre. They would indicate that diabetes is present in 78% of people with hypercholesterolemia, and even more incredibly, that 44% of people with normal cholesterol values are diabetic. These absurdly high rates of occurrence for diabetes would let us immediately know that these statistical expressions (or the basic data) cannot be trusted.

Consequently, if we still want to regard hypercholesterolemia as an antecedent maneuver that may cause diabetes, we need a more acceptable form of statistical expression. Because we assembled our patients as diabetics and nondiabetics, these groups can legitimately be used as denominators. We can then express the occurrence rates of hypercholesterolemia, exactly as we did before, as 26% (= 21/80) in the diabetic group and 8% (= 6/80) in the controls. These rates in the two groups would now represent the backward prevalence of hypercholesterolemia as an antecedent maneuver rather than its longitudinal prevalence as an outcome.

The rates just cited would be entirely appropriate statistically, because the proper denominators have been used. The rates would also be appropriate clinically, because these prevalences of hypercholesterolemia might reasonably be found in a group of diabetics and in a control group selected at a medical setting in which the research was being done. For cause-effect reasoning, however, the rates would now be structured as M/F vs. M/$\overline{F}$; and this statistical structure would create a drastically new mathematical arrangement of scientific thought. The outcome events—diabetes or its absence—would be counted in the denominators; and the imposed maneuvers—hypercholesterolemia or its absence—would be counted in the numerators. Despite the mathematical legitimacy of the statistical calculations, the results can discombobulate a reader's customary common-sense ideas about occurrence rates, because the calculated rates are now for prevalence of maneuvers per outcome, not for incidence or even for longitudinal prevalence of outcomes per maneuver.

If we wanted to know the risk of an obstetric complication when a baby is delivered by a midwife, we would look at how many complications occurred among babies delivered by midwives. Information about the prevalence of midwife deliveries in babies with obstetric complications would be confusing as well as useless for answering the question. Similarly, if we wanted to know the chance that flying in an airplane would lead to accidental death, we would not be helped by a prevalence rate for the proportion of accidental deaths that were due to airplane crashes. For therapeutic estimates of the relative frequency with which aspirin produces prompt relief of a headache, we could not use data showing the prevalence of antecedent aspirin usage in people with promptly relieved headaches.

The rates of antecedent prevalence for a maneuver are probably the single greatest source of difficulty for readers trying to appraise the cause-effect implications of cross-sectional data structures. Evaluating the chances of good or bad things that can follow a maneuver, people always think about occurrence rates that are incidences or perhaps longitudinal prevalences. For these rates, the compared maneuvers are put in the denominators and the outcomes in the numerators. When this well-established, traditional logic is violated, with the inversions that use outcomes as denominators and maneuvers as numerators, the destruction of a habitual pattern of reasoning may leave the reader too bewildered to retain any further capacity for critical appraisal. Backward reels the mind, confused become the thoughts, and insecure becomes the intellect as the reader struggles with the strange statistics to try to figure out what the figures really represent.

The M/F vs. M/$\overline{F}$ comparison of antecedent prevalence for a maneuver is a unique characteristic of retrospective case-control studies. The statistical structure is legitimate; and the research structure is often the best (or only) way to study the effects of maneuvers that cannot be investigated with cohort architecture. Nevertheless, the peculiarity of the statistical expressions is often a formidable intellectual barrier that stops a reader from taking the crucial first step in penetrating beneath the statistical expressions.

20.2.2. *Reversal in Diagnostic Marker Studies*

An alternative way to think about the cross-sectional case-control study in Table 20–1 is to regard it as process research rather than cause-effect research. In this situation, we would contemplate hypercholesterolemia not as a cause or effect of diabetes, but as a diagnostic marker for diabetes. With this approach, a clinician might examine serum cholesterol levels for the purpose of diagnosing diabetes when the test is positive (i.e., hypercholesterolemia) and ruling out diabetes when the test is negative (i.e., normocholesterolemia).

If hypercholesterolemia is to be used as a diagnostic marker for diabetes, the data in Table 20–1 would customarily be cited in two statistical indexes: The nosologic *sensitivity* of hypercholesterolemia as a positive marker in diabetic patients would be $21/80 = 26\%$. The nosologic *specificity* of normocholesterolemia as a negative marker in nondiabetic patients would be $74/80 = 93\%$. These two standard indexes are correctly constructed statistically because their denominators consist of the 80 patients chosen for each of the two groups in the study; but the values cited in the nosologic indexes have reversed the clinician's orientation in thinking about diagnosis. A clinician using cholesterol level as a diagnostic test for diabetes wants to know the diagnostic accuracy of positive or negative results for hypercholesterolemia. The denominators needed for these values come from marginal totals for the rows rather than the columns of Table 20–1. Diabetes was correctly identified in $21/27 = 78\%$ of patients with hypercholesterolemia; and the absence of diabetes was correctly identified in $74/133 = 56\%$ of patients with normocholesterolemia.

What the clinician really wants to know for the test procedure are the 78% and 56% values that respectively represent its *diagnostic* sensitivity, i.e., predictive accuracy of a positive result, and *diagnostic* specificity, i.e., predictive accuracy of a negative result. Instead, however, the customarily cited indexes are for *nosologic* sensitivity and *nosologic* specificity, using disease or nondisease groups as the denominators.

There are two main reasons for this reversal of orientation. First, because the groups of patients were assembled according to their attributes as diseased or nondiseased, the statistical calculations gain legitimacy if these attributes define the denominators of the indexes. Secondly, it is generally believed (as further discussed in Chapter 25) that nosologic sensitivity and nosologic specificity are *constant* properties of the diagnostic marker's identification of diseased and nondiseased groups. The indexes of diagnostic sensitivity and diagnostic specificity, however, are not constant properties of the marker. The reason for this variability will be shown in Section 20.3.3.

For the moment, the main problem to be noted is that a clinician cannot use the customary indexes of nosologic sensitivity and specificity that are provided by a marker study. To be applied clinically, the indexes must be converted by subsequent techniques, described in Section 20.3.3, that greatly increase the difficulty of understanding what is taking place.

20.2.3. *Reversal in Other Marker Studies*

In studies of spectral and prognostic markers, the problem of reversed statistics becomes particularly prominent when the dimensional data of the marker are expressed in central indexes for each part of the disease spectrum. For example, suppose we are evaluating serum omphalase level as a spectral marker to distinguish stages I and II of a particular disease. The results might be reported as follows:

Stage of Disease	Number of Patients	Serum Omphalase Levels (Mean ± s.d.)
I	17	6.1 ± 2.9
II	14	15.4 ± 6.2

Although the significant relationship between the stage of cancer and the level of omphalase shows its role as a spectral marker, the information is not reported in a clinically useful manner. Observing future patients with omphalase levels of 7.1, 10.9, or 14.7, the clinician will not know the diagnostic probabilities for locating each patient in stage I or II. For this decision, the data for the 31 patients in the spectral marker study would need a structural format that resembles the following arrangement:

Value of Serum Omphalase	Number of Patients with Stage of Disease	
	I	*II*
≤5	6	0
6–9	6	2
10–13	3	3
≥14	2	9
Total	17	14

This arrangement is suitable for clinical diagnostic usage. The chances of being in stage I are 75% (= 6/8) for a patient with an omphalase level of 7.1, 50% (= 3/6) for a level of 10.9, and 18% (= 2/11) for a level of 14.7.

This type of "pre-spective" statistics provides an estimate of clinical condition per marker result rather than the "post-spective" arrangement of marker result per clinical condition.

20.2.4. *Ambiguity in Ecologic Cross-Sections*

If forced to choose a directional orientation for the research presented in Table 20–1, most clinicians would probably make the assumption that diabetes leads to hypercholesterolemia rather than vice versa; and the clinicians would have no reluctance to accept 26% and 8% for the longitudinal prevalence rates of hypercholesterolemia in patients with and without diabetes. On the other hand, if presented with better data for longitudinal prevalence, clinicians might be willing to entertain the alternative proposal that hypercholesterolemia leads to diabetes. When we rejected longitudinal prevalence rates suggesting that diabetes occurs in 41% of normal people and in 78% of people with hypercholesterolemia, we were troubled more by the clinical absurdity of the rates than by their statistically illicit denominators.

A more acceptable set of denominators and rates of longitudinal prevalence could be obtained if the cross-sectional data came not from arbitrarily selected cases and controls, but from an entire community. Suppose we were able to do the research that allowed us to examine 10,000 people in a community and to determine whether each person had diabetes mellitus and/or hypercholesterolemia. Because each person was directly examined for both of the main variables, this study would be fully homodemic, in contrast to the semi-homodemic structures described in Section 18.4.1. The data would obviously be cross-sectional, and the study would be called *ecologic* because its group contains the members of a community. (Because the word *ecologic* has many modern connotations beyond residence in a particular locality, I would prefer to call such studies *communal, regional,* or *geographic* rather than *ecologic* cross-sections, but *ecologic* has become the customary adjective. Because the word may be passively jarring but not actively misleading, I shall not fight about it.)

A homodemic ecologic cross-section is a relatively unique form of cross-sectional research, not because the assembled group contains community people rather than clinical patients, but because only one group is assembled. For most of the research in which cross-sectional data are compared to study processes or cause-effect relationships, the investigator assembles two groups of people who become the cases and controls. In a homodemic ecologic cross-section, there is one group of people; and the data acquired when each person is examined will determine where that person is placed in the fourfold table of statistical results.

This distinctive method of assembling one group rather than two or more groups has some important scientific consequences that will be discussed in Section 21.4. At the moment, our main concern is with statistical problems in expressing the orientation of the results. Let us assume that the study of diabetes and hypercholesterolemia has again been conducted impeccably and that it yielded the results shown in Table 20–2.

The marginal totals of Table 20–2 show that diabetes was present in about 5% (= 497/10,000) of this population and that an elevated cholesterol level was present in about 8% (= 843/10,000). These results are clinically quite plausible. Furthermore, if we do some easy calculations, we can quickly see that the data show a distinctive relationship between diabetes and hypercholesterolemia. If the two events are unrelated in this group, we would expect their rate of concomitant occurrence to be the product of their individual occurrence rates, i.e., (843/10,000) × (497/10,000) = 0.0042. Instead of the expected 42 people, however, the upper left-hand cell shows 130 people. The observed concurrence rate, 0.0130 (= 130/10,000), is about three times higher (0.0130/0.0042 = 3.02) than would be expected if no relationship exists. (With this huge group of 10,000 people, we can anticipate that the value of chi square would be enormous, and it is: X^2 = 212.9. My available statistical tables go only as far saying that when X^2 in a fourfold table exceeds 30, P<0.000001. For X^2 of 212.9, P is even smaller.)

We now can feel pretty sure that hypercholesterolemia and diabetes are definitely related in this group of people, but we also have the pathoconsortive uncertainty described in Section 18.3.3.4. Which way does the causal direction go? Because we assembled only one group of people rather than two or more groups, we need have no statistical inhibitions about what to put into the denominator of any comparison of rates. We can go either way. It is legitimate to use a diabetic demarcation of denominators and to compare the longitudinal prevalences of hypercholesterolemia as 26% (= 130/497) and 7.5% (= 713/9503) for people with and without diabetes. It is also legitimate to use a hypercholesterolemic demarcation of denominators and to compare the longitudinal prevalences of diabetes as 15% (= 130/843) and 4% (= 367/9157) in people with and without hypercholesterolemia. Both sets of rates are also quite reasonable and should raise no clinical problems about plausibility. We could therefore use this evidence to support a causal claim that goes in either direction, without being constrained by either the statistical structure or the clinical plausibility of the data—but which way should we go?

A different problem arises if we want to compare the results by using the ratios and increments that express a statistical contrast. If we calculate the indexes of contrast for

Table 20–2. FOURFOLD TABLE SHOWING HYPOTHETICAL RESULTS IN AN ECOLOGIC CROSS-SECTIONAL STUDY

| Persons Found to Have Hypercholesterolemia | Persons Found to Have Diabetes: | | Total |
	Yes	No	
Yes	130	713	843
No	367	8790	9157
Total	497	9503	10,000

26% and 7.5%, the ratio is 3.47 (= 26/7.5) and the increment is 18.5%. If we use 15% and 4% for the same calculations, the ratio rises to 3.75, but the increment drops to 11%. The ecologic cross-section has thus produced a splendid set of statistical results, but we are left with the uncertainty of not knowing which causal direction to choose and how to express the observed contrast.

20.3. **PROBLEMS IN COMPOSITE STATISTICAL INDEXES**

To be expressed statistically, data are reduced into indexes that summarize such attributes as central tendency, spread, trend, concordance, or contrasts. To facilitate further interpretation of the data, two or more of these indexes are often further reduced by being combined into a single composite index.

For example, the index of relative dispersion (or coefficient of variation) that was discussed in Section 7.6.1 is obtained by dividing an index of spread by an index of central tendency. Thus, if the standard deviation of a set of data is 0.72 and the mean is 2.1, the index of relative dispersion is 0.72/2.1 = 0.34. All indexes of contrast are obtained in this composite manner by subtracting or dividing two single indexes of central tendency to form the increments, ratios, or porportionate increments that describe the contrast. This same tactic is often used scientifically with individual items of data rather than with statistical indexes. Thus, the albumin/globulin ratio for an individual patient's serum might be determined as 1.43 if the serum albumin level is 4.0 and the globulin level is 2.8.

The attractiveness of these composite expressions is obvious. They can reduce the work load of interpreting data by allowing the reader to focus on one expression rather than two. When used for two individual variables of data rather than for statistical indexes, the composite expressions often provide a better summary of a particular phenomenon than either variable alone. Thus, the Quetelet index, which contains a composite of height and weight, is often a better way of denoting obesity than either weight alone or height alone.

Nevertheless, when a composite index is formed, the individual components of data are lost. The loss can be particularly important if a reader needs to know each component to understand what the data show. For example, despite its popularity a generation ago, the albumin/globulin ratio is seldom calculated today. A clinician evaluating a patient's condition wants to know the individual values of albumin and globulin. During this evaluation, the clinician may mentally consider their ratio, but the ratio alone, without the component constituents of albumin and globulin, would be an unsatisfactory communication of data.

Similarly, the index of relative dispersion is a useful way of contemplating the compactness of a set of data, but cannot substitute for the individual indexes of central tendency and spread. For example, the value of 0.34 cited earlier as an index of relative dispersion was obtained by dividing two values as 0.72/2.1. It could also have been obtained from 47/139. If given only the value 0.34 for relative dispersion, however, we would not know whether the central index of the data is located at 2.1 or at 139.

In trying to understand a contrast of data, we need two separate statistical indexes of contrast: an increment and a ratio (or a proportionate increment) as noted in Chapter 8. We cannot fully evaluate a contrast if given only an increment or a ratio but not both. Because single composite expressions are so statistically attractive, however, they have regularly been created for various phenomena in clinical epidemiology. In exchange for this statistical appeal, the composite expressions produce two major hazards in communication and interpretation. A reader may not understand what is meant by the unfamiliar expression; and even if it is understood, the reader may not be given the component elements that are needed for thoughtful interpretation. The most popular composite expressions that produce these intellectual benefits and risks in clinical epidemiology are the risk ratio, the odds ratio, Bayes theorem, the likelihood ratio, and data that have been adjusted or standardized. These five types of composite expressions are individually discussed in the sections that follow.

20.3.1. *The Risk Ratio*

Many clinical readers are confused by the statistical usage of the word *risk* because they think of it as a single expression, such as 4% or 0.04. In fact, however, a statistical *risk* is a quotient, or rate, that has a distinctive numerator and denominator. The term might be less confusing if we called it a *risk rate* rather than *risk*.

In Table 20–2, suppose we contemplate hypercholesterolemia as a risk factor for diabetes mellitus. The risk of diabetes in normocholesterolemic patients is 367/9157 = 0.040, or 4.0%. The risk of diabetes in hypercholesterolemic patients is 130/843 = 0.154, or 15.4%. These two risks are simple proportions or occurrence rates. Their indexes of contrast consist of a direct increment, which is 15.4% − 4.0% = 11.4%, and a ratio, which is 15.4/4.0 = 3.85.

Because the contrast refers to two risks, a special name can be given to their ratio. As noted in Chapter 8, this ratio is often called the *relative risk, relative risk ratio,* or *risk ratio.* Because all three of these commonly used terms refer to exactly the same thing, readers are sometimes confused by the excess of jargon alone. For simplicity (and consistency), only the term *risk ratio* will be used here.

Although perfectly adequate as an index of contrast for two risks, the risk ratio may create confusion for readers who do not understand its meaning and components. A clinical reader seeing a quotient such as 130/843, and realizing that all such quotients can be regarded as ratios, may become confused about the distinction and may think that 130/843 is a *risk ratio,* when it is merely a *risk* or *risk rate.* A risk ratio really consists of four numbers, not two. The actual numbers that produced the foregoing risk ratio of 3.85 are (130/843) ÷ (367/9157).

The greatest scientific risk of the risk ratio, however, is not what it contains but what it omits. It does not indicate the increment of the contrasted risks, and it does not indicate the basic risk that is being incremented. If cited as the only index of contrast, a risk ratio of 3.85 does not tell us whether the component risks are 0.04 and 0.154, or 0.0004 and 0.00154, or 0.20 and 0.77. To interpret the ratio, however, we need to know whether its constituent elements are 77%/20%, or 15.4%/4%, or 0.154%/0.04%.

20.3.2. *The Odds Ratio*

In Section 20.2.4, we had a substantial problem in deciding which indexes of contrast to use for expressing the results of Table 20–2. Because of the ambiguous orientation of the data, we did not know which set of denominators was correct for calculating the indexes. If we used cholesterol for the denominators, the indexes of contrast were 3.85 for the ratio and 11.4% for the increment. If we used diabetes for the denominators, the indexes of contrast were 3.49 for the ratio and 18.7% for the increment.

This type of statistical ambiguity can arise in any fourfold table, regardless of whether the table was constructed from an ecologic cross-section or from separate groups of cases and controls. Although the two sets of indexes of contrast were not widely disparate in the ecologic cross-section data of Table 20–2, the disagreements can be quite striking if we determine the same pair of indexes for the data of Table 20–1.

In Table 20–1, if diabetes demarcates the denominators, the occurrence rates of hypercholesterolemia are 26% and 8%, yielding 3.25 as the ratio and 18% as the increment. With hypercholesterolemia demarcating the denominators, the occurrence rates of diabetes are 78% and 44%. For this pair of rates, the contrast ratio is substantially lowered to 1.8 (= 78/44), but the increment is substantially raised to 34%.

This is an unpleasant state of affairs. According to an arbitrary choice of denominators, we can get two different sets of indexes of contrast from exactly the same collection of data. The problem might seem to be an unresolvable dilemma, but the ingenuity of statistical expressions provides a way out.

20.3.2.1. **ADVANTAGES OF THE ODDS RATIO**

The foregoing dilemma can be neatly avoided if we get rid of the denominators and use the odds ratio that was described in Section 8.5.3. Although applicable to any fourfold table, the odds ratio is a particularly ideal expression for citing results in pathoconsortive data structures. The elimination of denominators allows the odds ratio to go both ways and to give the same result either way. In Table 20–2, the odds ratio can be calculated as (130/367) ÷ (713/8790) to yield a result of 4.37. In this calculation, the values of 130/367 and 713/8790 each gave the odds respectively of finding hypercholesterolemia in people with and without diabetes. If we wanted to go in the other direction, the respective odds for finding diabetes in people with and without hypercholesterolemia are 130/713 and 367/8790. The ratio of these two odds is (130/713) ÷ (367/8790), and the odds ratio is exactly the same 4.37 that we found when looking in the opposite direction. The odds ratio has thus eliminated the problem of choosing a direction. It gives the same result no matter which direction we choose.

Furthermore, in a fourfold table arranged with the basic interior cells of $\begin{Bmatrix} a & b \\ c & d \end{Bmatrix}$, such as the $\begin{Bmatrix} 21 & 6 \\ 59 & 74 \end{Bmatrix}$ of Table 20–1, we need not go through the process of writing or calculating the odds ratio as (a/b) ÷ (c/d) or as (a/c) ÷ (b/d). Either one of these arrangements becomes algebraically reduced to the simple structure: ad/bc. Because we can determine the odds ratio quickly and simply by multiplying the two terms of each inner diagonal and then dividing their products, the odds ratio is also called the *cross-product ratio*. The sequence of operations in a fourfold table is to multiply a × d and then b × c and then divide the products.

20.3.2.1.1. *Focal Arrangement of an Odds Ratio*

Although the odds ratio is bidirectional, the table that produces it must be suitably arranged to let the ratio focus on the particular relationship that is under consideration. Suppose we have found the following data:

| Presence of: | | Number of |
Variable X	Variable Y	People
Yes	Yes	a
Yes	No	b
No	Yes	c
No	No	d

When we set up a fourfold table for this information, we can put the X variable in the rows and Y in the columns, or vice versa. We can also let the *Yes* responses precede the *No* responses, or vice versa. Because the *a* and *b* results each represent a *Yes* response in variable X, they must always appear either in the same row or same column. The c and d results, representing a *No* response in X, must also be in the same row or column, opposite to that of a and b. Because a and c both represent a *Yes* response in variable Y and because b and d represent a *No*, these two pairs have an analogous relationship. The quartet of $\begin{Bmatrix} a & b \\ c & d \end{Bmatrix}$, somewhat like the optical isomers of a chemical structure, will therefore always maintain its basic spatial arrangement, regardless of how the pattern is rotated or put into mirror images, such as $\begin{Bmatrix} b & a \\ d & c \end{Bmatrix}$.

In half of the spatial arrangements, however, the criss-cross multiplication that produces the odds ratio will yield ad/bc, and the other half will yield the reciprocal value of bc/ad. Thus, if Table 20-1 were arranged as $\begin{Bmatrix} 6 & 21 \\ 74 & 59 \end{Bmatrix}$, rather than $\begin{Bmatrix} 21 & 6 \\ 59 & 74 \end{Bmatrix}$, the tabulation would still be quite correct as a table, but the odds ratio would be $(6 \times 59)/(21 \times 74) = 0.228$, instead of the 4.39, which is 1/0.228, that is obtained with $(21 \times 74)/(6 \times 59)$.

Some further analysis of the possible patterns will show that the ad/bc arrangement occurs whenever the two Yes-Yes and No-No cells, i.e., a and d, appear in the $\searrow$ diagonal that goes from upper left to lower right, regardless of whether a or d is on top. The bc/ad arrangement occurs whenever a and d cells are in the $\nearrow$ diagonal, going the opposite way.

Because the *Yes-Yes* concurrence of events (as for patients with both diabetes and hypercholesterolemia) is usually the main focus of the fourfold table, the ambiguity can always be prevented if the *Yes-Yes* cell is put in the upper left corner. The *No-No* cell will then automatically appear in the lower right corner. Regardless of whether the X or Y variable is chosen to be row or column, the odds ratio will then represent the focal value that is desired for ad/bc.

20.3.2.1.2. *Underlying Algebra of an Odds Ratio*

The odds ratio is so valuable in cross-sectional statistics that a bit of relatively nontraumatic algebra seems warranted to show how it works its magic.

Let us assume the X and Y represent two different binary response variables, each having the responses *Yes* and *No* (or *Present* and *Absent*), as shown in Table 20-3. Thus, X might be hypercholesterolemia and Y might be diabetes mellitus. For a total group of N people, let us assume that the result in X is *Yes* for n_1 people and *No* for n_2 people. We are interested in knowing the proportionate rate, or prevalence, with which a *Yes* in variable Y occurs in these two groups. Let us call these two proportions p_1 and p_2 respectively. Thus, there will be $n_1 p_1$ people who are positive for Y in the X-positive group and $n_2 p_2$ people who are positive for Y in the X-negative group. Using the customary notation that $q_1 = 1 - p_1$ and $q_2 = 1 - p_2$, the numbers of people who are negative for variable Y will be $n_1 q_1$ in the X-positive group and $n_2 q_2$ in the X-negative group. We have now produced the four basic cells of Table 20-3. The row totals will be n_1 and n_2; and for convenience of notation, let us represent the column totals as $f_1 = n_1 p_1 + n_2 p_2$ and $f_2 = n_1 q_1 + n_2 q_2$.

Now let us consider what happens when we calculate the conventional indexes of contrast, using the conventional arrangements. With variable X supplying the denominators for the contrast, the rates of occurrence for a positive result in Y are $n_1 p_1/n_1 = p_1$ and $n_2 p_2/n_2 = p_2$. The indexes of contrast will be $p_1 - p_2$ for the increment and p_1/p_2 for the ratio. With variable Y supplying the denominators for

Table 20-3. ALGEBRA FOR THE ODDS RATIO

Variable X	Variable Y		
	Yes	*No*	**Total**
Yes	$n_1 p_1$	$n_1 q_1$	n_1
No	$n_2 p_2$	$n_2 q_2$	n_2
Total	$n_1 p_1 + n_2 p_2 = f_1$	$n_1 q_1 + n_2 q_2 = f_2$	N

the contrast, the rates of occurrence for a positive result in X will be n_1p_1/f_1 and n_1q_1/f_2 respectively. The increment will be $(n_1p_1/f_1) - (n_1q_1/f_2)$ and the ratio will be $(n_1p_1/f_1) \div (n_1q_1/f_2) = p_1f_2/q_1f_1$. These two indexes are quite different from the previous increment and ratio.

To compare the two increments, we can use some additional algebra (which the reader will be spared) to show that $(n_1p_1/f_1) - (n_1q_1/f_2)$ becomes converted to $(p_1 - p_2)(n_1n_2/f_1f_2)$. Because the other increment was $p_1 - p_2$, the two increments will always differ unless $n_1n_2/f_1f_2 = 1$, or $p_1 - p_2 = 0$. In the latter instance, the proportional rates of occurrence will be identical; and the variables X and Y will have no "relationship." To compare the two ratios, we can note that one is p_1/p_2 and the other is p_1f_2/q_1f_1. These two values will always differ unless $p_2 = q_1f_1/f_2$.

On the other hand, when we eliminate the total denominators from the calculations, the positive occurrence of variable Y has an odds of $n_1p_1/n_1q_1 = p_1/q_1$ in the X-positive group and an odds of $n_2p_2/n_2q_2 = p_2/q_2$ in the X-negative group. The odds ratio will be p_1q_2/p_2q_1. Looking in the other direction, the positive occurrence of variable X has an odds of $n_1p_1/n_2p_2 = p_1/p_2$ in the Y-positive group and $n_1q_1/n_2q_2 = q_1/q_2$ in the Y-negative group. The odds ratio will again be the same: p_1q_2/p_2q_1. This value will differ from the p_1/p_2 ratio that was found with one arrangement of denominators, and the p_1f_2/q_1f_1 that was found with the other—but the odds ratio will be the same in either direction.

20.3.2.1.3. *The Odds Ratio in Cross-Sectional Sampling*

In addition to the statistical virtue of being unaffected by the denominators and orientation of two contrasted variables, X and Y, the odds ratio in a fourfold table has yet another immensely appealing attribute. If the groups contained in a case-control study suitably represent the parent ecologic community, a case-control study and an ecologic cross-section should produce similar odds ratios.

For example, let us first assume that the 80 people with diabetes in Table 20–1 are a random sample of the 497 diabetics in Table 20–2. With this sampling fraction, which is $0.161 (= 80/497)$ of diabetic people in Table 20–2, we would expect to find hypercholes-terolemia present in $(0.161) \times 130 = 21$ and absent in $(0.161) \times 367 = 59$ of the diabetic cases in Table 20–1. Now let us assume that the 80 nondiabetic people in Table 20–1 are a random sample of the 9503 nondiabetic people in Table 20–2. With this sampling fraction, which is $0.00842 = 80/9503$, we would expect to find hypercholesterolemia present in $(0.00842) \times (713) = 6$ and absent in $(0.00842) \times (8790) = 74$ members of the control group in Table 20–1. Looking at Table 20–1 (which, of course, has been "rigged" to show this point), we see that these expectations are confirmed.

You may now recall that when we used denominators to calculate conventional indexes of contrast for Tables 20–1 and 20–2, the two sets of indexes for each table were different within and between the tables. Thus, the two possible ratios to express Table 20–1 were 3.25 and 1.8; and they were 3.47 and 3.75 for Table 20–2. All this disparity vanishes, however, if we calculate the odds ratios. The odds ratio is $(21 \times 74)/6 \times 59) = 4.39$ in Table 20–1 and $(130 \times 8790)/(713 \times 367) = 4.37$ in Table 20–2. (The slight difference is due to the difficulty of getting fractions of people to appear in real-world research. For the odds ratios to be identical, we would need $(80/497) \times 130 = 20.93$ rather than 21 people in the upper left cell of Table 20–1 and $(80/9503) \times 713 = 6.002$ rather than six people in the upper right cell.)

This attribute of the odds ratio is glorious. We ordinarily think about representativeness as requiring one process of random sampling, not two. If we used two processes, with two different sampling fractions, we would worry that something would surely go wrong in the ultimate statistics. Nevertheless, we can use two distinctively different random samples—one having a sampling fraction of 0.161 for the cases and the other having a sampling fraction of 0.00842 for the controls—and the odds ratio for the case-control study will yield the same results as for the ecologic cross-section.

20.3.2.1.4. *The Odds Ratio as a Substitute for a Cohort Risk Ratio*

Beyond all these other delicious things, the odds ratio has one surpassing virtue that has made it irresistible for retrospective case-control studies: In suitable circumstances, the odds ratio can give an excellent approximation of the risk ratio that would be found in a cohort study of etiology.

To appreciate this virtue, which was first pointed out by the late Jerome Cornfield,[1] we need to have another look at Table 20–3. Let us assume in that table that variable X represents exposure to a maneuver and that variable Y represents the outcome event. In a cohort study, the risk (or rate of risk) is $n_1 p_1/n_1 = p_1$ for the probability that the exposed group will develop the outcome event. The corresponding risk in the nonexposed group is p_2. The *risk ratio* we would calculate in a cohort study is p_1/p_2.

If this research were done as a case-control study (with cases being the *Yes* group for the outcome event in variable Y and controls being the *No* group) the odds ratio would be $p_1 q_2/p_2 q_1$. Thus, the p_1/p_2 that we would like to find as the risk ratio has been multipled by q_2/q_1. Cornfield looked at this q_2/q_1 factor, realized that it was $(1 - p_2)/(1 - p_1)$, and realized further that p_2 and p_1 are usually quite small in studies of etiology of disease. Most of the chronic diseases that are investigated with trohoc research occur in the community at rates much lower than 0.1. We would therefore get a risk ratio such as 5 from data such as $p_1 = 0.05$ and $p_2 = 0.01$ so that $p_2/p_1 = 0.05/0.01 = 5$. In this situation, however, $1 - p_2$ and $1 - p_1$ will each be quite close to 1, and their ratio will also be quite close to 1, because $1 - p_2 = 0.99$, $1 - p_1 = 0.95$, and $0.99/0.95 = 1.04$. The odds ratio will therefore be $5 \times 1.04 = 5.2$ and will closely approximate the risk ratio. Thus, when p_1 and p_2 are small, the odds ratio approximates the risk ratio. The usual way of writing this approximation is

$$\frac{p_1 q_2}{p_2 q_1} \simeq \frac{p_1}{p_2}$$

For the situation in Table 20–2, the odds ratio, calculated as $p_1 q_2/p_2 q_1$ was 4.37 and did not closely coincide with the risk ratio of 3.85 calculated as p_1/p_2. The reason for the disparity was the relatively high rate of p_1. It was $130/843 = 0.154$ for the occurrence of diabetes in people with hypercholesterolemia. The rate of p_2, however, was suitably low: $367/9157 = 0.04$ for the occurrence of diabetes in the normal population. For these values, the q_2/q_1 factor was $0.96/0.845 = 1.13$. When this factor multiplied the p_1/p_2 factor of $0.154/0.04 = 3.85$, the odds ratio rose to $3.85 \times 1.13 = 4.37$. Except for this type of problem, in which the rates of outcome events have high levels, i.e., above 0.1, the odds ratio can closely approximate the risk ratio.

This final virtue of the odds ratio is so majestic that it is mindboggling. It implies that a simple, small-group, short-duration, inexpensive trohoc study can yield almost the same risk ratio produced by a complicated, huge-group, long-duration, expensive cohort study.

In describing the splendor of the pattern of normal distribution in a Gaussian curve, Sir Francis Galton, the father of modern biometry, once said that the curve was so magnificent that ancient Greeks would have deified and worshiped it if they had known about it. Neither Galton nor the ancient Greeks knew about the odds ratio. In *descriptive* statistics today, the Gaussian curve is less important than it used to be, because dimensional data are often better summarized with median and inner percentile ranges than with Gaussian-based means and standard deviations. The Gaussian curve is still splendid, but its most vital contributions today are in inferential rather than descriptive statistics. For composite descriptive summaries of the contrasts shown in fourfold tables, there is nothing more mathematically divine than the odds ratio. It may not yet have become deified and worshiped by epidemiologists, but it has surely been a major factor in the sanctification that has permitted retrospective case-control studies to substitute for cohort studies and to become so ascendant[2] in modern epidemiologic research.

20.3.2.1.5. *Estimation of Populational Risks*

Once we have accepted the idea that the odds ratio approximates the risk ratio of a cohort, our statistical horizon becomes even larger. We can now make all kinds of further estimates, although we have not examined a cohort and have no denominator data for calculating either the actual risks or the increments and ratios of risks. Liberated from the unpleasant demands of at-risk denominators, we can estimate certain aspects of risk not merely for the unexamined cohort but for the entire unexamined population.

If p_1 is the rate of risk in the exposed people and p_2 is the corresponding risk in the unexposed people, we know that we can use o, the odds ratio, to estimate the risk ratio of p_1/p_2; but we do not know the incremental risk of $p_1 - p_2$, which is often called the *attributable risk*. If we divide this value by p_2, however, we get $(p_1 - p_2)/p_2 = (p_1/p_2) - 1$. This is the proportionate increment in risk, and we can estimate it as o $-$ 1. If we calculate the proportionate increment by using the exposed group as the denominator, we would have $(p_1 - p_2)/p_1 = 1 - (p_2/p_1)$. Substituting the odds ratio value for p_1/p_2, we can estimate this latter expression as $1 - (1/o) = (o - 1)/o$. This term would tell us the *attributable risk per cent for the exposed group*—an entity that is regularly called the *etiologic fraction*. We can estimate it simply by subtracting 1 from the odds ratio and dividing by the odds ratio. Thus, by ablating the true denominators, we can find something as impressive as an etiologic fraction from our simple retrospective case-control study.

We can even go a step further. Suppose that exposure to the maneuver occurs in a proportion, e, of the total population. Nonexposure will occur in the proportion, $1 - e$. Because exposed people get the disease at rate p_1 and nonexposed people get it at rate p_2, the total occurrence rate for the disease will be $ep_1 + (1 - e)p_2$. In this total occurrence rate, p_2 will represent what would be expected in nonexposed people and all the rest is the excess attributable to exposure. Thus, the attributable populational risk would be $ep_1 + (1 - e)p_2 - p_2 = e(p_1 - p_2)$. If we divide this attributable population risk by the total population risk, we get $e(p_1 - p_2)/[ep_1 + (1 - e)p_2]$. The result, which is called the *population attributable risk per cent*, is $e(p_1 - p_2)/[e(p_1 - p_2) + p_2]$. Because we can substitute $p_1 \sim op_2$, this equation becomes $e(o - 1)/[e(o - 1) + 1]$.

Although we still do not know e, p_1, or p_2, we can solve this equation from the simple $\begin{Bmatrix} a & b \\ c & d \end{Bmatrix}$ results of our case-control study. We can estimate e, the proportion of exposure in the total population, by using the proportion of $b/(b + d)$ that was found in the control group. We can calculate o $=$ ad/bc. If we make these substitutions and work through the algebra, we will find that the population attributable risk per cent can be calculated as $(ad - bc)/[d(a + c)]$, or as $1 - [c(b + d)/b(a + c)]$. For example, if we seriously believe that hypercholesterolemia is a cause of diabetes mellitus, and if we seriously believe the results obtained with the 160 people in Table 20–1, we can determine the population attributable risk per cent as $1 - [(59)(80)/(74)(80)] = 1 - 0.797 = 0.203$. In other words, we can estimate that if we were able to eliminate hypercholesterolemia, we would eliminate about 20% of the cases of diabetes that now occur in the total population.

Seldom in the history of biologic statistics has so powerful a quantitative estimate been possible with so little effort expended in counting numbers.

20.3.2.1.6. *Estimation of Dose-Response Gradient*

In the bioassay activities discussed in Section 11.5.1, we could demonstrate the action of a particular stimulus by showing an increased gradient of response with increasing doses of the stimulus. This same dose-response tactic is frequently used in retrospective case-control studies to show the causal impact of a particular maneuver whose exposure is expressed in dosage, duration, or a combination of the two. Although we have not actually observed people who are placed at risk by the different exposures, the odds-ratio strategy can be used to estimate those risks and to produce evidence of a causal gradient.

The procedure can be illustrated with data taken from the famous Doll-Hill retrospective case-control study[3] of smoking and carcinoma of the lung. In 649 men with lung cancer and in a similar number of matched controls without lung cancer, the investigators found the following data for antecedent smoking of cigarettes:

Average Number of Cigarettes Smoked per Day	Cases with Lung Cancer	Controls without Lung Cancer
0	2	27
1–4	33	55
5–14	250	293
15–24	196	190
≥25	168	84
Total	649	649

For these data, the risk in nonsmokers is arbitrarily assumed to be 1. All other risks can then be compared as odds ratios versus the results in the nonsmokers. Thus, for smokers of 1 to 4 cigarettes per day, the odds ratio is $(33 \times 27)/(2 \times 55) = 8.1$. The corresponding odds ratios are $(250 \times 27)/(2 \times 293) = 11.5$ in smokers of 5 to 14 cigarettes per day, $(196 \times 27)/(2 \times 190) = 13.9$ for 15 to 24 cigarettes, and $(168 \times 27)/(2 \times 84) = 27.0$ for ≥ 25 cigarettes. The monotonic increase in the gradient is clearly evident when the odds ratios are all referred to the 29 nonsmoking cases and controls.

A somewhat puzzling feature of the gradient, however, is its erratic behavior between one dosage group and the next. If we refer each odds ratio to the preceding lower category of smoking, rather than to the nonsmokers, the largest odds ratio is the value of 8.1 noted for nonsmokers versus smokers of 1–4 cigarettes per day. For 1–4 versus 5–14 cigarettes per day, the odds ratio drops to $(250 \times 55)/(33 \times 293) = 1.42$; and for 5–14 versus 15–24 cigarettes per day, the odds ratio drops further to $(196 \times 293)/(250 \times 190) = 1.2$. At ≥ 25 versus 15–24 cigarettes, however, the odds ratio rises to $(168 \times 190)/(196 \times 84) = 1.9$. Some of this erratic behavior may be due to the fragility produced by having only 2 nonsmokers in the case group.

20.3.2.2. DISADVANTAGES OF THE ODDS RATIO

Like most other things that can produce extraordinary benefits, the odds ratio also produces extraordinary hazards. The mathematical ingenuity that creates the epidemiologic appeal of the odds ratio also creates some major problems in its comprehension, and some enormous demands on what is required scientifically for the odds ratio to be accepted as a credible measurement of reality.

20.3.2.2.1. *Problems in Comprehension*

Readers who use or see the words *odds* and *risk* in daily life are often quite confused by the epidemiologic usage of *odds ratio* and *risk ratio*. In the confusion about *risk* and *risk ratio*, as discussed in Section 20.3.1, a reader may not realize that a risk ratio contains four numbers, with two different rates of risk, coming from two sets of numerators and denominators. Similarly, most people in daily life think of *odds* as a ratio, such as 5 to 1 or 3 to 5. The term *odds ratio* then seems to be a formal designation for this idea. Instead, however, the *odds ratio* is actually another four-number expression: it is a quotient (or ratio) of two ratios, each of which is an *odds*.

After overcoming the initial difficulty of understanding this distinction, a reader may then have another important intellectual problem. While untangling the ingredients and meaning of the numerical collage, the reader either may become too discouraged to continue with the analytic reasoning or may lose track of the fact that the actual risks have become obliterated in the *risk ratio* or *odds ratio* used to express their quotient.

20.3.2.2.2. *The Absent Evidence of Risk*

To think about a spectrum of data, we need two indexes: for central tendency and for spread. To decide about a contrast, we also need two indexes: for the increment and the ratio. As noted in Section 8.2, we cannot evaluate the importance of the contrast unless we know both of these features. If someone wants to make a bet that will double his money, the ratio of 2 is important, but the incremental difference will determine whether he bets \$1 or \$10,000. Conversely, a ratio of 1.13 may seem initially unimpressive, but it can be quite clinically important if a new treatment increases survival from 80% to 90%.

The risk of death in an airplane crash may be 5 times higher on airline A than on airline B, but if the rates of death in crashes are 5 per billion miles flown on airline A and 1 per billion miles flown on airline B, most people will choose their airline on the basis of timing, convenience, and service rather than the small incremental risk. Conversely, if the risk of being physically attacked is only 1.06 times greater if we take an evening walk in region C than in region D, most people will avoid both regions if the rates of mugging are 19 per 20 walks in neighborhood C and 18 per 20 walks in neighborhood D.

Without knowing the actual rate of baseline risk and the actual rate of incremental risk, we cannot make sensible decisions in daily life or in medical research. The odds ratio can be a splendid substitute for the risk ratio, but the risk ratio cannot be a splendid substitute for evidence and thought. In the foregoing examples, nothing will be clinically or scientifically sensible unless we have absolute values for baseline risks and increments, not just ratios. A ratio of 1.13 for the risk of survival has no meaning unless we know that survival changed in absolute values from 80% to 90% rather than from 8% to 9%. A ratio of 5 for the risk of death in airplane crashes also has no meaning until we learn that the incremental change is from 1×10^{-9} to 5×10^{-9}. A ratio of 1.06 for the increased risk of walking in neighborhood C seems hardly worth concern, until we learn that the incremental risk of muggings per walk is 1/20 and that the baseline risk is 18/20 in neighborhood D.

Fascinated by the elegant mathematical achievements of the odds ratio, we may forget that scientifically it is a gross underachiever. In substituting for the risk ratio, the odds ratio provides only a ratio. It does not tell us the baseline risk or the incremental risk. These attributes have allowed the odds ratio to be perfectly suited to the data of trohoc research, because a retrospective case-control study cannot give any information about baseline risk or incremental risk. No cohorts were studied to determine risk. If we want information about risk, we have to seek it elsewhere. For purposes of scientific thought about risk, therefore, the odds ratio in a trohoc study is somewhat like a Potemkin village. Its mathematical exterior gives a dazzling display of an imitation risk ratio, but there are no real risks behind it.

20.3.2.2.3. *Overestimation of the Risk Ratio*

In the p_1q_2/p_2q_1 structure of the odds ratio, we usually focus on the p_1/p_2 component, because it represents the desired risk ratio. The ignored value of q_1 is particularly important, however, because it appears in the denominator of q_2/q_1 and because q_1 gets smaller as p_1 gets bigger. The enlargement of p_1 is thus accompanied by an enlargement of the q_2/q_1 factor. Consequently, if p_1 is too large to fulfill the criterion for allowing $1 - p_1$ to be regarded as ~1, the odds ratio will inflate the value of the risk ratio.

We saw this problem in Table 20–2, when the actual rates of risk were $p_1 = 0.154$ and $p_2 = 0.04$. The correct value of p_1/p_2 was 3.85, but q_2/q_1 was 1.13, and the odds ratio was raised to 4.37, which fallaciously elevated the true risk ratio. The problem is important if we seriously want to use odds ratios for estimating risk ratios in the many chronic diseases whose true rates of occurrence are substantially higher than the rates calculated from death certificate data. For example, certain cancers and arteriosclerotic ailments are regularly found at autopsy with rates that are much higher than the customary rates of reported detection. Thus, if $p_1 = 0.04$ and $p_2 = 0.01$, the odds ratio creates little change in the correct value of $p_1/p_2 = 4$, because $q_2/q_1 = 0.99/0.96 = 1.03$. On the other hand, if $p_1 = 0.4$ and $p_2 = 0.1$, the correct value of p_1/p_2 is still 4, but it will be substantially inflated by the odds ratio, because $q_2/q_1 = 0.9/0.6 = 1.5$. The odds ratio will then imply that the risk ratio is 6 instead of 4.

20.3.2.2.4. *Problems in Statistical Fragility*

Because the odds ratio allows important decisions to be made from small groups, investigators seeking to limit the costs of research will usually try to keep these groups as small as possible. Special formulas are regularly used to calculate the minimum sample size that can achieve statistical significance while showing the desired distinction.

The results of the inexpensive and significant research, however, may be extremely fragile in their statistical stability. A change of one or two patients from one cell to another in the fourfold table can produce substantial changes in the odds ratio and also in the statistical significance. For example, an investigator doing a trohoc study with 10 cases and 10 controls may find that six cases and one control were exposed to the suspected etiologic The fourfold table will be $\begin{Bmatrix} 6 & 1 \\ 4 & 9 \end{Bmatrix}$, which produces both stochastic significance (P = 0.029; one-tail Fisher Test) and the impressive odds ratio of 13.5 [$= (6 \times 9) \div (4 \times 1)$]. If one of the control patients had been more thoroughly interviewed and classified as *exposed*, however, the table would change to $\begin{Bmatrix} 6 & 2 \\ 4 & 8 \end{Bmatrix}$. The odds ratio would drop to 6, and the stochastic significance would vanish (P = 0.08; one-tail Fisher Test). Furthermore, if one of the cases was interviewed too aggressively and was erroneously classified as exposed, the table would change to $\begin{Bmatrix} 5 & 2 \\ 5 & 8 \end{Bmatrix}$. The P value would become still higher and more nonsignificant, and the odds ratio would drop to 4.

The stability of any statistics will usually be strengthened, of course, by large sample sizes, but big groups will not always solve the problem. For example, in a recent study[4] that contained a respectable sample size—367 cases and 643 controls—statistical significance would vanish and the odds ratio would become 1 with certain changes in classification,[5] which could be reasonably anticipated on a clinical basis, for 17 members of the case group and for 18 members of the control group.

Perhaps the best way to appraise the fragility of the statistics contained in an odds ratio is to examine the associated confidence interval. It is almost always calculated as an act of inferential statistics and is presented as evidence of the stochastic significance of the ratio. Thus, if the 95% confidence interval does not include the neutral value of 1, the investigator can claim stochastic significance at the level of $P < 0.05$.

The confidence interval can also be used, however, as an item of descriptive statistics, to show the fragility of the observed value. Thus, if the odds ratio is 4.3 with a tight confidence interval that extends from 3.9 to 4.7, the result is much less fragile than a similar odds ratio with a confidence interval that goes from 1.1 to 23.7. In the latter instance, because the true value of the odds ratio might be as low as 1.1, we might be less inclined to be impressed with the observed ratio of 4.3.

20.3.2.2.5. *Calculation of Confidence Interval*

The main difficulty in trying to use the confidence interval as a descriptive statistic is the problem of deciding how best to calculate it.[6] One immediate problem is the imbalance of possible ranges for the interval. If the odds ratio exceeds 1, it can go anywhere from 1 to infinity, but if below 1, the range is restricted to the interval from 0 to 1. For this reason, many mathematical approaches employ the odds ratio's logarithm, which will be zero if the odds ratio equals 1, and which can extend to $+\infty$ for values above 1 and to $-\infty$ for values below 1.

Among the plethora of available mathematical strategies for calculating confidence intervals, a method proposed by Cornfield[7] appears to have the current status of definitive standard, but the calculations are cumbersome, requiring an iterative procedure for solving several equations. Although the procedure can be performed with a special program in an electronic calculator, the strategy is seldom used. If we use the letter o to represent the observed odds ratio, the simplest method of getting a confidence interval is based on a proposal by Fleiss[8] to calculate the standard error as s.e. (o) $= o\sqrt{(1/a)+(1/b)+(1/c)+(1/d)}$. For the data in Table 20–1, o $= (21 \times 74)/(6 \times 59) = 4.39$ and the other term is $\sqrt{(1/21)+(1/6)+(1/59)+(1/74)} = \sqrt{0.245} = 0.495$. For a $1-\alpha$ confidence interval, we let $Z_\alpha = Z_{0.05} = 1.96$. The confidence interval would be calculated as $4.39 \pm (1.96)(4.39)(0.495)$, and it would extend from 0.12 to 8.66.

This easy approach is reasonably satisfactory when the fourfold table has large values in all four cells. For most circumstances, however, a better method derived from Woolf[9] works with the natural logarithm of the odds ratio, ln(o). For this purpose, the odds ratio is best estimated as o′ $= [(a + 0.5)(d + 0.5)]/[(b + 0.5)(c + 0.5)]$. If L′ $= $ ln(o′), the standard error of L′ is estimated as s.e.(L′) $= \sqrt{[1/(a+0.5)] + [1/b+0.5)] + [1/c+0.5)] + [1/(d+0.5)]}$. For the data of Table 20–1, o′ $= (21.5 \times 74.5)/(6.5 \times 59.5) = 4.14$, L′ $= $ ln 4.14 $= 1.421$, and s.e.(L′) $= \sqrt{(1/21.5) + (1/74.5) + (1/6.5) + (1/59.5)} = \sqrt{0.2305} = 0.480$. The 95% confidence interval around L′ would be $1.421 \pm (1.96)(0.480) = 1.421 \pm 0.941$; and it extends from 0.48 to 2.362. Because these values are logarithms, we need to convert them back to the original values by raising each one to the appropriate power of e. Thus $e^{0.48} = 1.62$ and $e^{2.362} = 10.61$. The confidence interval around the estimated odds ratio of 4.25 would therefore extend from 1.62 to 10.61.

Yet another approach, which seems to be the current favorite for calculating the confidence interval of an odds ratio, is a test-based method introduced by Miettinen.[10] It depends on the value of X^2 found in the 2×2 table. (When the numbers are small, X^2 should be calculated as X_c^2, with Yates correction.) The $1 - \alpha$ confidence interval will be the antilog of $[1 \pm (Z_\alpha/\sqrt{X^2})]$ln(o). For example, in Table 20–1, $X^2 = 10.025$ and $\sqrt{X^2} = 3.166$. Taking $Z_\alpha = 1.96$, we find $1.96/3.166 = 0.619$. The value of 1 ± 0.619 extends from 0.381 to 1.619. Because the odds ratio is 4.39, ln 4.39 $= 1.48$. The confidence interval for the ln(o) will extend from (0.381)(1.48) to (1.619)(1.48), which is 0.564 to 2.396. Taking the antilogs of these two numbers by raising e to the appropriate powers, we find that the actual confidence interval runs from 1.76 to 10.96. The results are similar, but somewhat narrower than what was found with the Woolf method.

Because natural logarithms are used in both the Woolf and Miettinen methods, the reader should be warned that the upper and lower limits of the confidence interval will not be symmetrically placed around the observed value of the odds ratio. Thus, in previous calculations in Chapter 7, the confidence intervals were symmetrical around the central index because of the $\bar{X} \pm Z_\alpha s_{\bar{x}}$ formula. With the logarithm procedures symmetry seldom occurs. Thus, for an odds ratio of 4.39, the confidence limits went from roughly 1.7 to 11.3.

20.3.2.2.6. *The Incalculable Odds Ratio*

Whenever one of the cells in the fourfold table is zero, the odds ratio cannot be calculated directly. Because the formula for the odds ratio must hold true for either the ad/bc or bc/ad arrangement, a value of 0 in one of the cells would necessitate the mathematical malpractice of dividing by 0. To avoid this dastardly act, the value of 0.5 is added to each of the four cells; and the odds ratio is estimated as $[(a+0.5)(d+0.5)]/(b+0.5)(c+0.5)]$. Because the cell with a zero in it will become 0.5, the value of $1/0.5 = 2$ will make the standard error quite large when the reciprocal values of the cells are used for the calculation.

For example, in a case-control study of the relationship between diethylstilbestrol and clear cell vaginal adenocarcinoma, Greenwald and coworkers[11] found the following data:

	Cases	Controls
Exposed	5	0
Nonexposed	0	8

The odds ratio here would be $(5+0.5)(8+0.5)/(0+0.5)(0+0.5) = (5.5)(8.5)/(0.5)(0.5) = 187$.

20.3.2.2.7. *The Problem of Suitable Representation*

When the odds ratio of a case-control study is used to substitute for the odds ratio of an ecologic cross-section or to estimate the risk ratio of a cohort study, the authenticity of the results depends on two fundamental requirements in statistics and science. Statistically, the case-control groups must be a proper sample of the population from which they are drawn. Unless the sample is chosen without bias, we have no assurance that the selected cases and controls suitably represent the available parent population of cases and controls.

Scientifically, the available parent population of cases and controls must suitably represent the scientific reasoning of the cause-effect relationship under study. If the study has a pathodynamic hypothesis, the available parent population should suitably represent the outcomes that follow the disease under investigation. If the study has an etiologic hypothesis, the parent population should suitably represent the occurrence of the disease as an outcome of the exposure or nonexposure to the suspected etiologic agent. If the study has a therapeutic hypothesis, the available population should suitably represent the good or bad things that can occur after the assignment or nonassignment of a particular treatment to the people eligible to receive it for a particular clinical condition.

These two sets of statistical and scientific demands are not unique to the odds ratio. The demands occur whether the results of cross-sectional studies are expressed in an odds ratio or in any other mode of statistical citation. The demands arise from principles of both the statistical and scientific inferences that must be satisfied to allow the results of any small cross-sectional collection of people to substitute for both a larger collection of people and a distinctive longitudinal sequence of events.

As noted in the other parts of this chapter and in several subsequent chapters, however, neither of these two sets of statistical and scientific requirements is regularly or even frequently fulfilled in the diverse types of case-control studies used for cross-sectional research. Statistically, the cases and controls are never obtained by random sampling and are almost never checked for the suitability with which they represent their parent population of cases and controls. Scientifically, the cases and controls are seldom chosen to fulfill the specific architectural distinctions they must satisfy for the cause-effect or other research hypothesis that is being tested.

For example, in a randomized trial, the different dosages of the compared agents would be assigned to groups of people whose baseline susceptibilities to the outcome event are made (reasonably) similar by the randomization. If members of these groups later decide to change either the original agents or dosages of the same agent, the reasons for the decisions would be suspected as possible sources of bias and would be carefully analyzed. In an intention-to-treat analysis, as discussed in Chapter 29, none of the changes would be acceptable; and the outcome events would be associated only with the originally assigned agents. Although these issues receive prominent attention when statistical arrangements are made to avoid bias in experimental trials, the scientific sources of problems in susceptibility and performance are almost never considered when odds ratios are calculated for dose-response curves or other comparisons in case-control studies.

Because the fundamental requirements of statistics and science are satisfied so infrequently, the odds ratio and other splendid indexes of mathematical expression must always be appraised with cautious skepticism, despite their quantitative grandeur.

20.3.3. *Bayes Theorem*

In Section 20.2.2, when we considered the data of Table 20–1 as a diagnostic marker study, the results were expressed with indexes of nosologic sensitivity and specificity. When we examined the table more carefully, looking at the rows rather than the columns, we readily noted the alternative expressions that a clinician would want for the diagnostic accuracy of the test. Despite their desirability, however, these alternative expressions are clinically unstable because they depend on the relative sizes of the diseased and nondiseased groups chosen for the study.

This section is concerned with that problem of relative prevalence, and with the mathematical strategies needed to convert the stable nosologic indexes into useful diagnostic indexes. The discussion will begin with a relatively simple algebraic demonstration of the problems. A reader who is willing to slog through the algebra, which is not difficult to understand, will then be ready to comprehend its transformation to one of the most inscrutable statistical expressions used in modern medicine: Bayes theorem.

To illustrate the procedure, we can use the pragmatic data shown in Table 20–1, but we also need some algebraic symbols to demonstrate what is going on. The basic algebraic symbols are shown in Table 20–4. Some additional symbols will be introduced as we proceed.

For the diagnostic marker study shown in Table 20–4, the customary nosologic indexes are *nosologic sensitivity* $= g = a/n_1$; and *nosologic specificity* $= f = d/n_2$. These two indexes are usually regarded as stable indicators of the performance of the marker test in the nosologically diseased and nondiseased groups under study. The indexes we would really like to know, however, refer to diagnostic rather than nosologic accuracy. These diagnostic indexes are *diagnostic sensitivity* $= v = a/m_1$ and *diagnostic specificity* $= u = d/m_2$. The index of diagnostic sensitivity is often called the predictive accuracy for a positive test result, and the index of diagnostic specificity is called the predictive accuracy for a negative test result.

Table 20–4. FOURFOLD TABLE SHOWING HYPOTHETICAL DATA IN A DIAGNOSTIC MARKER STUDY

Test Result	Diseased Group	Control Group	Total
Positive	a	b	m_1
Negative	c	d	m_2
Total	n_1	n_2	N

Table 20–5. SAME STUDY AS TABLE 20–1, BUT WITH CONTROL GROUP QUADRUPLED IN SIZE

| Presence of Hypercholesterolemia | Number of Persons In: | | Total |
	Diabetes Group	Control Group	
Yes	21	24	45
No	59	296	355
Total	80	320	400

In Table 20–1, the values for these four indexes were g = 21/80 = 0.26, f = 74/80 = 0.93, v = 21/27 = 0.78, and u = 74/133 = 0.56. The instability of the diagnostic indexes, v and u, would become apparent if we had quadrupled the size of the control group studied in Table 20–1. The results of this same study, performed with a control group containing 320 rather than 80 patients, are shown in Table 20–5. In Table 20–5, the nosologic indexes have the same values they showed in Table 20–1: g = 21/80 = 0.26 and f = 296/320 = 0.93. The diagnostic indexes, however, are dramatically different: v = 21/45 = 0.47 and u = 296/355 = 0.83. Simply by increasing the size of the control group, we produced a substantial fall in diagnostic sensitivity, and a substantial rise in diagnostic specificity.

The reason for this change becomes apparent if we consider the internal algebra that is needed in Table 20–4 to convert sensitivity from its nosologic value, $g = a/n_1$, to its diagnostic value, $v = a/m_1$. To do this conversion, we need some further ideas and symbols. Let $p = n_1/N$ represent the prevalence of the diseased group in the total group under study. Then $q = 1 - p = n_2/N$ will represent the prevalence of the nondiseased group. Let $t = m_1/N$ represent the prevalence of positive results for diagnostic test, and let $w = 1 - t = m_2/N$ represent the prevalence of negative results.

We can now start algebraically with the statement that $g = a/n_1$. Substituting $n_1 = pN$, we get $g = a/pN$, which can be rearranged to yield $a = gpN$. We also know that $v = a/m_1$ and that $m_1 = tN$. We can rearrange this relationship to yield $a = vtN$. We can now equate the two expressions for a to produce $a = gpN = vtN$, which leads to $gp = vt$. We can solve this equation for v to produce

$$v = \frac{gp}{t} \qquad [20.1]$$

This formula tells us how to convert the nosologic sensitivity of a test into its true diagnostic sensitivity or accuracy for positive prediction. We multiply g, the nosologic sensitivity, by the ratio of the two prevalences, p and t, for disease and positive tests, respectively, in the studied groups.

Thus, for the data in Table 20–5, g = 21/80 = 0.26; p = 80/400 = 0.2; and t = 45/400 = 0.11. The value of v is (0.26)(0.2)/0.11 = 0.47. Alternatively, of course, we could have obtained this value directly from Table 20–5 as v = 21/45 = 0.47. The analogous results for v in Table 20–1 show how diagnostic sensitivity is affected by the prevalence associated with nosologic sensitivity. In Table 20–1, g = 21/80 = 0.26; p = 80/160 = 0.5; and t = 27/160 = 0.17. Thus v = (0.26)(0.5)/(0.17) = 0.76. By direct inspection, we could also calculate v directly as 21/27 = 0.78. (Because of rounding during the calculations, the calculated values of v differ slightly from their direct values.)

With a similar algebraic development, it can be shown that nosologic specificity, f, is converted into diagnostic specificity, u, by an analogous equation, which is

$$u = \frac{fq}{w} \qquad [20.2]$$

Thus, the value of u was obtained directly in Table 20–1 as 74/133 = 0.556. It could have been calculated alternatively from f = 74/80 = 0.925, q = 80/160 = 0.5, and w = 0.831, to yield u = (0.925)(0.5)/0.831 = 0.556. In Table 20–5, in which q = 320/400 = 0.8 and w = 355/400 = 0.888, the value of u changed to a directly calculated result as 296/355 = 0.83 and to an indirect calculation of (0.925)(0.8)/0.888 = 0.83.

Because $p = n_1/N$ and $t = m_1/N$, $p/t = n_1/m_1$. Because $q = n_2/N$ and $w = m_2/N$, the indirect calculations could be eased if equation 20.1 were altered to $v = g \times (n_1/m_1)$ and $u = f \times (n_2/m_2)$. Although the values of m_1, m_2, t, and w appear in these formulas, they are really not needed. We can determine those values if we are given only the three results for nosologic sensitivity, nosologic specificity, and prevalence of disease. If given the value of g, f, and p, we can do the following algebraic caper: $m_1 = a+b = gn_1+(1-f)n_2$. Because $n_1 = pN$, $n_2 = qN$, and $t = m_1/N$, we can substitute appropriately to get $t = gp+(1-f)q$. Consequently, equation 20.1 can be written as

$$v = \frac{gp}{gp+(1-f)q} \qquad [20.3]$$

By a similar set of algebraic conversions, we can convert equation 20.2 into

$$u = \frac{fq}{fq+(1-g)p} \qquad [20.4]$$

The formulas cited in equations 20.3 and 20.4 are straightforward algebraic truisms. They tell us how the stable indexes of nosologic sensitivity and nosologic specificity can be converted, as soon as a clinician knows about prevalence of disease, to the desired values of predictive accuracy for the indexes of diagnostic sensitivity and diagnostic specificity. For example, if we wanted to use hypercholesterolemia as a screening test for diabetes, we might be moderately impressed by its diagnostic sensitivity of 0.78 in Table 20–1, in which p = 0.5. Our enthusiasm might be reduced as the diagnostic sensitivity fell to 0.47 in Table 20–5, in which p = 0.2. If we took this screening test into the community, as shown in Table 20–2, our enthusiasm would disappear. In the community, where diabetes is less prevalent than in the groups we assembled for the studies reported in Tables 20–1 and 20–5, the value of p would drop to 0.0497, and diagnostic sensitivity would drop to 0.15 (= 130/843). The changes in prevalence of disease would therefore produce three different results for diagnostic sensitivity even though nosologic sensitivity and specificity have retained the respective values of g = 0.26 and f = 0.93 in all three of the studies.

The relationships cited in the formulas of equations 20.1 through 20.4 were first noted in the 18th century by a British clergyman, Thomas Bayes, who perished before he published; and his work was reported posthumously by a friend. The algebraic relationships have been immortalized, however, under the eponym of *Bayes theorem*.

In Bayes' original work, the formulas were developed to show certain features of conditional probability; and so probabilistic symbols are still commonly used to cite the algebraic relationships. In those symbols, the prevalence of the disease, p, is written as $P(D)$. The prevalence of nondisease, q, is written as $P(\bar{D})$. The nosologic sensitivity is written as $P(T \mid D)$, which means the probability of a positive test result, given that the patient has the disease. The corresponding nosologic specificity of the test, f, is $P(\bar{T} \mid \bar{D})$.

The diagnostic sensitivity is then written as $P(D \mid T)$, which is the probability of having the disease, given that the patient has a positive result in the diagnostic test.

When all of these symbols for probabilities and conditional probabilities are appropriately substituted into equation 20.3, it becomes converted into one of the medical literature's greatest communicative terrors, which expresses Bayes theorem as

$$P(D|T) = \frac{P(T|D) \times P(D)}{[P(T|D) \times P(D)] + \{[1 - P(T|\overline{D})] \times P(\overline{D})\}} \qquad [20.5]$$

for the diagnostic sensitivity of a marker test. A similar set of probabilistic symbols converts equation 20.4 into

$$P(\overline{D}|\overline{T}) = \frac{P(\overline{T}|\overline{D}) \times P(\overline{D})}{[P(\overline{T}|\overline{D}) \times P(\overline{D})] + \{[1 - P(T|D)] \times P(D)\}} \qquad [20.6]$$

for the diagnostic specificity of the marker test.

The algebraic expressions of equations 20.3 and 20.4 might give medical readers a chance of understanding the "music" that is being communicated, but equations 20.5 and 20.6—which is the way in which the formulas are usually presented in medical literature—are a clashing cacophony of mathematical cymbals. After the latter equations (or some of their congeners) appear in the text, most medical readers are usually lost beyond recovery. Nevertheless, as noted in Chapter 25, the underlying assumptions, groups, and data of diagnostic marker tests are far more important than their Bayesian mathematical expressions, and require careful scientific attention that will be omitted if the reader drops out at this stage in the communication of evidence.

20.3.4. *The Likelihood Ratio*

The likelihood ratio, which is a recent, popular entry in the sweepstakes for creating indexes of diagnostic marker tests, can be viewed either as a type of risk ratio or odds ratio. Using the symbols of Table 20–4, the likelihood ratio is expressed as $(a/n_1) \div (b/n_2)$. It represents the probability of obtaining a positive test result in a patient with disease, divided by the probability of obtaining a positive test result in a patient without the disease.

If viewed as a quotient for the risks of having a positive test in patients with and without the disease, the likelihood ratio is analogous to a risk ratio. On the other hand, if we rewrite the likelihood ratio as $(a/b) \div (n_1/n_2)$, the expression represents the quotient of two odds for disease vs. controls: in the group with a positive test, and in the total. With the latter expression, the likelihood ratio becomes an odds ratio. It shows the odds for the chance that a particular test result comes from someone who actually has the disease for which the test was ordered. In Table 20–1, the likelihood ratio for a positive test is $(21/80) \div (6/80) = 3.5$. The likelihood ratio for a negative test is $(59/80) \div (74/80) = 0.797$.

Because $a/n_1 = g$ and $b/n_2 = 1 - f$, the likelihood ratio for a positive test result can be written as

$$L_{pos} = \frac{g}{1 - f}, \qquad [20.7]$$

and it is independent of prevalence. Similarly, the likelihood ratio for a negative test result is $(c/n_1) \div (d/n_2)$, which can be written as

$$L_{neg} = \frac{1-g}{f} \qquad [20.8]$$

Because the two likelihood ratios are independent of disease prevalence, they are desirable expressions of the statistical accomplishments of a diagnostic marker table, but they require *two* expressions rather than one. Furthermore, to be used in practical clinical activities, they must be converted to indications of diagnostic accuracy; and these conversions require the use of prevalence. Thus, with some additional algebra (which is not shown here), it can be demonstrated that the index of diagnostic sensitivity is

$$v = \frac{L_{pos} \times p}{(L_{pos} \times p) + q} \qquad [20.9]$$

and that the index of diagnostic specificity is

$$u = \frac{q}{q + (L_{neg} \times p)} \qquad [20.10]$$

For example, in Tables 20–1, 20–2, and 20–5, the values for L_{pos} are all the same. They are $g/(1-f) = 0.2625/(1-0.925) = 3.5$. The values for L_{neg} are also all the same: they are $(1-g)/f = 0.7375/0.925 = 0.797$. To obtain the diagnostic indexes for Table 20–1, we use expression 20.9 to calculate $v = 3.5 \times 0.5/[(3.5 \times 0.5)+0.5] = 0.78$. This is the same result obtained directly from the table as $v = 21/27 = 0.78$. Furthermore, we can use equation 20.10 to calculate $u = 0.5/[0.5+(0.797 \times 0.5)] = 0.56$, which is the same as the result obtained directly from the table as $u = 74/133$. Similarly, in Table 20–5, $v = 3.5 \times 0.2/[(3.5 \times 0.2)+0.8] = 0.47$, which is the same as $v = 21/45$. Also in Table 20–5, $u = 0.8/[0.8+(0.797 \times 0.2)] = 0.83$, which equals 296/355.

The great virtues of the likelihood ratios are that they are independent of prevalence and they are simpler than Bayes theorem for calculating diagnostic indexes of sensitivity and specificity. Equations 20.9 and 20.10 are obviously easier to understand than the corresponding Bayesian expressions in equations 20.5 and 20.6. Whether equations 20.9 and 20.10 are easier to understand than the corresponding equations 20.3 and 20.4 will be left to the reader's decision.

One major advantage of the likelihood ratios is that they do not require a 2×2 table for the results of a marker test. Consider the table shown in Section 20.2.3 for the value of different levels of serum omphalase in discriminating between patients in stage I or II of a particular disease. For the total of 17 patients in stage I and 12 patients in stage II, an omphalase value of 6-9 identified six patients in stage I and two in stage II. For these data, the n_1/n_2 ratio is $17/12 = 1.42$, and the a/b factor is $6/2 = 3$. The value for L_{pos} would be $3/1.42 = 2.1$ for this level of omphalase. When the omphalase value was ≥ 14, the test identified two patients in stage I and nine in stage II. For this result, the a/b factor would be $2/9 = 0.222$ and L_{pos} would drop to $0.222/1.42 = 0.16$. We could thus promptly see the relative diagnostic value of different levels of the omphalase test, without having to convert the results into the 2×2 table that is needed for Bayes theorem or for some of the other tactics described in Chapter 25.

The main problem with likelihood ratios is that they are often described with an exuberance of probabilistic jargon that can remove or impair whatever understanding a medical reader may have managed to achieve. The odds of n_1/n_2 can be regarded as the pre-test odds that a patient in the studied groups has the disease, without any additional marker tests having been done. After the marker test is performed, a positive result has the post-test odds of a/b; and a negative result has the post-test odds of c/d. The relationship may then be expressed as

$$\frac{\text{Likelihood}}{\text{ratio}} = \frac{\text{Post-test odds}}{\text{Pre-test odds}}, \qquad\qquad [20.11]$$

which can also be cited as

$$\text{Post-test odds} = \text{Pre-test odds} \times \text{Likelihood ratio} \qquad\qquad [20.12]$$

The relationship noted in equation 20.12 happens to be quite important for the statistical inferences performed by members of the Bayesian or likelihood schools of statistical reasoning. As items of communication in descriptive statistics, however, equations 20.11 and 20.12 may do more harm than good. By the time a medical reader has worked through all the convolutions of all the odds and ratios, the basic goals of a diagnostic marker test and the basic function of diagnostic indexes may be irretrievably lost.

Further ramifications of likelihood ratios in diagnostic marker studies are discussed in Chapter 25.

20.3.5. *Composite Indexes for Marker Tests*

Unlike the individual risk ratio and odds ratio, which compress the results of a fourfold table into a single composite index, the results that emerge from Bayes theorem and the likelihood ratios in diagnostic marker studies are indexes of transformation rather than compression. Bayesian or likelihood indexes are used to convert the clinically unsatisfactory nosologic indexes of sensitivity and specificity into clinically useful diagnostic indexes. During the conversions, the two old (nosologic) indexes are transformed into two new ones.

The statistical penchant for obtaining a single composite index in a fourfold table was used in the past, however, to produce two different composite expressions—the index of validity and Youden's J—which are sometimes still encountered in the medical literature of diagnostic marker studies.

20.3.5.1. THE INDEX OF VALIDITY

An old method of combining the two ideas of sensitivity and specificity into a single composite index is to cite the proportion of correct diagnoses in a fourfold table as $(a+d)/N$. This quotient has been called the *index of validity*. For the data of Table 20–1, the index of validity is $(21+74)/160 = 0.594$. Because $a = gn_1$ and $d = fn_2$, the index of validity can be rewritten as $(gn_1 + fn_2)/N = (g)\left(\dfrac{n_1}{N}\right) + f\left(\dfrac{n_2}{N}\right) = gp + fq$. The latter formula immediately indicates what is wrong with the index of validity. Its value is greatly affected by the prevalence of disease in the group under study. Thus, although g and f remain the same, the index of validity rises in Table 20–5 to $(21+296)/400 = 0.79$. In Table 20–2, in which g and f were the same as in Tables 20–1 and 20–5, and in which the diagnostic sensitivity was so low as to make the marker test worthless, the index of validity rises even higher to $(130+8790)/10,000 = 0.89$.

Because the properties of nosologic sensitivity and specificity should be inherent in the marker test, a composite index that varies with the prevalence of disease in the study is grossly unsatisfactory. The index of validity is seldom used today because it is generally regarded as having no validity.

20.3.5.2. **YOUDEN'S J**

A composite index that is independent of prevalence was proposed by Youden,[12] who suggested a formula that ultimately becomes J = nosologic sensitivity + nosologic specificity − 1. For the data in Tables 20–1, 20–2, and 20–5, J = 0.26 + 0.93 − 1 = 0.19.

Youden's J has the major advantage of avoiding prevalence, but its additive result obliterates the distinctiveness of individual differences for sensitivity and specificity. Thus, if the values were reversed, with nosologic sensitivity = 0.93 and nosologic specificity = 0.26, the marker procedure would have a quite different set of implications for clinical usage, but Youden's J would still be identical at 0.19.

Because important clinical distinctions are obliterated by the statistical compression, Youden's J is also an unsatisfactory index. It seldom appears in modern literature.

20.3.6. *Indexes of Adjustment and Standardization*

Epidemiologic data often receive statistical adjustments that are intended to remove or reduce the effects of unfair comparisons. Although used in both cohort and cross-sectional data, the adjustments may be particularly hard to understand in cross-sectional studies.

Certain comparisons of numbers can be immediately recognized as unfair because they lack a reference denominator. For example, the number of deaths in New Haven is smaller each year than in New York. If someone in New Haven uses this information to claim that New Haven is a healthier city than New York, you would promptly recognize the fallacy of the comparison. Because New Haven has a much smaller population than New York, the deaths should be compared as occurrence rates, expressed as number of deaths per total population, not just total number of deaths.

Even when a denominator is used to calculate and compare a rate, however, the contrast of two rates may still be unfair because the denominator groups have a different composition. For example, suppose we contrast the results of treatment for a particular disease at a relatively small suburban community hospital, A, and at a municipal hospital, B. Because hospital B is associated with a high-powered academic medical center, we may be dismayed to discover that the suburban hospital has a success rate of 63% (= 124/198), which is substantially higher than the 44% rate (= 222/502) found at hospital B. Before concluding that something is drastically wrong in academia, however, we might give some thought to the types of patients being treated at the two institutions. The municipal hospital may have worse results because it is treating a sicker group of people than the suburban hospital.

To check this suspicion, we can categorize each patient in one of the three stages of clinical severity for this disease, where stage I is best, stage II is next best, and stage III is worst. We can then see how the patients in each stage were distributed proportionately among the two hospital cohorts.

The results, which are shown in Table 20–6, demonstrate that our suspicion was correct. The cohorts were apportioned so that the favorable stage I provided 49% of the 198 patients in hospital A but only 10% of the patients in hospital B. The unfavorable stage III, on the other hand, occupied 60% of the spectrum in hospital B but only 26% in hospital A. Because of these disparities, a comparison of the crude success rates of 63% versus 44% for the two hospitals is unfair and misleading. To get a better idea of what really happened, we need to examine the success rates within each of the three subgroups, or *strata*, of stages. This examination, which is performed in Table 20–7, shows that the two hospitals actually have identical rates of success within each stage. Each hospital had

Table 20–6. SEVERITY OF ILLNESS AND DISTRIBUTION OF PATIENTS AT TWO HOSPITALS

Stage for Severity of Illness	Hospital A	Hospital B	Total
I	98 (49%)	49 (10%)	147 (21%)
II	48 (24%)	151 (30%)	199 (28%)
III	52 (26%)	302 (60%)	354 (51%)
Total	198 (100%)	502 (100%)	700 (100%)

82% success in stage I, 58% in stage II, and 31% in stage III. The rates in the overall totals for the two hospitals were different only because of the disproportionate distribution of the constituent strata.

For purely clinical purposes, Table 20–7 tells us what we wanted to know; and we might be quite satisfied to compare the results it provides within each of the three stages. For many epidemiologic and statistical purposes, however, we might want to have a single value that summarizes the total results for each hospital while correcting the imbalance in the component groups. To compare the two hospitals, we would want to contrast one suitably calculated rate for each hospital, not three sets of rates for the three stages.

The role of statistical adjustments is to make these corrections. The adjustment process can take place in two different ways. In one technique, called *standardization,* the results of any observed group are adjusted to reflect what would happen in a selected reference group that is called the *standard.* In the other techniques of adjustment, the results are altered according to attributes noted within the data.

20.3.6.1. **TECHNIQUES OF STANDARDIZATION**

In Table 20–7, the stratum death rates provided the data we needed, but the imbalance in stratum proportions created the problem. To deal with this problem, we can adjust the stratum proportions for hospitals A and B so that both institutions have the same proportions in their strata. The set of proportions that we decide to choose for this purpose provides the standardization.

To demonstrate the process, we can use some algebraic symbols, illustrated with the foregoing data. Let us begin with hospital A. Each of its strata, as shown in Table 20–6,

Table 20–7. SUCCESS RATES ACCORDING TO SEVERITY OF ILLNESS IN THE TWO HOSPITALS SHOWN IN TABLE 20–6

Stage for Severity of Illness	Hospital A	Hospital B	Total
I	80/98 (82%)	40/49 (82%)	120/147 (82%)
II	28/48 (58%)	88/151 (58%)	116/199 (58%)
III	16/52 (31%)	94/302 (31%)	110/354 (31%)
Total	124/198 (63%)	222/502 (44%)	346/700 (49%)

contains n_1 members, so that $n_1 = 98$, $n_2 = 48$, and $n_3 = 52$. The total number of people in the group is $n = \Sigma n_i = 198$. The proportions of the cohort occupied by each stratum are $p_i = n_i/n$, so that (as also shown in Table 20–6) $p_1 = 0.49$, $p_2 = 0.24$, and $p_3 = 0.26$. The rates of the outcome event in each stratum are $r_i = t_i/n_i$, so that (as shown in Table 20–7) $r_1 = 80/98 = 0.82$, $r_2 = 28/48 = 0.58$, and $r_3 = 16/52 = 0.31$. The crude outcome rate is $r = t/n = \Sigma t_i/n = 124/198 = 0.63$.

It can easily be shown algebraically that this crude rate equals $\Sigma p_i r_i$. Thus, the crude success rate value of $r = 0.63$ could also be calculated as

$$p_1 r_1 + p_2 r_2 + p_3 r_3 = r$$

Using the available values from Tables 20–6 and 20–7, we can substitute to get

$$(0.49)(0.82) + (0.24)(0.58) + (0.26)(0.31) = 0.62,$$

which differs from 0.63 because of rounding. If we used the original numbers to calculate these results in full arithmetical splendor, they would be

$$\left(\frac{98}{198}\right)\left(\frac{80}{98}\right) + \left(\frac{48}{198}\right)\left(\frac{28}{48}\right) + \left(\frac{52}{198}\right)\left(\frac{16}{52}\right), \text{ and}$$

we would get 0.63 rather than 0.62. In fact, if you examine the foregoing terms, you can see how appropriate numerator and denominator entities would cancel to produce

$$\frac{80}{198} + \frac{28}{198} + \frac{52}{198} = \frac{124}{198} = 0.63$$

The formula of $\Sigma p_i r_i$ for the crude success rate is enlightening because it lets us know how to make the desired adjustment. The values to be maintained are the r_i results for each stratum. The distorted values to be adjusted are the p_i proportions for each stratum. If we can obtain a standard set of P_i values to replace the existing p_i values, we can use the P_i factors throughout each group to make the necessary adjustment in the rate for that group. For this standard set of P_i values, we could use the p_i values from hospital A or the ones from hospital B throughout both groups, but a better compromise choice is to derive the standard proportions from the totals of the two hospitals. Thus, as shown in the far right column of Table 20–6, we can obtain a standard set of proportions as $P_1 = 147/700 = 0.21$; $P_2 = 199/700 = 0.28$; and $P_3 = 354/700 = 0.51$. If we multiply the observed stratum success rates by these standard proportions, we would obtain the adjusted rate in each cohort as

$$\Sigma P_i r_i = P_1 r_1 + P_2 r_2 + P_3 r_3$$

For hospital A, this formula would produce

$$\left(\frac{147}{700}\right)\left(\frac{80}{98}\right) + \left(\frac{199}{700}\right)\left(\frac{28}{48}\right) + \left(\frac{345}{700}\right)\left(\frac{16}{52}\right) = 0.49$$

as the standardized, adjusted rate of success. For hospital B, the corresponding result would be

$$\left(\frac{147}{700}\right)\left(\frac{40}{49}\right) + \left(\frac{199}{700}\right)\left(\frac{88}{151}\right) + \left(\frac{345}{700}\right)\left(\frac{94}{302}\right) = 0.49$$

The fact that the two hospitals have identical success results in the individual strata would now be reflected in an identical result for their standardized rates.

20.3.6.1.1. *Direct Standardization*

Public health epidemiologic data are regularly standardized according to the principle just described, but the process may differ in three minor ways: (1) The denominator groups usually represent a regional locality (such as a county, city, state, or nation) rather than a medical setting. (2) The particular variables used for the standardization are usually age and gender rather than severity of disease. (These variables are responsible for such phrases as *age-adjusted or age-gender standardized* to describe the subsequent rates.) (3) The standardizing population is usually obtained from the proportions of the appropriate strata noted in the most recent national census.

An example of this process can be shown if we compare the crude death rates of two cities—Houston, Texas, and the Tampa–St. Petersburg region in Florida. In Houston, which is not known for its salubrious climate, the death rate was 7.0 per thousand in 1970. In Tampa–St. Petersburg, the corresponding rate was 14.1. We can conclude either that Florida is a dangerous place to live or that the populations have a different composition. The latter distinction is shown in Table 20–8.

The stratum death rates in Table 20–8 are reasonably similar for the two cities in each stratum of age. The most striking difference is in the stratum proportions. Senior citizens (at age $\geqslant 65$) occupied 0.203 of the cohort in the Florida region but only 0.06 of the cohort in Houston. Because the death rate is highest in this oldest age group, the disparity might readily account for the difference in the crude rates even though the death rate among senior citizens was actually lower in Florida than in Houston.

If we wanted a single number with which to compare death rates in the two regions, we could standardize each region by using stratum proportions from the population of Houston, from the population of Tampa–St. Petersburg, or from a combination of the two populations. A more standard and traditional adjustment, however, uses stratum proportions for the population of the United States. This information, as shown in Table 20–9, would provide five values for our standardizing proportions. They would be $P_1 = 0.084$, $P_2 = 0.375$, $P_3 = 0.236$, $P_4 = 0.206$, and $P_5 = 0.099$.

Table 20–8. COMPOSITION OF POPULATION AND RATES OF DEATH IN TWO REGIONS OF THE UNITED STATES

	Houston				Tampa–St. Petersburg			
Age (Years)	Population ($\times 10^3$)	Number of Deaths	Stratum Death Rate ($\times 10^{-3}$)	Stratum Proportion	Population ($\times 10^3$)	Number of Deaths	Stratum Death Rate ($\times 10^{-3}$)	Stratum Proportion
<5	189.4	985	5.2	0.095	67.6	398	5.9	0.067
5–24	777.4	648	0.8	0.391	311.8	228	0.7	0.308
25–44	540.4	1389	2.6	0.272	203.3	552	2.7	0.201
45–64	357.9	4264	11.9	0.180	224.9	2871	12.7	0.222
$\geqslant 65$	119.9	6581	54.9	0.060	205.1	10,235	49.9	0.203
Total	1985.0	13,867	7.0	1.000	1012.7	14,284	14.1	1.000

Source of data: (a) U.S. Bureau of the Census. Census of Population 1970. Vol. 1. Characteristics of the Population. Part 1, United States Summary, Section 1. Washington, D.C., U.S. Government Printing Office, 1973; (b) National Center for Health Statistics. Vital Statistics of the United States 1970. Vol. 2. Mortality, Part B. Rockville, Maryland, National Center for Health Statistics, 1974.

Table 20–9. COMPOSITION OF POPULATION AND RATES OF DEATH FOR THE UNITED STATES, 1970

Age (Years)	Population ($\times 10^6$)	Number of Deaths ($\times 10^3$)	Stratum Death Rate ($\times 10^{-3}$)	Stratum Proportion
<5	17.2	57.8	3.4	0.084
5–24	76.2	39.9	0.5	0.375
25–44	48.0	78.4	1.6	0.236
45–64	41.8	327.5	7.8	0.206
≥65	20.0	756.2	37.8	0.099
Total	203.2	1259.8	6.2	1.000

Source of data: (a) U.S. Bureau of the Census. Census of Population 1970. Vol. 1. Characteristics of the Population. Part 1, United States Summary, Section 1. Washington, D.C., U.S. Government Printing Office, 1973; (b) National Center for Health Statistics. Vital Statistics of the United States 1970. Vol. 2. Mortality, Part B. Rockville, Maryland, National Center for Health Statistics, 1974.

Using the formula $\Sigma P_i r_i$, the standardized death rate for Houston would be $(0.084)(5.2) + (0.375)(0.8) + (0.236)(2.6) + (0.206)(11.9) + (0.099)(54.9) = 9.24$ per thousand. The standardized death rate for Tampa–St. Petersburg would be $(0.084)(5.9) + (0.375)(0.7) + (0.236)(2.7) + (0.206)(12.7) + (0.099)(49.9) = 8.95$ per thousand. The Florida chamber of commerce can now relax because the adjusted death rates become quite similar, although both of them exceed the national average of 6.2 per thousand.

This type of standardization process is commonly used to adjust for the demographic disparities of age and gender that may distort epidemiologic comparisons of regional rates of morbidity and mortality. The process is seldom used by clinicians because the key variables in clinical mortality for disease usually depend on severity of disease rather than demography, and besides, clinicians usually want to see the rates in each stratum rather than a single adjusted rate.

20.3.6.1.2. *Indirect Standardization*

The type of standardization that we performed in Section 20.3.6.1.1 is called *direct* because it uses the observed outcome rates in the strata and multiplies them by a standard set of stratum proportions. A different type of standardization is called *indirect*. It is used when we do not have the data we would want for the outcome rates in the observed strata. The strategy is to take the observed stratum proportions and multiply them by a standard set of stratum outcome rates.

Suppose we knew the populational distribution and the crude death rate of Houston but did not know the death rates in each stratum. In other words, we know that $p_1 = 0.095$, $p_2 = 0.391$, . . ., $p_5 = 0.060$, and that the crude death rate is 7.0 for Houston, but we do not know the associated values of $r_1 = 5.2$, $r_2 = 0.8$, . . ., $r_5 = 54.9$. If the people in Houston died at the same rate as people in the total U.S. population, the stratum death rates (from Table 20–9) would be $R_1 = 3.4$, $R_2 = 0.5$, . . ., $R_5 = 37.8$. Thus, the *expected* death rate in Houston would be $\Sigma p_i R_i$, which would be calculated as $(0.095)(3.4) + (0.391)(0.5) + (0.272)(1.6) + (0.180)(7.8) + (0.060)(37.8) = 4.63$. When the observed crude death rate of 7.0 in Houston is divided by the expected value of 4.63, we get an entity called the *Standard Mortality Ratio,* which is often abbreviated as SMR. In this instance, SMR = 7.0/4.63 = 1.51. It tells us the relationship of the observed crude death rate to what is expected from the indirect standardization. The observed rate in Houston is 1.51 times higher than what would be expected if its inhabitants were dying at the same rate as their standard counterparts. For the final standardized result to emerge, we multiply the SMR of Houston by the national standard death rate of 6.2. The product gives us the indirect standardized death rate for Houston, which is $1.51 \times 6.2 = 9.36$. (In this instance, the results of the direct and indirect standardizations are quite similar. They will not always be so, although we may not always be able to tell the difference, because we lack the necessary data. If the observed stratum rates for Houston were available, we would use them directly and would not need to calculate the indirect adjustment.)

20.3.6.1.3. *Hazards of Standardization*

The main hazards of standardization are that the results depend on whatever was chosen as the standardizing population. The observed results come from $\Sigma p_i r_i$. The standardizing population's results come from $\Sigma P_i R_i$. In the cross-over of the standardizing process, we get $\Sigma P_i r_i$ for the directly standardized results and $\Sigma p_i R_i$ for the expected value of the indirectly standardized results.

With either method, the value of the standardized results depends on the individual values of P_i and R_i that are found in the standardizing population. Unless the *same* standardizing population has been used for each of the compared values, the comparison of standardized results can be highly deceptive.

20.3.6.2. THE MANTEL-HAENSZEL ADJUSTMENT PROCEDURE

In the standardization procedures just described, we began with individual rates for cohort or cross-sectional denominator groups that were at risk for the outcome events; and we could do the standardization for each rate by using the results of a national population.

In case-control and in certain other cross-sectional studies, neither of these options is regularly available. The occurrences we determine may refer to antecedent exposures rather than subsequent outcomes; we may not know the results for the national population; and besides, the statistical adjustment is often aimed not at the separate rates of occurrence in individual groups but at a single odds ratio, which quantifies a contrast of two groups.

The adjustment becomes desirable if we suspect the odds ratio of being affected by certain important attributes that are disproportionately distributed in the compared groups. We could deal with these attributes, as we did in Table 20–7, by stratifying the results appropriately and by examining the odds ratios in each stratum. Thus, instead of drawing a conclusion from the crude odds ratio, we could stratify the groups under study and examine the odds ratios separately in men and in women or in the strata of young men, old men, young women, and old women, or in whatever other strata are suspected as being a source of bias. To draw a final conclusion about the odds ratio, however, we would need a mechanism that recombines the results of these individual strata into a single adjusted value.

A simple, elegant process for performing this adjustment was proposed by Mantel and Haenszel.[13] To illustrate the process, consider the results of the diabetes-hypercholesterolemia relationship cited as $\begin{Bmatrix} 21 & 24 \\ 59 & 296 \end{Bmatrix}$ in Table 20–5. When we examine things more closely, we discover that the group of 400 people contained 229 men and 171 women. If the odds ratio differs in men and in women, the higher proportion of men in the total group may distort the overall results. We therefore want to see whether the odds ratio of 4.39 is similar in men and in women. The answer to our question is provided by

Table 20–10. RESULTS OF TABLE 20–5 STRATIFIED FOR GENDER

Hypercholesterolemia	Men Diabetes Yes	No	Total	Women Diabetes Yes	No	Total
Yes	9	13	22	12	11	23
No	23	184	207	36	112	148
Total	32	197	229	49	123	171
Odds ratio:	$(9 \times 184)/(13 \times 23) = 5.54$ $X^2 = 14.7$			$(12 \times 112)/(11 \times 36) = 3.39$ $X^2 = 7.6$		

the stratified results in Table 20–10, which shows a substantial difference in odds ratios: 5.54 for men and 3.39 for women. This disparity would make us worry about the crude odds ratio of 4.39 in the unstratified data. This overall crude value of the odds ratio may be biased because of its higher value in men and the higher proportion of men in the total group. The Mantel-Haenszel method of adjusting for this bias is to recalculate the total odds ratio by giving appropriate weights to each of the component groups.

The reasoning works as follows: Let us assume that each of the groups in the stratified tables contains n_i members and is constructed as

$$\begin{Bmatrix} a_i & b_i \\ c_i & d_i \end{Bmatrix}$$

In the total overall table, the odds ratio will be $(\Sigma a_i \Sigma d_i)/(\Sigma b_i)(\Sigma c_i)$, but in each of the stratified tables, the odds ratio will be $a_i d_i/b_i c_i$. For example, in the stratification of Table 20–10, the respective values for men and women are $n_1 = 229$ and $n_2 = 171$. The respective odds ratios are $(9 \times 184)/(13 \times 23) = 5.54$ for $a_1 d_1/b_1 c_1$ and $(12 \times 112)/(11 \times 36) = 3.39$ for $a_2 d_2/b_2 c_2$.

We can make the appropriate adjustment by weighting each component odds ratio according to the n_i value from which it is derived and by then adding these components and dividing their sums. For the men, we would use $a_1 d_1/n_1 = (9 \times 184)/229 = 7.23$; and for the women, we would use $a_2 d_2/n_2 = (12 \times 112)/171 = 7.85$. Their sum would be 15.08. The corresponding values for $b_i c_i/n_i$ would be $(13 \times 23)/229 = 1.31$ for the men and $(11 \times 36)/171 = 2.32$ for the women, yielding a sum of 3.63. When we divide these two sums, we get $15.08/3.63 = 4.15$. This is the Mantel-Haenszel adjusted value of the odds ratio. Its value, as we would expect, lies between the 5.54 for men and the 3.39 for women. It also has lowered the overall value from 4.39 to 4.15, thus adjusting for the disproportionately high number of men.

The symbol for the Mantel-Haenszel adjusted odds ratio and the algebraic formula for the calculation are

$$O_{M-H} = \Sigma(a_i d_i/n_i)/\Sigma(b_i c_i/n_i)$$

Because of the imbalance in distribution of the men and women, the overall value of X^2 may also be distorted. It was 21.9 in Table 20–5, but the component values are 14.7 and 7.6 in Table 20–10. Mantel and Haenszel have also proposed a method for adjusting the value of X^2. The calculations of the adjusted X^2_{M-H} and of other strategies proposed for the adjustment can be found in more detailed statistical discussions[8, 14, 15] of this topic.

The stratification process (and the adjustments) are not restricted to the single variable shown in Table 20–10. The men and women could be further divided into old and young groups; and the old and young groups of men and women could be further divided according to categories of functional status and so on. An example of additional stratification for the data of Table 20–10 is presented in Exercise 20.9 at the end of the chapter.

20.3.6.3. MULTIVARIATE ADJUSTMENT PROCEDURES

Because many diverse attributes can be observed in the people under study, and because each attribute can be suspected as a possible source of distortion, many adjustment procedures contain multiple variables rather than clinical severity alone (as in Table 10–5), age alone (as in Table 10–8), or gender alone (as in Table 10–10). The adjustments may use combinations of two, three, or a multitude of different variables. The statistical methods of doing these multivariate analyses were briefly discussed in Chapter 10. Our main concern now is with the problems of trying to interpret the results of the adjustments.

20.3.6.3.1. *Problems in Multivariate Communication*

For medical readers, the first problem in multivariate communication is to understand what was done, how it was done, and what it produced. The vocabulary itself, let alone the operation of the mathematical model, may be a fundamental barrier to this comprehension. A reader who has illuminated the mystery of a simple *regression coefficient* may fall into instant darkness when confronted by a *standardized coefficient of partial regression*.

Beyond this superficial difficulty, however, lies the deeper difficulty of determining what has happened in a multivariate mathematical model that shows a calculated equation rather than an array of evidence. When data are presented in stratified tabulations, as in all the tables shown in this chapter, the reader can immediately see what was observed in the research. In the "number crunching" done by many of the multivariate models, however, the original evidence is transformed into diverse indexes of association. Thus a reader who wants to know what happened to **tall old men** can find the result in a table that presents multivariate evidence stratified for *height, age,* and *gender*. The actual evidence is not shown, however, when the mathematical model converts the data for these three variables into partial regression coefficients. Even if the reader successfully manages to understand the meaning of these coefficients, they remain indirect indexes of association rather than direct displays of evidence.

Consequently, to aid the understanding of both investigators and readers, a stratified tabulation of results can be quite helpful. If all of the analyzed variables were included, however, the tables would become unwieldy, and many of the multivariate categories would contain no members. This problem can easily be avoided by reducing the total number of variables to those that are most cogent and by forming composite categories, using methods discussed elsewhere.[16] For example, if we were studying patients with cancer, we could express the data with many individual variables that describe metastasis to every individual site in the body, such as adjacent lymph nodes, skin, bone, brain, liver, and so on. The many variables required for this description can be greatly reduced by using the composite categories of *regional metastasis* and *distant metastasis*.

20.3.6.3.2. *Delusions of Multivariate Adjustments*

Regardless of whether multivariate analyses are performed with or without a stratified display of the actual evidence, the main hazard of the procedure is the frequently erroneous belief that it has adjusted whatever distortions (or "confounders") are contained in the research. This belief is sometimes justified but is often a delusion.

If all the appropriate sources of distortion have been suitably recognized and entered into the multivariate analyses, they can often serve this adjusting function quite well. If important sources of distortion have been overlooked, omitted, or excluded from the analyzed evidence, however, no amount of mathematical manipulation can purge or purify the fundamental defects in the data and compared groups. Because the determination of what has been overlooked, omitted, or excluded requires scientific rather than mathematical decisions, a medical reader can usually make these judgments easily—but the reader may never reach this stage of reasoning if the claim of multivariate adjustment is credulously accepted without further evaluation. For cautious scientific appraisals, the main problems in most multivariate analyses are the biases that have not received suitable attention and the variables that have been omitted from the analyzed data.

20.4. THE ABSENCE OF REFERENCE DENOMINATORS

The indexes that create the risk ratio, odds ratio, nosologic sensitivity, nosologic specificity, and likelihood ratios all have one attribute in common: They ablate or ignore the pertinent denominators needed for their clinical comprehension and application.

A risk ratio, to be intelligible, must be supplemented by additional data to indicate the baseline risk and the incremental risk. An odds ratio, when used to denote risk, must be supplemented not only by baseline risk and incremental risk, but also by evidence that validates the odds ratio's accuracy in approximating a risk ratio. For clinical decisions, the indexes of nosologic sensitivity and specificity cannot be used directly and must be supplemented by denominator data, referring to prevalence, that permit their transformation into indexes suitable for diagnostic reasoning. The likelihood ratios require the other types of supplementation discussed in Chapter 25.

A medical reader is thus confronted not only with problems of understanding the basic statistical indexes of expression for cross-sectional studies, but also with the need to find additional data that enable the indexes to be interpreted. The additional data, however, may or may not be provided in the same cross-sectional study that yielded the statistical results. For example, suppose Table 20–1 is the product of a retrospective case-control study. To decide whether the odds ratio of 4.39 is a reasonably accurate approximation of the risk ratio, we would need to know the occurrence rate of diabetes in patients with hypercholesterolemia. This information is not contained in the case-control study that produced Table 20–1.

If we suppose that Table 20–1 is a diagnostic marker study, we can calculate 0.26 and 0.93, respectively, as the indexes of nosologic sensitivity and specificity for hypercholesterolemia in diagnosing diabetes mellitus. To determine how well hypercholesterolemia would perform clinically as a screening test for diabetes, however, we would need to know the prevalence of diabetes in the screened population. This information is also not provided by the case-control study of Table 20–1.

20.5. ERRORS DUE TO ATTRITION OR AUGMENTATION OF COHORT

All of the problems cited in Sections 20.1 to 20.4 deal with the reader's problems in understanding and interpreting the statistical evidence of cross-sectional studies. A quite different set of problems involves the trustworthiness of the statistical evidence itself. Whenever a cross-sectional study is used to substitute for a cohort study, the occurrence rates noted in the cross-section will almost always be an inaccurate representation of what happened in the cohort. The inaccuracies occur because the cohort will lose (or gain) various members between its inception and the time it reaches the cross-section that is studied by the investigator.

Because the maneuvers have already been imposed on the groups assembled in a cross-sectional study, the investigator collects the equivalent of a residue cohort. This residue consists of what remains after the original cohort has been altered by attrition or by augmentation. Some of the original members of the cohort may have died; others may have left the zone in which the cohort is under observation; yet others may have entered that zone by self-selection or by referral. Unlike a cohort study, however, cross-sectional research contains no data to let the investigator (or reader) know the composition of the original inception cohort or to determine how the original cohort has been changed.

By suitable inquiry, the investigator can ascertain and can exclude the members of the cross-section who have migrated into the original cohort, but the investigator cannot determine who has left it. The people are not there to be interviewed; and the investigator does not know who they are, how many of them are missing, or why they are missing. Unless the investigator can find a roster or other source of information to indicate what the original cohort should have been, there is no way to check whether the attritions or unrecognized augmentations have created a major or minor distortion of the results. If the necessary evidence is not available and cannot be acquired without performing the cohort study for which the cross-section is being substituted, the effects of the substitution must be evaluated with scientific judgment.

The scientific judgment depends not on the statistical information but on the type of maneuvers being investigated, the circumstances surrounding the imposition of the maneuvers, and the events that can occur during the elapsed serial time between a person's entrance into the cohort and appearance in the cross-section. In a study of biodynamic phenomena (such as normal growth and development in healthy people), attritions due to death are not as likely to occur as in studies of pathodynamic phenomena. In studies of pathodynamic phenomena (such as the development of complications or recurrences of a disease), the severity of the disease will affect the proportion of the cohort lost by death; and the characteristics of the medical setting (or zone) in which the study is done will affect both the cohort's losses due to nonlethal causes and the augmentations due to selective referral of patients. In case-control studies of etiologic or therapeutic agents, the residues assembled as cases and controls will have been potentially affected by all of the biases that can enter a nonexperimental study of cause-effect maneuvers.

20.5.1. *Illustration of Hypothetical Problems*

The problems can be illustrated if we think about their effects in a biodynamic and in a pathodynamic cross-sectional study.

For the biodynamic study, let us consider the way pediatricians construct the curves of annual growth in height and weight for normal children from ages 1 to 10. In a cohort study, we would assemble a single large group of children at age 1. We would follow them at annual intervals thereafter. The results obtained at those annual examinations until age 10 would show the changes in the cohort.

Because such a study is not easy to do, a simpler approach is to perform it as a set of longitudinal cross-sections. We find one group of normal children at age 1 and determine their spectrum of height and weight. We assemble another group of normal children at age 2 and determine their spectrum. We find similar groups and collect similar data for children at ages 3, 4, 5, and so on through age 10. The results found in these cross-sectional groups are then arranged longitudinally to form the normal growth curves used in daily practice by pediatricians throughout the world. The results seem reasonable as a substitute for cohort research, because we need not fear that substantial proportions of otherwise healthy children may die between one year and the next.

Now suppose we want to do another biodynamic study, determining the curves of quadrennial change in serum cholesterol and triglycerides for healthy adults between ages 60 and 80. In the cross-sectional approach, we would assemble groups of healthy adults at ages 60, 64, 68, 72, 76, and 80. The longitudinal curves drawn from the cross-sectional spectrums in these age groups might not be as readily acceptable as those obtained in the children. The original cohort will surely have lost many of its members by the time we meet the residue of survivors in the cross-sections at ages 76 and 80. If the people with high levels of cholesterol and triglycerides tend to die sooner than those with low levels, we may reach the quite erroneous conclusion that a fall in lipids is a physiologic concomitant of normal aging.

For a pathodynamic study, suppose we want to determine the occurrence of diabetic retinopathy during 10 years and 20 years after the detection of diabetes mellitus in adults. In a cross-sectional study, we would assemble a group of patients who have had diabetes for 10 years and another group who have had it for 20 years. This investigation has a strong potential for producing misleading results in the survivors who remain after members of the original cohort are removed by death. To demonstrate the problem, let us assume that the following things happen to the members of the original inception cohort:

1. During the first 10 years after detection of the diabetes mellitus, 10% of the cohort die. Retinopathy occurs in 20% of those who die and in 5% of the survivors.

2. During the next 10 years, death occurs in 20% of those who already have retinopathy. In those who did not yet have retinopathy, it develops in 16%; and of these "newly" retinopathic patients, 10% die. Among the remaining nonretinopathic patients, 5% die.

If we apply these conditions to an inception cohort of 10,000 persons with newly detected diabetes mellitus, 1000 would die in the first 10 years, and 200 of these would have had retinopathy. Of the 9000 survivors, 450 would have retinopathy. A cohort study would show the rate of retinopathy to be 650/10,000 = 6.5% at the end of 10 years. A cross-sectional study of the 9000 survivors would show this rate to be 450/9000 = 5%.

During the next 10 years, 90 ($= 0.20 \times 450$) of the retinopathic patients would die. Retinopathy would newly develop in $(0.16)(8550) = 1368$ patients, and of these, 137 would die. Among the remaining 7182 patients, 359 ($= 0.05 \times 7182$) would die. The total occurrence rate for development of retinopathy in the original cohort at the end of 20 years would be $(200 + 450 + 1368)/10,000 = 20\%$. In a cross-sectional study of the survivors at the end of 20 years, we would have $1368 - 137 = 1231$ patients with retinopathy and $7182 - 359 = 6823$ patients without it. We would conclude that the occurrence rate of retinopathy is $1231/(1231 + 6823) = 15\%$. The two sets of studies would thus show the following rates for the occurrence of retinopathy:

	Cohort Rate	Cross-Sectional Rate
At 10 years	6.5%	5%
At 20 years	20%	15%

A cross-sectional study of a longitudinally occurring phenomenon will almost certainly produce inaccuracies of this type. The basic results may be correct in demonstrating the general trend of the occurrence rates, but the individual rates may be inaccurate. The judgmental challenge in evaluation is to determine whether the rates are merely inaccurate quantitatively, as in the foregoing diabetic example, or whether they actually misrepresent or distort the phenomenon, as in the example of changes in lipids with aging.

20.5.2. *Examples of Real Problems*

Because relatively few long-term cohort studies of clinical phenomena have been conducted and compared with longitudinal cross-sectional studies, the magnitudes and effect of the efforts are difficult to demonstrate with real-world data. In one of three excellent examples, Weiss reviewed the risks associated with occupational exposures and showed the fallaciously distorted rates that can occur when a longitudinal cohort is assessed with repeated cross-sectional collections of data. In each of several published instances cited by Weiss,[17] the cross-sectional rates of an adverse outcome event (such as a cancer) were substantially elevated above the correct rate in the inception cohort.

In a second example of the problem, Henderson and Reinke,[18] studying factors affecting the duration and outcome of pregnancy, noted three types of bias that could arise from cross-sectional appraisals of longitudinal data. In one bias, the women who registered at a clinic early in pregnancy had a higher rate of prematurity than those who registered late. The distinction would have been missed if the rate of prematurity was examined only cross-sectionally without regard to the stage of pregnancy when follow-up began. A second bias arose because patients included in a cohort of pregnant women may drop out of the cohort later on. If not suitably compensated in the analyses, these losses can falsely elevate the rate of prematurity found in women who continue to be followed.

The third bias can arise from the secular timing of the study. When pregnant women are enrolled in cohort research, their pregnancy has an antecedent duration before they enter the cohort. If the admissions take place during a defined secular interval, the people enrolled at the earlier secular period, when the study begins, will contain a relatively high proportion of women who are close to delivery. The admissions toward the end of the secular period will tend to exclude pregnancies delivered early and will thereby seem to lower the rate of prematurity. These biases can be avoided if the study is confined to an inception cohort of women followed from very early in pregnancy until all women in the group have been delivered.

A third example, showing a quite different type of problem in longitudinal cohort versus longitudinal prevalence data, appeared in a study of spirometry by Glindmeyer and coworkers.[19] After obtaining spirometric function tests for 52 men on five annual occasions during a 5-year period, the investigators examined the longitudinal changes in two different ways. For cohort analysis, each person's changing values over time were fitted with a straight line, and the group's change as a cohort was determined as the average slope of the 52 lines. For longitudinal-prevalence analysis, the trend was examined in the mean values determined for the spectrum of cross-sectional results at each annual visit. After noting striking disparities in certain types of data, the investigators concluded that "it is unwise to use cross-sectional age coefficients as benchmarks for the evaluation of annual change in lung function determined by longitudinal study." The findings are particularly pertinent for issues in the serial range of normal, discussed in Chapter 28.

20.5.3. *Problems in Retrospective Case-Control Studies*

In the examples cited in Section 20.5.1 for biodynamic and pathodynamic maneuvers, the occurrence rates obtained in the cross-sectional studies were longitudinal prevalence rates. They could be compared directly (as 5% vs. 6.5% or as 15% vs. 20%) for their accuracy in representing the incidence rates that would be found in a cohort study; and, if the accuracy seems satisfactory, the longitudinal prevalence rates might be used as substitutes for incidence rates.

If the longitudinal phenomena involve a comparison of etiologic or therapeutic maneuvers, however, and if the cross-sectional research structure is a retrospective case-control study, the rates that emerge indicate an antecedent prevalence of maneuvers rather than a longitudinal prevalence of outcomes. For reasons cited earlier, these rates of antecedent prevalence cannot be compared with incidence rates and cannot be used as substitutes for them.

In the judgmental evaluation of trohoc evidence, therefore, the main problems to be considered are gross distortions due to bias rather than quantitative issues in the accuracy with which a longitudinal prevalence rate can substitute for an incidence rate. The scientific problems of bias in retrospective case-control studies will be discussed further in Chapters 21 to 23.

20.6. ABSENCE OF DESCRIPTIVE RESULTS

Although medical readers may often have difficulty in interpreting statistical indexes of description rather than the actual statistical evidence, the ultimate problem in communication of results occurs when neither the evidence nor the descriptive indexes are presented. To satisfy the demands of an editor, the results of the research may appear only in charts or graphs from which crucial data have been omitted; and the statistical indexes may cite a relationship whose direction is omitted. Thus, the investigator may say that "a relationship was noted between height and survival" but may not indicate whether survival rose or fell as height increased. Finally, the statistical evidence and descriptive indexes may have been completely replaced, as noted earlier, by P values and other symbols of statistical inference.

20.7. SYNOPSIS

The unfamiliar statistical expressions that appear in published literature are often a major impediment to a medical reader's understanding of the evidence.

Because of the temporal versatility of cross-sectional studies, the data in the statistical structures may be oriented in directions that reverse or confuse ordinary patterns of scientific thought. For analytic convenience, the components needed in scientific evaluations may be fused into a single composite index that provides a useful summary of the results, but that cannot be adequately interpreted without a knowledge of the missing components. The *risk ratio,* for example, shows the distinction noted in the quotient of two rates of risk but does not indicate crucial information about the baseline risk or the increment of attributable risk.

The odds ratio in a cross-sectional or case-control study has some major advantages. It can avoid problems in directional orientation, eliminate choices between row and column denominators, allow two different sampling fractions, and approximate the risk ratio that would be found in a cohort study. The odds ratio has the disadvantage of confusing readers who do not realize it comes from four numbers rather than two. It also overestimates the risk ratio when the true occurrence rates are relatively high (i.e., >0.1), and it encourages studies of small groups whose results are statistically fragile, despite stochastic significance. The fragility of the odds ratio can be evaluated from its confidence interval, but the implications of a wide confidence interval are not always carefully considered. The main problem in the odds ratio (or in other composite ratios), however, arises not from the mathematical structure of the ratio, but from the frequent failure of the underlying research to fulfill statistical requirements in sampling and scientific requirements in the architectural distinctions of groups and data.

In the cross-sectional or case-control research used for diagnostic marker studies, the conventional statistical indexes refer to a nosologic sensitivity and nosologic specificity that are not useful for clinical application of the results and that may be misleading because they ignore the prevalence of the disease in the group under study. To achieve clinical pertinence, the nosologic indexes must be transformed into predictive indexes of diagnostic sensitivity and diagnostic specificity. Although this transformation can be easily shown with simple algebra, it is often expressed in the complex symbols of Bayes theorem. A different method of achieving the transformation is to use likelihood ratios. They are easier to understand than the Bayesian symbols and they can avoid the need for converting dimensional measurements into binary categories, but they involve complex ratios of odds that must be dissected and reconstructed into probability values to make the results clinically cogent.

Statistical adjustments are commonly used to remove or reduce the possibilities of distortion due to confounding variables that are disproportionately distributed in the compared groups. The adjustments are easy to understand when the evidence is stratified and presented in tabulations for the attributes that are maldistributed. For many comparisons, however, the stratified results are recombined into a single index for each group. Mortality and morbidity rates for an ecologic region are often adjusted in this manner by being standardized for a selected population, which is usually the entire nation. The standardization is direct when it depends on the proportionate distribution of the standard strata, and indirect when it depends on the outcome rates in the standard strata. In case-control studies, the Mantel-Haenszel procedure of weighting the results in component strata is commonly used to adjust the odds ratio for groups in which the strata may be maldistributed.

Although stratified tabulations have the advantage of displaying the evidence directly, the display may be unwieldy for a large number of variables. The multiple variables can be reduced and combined into cogent composite categories, but many data analysts prefer to use multivariate mathematical models that depend on the addition of weighted combinations of variables. The results of these models are often confusing because readers do not understand the strategies behind the "number crunching" and because the basic evidence is obscured when reported indirectly as indexes of multivariate association. Regardless of whether the multivariate adjustments are done with stratified tables or additive models, however, their main hazard is the frequently erroneous belief that adjusting a multiplicity of variables has purified the results, although major sources of bias may not have been considered in the research or included in the analyzed data.

A fundamental problem in all cross-sectional studies is the unknown attrition or augmentation of the inception cohort that would have been investigated in ideal circumstances. According to the way these attritions or augmentations occur, the cross-sectional results can be a suitable substitute or a gross distortion for what would have been found in the appropriate cohort.

EXERCISES

[For classroom usage, these exercises are divided into two parts. Exercises 20.1 through 20.4 refer to the text up to Section 20.3.6. Exercises 20.5 and thereafter refer to the text from Section 20.3.6 to the end of the chapter.]

Exercise 20.1. In 1983, Goldacre and coworkers[20] reported results of a case-control study testing the hypothesis that vasectomy may predispose men to cardiovascular disease. The cases consisted of men, below age 55, who had been hospitalized or who died with diagnoses of myocardial infarction, stroke, or hypertension. The controls for hospitalized cases were chosen from acute care medical and surgical discharges at the same hospital. The controls for men who died without being hospitalized were chosen from control death certificates. Two controls were chosen for each case and matched for age (within 5 years), admission date (within 6 months), and district of residence. Men with certain chronic diseases (e.g., multiple sclerosis) or with cardiovascular diseases were excluded from the control group. For each patient, the performance of antecedent vasectomy was sought and checked when necessary in records examined without any knowledge of whether the patient was a case or control.

The overall results showed the following numbers:

Previous Vasectomy	Cases	Controls
Yes	36	81
No	1476	2943
Total	1512	3024

Without further consideration of scientific quality in the design and analysis of this study, please answer the following questions about the statistical results.

20.1.1. What are the odds that a control patient had received vasectomy?

20.1.2. What are the odds that vasectomy had occurred in a case?

20.1.3. What is the odds ratio for the table?

20.1.4. What is the confidence interval for the odds ratio? What do you conclude from its result?

20.1.5. What is the risk of cardiovascular disease in a man who has had a vasectomy?

20.1.6. What is the risk of cardiovascular disease in a man who has *not* had a vasectomy?

20.1.7. What is the risk ratio?

Exercise 20.2. In 1971, Herbst and coworkers[21] reported the following results for a case-control study of the relationship between clear cell vaginal cancer and in utero exposure to diethylstilbestrol.

	Cases	Controls
Exposed	7	0
Nonexposed	1	32

After showing what you did to determine whether this result is stochastically significant, calculate the odds ratio and its confidence interval for these data. Please use at least three different methods for calculating the confidence interval to see how well the results agree.

Exercise 20.3. As a diagnostic marker for acute myocardial infarction, creatine phosphokinase (CPK) showed the following results:[22]

	Number of Patients with Myocardial Infarction	
Value of CPK	Yes	No
≥280	97	1
80–279	118	15
<80	15	114

20.3.1. If you set 80 as the boundary for an abnormally high CPK, what are the values for the nosologic sensitivity, nosologic specificity, diagnostic sensitivity, diagnostic specificity, positive likelihood ratio, and negative likelihood ratio of the test?

20.3.2. With symbols as defined in the text, what are the numerical values of $P(D)$, $P(D|T)$, $P(T|\bar{D})$, and $P(\bar{D}|\bar{T})$ that can be found in the fourfold table of Exercise 20.3.1? Calculate the value of $P(D|T)$ using appropriate substitutions into Bayes theorem.

20.3.3. Now set 280 as the boundary for an abnormally high CPK and reconstruct the fourfold table for these data. What happens to the values of the six indexes you determined in Exercise 20.3.1?

20.3.4. Without converting the cited data to a fourfold table, what simple method can you use for expressing the results of the test?

20.3.5. A clinician tells you he does not understand the index(es) you provided in Section 20.3.4. He wants you to explain it to him in simple terms. What would you say?

Exercise 20.4. An investigator wants to use the white blood count (WBC) to differentiate streptococcal from nonstreptococcal causes of sore throat. A group of 100 cases with culture-proved group A streptococcal sore throats is assembled; and the patients are matched individually in age, race, and gender, with a control group of patients whose sore throats were culture-negative. The mean and standard deviation values for WBC are 9265 ± 487 in the cases and 8130 ± 640 in the controls. After showing that the results are stochastically significant, the investigator concludes that the white blood count offers a useful index for discriminating between streptococcal and nonstreptococcal pharyngitis.

20.4.1. Please verify the investigator's conclusion about stochastic significance.

20.4.2. Are you satisfied with the presentation of the data? If not, why not?

20.4.3. Do you agree with the investigator's conclusions? If not, why not?

Exercise 20.5. Suppose you know the stratum proportions for hospital A as shown in Table 20–6 and you know the crude success rate of $124/198 = 63\%$ in that hospital, but you do not know the stratum-specific success rates. You have been asked to perform an *indirect* standardization for the results of hospital A, using the results of hospital B (in Table 20–7) as the standardizing population. What would you do and what would your answer be?

Exercise 20.6. What is the direct standardized death rate for Houston in Table 20–8 if you use the Tampa–St. Petersburg data as the standardizing population?

Exercise 20.7. The results of the annual death rate per thousand people in the United States at various point in secular time can be approximated as follows:

	1920	1940	1960	1980
Method A	14.4	10.6	7.5	5.2
Method B	12.5	10.6	9.1	8.9

One of these methods shows the crude death rate. The other method shows the directly standardized death rate, according to the population noted at one of the census years.

20.7.1. Which year was used for the standardization?

20.7.2. Which method shows the crude death rates? What is the reason for your answer?

Exercise 20.8. In 1974, the Royal College of General Practitioners[23] reported the results of a cooperative prolective cohort study investigating the relationship of subsequent morbid events and type of contraception in about 47,000 women. About 23,000 women were cited as takers, i.e., users of oral contraceptives; and the remaining women were either former users (i.e., ex-takers) or nonusers (i.e., controls). The occurrences of certain morbid events were presented as rates of occurrence for each of these three maneuvers, and a "standardised rate per thousand women years" was listed for each morbid event. The following is an exact replica of the text describing the standardization process:

The morbidity data are simultaneously standardised for age, parity, social class, and cigarette consumption. The indirect method of standardisation is used. The morbidity rates in the total Study population are used as standard.

Seven sub-groups are used for both age and social class, and six sub-groups for both parity and cigarette smoking. This results in 1,764 cells in each of the three contraceptive groups—Takers, Ex-Takers, Controls.

The relationship of the Takers, the Ex-Takers, and the Controls is dynamic, in that there is constant movement of subjects between the groups. The advantage of basing standardisation upon cumulative experience is that it makes allowance for all changes in group characteristics which have occurred up to that date.

Information on the four characteristics used for standardisation is not complete for all 47,000 subjects. The age is known for all, but 13 subjects have no parity recorded, and these are entirely excluded from the standardised data. The 135 subjects whose social class was indeterminate have been classified with "other." The daily cigarette consumption of 148 subjects who smoked was not recorded, and they were included in the middle of the five ranges of cigarette consumption. Any errors due to incorrect coding of these few subjects would, of course, have no material influence on the results of the standardisation procedure.

In general, the standardisation procedure has resulted in only small adjustments to the non-standardised rates.

20.8.1. How did the "1764 cells" arise?

20.8.2. Do you understand what was done for the standardization? If so, please write a brief set of directions that would tell a computer programmer or a research assistant how to work with the data to do the job.

20.8.3. Why do you think the investigators used an indirect rather than a direct standardization?

20.8.4. Do you agree that this multivariate standardization process is reasonable? Do you believe it takes care of the major biases that might be present in this study?

Exercise 20.9. The investigator who did the work cited in Tables 20–5 and 20–10 of the text has given you some additional information about the people. It shows the following:

Presence of Hypercholesterolemia	Old Men		Young Men		Old Women		Young Women	
	Yes	No	Yes	No	Yes	No	Yes	No
Yes	5	6	4	7	7	5	5	6
No	13	104	10	80	12	40	24	72

(Presence of Diabetes in)

20.9.1. Does this information change your previous opinion about the cited relationship? (Indicate whatever calculations you did to check the situation.)

20.9.2. What are the overall odds ratios in this study, irrespective of gender, for old and young people?

20.9.3. Calculate an odds ratio that would adjust the results of this study for any disproportions concomitantly noted in age and gender.

Exercise 20.10. You want to do a cross-sectional study of a new diagnostic test for cancer. You plan to choose cases and controls from a hospital population and to study their corresponding levels of *neoplasmognome,* the chemical substance that may denote the presence of a cancer. Name at least one main *chronologic* difficulty that may distort the results because your study is cross-sectional rather than longitudinal.

Exercise 20.11. A cohort of diabetic patients, all of them free of retinopathy, will be assembled at age 15. The cohort can be divided into two strata having a high risk and low risk for the future development of retinopathy and death. The subsequent incidence rates with time for the two strata can be shown as follows:

	High-Risk Stratum		Low-Risk Stratum	
	From Age 15 to 34	*From Age 35 to 55*	*From Age 15 to 34*	*From Age 35 to 55*
Alive, no retinopathy	55%	27%	84%	68%
Alive, with new retinopathy	20%	25%	8%	12%
Dead, with new retinopathy	15%	30%	6%	14%
Dead, without retinopathy	10%	18%	2%	6%
Alive, with old retinopathy	—	60%	—	82%
Dead, with old retinopathy	—	40%	—	18%

If the cohort contains 75% high-risk patients and 25% low-risk patients, what would be the cohort incidence rates for retinopathy at ages 35 and 55? What would be the longitudinal prevalence rates for retinopathy if the available members of the cohort are examined cross-sectionally at ages 35 and 55? (Hint: Although all of this can be worked out algebraically, the calculations may be easier if you assume that the cohort begins with 20,000 patients at age 15.)

CHAPTER REFERENCES

1. Cornfield, 1951; 2. Cole, 1979; 3. Doll, 1952; 4. MacMahon, 1981; 5. Feinstein, 1981; 6. Fleiss, 1979; 7. Cornfield, 1956; 8. Fleiss, 1981; 9. Woolf, 1955; 10. Miettinen, 1976; 11. Greenwald, 1971; 12. Youden, 1950; 13. Mantel, 1959; 14. Schlesselman, 1982; 15. Kleinbaum, 1982; 16. Feinstein, 1972; 17. Weiss, 1983; 18. Henderson, 1966; 19. Glindmeyer, 1982; 20. Goldacre, 1983; 21. Herbst, 1971; 22. Department of Clinical Epidemiology (McMaster), 1983; 23. Royal College of General Practitioners, 1974.

Scientific Decisions in Choosing Groups

Beyond the statistical issues cited in Chapter 20, cross-sectional studies contain a more important set of problems that are scientific rather than mathematical. The problems arise because cross-sectional studies allow the investigator to make many arbitrary decisions in choosing groups and getting data, and because no well-established, consistently applied scientific standards have been developed for making the decisions.

After the research hypothesis is stated for a cohort study, the groups to be examined are defined by the maneuvers under comparison. The maneuvers may or may not have been allocated experimentally, and they may or may not have been observed with preplanned methods of data collection—but no one has any doubt about which maneuvers are being investigated or whether the maneuvers preceded the outcomes.

In cross-sectional research, however, everything has already happened before the investigator reaches the scene. In each person selected for the study, the baseline states, maneuvers, and outcomes under investigation have already occurred. If the cross-sectional study is concerned with etiologic or therapeutic maneuvers, the people who enter the study are *not* chosen according to their baseline state, as in a randomized trial, or according to their baseline state and imposed maneuvers, as in an observational cohort study. In many instances, the cross-sectional groups are chosen according to their directly known outcomes, as cases or controls; and the investigator then ascertains each person's antecedent baseline state and maneuvers. In other instances, the cross-sectional groups are assembled as a single collection of people; and the investigator then obtains the data that allow each person to be classified simultaneously for baseline state, maneuvers, and outcome.

The cross-sectional research has a forward direction in biodynamic and pathodynamic studies in which the basic groups are chosen according to the maneuvers of health and disease. Because the groups are not assembled in a premaneuver baseline state, the research usually begins long after imposition of the maneuvers, which are represented by the diseased cases, nondiseased controls, or other groups under contrast. The scientific accuracy of the research will obviously depend on whether the chosen groups and their observed outcomes accurately represent the spectrum of clinical conditions that are the contrasted maneuvers. An analogous situation occurs in the cross-sectional evaluation of marker tests and other processes. Here, too, the selected groups of patients represent a spectrum of health and disease that must be suitable in its scope and proportional constituents.

These distinctions create major scientific difficulties at the very onset of a cross-sectional study, when the investigator chooses the basic groups to be investigated. In cohort research, the choice is made with a simple scientific standard. The groups are demarcated according to their baseline state, before imposition of the maneuvers. In cross-sectional research, however, the groups are already in an outcome state. The maneuvers may not be discovered until the groups are chosen; or the previous effects of biodynamic and pathodynamic maneuvers may have distorted the spectrum of people available to form the groups. Lacking a straightforward standard for choosing the fundamental groups, the cross-sectional investigator has no clear scientific guidelines for the strategy. In the absence of rigorous scientific standards, the remarkable versatility of cross-sectional research has been accompanied by a remarkable diversity of methods not only for choosing groups but also for collecting data and interpreting the results.

The rest of this chapter is concerned with the problems of bias in choosing a basic framework for cross-sectional research and demarcating the basic groups under study. The next chapter will be devoted to the collection of data and management of subsequent hypotheses. Many of the main scientific problems in cross-sectional studies arise from the opaque shields that nature may erect to keep its secrets from being revealed, but many other major problems are due to the clouded vision we may produce in ourselves while searching for the revelations.

21.1. EFFECTS AND SOURCES OF BIAS

In all of the cohort and cross-sectional structures of homodemic research, the maneuvers and outcomes can be shown as the two main axes of a fourfold table that appears as:

Exposure to Principal Maneuver	Presence of Outcome Event	
	Yes	*No*
Yes	a	b
No	c	d

In representing the effects of the compared maneuvers, the numerical values of $\begin{Bmatrix} a & b \\ c & d \end{Bmatrix}$ in this table can be distorted internally or externally. The internal problems create an unfair or *biased comparison.* The external problems, which were previously discussed as *distorted assembly,* produce results that do not adequately represent the intended population, even if the internal comparison is unbiased.

A reader (or investigator) can readily discern the existence of an externally distorted assembly. By examining the characteristics of the investigated groups, we can promptly decide whether they suitably represent the people to whom the results will be externally applied. For example, the investigator may have compared several antibiotics in the treatment of urinary tract infections in young women living in the northeastern United States. Unless we have some reason to believe that these women are unique, the results can presumably be extended to apply to the treatment of urinary tract infections in young women living in many other parts of the world. On the other hand, the results may not necessarily pertain to urinary tract infections in older women or in men.

The existence of internal biases is much more difficult to recognize. As discussed in earlier chapters, subtle problems can arise in every architectural component of comparison when the maneuvers are actually performed and when data are later collected to show the results. If these problems are not prevented or suitably managed, the members of the four cells in the table will be accrued in disporportionate numbers that create biased results for the internal comparison of the maneuvers.

21.1.1. *Architectural Effects of Bias*

The four main locations for bias in the architecture of a cause-effect relationship were shown earlier as susceptibility in baseline states, performance of maneuvers, detection of outcomes, and transfer of groups or data. These effects will produce values for a, b, c, and d (or more elaborate enumerations) that distort what should have happened in a fair comparison of the two maneuvers.

The role of an experimental trial is to act as an artificial investigational structure that uses special tactics to try to thwart the effects of these biases. When cause-effect research is not conducted as an experimental trial—and sometimes even when it is—the investigator and reader must beware of distortions produced by these biases. The scientific credibility of the results will depend on how well the investigator has taken precautions to avoid the biases or to adjust the data appropriately.

The types of precautions that can be used in cohort research were discussed in Chapters 15 to 17. In cross-sectional research, the opportunity for bias—particularly in the transfer from actual to counted groups—is substantially greater than in cohort research because an inception cohort is seldom identified and because all of the data collections and enumerations occur *after* the maneuvers and outcome events have already transpired.

21.1.2. *Sources of Innate Bias*

The terms *susceptibility, performance, detection,* and *transfer* refer to the effects of bias occurring at different locations in the causal pathway. These effects can have many different sources, which can be catalogued in two main groups: the *innate* biases that arise during the actual imposition and consequences of maneuvers; and the *investigative* biases that occur during the subsequent research. This section contains a brief review of sources of innate bias.

Susceptibility bias can have at least six innate sources. It is most commonly produced by *allocation bias,* when maneuvers are either self-selected or clinically assigned for people with major prognostic differences in susceptibility to the outcome event. Because of these selections, people receiving maneuver A may not fulfill the same admission criteria as those receiving maneuver B and may have striking differences in prognostic expectations for the outcome event. Susceptibility bias can also be created, as discussed in Sections 16.2.3.2 and 16.2.4.2, when people with different prognostic expectations refuse or abandon the maintenance of a particular maneuver because they have difficulty in suitable *compliance* or suitable *regulation* for that maneuver.

The problems of *vulnerability* (see Section 15.5.2.3) can produce susceptibility bias if the recipients of a maneuver are either excessively or inadequately susceptible to its action. A fifth source of susceptibility bias, which is discussed further in Section 21.2.2.1.3, is the existence of a *protopathic* problem in temporal precedence when the maneuvers are chosen. This type of problem arises when the outcome event, although often not yet identified, has already occurred at baseline. The clinical manifestations of the event may then affect the choice of the baseline maneuver with which the outcome is later associated. The sixth source of susceptibility bias arises because of patterns of *referral* or *migration* (see Section 15.5.2.7) that may bring people with unusually good (or poor) prognoses to a particular location, such as a hospital or geographic region, which may then seem to have particularly good (or poor) rates of outcome events when compared with other locations.

Performance bias has two main innate sources, which are intrinsic and extrinsic. Intrinsically, the maneuvers may not have been given or received with appropriate proficiency. Extrinsically, the action of the compared maneuvers may have been contaminated by the action of various co-maneuvers.

Detection bias arises from natural phenomena that lead to differences in the medical surveillance, ordering of tests, or interpretation of outcome evidence for the recipients of different maneuvers. Aside from expectations that make people anticipate good or bad results from a particular maneuver, the detection bias problem can also be produced, as discussed in Section 17.4, by intensive attention to a new maneuver, by the existence of a co-morbid disease that evokes increased medical surveillance, or by a maneuver's production of incidental co-manifestations, which lead to tests that detect an otherwise silent coexisting disease.

Transfer bias occurs innately if the different types of outcomes for a particular maneuver are not suitably represented in the collected data. The outcome events may have led to disproportions in people who become lost to follow-up or who are referred afterward to the sites at which the research groups are accrued. The different sources and effects of *referral bias* will be discussed later in Section 21.2.2.5.

21.1.3. *Sources of Investigative Bias*

Because the innate biases that are inherent in the human events under investigation can be eliminated only in special experimental circumstances, a plan for nonexperimental research must anticipate the biases and deal with them appropriately. The origin of a different set of biases, however, is investigative rather than innate.

Because cross-sectional research begins after the various innate biases have already occurred, an investigator either can passively allow these biases to persist or can actively try to correct them. The investigative efforts, however, may lead to certain transfer phenomena that augment the existing biases or create new ones. The investigative phenomena are transfer biases in their source, but their effects can appear at the susceptibility, performance, and detection locations in the pathway of causal comparisons.

As discussed later, analogs of susceptibility bias or detection bias can be produced by various transfers that arise from the investigator's decisions about which groups to include in the research. Similar effects in susceptibility and detection can be produced by the participation bias of people who are solicited to volunteer their data. An analog of performance bias can arise when data are excerpted from archival records or when people are interviewed to determine their antecedent exposure to maneuvers. These transfer phenomena during the investigative activities can alter the results of purely descriptive research and can distort the proportions or other evidence contrasted in comparative research.

The rest of this chapter and part of Chapter 22 are concerned with the diverse sources of innate and investigative biases in cross-sectional research and with mechanisms that can be used to avoid the biases.

21.2. **OPPORTUNITIES FOR BIAS IN CROSS-SECTIONAL RESEARCH**

Because cross-sectional research can be used for purely descriptive purposes as well as for studying processes and cause-effect relationships, different kinds of bias can occur to distort the results.

In descriptive research, there are no compared maneuvers to be checked for biases in susceptibility or performance. The main problems are in transfer and in detection. The transfer problem is reflected in the spectrum of the group under study and the detection problem appears when the selected characteristics of the group are ascertained. These problems are well illustrated by long-standing difficulties in the decennial cross-sectional study that is called a *national census*. The scope of the studied population may be impaired by the census taker's inability to reach all members of certain ethnic groups; and the interviewed persons may be reluctant to give accurate answers about certain questions relating to income, sex, life style, or other sensitive features of behavior.

In process research, analogous but somewhat different problems arise in scope and detection. The groups chosen for comparison in the research may not contain an adequate scope of conditions to challenge the procedure being tested; and the output produced by one procedure may not be suitably blinded to keep its results from biasing the output of the other procedure. Other sources of bias, discussed in Chapters 25 to 27, can arise when the framework of comparison is chosen during the basic planning of the study.

In cause-effect research, when a logistically easy cross-sectional structure is substituted for a logistically difficult cohort structure, we might expect special attention to be given to the problems produced by the four different forms of bias. Surprisingly, however, these biases often receive much less attention in cross-sectional research than they do in cohort research.

The problems of bias in cross-sectional studies will be discussed separately for biodynamic and pathodynamic research, and for etiologic and therapeutic research.

21.2.1. *Biodynamic and Pathodynamic Studies*

In explicatory studies of physiologic, pharmacologic, and pathophysiologic phenomena, the main issue in susceptibility bias arises from the scope of the spectrum of healthy and diseased people under investigation. The responses to certain physiologic or pharmacologic stimuli in normal people are often analyzed as though they represented health, but the responses found in small groups of healthy volunteers may not adequately represent what would be found in a group containing a broader scope of age, gender, race, or ethnic background.

In explicatory studies of pathophysiology in diseased groups, the spectrum of the disease is particularly important. Because every human ailment has a broad spectrum of different manifestations, chronometric durations, auxometric rates of progression, co-morbid associated ailments, and severity of functional effects,[1-3] people in different parts of the spectrum of the ailments may have strikingly different responses to the explicatory stimuli used during the research. The results, however, may be analyzed as though the handful of studied volunteers represented the disease.

The problems are illustrated in Figure 21–1. Let us assume that the spectrum of disease severity is distributed as shown in the top two circles so that 20% of patients are *mild,* 40% are *moderate,* and 40% are *severe.* Let us also assume that the responses to a test stimulus are generally **low** in the *mild* group, **medium** in the *moderate* group, and **high** in the *severe* group. To make these numbers more specific, let 5 units be a low response, 10 units be moderate, and 20 units be high. In a properly distributed spectrum, we would expect the average response to be $(0.20 \times 5) + (0.40 \times 10) + (0.40 \times 20) = 13$ units.

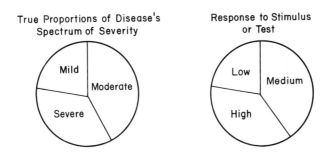

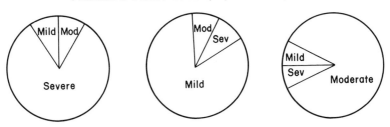

Figure 21–1. Disproportional spectral groups as sources of biased results in biodynamic or pathodynamic studies. (For further details, see text.)

The three circles in the bottom group of Figure 21–1 show what can happen if the investigator assembles a disproportionate spectrum of the disease. In the left-hand circle, in which the patients are distributed as 10% mild, 10% moderate, and 80% severe, the average response will be $(0.10 \times 5) + (0.10 \times 10) + (0.80 \times 20) = 17.5$ units. In the middle circle, the respective distribution for mild, moderate, and severe groups is 80%, 10%, and 10%. The average response will be $(0.80 \times 5) + (0.10 \times 10) + (0.10 \times 20) = 7$ units. In the right-hand circle, with respective distributions of 10%, 80%, and 10%, the average response will be $(0.10 \times 5) + (0.80 \times 10) + (0.10 \times 20) = 10.5$ units. All three of these investigated groups of cases will yield the wrong average results, but no one may know what has happened because the role of spectral distinctions was not adequately considered.

21.2.1.1. SPECTRUM IN PATHODYNAMIC STUDIES

Because only small numbers of patients can be studied in the explicatory experiments of pathophysiology, the investigator can seldom examine a wide or representative spectrum of disease. In other forms of pathodynamic research, however, the patients are not exposed to any experimental stimuli. With relatively modest effort, the investigator can usually obtain a broad spectrum of the cases and controls needed to demonstrate that the observed distinctions are due to the disease itself rather than to different susceptibilities created by different parts of the disease's clinical spectrum, by co-morbidity, or by demographic variations in age, gender, or genetic differences. Nevertheless, the need for this type of spectral discrimination is commonly overlooked in pathodynamic studies. Because the problems of spectral discrimination are similar in pathodynamic and in diagnostic marker studies, this issue will be reserved for further discussion when we reach diagnostic marker research in Chapter 25.

21.2.1.2. SUSCEPTIBILITY TO RECURRENCES OF DISEASE

An interesting type of susceptibility bias that is distinctive to pathodynamic research arises when cross-sectional rather than cohort studies are used to determine the effect of repeated episodes of a particular disease—such as asthma, epilepsy, or pneumonia. Although susceptibility to recurrences may be determined by the patient's condition after the first episode, the changes noted in a cross-sectional group of recurrences may be fallaciously attributed to the pathodynamic effects of the recurrences rather than to the patient's underlying susceptibility before the recurrence.

To illustrate this problem, suppose that episodes of asthma tend to recur almost exclusively in people who already have chronic pulmonary disease, but suppose we do not know this fact when we do cross-sectional studies to determine whether recurrent asthmatic attacks cause chronic pulmonary disease. If we studied a group of people with first episodes of asthma, we might find that 50% have otherwise normal lungs and 50% have evidence of chronic pulmonary disease. In a group of people with second episodes of asthma, we might find that almost 100% have chronic pulmonary disease. Not knowing about the susceptibility distinction, we might then arrive at the false conclusion that recurrent episodes of asthma create chronic pulmonary disease in patients who were previously free of it.

21.2.1.3. TRANSFER BIAS IN LONGITUDINAL CROSS-SECTIONS

Another source of error in biodynamic studies is the transfer bias, discussed in Section 20.5, that can arise when members of the original cohort are lost by attrition and do not appear in later cross-sectional studies. Conversely, the original cohort may have been augmented by people who migrated into the group available for the cross-section.

This type of problem is particularly likely to occur in longitudinal cross-sections of pathodynamic phenomena rather than normal growth and development. Because the in-migration and ex-migration of cohort members will often depend on their spectral characteristics for the disease, the transfers may produce biased results about the long-term behavior of the disease unless adequate attention is given to the spectral distinctions.

21.2.2. *Etiologic and Therapeutic Studies*

The classic epidemiologic case-control model for etiologic and therapeutic research was developed from the investigation of a common source outbreak. When manifestations of food poisoning appear in a group of people who shared a common meal at some public occasion, such as a community picnic or dinner, the individual items on the menu each become suspected as the etiologic culprit. All people who attended the meal are asked about their ingestion of each individual item on the menu. The prevalence of antecedent ingestion for each item is then compared in the cases, i.e., people who became sick, and in the controls, i.e., those who remained well. The item with the most distinctively different prevalence in the two groups usually becomes suspected as the cause of the outbreak.

Because of frequent success in solving these etiologic mysteries, the retrospective case-control technique has been applied to other cause-effect relationships. During this application, the investigators often overlook the distinctive clinical situation that makes the case-control method so successful in determining the etiology of common source outbreaks. There is a defined closed cohort comprising the single group of people who ate the meal. The outbreak begins relatively soon after the meal, and the manifestations of gastroenteritis (or whatever malady occurs) are usually clearly evident. The toxin is usually quite potent, so that it produces the malady in most of the people exposed to it. The interval between the investigation and the antecedent events is relatively short, so that most people can still clearly remember afterward which items they did or did not eat at the meal. The interval between the events and the investigation may even be so short that some of the leftover food is still available for laboratory examinations that can confirm the presence of the offending microbial agent.

This distinctive situation—a closed cohort with almost universal susceptibility, a clearly defined sequence of events, and a potent maneuver with a high attack rate for a clinically overt outcome that occurs shortly after the imposed maneuver—has made the case-control technique effective for investigating etiology of common source outbreaks. None of these distinctions is present, however, for the noncohort, nonacute, noninfectious, low-potency, low–attack-rate, long-duration, nonclinically overt outcomes to which the case-control method has subsequently been applied in etiologic and therapeutic research. An investigator using this research structure therefore has the difficult job of getting and analyzing a collection of cross-sectional data that must account for the entire medical itinerary that would occur from baseline state through imposition of maneuvers to discernment of outcome events.

21.2.2.1. SUSCEPTIBILITY BIAS

Although the establishment of rigorously specified criteria for admission has been a fundamental requirement of scientific plans for the evaluation of maneuvers, and although the prevention or reduction of susceptibility bias is the single outstanding scientific accomplishment of randomized allocation, neither one of these two major scientific principles receives thorough attention in most retrospective case-control studies. The baseline *clinical* status of the people receiving the maneuvers is generally ignored. The cases and controls are usually classified according to the ailments present in their outcome status and according to certain demographic attributes—such as age, race, and gender—that were present in the outcome status but also at baseline. Attention is seldom given to the roles of premaneuver admission criteria and randomized allocation of maneuvers in preventing susceptibility bias in the compared baseline states.

21.2.2.1.1. *Ascertainment of Baseline Status*

The usual explanation for the neglect of susceptibility bias in retrospective case-control research is that the investigative comparison is concerned with cases and controls at the outcome end of the causal pathway, not with an exposed and nonexposed cohort at the beginning. As a description of the research structure, this explanation is quite correct, but it cannot justify the scientific reasoning of the research hypothesis. Because the scientific inference refers to the effects of maneuvers in an exposed and nonexposed cohort, a research plan that ignores the scientific requirements of this inference cannot produce satisfactory evidence.

Although the case-control structure necessitates a retrospective categorization of events, the premaneuver baseline status can usually be ascertained if the investigator makes the effort. The effort is often omitted because of the belief that an interviewed person will not remember details of a long-ago baseline state. Nevertheless, if the person's memory can be trusted to recall long-ago maneuvers, it can also be trusted to recall why the maneuvers were taken and what kind of illness (if any) they were aimed at. If the person's memory cannot be relied upon for data about both maneuvers and baseline state, other sources of information must be used to verify or supplement the data. For maneuvers that were prescribed therapeutically, the records of the prescribing clinician will contain information about both the baseline state and the maneuvers. For maneuvers that were not prescribed, additional data about baseline state (and maneuvers) can be obtained from family, friends, or diverse archival sources.

A classification of baseline state is particularly important for noting the clinical indications for therapy or the other premaneuver phenomena that can be important sources of susceptibility bias. If this information is omitted or ignored, the subsequent scientific inference from the results of the research will contain a striking disparity between data and reasoning. The clinical attributes of the baseline state—a fundamental "parameter" in the scientific inference—are disregarded.

21.2.2.1.2. *Baseline Features in Susceptibility*

In studies of etiology, the investigator must deal with all the problems of nature and nurture that have been traditional sources of uncertainty in scientific reasoning. In view of the customary epidemiologic concern with environmental impact, the current focus on etiologic agents or risk factors has usually emphasized a person's nurture: dietary intake, smoking, alcohol, physical exercise, education, socioeconomic status, environmental pollution, industrial toxins, and pharmaceutical agents. The role of nature has usually been confined to such individual constitutional factors as blood pressure, serum lipids, blood glucose, and bleeding and clotting mechanisms.

Other major natural factors, however, have received limited or unsatisfactory attention for their potentially important contributions in susceptibility to such outcome events as coronary artery disease, stroke, or manifestations of atherosclerosis. In studies of etiology, the genetic role of familiar longevity is usually ignored despite the general clinical impression that the best way to ensure a long life span is to choose long-lived ancestors. The important role of the human psyche has been classified in a remarkably primitive manner. Although serum lipids are catalogued in an elaborate set of categories, the intricacies of the human psyche have been crudely divided into two coarse groups: Type A and Type B.

In studies of therapy, retrospective case-control investigations have seldom used the rigorous scientific precautions needed for unbiased evaluations of the actions of therapeutic maneuvers. Criteria are almost never established for the baseline clinical features that would have made patients eligible for admission to a cohort study of therapy; and little or no attention is given to the susceptibility bias that may have been created when the therapeutic agents were chosen or assigned without randomization.

21.2.2.1.3. *Protopathic and Other Sources of Susceptibility Bias*

Beyond these baseline differences in prognosis, various other sources of susceptibility bias are also regularly overlooked in cross-sectional research. When investigators perform dose-response analyses by examining the amounts and durations of antecedent maneuvers, attention is seldom given to the effects of compliance-determined susceptibility bias or regulation-determined susceptibility bias in altering the quantities in which the maneuvers were chosen, maintained, or changed. The timing of onset for maneuvers and co-maneuvers is seldom checked for vulnerability bias; and the immense problems of referral bias—which will be discussed later for their effects not only in susceptibility but also in detection and transfer—are frequently ignored.

A particularly striking problem in case-control research is the protopathic bias that can arise if a particular maneuver was started, stopped, or otherwise changed because of a baseline manifestation caused by a disease or other outcome event that is later associated with the altered use of that maneuver. The outcome event may or may not have been formally recognized when the maneuver was altered.

For example, women with benign cystic mastitis are regularly told to avoid using oral contraceptive pills (OCP) because the hormones may adversely affect the breast disease. In a subsequent case-control study of the relationship between oral contraceptive pills and benign breast disease, the antecedent prevalence of OCP usage will therefore be lower in the cases than in the controls. The "pill" may then be fallaciously thought to have protected against benign breast disease. Conversely, if women with benign breast disease appear in the control group for a study of the relationship between OCP and breast cancer, the lower prevalence of OCP usage in the controls will fallaciously suggest that OCPs cause breast cancer.

The results of retrospective case-control or other observational studies can be substantially biased if protopathic difficulties are not recognized and suitably managed.

21.2.2.2. **PERFORMANCE BIAS**

For issues in performance bias, the effects of co-maneuvers must be recognized, disentangled, and properly analyzed in both cohort and cross-sectional research. Two other problems in performance of maneuvers, however, are much more prominent in cross-sectional than in cohort research. Because of the retrospective ascertainment process, the most obvious scientific challenge is to obtain an accurate and unbiased account of the maneuvers that each person actually received. A more subtle scientific problem arises because the ascertainment process is aimed at the actual rather than the intended use of the maneuvers. In a randomized trial, an intention-to-treat analysis can deal with the difficulties in vulnerability, compliance, intermediate regulation, and other sources of retrograde susceptibility bias that did not become apparent until after the recipients had been exposed to the maneuvers. In cross-sectional research, however, little or no attention is given to these biases in affecting the quantity, continued maintenance, or cessation of the received maneuvers.

21.2.2.3. **DETECTION BIAS**

Although necropsies are performed much less frequently today than before and are also less frequently attended by clinicians, every observant clinician has had a chance to see the many cancers, infarctions, atherosclerotic arteries, occluded veins, stones, acute inflammations, and chronic inflammations that were first discovered at necropsy, having been undiagnosed or unsuspected during the patient's lifetime. In some instances, the disease detected at necropsy was responsible for the patient's demise but was incorrectly or imprecisely diagnosed. In other instances, the disease escaped detection during life because it was either symptomless or noncontributory to the fatal ailment. In yet other instances, the disease would formerly have escaped detection—even at necropsy—because the site was not examined in the same way, the specimens of tissue were not prepared with the same methods used today, or the disease cannot be diagnosed from morphologic evidence.

The occurrence of this large community reservoir of previously undetected disease has been demonstrated in several reports of necropsy-centered research.[4, 5] The reservoir is usually quantified, however, only for the necropsy proportions of previously diagnosed and previously undiagnosed instances of the disease. Thus, the investigators may state that about 20% of the lung cancers noted at postmortem examination were previously undiagnosed during life.[4, 5] The investigators seldom perform the additional quantification of converting the newly detected instances of disease to an occurrence rate for the community at large. The necropsies in which a particular disease was unsuspected can be used as a denominator for this rate, and the instances of new discovery can be used as a numerator. When such calculations are performed, the occurrence rate of unsuspected disease may be substantially greater than the usual rates cited for either the reported incidence or prevalence of the disease.[6] Certain ailments, such as coronary artery disease, may be found in one of every two people closely examined at necropsy,[7] and other diseases, such as cancer of the prostate, may be almost ubiquitous, being found in about 75% of prostate glands subjected to careful sectioning and microscopic inspection.[8]

Although this large reservoir of undetected disease is readily available for discovery by improved methods of diagnostic technology, the impact of the phenomenon seldom receives careful attention in research in which the outcome event is detection of a particular disease. The attention is essential because the maneuver under investigation can often play an important role in evoking the use of the requisite diagnostic technology and in affecting the interpretation of the technologic data. The detection-of-disease problem is particularly cogent in retrospective case-control research, because the trohoc procedure has been commonly employed to study the etiology of disease and to investigate the risks rather than the benefits of therapy. Because the occurrence of a previously undiagnosed disease is usually the outcome of the maneuvers investigated in such research, the avoidance of detection bias is a crucial (although often neglected) component of the requirements that must be fulfilled for the observed evidence to be used in scientific inference.

21.2.2.4. **PUBLICITY BIAS IN DIAGNOSIS AND REPORTING**

As an innate event that occurs before the research is begun, publicity bias can have two important effects. The publicity given to a particular relationship of maneuver and outcome can create a detection bias in the original diagnosis of the disease for suitably exposed persons, and also a transfer bias in the likelihood that exposed cases will be reported to a registry.

An example of detection bias is shown by the diagnostic problem of a pediatrician examining a child who is severely ill with an unknown febrile ailment for which aspirin treatment was given early in the ailment. Because of the extensive publicity about an alleged relationship between aspirin and Reye's syndrome, the pediatrician may be particularly inclined to make a diagnosis of Reye's syndrome. For another patient, with exactly the same clinical manifestations but without a history of aspirin ingestion, the pediatrician may make some other diagnosis.

The existence of this type of diagnostic bias was dramatically demonstrated in a special study[9] in which practitioners making a diagnosis from the clinical manifestations of a written case vignette regularly diagnosed toxic shock syndrome when the patient was also cited as a menstruating tampon user, but not when information about catamenial status was omitted.

Another recent study[10] has demonstrated the transfer bias produced by reporting bias if publicity about a suspected maneuver-outcome relationship induces physicians to submit appropriate case reports but to omit sending inappropriate case reports to a registry where the relationship is being studied. Both of these effects of publicity bias, in the original diagnosis and subsequent reporting of a maneuver-outcome relationship, create innate biases in the fourfold table by disproportionately increasing the table's *a* cell, which shows the group having a coexistence of maneuver and outcome.

21.2.2.5. OTHER TRANSFER BIASES

Although any cross-sectional study is prey to the quantitative hazards, described in Section 20.5, that may produce an attrition of the cohort between the imposition of the maneuvers and the transfer of members to the counted results, the structure of the retrospective case-control study encourages several other forms of transfer bias. They can arise during the clinical decisions that are made when patients are referred for diagnostic tests or hospitalization, and when investigators choose the particular people who will be admitted to the study as cases or controls.

21.2.2.5.1. *Berkson's Bias in Hospital Referral*

An intriguing feature of referral patterns that can lead to transfer bias was originally described by Joseph Berkson.[11] The problem is often called *Berkson's bias*, despite his preference for some other title (such as *Berkson's paradox*) and despite the fact that the bias can be produced by two different sources: mathematical and clinical. Berkson, thinking about the mathematical issues, noted that people with two different diseases would have a higher probability of being hospitalized than people with only one disease. If the rates of hospitalization are different for the two diseases, however, their concurrence in a hospitalized group will misrepresent the rate of their true concurrence in the community population.

To illustrate this point, let us assume that coronary disease occurs at a rate of 0.1 and peptic ulcer disease occurs independently at a rate of 0.02 in the general population. If the two diseases are unrelated, their rate of concurrence should be $0.1 \times 0.02 = 0.002$. In a population of 100,000 people, as shown in Figure 21–2A, we would have 10,000 people with coronary disease and 2000 people with peptic ulcer. Among the 10,000 people with coronary disease, 200 would also have peptic ulcer and 9800 would have coronary disease alone. Among the 2000 people with peptic ulcer, 200 would also have coronary disease and 1800 would have peptic ulcer alone.

Now let us assume that persons with coronary disease are hospitalized at a rate of 0.2 and that persons with peptic ulcer are hospitalized at a rate of 0.05. Hospitalization will occur for 1960 of the 9800 people with coronary disease alone and for 90 of the 1800 people with peptic ulcer alone. In the 200 people with both coronary artery disease and peptic ulcer, the two forces of hospitalization will act concurrently. Of these 200 people, 40 will be hospitalized at the rate of 0.2 for coronary disease; and of the remaining 160 people, 8 will be hospitalized at the rate of 0.05 for peptic ulcer. (The same number of 48 people would be hospitalized with both diseases if we did the calculations alternatively as $0.05 \times 200 = 10$ hospitalized because of the peptic ulcer diagnosis and $(200 - 10)(0.2) = 38$ hospitalized with the coronary diagnosis.)

The hospitalized group, as shown in Figure 21–2B, will thus contain 1960 people with coronary disease alone, 90 people with peptic ulcer alone, and 48 people who have both

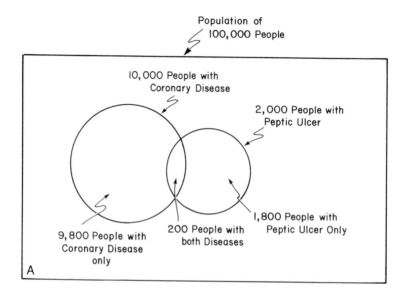

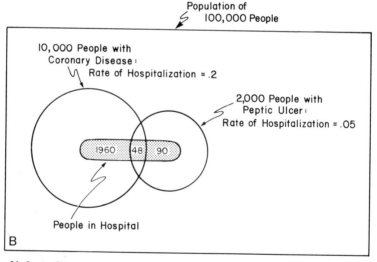

Figure 21–2. *A,* Concurrence of two diseases in a general community population. *B,* Effects of different rates of hospitalization on concurrence of two diseases in the hospital serving the general community. (For further details, see text.)

diseases. The total number of patients with peptic ulcer will be 138 ($= 90 + 48$); the total number of patients with coronary disease will be 2008 ($= 1960 + 48$). Among patients with coronary disease, the concurrent co-morbid prevalence of peptic ulcer will be 48/2008 = 0.024, which is a slight exaggeration of its true concurrence rate of 0.02 in the community. Among the 138 patients with peptic ulcer, however, the concurrence of coronary disease will be 48/138 = 0.35, which is 3.5 times greater than its concurrence rate of 0.1 in the community. If we did not know the true state of affairs in the community, we would not be aware of this fallacious elevation in the concurrent hospital rate. Impressed by its relative magnitude, we might then conclude erroneously either that peptic ulcer can pathodynamically lead to coronary disease or that coronary disease is an etiologic factor in predisposing to peptic ulcer.

21.2.2.5.2. *Clinical Sources of Hospital Referral Bias*

In being concerned only with the additional mathematical probabilities of hospitalization created by the concurrence of two diseases in the same person, Berkson's demonstration was based on the assumption that the two diseases had independent but additive effects. In Berkson's model, a person with both coronary disease and peptic ulcer would be hospitalized at a rate that is the probabilistic union of the two individual rates of hospitalization, i.e., $(0.2) + (0.05) - (0.2 \times 0.05) = 0.24$. Although the model depends on the reasonable idea that people with different clinical conditions will have different rates of referral to hospitals, no provision is made for the distinctive clinical reasons why patients are hospitalized and what happens after they get there. These clinical decisions can greatly alter the mathematical probabilities calculated in Berkson's model. For example, in patients with overt manifestations of both coronary disease and peptic ulcer, the total clinical severity of illness may lead to hospitalization at a rate of 0.75 rather than a probabilistic rate of 0.24. In a patient admitted only for treatment of a known peptic ulcer, silent coronary disease may be detected in a routine screening electrocardiogram.

For these reasons, the phenomenon described by Berkson can be generically called *hospital referral bias*, but its appropriate analysis and management requires attention to clinical referral decisions rather than enhanced mathematical probabilities alone.

Although the hospital referral–bias phenomenon was ignored for many years because it had been conjectured by Berkson but not actually documented, several empiric demonstrations have now been provided.[12-14] In some relationships, relatively little bias was noted; but other relationships showed striking distortions in which the odds ratios in nosocomial groups were 17 times higher or 0.2 times lower than the corresponding true value in the community population. Because hospital referral bias may arise whenever the likelihood of hospitalization is affected by the concurrence of diseases and/or maneuvers, the clinical sources of hospital referral must be suitably analyzed in any cross-sectional study in which the cases or controls or both are derived from a hospitalized population.

As noted in the next few sections, the patterns of clinical referral can be a source of innate bias in hospitalized patients and also a source of investigative bias when efforts are made to compensate for the innate biases.

21.2.2.5.3. *Co-Manifestation Problems in Referral for Diagnostic Procedures*

A patient can be referred to a hospital for many different reasons. In some instances, the main diagnosis is already known, and hospitalization is intended only for treatment. In other instances, when a principal diagnosis has not yet been established, the patient is admitted for diagnostic procedures as well as treatment. In yet other instances, a patient with a disease of interest to an investigator may have been hospitalized only because of clinical phenomena associated with an unrelated co-morbid disease. Regardless of the patient's pre-admission diagnostic status, many previously undiscerned diseases can be detected during the multiple tests that are often ordered today as acts of differential diagnosis or as case-finding screening procedures.

Although performed because of the referral process that led to hospitalization, the diagnostic procedures can produce detection bias if certain diseases become preferentially revealed in association with certain maneuvers. One source of this problem, as discussed in this section, arises if an innocent maneuver produces an innocent side effect that resembles the manifestations of an important disease, which can often remain silent and undetected during life. When patients with the appropriate clinical manifestations receive diagnostic testing, the tests will reveal many cases in which the important disease was responsible for the manifestations. The test procedures, however, may also reveal many instances in which the revealed important disease was silent and the clinical manifestations were due to the maneuver alone. The newly diagnosed silent cases, which would otherwise have remained undetected, may then fallaciously be ascribed to the antecedent maneuver.

Several examples of this problem have already been cited. A laxative that produces benign gastritis and the side effect of hematemesis may be falsely deemed responsible for the silent gastric ulcers or cancers revealed during the diagnostic work-up of the hematemesis. The bleeding produced as a side effect of the endometrial hyperplasia in patients receiving postmenopausal estrogen therapy may be held responsible for silent endometrial carcinomas discovered during the diagnostic dilation and curettage.

As noted later, the adjustment of co-manifestation problems is relatively easy if the side effect of a maneuver is a functional manifestation (such as insomnia or flatulence) rather than both a separate disease and its associated manifestation (such as gastritis and hematemesis or endometrial hyperplasia and vaginal bleeding). If the exposure leads to an incidental disease that then produces the co-manifestation, the adjustment process is more difficult.

21.2.2.5.4. *Co-Morbidity Bias in Selected Control Groups*

Because of the biases produced by differential rates of hospital referral, studies of coexisting diseases are best conducted in a community population and should be avoided in hospitalized patients. For case-control studies of maneuver-disease rather than disease-disease associations, the potential biases of co-morbidity can occur if diseases bearing a distinctive relationship to the investigated maneuvers are used as control groups for the research.

In the scientific logic of cause-effect reasoning, the outcome event in a cohort comparison of etiologic maneuvers is the occurrence of a particular target disease. The alternative (or nonoutcome) event is the absence of that disease. When this logic is inverted for the structure of a retrospective case-control study, the people who have developed the target disease are eligible to become the cases. Everyone else, who has not developed the target disease, should then be eligible to be the controls.

Despite its intuitive appeal, this logic is often discarded in case-control studies. Sometimes the reason is convenience. It may be much easier to obtain the control group from the same available framework as the cases rather than trying to obtain representatives of "everything else." At other times the reason is scientific. The problems of susceptibility bias and detection bias cannot be managed if the control group merely represents "everything else" and is chosen without precautions that will give the controls the same degrees of susceptibility and detection as the cases.

Regardless of the reasons for avoiding a general selection of "everything else," the control group is often chosen from people who have a particular disease or group of diseases. This choice can make the research especially convenient if people with the selected control condition(s) are abundant and readily available to the investigator.

Table 21–1. HYPOTHETICAL EFFECTS OF EXCELLITOL IN A COMMUNITY COHORT

People Exposed to:	Lung Cancer	Occurrence of: Other Cancer	No Cancer	Total
Excellitol	125	571	24,304	25,000
No Excellitol	75	429	74,496	75,000
Total	200	1000	98,800	100,000

The choice is often quite satisfactory if the maneuver under investigation has no distinctive etiologic relationship to the control condition(s). A problem in *co-morbidity bias* will arise, however, if the maneuver has either a distinctly positive or negative etiologic association with the control condition(s). If positive, the co-morbid association can obscure a positive relationship between the maneuver and the target disease. If the maneuver-control association is negative, a false-positive relationship can be produced between the maneuver and the target disease.

To demonstrate this problem, consider a hypothetical relationship between lung cancer, other cancers, and a suspected causal agent, Excellitol. The data for the community relationships are shown in Table 21–1. If we assume that lung cancer occurs in the general population at a rate of 2 per thousand ($= 0.002$) and that other cancers occur at the rate of 0.010, the community population of 100,000 will contain a total of 200 cases of lung cancer and 1000 cases of the other cancers. Now let us assume that Excellitol is a common enough substance so that 0.25 of the people have been exposed to it. Of the 100,000 people, 25,000 would be exposed and 75,000 would be unexposed. If we further assume that lung cancer is five times more likely to occur in Excellitol-exposed people than in those who were not exposed, the occurrence rates of lung cancer would be $125/25,000 = 0.005$ in the exposed group and $75/75,000 = 0.001$ in the unexposed group. If other cancers are four (rather than five) times more likely to occur with Excellitol than without it, their respective rates of occurrence will be $571/25,000 = 0.023$ in the exposed and $429/75,000 = 0.0057$ in the nonexposed groups.

Now suppose we do a case-control study in which we assemble all 200 cases of lung cancer and a proportional group of 200 controls from the noncancer population. The results will show a fourfold table of $\begin{Bmatrix} 125 & 50 \\ 75 & 150 \end{Bmatrix}$ and the odds ratio will yield the correct value of 5. If we use a proportional group of 200 people with the other cancer as a control group, however, the fourfold table will be $\begin{Bmatrix} 125 & 114 \\ 75 & 86 \end{Bmatrix}$. The odds ratio will be an unimpressive value of 1.26, and we will fail to note the distinctive causal impact of Excellitol in both groups.

Now let us consider a different set of relationships, shown in Table 21–2, for a community in which 25% of the people are again exposed to Excellitol, with the total occurrence rates again being 0.002 and 0.010 respectively for lung cancer and for other cancers. In this situation, however, Excellitol has no effect on lung cancer, which occurs in $50/25,000 = 0.002$ of the exposed and in $150/75,000 = 0.002$ of the unexposed people. Conversely, Excellitol does have a protective effect against other cancers. In exposed people, other cancers occur at a rate that is one-fourth their rate of occurrence in nonexposed people. This distinction is shown by the respective rates of $77/25,000 = 0.003$

Table 21–2. A DIFFERENT SET OF HYPOTHETICAL EFFECTS OF EXCELLITOL IN A COMMUNITY COHORT

People Exposed to:	Lung Cancer	Occurrence of: Other Cancer	No Cancer	Total
Excellitol	50	77	24,873	25,000
No Excellitol	150	923	73,927	75,000
Total	200	1000	98,800	100,000

and 923/75,000 = 0.012 for occurrence of other cancers in the exposed and nonexposed people in Table 21–2.

If we perform a case-control study and again find proportional representation in the 200 people of the control groups, the results of the fourfold table will be $\begin{Bmatrix} 50 & 50 \\ 150 & 150 \end{Bmatrix}$ if the controls come from the noncancer population. The odds ratio will show its correct value of 1. If 200 people with other cancers become the control group, however, the fourfold table will be $\begin{Bmatrix} 50 & 15 \\ 150 & 185 \end{Bmatrix}$. The odds ratio will produce an impressive value of 4.1 and will be stochastically significant. We may then conclude erroneously that Excellitol is causally associated with lung cancer.

These examples demonstrate that co-morbidity bias is a unique type of transfer bias. It occurs only in case-control studies and not in other research structures. The problem arises when the main maneuver under investigation has a distinctive co-relationship, in either causal or protective directions, to the outcome rate of the other morbid condition(s) chosen as the control group. The problem is not easy to manage in case-control studies because certain maneuvers may be suspected of having so many additional co-morbid relationships that a suitable control group may be hard to find. Conversely, if certain control groups are rejected because of false-positive suspicions about a co-morbid relationship, the results may be biased by the inappropriate exclusion of an appropriate control group.

For example, as noted later, many patients with cardiovascular disease were excluded as possible controls in a case-control study of the relationship between reserpine and breast cancer. Because reserpine was prescribed for hypertension but did not etiologically create it, the presence of cardiovascular disease in the control group would not have led to comorbidity bias. Instead, the exclusion of patients with cardiovascular disease created a different transfer bias (as noted later) that produced a falsely low proportion of antecendent reserpine usage in the control group.

21.2.2.5.5. *Choice of Incidence vs. Prevalence Cases*

In a cohort study of etiologic action for a particular maneuver, the outcome event is an incidence phenomenon: the new occurrence of the target disease in a person who was previously free of that disease. In cross-sectional research, however, the investigator will find the disease in both incidence and prevalence cases. The prevalence cases are usually people in whom the disease had occurred and was diagnosed at some previous occasion, and who are still alive and available for the research. The incidence cases will be people in whom the disease has been newly detected.

Both types of cases can create problems in bias. For prevalence cases, the problem is obvious. As the residue of an unidentified inception cohort (or cohorts), the prevalence cases are quite likely to contain transfer bias due to attrition or augmentation of the original cohort(s). For this reason, the cases in a case-control study are often restricted to incidence cases.

The incidence cases, however, have a more subtle problem. Their disease may have been new in detection but not new in occurrence. For example, a screening campaign will discover many instances of prevalent cases whose asymptomatic or subclinical disease is not new but is newly detected by the screening test. If such people are categorized as incidence cases, the results will create problems in both heterodemic and case-control research. In heterodemic research, the numerator data will be inaccurate for the true incidence of the disease in the denominator population. In case-control research, the hazard of protopathic bias, as discussed earlier, will arise if early manifestations of the outcome disease affected the choice of the baseline maneuvers that are later associated with the disease when it is eventually detected as an outcome event.

21.3. CHOICE OF A FRAMEWORK

The many biases that have just been discussed constitute the scientific risks that accompany the logistic benefits of a cross-sectional research structure. A case-control or other cross-sectional study may be much easier to carry out than an observational cohort study or randomized trial, but the investigator must worry about creating biases during the research while simultaneously trying to remove or reduce the many forms of innate bias that will have been incorporated into the available groups and data. The investigator's scientific challenge is to establish methods for demarcating the groups and collecting the data in a way that will eliminate or sufficiently reduce those biases to make the results acceptable as scientific evidence.

The problems of collecting cross-sectional data will be discussed in Chapter 22. The rest of this chapter is concerned with the demarcation of groups. The first step in choosing groups for a cross-sectional study is to select a basic framework that can avoid the scientific hazards of transfer bias.

21.3.1. *Frameworks Available for Selection*

Statisticians often use the term *sampling frame* to refer to the basic group of people from whom a sample will be chosen for a study. The sampling frame may consist of all people living in New Haven during a particular week, or all people who visit the Eiffel Tower on a particular day, or all patients admitted to Megalopolis Hospital during a particular year. From this sampling frame, a selection process (which usually involves random choices) provides the actual sample that will be investigated during the study.

Because the groups studied in medical research are seldom obtained by random sampling, the term *framework* can be used to denote the medical counterpart of a *sampling frame*. Regardless of whether the research is done as an experimental trial, an observational cohort, or a cross-sectional study, the framework of the research is the entity chosen as the source of the people under investigation. This source can be either a zone or a registry. A *zone* is defined by its ecologic, occupational, or nosocomial characteristics. It can be a particular community or geographic region; a school or factory; or a hospital, clinician's office, or other medical setting. A single zone can also be formed as a composite of several individual zones, which are joined for the purpose of a particular investigation. A *registry* is a collection of data about a particular group of people who share a common personal characteristic, which may have been exposure to the same agent, development of the same disease, birth, marriage, or death.

The people found in the *zones* studied in medical research are seldom previously differentiated according to any special personal attributes. They are in that zone because they live, work, go to school, or were sick there. Some of the people may have been selected for certain jobs because of special qualifications, or they may have been chosen (or referred to) certain doctors or hospitals because of reasons related to gender, religion, disease, or socioeconomic status—but a zone usually contains a relatively general group of people. By contrast, all of the people found in a medical *registry* had their data selectively accrued there because of a specific purpose for which the registry was established. Some of the registries—such as those that collect certificates of marriage, divorce, birth, or death—may be quite general in their target population, but others are concerned with specific diseases, such as cancer; and yet others are established for *ad hoc* collection of medical information related to infections, adverse drug reactions, exposure to suspected noxious agents, or diseases receiving special investigative attention.

After a framework is chosen, the investigator must develop an access to the people who are potential candidates for the research. If the selected framework is a registry, the names of the people who might be chosen are already recorded in the registry's archives. If the framework is a zone, the investigator can find candidates by public appeals or by using rosters. The rosters may contain names for everyone in the zone and also for selected subgroups. For example, hospital rosters may be available to show all patients who have been admitted or discharged, who have attended certain clinics or services, or who have received certain tests, procedures, and treatments. Hospitals may also maintain rosters that resemble registries in containing lists of people with diagnoses of individual diseases.

This very first step in the research, before anything else happens, can be a major source of bias because of the referral process that brought people to the particular rosters or registries used as the framework. At a general hospital, the roster of admissions and discharges may suitably represent the events occurring in the general community, but special hospitals may acquire an unrepresentative collection of people and events. Within a particular hospital, collections of patients with the same disease may have different spectrums if obtained from rosters of medical or surgical services. Although a roster is representative and complete, the results may be biased by the mechanism used to retrieve medical records or to obtain follow-up data for people cited in the roster.

In an ecologic zone, the investigator may use diverse forms of publicity to induce people to volunteer for the study. If the maneuvers have already occurred before the people volunteer, the effects of certain outcomes may bias the composition of the volunteer groups. If the maneuvers are imposed after the people volunteer (as in a randomized trial of a public health intervention), the volunteer group may not suitably represent the intended population. For example, in a recent randomized trial of multiple-risk–factor interventions in healthy volunteers,[15] the mortality rates in both the actively treated and control groups were substantially lower than the investigators had anticipated from general population data.

If the framework is a registry that collects instances of a particular clinical condition, the opportunities for bias are substantially increased. If active surveillance is maintained in a particular region, the registry may collect all the pertinent cases for that region. For example, by thorough liaison and ongoing communication with pertinent sources of data, the Connecticut State Tumor Registry has become an effective and reasonably complete repository of information for cancers diagnosed in the state of Connecticut. On the other hand, if the registry is a passive recipient of case reports, appealing for information but performing no active solicitation and surveillance, the clinicians or other people who decide to respond to the appeals may send information that is both incomplete and biased in representing the groups and events that have actually occurred. Thus, the types and proportions of adverse drug reactions casually reported by clinicians to a federal registry may indicate merely the vicissitudes of the reporting clinicians rather than the occurrence of the adverse reactions.

When a registry is established to collect cases in which a particular disease and maneuver have been associated, the publicity used to announce the registry may bias the collection of data. People who have the disease without the maneuver, or the maneuver without the disease, may be much less likely to be reported to the registry than those who have both the disease and the maneuver. We saw an example of this problem in Section 17.6.3 for the inception and non-inception cohorts assembled in the DESAD project[16] studying the subsequent course of women who had received in utero exposure to diethyl-stilbestrol (DES). An analogous problem has been suspected[9] in the data collected by registries established to study the relationship of tampons and toxic shock syndrome.

21.3.2. *Uni-Group vs. Conjoined Frameworks*

The people under investigation in a cohort or cross-sectional study can be originally assembled as a single group or as a conjunction of two or more groups. In a single-group arrangement, the people are assembled according to certain eligibility criteria that do not involve either the maneuvers or the outcomes in the group. The occurrences of maneuvers and outcomes for each person are determined *after* the single group has been chosen. In the conjoined arrangement, the people are assembled according to eligibility criteria that demarcate groups with different maneuvers or different outcomes. These different groups are then conjoined to form the apparently single collection of people under study. If the groups were chosen according to maneuvers, the investigator ascertains their subsequent outcomes. If the groups were chosen according to outcomes, the investigator ascertains their antecedent maneuvers.

The effects of the uni-group and conjoined arrangements will be considered separately for cohort and for cross-sectional studies.

21.3.2.1. **COHORT STUDIES**

In an experimental trial, a single group of people who fulfill the admission criteria receive maneuvers that are assigned by randomization or by some other mechanism that produces an unbiased allocation. The people are then followed to ascertain their outcome events. The sequence of collection and demarcation of groups is shown in Figure 21–3.

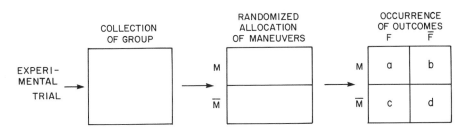

Figure 21–3. Formation of subgroups in a randomized trial.

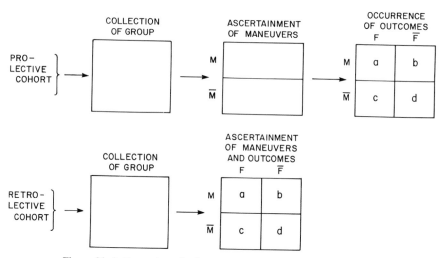

Figure 21–4. Formation of subgroups in two types of cohort research.

The diagrams of Figure 21–4 show the sequence of events in cohort studies performed without randomization. The top diagram of Figure 21–4 demonstrates the formation of a uni-group prolective study of an inception cohort. Except for the need to ascertain rather than allocate maneuvers, the investigator uses a procedure identical to that of the randomized trial in Figure 21–3. The maneuvers and outcomes are determined after the single group is assembled.

The second row of Figure 21–4 shows the collection of a uni-group retrolective cohort study. After choosing the single group, the investigator checks the archival data to ascertain the maneuvers and outcomes that have already occurred.

In Figure 21–5, the cohort studies are performed with conjoined rather than single groups. In the top diagram, the maneuvers are compared concurrently but not co-zonally. This situation occurs when the results obtained after use ⁵ the principal maneuver at one medical setting are compared with the results of a comparative maneuver used concurrently at some other medical setting. The middle row of Figure 21–5 shows the situation for a historical control study. The outcomes ascertained in the group receiving the principal maneuver are compared against the already known outcomes in a group who previously received a comparative maneuver. In the bottom row of Figure 21–5, dotted lines show the use of a contrived control group assembled by mathematical manipulation of data from various collections of vital statistics.

21.3.2.2. CROSS-SECTIONAL STUDIES

Cross-sectional studies can also be performed with uni-group or conjoined group arrangements. In an ecologic cross-section, the investigator assembles a group of people in a community and then determines each person's status as having been exposed or nonexposed to the maneuver and having attained or not attained the outcome event. This is the type of study that produced the data shown earlier in Table 20–2. In a nosocomial cross-section, the investigator may assemble a consecutive series of patients admitted to a hospital and may then determine their status for antecedent maneuvers and existing

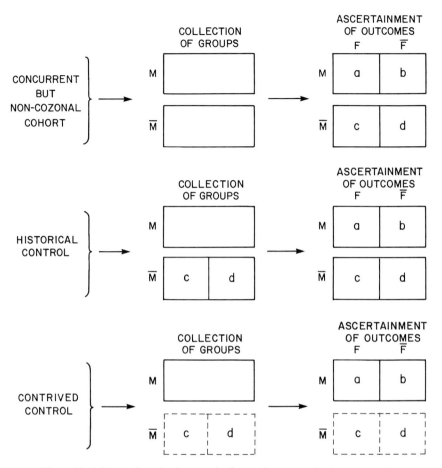

Figure 21–5. Formation of subgroups in three other types of cohort research.

outcomes. (For diagnostic marker or other process studies to be discussed later, a uni-group nosocomial cross-section may be assembled as a consecutive series of people receiving a particular diagnostic procedure.) The arrangement of uni-group cross-sectional studies is shown in the top diagram of Figure 21–6.

In case-control studies, the conjunction of two or more groups is indicated by the name *case-control*. In a pathodynamic case-control study, as shown in the middle row of Figure 21–6, the investigator conjoins a group of diseased cases with a group of nondiseased controls, and then determines the occurrence of retinopathy or some other suspected consequence of the disease in each group.

A retrospective case-control study, as shown in the bottom row of Figure 21–6, has a unique diagram that befits its other unique distinctions in epidemiologic research. The two (or more) groups that are collected to form a retrospective case-control study are split along the vertical axis of outcomes rather than along the horizontal axis of maneuvers. After the groups are chosen and joined for their outcomes as diseased cases or nondiseased controls, the investigator ascertains the antecedent maneuvers in the groups.

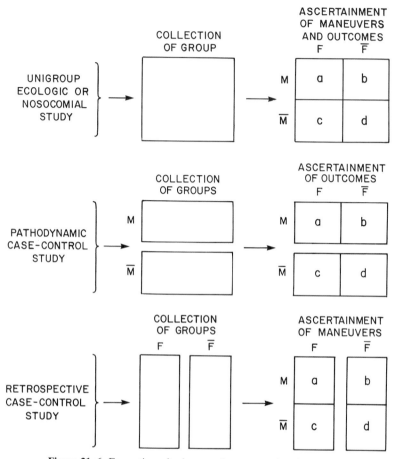

Figure 21–6. Formation of subgroups in cross-sectional research.

21.3.2.3. THE HAZARD OF CONJOINED FRAMEWORKS

When the universe under analysis in a fourfold table is formed as a conjoined clump of groups rather than as a unitary whole, the investigator has several excellent opportunities to create biases beyond any that were produced innately by ordinary events alone. The fourfold table that expresses the research results has two basic axes: one for maneuvers and the other for outcomes. In a uni-group selection, the investigator first chooses the people and then ascertains each person's data for both axes. In a conjoined selection, however, the groups are chosen according to their known data for either the maneuvers or outcomes in one of those basic axes. After the people are chosen, the investigator ascertains the unknown data for the outcomes or maneuvers in the other axis. If the initially known data define the *basic entity* and the ascertained data define the *focal entity*, the conjoined method of selection allows the investigator to create bias in delineating the basic entity and in ascertaining the focal entity. This opportunity occurs because the basic groups of a conjoined study can be formed and identified by several different processes rather than by the same single process used in a uni-group study.

For example, in a case-control study, the cases have all received the particular diagnostic procedures needed to demonstrate the disease that made them *cases*. The control group, however, may consist merely of people in whom that disease has not been identified; and so the controls may not have received the same diagnostic procedures as the cases. In a uni-group cross-sectional study, when outcomes and maneuvers are ascertained at the same single examination of each person, the ascertainment process is much less likely to be biased than in a conjoined case-control study, in which the investigator, knowing the person's status as a case or control on one axis of the fourfold table, can make subtle use of this knowledge while ascertaining the outcome event or antecedent maneuver that determines the same person's status on the other axis.

The existence of a conjoined arrangement of groups does not imply that investigative bias is present, nor does a uni-group selection eliminate the possibility. The conjoined arrangement, however, should act as a warning to both investigator and reader that investigative bias has had an additional chance to occur when groups were demarcated and when focal events were checked to ascertain the outcomes or the antecedent maneuvers.

21.3.3. *Desirability of Different Cross-Sectional Frameworks*

The basic framework for a cross-sectional study can be either a uni-group source that will provide both of the basic groups under selection or a single source of the case group, which will then be conjoined with controls taken from another source.

21.3.3.1. UNI-GROUP FRAMEWORKS

Although any of the cited zones or registries can be used as a uni-group framework for cross-sectional research, the desirability of a particular framework will depend on the relationship under study.

To study the community effects of infections or vaccinations, an ecologic zone is the preferred and commonly used framework in infectious disease epidemiology. To study the intrahospital transmission of infections, a nosocomial zone is the obvious framework; and this type of research has led to a modern version of the nosocomial epidemiology that was introduced by Semmelweis a century ago.

To study diseases that have a relatively low rate of occurrence, an ecologic zone is usually unsatisfactory because too many people would have to be investigated to find the relatively few cases of the target disease. In certain special circumstances, however, when all the cases can readily be identified from a defined community or catchment area, the rest of the ecologic region can be used as a source of the controls.

Except for the uncommon situations, described in Section 18.6.2, that permit this type of population-based or closed cohort approach, the main framework for most studies involving diseased cases and nondiseased controls is a nosocomial zone or registry where an ample number of cases of the disease has been collected. Such a framework can be used in a uni-group selection process if both the cases and controls come from the same roster for the same secular interval. At a hospital, this type of framework would be provided by a roster of successive admissions or a roster of people who received a particular diagnostic procedure. At a registry, the roster would consist of all people whose descriptions were acquired by the registry for the selected secular interval. After the diseased cases are identified on the framework roster, everyone else listed on that roster is eligible for consideration as a control.

21.3.3.2. **CHOICE OF A CASE FRAMEWORK**

If both the cases and controls come from a single roster of nosocomial admissions, nosocomial diagnostic procedures, or reports submitted to a registry, the control group may not always be satisfactory because of co-manifestation bias or co-morbidity bias, but the problem of referral bias will be reduced, because everyone will have been referred to the same source that provides the single roster. (The management of co-manifestation and co-morbidity bias is discussed in Section 21.4.2.)

If a two-group framework is used, the problems of referral bias are particularly likely to occur when one roster is used to choose the cases and another roster is used for the controls. The case roster will usually be a list of people with a main disease under investigation; but the control roster may be a list of people admitted to selected parts of the hospital, or people having a selected group of diseases, or persons chosen from sources outside the hospital. In these circumstances, the different reasons that brought the cases to one roster and the controls to another can be a major source of referral bias.

This problem is particularly difficult to manage if the cases come from a registry and the controls come from some other source. If the registry conducts vigorous surveillance for a particular zone (such as a state tumor registry or a federal registry of death certificates), the assembled data can be regarded as reasonably complete and unbiased for the identified cases. If the registry does not conduct active surveillance or if the registry was established for *ad hoc* study of a particular causal relationship, the collection of cases will almost surely be distorted by transfer bias. Furthermore, the investigator will have no uni-zonal mechanism available to help reduce the bias. Because of this problem, a dual framework for cases and controls will have particular difficulty avoiding the hazards of transfer bias if the cases come from either a passive surveillance registry or an *ad hoc* research registry.

21.3.3.3. **CHOICE OF A CONTROL FRAMEWORK**

In case-control studies in which the cases come from one framework and the controls from another, a large diversity of sources has been used as the control framework. The nosocomial sources of controls include the following: other people hospitalized with similar diseases (e.g., patients with cancer of the lung as a control group for cases with cancer of the stomach); other people admitted by the same physician who attended the cases; other people admitted to the same hospital service as the cases; people admitted to other services of the same hospital; people admitted with a selected disease or group of other diseases; any other people admitted to the same hospital; and people receiving the same diagnostic tests as the cases. (In some of these examples, an appropriate single roster can be used to provide both the cases and controls.) In pathodynamic case-control studies, the nosocomial control groups have included healthy volunteers, apparently healthy patients seen in ambulatory locations of the hospital, or patients treated in diverse ambulatory clinics.

When controls are chosen from the community, the sources have been the following: friends identified by the cases; neighbors of the cases; other people randomly chosen from the same community; people living in a retirement community or other congregate setting; and people obtained by random-digit dialing of telephones in the same community. In addition to these techniques, community control groups have sometimes been contrived from various arrangements of data contained in compendia of vital statistics.

The main rationales offered for these diverse choices usually rest on arguments about whether the hospital or the community is the best choice of the control framework[18] and on conjectures about the best way of obtaining an unbiased selection of the potential controls contained in the chosen framework. The many discussions of these rationales seldom consider the more basic scientific function of the control group. Its statistical role is to provide comparative data; but its scientific role is to help reduce the innate biases in susceptibility, performance, detection, and transfer that will have accrued in whatever cases and controls are available for selection at the end of the causal pathway. Because this scientific role is seldom considered, the choice of the second framework has been approached mainly as a statistical activity in sampling a control group from people who do not have the disease present in the cases, rather than as a scientific activity in reducing or adjusting the inevitable innate biases that are present for the contrast with nondiseased people.

21.4. SCIENTIFIC PRINCIPLES IN FRAMEWORK SELECTION

In a pathodynamic study, the control group must fulfill the scientific requirements of the spectral contrast that is further discussed in Chapter 25. In a retrospective case-control study of etiology or therapy, a scientific approach to the choice of a framework would be to recapitulate the itinerary that would occur in the basic architecture of a comparison between exposed and nonexposed people. The characteristics noted in the persons who would emerge as the case and control groups after such a comparison could then be used as the framework for choosing such groups retrospectively. Because a randomized clinical trial offers the most unbiased architectural structure for a scientific study of this comparison, the experimental principles used to admit, observe, and identify groups in a randomized trial can be used to provide the framework for choosing the control as well as the case group in a retrospective case-control study.

21.4.1. *Population-Based (Closed-Cohort) Studies*

In a randomized trial, we would begin with a defined population or cohort of people at risk for the outcome event. This approach, which offers a particularly effective way to avoid transfer bias, is used in case-control studies that are often called *population-based* or *closed-cohort* research.

The cases may be chosen from a population-based registry or roster that includes such events as all cases of sudden death, birth deformity, or detected cancers occurring in a demarcated ecologic region. If such a registry or roster has not been maintained, data collected from all the appropriate nosocomial sources in the region may be combined to form a single number that represents the occurrence of the selected events in the region's population. In heterodemic research, this number can become an occurrence rate when divided by the estimated eligible population in the region. In case-control research, the enumerated group of cases can be joined by a comparative control group chosen from the same population. If the registry or roster was established beforehand for the entire region and if all cases in that region have been appropriately reported, we need not worry too much about the transfer bias that can occur when a registry is created *ad hoc* to study an individual clinical condition or relationship. The main problem is to choose an appropriate control group.

The easiest way to choose a population-based control group is to use some other condition that has been collected at the same registry. Such choices would provide contrasts between cases of sudden death and controls who did not die suddenly; cases with one type of birth deformity and controls with some other type of birth deformity; cases with one type of cancer and controls with other types of cancer; cases acquired as confirmed reports of toxic shock syndrome and controls acquired as submitted reports in which toxic shock syndrome was not confirmed. These choices are attractive because they will allow both the case and control groups to be population-based, but the subsequent results, as noted earlier, may not always be appropriate for the scientific inference. When we think about the outcomes that follow whatever maneuver is under investigation, the cases will be suitable for the outcome, but the controls may not be. For example, if we wonder whether a gestating woman's use of Excellitol causes certain birth deformities, the appropriate alternative outcome is the absence of those deformities, not the occurrence of some other types of deformity. Similarly, if a particular maneuver predisposes to sudden death or protects against it, the appropriate outcome event is the absence of sudden death, not the occurrence of non-sudden death.

Unless the alternative outcome event suitably represents what we are looking for, the population-based registry or roster may be an unsatisfactory source of the control group. The investigators may therefore have to use some other framework for finding that group. Because the population of the region represents the cohort from which the cases emerged, the trohoc-cohort hybrid described in Section 18.6.2 may be an excellent way to find a population-based control group. The controls can be chosen from all other eligible people in that region who did not experience the outcome event that defines the cases.

In this population-based technique for choosing cases and controls, the cohort is defined and closed by an enumeration of all people who are at risk for the outcome event and who are eligible to receive the maneuver under study. According to the investigated relationship, the cohort can consist of all people living in a particular region, all people who have received a screening test, all children born in a particular region, or all patients admitted to a hospital with a particular disease. The people in the cohort who develop the outcome event are candidates as cases; all the other people in the cohort are candidates to become the controls. The situation is depicted in Figure 21–7. The first step in the research is to identify the closed cohort of eligible people. The next step is to identify the members of this cohort who have had the outcome event that makes them cases. The remaining members of the cohort are then available as controls.

Although used for case-control studies of disease etiology in the research described in Section 18.6.2, the closed-cohort approach can also be applied to evaluate therapy. For example, Horwitz and coworkers have used this technique to study the value of anticoagulant[19] and of lidocaine[20] treatment in patients with acute myocardial infarction. The closed-cohort approach is readily applicable for studying therapy when all the candidate patients can be identified from appropriate rosters (such as admissions to a special-care

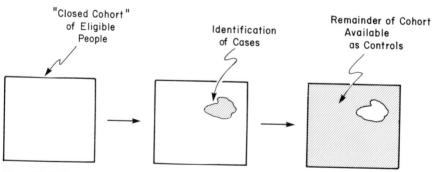

Figure 21–7. Sequence of procedures for choosing cases and controls in a closed cohort study.

unit), when all the outcome events can be detected, and when the investigated therapeutic agents have been available for common usage. The technique is obviously inapplicable for studies of new therapeutic agents or for circumstances in which a suitable cohort roster cannot be obtained or outcome events fully discerned.

In studies of public health maneuvers in a community, the community can serve as a population base, but the outcome events may be dispersed at different nosocomial locations, so that the total outcomes of the cohort are uncertain. This problem often makes the closed-cohort approach unfeasible for studies of disease etiology, and necessitates the alternative frameworks discussed in the next few sections.

21.4.2. *Compensations for Innate Biases*

Regardless of whether a closed cohort can be obtained as a single framework of candidates for the research, the particular people who become selected as cases or controls must often fulfill many other scientific functions. The most important functions are to help provide adjustments or compensations for the innate biases that can be anticipated in the research. These compensations can sometimes be obtained in the selected framework; or the necessary adjustments can be applied after the candidate members are selected from the framework.

21.4.2.1. **ADJUSTMENTS FOR SUSCEPTIBILITY BIAS**

Because a person's susceptibility to the outcome event cannot be determined until the person has become identified as a potential member of the control group, the adjustments needed for the customary sources of susceptibility bias are made with information assembled after the control framework has been chosen. They do not affect the basic choice of the framework. The adjustments needed to deal with protopathic bias or problems in vulnerability are also not framework problems, because the adjustments are made (as noted in Chapter 22) with data attained after the candidates are chosen.

21.4.2.2. **COMPENSATION FOR PERFORMANCE BIAS**

In case-control research, performance bias can occur in two main ways. The first source arises in a conventional manner if the principal maneuver is held responsible for effects that are really caused by a co-maneuver. This problem, which does not affect the choice of a framework, would be managed during the acquisition of data by obtaining suitable information about exposure to agents that might act as co-maneuvers, and by appropriate analysis of the information.

The second source of performance bias is distinctive to case-control studies in which the antecedent maneuver is ascertained from interviews. As discussed in Chapter 22, the ascertainment may be biased by a difference in the intensity with which the cases and controls have recalled or ruminated about antecedent exposure. To compensate for recall bias, the control group can be chosen to have a clinical condition that would evoke equal efforts in recollection of previous exposures. Although compensating for recall bias, however, this choice may introduce co-morbidity bias if the control group has also been affected by the maneuver.

21.4.2.3. **COMPENSATION FOR DETECTION BIAS**

If detection bias is potentially a major problem in the research, it cannot be suitably adjusted unless both the cases and controls have received the appropriate diagnostic procedure needed to identify the target disease. In such circumstances, the best framework for the study may be a roster of people who have received that diagnostic procedure. Such a roster can eliminate the disparities of detection bias while providing a uni-group framework for the study. The people with positive results in the diagnostic procedure become candidates as cases, and those with negative results become candidates as controls. The main hazard of this compensation is that a diagnostic roster may also introduce separate problems of co-morbidity bias. These problems can be managed as noted in the next section.

21.4.2.4. **COMPENSATION FOR CO-MORBIDITY BIAS**

In the proposed compensations for recall bias or detection bias, we take the chance of creating co-morbidity bias if the selected control group has a distinctive etiologic relationship to the principal maneuver. This hazard can be avoided, however, if we do not allow the control group to contain any diseases for which an etiologic relationship is suspected.

For example, if we believe that recall bias or detection bias can affect data for a causal relationship between Excellitol and lung cancer, patients with chronic pulmonary disease would not be a suitable control group if Excellitol is also suspected of causing (or preventing) chronic pulmonary disease. If Excellitol causes chronic pulmonary disease but not lung cancer, the group of lung cancer cases will be biased if it contains patients who have both diseases. In patients with both diseases, the Excellitol that caused the co-morbid disease but not the main disease would be falsely accused of causing the main disease if the co-morbid ailment has been excluded from the control group.

When done without suitable compensatory reasons, co-morbid exclusions can produce the type of bias discussed in Section 21.2.2.5.4. When done appropriately, co-morbid exclusions in the case group usually require information obtained after the candidate cases have been selected. The procedure is described further in Chapter 22.

21.4.2.5. **COMPENSATION FOR CO-MANIFESTATION BIAS**

If the maneuver causes an additional disease that produces the same manifestations as the main disease, the problem of co-manifestation bias can be compensated if people with the additional co-morbid disease are excluded from both the case and the control groups, as described in the previous section. For example, because postmenopausal estrogen therapy regularly produces endometrial hyperplasia and because the hyperplastic endometrium regularly produces the bleeding that evokes suspicions of endometrial cancer, patients with endometrial hyperplasia should be excluded (or analyzed separately) in a study of the relationship between endometrial cancer and postmenopausal estrogens.

If the maneuver creates its co-manifestation without producing a specific disease, the problem of co-manifestation bias will require different management. The available cases and controls should be stratified according to the particular clinical manifestation(s) that evoked the diagnostic procedure. These manifestations can usually be classified as typical, atypical, or none. For example, in patients with gallbladder disease, the typical clinical manifestations are appropriate forms of abdominal pain or jaundice. The atypical (and dubiously pathodynamic) manifestations are various types of bloating, belching, or other symptoms sometimes regarded as dyspepsia. If tea drinking produces dyspeptic manifestations that lead to the diagnostic detection of otherwise silent gallstones, the odds ratio for the tea drinking/gallstones relationship will be biased in the stratum of patients with dyspepsia but not in the other strata. Consequently, an unbiased odds ratio should be available in the stratum of patients who had either typical or no clinical manifestations of gallstones. Because postmenopausal estrogens produce the side effect of bleeding, which is a typical manifestation of endometrial carcinoma, a compensation for co-manifestation bias in this relationship would require examining the odds ratio in people who did *not* have bleeding as a stimulus leading to the diagnostic procedure.

21.4.3. *Use of Multiple Frameworks*

The cited compensations or adjustments will usually require a sophisticated clinical knowledge of the medical itinerary for the events that can occur between baseline states, exposure to maneuvers, detection of outcome events, and collection of research data. Without careful consideration of the particular phenomena and decisions that affect the natural course of events for a suspected cause-effect relationship, we cannot follow a conventional arbitrary ritual for obtaining groups and data, and then hope that the innate biases contained in those events will somehow be suitably recognized and managed.

Because each cause-effect relationship will have its own medical itinerary, a general set of principles cannot be stated for choosing each case or control group. The need to suspect and manage different biases will depend in each instance on the particular maneuver regarded as a cause and on the particular outcome (or disease) regarded as the effect. When reasonable suspicions can be raised about possible biases, the demands of scientific inference require suitable attempts to compensate or adjust for the biases. Because we cannot be sure that the compensations will always be satisfactory, a useful approach is to obtain control groups (and sometimes case groups) from several distinctly different frameworks.

The frameworks should differ in their defining characteristics, not merely in their locations. For example, the results found at three differently located registries or general hospitals may all be similar merely because each framework contains the same innate biases. The similarity of results would be more convincing if data from a registry, a general hospital, and an ecologic zone all show the same distinctions. Within a single institution, different frameworks can be used to obtain control groups from a general admissions roster, a particular service roster, a diagnostic procedure roster, or a diagnosed disease roster.

When results from suitably different frameworks are similar, the similarity can sometimes be used to sustain the correctness of decisions made in various compensations and adjustments. In other instances, the different results found from multiple frameworks may also sustain these decisions by demonstrating the actual biases that can occur. For example, when the odds ratio is substantially elevated in a community control group but is 1 in a control group chosen to compensate for recall bias, the investigator might be justified in claiming that the compensatory control group has given the right answer and that the problem of recall bias has been directly demonstrated.

On the other hand, a similarity of results will not always prove that the research was correct, because the same innate bias may have been left undiscerned and unadjusted in each framework. Furthermore, a dissimilarity in multiple results may not always prove that one framework was biased and the other was suitably compensated, because the compensation process may have produced its own errors.

Perhaps the main points to be noted as we conclude this section are that the easy simplicity of the case-control technique is accompanied by a complexity of difficult scientific problems in choosing suitable frameworks, and that the solution of the problems almost always involves subtle knowledge of clinical medicine rather than statistics.

21.5. ADDITIONAL INVESTIGATIVE SOURCES OF BIAS

Instead of using the scientific principles that would include or exclude people in a randomized trial, the investigator may choose a control group because of its convenient availability, because of arbitrary decisions about the cause-effect relationship, or even (in at least one notable instance) because a previously chosen control group gave results that were regarded as unsatisfactory.

Because these decisions affect the control group and may not be applied equally to the case group, all of the decisions can add a transfer bias beyond whatever innate bias was present in the available evidence.

21.5.1. *Convenient Source of the Control Group*

To have the disease that is a major focus of the investigation, the cases of a case-control study will almost always be chosen from a nosocomial location or from a registry where instances of the disease are collected and identified. If either of these sources also contains data for other people who do *not* have the focal disease, the other people become a convenient source of a control group. Their availability makes things particularly easy for the investigator, who can then conduct the entire project at a single site, without having to look elsewhere for controls.

This strategy can be justified with the argument that the members of the case group had to become suitably "medicalized" before their data could be collected at the nosocomial location or registry. Therefore, if the same source is used for choosing the control group, its members will have received a similar degree of medicalization. The argument is attractive, but it relies on the concept of medicalization to take care of many events that it cannot account for. The important principles of scientific analysis deal with a complete cause-effect pathway, which is a full medical itinerary, not just the particular single-state endpoint of medicalization that led to the person's location in a nosocomial roster or registry.

For example, if we suspect that exposure to Excellitol causes cancer of the lung, the outcome events of this relationship are *lung cancer* and *not lung cancer*. If the relationship is being investigated with a case-control study conducted at a tumor registry, the control group will contain people with *other cancers*. This control group may or may not represent the natural control group, which would contain a mixture of people who are healthy, who have diverse noncancer diseases, and who have other cancers. If the *other cancer* group is suitably representative of the non–lung cancer outcomes, the substitution may be satisfactory. If a co-morbidity problem is present, however, we may get the distortions shown earlier in Tables 21–1 and 21–2 and in Section 21.2.2.5.4. Thus, if Excellitol causes other cancers, the entire relationship may be obscured because the antecedent prevalence of Excellitol may be elevated in both the case and control groups. Conversely, if Excellitol protects against the development of other cancers but has no effect on lung cancer, the case-control study will suggest that Excellitol causes lung cancer. The prevalence of Excellitol will be normal in the lung cancer group and substantially below normal in the other cancer group, so that the odds ratio will be falsely elevated.

These problems are less likely to occur when the source of controls is a community or a general nosocomial zone rather than a registry. The people admitted to a general hospital are more likely to contain suitable representation from the world of noncases than the people found at a registry or special hospital.

21.5.2. *Arbitrary Unilateral Exclusions*

Regardless of how the case and control frameworks are chosen, many of the candidates encountered in those frameworks may be excluded from admission to the study, just as many candidates are excluded from admission to randomized trials. The case-control exclusions are done, as discussed previously and also in Chapter 22, to eliminate or compensate for the specific biases that have been identified in the foregoing discussion. Sometimes, however, the investigator may use various reasons of plausibility to exclude certain otherwise eligible people from the case group or the control group. The stated justification for the exclusions may be diverse features of age, race, gender, co-morbidity, or co-medication for the relationship under study. If carried out equally in both the case and control groups, such exclusions may not produce any bias, but a transfer bias can arise if the exclusions are applied unilaterally in one group or the other but not in both.

For example, suppose we wanted to study the etiology of toxic shock syndrome. If both the case and control groups are confined to women of menstrual age, we might not be able to discern an etiologic relationship for the toxic shock syndrome that occurs in men, children, and nonmenstruating women, but the fourfold table would itself be unbiased in its basic formulation. If we decided, however, to include men, children, and nonmenstruating women in the case group but to exclude them in the controls (or vice versa), the transfer bias would substantially distort the subsequent results noted for antecedent use of tampons.

This type of unilateral exclusion can produce transfer bias whenever the excluded group has a disproportionately high or low rate of occurrence for the focal event. The use of unilateral exclusions has been suspected[21] as a cause of the now discredited[22] relationship that was initially found in case-control studies of reserpine and breast cancer. In that study, many patients with cardiovascular disease, who could have been expected to have a disproportionately high antecedent prevalence of reserpine usage, were excluded from the control group but not from the cases.

21.5.3. *Retroactive Alteration of the Control Group*

In one notable case-control investigation[23] of the relationship between reserpine and breast cancer, the investigators used a cancer registry framework to select a case group of breast cancers and a control group from people with all other cancers. After ascertaining the antecedent usage of reserpine in both groups, the investigators found that the odds ratio was slightly elevated but not quantitatively impressive or stochastically significant. With a rationale based on an unproved conjecture that reserpine might be related to certain other cancers, the investigators then decided to exclude these suspect cancers from the control group. The newly created second control group, containing the other cancers remaining after exclusion of the previous batch, yielded an odds ratio that was twice as high as before and that was stochastically significant.

The investigators were commendably forthright in openly describing all the details of their methods, and the work was accepted for publication in a highly respectable journal. Because a retroactive alteration of the control group to fit the research hypothesis is not a generally accepted principle in other branches of medical science, the violation of the principle may not have been recognized by readers unfamiliar with the investigative creativity permitted in case-control research.

21.6. **ENTERING THE FRAMEWORK**

Regardless of the basic framework(s) chosen for a cross-sectional survey or case-control study, the investigator must enter the framework(s) to acquire the individual people who will be investigated.

At this point in the research, after the initial choice of a framework, each framework is an announcement, a map, or a list. In an ecologically based study, the investigator may solicit volunteers through announcements in the media, direct solicitation of people at their homes, or requests contained in letters or telephone calls. A nosocomially based study usually depends on several types of rosters. The roster may be simply an unedited collection of patients' medical records in a private practitioner's office or a special list, maintained at a hospital, that shows admissions, diagnoses, procedures, and other activities. In a registry-based study, the registry will have its own collection of data, organized with various types of indexing.

Regardless of the framework, the research contains events for a selected secular interval. This interval will demarcate the eligible dates for events recorded in archival data or the period of time used for solicitation of individual people whose events will be noted after they are examined. In addition to this secular choice of a time period, the investigator will also establish some coarse screening criteria that can be promptly and easily used to exclude potential candidates from consideration for admission. For example, if the study is concerned with men who do not have coronary disease, the screening criteria would exclude women or any men known to have angina pectoris or myocardial infarction. These screening criteria can be either stated during the announcements or interviews with which people are solicited, or the criteria can be applied when suitable rosters are examined. The screening criteria can then be re-applied when volunteers appear or medical records are obtained.

These secular and screening criteria will reduce the basic framework to an operational framework that provides the people eventually admitted to the study either directly or as persons described in recorded data. The candidates who pass the secular and screening criteria must also pass the subsequent admission criteria before they actually enter the formal study—but the investigator must first choose a mechanism for inviting candidates and deciding how many to invite. If a sample size has previously been calculated, candidates who volunteer can be successively asked to join until the required group size has been obtained. If the candidates are solicited from a roster, and if the roster seems to contain a surplus of candidates, the investigator can (and should) choose the desired number randomly from those listed on the roster. If the roster indicates that not enough candidates will be available, the investigator may either abandon the research or extend its confines by expanding the secular period, relaxing the screening criteria, or adding another framework to the project.

In many instances, a sample size is not calculated before a project begins, because the investigator may not know the details required for the calculations. In fact, when asked to supply the expected rates of events in the compared groups so that a statistically significant sample size can be determined, the investigator may reply that if those rates were known, the research would not be necessary. In such circumstances, the investigator will usually try to acquire all the people who fulfill the appropriate eligibility requirement and will fervently hope that they turn out to be enough.

Aside from these problems in the investigator's decisions about how many people to obtain and how to obtain them, a separate transfer bias may be created when the solicited people decide to accept or reject the invitation to participate. If the research depends exclusively on archival data, all the necessary information can be acquired from the archives, without any direct personal interviews. If the selected cases and controls must be interviewed to learn about their antecedent maneuvers or coexisting events, however, a transfer bias may arise due to disproportionate participation in the interviews. The members of the four cells in the fourfold table may not be available in the same proportions in which they occur in the table. Because this bias arises during attempts to collect data, it will be discussed in Chapter 22.

21.7. ADJUSTMENTS PRODUCED BY MATCHINGS, STRATIFICATIONS, AND MULTIVARIATE SCORES

When the results of the research ultimately appear in a fourfold table that relates maneuvers and outcomes, we will want to be sure of at least two things: the total group under study should adequately represent the external spectrum to be investigated; and the internal comparisons performed within the table should be unbiased. Although the various strategies discussed in this chapter can be used to help achieve these goals when the basic groups are selected, many other attempts to reduce bias are made after the data have been collected. In these activities, the investigator tries to equalize or adjust features that are dissimilar in the compared groups. The mechanisms used for producing these similarities depend on such adjustment tactics as matchings, stratifications, or multivariate scores. In the matching techniques, the control person (or persons) for each case is chosen to match the individual case in certain selected attributes. They are usually demographic features, such as age and gender. After the focal event is ascertained for each case and control, the results can be compared for each pair (or other combination) of the demographically matched cases and controls.

In the stratification techniques, no attempt is made to match individual people. Instead, the cases and controls are divided into subgroups or strata whose members all possess similar attributes, such as being *old white women*. Results for the focal event are then compared within similar strata of cases and controls. In the multivariate score technique, each person is given a score derived from a numerical mathematical weighting of selected attributes. Results for cases and controls can then be compared according to diverse mathematical analytic tactics, or within subgroups of people who have identical scores, or within strata defined by people who have a similar range of scores.

The adjustment techniques are often applied, after the research is completed, to try to improve the similarity of compared groups. To ensure that certain desired similarities will indeed occur, however, the techniques are often used when the cases and controls are initially chosen for the study. Because the case group is chosen first, the techniques are then applied to select members of the control group from its framework.

If the strata or scores of the case group are promptly identified, the controls can be enrolled successively until their total numbers in each stratum or score reach the sizes that correspond to the numbers noted in the cases. Because this awkward procedure is seldom used, almost all of the stratified- or multivariate-score analyses in case-control studies are conducted, after the research is completed, for control groups that were chosen in a relatively unconstrained manner.

The demographic matching process is relatively easy to do, however, and is commonly used to choose a control group that is matched to the cases. Because the nosocomial rosters of potential cases and controls often indicate each person's date of admission to the roster as well as the person's age, gender, and (perhaps) race, these demographic attributes can readily be used in the matching procedure. After each case is identified, the corresponding date of admission is found in the roster of controls. The list of controls is then scanned incrementally forward and backward in time until someone is found who matches the case in gender, in race (if pertinent), and in age. To ease the process, the ages are regarded as suitably matched if within several years of one another rather than identical. The secular constituent of the matching process in the roster also avoids the cumbersome process of trying to choose controls randomly, because the control member for each case can be chosen as the appropriately matched person whose date of admission is nearest that of the case. (If several suitably matched controls are available, the choices among them can be made randomly.)

21.7.1. *Scientific Issues in Matching*

In the tactic just described, the matching process offered a convenient mechanism for obtaining a control group that would resemble the cases in secular and demographic attributes. A more important issue in matching (or other forms of adjustment) is the scientific role of the procedure. In the scientific architecture of a randomized trial, two people about to be exposed to contrasting maneuvers would be matched if they have similar prognostic susceptibilities for the outcome event. We would match a good prognostic risk with another good prognostic risk, or a stage II cancer with another stage II cancer. If the matched people are not prognostically similar, a matching based on other attributes would be unsatisfactory.

For example, if we match two people who are each white men, age 55, of normal weight and height, for a comparison of medical versus surgical treatment of coronary artery disease, the match would be unsatisfactory if one of the men is asymptomatic with single-vessel involvement and the other man has severe angina, intractable congestive heart failure, and four-vessel involvement. Similarly, despite identical values in the five demographic variables of race, gender, age, weight, and height, the match for a comparison of cancer therapy would be grossly inadequate if one of the people is in TNM stage I and the other is in TNM stage III.

Since the choice of suitable prognostic variables was discussed earlier, the main point to be noted now is that the prime scientific role of the matching procedure is to achieve prognostic similarity before the maneuvers are imposed, and that the prognostically cogent variables for a patient's baseline clinical condition are almost always very different from those that might predict the risk of development of a disease in a healthy person. In public health epidemiologic studies of the risk of disease in healthy people, the customary variables used for matching or other adjustments are such demographic features as age, race, gender, and ethnic background. As noted earlier, these variables may not be ideal, but some of them are reasonably cogent predictors of the morbidity or mortality that constitutes the outcome variable in the research. In clinical epidemiologic studies of the impact of therapy, however, the most cogent predictors of prognosis are found in clinical, morphologic, and laboratory variables, not in purely demographic data. Yet the demographic information is often the main or the only source of variables used for adjustments in these studies.

Because of this defect, the statistical process of adjustment may omit the crucial variables needed to fulfill its scientific function. The matchings, stratifications, and multivariate scores may give the work an impressive air of statistical panache; and the investigator may be convinced that all the important variables or biases have been accounted for; but the procedure's scientific superficiality may negate its mathematical profundity.

21.7.2. *Statistical Issues in Matching*

Regardless of the scientific quality of the matching process, an unresolved mathematical dispute has developed about whether a matched or unmatched format should be used to analyze the data in a study in which the controls were individually matched to the cases.

For example, suppose an investigator has completed a case-control study in which 100 cases and 100 controls were each asked about exposure to a maneuver suspected as a possible cause of the disease. At the end of the study, the investigator finds the following data:

	Cases	Controls	Total
Exposed	30	15	45
Nonexposed	70	85	155
Total	100	100	200

The odds ratio for these data is 2.4 $[= (30 \times 85) \div (15 \times 70)]$ and because $X^2 = 6.45$, the results are stochastically significant at $P < 0.025$.

A critical reviewer, however, having noted that the controls were selected by matching, claims that this format of presentation is incorrect and that a matched arrangement should be used. In response, the investigator prepares the following table for the matched results:

Exposure	Exposure in Controls		Total
in Cases	Yes	No	
Yes	10	20	30
No	5	65	70
Total	15	85	100

The agreement matrix of this matched-analysis table has an odds ratio of $20/5 = 4.0$. The value of the uncorrected X^2 is calculated as $(20-5)^2/(20+5) = 9.0$, and P is <0.005. In this second table, everything is still consistent with the unmatched results. The numbers are still stochastically significant and the odds ratio still shows that exposure is associated with an elevated risk, but what is the magnitude of that risk? Is the odds ratio really 2.4 or is it 4.0?

This problem arises because the matched arrangement, as just described, permits a special form of statistical analysis that cannot be used with unmatched data. To show the algebra of this arrangement, suppose we have determined the results of the focal event, such as exposure or nonexposure to an antecedent maneuver, as *Yes* or *No* for each member of the matched case-control pairs. The four possible types of responses could be enumerated as follows:

Exposure Noted in:		
Case	*Control*	**Number of Pairs**
Yes	Yes	a
Yes	No	b
No	Yes	c
No	No	d

Total number of pairs   N

These results could then be tabulated in an agreement matrix as follows:

	Controls		
Cases	Yes	No	Total
Yes	a	b	f_1
No	c	d	f_2
	g_1	g_2	N

For these data, the odds ratio is determined as b/c, and X^2 (uncorrected) can be calculated with the McNemar formula as $X_M^2 = (b-c)^2/(b+c)$. If the numbers are small, a Yates-like type of correction is sometimes employed to do this calculation as $X_M^2 = (|b-c|-1)^2/(b+c)$.

If the data are arranged in an unmatched fashion, the N pairs of cases and controls become a total of 2N people, and the marginal totals of the agreement matrix become the interior cells of the fourfold table. Thus, the conventional fourfold table would be

Exposure	Cases	Controls	Total
Yes	$a+b$	$a+c$	f_1+g_1
No	$c+d$	$b+d$	f_2+g_2
Total	f_1+f_2	g_1+g_2	2N

The odds ratio for this table would be $(a+b)(b+d)/(a+c)(c+d)$. The value of X^2 would be $[(a+b)(b+d)-(a+c)(c+d)]^2 \times N/[(f_1+f_2)(g_1+g_2)\ (f_1+g_1)(f_2+g_2)]$.

The different formulas for the calculations immediately show why the two sets of arrangements for the same set of data will not always give the same results for the odds ratio and the X^2 test of stochastic significance. Arguments may then ensue about which arrangement should be used, particularly if one arrangement is more favorable than the other for the investigator's hypothesis. Because both sets of arguments can be justified, the investigator should always present the results of both analyses and let the readers take their choice.

In general, because of the way the McNemar X^2 calculation is done, the matched arrangement is more likely to produce a stochastically significant P value than the unmatched arrangement. The matched arrangement is also particularly desirable to confirm the results found in an unmatched arrangement if certain individual cases or controls have been excluded from analysis because of special eligibility criteria that were imposed after the cases and controls were originally selected.

The unmatched arrangement has the major virtue of being easier to understand. When the interior cells appear as four individual numbers (rather than in the more elaborate algebraic symbols used for illustration here), the reader can promptly see what really happened and can readily determine the particular increments, ratios, or other expressions that will help denote the quantitative significance of the results. This evaluation of evidence is much more difficult when the data appear in the unfamiliar arrangement of the agreement matrix. Most readers are accustomed to seeing agreement matrixes for the results of process research, which is aimed at evaluating agreements, but not for the relationships of maneuvers and outcomes that are studied in cause-effect research.

If the matching process were always used for an important scientific role, with substantial attention given to identifying and matching for the major innate biases in the data, the matched pairs would then have a scientific sanctity, which might shield them from being disrupted into an unmatched arrangement. This scientific function occurs when the attributes selected for the matching refer to susceptibility bias or other major sources of innate bias in the analytic comparison. In many instances, however, the matched attributes are demographic features of age and gender that are easily determined from the framework list, and that do not have a cogent effect on clinical susceptibility or other major biases. In these circumstances, the demographic matching is used mainly as an act of convenience that eases the choice of controls and that facilitates subsequent comparisons. Because the matching is used mainly for the convenience of the investigator, its results can also be easily rearranged for the convenience of the reader.

My own preference, therefore, is to rely mainly on the unmatched results. Because the matched odds ratios for each table should also be cited in the accompanying legend or in a footnote, they can serve as confirmation of the unmatched odds ratios. The unmatched data are easier to understand; and, because the numbers are larger, the results are less fragile statistically. In addition, the odds ratio calculated for the unmatched results accounts for all four cells in the agreement matrix rather than the possibly unstable conclusions that may be obtained when only the b and c cells are analyzed in the matched data. For example, if $\begin{Bmatrix} a & b \\ c & d \end{Bmatrix}$ is the format of a matched agreement matrix, the previous matrix

$\begin{Bmatrix} 10 & 20 \\ 5 & 65 \end{Bmatrix}$ yielded an odds ratio of 4.0 and a X^2 value of 9.0 in its matched form but corresponding values of 2.4 and 6.45 in unmatched form. With a larger sample size of 300 rather than 100 matched pairs, the agreement matrix of $\begin{Bmatrix} 75 & 20 \\ 5 & 200 \end{Bmatrix}$ would also yield a matched odds ratio of 4 and a X^2 value of 4.5, but the unmatched arrangement would have the form $\begin{Bmatrix} 95 & 80 \\ 205 & 220 \end{Bmatrix}$. For all 600 people in the study, the unmatched results would be statistically unimpressive. The odds ratio would be $(95 \times 220)/(80 \times 205) = 1.3$, and X^2 ($= 1.8$) would not be significant. A significant result would be obtained only with the matched arrangement, which would depend exclusively on data found in the 25 discordant pairs, ignoring the preponderant evidence of the 275 ($= 75 + 200$) concordant pairs.

For the previous sample size of 100 pairs, an agreement matrix of $\begin{Bmatrix} 35 & 20 \\ 5 & 40 \end{Bmatrix}$ would yield the same matched odds ratio of 4.0 and X^2 of 9.0, but its unmatched format would lower the odds ratio to 1.83 and the X^2 value to 4.5. Furthermore, again for a group of 100 pairs, the agreement matrix $\begin{Bmatrix} 40 & 16 \\ 4 & 40 \end{Bmatrix}$ would also yield a matched odds ratio of 4, which is stochastically significant, but the unmatched odds ratio would be 1.6 and would *not* be stochastically significant. (The proof of the latter two sets of assertions is left for Exercise 21.8 at the end of the chapter.)

21.7.3. *Number of Controls per Case*

In most case-control studies, the cases are harder to find than the potential controls; and the investigator will usually try to obtain all the cases that can be located within the selected framework. After the size of the case group is determined, a decision must be made about how many controls to choose. No general standards have been established for this decision, and no general agreement exists in the diverse statistical discussions of the problem.

According to statistical principles, we would want to avoid numerically fragile results. We therefore try to obtain a large control group. According to scientific principles, we would want to avoid the potential bias of a single separate framework for controls. We would therefore try to obtain control groups from several different frameworks. With either approach, the total number of controls might be the same, but one decision would depend on the purely quantitative strategies of statistics and the other depends on qualitative strategies of science. The qualitative strategies will be further discussed in Chapter 23.

In quantitative strategies, if the case group is too small, an oversized control group may be useful in producing stochastic significance for results that otherwise fail to achieve it. For example, suppose we can find only 14 cases of a particular disease. Whatever quantitative estimate we make from only 14 cases may be relatively fragile. If we also obtain 14 controls and then learn that antecedent exposure occurred in eight cases and in four controls, the fourfold table would show $\begin{Bmatrix} 8 & 4 \\ 6 & 10 \end{Bmatrix}$. The odds ratio would be a reasonably impressive value of 3.3, but it is not stochastically significant ($X^2 = 2.3$, P >0.05). If we quintupled the size of the control group (obtaining five controls for every case) and if the proportionate distinctions remained the same, the fourfold table would not show $\begin{Bmatrix} 8 & 20 \\ 6 & 20 \end{Bmatrix}$. The odds ratio would still be 3.3, but X^2 would rise to the stochastically significant value of 4.3. Thus, although the case group is still as fragile as before, the larger-sized control group will have pulled the results across the border into the promised land of statistical significance.

If the case group has a reasonable size, many investigators prefer the simple quantitative strategy of choosing a number of controls equal to the number of cases. If the controls are chosen from a roster according to the demographic principles noted earlier, the one-to-one matching has the advantage of making the subsequent statistical analyses relatively simple for either a matched or unmatched analysis of data. If the controls are matched in a 2:1 proportion or higher, the unmatched analysis is still simple, but the matched analysis becomes statistically much more complex.

If many controls can be expected to be excluded from admission after their other qualifying characteristics are noted, a many-to-one matching may be desirable to ensure that enough controls are available for analysis after the excluded choices are removed from the study.

21.8. **SYNOPSIS**

The framework used to choose people for admission to an observational study can be either the *zone* of an ecologic, occupational, or nosocomial setting, or a special *registry* formed to collect data about clinical conditions or personal attributes. The mechanism used for selecting the individual people can be operated in a uni-group or conjoined manner. In a uni-group selection, the candidates are chosen from a single framework, and both of the main variables under contrast (i.e., for maneuvers and outcomes) are ascertained *after* the candidates are admitted. In a conjoined arrangement, the basic groups (i.e., diseased cases and nondiseased controls) are chosen from two frameworks, and one of the main variables (e.g., presence or absence of the outcome disease) is known at the time of admission.

When a registry is established *ad hoc* to study a specific relationship, the associated publicity can bias the original diagnoses for exposed patients and can lead to disproportionate referral of data for exposed and diseased people. At a hospital setting, the proportions of exposed and diseased people can be distorted by both mathematical probabilities and clinical practice in patterns of referring patients to hospitals. If the investigator chooses prevalence cases rather than incidence cases, the case group can be distorted by the transfer biases occurring in the residue of an unspecified cohort.

Although certain registries or zonal rosters offer the advantage of a uni-group selection mechanism for both cases and controls, the outcome events in the selected control group may not be appropriate for the intended scientific inference. If the maneuver has a specific positive or negative (rather than neutral) relationship to the condition(s) contained in the control group, co-morbidity bias can distort the calculated relationship between the maneuver and the case group. If the maneuver produces clinical side effects that resemble features of the main disease, co-manifestation bias can lead to a preferential diagnostic detection of the disease in people receiving the maneuver. A particularly desirable uni-group framework is a population-based study in which the cases and controls are chosen, when possible, from a closed cohort of people in a defined ecologic region or nosocomial setting. When two (or more) frameworks are used for a conjoined selection of case and control groups, a prior knowledge of one of the main variables (e.g., a person's identity as a case or control) and preconceptions about the cause-effect relationship can lead to biased exclusions of eligible candidates or biased ascertainment of the other main variables (e.g., exposure to maneuvers).

The scope of spectrum in the cross-sectional groups under study may be quantitatively inadequate in descriptive studies, such as a national census, and the scope can be qualitatively inadequate or biased in process research and in biodynamic and pathodynamic studies. In cross-sectional or case-control studies of etiology and therapy, the premaneuver baseline conditions are seldom adequately identified or investigated as sources of susceptibility bias; and the impact of detection bias is often ignored. Both of these biases can be managed or adjusted by choosing control groups not for their investigative convenience or statistical merits, but for their scientific location and function in a complete cause-effect itinerary.

Although matchings, stratifications, or multivariate models can be used to adjust for disproportionate bias in the subgroups under analysis, the adjustment processes seldom include data for the cogent clinical attributes and indications that are prime sources of susceptibility bias in choice of maneuvers. Because of this omission, the desirable convenience offered by the matching process in choosing control groups is often scientifically superficial, and the matched arrangement need not always be preserved in the statistical analysis. If matched and unmatched analyses disagree, both sets of results should be reported, although the main statistical tabulations should be presented in whatever format will aid the reader's understanding.

EXERCISES

Exercise 21.1. Using appropriate sources in published medical literature (or help from an instructor), find examples of the following types of research:

> **21.1.1.** A cross-sectional descriptive study conducted in a single zone.
> **21.1.2.** A pathodynamic (or pathoconsortive) study.

For each study, discuss the quantitative and qualitative adequacy of the spectrum of people under analysis. If you have noted any inadequacies, what types of problems or biases do they produce in interpreting the results of the research?

Exercise 21.2. Again using appropriate sources, find examples of the following types of research:

> **21.2.1.** A community or other nonhospital-based cross-sectional survey of a cause-effect relationship.
> **21.2.2.** A retrospective case-control study of an etiologic risk in healthy people.
> **21.2.3.** A retrospective case-control study of adverse consequences of therapy.

For each study, describe the particular framework used to acquire the investigated groups, and discuss any transfer bias that may have been produced by the framework itself. Describe any investigative biases that may have occurred when groups were selected within the framework. Discuss the adequacy of the mechanisms (if any) that were used to deal with susceptibility bias. (Please do not consider biases in detection of outcome events or ascertainment of maneuvers. They will be sought in other exercises in later chapters.)

Exercise 21.3. In 1982, Siscovick and coworkers reported a case-control study on physical activity and primary cardiac arrest.[24] Through a special emergency service that covered Seattle and its suburban King County, the investigators found reports of all people at ages 25 to 75 who died with out-of-hospital primary cardiac arrest during December, 1979, to January, 1981. Candidates were excluded if they had a history of prior heart disease, major co-morbidity, or no spouse; if the surviving spouse reported that the candidate previously had a clinical condition that limited his usual activity; or if the spouse refused a more detailed interview. In the detailed interview, the candidate's spouse was asked questions to allow a special rating of the candidate's customary expenditure of energy in physical activities.

A control group was identified from the community using random-digit dialing. Control subjects were matched to each case for age (within 7 years), gender, marital status, and urban or suburban residence. Potential controls with prior heart disease or co-morbidity that limited their usual activity were excluded. In the telephone calls, spouses of the controls received the same detailed inquiry about energy expenditure that was used for spouses of the cases. After finding that the control group had significantly higher values of high-intensity leisure time activities than the cases, the authors concluded that persons who engage in high-intensity leisure time activities have a reduced risk of primary cardiac arrest.

21.3.1. Using the taxonomy described in this chapter (or earlier), classify the structure and framework of this study.

21.3.2. Of the various innate biases discussed in this chapter, which ones would you be most concerned about in accepting the authors' contentions?

Exercise 21.4. In young patients with first attacks of rheumatic fever, the prevalence of distinctive cardiac damage is about 42%. In young patients with recurrences of rheumatic fever, the prevalence of distinctive cardiac damage is about 80%. This difference in rates was interpreted for many years as indicating that recurrent attacks of rheumatic fever regularly created cardiac damage in patients who initially escaped it in a first attack. What kind of survey is represented by these data? What might be wrong with the stated interpretation? How might you check whether the interpretation is correct?

Exercise 21.5. For the past 10 years, interest has arisen in the possible association between amphetamine use and homicidal violence. In certain animal models of aggression, amphetamine has been shown to have a calming action. Because endogenously produced phenylethylamine is similar to de-amphetamine, psychiatrists have recently studied its relationship to aggressive behavior.

In a study reported in The Lancet,[25] 10 male prisoners who committed violent crimes were matched for age, height, and weight with 10 other male prisoners who committed nonviolent crimes. The men in both groups were aged 24 to 59 years; time spent in prison for the current sentence ranged from 12 to 30 months. The authors reported that plasma concentrations of free and conjugated phenylacetic acid (a metabolite of phenylethylamine) were significantly higher in the aggressive group than in the controls (876 ng/ml vs. 493 ng/ml, $P<0.025$). The authors concluded that phenylethylamine overproduction may represent a compensatory response by the body in its attempt to curb aggressive tendencies present as a result of as yet unknown functional derangements.

What kind of study is this? Does it permit the inference stated by the authors? If not, what kind of practical study would you propose? Are you satisfied with the choice of controls? If not, what would you do differently?

Exercise 21.6. Several observational studies have provided conflicting evidence of an association between colonic cancer and antecedent treatment with alpha methyldopa for hypertension. You want to resolve this question with a well-designed retrospective case-control study. The case group will consist of all patients with newly diagnosed colonic cancer at the County General Hospital during the past 5 years. Which of the following groups would you choose as controls, and why? Can you suggest any better choices for control groups?

a. Neighbors of the cases, matched with the cases by age and gender.
b. Patients undergoing elective surgery at County General Hospital during the past 5 years—excluding patients with liver, cerebrovascular, kidney, and cardiac disease—matched with the cases by age, gender, and year.
c. Patients undergoing colonoscopy at Suburban Hospital during the past 5

years, found not to have cancer and matched with the cases by age, gender, and year.

d. Patients randomly chosen from those with a discharge diagnosis of anemia at County General Hospital during the past 5 years.

e. All siblings of the case group.

Exercise 21.7. Here is an exercise that will allow you to observe and calculate the effects of Berkson's bias. Assume that Excellitol and cancer have the community relationships shown in Table 21–2. Now assume that people with lung cancer are hospitalized at a rate of 0.8, that people with other cancers are hospitalized at a rate of 0.5, and that all other people are hospitalized at a rate of 0.03. Because of close surveillance and/or noncarcinogenic side effects of Excellitol, assume that people receiving it are hospitalized at a rate of 0.1. If you work at the hospital that is the sole nosocomial location for this community, what will be the numbers of patients you encounter for each of the six subgroups of Table 21–2? What will be the odds ratio for the Excellitol/lung cancer relationship if the control group is chosen from patients with other cancers, with noncancers, or with anything other than lung cancer?

Exercise 21.8. The very end of Section 21.7.2 contains $\begin{Bmatrix} 40 & 16 \\ 4 & 40 \end{Bmatrix}$ as an agreement matrix having a matched odds ratio of 4. The text asserts that this odds ratio is stochastically significant, and that the unmatched odds ratio is 1.6 and not stochastically significant. Please do the calculations that will confirm (or refute) these assertions.

Exercise 21.9. (Optional exercise) Here is an interesting challenge if you like to play with algebra. Under what circumstances will the odds ratio be identical in a matched and unmatched arrangement of data for the same basic fourfold agreement matrix? Under what circumstances will the two sets of odds ratios show striking disagreements?

CHAPTER REFERENCES

1. Feinstein, 1974; 2. Feinstein, 1970; 3. Charlson, 1980; 4. Heasman, 1966; 5. Bauer, 1972; 6. Horwitz, 1981 (Lancet); 7. Beadenkopf, 1963; 8. Franks, 1954; 9. Harvey, 1984; 10. Jason, 1982; 11. Berkson, 1946; 12. Roberts, 1978; 13. Conn, 1979; 14. Gerber, 1982; 15. MRFIT, 1982; 16. Labarthe, 1978; 17. Harvey, 1982; 18. Stavraky, 1983; 19. Horwitz, 1981 (J Chron Dis); 20. Horwitz, 1981 (JAMA); 21. Horwitz, 1981 (Circulation); 22. Labarthe, 1979; 23. Armstrong, 1974; 24. Siscovick, 1982; 25. Sandler, 1978.

Scientific Decisions for Data and Hypotheses

The results of a cause-effect study are usually presented as a relationship of two critical variables. One of these is the basic or *grouping* variable. It indicates the main groups under study: the people who did or did not receive the principal maneuver; or the cases who did and the controls who did not develop the disease (or other outcome event). The second is the *focal* variable, which indicates the presence, absence, or magnitude of a focal event in each group.

In a cohort study, the grouping variable indicates the compared maneuvers, and the focal variable indicates the outcome. In a cross-sectional study, the grouping and focal variables can denote either maneuvers or outcomes, according to the structure of the study. In a pathodynamic study, the grouped cases and controls represent maneuvers, and the focal variable represents outcomes. In a retrospective case-control study, the grouped cases and controls represent outcomes, and the focal variable represents maneuvers. In a pathoconsortive study, the investigator is not sure which is which.

If the study has a uni-group framework—as in a randomized trial, ecologic survey, or nosocomial base for a cross-sectional survey or concurrent cohort study—the data about maneuvers and outcomes are collected after the single group is assembled. If the study has two or more frameworks, the data for the focal variable are obtained in the assembled groups. The process of obtaining this additional information is usually called *ascertainment*. It includes the acquisition of data for the focal variable and for other variables that may describe baseline status, co-maneuvers, or other features pertinent to the cause-effect analysis.

After the ascertained data are collected, the basic results of the research are at hand. The results will be arranged into appropriate statistical expressions, which are then reviewed. During this review, the investigator decides whether the statistical evidence does or does not support the original hypothesis of the research. If the original hypothesis is not supported, or if a hypothesis was not clearly established before the research began, the investigator may draw conclusions as a hypothesis that is formed retrospectively.

This chapter describes the problems of maintaining scientific principles in the collection of focal data and in the formulation of retrospective hypotheses or conclusions.

22.1. ESTABLISHMENT OF FOCAL TIME

In cohort studies of compared maneuvers, zero time has a crucial scientific role. It indicates the time of onset for the maneuver and the zero state (or baseline state) on which the maneuver is imposed. In an observational study, zero time for each person is the date at which the compared maneuvers were (or might have been) begun. In a randomized trial, zero time can be the initial date of imposition for maneuvers, but is more commonly chosen to be the date of randomization.

Because case-control studies are conducted in retrospect, after the compared maneuvers have already been received, a date of zero time cannot be demarcated in the same way as in a cohort study. What is chosen, instead, is a date of *focal time,* which corresponds to zero time in a cohort study. In a retrospective case-control study, focal time represents the time at which the principal maneuver was (or might have been) initiated. The person's focal state at focal time corresponds to the pre-maneuver baseline state.

22.1.1. *Focal State Eligibility*

Information about focal state will be used to determine each person's eligibility for admission to the study. For example, people who are not appropriately qualified to receive all of the compared maneuvers would be excluded from a randomized trial and should be excluded from a case-control study. People who are not appropriately vulnerable to the maneuvers would be excluded from both types of research.

In a randomized trial, people who begin with maneuver A at zero time and who later change to maneuver B would not be counted along with people who received maneuver B initially. The changeover group would be either analyzed separately or counted as though they had received maneuver A. This same type of analytic consideration should be applied in a case-control study. If people receive *no* maneuver at focal time and then later receive a specific maneuver, a susceptibility bias can be created if the person's prognostic state has changed between focal time and the onset of the maneuver.

Beyond these features of eligibility for admission and susceptibility to maneuvers, the focal state data will later be used analytically, as discussed in Chapter 23, for the adjustments needed to eliminate or reduce the susceptibility bias that can be expected when the compared maneuvers are assigned without randomization.

22.1.2. *Effects of Secular-Focal Interval*

Because case-control studies are done after the investigated events have already occurred, a substantial period of time may have elapsed as the *secular-focal interval* between the secular date at which the research is done and the antecedent secular date at which each person's focal time occurred. If the focal state data are available in suitably recorded archives, the problems of human memory can be avoided. If the focal state data are acquired through conversation at a later secular date, however, the interviewed person may have great difficulty remembering exactly what happened a long time ago.

If the focal event consisted of smoking, dietary habits, occupation, or some other maneuver that was maintained continuously for a long time before the occurrence of the outcome event, the identity and timing of the maneuver can be recalled reasonably well. If the maneuver was a single exposure, such as use of a particular medication, that was followed shortly afterward by an outcome event, such as an acute disease, the problems of identity and timing can be formidable if both the exposure and the outcome occurred long before the interview.

An additional problem in the timing of acute events arises when members of the control group are interviewed. To avoid a nonconcurrent comparison, the control persons should be asked about their possible exposure at a secular date that corresponds to the secular date of possible exposure for the cases. Not having had an outcome event that might stimulate the recall of exposure, the members of the control group may not clearly remember what happened. The difficulties of distant recall for acute exposures and acute outcomes can be reduced if members of the case and control groups are interviewed almost immediately after the outcome events took place, but such research would have to be conducted with intense surveillance and advance plans. The efforts needed to find appropriate cases and controls near the time of the acute illness would sharply curtail the convenient ease of retrospective case-control research.

If the investigated relationship is between a chronic exposure (such as diet) and a nonacute outcome event (such as cancer), the sequence and timing of distant phenomena are less likely to produce important errors. The main problems in chronic relationships will usually be the demarcation of exposure for the chronic maneuver and the contributory roles of co-maneuvers, co-morbidity, and diagnostic detection during the long incubation period between the onset of the main maneuver and the identification of the outcome.

22.1.3. *Problems of Temporal Precedence*

The interviewee may have trouble remembering not only the identity of the exposure but also its sequential location in time. The problem of temporal precedence is particularly important if the outcome event is an acute ailment such as Stevens-Johnson syndrome, Reye's syndrome, toxic shock syndrome, or some other condition that is defined as a cluster of manifestations. These ailments can often begin with a prodrome of symptoms that may then evoke or affect the use of a particular agent. When the full-fledged syndrome later becomes apparent, the antecedent agent may be associated with the outcome and regarded as a contributory cause. This type of protopathic bias produced the fallacious indictment, about 15 years ago, of sulfamethoxypyridazine as a possible cause of Stevens-Johnson syndrome.[1] Similar or analogous problems in temporal precedence have been recently suspected in the alleged relationships between aspirin and Reye's syndrome and between tampons and toxic shock syndrome.[2]

Even in nonacute relationships, however, the role of temporal precedence can still produce important problems in protopathic bias. Like an acute disease, a chronic disease can also have early manifestations that evoke or affect the use of a particular agent. When eventually detected or used as a grouping variable in a case-control study, the disease may then be associated with the later rather than earlier use of the agent. The results will distort the antecedent prevalence of certain agents in either the case or control groups and may then yield fallacious odds ratios for the investigated relationship. This type of protopathic bias[3] has been regarded as responsible for the false demonstrations that oral contraceptive pills could cause prolactinomas or protect women from benign breast disease, and that coffee could cause pancreatic cancer.

The problem of protopathic bias can be avoided by noting each person's focal (baseline) state at the time of the putative exposure and by determining any specific indications or contraindications that may have affected the use of the focal maneuver. Such patients can then be excluded from the research (as they would be in a randomized trial). The necessary information about baseline state and clinical indications may be available in archival data if the maneuver is a therapeutic agent, but may be difficult to obtain and unreliable if it depends exclusively on an interviewed person's recollection of long-distant events.

22.2. ASCERTAINMENT OF DATA FOR FOCAL VARIABLE

In cohort research, the role of double-blinding or other forms of objective discernment of the focal variable has received considerable scientific attention. The need for such attention seems obvious, because someone who knows both the research hypothesis and a person's status for the grouping variable (i.e., the maneuvers) may be biased in observing the focal event (i.e., the outcome). In cross-sectional research, however, similar scientific precautions are not always used when the focal event is ascertained, particularly in retrospective case-control studies in which both the patients and the interviewers know the patient's identity as a case or control.

If the focal event is an objectively performed laboratory measurement—as in many pathodynamic and some etiologic case-control studies—there is no major need to "blind" the observer. If the focal event, however, is reported subjectively by one person who is interviewed subjectively by another person, both people have an excellent opportunity to be biased. The collection of doubly subjective data—acquired during a conversation between two persons—occurs most often in retrospective case-control studies, but the problems to be discussed will pertain whenever subjective information is collected in any non-cohort research structures.

22.2.1. *Interviewer Bias*

An interviewer's attitude and mode of interrogation can substantially affect the response of a person who is asked to recall a medication, a dosage regimen, or some other antecedent exposure. The interviewer's suggestions can readily encourage certain responses or inhibit others. When the person is asked to describe details of dietary intake, exercise, life style, or other antecedent activities, the interviewer's preconceptions can also affect the choice of higher or lower categories in the recorded scale of classification.

This type of problem can be avoided in cohort studies if both the interviewer and the interviewee are kept unaware, i.e., double-blind, of the identity of the maneuver. In cross-sectional research, however, the outcome event has already occurred, and the case or control status of the interviewed person is usually known to that person when the investigative inquiry occurs. During the procedures used to identify suitable people and to solicit their participation in the research, the research hypothesis may even have been described to each person. If the interviewer also knows both the research hypothesis and the interviewed person's status as a case or control, the biases of both people can be reinforced during the interview process.

If data about the focal event are obtained from an archival source, the *interviewer* is the person who reviews the data to excerpt the pertinent information. According to the bias of the data excerpter, this review can be performed with different degrees of intensity and with different criteria for acceptance or rejection of information that is ambiguous or uncertain.

22.2.2. *Anamnestic (Recall) Bias*

The interviewed person has two different tasks. The first is to try to recall, as accurately as possible, what actually happened in the past. The second task is to make this anamnestic effort with adequate vigor, regardless of personal status as a case or control.

Although the accuracy with which people can recall past events is a crucial scientific issue when the investigation depends on such recollections, the issue has received relatively little attention in pertinent forms of case-control research. Investigators seldom report the results of either large or small studies in which interviews were repeated, at some suitable time after the original encounter, to determine the variability of responses to the same set of questions.

The few studies that have been conducted have shown some striking disparities in results. In one study[4] a group of women were asked in the last trimester of pregnancy to specify the medications they had received during the pregnancy. Several months after the pregnancy was completed, the women were interviewed again and asked for the same information. The subsequent responses showed many major disagreements with the original answers. In a different study, a group of people in a case-control investigation of etiology for cancer of the lip, when asked about their previous employment in the occupation of professional fisherman, gave substantially different responses according to the way in which the occupational question was asked on two different occasions.[5, 6] In a case-control study of toxic shock syndrome, when 22 women were interviewed twice, the use of a particular tampon brand was reported by seven in the first interview and by 11 in the second.[7]

Readers who wonder about the problem of accurate recall for distant events are invited to pause in the text right now and to describe what they ate for their evening meal three nights ago, to characterize what clothing they wore to a party three weeks ago, and to state what team was the winner of an outstanding sporting event (such as the Super Bowl in football, or the World Cup in soccer) three years ago. If you feel generally competent in mental activities but had difficulty with these recollections, you can appreciate the plight of persons who are suddenly asked to recall events of a distant past.

In addition to its basic anamnestic challenge, the recall process can be biased by the person's status as a case or control or by the investigator's role in the interview process. A woman who has given birth to a deformed child is much more likely than a woman with a normal baby to ruminate about everything that transpired immediately before and during the pregnancy. If a woman delivers twins, an intensive inquiry may be conducted to determine whether she used a fertility agent in becoming pregnant. The inquiry is likely to be less intensive, or may be omitted, if the pregnancy produced a single child.

Because research methods are seldom reported with sufficient detail, relatively few publications contain enough information to allow a reader to discern potential sources of biased ascertainment. One good example is apparent in the methods of a special project[8] established to study the relationship of DES and vaginal adenocarcinoma. The investigators accepted, without further question or attempts at verification, a physician's letter stating that DES had been used during the pertinent pregnancy. If the use of DES was denied, however, the physician's affirmation of nonexposure was not accepted, and a more intensive inquiry was conducted before the negative result was allowed to stand.

22.2.3. *Specification Bias*

A different problem in accuracy and bias can arise if the focal maneuver is not well specified during the collection of data. For example, certain common pharmaceutical substances, such as aspirin, or other readily available agents, such as food additives, can often be used without the recipient being aware of their usage. Unless the investigator has established a complete list of all the ways in which exposure to this agent might have occurred, and unless the interviewed person is asked about all the possibilities, the occurrence of an exposure may not be recognized. If these listings and other methods of inquiry are not applied equally for all persons in the research, regardless of their status as cases or controls, the results may be biased by the answers received during the disparate types of specification.

22.3. REDUCTION OF ASCERTAINMENT BIAS

The reduction or prevention of ascertainment bias is a difficult job, particularly in a case-control study in which the grouping variable may be known to each case and control, and also to the person who ascertains the focal variable. Nevertheless, several relatively easy precautions against bias are available to investigators who recognize the importance of the scientific principle and who are willing to make the necessary efforts.

22.3.1. *Hiding the Research Hypothesis*

Perhaps the best way to prevent ascertainment bias is for the research hypothesis to be hidden both from the people who are under investigation and from the people who do the ascertainment. If neither the interviewers nor the interviewees know exactly what maneuver the investigator is interested in, the opportunity for biased ascertainment will be sharply reduced.

The hiding of a research hypothesis is not easy. The investigator may have to establish one or more decoy hypotheses about focal variables that will receive considerable attention in the ascertainment process along with the main focal variable. For example, if the investigator suspects that tea drinking is a causal maneuver for gallstones, the inquiry in a case-control study can also include smoking, coffee drinking, and ingestion of alcohol. If the investigator suspects that estrogen replacement therapy causes gallstones, the inquiry can include information about tranquilizers, analgesics, or other pharmaceutical substances.

As long as several other focal variables receive at least as much attention as the main variable suspected as the principal maneuver, the investigator can try to avoid making an open statement of the research hypothesis. When informed consent is solicited from the participants, and when instructions are given to the research assistants who acquire the data, the investigator can say merely that the study is being conducted to determine the relationship between gallstones (or whatever disease is being investigated) and various aspects of antecedent nutrition, medication, and life style.

No one will be misinformed by the statement, because it is true and because information about these attributes is almost always solicited in retrospective case-control studies, regardless of whether any of the attributes are suspected as principal maneuvers. Human investigation committees should have no trouble in approving either the research or the statement, because the research process consists only of an inquiry. The subjects of the research are not exposed to anything more hazardous than an interview or a letter.

The ascertainment process will also be relatively unbiased if it is performed *before* a research hypothesis has been established, without anyone knowing which maneuvers and outcomes will subsequently be suspected as being related. For example, in the Boston Collaborative Drug Surveillance Project,[9] all hospitalized patients were interviewed shortly after admission to ascertain their antecedent usage of medications. Because the information was not used until later for various case-control or other studies whose hypotheses were not evident at the time of the interviews, the interview process could be regarded as relatively unbiased.

On the other hand, if a causal maneuver has already been suspected and a research hypothesis has already been established for a case-control study, perhaps the best way to *ensure* ascertainment bias is to have the interviews performed not by a research assistant but by the investigators themselves. The scientific precaution of keeping the investigator out of the ascertainment process may sometimes be overlooked when the research is conducted in great haste because the topic under study seems particularly urgent. For example, in case-control studies of the use of tampons in toxic shock syndrome and of aspirin in Reye's syndrome, this elementary scientific precaution was omitted. The investigators, knowing the etiologic agent that was suspected as the cause of the disease, and knowing each interviewed person's status as a case or control, often conducted the interviews themselves.

22.3.2. *Hiding the Investigated Person's Identity*

If the case-control study has a nosologic framework, so that each case and control patient was admitted to a medical institution, the identify of the patients as cases and controls can usually be hidden not only from the interviewers, but also from the patients themselves.

All that is necessary is for the mailed or spoken solicitation to contain no identification of a specific disease. The solicitation can be phrased in a statement such as, "We are doing a study of people who have the condition for which you were admitted to hospital X on date Y." The statement is correct, but it provides no special focus to indicate either the patient's disease or the particular disease that is under investigation. Because the statement is true and can do no harm to either patients or data collectors, it should also be readily acceptable to human investigation committees.

In fact, a statement of this type is probably the best way to describe the research not only to patients but also to the research assistants who collect the data. The data collectors can be told only that the research is being done to investigate the relationship between various clinical conditions and their antecedent (or subsequent) events. The likelihood of interview bias can be substantially reduced if the investigator can use this approach to keep the identity of cases and controls hidden from the data collectors, particularly if the sequence of interviews (or archival excerptions) occurs in a reasonably random mixture of cases and controls, rather than in the usual pattern whereby all the cases are interviewed, followed by all the controls, or vice versa.

On the other hand, the likelihood of anamnestic bias becomes particularly high if the investigated people are told their identity as cases or controls and are even told (as in some studies) exactly which antecedent maneuver is under suspicion.

22.3.3. *Formats for Data Acquisition in Interviews*

Another way of trying to reduce interviewer bias is to establish a rigorous and relatively rigid format for data acquisition. The interviewer should always be allowed the flexibility needed for courteous and civilized discourse with the interviewed persons, but the phrasing of serious questions, i.e., those whose answers provide crucial research information, and the methods of recording the answers should be relatively inflexible and uniform for all interviews.

The format should include an opportunity for each pertinent positive response to be followed by additional questions that also have a uniform arrangement for phrasing and responses. Certain types of information that might reveal the interviewed subject's identity as a case or control can be placed at the end of this format, after the other sensitive data have already been collected and recorded.

Because the format used for the interviews is the most important scientific instrument of many case-control studies, the format itself is a vital ingredient of the research and should be displayed, or made available for display, to any reviewer who wishes to see it. The format should preferably be published, as an appendix or internal constituent of the text, along with the report of the research itself. If editors are unwilling to supply additional space for this purpose, the investigators should outline the format in their account of *methods* and should indicate how interested readers can obtain copies for inspection.

In a particularly well-conducted study, the investigator may make additional attempts to check the consistency and accuracy of the interview process. To check the interviewers, a second person can re-interrogate each member of a selected subset of patients shortly after the first interview was conducted. To check the patients, interviews can be repeated at a subsequent date several months later. The accuracy of the information can be checked by interviewing a spouse or someone else who knows the patient's past history and by reviewing pertinent information that might have been noted in archival records.

Social scientists are very familiar with these scientific necessities in interview research, and the social science literature contains many discussions of the necessary requirements and techniques. The omission of these scientific principles has been so pervasive in epidemiologic research, however, that one of the current leaders[10] in the field recently decried the "extremely sketchy" ways in which data-gathering is conducted and reported. He concluded that epidemiologists have paid "inadequate attention to the quality of the data obtained in our investigations" and that the need for improving "the validity of the data is particularly urgent."

22.3.4. *Reducing or Compensating for Anamnestic Bias*

Despite all efforts made to keep the data collector unbiased and to hide the identity of cases and controls from even themselves, the data obtained in an interview ultimately depend on the memory and responses of the interviewed person.

An important first step in the procedure, therefore, is a crude assessment of the interviewee's sensorial competence. Either the ailment that led to the interviewee's selection for the study or a subsequent medical problem may have caused difficulties in the ability to understand questions, remember events, or respond accurately. If the interviewer does not discern that the answers are untrustworthy, grossly erroneous data may be entered into the research.

For people who are sensorially competent, the interviewer may make various efforts to stimulate memory. The patient may be reminded of occasions on which exposures may have occurred, supplied with lists of commercial names of possible agents, or even, in a personal interview, shown pictures of pharmaceutical tablets or other pertinent substances. This type of multiple-choice question is best delayed, however, until after the patient responds to an open-ended question about exposure. If the patient can spontaneously name a particular agent, citing it by commercial brand, the information is more likely to be reliable than a choice made from a multiple listing.

While trying to improve a person's recall, however, a zealous investigator (or interviewer) may use tactics that are more likely to create bias than to improve accuracy. For example, in a case-control study[11] of the etiology of toxic shock syndrome in menstruating women, the investigators had previously established the hypothesis that the causal agent was tampons, particularly the Rely brand of tampons. Oriented to this preestablished hypothesis, the questionnaire concentrated almost exclusively on gynecologic and catamenial events, with no attention given to antecedent or concomitant co-morbidity, co-medication, nutrition, or other factors that might have been explored if the etiology of the disease were regarded as uncertain.[12] The questionnaire also contained no mention of any specific brands of tampons, except for Rely, which was asked about not only by brand name but emphasized with reminders that it may have been received as a free sample.

When not produced by this type of prejudiced inquiry, anamnestic bias can arise spontaneously and can sometimes be too great to be reduced or eliminated merely with efforts to stimulate the patients' memories. As noted in Chapter 21, this problem can be approached by choosing a control group that can compensate for the recall bias in the cases by containing people who are likely to have reviewed their past events with a similar vigor. For example, in case-control studies of certain birth defects suspected of being related to in utero exposure to estrogens, patients with other (presumably unrelated) congenital anomalies were chosen as a control group.[13] The mothers of the control children could be expected to have also ruminated vigorously about prenatal events.

22.3.5. *Information from Archival Sources*

Perhaps the best way to avoid an interviewed person's inaccurate or biased recall, however, is to avoid obtaining the data from interviews. If suitable information about exposure was recorded in archival documents, the archival data, despite all their attendant defects, can often be more trustworthy than a fallible or prejudiced human memory.

If the archival information about exposure was recorded before any suspicions about the condition that made the patient a case or control, the information itself was probably obtained and inscribed without bias. The archival data, of course, can be incomplete or misused. When desired details are absent, the investigator may erroneously regard an absence of information as indicating *no exposure*. When details have been recorded, bias may be produced when the information is excerpted during the research process.

22.3.5.1. **BIAS IN PREVIOUS RECORDING OF DATA**

In many medical records, particularly in such specialties as ophthalmology, orthopedics, gynecology, obstetrics, and urology, the clinicians may confine their notes to information about the particular clinical condition that evoked medical attention. Such records may not contain the data about past history, life style, or antecedent exposures that are usually asked about and inscribed in the more compulsively detailed records maintained by pediatricians, internists, or family physicians.

If the archival information about exposure was recorded *after* development of the pertinent clinical condition, however, the intensity of the interrogation may reflect the prevailing belief about the relationship of exposure and disease. Clinicians who are unaware of a relationship, or unconcerned about the possibility, may not record any data about the pertinent exposure. For example, information about the antecedent use of replacement estrogens is commonly solicited and recorded as part of the *present illness* when a postmenopausal woman is admitted to a medical service with a diagnosis of endometrial cancer, osteoporosis, or stroke. If the diagnosis is pneumonia, however, information about estrogen usage may not appear anywhere in the record. A patient's previous exposure to a suspected causal agent may thus be asked about and recorded if the patient has the "right" disease, but may be left as unknown if the patient has the "wrong" disease.

22.3.5.2. BIAS IN EXCERPTION OF DATA

Because the same biases that can occur during interviewing can also occur when information is excerpted from archival data, the data collector should preferably be kept unaware of the research hypothesis and of the patients' case/control identity, even if the basic source of information is an inanimate medical record. This type of blinding can be attained or approximated with some of the previously discussed strategies for "hiding" the particular disease or exposures that are prime targets in the investigated relationship.

In addition to (or instead of) this strategy, the investigator can use the previously mentioned process of differential xeroxing (see Section 17.4.1). For this process, a person who is unaware of the research hypothesis goes through the archival information and replicates the particular page or pages that contain the pertinent data about exposure. A person who is aware of the research hypothesis then reviews these excerpts to see whether they contain any potentially biasing material about the patient's disease. After this material is removed, the remaining information is rearranged to form the collection that is given to the person who will actually excerpt the data.

22.3.5.3. PROBLEMS IN MULTIPLE SOURCES OF DATA

Because so little attention has been given to scientific standards for data collection in case-control research, very few studies are available to demonstrate the problems that can arise and that require resolution when several sources are used for ascertainment. The most commonly used sources of data, beyond individual interviews, are the archival records maintained by hospitals, individual practitioners, and pharmacists.

When these diverse sources produce conflicting evidence, the investigator must decide what to do about the conflicts; and the decisions can strikingly affect the results of the research. In one case-control study,[14] for example, the odds ratio varied from 2.8 to 4.1 to 5.8 when based respectively on interview data alone, medical record data alone, or a combination of data from the two sources. In another study,[15] however, the odds ratios showed a fall, rather than a rise, when calculated from combined rather than individual sources of data. To avoid these problems, the data from separate sources can be segregated rather than combined, and odds ratios can be calculated separately for the results found with each source of data.

22.3.6. *Biases Produced During Analysis*

Although the basic information may be collected without distortion or prejudice, bias can arise when the information is analyzed. The opportunities for biased analysis occur when the investigator makes decisions about managing unknown data and when exposure is demarcated after the results have been inspected.

22.3.6.1. **MANAGEMENT OF UNKNOWN DATA**

The investigator's decisions about what to do with unknown data are important. If the absence of information about a particular exposure is regarded as evidence of nonexposure, a substantial bias may be produced if the cases were admitted mainly to a pediatric or medical service and if the controls came from other services where the appropriate information is often missing. The same problem arises if the cases had a disease previously suspected of being related to the exposure, but the controls did not. For example, in a recent case-control study[16] of the relationship of antecedent estrogen therapy to breast cancer, the odds ratio was 3.3 when unknown information about exposure was regarded as negative, but the odds ratio dropped to 0.9 when the people with unknown exposures were removed from analysis. For this reason, unknown data should not be used as evidence of nonexposure, and the report of the research should indicate how the unknown data problem was managed.

22.3.6.2. **RETROACTIVE DEMARCATION OF EXPOSURE**

In a randomized (or nonrandomized) planned comparison of maneuvers in a cohort, the maneuvers form the grouping variable, and their identity would be specified beforehand. In case-control studies, however, the maneuvers may be ascertained as the focal variable.

When the suspected agent is a substance that had to be given at a certain level of proficiency (in the amount and duration of exposure) to produce its alleged effect, the specification of what is meant by *exposure* may be delayed until after the data are analyzed rather than established beforehand. Occasionally, the specification of exposure may be even omitted from the published results. For example, in most of the case-control studies devoted to the possible relationship of endometrial cancer and postmenopausal estrogen replacement therapy, no stipulations were reported for the type, amount, and duration of estrogen that would qualify as an exposure.[17]

The absence of previous specifications, before the research is done, allows the results to contain a possibly biased demarcation of exposure. McDonald and coworkers[18] have shown how dramatically different results can be created in the same set of data—with odds ratios ranging from 0.9 to 7.9—according to the investigator's choice of criteria for demarcating exposure to estrogens. If these criteria are established *after* the data have been analyzed, the investigator can easily achieve whatever odds ratio is desired. The problem can be avoided if criteria for exposure are stipulated before the research begins.

22.4. **OTHER FEATURES OF ASCERTAINMENT**

In a case-control study, the choice of frameworks will indicate the candidates to be considered as cases and controls. With the grouping variable selected by this decision, the main role of the ascertainment process is to identify the focal variable as the outcome event in a pathodynamic study or as an antecedent maneuver in a trohoc study.

Several other important items of information, however, may also be ascertained along with data about the focal variable. Some of this information will determine the person's eligibility as a case or control. For example, until the patient's medical history is learned during an interview or excerption of archival data, we will not know whether the person is an incidence or prevalence case of the target disease, whether a diagnostic procedure was ordered because of co-manifestation problems, or whether the person has a disease that can produce co-morbidity bias.

The additional data obtained during the ascertainment process will also demarcate the person's pre-maneuver baseline state (and therapeutic indications if any existed). The information will be needed for suitable analysis of issues in susceptibility bias and protopathic bias. If detection bias is a potential problem, and if the problem was not managed by choice of an appropriate framework, information about detection procedures will also have to be acquired during the ascertainment process.

Because the use of this additional information will be discussed in Chapter 23, the main point to be noted now is that an objective, unbiased ascertainment is just as essential for all the additional data as for the focal variable.

22.5. BIAS IN PARTICIPATION OF GROUPS

When a case-control study begins, the groups involved in the investigated relationship form a fourfold table whose proportionate contents may already have been distorted by the innate biases described previously. The investigator is then scientifically challenged to choose cases and controls in a way that can compensate for those biases. Regardless of how well that basic challenge is managed, the investigator may have additional problems if people must be recruited to participate in interviews. Disproportionate losses of potential participants can produce further distortions in the four cells of the table. Some of the eligible people may be lost because they are dead, too sick to participate, or refuse to volunteer; others may be left out because information about the focal variable is unknown.

Either source of omissions can create a major transfer bias in the results. Although the people studied in any form of medical research must be willing to participate in the study, and although the problems of volunteer bias have received considerable attention in other forms of scientific investigation, the issue has seldom been discussed for case-control studies. When the investigator prepares the lists of people who will be invited to participate as cases and controls, the fourfold table that is envisioned has the following true structure.

Exposed	Cases	Controls
Yes	A	B
No	C	D

After these people are solicited for interviews or acquired as data from archival records, the omission of persons who are not included in the anticipated table will give the following structure for the results that are actually collected:

Exposed	Cases	Controls
Yes	a	b
No	c	d

The correct odds ratio in the anticipated groups is AD/BC, but the odds ratio calculated for the participating groups will be ad/bc. Unless the participation proportions are the same in all four cells, so that $a/A = b/B = c/C = d/D$, or unless the distortions in certain cells are appropriately compensated in other cells, the results can be substantially biased.

In one of the few studies that have been devoted to the magnitude of this problem in case-control research, Horwitz and coworkers[15] determined the values of A, B, C, and D from information contained in the medical records data of cases and controls, and then compared the values of a, b, c, and d in patients who were available for interviews. The results of a/A, b/B, and so on—which simply reflect proportionate availability for interviews and not any changes in exposure status reported during the interviews – are shown in Table 22–1.

The data of Table 22–1 show striking disparities in the proportionate availability of people in different cells of the fourfold table. The marginal totals show that cases of endometrial cancer were more likely to be available for interview than controls; and that women exposed to estrogen were more available than nonexposed women. In the interior four cells of the table, the a cell, containing exposed cases, showed an availability proportion of 91%, which was almost twice as high as the 56% proportion of availability in the d cell, containing nonexposed controls. Fortunately, in this particular instance, the two extreme disparities provided a relatively good internal compensation for bias in the odds ratio. Thus, the odds ratio factor for the distortion produced by disparate availability would be $(0.91)(0.56)/(0.70)(0.61) = 1.2$. In other words, the odds ratio calculated from the people available for interview would be $(40 \times 71)/(16 \times 64) = 2.8$. This value is about 1.2 times the value of $(44 \times 126)/(23 \times 105) = 2.3$, which would be calculated as the odds ratio in the medical record group.

In an analogous later study of response rates and odds ratios, Austin and coworkers[19] also found consistent patterns of biased participation associated with the risk factors and outcome events in a population-based survey of cardiovascular disease. In the Austin study, the rate of participation was also higher in people having the risk factor, but the rate was lower in people having the target disease, thus producing an increased response proportion in the "worried well" members of cell b of the fourfold table. These investigators also found, however, that the biases of response in individual cells were often cancelled out in an internal compensation when the four numbers in the cells were multiplied and divided to form the odds ratio. Although the investigators proposed a mathematical model in which these cross-cancellations might regularly be expected to yield an unbiased odds ratio, the model requires assumptions that may not regularly apply, particularly in the many epidemiologic studies in which response rates are low.

Because an internal compensation cannot be relied upon to produce an undistorted odds ratio, the effects of nonparticipation bias create a difficult and currently unresolved problem in case-control studies. Since the problem has received so little attention, its magnitude and effects are uncertain; and no general standards have been proposed for its

Table 22–1. PROPORTIONS AVAILABLE FOR INTERVIEW AMONG PEOPLE IDENTIFIED FROM MEDICAL RECORDS AS POTENTIAL PARTICIPANTS IN A CASE-CONTROL STUDY

Recorded History of Antecedent Exposure to Estrogen Therapy	Cases (Women with Endometrial Cancer)	Controls (Women Tested and Found Not to Have Endometrial Cancer)	Total
Yes	40/44 (91%)	16/23 (70%)	56/67 (84%)
No	64/105 (61%)	71/126 (56%)	135/231 (58%)
Total	104/149 (70%)	87/149 (58%)	191/298 (64%)

Each denominator indicates the status of patients, as identified in medical record information. Each numerator indicates the corresponding number of patients who were willing to be interviewed regarding antecedent exposure. The data are adapted from Table 3 of Horwitz and coworkers.[15]

management. If the proportions of nonparticipation are small, the impact may also be small; but if the proportions are high, the investigators may need to calculate and analyze odds ratios separately for the groups demarcated by the archival data and for the groups available as interviewed participants.

22.6. RETROSPECTIVE HYPOTHESES, MULTIPLE CONTRASTS, AND POOLED DATA

In the customary design of cause-effect research, the hypothesis is stated prospectively as the first step in outlining the plan of the project. The compared maneuvers and the target outcome are identified; and they determine the subsequent structure of groups and collection of data.

A common problem in prospective specification of the hypothesis is that the investigator may be qualitatively precise in stipulating baseline states, compared maneuvers, and outcomes, but quantitatively imprecise about the direction and magnitude of the expected relationship. Thus, the hypothesis may be stated symbolically as F/M vs. $F/\bar{M}$, rather than as $(F/M) > (F/\bar{M})$, or as $(F/M) = 0.6(F/\bar{M})$, or $(F/\bar{M}) = (F/M) + 10$. When those initial specifications about direction and magnitude have been omitted, the distinctions noted in the subsequent data will not have been anticipated. Various statistical squabbles may then ensue about whether stochastic significance should be tested with one- or two-tailed standards, whether a stochastically significant result is quantitatively significant, and whether the group sizes are large enough to conclude that a stochastically nonsignificant result is quantitatively insignificant.

A quite different problem arises when the observed results, in coinciding with or departing from the expectations of the original hypothesis, are received with different degrees of happiness by the investigator. The investigator's response to the results will usually depend on whether they are anticipated or unanticipated, welcome or unwelcome, passively disappointing or actively repugnant.

If unhappy with the results, the investigator usually has two recourses available: the original hypothesis can be rearranged to fit the observed data; or the observed data can be rearranged, augmented, or submitted to auxiliary analyses that are done to support the original hypothesis. The rearrangement of data and reasoning to form or support these retrospective hypotheses is a legitimate scientific activity, because science depends on conclusions that are supported rather than contradicted by the available evidence. On the other hand, the activity itself creates two sets of major scientific problems.

The first set of problems deals with the credibility of the evidence that generates a retrospective hypothesis. Is the observed relationship real or merely a statistical artefact created during the auxiliary analyses? Beyond the statistical distinctiveness of the observed results, do the groups and data allow a scientific inference that the results are acceptable evidence of the proposed relationship? If the evidence is acceptable as neither a statistical nor a scientific artefact, the second set of problems deals with the degree of scientific confidence that can be placed in a retrospective hypothesis. Should the results be regarded as confirmatory support of a tested hypothesis; or should the hypothesis retrospectively generated by the data be viewed with the suspicion given to a screening test that often yields false-positive results and that has no real credibility until confirmed by a separate, more accurate test?

The rest of this section contains a discussion of the occurrence and management of these problems. They arise in all types of research structures, but are particularly common in cross-sectional studies.

22.6.1. *Incentives for Retrospective Hypotheses and Auxiliary Analyses*

The incentives for retrospective hypotheses and auxiliary analyses arise from six main types of relationship between the original hypothesis and the investigator's reception of the results. The six relationships are outlined in Table 22–2 and are further discussed in this section.

In the first four situations in Table 22–2, the result of the research is welcomed; the investigator's subsequent activity depends on the enthusiasm of the welcome and the unexpectedness of the results. In the first two situations, the results are anticipated because they coincide with the expectations of the original hypothesis. If the results provide strong support, i.e., both quantitative and stochastic significance, they will usually be welcomed enthusiastically. If the investigator performs auxiliary analyses of the data, the aim is to increase the precision and applicability of the results by identifying further distinctions in outcomes, maneuvers, or subgroups.

In the second situation, the results coincide with the hypothesis, but they are statistically weak. They may lack quantitative significance or stochastic significance or both. Welcoming the results, but disappointed by their weakness, the investigator may try to increase their statistical strength. The auxiliary analyses will be done in an effort to obtain that increased strength.

In the third situation, the result is welcome but comes as a surprise. The observed distinction is unanticipated but is quite acceptable to the investigator because it is consistent with either the original hypothesis or with a latent objective of the research. For example, if a new hormone fails in the goal of restoring a lost libido but has the unexpected side effect of curing baldness, the investigator will happily accept the unexpected results. If any auxiliary analyses are performed, the goal is usually to provide an explanation for the unexpected findings.

In a fourth situation, any positive result is welcome, because nothing was anticipated. The study was begun, without an established hypothesis, as a "fishing expedition" in which multiple analyses were done to screen the available data for anything significant that might emerge. In this circumstance, the main auxiliary analyses have already been performed as part of the process that produced the main results. The investigator's next step will create a retrospective hypothesis to fit the results.

Table 22–2. INVESTIGATOR'S RECEPTION OF RESULTS AND REASONS FOR ADDITIONAL AUXILIARY ANALYSES

Situation	Was Result Anticipated?	Was Result Welcome?	Investigator's Goal	Reasons for Additional Auxiliary Analyses
1	Yes	Yes	Keep hypothesis	Increase precision
2	Yes	Yes, but weakly supportive	Keep hypothesis	Generate support
3	No	Yes	Keep hypothesis	Provide explanation
4	No (No hypothesis)	Yes	Generate hypothesis	(Already performed)
5	No	No	Find new hypothesis	Generate hypothesis
6	No	No	Keep hypothesis	Generate support

The fifth and sixth situations are particularly unhappy for the investigator, because the results are both unexpected and unwelcome: the original hypothesis is not supported by the data and may even be refuted. If the undesirable results are too repugnant to be accepted, the investigator has two salvage options available. In one option, the initial hypothesis is abandoned, and auxiliary analyses are done in search of a positive relationship that can generate a new hypothesis. In the other option, tenaciously clinging to the original hypothesis, the investigator does auxiliary analyses, trying to find support for it. Because the salvage operations are usually conducted as acts of despair, they contain not only all the potential hazards of retrospective hypotheses and analyses, but also the hazard of self-delusion by a desperate investigator.

22.6.2. *Types of Auxiliary Analyses*

Two main types of procedure are available for the auxiliary analyses. In one procedure, data from other studies are joined to augment the "pool," i.e., the group size, of information entered into the statistical analyses. The "pooling" process, which is usually performed to strengthen a set of welcome but weak results, will be discussed further in Section 22.6.4.1. The second procedure is to perform multiple-contrast analyses of data arranged in various patterns of relationships for maneuvers, outcomes, and subgroups of patients.

If the multiple-contrast arrangements are organized as fourfold tables, the investigator can check the presence or absence of different outcomes for the same maneuvers, different maneuvers for the same outcomes, or combinations of different maneuvers and outcomes. In addition, the fourfold tables of maneuver-outcome relationships can be checked in patients demarcated into different subgroups formed by various attributes of age, gender, or diverse clinical and demographic attributes. These multiple-contrast analyses have certain hazards that are purely statistical, but other problems are distinctive to the situation in which multiple contrasts are employed. They will be further discussed as those individual situations are considered in the next few sections.

22.6.3. *Management of Unanticipated but Welcome Surprises*

The retrospective formulation of hypotheses to fit the good or bad things encountered as welcome surprises in the data is not unique to cross-sectional research and has occurred even in randomized clinical trials. For example, in the original hypothesis of the UGDP trial[20] of hypoglycemic agents for treatment of diabetes mellitus, the main outcomes to be considered were morbidity from cardiovascular, nephropathic, and neuropathic complications. When unexpectedly high rates of death were noted in the patients, however, the original hypothesis was changed to make mortality the main outcome event. In the original hypothesis of another randomized trial, sulfinpyrazone[21] was given for the outcome goal of preventing recurrent myocardial infarction. When sudden death occurred less frequently in the sulfinpyrazone-treated patients than in the control group, the initial hypothesis about sulfinpyrazone's efficacy was changed.

Cross-sectional research, however, provides a much greater opportunity than cohort research to explore a large number of diverse hypotheses. In a cohort study, the investigator is limited to the few focal variables that can be examined repetitively during follow-up. Because cross-sectional studies are much quicker and less expensive than cohort research, the investigator can obtain data for a large number of focal variables and can then analyze the relationship between each of those variables and the grouping variable that defined the cases and controls.

If satisfactory data are available for a uni-group study conducted in an ecologic or nosocomial zone, the research may be conducted as a screening test, without any previous hypotheses. The investigators can arrange to construct and analyze fourfold tables in which every variable that might be considered as a possible maneuver is related to every variable that might be considered as a possible outcome. For example, using a computerized nosocomial roster that contained data about pre-admission medication and discharge diagnoses for about 25,000 patients, the investigators[9] constructed a large series of fourfold tables of relationships between individual diseases and individual medications. Although the number of explored relationships was not cited, the accompanying publications[9, 22] mention at least 42 diseases and 32 agents. Consequently at least 1344 fourfold tables were evaluated. (One of the positive relationships that emerged from these explorations led to the now rejected idea that reserpine was a possible cause of breast cancer.[23]) Even without the aid of all the computerized information, a relatively brief interrogation in a retrospective case-control study can inquire about medications, smoking, nutrition, and life style, and can thereby yield the names of scores of substances that can be analyzed as etiologic suspects.

These explorations are sometimes called "fishing expeditions" or "data dredging" activities, but the procedures are not inherently unreasonable, particularly when used to search for etiology of disease rather than adverse reactions to drugs. If we do not know what causes a disease, we might as well examine any suspects we can think of. On the other hand, although data-dredging activities have the benefit of evaluating many etiologic suspects in a single study, there are also some major risks. The most obvious risk is obtaining factitious significance in the multiple statistical contrasts.

22.6.3.1. FACTITIOUS STOCHASTIC SIGNIFICANCE IN MULTIPLE CONTRASTS

By setting the α level at 0.05 for the stochastic contrast of a difference in results for two groups, we decide to take a 0.05 chance of drawing a false-positive conclusion if, in fact, the two groups are really similar. In this instance, the $1-\alpha$ chance of being correct, i.e., not drawing a false-positive conclusion, is 0.95. When a second comparison is conducted for another pair of results, the chance of avoiding a false-positive conclusion is also 0.95. The chance of avoiding a false-positive conclusion during the two comparisons is therefore $0.95 \times 0.95 = 0.90$. If a third comparison is conducted, the chance of avoiding a false-positive conclusion somewhere in all three comparisons is $0.95 \times 0.95 \times 0.95 = 0.86$. Thus, although the α level was set at 0.05 for the risk of a false conclusion in a single comparison, the chance of forming a false conclusion somewhere is raised to $1-0.86 = 0.14$ when three separate contrasts are conducted in the same basic set of data.

As noted in Section 9.8, the general formula for the chance of a false-positive conclusion during multiple contrasts is $[1-(1-\alpha)^k]$, where α is set at an individual level such as 0.05 and k is the number of contrasts. If we perform 30 contrasts, each at an α level of 0.05, the chance of drawing a false-positive conclusion is $[1-(0.95)^{30}] = [1-0.21] = 0.79$. If we perform 100 contrasts, the chance increases to $[1-(0.95)^{100}] = 1-0.006 = 0.994$; and we are almost sure to draw a false-positive conclusion somewhere along the line. In general, as a crude guideline, we can anticipate reaching one false-positive conclusion in every 20 stochastic contrasts performed at an α level of 0.05. Thus, the investigators who checked at least 1344 drug/disease relationships in their nosocomial roster could have expected to find about 67 that were stochastically significant by chance alone.

22.6.3.2. PREVENTION OF FALSE-POSITIVE CONCLUSIONS

The troublesome potential for obtaining factitiously positive results in the multiple statistical contrasts of a "fishing expedition" can be dealt with in two different ways: mathematically and scientifically. Mathematically, the decisive level of α for each comparison can be lowered substantially to account for the number of multiple comparisons. The choice of this lower level has evoked a series of ingenious proposals that have enriched the statistical literature with such eponyms as Bonferroni, Scheffé, Newman-Keuls, Duncan, Dunnett, and Tukey. The simplest proposal is to lower α to a level of α/k, where k is the number of contrasts. If we were performing 10 contrasts, the decisive level of α for each contrast would be set at $0.05/10 = 0.005$. The value of $[1-(0.995)^{10}]$ would then be $1-0.95 = 0.05$, and our ultimate α level for the 10 contrasts would be back at the desired boundary of 0.05.

No matter which mathematical strategy is used to choose the lowered level of α, however, a purely statistical approach does not deal with the investigator's scientific goals in examining multiple contrasts for the cited situation. The purpose of a fishing expedition is to catch fish or something that can be regarded as possible fish. Because the expedition is used like a diagnostic screening test, we want it to be highly sensitive, even if it sometimes gives false-positive results, since we do not want to miss anything important. With this goal, we clinically seek screening tests that will have high sensitivity; and we will accordingly withhold any permanent diagnostic decisions until we receive the results of a more accurate confirmatory test.

If a multiple-contrast fishing expedition is viewed in a similar manner—with no conclusions accepted until confirmed in subsequent research—the mathematical lowering of α to levels of 0.005 (or even lower) for individual comparisons would destroy the expedition's sensitivity as a screening test. The draconian demands for drastically low P values might make the investigator unable to demonstrate a significant relationship even when it is present.

A better scientific solution for the multiple-contrast problem, therefore, is to concentrate on the scientific structure of the research. This structure is often overlooked when the data-dredging activities are conducted merely as statistical examinations of fourfold tables. Because the explored outcomes and maneuvers can easily be cited as present or absent for each person, the manifold fourfold tables can quickly be constructed, examined, and annotated by a computer that has been programmed to do the work and ring a bell whenever something significant is found. Unfortunately, this purely statistical approach may not produce satisfactory architectural structures for drawing a scientific inference from the results.

Because each proposed relationship for each maneuver and each outcome may require a different set of criteria for suitability of cases, controls, and admissible data, the results that emerge as significant, according to quantitative and stochastic statistical criteria, may not be acceptable according to scientific criteria. The chance that led to the false-positive distinction may have been an artefact produced by innate bias in the contrasted evidence rather than by stochastic opportunities in multiple contrasts. Consequently, a cogent form of prophylaxis against false-positive results in the multiple-contrast screening process is not to lower the statistical demands for α but to raise the scientific standards for research architecture. The support for a hypothesis would depend not on the magnitude of an adjusted level of α but on the architectural evidence that sustains scientific inference for an appropriate comparison of baseline states, maneuvers, and outcomes in the proposed relationship.

22.6.4. *Management of Weak Support*

If the results of a study strongly support the investigator's original hypothesis, they may receive additional analyses to make the findings more precise. For example, after noting that treatment A has shown the anticipated (and desired) superiority to treatment

B in a randomized clinical trial of the main outcome of the original hypothesis, the investigator may compare treatment A versus treatment B for alternative outcomes or for subdivisions of the main outcome. Thus, if A is unequivocally better than B in a global score of improvement, the superiority of A may also be checked for costs, for adverse side effects, or for individual symptoms or other manifestations that were incorporated in the global score. Alternatively, or additionally, the investigator may check the accomplishments of A versus B in various subgroups of patients demarcated according to their clinical condition in the baseline state before therapy.

If the results of a randomized trial provide only weak support for the original hypothesis, however, an investigator who still has faith in the hypothesis can try to buttress its strength either by pooling additional data from other randomized trials or by searching within the existing data for subgroups that show statistically significant distinctions.

22.6.4.1. POOLING DATA FROM SEVERAL STUDIES

The strengthening of weak results by pooling data from several studies is more than just a legitimate scientific activity. It is the main basis for conducting collaborative clinical trials in which multiple institutions pool their data with the hope of achieving a stochastic significance that cannot be obtained from the results of a single institution alone. The pooling of data has therefore become a traditional, respectable activity in clinical epidemiologic science and statistics.

Unfortunately, because no principles have been established for the criteria that must be satisfied for pooling to be scientifically acceptable, its performance can be evaluated with many inconsistencies, and its results may create controversies. One possible requirement would be to insist that all the pooled data come from randomized trials. Although scientifically attractive, this requirement would eliminate the acceptability of results from the many collaborative studies that have been performed in observational circumstances in which randomization was impossible or unfeasible.

A second possible scientific principle would be the requirement that the pooled results comprise studies having homogeneous protocols, which would involve similar patients, examined and followed in similar manners after receiving the tested maneuvers. This homogeneous protocol principle would be violated if the pooling process is applied to data from randomized trials using different research protocols for groups of patients who did not meet the same criteria for admission.[24] This type of heterogeneous pooling recently produced stochastically significant efficacy for the pooled results[25] of individual randomized trials in which anticoagulant therapy had not been impressive in preventing mortality from acute myocardial infarction. Because the results in most of the pooled trials were generally favorable to anticoagulants, the pooling provided a statistical power that was not achieved with the sample sizes used in the individual studies.

Another possible scientific principle would be the requirement that results be generally similar for each of the individually pooled studies. If the component studies show major contradictions despite presumably similar protocols and similar patients, the absence of consistency would suggest that something has gone wrong. The requirement for similar component results has been a source of major controversy in at least two large-scale collaborative randomized trials in which results from the participating institutions were pooled for a single analysis despite some striking disparities in the components. For example, in the UGDP trial[20] of diabetic therapy, major distinctions in death rates of the compared agents were noted in only four of the 12 participating institutions, and the death rates, regardless of treatment, were strikingly higher at two institutions than at all the others. In the VA collaborative trial of surgery versus medical therapy for coronary artery disease, the pooled results for 3-year survival rates showed no significant difference in the treatments.[26] At one of the participating institutions, however, where surgery produced substantially better results than medical therapy, the investigators insisted that their data be published separately,[27] without being "drowned in the pool." A controversy then developed about the ethics of the investigators' decision to secede from the collaborating group, and to present a separate, individual report.

At federal regulatory agencies, the acceptability of pooled data may sometimes be judged by standards of source rather than scientific quality. If the information comes from a common protocol applied to similar patients by a consortium of academicians conducting a collaborative study, the pooling may be regarded as a satisfactory way to provide statistical significance. If the information comes from a common protocol applied to similar patients by a consortium of private practitioners under sponsorship of a pharmaceutical company, the pooling is often regarded as unacceptable, and a demand may be made that each practitioner's study produce statistically significant results. No data have been collected for the effects of this policy in escalating the costs of developing new pharmaceutical agents.

22.6.4.2. STATISTICAL SIGNIFICANCE IN SUBGROUP DATA

The disappointing results of a single trial may become joyful if statistical significance is found in the analysis of subgroup data for different components of the outcome events, or for different clinical conditions in the baseline state.

Beyond its obvious appeal for an investigator seeking statistical significance, this type of analysis may often be scientifically quite justified. The original outcome variable may have been too insensitive to show the treatment's major efficacy, and the efficacy may have been most prominent in certain clinical subgroups rather than in all patients who entered the trial. Although each such multiple-subgroup analysis must be judged on its own merits, the results are more likely to be convincing if the outcome events and clinical subgroups that produce significant results were identified in the research hypothesis (or protocol) that was prepared *before* the study began. If significant subgroups emerge only after multiple analyses of the data and also have no plausible explanation, the results may have difficulty escaping from the suspicion that they are statistical artefacts.

22.6.5. *Management of Unwelcome Results*

A randomized trial or a cross-sectional study produces unwelcome results if they are inconsistent with the distinction anticipated by the investigator. In this situation, the investigators in both types of studies may use multiple subgroup analysis in the hope of salvaging something positive. In a retrospective case-control study, however, the investigator has yet another kind of opportunity. The additional data gathered during the ascertainment process may provide multiple candidates as alternative maneuvers that can generate new hypotheses.

22.6.5.1. NEW HYPOTHESES FROM ANALYSIS OF MULTIPLE MANEUVERS

Beyond the demographic information gathered when data are collected during interviews with patients or from excerptions of archival records, the investigator in a case-control study may acquire additional information about many other attributes: smoking, occupation, education, alcohol, coffee, tea, nutrition, exercise, medications, psychic stress, antecedent diseases, and so on. Each of these attributes can then be analyzed as a possible principal maneuver if the main etiologic suspect fails to give a positive result.

For example, in a retrospective case-control study of the etiology of pancreatic cancer,[28] the principal maneuvers suspected in the original research hypothesis were smoking and alcohol. When the research data yielded negative results for these agents, the investigators checked many other candidate maneuvers as alternative suspects. When a positive relationship emerged for coffee, the retrospective hypothesis was presented as a possibly causal indictment, and the concept of coffee as a carcinogen received major publicity until the hypothesis was refuted when tested in subsequent studies.[29, 30]

22.6.5.2. HYPOTHESES SUSTAINED BY MULTIPLE-SUBGROUP ANALYSIS

In the problem just cited, a positive result is achieved by finding a new maneuver and a new hypothesis. A different type of problem is created when the investigator, trying to preserve a hypothesis that has not been sustained by the main results of the study, searches for support by analyzing multiple subgroups of people. Because the main maneuvers and outcomes were established before the research began, the items available for this type of analysis are characteristics of the investigated people.

The established maneuvers and outcomes can be checked in a large series of fourfold tables for people partitioned into univariate subgroups according to age, gender, smoking, and diverse clinical conditions. If nothing is found in these univariate analyses, the subgroups may be extended into bivariate or multivariate partitions. Eventually, if enough subgroups are checked, the investigator will usually find a fourfold table with positive results and may then claim that the hypothesis has been supported—at least in the cited subgroup.

This type of problem is also not unique to cross-sectional research. Whenever a large randomized trial yields unwelcome results, the investigators may have similar temptations and may undertake similar subgroup analyses. For example, when negative results were found in the recent MRFIT randomized trial of multiple risk factor interventions,[31] the investigators performed additional analyses for multiple subgroups. Some of these analyses showed favorable results for the interventions and others showed unexpectedly unfavorable results. An unresolved dispute[32] now exists about whether the unfavorable results arose from statistical chance as part of the multiple contrast problem, or from deleterious effects of the interventions.

The multiple-subgroup problem in retrospective case-control studies was well demonstrated in a recent large-scale investigation of the relationship of artificial sweeteners to cancer of the bladder.[33] The overall odds ratio found in the study was approximately 1, with a tight confidence interval that suggested no causal role for the artificial sweeteners. After multiple-subgroup analyses, however, a significantly elevated odds ratio was found in two subgroups of patients: white men who were heavy smokers, and nonsmoking white women who were not exposed to certain chemical substances. Because the overall results were so negative, the elevated risks in these subgroups could not be used to indict the artificial sweeteners. On the other hand, because of the elevated risks in those subgroups, the artificial sweeteners could not be completely exonerated. Therefore, after all the expense and effort of the large-scale study that was intended to resolve the etiologic question, the artificial sweeteners were left hanging under a cloud—neither fully exculpated nor adequately impeached.

22.6.5.3. RESULTS IN COMPLEMENTARY SUBGROUPS

Aside from the artefacts that can be produced during the analyses of multiple subgroups, the results may be presented in a misleading manner. Suppose the risk is not elevated in a total group, which is then divided into two complementary subgroups. If an elevated risk is found in one of those subgroups, then the risk is usually lowered in the other. What goes up in one subgroup goes down in the other.

For example, consider the following total results for a case-control study of 200 people:

Exposed	Total Group Cases	Controls
Yes	25	24
No	75	76
Total	100	100

The negative result of this study is immediately apparent. (If you insist on quantification, the odds ratio is 1.04, with a 95% confidence interval, by the Wolff method, extending from 0.56 to 2.00.)

The investigator may now partition these patients according to height and may find the following results in the subgroup of *tall* people.

Exposed	Tall People Cases	Controls
Yes	19	7
No	41	52
Total	60	59

The odds ratio for this subgroup is 3.4 and is stochastically significant ($X^2 = 6.8$, $P<0.01$). The investigator may now be delighted because the research hypothesis—that exposure was a risk factor—is supported in the tall people. The investigator may then propose various biologic mechanisms that make tall people particularly prone to the action of the etiologic agent.

In the meantime, however, the investigator may neglect to consider (or to report) what happened in the other part of the original group after the subgroup of tall people was demarcated for separate analysis. The results in the subgroup of non-tall people are as follows:

Exposed	Non-Tall People Cases	Controls
Yes	6	17
No	34	24
Total	40	41

The odds ratio for this subgroup is 0.25 and $X^2 = 7.0$, $P<0.005$. In other words, short people who were exposed to the maneuver were four times *less* likely to become diseased than short people who were nonexposed.

Thus, if indicted as a possible cause of the disease in tall people, the maneuver must be praised for its role in protecting short people. This type of complementary relationship should always be suspected when significant results emerge from the subgroup partitioning of nonsignificant results. Because many investigators and editors seem unaware of the problem, however, the results of the complementary subgroups may not be submitted for publication, or the editors may not request (or permit) enough reported details for a reader to be able to note the distinctions.

22.7. INTERPRETATION OF MODIFIED HYPOTHESES

Except for the first situation in Table 22–1, where auxiliary analyses are performed to increase the precision of results for a strongly supported hypothesis (and sometimes even in that situation, too), the conclusions that emerge from the research represent a modified hypothesis. It is different from what was expected in the original plans or in the original set of analyses.

22.7.1. *The Role of Preexisting Beliefs*

Having been evoked because of the investigator's previous beliefs in anticipating and welcoming the original results, the modified hypothesis will be reviewed by readers who also hold previous beliefs that affect their willingness to regard the surprises as reasonable expectations and to accept the conclusions as welcome. Because personal beliefs depend on preconceptions and prejudices, the interpretation of the conclusions becomes a matter of opinion for editorial policy, rather than principles for scientific "news." Because these opinions will differ among different people, the "news" itself will often seem to be controversial, but the controversies will really be provoked by differences in editorial policy.

For example, a major source of controversy in the UGDP randomized trial[20] of hypoglycemic agents for diabetes mellitus was the unwillingness of practicing diabetologists to accept the modified hypothesis that the oral agents were lethal. The clinicians were prepared to regard the agents as ineffectual in reducing vascular complications, but were ready to continue using the agents because of their potential value in preventing infections and because of their obvious appeal in avoiding the hypoglycemic reactions and discomforts of insulin therapy. Because these potential or definite benefits were not evaluated in the trial, the practitioners could argue that the trial had received an unfair design as well as unsuitable conclusions.

Many other clinicians, on the other hand, approached the UGDP trial with the belief that oral hypoglycemic agents were either unnecessary therapy for many patients whose blood glucose could be well regulated by diet alone, or an inadequate replacement for insulin in patients who really needed additional therapy. Because these clinicians anticipated no benefits from the oral agents, results that showed a lethal risk were readily acceptable.

Some of the controversy that has already developed over the public health trial of multiple risk factor interventions (MRFIT)[31, 32] depends on the evaluator's belief about what was to be expected from the interventions and what was to be welcomed in the results. This belief will even determine the decision about whether the investigators performed the auxiliary analyses because the original results were regarded as repugnant, or as weak but welcome.

In any study in which auxiliary analyses are done, the plausibility of statistically significant risks or benefits in certain subgroups will also depend on preestablished beliefs. These beliefs are more likely to be accompanied by satisfactory evidence for clinical than for public health maneuvers, because clinical experience provides the unquantified cohort observations that serve as historical control data. The clinical beliefs may be wrong or right, but they are usually based on direct homodemic observation of individual patients.

Public health interventions, however, are often applied to communities rather than to individual people, and the subsequent effects may be observed heterodemically. Consequently the observations are less direct and the conclusions are more difficult to prove. Thus, if someone claims that reducing the speed limit to 55 miles per hour prevents auto accidents on highways, the contention is usually sustained either by its plausibility alone, or by heterodemic data that are equivocal because the same gasoline problem that led to the lower speed limit may also have kept many cars off the road. On the other hand, if someone else claims that a reduction in the speed limit provides better gasoline mileage, people can check the claim "homodemically" by observing its effect in their own automobiles.

Better data are also generally available to denote susceptibility for prognostic outcome of an established clinical condition than for the chance of its development in healthy people. For example, physicians can more accurately predict how long a pregnancy will take than how long it will take to get pregnant. A clinical background of direct prognostic observations is available to provide plausibility for the subgroups that emerge as allegedly important in auxiliary analyses of therapeutic interventions, but may not be available for public health or etiologic interventions. Thus, if subgroup analyses show that a commonly used over-the-counter pharmaceutical agent provides significant *relief* for sore throats that are moderately painful, but not for extremely painful throats, the results in the clinical subgroups are consistent with well-established clinical prognostic expectations. If subgroup analyses show that daily use of the same pharmaceutical agent significantly *prevented* pancreatic cancer in white men ages 45 to 60, but not in other demographic groups, our knowledge of susceptibility to pancreatic cancer is so meager that the contention has no basis for plausibility.

22.7.2. *The Role of Scientific Inference*

Many difficulties in forming editorial opinions could be avoided if better standards were both more available and more frequently applied at the stage of scientific inference that precedes the editorial activities conducted as confirmatory decisions, explicatory hypotheses, and policy decisions. If scientific inference were used more carefully to determine what is acceptable as news and to eliminate consideration of modified hypotheses based on scientifically inadequate evidence, many fewer items of badly flawed news would pass through the pathway of reasoning to become disputes in the final stages of editorial opinion.

Few human beings, however, are able to bring a completely dispassionate objectivity to the appraisal of news, and whatever objectivity they begin with may be diverted by the allure or excitement of events in the editorial process. The thoughtful appraisal that should have been conducted as scientific inference may be hasty or biased, and the separate attention that should be devoted to confirmatory reasoning may not occur. Consequently, when the results of the modified hypothesis in a fourfold table fulfill statistical standards for quantitative and stochastic significance, relatively short shift may be given to the intricate reasoning needed for the scientific inference that the observed evidence is valid as news. The fulfillment of statistical standards alone may then be followed almost directly by the conclusion that the hypothesis has indeed been supported.

Because a modified hypothesis was, at best, generated by the research, it can hardly be immediately regarded as confirmed. Major problems about the confirmation decision will arise, however, if the modified hypothesis emerged from a vastly expensive, massively complex, randomized clinical trial that cannot be readily repeated to confirm its results. In this circumstance, because a repetition of the study is unlikely, relatively little can be done except to argue about the relative merits of the news and editorials. If the modified hypothesis is new, however, and if it arose from a case-control study or from other forms of research that can be repeated easily and inexpensively, the confirmation decision can always await the results of further research. The results of the modified hypothesis, if presented with suitable caution, will be worth reporting so that the relationship can be brought to the attention of the scientific community. Other investigators can then join in performing the subsequent studies needed for confirmation.

Despite obvious scientific advantages, a delay to await confirmation may not be acceptable if the proposed relationship elicits either great fears about risk or optimistic anticipations of benefit. The suspicion that a particular agent may kill people, cure cancer, deform babies, or prevent heart attacks will then take the evaluation out of the rationality of scientific discourse and into the political arenas of public policy. Although provoked by public concern, this transfer of reasoning may be abetted by certain patterns of behavior among the scientists. A particularly enthusiastic or zealous investigator may present the results in a manner suggesting that the modified hypothesis has been tested rather than merely generated. A particularly prejudiced reviewer, who avidly welcomes the results, may decide that the modified hypothesis has been confirmed.

22.7.3. *The Allure of Explicatory Hypotheses and Policy Decisions*

The two main causes that seduce otherwise rational scientists into these patterns of behavior are usually the devotion to either a particular explanation for the modified hypothesis, or to a particular policy that can be established as a conclusion.

22.7.3.1. **THE ATTRACTION OF EXPLICATORY HYPOTHESES**

Whenever a cause-effect relationship has been demonstrated, scientists always wonder about the mechanism that produces the relationship. How does the maneuver do its job? The answers to this type of question are responsible for all of the explicatory research performed in biomedical investigations; and the laboratory studies are usually designed to answer the questions directly.

When the observed relationship is found as an unexpected surprise in a study of groups of people, however, neither the investigator nor the reader may be prepared for the surprise; and there may be relatively little direct evidence available from previous research to provide a plausible explanation for the relationship. To make the relationship more acceptable, the investigator may then attempt to provide this plausibility by proposing various explicatory mechanisms that might account for the action of the maneuver. The creative intellectual energy that is consumed during these conjectures may be diverted from the energy needed earlier to evaluate the scientific quality of the evidence and inference.

An easy quantitative test can be applied in clinical epidemiologic research to identify the possible occurrence of this diversion. The test, which produces an *explicatory-diversion ratio,* is based on measuring the length of the text in certain portions of the *discussion* section of the published report. In preparing the discussion, the investigator usually comments on the reasoning process used for the scientific inference and on editorial interpretations of the results. The discussion of scientific inference from the news should indicate the potential biases that were contemplated in the groups and data, and should justify the investigator's reasons for believing that these biases were adequately managed. The subsequent editorial interpretations will usually include the investigator's speculations about the explicatory mechanisms by which the maneuver produces the outcome attributed to it.

In a scientifically cautious evaluation, the discussion of scientific inference can be expected to receive a substantially larger amount of text than the conjectures about explicatory mechanisms. The ratio of explication to inference in the printed contents of the discussion in the text should therefore be much smaller than 1. If this ratio is close to 1 or exceeds it, the reader (and investigator) should beware that an excessive amount of explicatory diversion has occurred.

In the report[22] of the retrospectively formed hypothesis that led to the false indictment of reserpine as a cause of breast cancer, the discussion of possible biases or inaccuracy in the results occupied 15.5 cm. of text. The discussion of mechanisms by which reserpine might produce its carcinogenicity for breast cancer occupied 21.8 cm. of text. The explicatory-diversion ratio was $21.8/15.5 = 1.4$, an impressively elevated value.

22.7.3.2. **RETROGRADE EFFECTS OF POLICY PREJUDICES**

Because the policy prejudices of the reviewer (or investigator) will often determine the reception given to a particular conclusion, these prejudices may have a retrograde effect on the antecedent reasoning with which the conclusions and the sustaining evidence are evaluated. If welcome, a conclusion may be readily accepted, regardless of the quality of the evidence. If unwelcome, the conclusions may be vigorously resisted, with major efforts made either to discredit the evidence, or to find various alternative explanations for the results. (Multiple-subgroup analyses and pooling data are two approaches to finding alternative explanations.)

In modern clinical epidemiologic research, these prejudices are often caused by ideologic beliefs about three sets of phenomena, regarding maneuvers, investigators, and risk-benefit appraisals. These ideologic prejudices occur regardless of the architectural structure used for the research; and they may be applied even when the investigation was performed with the "gold standard" of a randomized clinical trial. Because such trials are seldom available for most policy decisions, however, the prejudices have their main opportunity to appear in evaluations of data from cross-sectional and other non-cohort forms of research.

22.7.3.2.1. *The Noxiousness of Maneuvers and Motivations*

In industrialized, highly technologic Western society today, many people hold the belief that any substance produced by a profit-making commercial organization is inherently noxious until proved otherwise. Regardless of the available justification, this prejudice makes the believers quite willing or even excessively credulous about accepting the basic "guilt" of drugs, devices, or other commercially manufactured products while maintaining devout faith in the basic "innocence" of drugs, devices, or surgical procedures that are employed by academic or other entrepreneurs who do not seem to have overtly commercial motives.

An alternative consequence of this belief occurs when massive screening programs or other interventions are undertaken to provide public health "benefits" under governmental auspices. Without commercial sponsorship, the research is not subjected to a regulatory agency's demands for evidence of adverse side effects. Consequently, the "beneficial" campaigns may be conducted and reported without any attention to the stigmas or other problems produced by "labeling,"[34] the personal or familial frustrations of maintaining certain maneuvers, and other important adverse psychosocial effects of the interventions. On the other hand, side effects may be avidly sought when a deliberately noxious governmental intervention—such as atomic radiation or defoliant chemicals—becomes exposed to people for whom the noxious effects were not intended.

22.7.3.2.2. *The Integrity of Investigators*

A corollary of the preceding prejudice is the frequently held belief that objectivity and integrity are compromised in any investigator who works for a profit-making organization or who receives support from it. This prejudice may make a reviewer suspicious of any research conducted under such auspices, while maintaining steadfast assurance that truth has been sought dispassionately if the investigators are in federal, academic, or other noncommercial enclaves. Having no direct financial benefit from the research, the nonprofit investigators can obviously be relied upon to maintain a selfless, olympian approach that is oblivious to such alternative motivations as power, fame, reputation, promotion, space, retinue, and budget.

22.7.3.2.3. *Standards for Risk-Benefit Evaluations*

The third policy prejudice involves the use of different scientific standards to evaluate risks and benefits. If a cause-effect maneuver seems to produce a benefit, the results may be unacceptable unless the evidence comes from a randomized clinical trial. If the maneuver seems to produce no benefit or a risk, however, any type of evidence can receive serious attention, regardless of the scientific quality of the research structure and data.

The policy has many reasonable justifications. We generally want to be safe rather than sorry, and to protect people from major disasters that may occur in exchange for minor benefits. The classic example of such a disaster is the phocomelia that developed in the fetus while thalidomide was relieving the mother's nausea or anxiety in early pregnancy. On the other hand, a policy that vigorously emphasizes the removal of *any* potential unsafety can also produce the disasters that occur when someone shouts "Fire" on observing a match lit in a crowded theater.

For example, if replacement estrogens are indeed a cause of postmenopausal endometrial cancer, the estrogen-induced cancers seem to be relatively quite benign, with extraordinarily high survival rates occurring after hysterectomy in the affected women.[35, 36] The postmenopausal replacement estrogens, however, also have the benefit of preventing osteoporotic fractures of the hip or other major bones. Because the effects of the fractures may be much more chronic and difficult to remedy than an easily removed, relatively benign endometrial cancer, the shouts of "carcinogen" that lead to a cessation of otherwise desirable therapy may create the greater disaster of functional limitations and incapacitations caused by osteoporotic fractures.

The values and beliefs of the people who are direct recipients of the evaluated maneuvers, however, may not be suitably represented when the public policy deliberations occur. The policy makers, who presumably *do* represent those people, may receive relatively little input directly from their constituents; and the major clamor may come from self-appointed consumer advocates or from manufacturers of the product under evaluation. Because one group derives its power from publicity and the other from money, the atmosphere seldom encourages a careful weighing of evidence and suitably balanced decisions.

The itinerary that brings a particular topic into the arena of public policy decisions may also be affected by the same opinions noted previously about profit-making organizations. Thus, when a particular research study shows no benefit or possible risk from a commercially sponsored maneuver, an outcry may immediately arise to have the maneuver suitably castigated—removal from the market, addition of warning labels, and so on. On the other hand, when similar negative results emerge from a maneuver sponsored by public health or academic groups, no similar cries may be heard, and the results of the study may even be disregarded.

For example, when a large-scale randomized controlled trial showed no benefit for a commercially produced agent (tolbutamide),[20] vigorous efforts were made to have the agent impeached. When another large-scale randomized controlled trial showed no benefit for a public health–sponsored agent (multiple risk factor intervention),[31] the results were generally dismissed as being a fluke in the design or conduct of the research. When retrospective case-control studies showed a possible risk for commercially produced oral contraceptive agents in causing thromboembolism,[37, 38] the results received widespread publicity, and the hazards were noted as warnings on the labels of the purchased preparations. When some other retrospective case-control studies showed a possible benefit for oral contraceptive agents in preventing cancer of the uterus, ovary, and breast,[39] the results received relatively little attention, and no demands were expressed about the need to alert more women to this potentially major breakthrough in the prevention of cancer.

In a private entrepreneurial Western society, the existence of this double standard of policy decisions seems ironically peculiar, because it suggests that consistent rational judgments about the scientific risks and benefits of medical or public health maneuvers can be made only in countries where the economy is totally controlled by the government.

22.8. SYNOPSIS

The maneuvers and outcomes studied in a cause-effect relationship are identified with grouping variables and focal variables. After being identified, the basic groups are examined to ascertain the focal variables and other pertinent data.

In case-control studies, a date of focal time must be established as a counterpart of the zero time point when maneuvers are imposed in cohort studies. When each person is checked for qualifications for admission, the focal state data will be used in excluding candidates with protopathic alteration of maneuvers, in managing questions of appropriate vulnerability, and in prognostic analyses of baseline susceptibility. If determined from interviews conducted long after the actual events took place, the focal state information may be unreliable in both identification and timing of events.

The process of ascertaining focal state information can be biased if an awareness of the grouping variable affects the collection and analysis of data for the focal variables. In case-control studies, ascertainment bias can be caused by prejudices of the interviewer or data excerpter, and by preferential recall by the interviewed persons. Specification bias can occur if exposure is not well specified or is better described for one of the compared groups than for the other.

Ascertainment bias can be reduced by various strategies for keeping the interviewed persons and the data collectors unaware of the research hypothesis, by rigorously arranged formats for collecting data, by various reminder tactics to refresh memory, by choosing control groups with an equally strong incentive to recall antecedent exposures, and by relying on archival records, rather than interviews, as prime sources of data. A preferential avidity for certain relationships may have occurred, however, when the archival data were originally inscribed or later excerpted. Ascertainment bias can also arise during the analysis rather than acquisition of data because of the investigator's arbitrary choices regarding multiple sources of data, management of unknown data, and retroactive demarcation of the dose regarded as exposure to a maneuver.

In addition to data regarding antecedent maneuvers, the ascertainment process involves acquisition of suitable information about each person's eligibility for the research, pre-maneuver baseline state, and issues that may affect biases in susceptibility, protopathic alteration of maneuvers, co-maneuvers, co-morbidity, and detection of outcome events. The groups available for the research may be distorted by a transfer bias arising from the differential willingness of people to receive or volunteer for interviews.

After being obtained, the results of the research may or may not be welcomed by the investigator. If welcome, the results may receive auxiliary analyses to increase the precision or strength of the relationship or to provide explanation for unexpected findings. Auxiliary analyses can also be performed to generate a hypothesis where none existed, to find a new replacement hypothesis if the original hypothesis was unsupported, or to generate support that may help sustain an unconfirmed original hypothesis.

The auxiliary analyses may rely on data pooled from several studies, or the results of a single study may be appraised in multiple subgroups or other rearrangements of data formed from diverse combinations of outcomes, maneuvers, and baseline states. Although no standards currently exist for the conditions under which pooling is acceptable, the scientific acceptability of the process would be increased if the individual pooled studies were relatively homogeneous in their protocols and results. In multiple-subgroup analyses, the level of α can be lowered to prevent stochastic significance from arising fallaciously during the multiple contrasts, but false-positive results can be more effectively prevented by insisting on suitable standards of scientific inference for each proposed relationship. In addition to these precautions, no hypothesis should be regarded as suitably tested or confirmed by the same set of data that were used to generate the hypothesis; and a reverse-direction relationship should always be evaluated in complementary components whenever subgroup analysis reveals positive results not found in the total group.

EXERCISES

Exercise 22.1. What problems would you anticipate for ascertaining the *maneuver* in persons interviewed during case-control studies exploring the following cause-effect relationships: (Please confine your comments to ascertainment of the maneuver. Do not include other sources of troublesome bias.)

    22.1.1. Jogging as a prophylactic or provocative agent for sudden death.
    22.1.2. Use of tetracycline and subsequent development of stained teeth in children.
    22.1.3. Use of cephalosporin drugs and subsequent development of chronic pulmonary disease in adults.
    22.1.4. Use of fluoride toothpaste in childhood and occurrence of cancer in young adult life.
    22.1.5. Use of tranquilizers and subsequent development of pancreatic cancer.
    22.1.6. Exposure to general anesthesia and subsequent development of Alzheimer's disease.
    22.1.7. Visit to eastern Connecticut and subsequent development of Lyme disease.

Exercise 22.2. For each topic in Exercise 22.1, what could you do to verify the accuracy of the report obtained in personal interviews with each case and control?

Exercise 22.3. For each topic in Exercise 22.1, what is the single greatest innate bias that would worry you as something about which to take precautions?

Exercise 22.4. For each topic in Exercise 22.1, *briefly* outline the preexisting beliefs frmtthat would facilitate or impair acceptance of whatever conclusion is found in the research.

Exercise 22.5. Avoiding examples that have been cited in the text, find a published report for each of the following three types of research:

    22.5.1. Randomized clinical trial of a therapeutic agent.
    22.5.2. Retrospective case-control study of adverse effects (e.g., disease) of a public health maneuver (e.g., smoking, nutrition, occupation, etc.).
    22.5.3. Retrospective case-control study of adverse effects of a therapeutic maneuver (e.g, pharmaceutical agent or surgery).

For each study, examine the results to determine whether multiple auxiliary analyses were done in checking the original hypothesis or in proposing a new hypothesis. Briefly outline the research project and the auxiliary analyses. Why do you think they were done? How did they alter the original hypothesis? What did the investigators do statistically (e.g., lowered value of α) or scientifically (e.g., discussion of scientific inference) to justify the analyses and their conclusions?

Exercise 22.6. Can you name some medical or public health topics in recent years that seem to have been discussed much more in journalistic media and political enclaves than in scientific publications? Why do you think this has happened?

CHAPTER REFERENCES

1. Bianchine, 1968; 2. Horwitz, 1984 (Arch Intern Med); 3. Feinstein, 1981; 4. Klemetti, 1967; 5. Spitzer, 1975; 6. Chambers, 1977; 7. Davis, 1982; 8. Labarthe, 1978; 9. Boston Collaborative Drug Surveillance Program, 1973; 10. Gordis, 1979; 11. Shands, 1980; 12. Harvey, 1982; 13. Ferencz, 1980; 14. Mack, 1976; 15. Horwitz, 1980; 16. Horwitz, 1984 (Am J Med); 17. Horwitz, 1978; 18. McDonald, 1977; 19. Austin, 1981; 20. University Group Diabetes Program, 1970; 21. Anturane Reinfarction Trial Research Group, 1978; 22. Boston Collaborative Drug Surveillance Program, 1974; 23. Labarthe, 1979; 24. Goldman, 1979; 25. Chalmers, 1977; 26. Murphy, 1977; 27. Loeb, 1979; 28. MacMahon, 1981; 29. Goldstein, 1982; 30. Severson, 1982; 31. MRFIT, 1982; 32. Stallones, 1983; 33. Hoover, 1980; 34. Sackett, 1983; 35. Chu, 1982; 36. Wells, 1981; 37. Vessey, 1968; 38. Sartwell, 1969; 39. Centers for Disease Control, 1982.

PART FIVE

NON-COHORT STRUCTURES IN CAUSE-EFFECT RESEARCH

The scientific and statistical principles discussed in Chapters 18 to 22 pertain to any type of research structure, but they are particularly valuable for understanding and interpreting the many studies that are conducted without a cohort arrangement. The structures of non-cohort research may be strange and uncomfortable to clinical readers who are accustomed to the experimental methods of laboratory investigation, and to scientific reasoning that is based on a cohort design. If the non-cohort results are also reported in unfamiliar or incomprehensible statistical expressions, clinicians may try to escape the communicative difficulties by avoiding reading the report.

For several decades, clinicians have chosen this avoidance option not only because it eliminated the intellectual ardors of trying to understand epidemiologic studies, but also because the topics under discussion were not clinically appealing. The topics were often concerned with nutrition, life styles, occupation, socioeconomic factors, or other community and public health issues. Although pertinent to clinical practice, these issues often seemed less exciting than the pathophysiology, differential diagnosis, pharmacologic agents, and surgical interventions that have been a traditional focus of clinical instruction and attention.

In recent years, however, both the public health phenomena and the non-cohort research structures have become increasingly prominent in the expanded domain of clinical education, practice, and investigation. Even if clinicians today remain more concerned with remedial cure than with prophylactic prevention, they cannot escape inquiries from patients who seek advice, guidance, or evaluative appraisals for the nonmedical interventions that are frequently proposed for promoting health and avoiding disease. Thoughtful clinicians have also discovered (or have always understood) that they cannot practice good medicine merely as connoisseurs of applied pathophysiology, clinical pharmacology, and surgical procedures. To excel in the artful science of patient care, the clinicians must also know about their patients' life style, occupation, socioeconomic status, and other community variables.

Beyond the role of these nonmedical phenomena in the personal encounters of clinical practice, however, the clinicians' traditional investigative interests in pathophysiology, diagnosis, and therapeutic agents have also been invaded by methods once regarded as the exclusive domain of public health epidemiologists. Clinical questions are now often answered with case-control techniques that are applied in all three directions of temporal orientation: forward to study phenomena of pathophysiology, concurrently to study the efficacy of diagnostic technology, and backward to investigate adverse effects of drugs. The heterodemic research used for ecologic analyses of death certificates could formerly be clinically dismissed as part of the arcanum of public health epidemiology. In recent years, however, heterodemic data have been used for clinical decisions about the accomplishments of pharmacologic agents, coronary care units, and other therapeutic interventions.

This challenge from both patients and published literature eliminates the option of continuing to ignore the contents, structures, and methods of non-cohort forms of medical research. A clinician who wants a better understanding of today's literature, or a medical student whose practice will be conducted mainly in the 21st century, is herewith invited to pursue the discussion contained in the next two chapters.

Retrospective Case-Control (Trohoc) Studies

Many of the major modern triumphs ascribed to epidemiologic research have been initiated with evidence from retrospective case-control studies. The triumphs include the generally accepted indictment of cigarettes as a cause of lung cancer and the more disputed indictments of such alleged causal agents as DES for clear cell vaginal adenocarcinoma, replacement estrogen therapy for endometrial cancer, and tampons for toxic shock syndrome. Because the incriminated agents range from personal habits to pharmaceutical substances, the retrospective case-control technique obviously has wide scope and importance.

23.1. REASONS FOR USING TROHOC RESEARCH STRUCTURES

As noted in Chapter 18, retrospective case-control structures are sometimes used merely because they are relatively quick, simple, and convenient replacements for either experiments or observational cohort studies that might have been done almost as easily if the investigator were willing to add the extra effort. In most instances, however, the trohoc structure is used because it is the only feasible method of doing the research and because it is usually more convincing than the heterodemic structures, described in Chapter 24, that offer the main other epidemiologic approach.

Because many nonepidemiologists do not understand the reasons for using the scientifically peculiar case-control technique, the rest of this section indicates why more powerful research structures are seldom feasible and why retrospective case-control studies have become so popular.

23.1.1. *Problems in Experimental Trials*

Experimental trials can almost never be used to study agents suspected of causing noxious effects. As soon as the suspicion arises, it will create too many ethical, legal, and logistic difficulties in finding either enough people to volunteer for exposure to the agents, or enough investigators willing to do the research. If an experimental trial was originally conducted to study the benefits rather than risks of a particular agent, the people who participated in the trial may be recalled and reexamined many years later if the agent becomes suspected as harmful. This type of situation was described earlier (Section 18.1.2) for studying the long-term outcome[1,2] of patients originally investigated in a trial of short-term efficacy for diethylstilbestrol.[3] Except for these rare opportunities, randomized-trial data are unobtainable to study substances directly suspected as noxious.

23.1.2. *Problems in Prolective Cohorts*

For similar reasons, observational data are seldom obtainable prolectively from inception cohorts. If the agent is suspected as harmful, neither patients nor investigators may be willing to participate in the research. If the agent has *not* been suspected of harm, investigators may not want to do research that may possibly yield negative results.

Because a long incubation period may be needed for pathogenicity to be demonstrated, an investigator studying a harmless substance might have to invest years or decades of work before reaching the negative conclusion that the substance is harmless. Relatively few investigators have the combination of public altruism and scientific masochism needed to conduct such studies. The negative conclusion might be worthwhile for society, but it may not bring the investigator any of the acclaim, excitement, or other anticipated rewards that usually stimulate people to do research. Besides, a negative result for an *unsuspected* agent may not even be accepted for publication. The editors may not want to use their journal's space for uninteresting discoveries.

If the suspected agent does not have a potentially long incubation period, however, and if the initial suspicion of harm is either weak or uncertain, both patients and investigators may be willing to engage in a relatively short-term prolective study in an inception cohort. Such studies have been done, for example, to investigate whatever harm may follow the use of oral contraceptive agents.[4-6] Save for the exceptions just cited, suspected noxious agents have seldom been studied prolectively in an inception cohort. To use a prolective type of observational mechanism, an investigator may invite people to enroll in a study and to be followed thereafter, but the assembled group may not be an inception cohort and the observational mechanism may begin after rather than before the maneuver was imposed. The people who volunteer for the research will usually form a multi-serial cross-section whose maneuvers began at diverse times before they entered the cohort. In addition to containing all the transfer biases previously discussed for such groups, their data for the admission state and subsequent events may be obtained indirectly rather than by specific examination.

In the indirect approach, the members of the volunteer cross-sectional group are classified initially according to demographic and other information they submitted in questionnaires returned when they volunteered. Their subsequent outcome events are also determined indirectly from questionnaires, death certificates, or other information submitted to the investigator from the primary sources of observation. In the direct approach, the volunteers are specifically examined and followed by the investigators so that the research data are acquired with standardized investigative methods for making primary observations.

The indirect method of observing a volunteer multi-serial cohort was used by Doll and Hill[7] in the famous study that followed their previous case-control research[8] on cigarettes and lung cancer, and also by investigators who did the American Cancer Society study[9] of this same relationship. Except for these two multi-serial, indirectly prolective cohorts, all other multi-serial cohort studies[10-12] of the cigarette–lung cancer relationship cited in the original Surgeon General's report[13] were multi-serial and retrolective.

The direct method of forward observation of a volunteer multi-serial cross-section has been used in several well-known public health studies conducted in community laboratories[14] that are usually identified eponymically by their ecologic framework in such places as Bogalusa,[15] Bustleton,[16] Evans County,[17] Framingham,[18] Honolulu,[19] and Tecumseh.[20] In these studies, the investigators can try to manage the multi-serial problem by using the direct baseline examinations to find and exclude any patients who have already developed unsuitable diseases (such as those to be counted as outcome events). With the cohort restricted to healthy people, the groups can be stratified for age to adjust for problems of multi-seriality. The adjustment is not always totally effective, because healthy people of the same age might still have different durations of serial time in previous exposure to such maneuvers as smoking, diet, or exercise. Nevertheless, by excluding unhealthy people and by stratifying for age, the adjustment provides scientific precautions that cannot be obtained in other types of multi-serial cohort research.

In an intriguing effort to shorten the duration of long-term follow-up by using age as a surrogate for postmaneuver serial time, a group of investigators[21] performed a short-term multi-serial cohort study in the Framingham population. The assembled cross-sectional group was followed for 1 year rather than for 20 years, as in the larger, longer Framingham study. The compared results in the corresponding age strata of the short-duration and long-duration cohorts showed many similarities and a few disparities; but the protracted cross-section technique does not yet seem to have displaced the long-term cohort as a methodologic approach to the public health issues.

23.1.3. *Problems in Retrolective Cohorts*

Investigators who do retrolective public health studies can obtain inception cohorts from such sources as college enrollment and military records, but may encounter substantial problems in archival framework and volunteer recruiting. The framework must have a roster that can identify the people to be solicited and must contain satisfactory data to describe their baseline state. If the main outcome event has already occurred when the study begins, the identity of the outcome event may or may not be contained in the data available at the framework. If the main outcome event is not recorded in the archival data or if it has not yet occurred when the study begins, the investigator must be able to locate the cohort members and invite them to contribute their current data about outcome events. The people who are available to be found and the subset of volunteers who accept the invitation to participate will then form a residue cohort, with all of its potential transfer biases.

For clinically-based retrolective cohort studies of the outcome of patients with an established clinical condition or disease, the frameworks have been medical settings or special registries. The registries may have been established for general usage (such as cancer registries) or for an *ad hoc* project, such as the follow-up of people having clinical conditions associated with DES.[22, 23] For public health retrolective cohort studies of the outcome of healthy people exposed to various etiologic agents, the frameworks have been much more diverse. They include records from schools or colleges, from military or veterans groups, insurance companies, industrial sources, and the registries used for licensing people in various occupations, such as hairdressers and barbers.

If the outcome event is not recorded in the framework data, the ability to recruit participants is crucial to the success of such studies. The participation proportion will usually depend on the interval elapsed between the cohort's inception date and the date when the research begins, and on the way the solicited people perceive the seriousness of the research and any potential personal threats it may contain. Because of an ongoing relationship with a clinician, the members of a clinically-based cohort are usually easier to locate and may be more likely to participate, if urged by that clinician, than members of a public health cohort.

23.1.4. *Statistical Problems in Cohort Research*

A substantial statistical problem in either prolective or retrolective studies of cohorts is the size of the groups needed to provide stochastic significance in comparisons of results for the outcome event. For clinically-based cohorts, the outcome rates for events such as success or failure, alive or dead, are usually in the range of 0.1 to 0.9. Stochastic distinctiveness can therefore be found with groups that seldom need more than 400 people and that often contain less than 100. If the outcome phenomenon is a change in a measured dimension, such as weight or blood pressure, relatively small group sizes can still produce significant distinctions in measured indexes of central tendency.

On the other hand, in public health cohorts whose outcome events are diseases that develop at low rates of occurrence—such as 0.01, 0.005, 0.001, or even lower—huge sample sizes are often required for showing statistical significance; and doubts about statistical power may regularly arise if the results are negative. For example, when no cases of clear cell vaginal adenocarcinoma were noted in a retrolective inception cohort[24] of 819 women exposed in utero to DES, doubts arose about the likelihood of finding any cases in so relatively small a cohort group.

Retrolective studies of public health phenomena have the advantage of reducing the costs of obtaining and following a huge cohort prolectively, but also have two major disadvantages. If the outcome event must be discerned after the cohort is identified, the investigators are at the mercy of the transfer biases that can occur when the cohort members are solicited. More importantly, if the public health cohort study requires reliable data for blood pressure, serum lipids, electrocardiograms, or other paraclinical variables, the baseline state information may be unavailable or unreliable in the archives of the public health framework. To collect reliable baseline data for a public health cohort, the investigators would have to work prolectively and would then have the burden of following a huge number of people for a protracted period of time.

23.1.5. *Problems in Cross-Sectional Surveys*

The expense and effect of long-term prolective follow-up for a public health cohort can be avoided if an ecologic framework is used for a cross-sectional survey. At a single examination session for each eligible person in the community, the investigator can obtain data to identify both maneuvers and outcomes, and can then analyze the data with the type of fourfold structure shown in Table 20–2 or with more sophisticated mathematics. A suitable publicity campaign can enable the investigator to achieve a high rate of volunteer participation from the community members; and the incentive to volunteer may be increased if the people know they will be examined only once.

This type of cross-sectional survey eliminates the difficulty of having to do long-term follow-up examinations but not the difficulty of large sample sizes, because the group required to achieve stochastically significant distinctions for low-rate outcome events in a cross-sectional ecologic study will have to be just as large as in a prolective cohort study. The cross-sectional survey will thus save follow-up time but not sample size; and the saving of time will be accompanied by several major problems that are not present in a cohort.

One of these problems, discussed earlier as *pathoconsortive*, is the decision about sequence when two things are noted concomitantly. If a person is found to have both diabetes mellitus and hypercholesterolemia, or both psychic depression and cancer, which came first? A second problem is that certain types of transfer bias, due to attrition or other losses of cohort, are almost impossible to discern or to manage in a cross-sectional survey. When a multi-serial cohort of otherwise healthy people with hypercholesterolemia is assembled for follow-up examinations to detect subsequent coronary disease, the investigator may not know how long those people have had the hypercholesterolemia and how many members of their inception cohort have already died before the residue cohort was assembled for the cross-sectional research. On the other hand, the investigator can determine the outcomes associated with hypercholesterolemia for otherwise healthy people in each cross-sectional age group, and can use the follow-up results of a younger group to get an idea of how the attritions might have biased the composition of the people initially assembled in the next older age group.

In a cross-sectional survey, however, this compensating option is not available to check or adjust for transfer bias. If outcome events have produced a biased attrition in the available cross-sectional group, the investigator has no satisfactory way to check it without doing the cohort study that the cross-section was intended to avoid. Furthermore, people who already have the outcome event, and who are still alive and available, may be particularly likely to shun participation in the cross-sectional study. Already receiving medical attention for that outcome event, they may be unwilling to engage in the additional medicalization implicit in the research. Some of them, even if willing to participate, may be located in hospitals where their existence will be missed if the survey depends only on finding participants at their homes. In contrast to the cross-sectional investigator's precarious dependence on finding everyone who has the outcome event, the cohort investigator can deliberately exclude such people at the beginning of the research and can concentrate on the subsequent course of people who are relatively healthy on admission to the cohort.

23.1.6. *The Appeal of Trohoc Research*

Retrospective case-control research can eliminate all the cited difficulties in performing experiments, recruiting vast numbers of people, following vast numbers of people, or finding enough people with the outcome event. People with the outcome event are usually found easily, because the investigator begins with a list of cases contained in a nosocomial roster or other appropriate registry of clinical conditions. The group sizes can be relatively small, because the stochastic distinctions to be sought are in relatively high rates of prevalence for exposure to an antecedent maneuver. There is no follow-up to be performed, because the data collection is finished after the single cross-sectional act of ascertainment for antecedent events. There are no ethical qualms about randomization or experimentation, because whatever maneuvers the people received were imposed with their own volition and consent.

These splendid advantages give trohoc research its attractive appeal for investigating all types of cause-effect maneuvers. It has become eminent as an epidemiologic substitute for evaluating public health or even clinical maneuvers that would otherwise be too difficult to investigate with experimental trials, observational cohorts, and cross-sectional surveys. In exchange for these advantages, however, the trohoc investigator inherits all the innate biases that the other research structures were intended to prevent, and must then make plans to deal with those biases while avoiding the addition of new ones during the research.

23.2. SCIENTIFIC CHALLENGES IN TROHOC RESEARCH

Because a single acquisition of cross-sectional data in a retrospective case-control study must account for a complex medical itinerary that extends from baseline state to the enumerated outcome of a maneuver, the investigators must cope with all the innate biases that can arise as groups of free-living people move through that itinerary.

23.2.1. *Medical Itinerary for the Cases*

For the group of cases, who have developed the outcome event and who are the main focus of investigation in a case-control study, the medical itinerary is particularly important. In studies of public health maneuvers, such as cigarette smoking or tampons, the maneuver is self-selected by its recipients. In studies of clinical maneuvers, such as estrogen therapy or treatment with other pharmaceutical substances, the principal maneuver is first chosen by a clinician and then imposed on those recipients who acquiesce in the choice. These selective decisions and acquiescences usually occur without a consistent set of criteria to demarcate the people who are eligible for admission to receive the principal maneuver, and without any mechansm for equalizing baseline susceptibility in groups who do or do not receive it.

After the principal maneuver is (or is not) imposed, its subsequent degree and duration of maintenance depend on decisions made by the recipients and their clinical advisors; and the maintenance period may be accompanied by many events, related or unrelated to the principal maneuver, that elicit the addition of various co-maneuvers.

While the postmaneuver period is in progress, the recipients will receive various degrees of medical surveillance. In some situations, the surveillance may be nonexistent, as in healthy cigarette smokers or tampon users who have no regular plan for medical examinations. In other circumstances, for reasons that are related or unrelated to any of the maneuvers, baseline states, or subsequent events, the surveillance may be scheduled at regular intervals or sought *ad hoc* for various illnesses.

The examinations performed during the medical surveillance visits will vary with the customary routines of the clinician, with the particular stimuli that evoked surveillance, and with the clinician's responses to those stimuli. Some clinicians order many tests and extensive work-ups for few or weak stimuli; other clinicians are less vigorous in their activities.

Somewhere during this interval the outcome event may occur, with or without symptoms or other clinical manifestations that would evoke medical attention. If the routine or *ad hoc* surveillance examinations contain a procedure adequate for diagnosing the outcome event, and if the procedure gives a correct result, the occurrence of the outcome event will be noted. Otherwise, the outcome event will escape detection.

After being detected, the outcome event will or will not be recorded in a roster or registry that is used as a framework for the cases chosen by the investigator. Any outcome events that were not recorded in this framework will also escape detection in the research.

23.2.2. *Medical Itinerary for the Controls*

In a cohort study, the medical itinerary of the control group, i.e., the people receiving the comparative maneuver, can be described in a manner quite similar to the description just given for the people who become cases in a trohoc study. After receiving the comparative (or no) maneuver, the nonexposed people are followed with various degrees of surveillance; the test procedures are evoked (or not evoked) by various stimuli; and the occurrence or nonoccurrence of the outcome event is eventually recorded in an accessible framework of data.

In retrospective case-control studies, however, the control group consists of people in whom the outcome event has not been recorded. There is no way to describe the customary medical itinerary of these people, because it depends on what the investigator decides. If the investigator chooses the controls from presumably healthy people living in a community, many of the controls may have had none of the medical surveillance, test procedures, or other features of the itinerary experienced by the cases. If chosen from a nosocomial source, the controls will have a definite medical itinerary that brought them to the source, but the itinerary will depend on the particular clinical conditions that were chosen to demarcate the control group. With certain conditions, the control group will have an itinerary that resembles what happened in the cases. With other conditions, the itineraries may be drastically different.

For example, we can be reasonably sure that a case group of women with breast cancer will all have had their breasts carefully palpated at various times by themselves or by a clinician; many of them may also have received mammography; and all of them have had tissue surgically excised and histopathologically examined to establish a diagnosis of breast cancer. If the control group is chosen from women hospitalized for other conditions such as cataracts, dental disease, or hemorrhoids,[25] the additional mammographic or histologic examinations have probably not occurred at all; and regardless of how and whether these women examined themselves, their breasts may have received either no medical examinations or examinations that were too perfunctory to detect a small or asymptomatic lesion.

23.2.3. *Medical Itinerary and Innate Biases*

Figure 23–1 shows the events that are observed when an ordinary cohort study is performed for a cause-effect maneuver that has been imposed in the natural circumstances

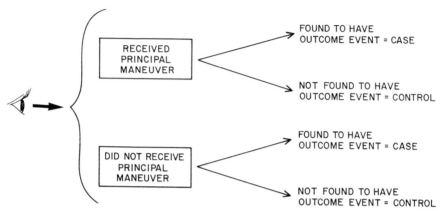

Figure 23–1. Medical itinerary for case and control outcome groups found in a cohort study.

of everyday life. The people who received or did not receive the principal maneuver are identified; and the occurrence or nonoccurrence of the outcome event is then noted. The end of the itinerary shows the four groups of exposed and nonexposed cases and controls who would appear in the fourfold table of results.

Figure 23–2 shows the events that are discerned when an ordinary retrospective case-control study is performed in these same observational circumstances. The cases and controls are noted; and the antecedent exposure or nonexposure to the principal maneuver is ascertained. The beginning of this itinerary at the left-hand side of the drawing shows the four groups of exposed and nonexposed cases and controls who would appear in the fourfold table of results.

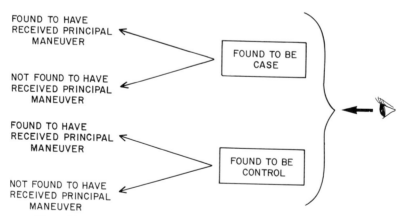

Figure 23–2. Investigative sequence in a retrospective case-control study.

The events occurring in these ordinary circumstances, however, can produce all the innate biases that were discussed in previous chapters. The principal maneuver may have been given to people who were not suitably eligible to receive it; the maneuvers may have been allocated in a way that created susceptibility bias, and maintained in a way that created performance bias; the outcome events may have been discerned with detection bias; and the information about outcomes and maneuvers may have been collected in a way that produced transfer bias.

Because a scientific architecture for research is intended to prevent, reduce, or compensate for these innate biases, the strategies of a scientifically planned cohort study are shown in Figure 23–3. The potential candidates are first screened to select those who fulfill admission criteria for the cohort under investigation. These candidates must not have the outcome event and must have no strong indications for either receiving or not receiving the principal maneuver. When the maneuvers are assigned, susceptibility bias is prevented by allocating the maneuvers randomly. Maneuvers that were not randomly allocated are examined with suitable prognostic analyses. Arrangements are then made for the compared maneuvers to receive a similar performance and to be analyzed with suitable adjustments for possible biases produced by differences in compliance, intermediate regulation, and co-maneuvers. The investigator then uses double-blinding or other strategies to provide an objective, equal detection of the outcome event in the compared groups. Finally, to prevent or reduce transfer bias, the investigator carefully examines the attrition of the two cohorts and suitably adjusts the losses that have occurred between the admission to the cohorts and the eventual counting of outcome events.

An experimental randomized trial has the scientific advantage of permitting all these innate biases to be removed or substantially reduced, but has the disadvantage of being unfeasible to carry out for many cause-effect investigations. A retrospective case-control study has the virtue of being easy to carry out, but has the scientific disadvantage of producing groups and data that incorporate all the potential innate biases. The candidate cases and controls that await the investigator who begins on the right-hand side of Figure 23–4, after all the events have occurred, will contain a mixture of people who are qualified and unqualified for admission to an unbiased study of the compared maneuvers. The compared maneuvers will have been received without randomization and without precautions to maintain similarity in performance. The outcome events will have been discerned without precautions to maintain similarity in detection; and the members of the eight outcome-state groups of qualified and unqualified cases and controls may have been transferred in unequal proportions from their outcome locations to their appearance in the investigator's collected data.

The scientific challenge for the trohoc investigator is to keep those many sources of bias from producing distorted results.

23.3. THE EXPERIMENTAL TRIAL MODEL

Sir Austin Bradford Hill, who helped inaugurate and develop the modern era of statistically planned randomized clinical trials, has emphasized the importance of experimental thinking in nonexperimental research. Hill's advice[26] was to plan observational studies with "the experimental approach firmly in mind" and to make the observations "in such a way as to fulfill, as far as possible, experimental requirements."

This policy offers the best scientific strategy for designing and evaluating a retrospective case-control study. When the research hypothesis is stated, before or after the study is done, a relationship is proposed between a particular maneuver and a particular outcome event. The statement of the hypothesis immediately allows us to ask how the proposed

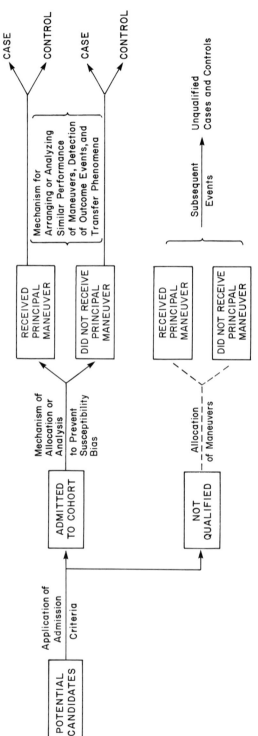

Figure 23–3. Scientific plans for avoiding bias in cases and controls of a cohort study. (For further details, see text.)

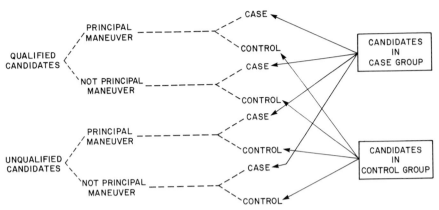

Figure 23–4. Qualified and unqualified candidates in a retrospective case-control study. (For further details, see text.)

relationship would be studied in a randomized clinical trial. The answer to that question will indicate the basic architectural components of the trial; and when we think further about the scientific role of each component, we can discern the things that must be accounted for in a retrospective case-control study.

We shall need to develop suitable admission criteria for the baseline state of people qualified to receive the compared maneuvers. We shall need prognostic analyses that can help reduce susceptibility bias arising in the absence of randomized assignment of maneuvers. We shall have to avoid two types of problems in performance bias: the problems that may have occurred when the maneuvers were actually received and those that may be produced later when the maneuvers are identified. We shall need to recognize and manage any detection bias that occurred while or after the compared maneuvers were administered. We shall have to deal with the problems produced by referral or other transfer biases in the postoutcome data. And while we do all those things to cope with the innate biases expected in the acquired groups and data, we must try to avoid adding any investigative biases during our own work.

By recapitulating the intellectual structure of a randomized trial as we think about the plans for the retrospective case-control study, we can incorporate most of the necessary components into the research design; and we can make suitable compensations or adjustments for whatever problems could not be addressed directly. In many comments about the design of case-control studies,[27-29] the research is regarded as a distinctive entity of its own, or its strategies are compared with those of observational cohort studies. In the principles of scientific inference, however, a retrospective case-control study is used as a substitute for an experimental randomized trial. As the scientific "gold standard" for the conclusions of cause-effect research, the experimental trial must also be used as the intellectual model for indicating the appropriate components of the research design—even when an experiment is not conducted and even when the research follows a backward rather than forward direction of observation.

23.4. TWENTY SCIENTIFIC PRINCIPLES FOR TROHOC RESEARCH

Because of the subtle features involved in any proposed cause-effect relationship between a particular maneuver and a particular outcome, the many things to be considered in individual research studies cannot be completely cited in a single general check list. Nevertheless, many such lists have been developed[30-32] and have made helpful contributions as guidelines for planning and evaluating the experimental cohort architecture of a randomized clinical trial. Although the best approach to thinking about a retrospective case-control study is to consider what would happen in a randomized trial, an analogous check list might be helpful as a "review of systems" that can be applied after a case-control study has received its initial appraisal.

Several years ago, Horwitz and I[33] suggested 12 features that might be used for this purpose, but several other features can be added after a consideration of the challenges cited in Chapters 21 and 22. Accordingly, the following 20 principles can serve as a check list for the scientific quality of a retrospective case-control study. The list is intended to augment, not replace, the primary evaluation done when the research components are considered according to the model of an experimental randomized trial. The first 13 principles in the list refer to acts of thinking and planning that take place before the research begins. The next two principles refer to the activities involved in collecting data. The last five principles refer to procedures that occur after collection of data but that can also be planned (and sometimes done) beforehand. The 20 principles are described briefly, as befits a check list. Most of the principles are explained or justified in the earlier text; but some will receive additional discussion in the rest of this section.

23.4.1. *Establish Research Hypothesis Beforehand*

The specific relationship to be investigated between maneuvers and outcomes should be stated as the research hypothesis before the work begins. The statement is needed to indicate whether the research is testing or generating hypotheses; to specify which hypotheses should be hidden (if necessary); to demarcate the components of the architectural reasoning; and to guide the development of objective methods for ascertaining data.

23.4.2. *Define Exposure Beforehand*

The specific entity or regimen to be regarded as the principal maneuver should be stipulated before the research begins, so that exposure is not defined afterward to coincide with what is found when the data are analyzed.

23.4.3. *Define Admission Criteria for Focal Time and Baseline State*

These criteria, which correspond to the analogous criteria that might be used in a randomized trial of the principal and comparative maneuvers, indicate the particular focal time, in each person's medical itinerary, at which the principal maneuver was (or was not) imposed. Each person's baseline (focal) state, at focal time, will then be checked to determine the characteristics that qualify the person for admission to the study. Although the information may be difficult to acquire, the criteria should contain the same principles of exclusion or inclusion that would have been used in a randomized trial. The baseline state data will also be used to check for the protopathic, vulnerability, and other susceptibility problems noted in the next three sections.

23.4.4. *Check for Protopathic Problems If Pertinent*

Note whether any of the features at focal time might have been early manifestations of the condition subsequently noted as the person's outcome state. If those manifestations might have mandated or contraindicated the use of the principal (or comparative) maneuvers, the person is ineligible for admission to the study. If a previously used agent was maintained but with dosage altered because of possibly protopathic focal state phenomena, the patient should also be excluded.

23.4.5. *Check for Vulnerability Problems If Pertinent*

Note whether focal time occurred at a point when each person was suitably vulnerable to the proposed action of the maneuver. If the maneuver was (or would have been) given before or after the appropriate period of vulnerability, the person is either ineligible for admission to the study or should be classified according to the maneuver used during the period of vulnerability.

23.4.6. *Check and Later Adjust for Prognostic Susceptibility Bias*

Many problems of prognostic susceptibility bias will be managed with suitable admission criteria that exclude persons whose co-morbidity, clinical severity, or other focal state attributes would have excluded them from a randomized clinical trial of the compared maneuvers. For the people admitted to the study, note the demographic, clinical, or other features that are cogent prognostic predictors of the outcome event. These cogent predictors will later be used for the prognostic stratifications (or other appropriate analyses) that compensate or adjust for the absence of randomization when the maneuvers were allocated.

23.4.7. *Choose a Framework for Unbiased Referral*

Consider the patterns of exposures, outcomes, and medical itineraries that might bias the referral (or availability) of people in the four cells of the basic statistical table of results. If antecedent publicity or customary practices in medical care might have distorted the proportions of that table, choose a framework that can prevent or compensate for the bias. These considerations will usually eliminate the choice of an *ad hoc* disease registry, unless the assembled material at the registry can be used as a satisfactory uni-group source of both cases and controls. A nosocomial framework will usually be necessary to find suitable cases of disease and can often also be used as a uni-group source of controls. The uni-group process becomes possible if the controls are selected not according to specific diagnoses but according to rosters of admissions to a hospital, admissions to a single service, or performance of diagnostic procedures. A purely ecologic framework can seldom be a satisfactory source of controls for therapeutic maneuvers, because the interviewed persons will seldom be able to provide adequate information about the pretherapeutic baseline state. An ecologic framework may yield satisfactory conjoined controls for studies of public health maneuvers if adequate data can be obtained about the date and state of the control group members at focal time.

23.4.8. *Choose a Compensatory Control Group If Pertinent for Anamnestic (Recall) Bias*

If the outcome event is likely to create anamnestic bias in interviewed cases, and if this bias cannot be overcome with suitable reminders during the interview of the controls, choose a control group with an outcome event that would also produce increased efforts at recalling previous exposures. To demonstrate that the anamnestic bias has been compensated, choose (and note the results in) an additional control group, selected without regard to the presence of a compensating condition.

23.4.9. *Choose a Compensatory Control Group If Needed for Detection Bias*

If the maneuver-outcome relationship can produce phenomena that would lead to bias in medical surveillance, ordering of diagnostic procedures, or interpreting diagnostic results, a control group must be chosen to compensate for the possibility of detection bias. The bias can be compensated and the study can have a uni-group framework if both the cases and controls emerge from the roster of an appropriate diagnostic procedure.

The use of a diagnostic procedure framework is further discussed in Section 23.5.

23.4.10. *Develop Strategy for Managing Co-Morbidity Bias If Pertinent*

If chosen to compensate for anamnestic bias or detection bias, the control groups may contain the co-morbidity bias discussed in Chapter 21. The latter problem can be managed by making advance decisions about which diseases might create co-morbidity bias and by excluding such diseases from both the case and the control groups. The review of diagnostic evidence (as described in Section 23.4.17) can be used to find the coexistence of unwanted co-morbid diseases in the case group.

23.4.11. *Develop Strategy for Managing Co-Manifestation Bias If Pertinent*

Despite the method discussed in Section 23.4.7 for choosing an unbiased framework, disproportional referrals can occur within that framework because of co-manifestation bias. To avoid this problem, the groups should be stratified according to the main types of presenting manifestations (see Section 21.4.2.5) and also, if necessary, according to diagnostic procedures.

23.4.12. *Choose Incidence Cases of Disease*

For reasons noted earlier, only newly detected incidences of a disease should be admitted to the study. This stricture applies to the diseased members of the case group and to any specific diseases that may have been deliberately selected for inclusion in the control group. If co-manifestation bias and detection bias are potential problems in the research, the different types of newly detected disease (with or without typical clinical manifestations) should be stratified and analyzed appropriately.

23.4.13. *Avoid Arbitrary Unilateral Exclusions*

Whenever people are excluded from admission for reasons cited in the foregoing sections or for any other reasons, the exclusions should be applied equally to the candidates for both the case and control groups. If applied to cases but not controls, or vice versa, the exclusions can create the transfer bias discussed in Section 21.5.2.

23.4.14. *Establish Unbiased Methods of Ascertainment*

Precautions should be taken to maintain objectivity in people who acquire data by interviews or by excerpting archival records. The methods that can be used for these precautions were described in Chapter 22.

23.4.15. *Use Precautions Against Anamnestic Bias*

Develop a format of operation that will contain objectivity and vigor in searching through archival data, or in conducting interviews that will enhance the person's rumination and memory about past events.

23.4.16. *Record Unknown Exposure as Unknown, Not Absent*

When no information is available to indicate whether a person was or was not exposed to a particular maneuver, exposure should be regarded as *unknown,* not as *absent* or *nonexistent.*

23.4.17. *Review Diagnostic Evidence for Cases and Controls*

The purpose of this review, which should be performed objectively, is to remove diagnostic interpretation bias that may have occurred when the original evidence was diagnostically designated by someone who was aware of the antecedent maneuvers. The review is particularly important when the diagnostic decisions require subjective interpretations. The review of evidence in the cases should almost always be possible and can be used not only to confirm the original diagnosis, but also to identify cases with coexisting co-morbid ailments that may require exclusion from the study. The review of evidence in the controls may be impossible if suitable diagnostic procedures were not performed. If detection bias is an issue in the research, the control group should be obtained by a mechanism that will arrange for them to have received such procedures, so that their diagnostic evidence can be objectively reviewed.

23.4.18. *Review Evidence for Reliability of Data Collection and Coding*

A mechanism should be established to determine the consistency (and if possible, the accuracy) with which information was collected during the interviews or excerptions. The process should include attention to the procedures with which raw information was transformed into categories of classification and coding.

23.4.19. *Establish Mechanism for Management of Multiple Data Sources*

When data are acquired from several different sources (such as interviews and archival excerpts), results from each source should be analyzed separately.

23.4.20. *Establish Mechanism for Management of Participation Bias*

If any of the identified candidates do not participate in the research, the characteristics of the participants and nonparticipants should be examined separately to determine whether nonparticipation has distorted the results. If archival data are suitable for characterizing all candidates, participation bias can be avoided by relying on the archival information.

23.5. ADVANTAGES OF A DIAGNOSTIC PROCEDURE FRAMEWORK

The most novel strategy proposed in Section 23.4 and in Chapter 21 is the use of a diagnostic procedure roster as a uni-group framework for choosing both the cases and controls. This strategy has seldom been used in retrospective case-control studies, despite the frequency with which such studies have been aimed at nonacute diseases that often occur in silent or lanthanic patterns for which detection bias becomes a major problem.

The strategy gets its uni-group framework because cases and controls are identified according to the results of the diagnostic procedure. For example, in a study of etiologic antecedents for lung cancer, patients with normal chest roentgenograms can be accepted, with reasonable confidence, as not having lung cancer. Persons with suitably abnormal lung fields may require further testing and almost always receive it. The results of the further tests will then identify the patient as having or not having lung cancer.

The main advantage of the diagnostic procedure strategy is the opportunity of eliminating all three components of the medical itinerary that can produce detection bias. The diagnostic evidence can be obtained and objectively reviewed to avoid biased interpretation. Because everyone will have been diagnostically tested, no one will have been deprived of getting the appropriate procedure because of surveillance bias or test-ordering bias.

The main disadvantage of the strategy is the possibility that it may lead to co-morbidity bias and/or co-manifestation bias. Co-morbidity bias can be eliminated, however, by the methods discussed in Section 21.4.2.4, and co-manifestation bias can be adjusted as noted in Section 21.4.2.5.

23.5.1. *Choice of a Diagnostic Procedure*

When several diagnostic procedures are available, a choice must be made about which one to use as the framework. For example, will the ordering of a chest x-ray suffice to eliminate detection bias in the diagnosis of lung cancer, or should we insist on sputum Pap smears or histologic evidence? If we insist on histologic evidence, must it come from pulmonary tissue? As another example, suppose we are interested in the morphologic entity of cerebral arteriosclerosis rather than the clinically overt entity of stroke. Should the diagnostic procedure framework for cerebral arteriosclerosis be chosen from people who have received skull x-rays, cerebral arteriograms (unilateral or bilateral), radionuclide scintiscans of the brain, or computer-assisted tomography of the head?

In general, the best diagnostic framework will be the coarsest possible screen that will detect almost all instances of the disease while still being generally applicable to a large number of people. For example, because very few instances of lung cancer are missed with chest x-ray, it would be a suitable framework for a study in which the cases are patients with lung cancer. Because the current form of flexible bronchoscopy also has high sensitivity in detecting lung cancer, a bronchoscopic roster might also be a good framework. A roster of patients who have received histologic examination of pulmonary tissue might not be satisfactory unless the framework can yield enough patients without lung cancer to be available for the control group.

23.5.2. *Opposition to a New Paradigm*

Perhaps the greatest difficulty encountered with a diagnostic procedure framework is paradigmatic rather than scientific. As a new operating policy in the methods of case-control research, the strategy can be expected to receive the opposition often accorded to any new method that is perceived as a threat to the validity of existing customs and concepts. Although the cause-effect relationships of many therapeutic maneuvers (particularly over-the-counter drugs) are regularly reevaluated because adequate proof of beneficial efficacy was lacking in earlier studies, many epidemiologists may be reluctant to contemplate the need for similar reevaluations of etiologic or therapeutic maneuvers in which adequate proof of noxious causality was compromised by previously unrecognized problems of detection bias. Because the prevention of detection bias, when pertinent, is a fundamental principle of scientific architecture in case-control studies, investigators who want to reject the diagnostic procedure framework should offer a constructive alternative to deal with the problem. In the absence of a constructive alternative, the new procedure seems much less likely to produce distorted results than the overt biases incorporated without suitable recognition or adjustment in the conventional technique.

23.6. SCIENTIFIC PROBLEMS IN CONVENTIONAL STRATEGIES

During the past few decades, many retrospective case-control studies have been conducted with a conventional paradigmatic strategy that differs substantially from the scientific principles that have been discussed in this chapter and in the preceding text. In the conventional paradigm, a retrospective case-control study is considered to be a separate, distinctive form of research, with its own objectives and operating principles. Because the research is not regarded as a scientific substitute for an experimentally planned cause-effect investigation, the studies are seldom planned or analyzed with architectural principles of scientific inference.

23.6.1. *Choices of Framework*

In the conventional paradigm, a retrospective case-control study is generally regarded as a sampling of suitable groups from the available cases and controls, not as an attempt to recapitulate the medical itinerary of people exposed or not exposed to the main maneuvers under study. Because the framework is not assigned the scientific functions discussed previously, the investigator's main concern in choosing a control group is its source and size rather than its scientific role in achieving a suitable medical itinerary for persons receiving the compared maneuvers.

Accordingly, most discussions about the framework of case-control studies are devoted to whether the control group should be chosen from a hospital or community population or both; what type of mechanism (matching, random selection, etc.) to use in choosing the controls; and whether the number of people in the control group should equal or exceed the size of the case group.

23.6.2. *Collection of Data*

In the conventional paradigm, a case-control study is not intended to recapitulate the scientific architecture of an experimentally designed trial. Consequently, retrospective case-control research is often conducted without the scientific principles used as precautions against biased observations. No attempt may be made to keep the data collectors unaware of the main hypothesis or to hide the identity of the cases or controls when crucial information is assembled about exposure to maneuvers. In addition, because the case-control study is not viewed as a substitute for a randomized trial, information is often omitted about a pre-maneuver baseline state, eligibility for admission to a qualified cohort, differential distinctions in susceptibility bias, problems in detection bias, or the attritions and referrals that can produce transfer bias.

23.6.3. *The Concept of Confounding*

Because the architecture of a cause-effect pathway is not considered in the conventional paradigm, the various sites of innate bias are not identified for discussion. In an architectural analysis, the sources of innate distortion are located in specific sites of the cause-effect pathway. They are identified as inappropriate admission, susceptibility bias, performance bias, detection bias, and transfer bias. In the alternative paradigm, the idea of distortion is sometimes cited under the title of *selection bias,* but most commonly the diverse sources of bias are lumped together under the name of *confounding.*

A confounding variable, or *confounder,* is usually defined as a phenomenon, external to the two main variables of maneuver and outcome, that can distort their relationship as calculated from a fourfold table or other statistical expression.[34, 35] Because of the vagueness of definition and architectural location, a confounder resembles an evil spirit, somewhat like the miasmas of ancient medicine, that must be guarded against; but no specifications are cited for where to station the guards or what they should look for. In the conventional paradigm, the investigator must use various intuitions to perceive the possibility of confounding variables, and to plan or analyze the research appropriately. In the architectural paradigm, the investigator can contemplate the biases by using the review of systems that identifies each possible source of problems in the architectural pathway.

23.6.4. *Concepts of Undermatching and Overmatching*

Without a specific architectural outline for the cause-effect pathway, the conventional paradigm contains no instructions for how to recognize and manage confounding. Instead, there is a general but nonspecific fear of either *undermatching,* when a confounder has not been accounted for, or *overmatching,* when problems are produced by a presumably misguided attempt to deal with confounding. Another effect of confounding is called *effect modification.* It occurs when something happens to produce an inappropriate alteration in the relative proportions of counted frequencies for the outcome event.[34, 35]

In the architectural paradigm, these problems can be specifically identified. For example, the failure to account for susceptibility bias is a major problem in undermatching; and the transfer bias produced when a maneuver's co-morbid diseases are included in the control group is a major problem in overmatching. In the conventional paradigm, however, the definitions of undermatching, overmatching, and effect modification have been difficult for many readers to understand; and no specific criteria have been cited for recognizing their existence.

In the absence of better scientific specifications, the complaint of undermatching or overmatching is often used as a source of confusion rather than enlightenment, whenever one investigator disagrees with what another investigator has done. For example, when suggestions are made that susceptibility bias and vulnerability bias have not been properly accounted for, i.e., undermatched, in case-control studies of the effects of various therapeutic agents in pregnancy, an adherent of the conventional paradigm may claim (erroneously) that such an adjustment would create overmatching.

23.6.5. *Scientific Consequences*

The greatest problem of the conventional paradigm, however, is that it does not use the opportunity to let scientific method act as an intellectual mechanism for solving scientific problems. The retrospective case-control study is regarded as a unique activity of its own—a type of sophisticated statistical art that is detached from the customary principles of method, architecture, and evidence that are applied in all other forms of scientific research. When this isolation from customary scientific standards is questioned, the critics may then be accused of not understanding the paradigm, somewhat in the way that nonbelievers may fail to comprehend or accept the basic tenets of a religious faith.

Because retrospective case-control studies are an irreplaceable scientific structure for evaluating cause-effect relationships that cannot be investigated with more powerful architectural formats, the scientific improvement of trohoc research is a fundamental challenge in clinical epidemiology. A first step in meeting that challenge is to improve the principles of scientific method and architectural reasoning that are used in the research.

23.7. CONFLICTS, CONTROVERSIES & SCIENTIFIC STANDARDS

Because retrospective case-control studies are conducted when randomized trials are unfeasible, the results are almost never directly confirmed by experimental evidence. The closest form of validation for trohoc research, therefore, is usually a cohort study of the same relationship. Because the cohort research may seldom be feasible, however, case-control studies have usually been checked with other case-control studies.

The seminal event for the prestige of case-control studies was their role in providing the first epidemiologic evidence[8] of a relationship between cigarette smoking and lung cancer. When the results were later confirmed in observational cohort studies of the same relationship,[7] the value of the case-control method seemed established; and it then became applied to investigate many other cause-effect questions. As noted earlier, however, these applications generally took place under an operational paradigm that liberated case-control studies from the need for external validation or scientific verification.

Not being evaluated as a substitute for more powerful scientific structures, a case-control study could be assessed with whatever standards seemed suitable to its practitioners. If the research was not intended to recapitulate the architecture of a scientifically planned comparison of maneuvers, it need not be subjected to the same scientific principles employed in experimental trials of those maneuvers. With this paradigmatic liberation from scientific constraints, retrospective case-control studies have been designed, conducted, and reported with a *laissez-faire* freedom that allows the investigators the extraordinary latitudes noted earlier in choosing cases and controls, obtaining data, and changing hypotheses.

23.7.1. *Contradictions in Case-Control Results*

In such *laissez-faire* circumstances, contradictory results would be inevitable; and conflicts can readily be found when the same relationship is investigated with two or more case-control studies or with a cohort study that precedes or follows a case-control study. In 1979, a casual survey[33] of case-control research disclosed 17 different cause-effect relationships in which the result of one or more case-control studies had been contradicted by other case-control studies or by cohort research. The diseases under investigation in those studies included myocardial infarction, cleft lip and palate, benign breast disease, and a variety of cancers. The agents investigated as causal factors were such public health maneuvers as normal lactation, circumcision, age at menarche, and coffee drinking; such diseases as tuberculosis, allergy, herpes infection, and benign prostatic hyperplasia; and such therapeutic agents as irradiation, appendectomy, oral contraceptive pills, aspirin, reserpine, and replacement estrogens. The twelve methodologic criteria that were used to appraise scientific standards in those case-control studies were noted to have been commonly violated in the research activities.

In a more extensive study[36] now in progress, the 1979 survey has been brought up to date. The investigators have found more than 100 additional cause-effect relationships in which the results of one or more case-control studies were contradicted by other case-control studies or by cohort research.

23.7.2. *Scientific Standards in an Excellent Study*

Although many retrospective case-control studies have not had high scientific quality, some have been outstandingly good. Despite the absence of overt scientific standards, individual investigators will often establish and apply appropriate principles. To demonstrate that scientific principles *can* be employed in trohoc research, I shall briefly outline a study that fulfills almost all the scientific requirements discussed in this chapter. (In searching for an exemplary study, I deliberately omitted consideration of any work done by myself or by investigators with whom I have been associated.)

In 1980, Ferencz and coworkers reported a retrospective case-control study of maternal hormone therapy and congenital heart disease.[37] The case group under study contained 110 infants, born during 1972–1975, with conotruncal malformations of the heart. The three control groups, which are described shortly, contained 186 matched controls, 110 random controls, and 20 disease controls. After obtaining ascertainment data by methods described in the comments that follow, the authors concluded that they had failed to show an association between maternal hormone intake and (conotruncal) congenital heart disease, and that the relative risk was unity uniformly throughout the population of cases.

Because an excess of conditions for which hormones are given was not found among case mothers, the authors also concluded that susceptibility bias had not produced the positive associations found in previous studies. The latter conclusion seems unconvincing, however, because of data contained in the authors' Table 6. The results for the case group, compared with random and matched normal controls in that table, show that the mothers of the cases had a much greater prevalence of bleeding episodes during pregnancy. The case mothers also had more flu in the first four lunar months, a higher maternal weight/height index, and a substantially higher familial history of congenital malformations.

Regardless of the way in which the investigators interpreted their results about susceptibility bias, the study was done with the following types of attention to the 20 methodologic principles cited in Section 23.4:

1. *Hypothesis:* Established beforehand: Although endocrine imbalance could affect fetal development at a time when the differentiation of conotruncal structures is in process, the suspected association may arise from susceptibility bias, i.e, an excess among case mothers of abnormalities for which hormones are given.

2. *Exposure:* Established beforehand as any exogenous (sexual) hormone intake in early pregnancy.

3. *Admission criteria:* Zero time was onset of pregnancy, and the candidates consisted of pregnant women who were mothers of the cases and controls. Although admission was not restricted to mothers having clinical reasons for use of hormones, a separate control group was matched to the cases for factors that might evoke such usage.

4. *Protopathic bias:* Not applicable. The outcome event (delivery of the malformed baby) cannot occur before exposure.

5. *Vulnerability bias:* To be classified as exposure, hormone intake was required to have occurred during the first four lunar months of pregnancy or during the extended period, which included the month prior to the last menstrual period.

6. *Prognostic susceptibility bias:* Prognostic susceptibility was determined with multivariate scores for reproductive and other factors predisposing to congenital malformations. Antecedent exposure was examined in people with similar scores, and the cases and one control group were matched (or

adjusted) for secular date of pregnancy and date of prenatal registration as well as maternal age, parity, and past fetal loss.

7. *Unbiased framework:* Population-based study. The cases were found via a roster of the Maryland State Intensive Care Neonatal Program. The controls were taken from all other members of Maryland's birth population. Of two control groups chosen from normal infants, one group was a random representative of the birth population; and the second group was matched to cases according to criteria for susceptibility. (A third control group was chosen to compensate for anamnestic recall, as noted in the next comment.)

8. *Control group for anamnestic bias:* This additional precaution was taken with a disease-control group chosen separately, in the same population, from children who were noted to have hypoplastic left heart syndrome, which is not suspected of an association with hormone taking. The authors reported no evidence of excess recall in the case or disease-control groups.

9. *Control group for detection bias:* Not applicable. Conotruncal malformations in cases are almost always clinically overt.

10. *Co-Morbidity bias:* Not applicable. (No control group was used for detection bias and the anamnestic control group had a condition not associated with hormones.)

11. *Co-Manifestation bias:* Not applicable. In this situation, hormone therapy produces no overt side effects as manifestations that would evoke diagnostic attention to the discovery of congenital heart disease.

12. *Incidence cases:* Yes. The congenital heart disease is evident at or shortly after birth.

13. *Unilateral exclusions:* None made.

14. *Unbiased ascertainment:* Although no comment was made about hiding the hypothesis or "blinding" the two trained interviewers, the interview instrument was a structured questionnaire with precoded choices. Results of interviews were checked with physician and hospital records.

15. *Reduction of anamnestic bias:* In addition to use of a special control group, the interviews were conducted personally; and the interviewed people were given diverse reminders, specifications, and photographs or displays of hormone medications.

16. *Recording of unknown exposure:* No description was cited in the published report. (Because of rigorous ascertainment methods, however, all exposures were probably determined as positive or negative.)

17. *Review of diagnostic classification:* Not attempted in random or matched control group. For the cardiac ailments of cases and disease-controls, investigators reviewed all data from catheterization, surgery, and autopsy. No comment was made about objectivity in this review, but data regarding maternal exposure to hormones were presumably not contained in the diagnostic evidence reviewed for each child.

18. *Review of data collection techniques:* The consistency of the research assistants was not checked, but physicians and mothers agreed in about 90% of instances regarding use or nonuse of hormones.

19. *Multiple data sources:* No comment was made about selection of data when physicians and mothers disagreed.

20. *Participation bias:* About 90% of the invited people participated in the study. The authors checked for this bias and reported that "nonparticipation did not alter . . . characteristics in the interviewed group."

You should review the published report yourself to see how these methods were used. The *analysis* of the acquired data is somewhat hard to understand because the investigators used complex multivariate tactics, but the *methods* section is clearly written and the strategies are readily discerned. Except for omitting a description of management of multiple-source and discrepant data, the investigators complied quite well with all of the scientific principles that were pertinent to the studied relationship. Having examined reports of the many case-control studies investigating the relationship of congenital anomalies and in-utero exposure to sexual hormones, I would regard this work as having the best scientific methods in the batch. I congratulate the investigators and thank them for providing this example of excellent scientific principles in epidemiologic case-control research.

23.8. RETROSPECTIVE CASE-CONTROL STUDIES OF THERAPEUTIC BENEFITS

An unusual scientific double standard in case-control research is its frequent acceptance for demonstrating the risks of therapeutic agents but its rejection (or neglect) as a possible method of demonstrating therapeutic benefits. Although many of the allegedly adverse effects of therapeutic agents have been documented only with trohoc evidence, the retrospective case-control method has seldom been employed if the therapy was suspected of producing a benefit rather than a risk. Several years ago, when postmenopausal estrogen treatment was shown to protect against osteoporotic fractures, the investigators found that they had performed the first case-control study in which the main research hypothesis[38] involved a benefit rather than risk of therapy.

Because the evaluation of a cause-effect relationship is either acceptable or not acceptable as an act of scientific research, and because a scientific evaluation does not depend on whether the effect is regarded as a risk or a benefit, the trohoc method can also be employed to investigate therapeutic benefits. The method is not applicable to study new therapeutic agents, because the cases and controls would have a nonexistent or minuscule prevalence of antecedent exposure, but trohoc research could be applied for studying benefits of old agents—particularly when randomized trials are unlikely to be conducted and when observational cohort studies might take too long or be too expensive.

For example, despite many previous randomized trials, the value of anticoagulant therapy remains controversial in patients with acute myocardial infarction. Because funding seemed unlikely for the new randomized trials that might be needed to resolve the dispute, the relationship was investigated in a case-control study.[39] The cases contained people who had died and the controls contained survivors of a closed cohort of patients with a diagnosis of acute myocardial infarction admitted to a hospital special care unit. Focal time was identified as the moment of admission to that unit; and focal state and exposure or nonexposure to anticoagulant therapy were determined from the recorded medical data, excerpted by research assistants who were kept unaware of the research hypothesis.

The focal state data were used to exclude patients who would have been ineligible for admission to a trial of anticoagulant therapy because they were moribund or because they had mandatory indications (e.g., deep vein thrombosis) or contraindications (e.g., bleeding peptic ulcer) for anticoagulant treatment. For cogent prognostic stratification, the qualified patients were divided into good-risk and poor-risk groups, according to the Killip classification[40] of the severity of the myocardial infarction at focal time. When the odds ratios showed no advantage for anticoagulant therapy in the good-risk group but a distinct advantage in the poor-risk group, the results helped resolve several long-standing controversies.

The previous randomized trials of anticoagulant therapy had failed to show stochastically significant differences not merely because the trials were undersized, as claimed in an analysis of their pooled data,[41] but because the poor-risk patients had either been excluded from the trials or admitted in too small proportions for their benefits to become evident. Because good-risk patients had no apparent benefit from anticoagulant therapy, its advantages for the poor-risk patients would not be shown in trials in which a prognostic stratification was omitted and in which good-risk patients were the dominant constituents of the cohort.

Another advantage of the type of trohoc study just cited is that it can be used to investigate several types of antecedent therapy in the dead cases and surviving controls. Thus, in addition to examining the effects of anticoagulant therapy in those groups, the trohoc investigators also checked the efficacy of lidocaine prophylaxis.[42] In previous randomized trials, lidocaine had been shown to prevent major arrhythmias, but the sample sizes were too small to demonstrate that the arrhythmias might be lethal and that their prevention might be life-saving. Because a randomized trial of this hypothesis was unlikely to be conducted, and because an observational cohort study might require a mammoth sample size, the investigators used their trohoc data to find that lidocaine prophylaxis seemed significantly efficacious in preventing arrhythmic deaths.

23.9. NONEPIDEMIOLOGIC CASE-CONTROL STUDIES OF ETIOLOGY

The last aspect of trohoc research to be discussed here is its frequent use as an act of clinical rather than epidemiologic investigation for etiology of disease.

Epidemiologists have regularly collected diseased cases and nondiseased controls to study public health maneuvers or antecedent clinical therapy as possible causes of the outcome events. Clinical investigators regularly use this same research structure to study the etiologic role of various biochemical, immunologic, or microbiologic phenomena. Being determined in the current status of cases and controls, the focal phenomena cannot always be routinely demonstrated to be antecedent events in a temporal sequence. Consequently, the investigators (and readers) often have difficulty deciding whether the focal phenomena preceded or followed the development of the associated clinical condition. The research may thus have a pathoconsortive rather than a clearly etiologic or clearly pathodynamic conclusion.

The structure of the research is similar, regardless of whether the relationship is regarded as pathoconsortive or clearly etiologic, and the results are usually much easier to understand and to accept than the data of conventional epidemiologic case-control studies. Because the focal phenomena are regularly measured with objective paraclinical technology, the data do not create problems in biased ascertainment, and because the assessments are regularly cited in dimensional scales, the results are reported in means or other average values of central tendency rather than in rates and fourfold tables.

Since the odds ratios and other customary statistical accoutrements of epidemiologic research are absent, readers may not recognize such work as being a retrospective case-control study. Nevertheless, the trohoc structure has been used in many reports that regularly appear in prominent general medical journals. For example, etiologic conclusions were drawn[43] when a stimulation index of cellular sensitivity to collagen had higher mean values in patients with thromboangiitis obliterans than in patients with arteriosclerosis obliterans or in a healthy control group. An etiologic conclusion was also proposed[44] when the geometric mean of IgG antibodies to a papillomavirus antigen was significantly higher in patients with anogenital warts or cervical neoplasia than in control groups. When the mean serum calcium levels were similar in hyperparathyroid patients with and without hypertension, hypercalcemia was regarded as an unlikely cause of hypertension in hyperparathyroidism.[45] When mean levels of mobilizable lead were higher in patients with hypertension who had reduced renal function than in those without renal impairment, the investigators concluded that lead may have an etiologic role in the renal disease of some patients usually designated as having essential hypertension.[46] Bacterially degraded bile salts, having been absorbed with higher median values in patients with adenomatous colonic polyps than in controls, were regarded as involved in the adenocarcinoma sequence of the colon.[47]

The nonepidemiologic trohoc studies have yet another advantage beyond trustworthy data and easy comprehension of results: The studies are easy to repeat. The work does not involve complicated techniques for soliciting participants, performing interviews, or excerpting information from archival sources. An investigator can often readily repeat the study by obtaining (if necessary) a few extra measurements on specimens already acquired from hospitalized patients.

Nevertheless, the research contains certain fundamental epidemiologic problems that are often ignored. The choice and demarcation of cases and controls can be just as challenging (and just as inadequate) in this type of research as in more conventional case-control studies, and the process of scientific inference is often more difficult. Because of the temporal problem in sequence of events, we may have great difficulty deciding which variables are to be regarded as outcomes and which as maneuvers. Unless the patient previously received appropriate tests, there may be no way to determine whether the focal phenomenon that is measured in blood, cells, or other body constituents occurred before or after the development of the associated disease.

Consequently, the spectrum of the investigated cases and controls becomes as important in this type of research as in pathodynamic or diagnostic marker studies. The spectrum of cases should include early instances of disease, to show that the etiologic agent is present when the disease is first found rather than being produced later by the disease's long-term pathodynamic consequences. The spectrum of controls should include people with suitable co-morbidity, to demonstrate that the etiologic agent is distinctive to the disease rather than to co-morbid ailments that may often accompany the disease. Because the selected cases and controls seldom have a suitable spectrum in these nonepidemiologic trohoc studies, however, a rigorous scientific inference is often impossible.

A separate statistical problem in this form of research is that the results may show a relationship but not an estimate of risk. When central indexes (such as means) are contrasted for the cases and controls, the statistics receive the retrograde citation that was discussed earlier in Section 20.2.3. Thus, we may be given persuasive evidence that the mean level of immunoglobulin zeta is elevated in patients with omphalosis and that the elevation has an etiologic role in leading to omphalosis—but we may have no idea of how much of an elevation constitutes a *risk* and how great that risk may be.

23.10. SYNOPSIS

In the clinical investigation of maneuvers regarded as beneficial, randomized trials or observational cohort studies are relatively easy to do. In public health or clinical research for maneuvers suspected as noxious, however, neither patients nor investigators may be willing to volunteer for randomized trials or for prolective cohort studies.

To investigate public health maneuvers or possibly noxious risk factors, observational cohort studies are particularly difficult to do and to interpret, because they require a very long period of observation for very large numbers of people. For prospective cohort research, the investigators usually begin not with an inception cohort but with a multi-serial volunteer cross-section. The multi-serial groups may contain diverse types of bias; and the data, if obtained indirectly, may have many scientific inadequacies. For retrolective cohort research, a suitable framework may not be available for the necessary baseline data; and prolective information about outcome events may be unreliable or affected by transfer bias in the volunteers who participate. In cross-sectional ecologic surveys, the problem of long-term follow-up is avoided but is replaced by other major problems in transfer bias.

Retrospective case-control studies have the strong appeal of being readily applied to explore cause-effect relationships that are impossible or too difficult to investigate with more powerful scientific structures. In exchange for investigative ease, however, the trohoc structure contains intricate challenges for the scientific inference that can be performed when the outcome status at a single point in time for the selected case and control groups is used as a substitute for a complete medical itinerary.

To approach the scientific quality of an experimental randomized trial, retrospective case-control studies should be planned by recapitulating the architectural components, reasoning, and analysis of an experimental trial. With such reasoning, the investigator can develop appropriate methods to choose groups and collect data that can avoid or reduce innate biases in susceptibility, performance, detection, and transfer. A set of 20 principles can be used as a scientific "review of systems" for choosing hypotheses, defining exposure, timing events and states, and managing diverse strategic problems when the investigator makes decisions in selecting groups, establishing criteria, obtaining data, and analyzing results. Although seldom applied in conventional case-control studies, a diagnostic procedure framework may be the best approach for dealing with the pervasive problem of detection bias, particularly if suitable adjustments are made for associated problems in co-morbidity and co-manifestations.

The current vagueness of epidemiologic concepts and terminology for *confounding, overmatching, undermatching,* and *effect modification* can be avoided by using specific architectural principles for scientific inference, and by considering specific biases that can occur at different architectural locations in the cause-effect pathway. Without such principles, the continued use of laissez-faire approaches in retrospective case-control studies may continue to add more uncertain and contradictory results to the many uncertainties and contradictions that have already been produced.

Although generally regarded as a research method of public health epidemiology, case-control studies are pertinent for three distinctively clinical types of investigation. The case-control structure has commonly been used for studying the adverse effects of therapeutic agents but can also be applied—with appropriate scientific standards and in suitable clinical circumstances—to investigate therapeutic benefits rather than risks. Case-control methods have also been frequently applied in clinical investigation of the etiologic roles of biochemical, immunologic, or microbiologic phenomena that can be measured easily and objectively, without epidemiologic problems in soliciting or interviewing volunteers. Although the main data are laboratory measurements, these nonepidemiologic case-control studies contain many overlooked epidemiologic problems in the spectrum of cases and controls, in temporal sequence of events, and in demarcating magnitudes of risk.

EXERCISES

Exercise 23.1. Using any one of the retrospective case-control studies that you chose for Exercises 21.2.2, 21.2.3, 22.5.2, or 22.5.3, evaluate that study *briefly* according to the 20 principles cited in Section 23.4.

Exercise 23.2. What clinical scenario would you give to involve susceptibility bias, protopathic bias, or vulnerability bias as an explanation for the following cause-effect relationships recently reported in retrospective case-control or other observational studies?

   23.2.1. Regular use of a mouthwash is a risk factor for oral cancers.[48, 49]
   23.2.2. A low serum cholesterol is associated with an elevated risk of subsequent cancer.[50]
   23.2.3. Digitalis therapy increases the risk of mortality after recovery from acute myocardial infarction.[51]
   23.2.4. Beta adrenoceptor blocking agents are a cause of retroperitoneal fibrosis.[52]
   23.2.5. Treatment with cimetidine may cause gastric cancer.[53]

Exercise 23.3. In a recently reported case-control study,[54] each of 81 gallbladder cancer cases was matched for age, sex, hospital, and admission date with a benign gallbladder disease control group who had been discharged with a diagnosis of cholelithiasis or cholecystectomy.

In the 37 cancer cases and 64 benign gallbladder controls for whom suitable data were available, the tabulated information was as follows for size of largest gallstone:

Size of Largest Stone (cm.)	Cancer Cases	Benign Gallbladder Controls	Odds Ratio
<1	8	23	1.0
1.0–1.9	5	25	0.6
2.0–2.9	10	12	2.4
≥3	14	4	10.1

(The odds ratios were calculated using patients with stones <1 cm. as having a value of 1.) From these results, the authors concluded that there was a strong association of gallbladder cancer with large gallstones.

Without considering any of the statistical features of the research, and without regard to the participation bias problems produced by patients for whom gallstone size was unknown, what type of reasonable clinical scenario can you envision that would either reduce the true magnitude of this association or that might even make the association an artefact produced by bias? What mechanism(s) would you propose to reduce or eliminate the problems you have cited?

Exercise 23.4. The Doll-Hill retrospective case-control study[8] on smoking and lung cancer has become an epidemiologic classic that is worth reviewing as a prototype for this form of research. Please read the study both for its historical value and also for considering any methodologic problems that it may contain. If you notice any problems, what suggestions would you offer for correcting them?

Exercise 23.5. Several of your colleagues have obtained laboratory evidence that estrogens produce supersaturated bile in premenopausal women. They ask you to help develop a protocol for a retrospective case-control study to determine whether women who take oral contraceptive pills have an increased risk of developing cholelithiasis. What are the principal sources of bias that might distort the results of such a study, and what research plan could you use to avoid or reduce those biases?

Exercise 23.6. Beta-blocking agents were being used for many years in Europe long before large-scale randomized trials were done to provide convincing evidence that the agents were efficacious in preventing recurrent myocardial infarction or death when given to patients who had recovered from an acute myocardial infarction. The head of a European national health agency, which does not have funds available for a large-scale randomized trial or cohort study, has come to you to solicit a plan for a case-control study of the efficacy of these agents in her country. *Briefly* outline the plan you would offer.

[For Exercises 23.7 to 23.9, the class can be divided into several groups who share parts of the various tasks. The total assignment is too long for any but the hardiest of readers to undertake in a single session.]

Exercise 23.7. The references that follow refer to a series of published investigations or commentaries on the relationship of reserpine and breast cancer. The first four items cite the three papers that were published concomitantly in a single issue of The Lancet, together with the accompanying editorial. Item 5 indicates letters and comments sent to The Lancet in response to these publications.

1. Boston Collaborative Drug Surveillance Program. Reserpine and breast cancer. Lancet 1974;2:669–71.
2. Armstrong B, Stevens N, Doll R. Retrospective study of the association between use of rauwolfia derivatives and breast cancer in English women. Lancet 1974;2:672–5.

3. Heinonen OP, Shapiro S, Tuominen L, Turunen MI. Reserpine use in relation to breast cancer. Lancet 1974;2:675–7.
4. Editorial. Rauwolfia derivatives and cancer. Lancet 1974;2:701–2.
5. Letters to the Editor: Rauwolfia derivatives and breast cancer. Lancet 1974;2:774–5, 883, 996–7, 1315–6.

Please pretend that you are the commissioner of the Food and Drug Agency (or the appropriate national analog in your country) as of the moment when these publications appeared. You are now besieged by two clamoring groups of people. Certain governmental and health-oriented noncommercial agencies have been conducting large-scale campaigns to persuade hypertensive people to start and maintain treatment. Because reserpine is one of the main drugs used for therapy (as of 1974), these agencies are reluctant to see reserpine labeled as dangerous. They want no action taken and want further time to evaluate the three studies. On the other hand, certain consumer advocate groups are claiming that reserpine has been shown to be a carcinogen and should be removed from the market. They say you are encouraging cancer with every minute of delay in allowing this drug to remain available for usage. In addition, the original academic investigators, feeling sure they have demonstrated a cause-effect relationship, are urging prompt regulatory action. On the other hand, the pharmaceutical manufacturers, stunned by the unexpected indictment of their previously well-accepted and "safe" product, claim that the research contains many problems, some of which were noted in comments of item 5. The manufacturers also want further time for evaluation of the data.

Given the pressure from these opposing forces and your need for some sort of action, please respond to the following:

23.7.1. As a scientist, prepare a brief statement, containing no more than 100 words, that summarizes the conclusions of your scientific appraisal of these papers and the putative relationship.

23.7.2. As the leader of a major health agency, what action would you take?

23.7.3. As a federal policy-maker, what strategy would you propose to avoid similar controversies in the future?

Exercise 23.8. After this first set of publications on reserpine/breast cancer appeared in 1974, at least 10 additional case-control studies were reported. Please briefly review these studies, which are cited in the following references, and then answer the questions of Exercises 23.8.1 and 23.8.2.

1. Mack TM, Henderson BE, Gerkins VR, et al. Reserpine and breast cancer in a retirement community. N Engl J Med 1975;292:1366–71.
2. O'Fallon WM, Labarthe DR, Kurland LT. Rauwolfia derivatives and breast cancer. A case-control study in Olmsted County, Minnesota. Lancet 1975;2:292–6.
3. Laska EM, Meisner M, Siegel C, et al. Matched-pairs study of reserpine use and breast cancer. Lancet 1975;2:296–300.
4. Lilienfeld AM, Chang L, Thomas DB, Levin ML. Rauwolfia derivatives and breast cancer. Johns Hopkins Med J 1975;139:41–50.
5. Armstrong B, White G, Skegg D, Doll R. Rauwolfia derivatives and breast cancer in hypertensive women. Lancet 1976;2:8–12.
6. Aromaa A, Hakama M, Hakulinen T, et al. Breast cancer and use of rauwolfia and other antihypertensive agents in hypertensive patients: A nationwide case-control study in Finland. Int J Cancer 1976;18:727–38.
7. Kewitz H, Jesdinsky HJ, Schroter PM, Lindtner E. Reserpine and breast cancer in women in Germany. Europ J Clin Pharmacol 1977;11:79–83.
8. Christopher LJ, Crooks J, Davidson JF, et al. A multicentre study of rauwolfia derivatives and breast cancer. Europ J Clin Pharmacol 1977;11:409–17.
9. Williams RR, Feinleib M, Conner RJ, Stegens NL. Case-control study of antihypertensive

and diuretic use by women with malignant and benign breast lesions detected in a mammography screening program. J Natl Cancer Inst 1978;61:327–35.
10. Kodlin D, McCarthy N. Reserpine and breast cancer. Cancer 1978;41:761–8.

23.8.1. Although these studies contradict the previous relationship, is their scientific quality superior to the previous studies? Which ones of this second batch of case-control studies do you think are superior to the first? Why?

23.8.2. Which of the second batch of studies do you think is scientifically inferior to those in the first? Why?

Exercise 23.9. In 1979, Labarthe wrote a summary of methodologic problems in the reserpine/breast cancer case-control studies; and in 1980, Labarthe and O'Fallon reported results of a cohort study. These two publications, which are currently regarded as the "last word" on this subject, are cited below. Do you agree with the conclusions that were reached? If not, what conclusions or actions would you recommend?

1. Labarthe DR. Methodologic variation in case-control studies of reserpine and breast cancer. J Chron Dis 1979;32:95–113.
2. Labarthe DR, O'Fallon WM. Reserpine and breast cancer: A community-based longitudinal study of 2,000 hypertensive women. JAMA 1980;243:2304–10.

CHAPTER REFERENCES

1. Bibbo, 1977; 2. Bibbo, 1978; 3. Dieckmann, 1953; 4. Royal College of General Practitioners, 1981; 5. Ramcharan, 1981; 6. Vessey, 1981; 7. Doll, 1964; 8. Doll, 1952; 9. Hammon, 1958; 10. Dorn, 1958–1959; 11. Dunn, 1960; 12. Best, 1961; 13. Advisory Committee, 1964; 14. Kessler, 1970; 15. Frerichs, 1979; 16. Cullen, 1983; 17. Cassel, 1971; 18. Dawber, 1980; 19. Yano, 1983; 20. Francis, 1965; 21. Gillum, 1976; 22. Herbst, 1972; 23. Labarthe, 1978; 24. Lanier, 1973; 25. Boston Collaborative Drug Surveillance Program, 1974; 26. Hill, 1953; 27. Sartwell, 1974; 28. Jick, 1978; 29. Cole, 1979; 30. Mahon, 1964; 31. Lionel, 1970; 32. Chaput de Saintonge, 1977; 33. Horwitz, 1979; 34. Miettinen, 1981; 35. Kleinbaum, 1982; 36. Mayes and Horwitz, personal communication; 37. Ferencz, 1980; 38. Hutchinson, 1979; 39. Horwitz, 1981 (J Chron Dis); 40. Killip, 1967; 41. Chalmers, 1977; 42. Horwitz, 1981 (JAMA); 43. Adar, 1983; 44. Baird, 1983; 45. Daniels, 1983; 46. Batuman, 1983; 47. Werf, 1982; 48. Blot, 1983; 49. Wynder, 1983; 50. Taylor, 1983; 51. Moss, 1983; 52. Pryor, 1983; 53. Colin-Jones, 1982; 54. Diehl, 1983.

Chapter 24

Heterodemic Studies

All of the cause-effect studies discussed so far have been *homodemic,* i.e., involving the same people. When a maneuver and an outcome were associated to form a statistical structure such as F/M or M/F, each person who appeared in a denominator was also represented in the corresponding numerator, regardless of whether the research structure was a forward-directed cohort, a concurrent cross-section, or a backward-directed trohoc. Each person in each group was individually examined, counted, and suitably represented in each mean, rate, or other statistical expression for the numerators and denominators of the groups.

In a homodemic study, when we report that the 5-year survival for treatment A is 10%, we imply that the cohort had a denominator of people who all received treatment A, who were all followed thereafter, and who were all noted to be alive or dead for the numerator event 5 years later. If we report that 70% of doctors prescribe Excellitol for athlete's foot, the implication is that all of the doctors in this cross-sectional survey were asked about their preferred treatment and that 70% chose Excellitol. If we find that the mean serum bilirubin was 3.7 mg./dl. in cirrhotic patients with gastrointestinal bleeding and 1.2 mg./dl. in cirrhotic patients who did not bleed, we have presumably obtained a bilirubin value for each of the cirrhotic bleeders and nonbleeders, summed those values, and calculated the respective means.

The statistical data of a homodemic study thus have five distinguishing characteristics:

1. The basic biologic unit examined in the research is an individual person.

2. The basic statistical units are individual measurements in each person. The final results are quantified summaries of the individual measurements.

3. The groups who form the denominators consist of people whose data were individually obtained by the investigator, and who fulfilled specific investigative criteria for admission to each group.

4. The entities that appear in the numerator were specifically checked for each of the people who constitute the denominator.

5. If a particular person was unavailable for examination or if data for a particular variable are unknown, the denominators and numerators are adjusted accordingly. In cohort studies, actuarial procedures can be used when numerator data are not available, but the most common tactic for people with unavailable data in homodemic research is to omit those people from both the numerator and the denominator. Thus, if we know age for each of 24 patients who had an episode of gastrointestinal bleeding, but if we have serum bilirubin data for only 22 of those patients, the mean age of the group could be calculated with 24 people in the denominator and the mean serum bilirubin could be calculated with 22. The adjustments might not make use of all the data and might sometimes produce misleading results, but the adjustment process itself is straightforward, with everyone accounted for.

These homodemic principles are so familiar in the architecture of scientific research that their specifications may seem redundant. The specifications are necessary, however, because none of them is fulfilled in the heterodemic studies that are a traditional form of research in public health epidemiology and that often seem so unattractive when first described to medical students. If heterodemic research were applied exclusively to evaluate public health maneuvers, clinicians might want to continue their tradition of viewing the results with apathy or scorn—but heterodemic studies are now being used to draw cause-effect conclusions about such clinical maneuvers as therapy for asthma, treatment of hypertension, the effects of screening for cancer, and the value of intensive care for acute myocardial infarction. Because the products of heterodemic research can no longer be clinically avoided, it is worth learning about the structures from which they come.

24.1. **DISTINCTIVE PRINCIPLES OF HETERODEMIC RESEARCH**

For heterodemic research, the five principles that were just described for people, statistics, denominators, numerators, and unknown data can be listed as follows

1. The basic biologic unit examined in heterodemic research is a group of people.

2. The individual statistical elements consist of the total results found collectively in three different groups of data. Two of these counted groups are arranged as numerators and denominators to form the rates of an outcome (or focal) event. These rates are then statistically associated with data for a different phenomenon enumerated in a third group. For example, if the mortality rate in different countries is associated with the sale of sugar in those countries, the national census count provides denominators for the mortality rate; death certificate counts provide the numerators; and data from sugar manufacturers provide information about sales. Although two variables seem to be compared, three variables were actually counted or estimated.

3. Although groups of people are the focus of the research, the people who form the denominators in the statistical rates were *not* specifically examined by the investigator, and any admission criteria are applied in a "second-hand" way to the summaries supplied by the source of the denominator data.

4. The separate collections of people who form the numerators were also not specifically examined by the investigator and are also admitted with second-hand criteria, applied to summaries from the separate source of numerator data. If the rates formed by the numerators and denominators are associated with an exterior third variable, the information about that variable is obtained from a third source of data, also derived without specifications from the investigator.

5. Because no individual data are assembled for individual people, there are no problems in managing lost or unknown information for a group's constituents. The investigator's main challenge is to decide whether the acquired information is satisfactory for analysis of the group. Although no general principles have been established for this decision, certain criteria are sometimes applied. For example, an epidemiologic standard of satisfactory scientific quality in a particular nation's death certificate data is that no more than 15% of the deaths should be ascribed to unknown or nonspecific causes.[1] If this criterion is not fulfilled, the cause-specific mortality rates from that nation are not accepted as admissible evidence.

24.2. **SOURCES OF DATA**

Of the three sources of data commonly used in heterodemic research, two sources supply the numerators and denominators for the statistical rates, which usually represent an outcome variable. The third source supplies information for the variable that becomes regarded as the maneuver associated with the outcome rates.

24.2.1. *Sources of Denominator Data*

The denominators for heterodemic studies usually come from information assembled by the census bureau to describe (and count) the general population of a particular ecologic region at a particular point in time. The information can then be used to construct a denominator group consisting, for example, of all 35- to 64-year-old women living in New Haven in 1984. The counted size of this group would be derived from data acquired in the 1980 census and then modified to adjust the 1980 magnitude to its estimated value in 1984.

The ecologic estimations usually depend on data for annual births and deaths in the region, together with an index of the region's in-migration and out-migration. One such migration index is based on school census data. For example, suppose town A has a population of 10,000 in the 1980 census, of whom 1500 are children of ages 4 to 14. If no deaths occurred in this age group, 1 year later we would expect to find 1500 children of ages 5 to 15 in school. If the school census shows 1575 children in that age group, the children's cohort has increased by 75/1500, or 5%. We then assume that the town has had a total in-migration rate of 5%. Consequently, if the town had 400 deaths and 200 births in 1981, and if we estimate its net in-migration for that year as 5% of 10,000 (or 500), the estimated 1981 population will be $10,000 - 400 + 200 + 500 = 10,300$. (Readers who feel uncomfortable about these estimation procedures are invited to propose a superior substitute.)

Because of the way the denominator data are collected for an ecologic region, only a limited number of characteristics can be used to demarcate the groups that are directly compared. The characteristics are usually nonclinical and are summarized in the classic epidemiologic phrase "person, place, and time." The data about *persons* consist of demographic information—such as age, gender, race, and occupation—that are readily available from the census bureau's collected counts. The census bureau may also have information about socioeconomic status and about birthplace or other indexes of geographic migration for each person or the person's parents. The *places* consist of geographic regions that are demarcated for census counts and for other collections of mortality and morbidity data. The *times* consist of secular dates on the calendar, usually divided at annual or monthly intervals.

24.2.2. *Sources of Numerator Data*

According to the question asked in the research, the numerator information for an ecologic denominator group can be obtained from a registry of death certificates, a hospital, a diagnostic laboratory, or some other suitable source of data. Thus, we could collect the Connecticut death certificates for 1984; find and count the deaths that were noted for 35- to 64-year-old women whose address was listed as New Haven; and divide this number by the corresponding ecologic denominator. The result would be the annual mortality rate for that particular general population group in New Haven in 1984.

A similar mechanism would be employed if we determined all the new cases of systemic lupus erythematosus (SLE) that were noted in women of this age group at all of the hospitals in New Haven during 1984. Dividing this number by the corresponding ecologic denominator would let us estimate the annual incidence of (hospitalized) SLE in this particular population in 1984.

The information available on numerators and denominators can then be arranged to provide a series of descriptive rates and comparisons. Thus, by letting the general U.S. population be the denominators at different annual intervals and by noting the associated annual deaths ascribed to coronary heart disease, we can create a comparison that shows the secular trend in mortality for coronary heart disease in the U.S. from 1940 to 1980. With analogous arrangements, we could make geographic (or national) comparisons of the mortality rates for coronary heart disease in 1980 in the U.S., the United Kingdom, Finland, and Italy. With a different set of arrangements, we can make demographic comparisons, at a particular time and place, of mortality rates in men and women of different ages and races. We can also note the secular trends of geographic differences in these demographically partitioned mortality rates.

These comparisons, however, are seldom performed merely for descriptive purposes. The investigator either starts with an analytic cause-effect motive in making the comparisons or develops analytic ideas after inspecting the results. The cause-effect motives and ideas refer to the possibility that an exterior agent may be causing the trends or differences found in the compared rates. The suspected causal maneuver is a concomitant entity that occurred not in the specific members of the group under study but in the milieu of that group's corresponding place and time.

24.2.3 *Sources of Data About Maneuvers*

When a particular exterior entity is suspected as a causal maneuver, its occurrence must be documented in the group-place-time milieu that is under consideration.

This documentation may be available from the previous two sources of data. For example, data about socioeconomic status, occupation, and geographic migration might be sufficiently well recorded in census information and in death certificate data so that these variables can be analyzed successfully without recourse to any additional sources of information. Sometimes the exterior maneuver is a single event, introduced at a single point in time or in a single ecologic milieu, and no additional information may be needed. For example, in Section 6.6.3, we contemplated the possibility that the financial depression of the 1930s may have caused a change in secular increments of population growth, and that the introduction of antibiotics in the 1940s may (or may not) have been responsible for the subsequent decline in secular mortality from tuberculosis.

In most instances, however, the suspected exterior maneuver is an agent whose respective levels are to be associated with the calculated rates of disease; and data then must be obtained about the levels of that maneuver. The maneuvers include such public health phenomena as ingested commodities (e.g., water, milk, alcohol, individual foods), inhaled commodities (e.g., cigarette smoke, atmospheric substances and pollutants), atmospheric agents (e.g, rainfall, ambient temperature, season of year, barometric pressure), and economic conditions (e.g., employment rate, gross national product, welfare arrangements, taxation policies). In recent years, the suspected exterior maneuvers have included such medical activities as screening programs, diagnostic procedures, pharmaceutical agents, and intensive care units.

Information about a suspected exterior agent is obtained from yet another source of data. Thus, a national bureau of nutrition (or commercial manufacturers) may tell us about changes in the "fortification" of bread; the tobacco industry may provide data on sales of cigarettes; the weather bureau can supply information about atmospheric features; and the pharmaceutical industry can indicate the magnitude of sales of various drugs. These exterior data about maneuvers can then be associated with the changes noted in the events or rates obtained from the other sources of data.

24.3. ORGANIZATION OF DATA

The available information is usually organized according to place, time, or a mixture of the two.

24.3.1. *Ecologic Surveys*

In an ecologic survey, the different rates of events in a series of different ecologic regions are associated with the concomitant occurrence of a maneuver, such as water or air, in that region. Surveys of this type have been the basis for data (and current controversies) about the relationships between "soft" water and coronary disease, and between air pollution and a variety of major ailments. Ecologic surveys have also shown a positive correlation between consumption of animal protein and lymphoma mortality[2] and rising rates of cardiovascular mortality with increasing prevalence of use of oral contraceptives in young women.[3]

In the characteristic display of data, as shown in Figure 24–1, the ecologic regions act as points on the graph. The data for the maneuver are placed on the abscissa (X-axis), and the data for the outcomes become the ordinates (Y-axis). The ecologic zones may be labeled with numbers, as shown in Figure 24–1, or with letter abbreviations, as shown in an analogous study in Figure 24–2.

24.3.2. *Secular Surveys*

In a secular survey, the time trend in the observed rates is associated with the introduction, cessation, or level of change of the suspected causal maneuver in a single ecologic region. For example, a rise in the rate of sales of alcoholic beverages might be secularly associated with a similar trend in mortality from cirrhosis. A secular fall in the consumption of eggs might be associated with a concomitant fall in coronary death rates. The secular trends need not be concurrent. Thus, if the maneuver is believed to have a delayed action, the trends of the outcome event might be shown for a secular era that is several years later than the secular trend shown for the maneuver. A graphic demonstration of this type of delayed secular association process is shown in Figure 24–3. Because the authors[1] were trying to show a time lag between ischemic heart disease and the antecedent consumption of certain commodities, such as sugar, the secular dates in the upper graph of Figure 24–3 correspond to secular dates 9 years later in the two lower graphs.

The suspected maneuver may be inferred from certain secular trends rather than demonstrated from specific external data. For example, when complex ventricular septal defects showed a strong tendency to occur secularly (and ecologically) in children born in

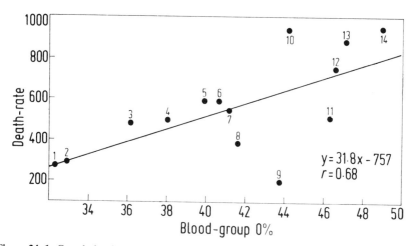

Figure 24–1. Correlation between blood groups and death rates per 100,000 from ischemic heart disease in men aged 55 to 64 in various countries. 1, Yugoslavia; 2, Poland; 3, Austria; 4, Sweden; 5, Norway; 6, Denmark; 7, West Germany; 8, Switzerland; 9, France; 10, U.S.A.; 11, Netherlands; 12, U.K.; 13, New Zealand; 14, Australia. (From Mitchell JRA. An association between ABO blood-group distribution and geographical differences in death-rates. Lancet 1977;i:295–7 (Feb 5).

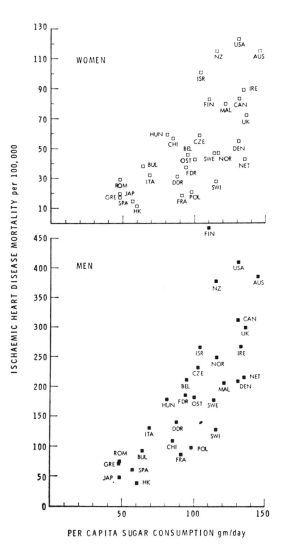

Figure 24–2. Male and female ischemic heart disease mortality plotted against sugar consumption in 30 countries. (From Armstrong BK, et al. J Chron Dis 1975; Chapter reference 1.)

summer and in urban regions, the investigators concluded that the defects may be caused by an environmental agent more prevalent in early winter and in cities.[4]

24.3.3. *Other Arrangements*

In certain other arrangements, information about the maneuver does not come from an external source and is obtained instead from one or both of the other two sources that produced data for the outcome rates. An example of this arrangement was the examination of a demographic characteristic—geographic migration—as a heterodemic maneuver. When migrants to Ohio were found to have substantially higher death rates for cancer than their

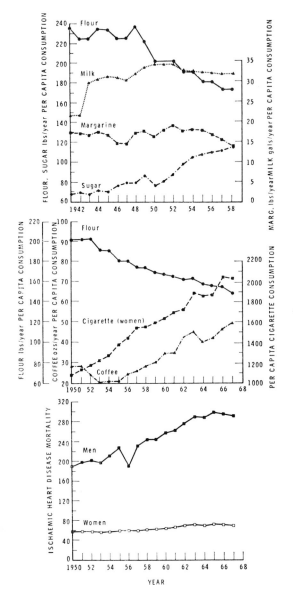

Figure 24–3. Age-standardized ischemic heart disease mortality in men and women aged 35 to 64 in England and Wales (1950–1967) and consumption of highly correlated commodities in the same year and nine years previously. (From Armstrong BK, et al. J Chron Dis 1975; Chapter reference 1.)

demographic counterparts who had been born in Ohio, the investigators suggested that the migrants get the least desirable jobs and are thus exposed to more industrial carcinogens.[5]

24.3.4. *Display of Data*

In a secular study, the data for the outcome event and the maneuver can be portrayed as two curves having similar (or different) patterns in time. Alternatively, the data for outcome event and maneuver at each secular point can be plotted simultaneously on a single graph. Because the geographic regions in an ecologic study do not have a ranked order that permits them to be easily graphed, the outcome rates can be plotted against the maneuver data for each identified ecologic location, as shown in Figures 24–1 and 24–2.

24.4. THE APPEAL OF HETERODEMIC RESEARCH

Although retrospective case-control studies are relatively quick, easy, and cheap, heterodemic research is even quicker, easier, and cheaper. The hard work of obtaining the basic data has already been done, before the investigator begins, by the efforts of governmental or commercial agencies. If the collected information is made available in published compendia or computer tapes, suitable groups of data can often be found to show outcome rates and the associated changes in a selected maneuver. The investigator can then do the research at a desk or in an armchair, with no cost or effort beyond the time needed to find the collected data, plot the corresponding points on a graph, and process the statistical associations.

Epidemiologists often use the term "armchair" research to distinguish this type of investigation from the "shoe-leather" research with which homodemic information is obtained by direct examination of the people under study. "Shoe-leather" epidemiologists examine prolective cohorts and ecologic cross-sections, conduct semihomodemic ecologic studies, or do the detective work involved in pursuing the people and phenomena of an unusual outbreak of disease.

Heterodemic research is so simple and easy that it can be (and has been) used for almost any topic that might strike the fancy of a person who can find appropriate data. Armed with a copy of mortality rates for different regions or with a national abstract of statistical data, anyone can become an investigator by putting anything together. Exercise 24.5 at the end of the chapter contains a challenge for the reader to create both a bizarre and a plausible relationship to augment the many bizarre and plausible relationships that have already been created in heterodemic research.

As might be expected, when the research is so easy to do, it will also have some major disadvantages. For heterodemic research, the main disadvantage is the difficulty of fulfilling scientific standards that would allow the results to be regarded as anything more than a dubious manipulation of dubious statistics. The investigative activities fulfill so few of the most elemental principles of scientific inference that an important challenge in heterodemic research is to find circumstances in which the results warrant serious attention and scientific credibility.

Before that challenge is considered, we need to understand some of the ways in which the data are statistically manipulated. The elaborate mathematical procedures applied to heterodemic information may sometimes be so awesome or baffling that readers may forget to think about the basic scientific principles involved (or neglected) in the statistical expressions.

24.5. STATISTICAL OPPORTUNITIES AND HAZARDS IN HETERODEMIC RESEARCH

The analysis of heterodemic data offers unparalleled opportunities for statistical creativity and scientific error in choosing among multiple candidates, demarcating distributions, applying standardizations, substituting indexes, and performing multivariate explorations. Because of all the things that can be done and examined, an investigator who cannot find support for any proposed hypothesis has really not looked very carefully.

24.5.1. *Choosing Among Multiple Candidates*

In deciding what relationships to check and how to check them, an investigator can choose among a cornucopia of maneuvers, outcomes, and ecologic or secular linkages. The suspected maneuvers can be anything for which suitable data can be obtained. The selected outcome events can be total mortality, mortality attributed to individual diseases, occurrence of individual diseases, or any other phenomena cited in available data. Aside from all the maneuvers and outcomes that can be co-related, the associations can be established from data linked in diverse ecologic zones and in diverse secular periods. The ecologic zones can consist of different countries, large regions within a country, and smaller regions within a larger one. The points of time checked in secular trends can be individual months, groups of months, individual years, or groups of years. If the relationships noted for these outcomes, maneuvers, places, and times do not produce what the investigator is looking for, the data of persons can lead to other opportunities. The evidence can be checked in various subgroupings formed by age, race, gender, and other demographic attributes.

Because so many hypotheses can be generated or tested with this information, the exhaustion of an armchair investigator has usually been the main deterrent to unrestrained acts of data dredging. Even though no work is needed to gather data from individual people, heterodemic associations have usually required investigative effort in finding collections of data, excerpting the appropriate numbers, and doing the statistical calculations. In an age of computers, however, this deterrent is gradually vanishing. Because the heterodemic data are now frequently stored in computerized arrangements, even the armchair labor can often be avoided. The computer can be programmed to examine everything against everything in every possible way; and the only exhaustion that might restrain the investigator is the task of examining the myriads of tabulations and other printouts produced by the computer.

The main hazard of all these opportunities in data dredging is the problem of interpreting the many significant relationships that will inevitably emerge by chance when enough things are examined. The investigators and readers will have to decide how many of the relationships are artefacts of stochastic fate, which ones can be regarded as plausible, and which ones fulfill the architectural standards that can allow acceptance for scientific inference in cause-effect reasoning.

A second prominent hazard occurs when an investigator chooses support from the vast hordes of available data. Infatuated with a research hypothesis, the investigator may choose information that is consistent with the hypothesis while ignoring other data that are inconsistent. The selected results may then show the pattern of a persuasive relationship only because the unpersuasive points have been omitted from the data. For example, the current cholesterophobic era—in which coronary artery disease is attributed to abnormalities in cholesterol or other lipids—was inaugurated epidemiologically with data from a heterodemic association.[6] The death rates for "arteriosclerotic and degenerative heart disease" in six countries showed a strong, almost linear positive relationship to the proportion of fat calories available in the respective national diets. Many years later, however, it was learned that those six countries had been highly selected. The relationship between dietary fat and heart disease would have almost disappeared in the heterodemic data if the original evidence had included 16 additional countries that might quite properly have been analyzed along with the selected group of six countries.[7]

24.5.2. *Demarcating Distributions*

Any collection of data for the occurrence of a particular event will show a spectrum of distribution. If the event is a person's height, some people are taller and others are shorter than those in the middle. If the event is a rate of death or some other phenomenon found in different places or eras, the distribution will also show certain places at the high end of the spectrum and other places at the low end.

In Chapter 28, we shall consider the problems of demarcating a spectrum of data to determine a range of normal for individual people. Regardless of whatever statistical strategies are used for this demarcation, a clinical reader can always employ principles of health, rather than statistics, to decide whether a particular high or low value is truly abnormal. In epidemiologic rates of outcome events in different ecologic places or secular times, however, there are no concomitant clinical principles for deciding what is too high or too low. The decision about where to draw the boundaries and to proclaim something as egregiously deviant depends entirely on what the investigator wants to do. The rates for a particular locality can thus be branded as dangerously high or exalted as enviably low, according to the investigator's ideology, hypothesis, or goal in making the decisions.

The obvious scientific hazard in this activity is the absence of any scientific standards. The demarcations and designations depend entirely on the beliefs, whims, or prejudices of the investigator. Several places clustered together at the high or low ends of the spectrum may have relatively tiny differences in their individual rates, but a particular region may be singled out for the title of *highest* or *lowest* if its other characteristics conform to the investigator's preconceptions.

A second hazard is that the hypotheses or conclusions may be oriented in only one direction. Thus, when a particular region is found to have the highest rate of cancer in a spectrum of regions, considerable speculation, additional analyses, and extensive publicity may be given to the plight of the inhabitants of that region and to the search for its environmental carcinogens. On the other hand, when some other region is found to have the *lowest* rate of cancer in the spectrum, no attention may be given to the healthful virtues of the region or to a search for the features that help it protect against cancer.

A third hazard is the frequency with which statistical demarcations and biologic preconceptions can be joined in a *folie à deux* that produces major scientific blunders, somewhat like the error (see Section 19.4.5) of regarding high atmospheric pressure as a cause of cholera. For example, a state of panic developed not too long ago when the National Center for Health Statistics reported that the national cancer death rates had strikingly increased from 168 to 176 per 100,000 during the first six months of 1975. Agencies doing cancer research were alarmed because the data seemed to refute their apparent progress. Consumer advocates, shouting "Hunt the carcinogen," wanted to round up the usual suspects in nuclear radiation, food additives, or widely used drugs. After further thought, data, and analysis, however, the apparent upsurge in cancer was dismissed as fallacious[8, 9] and was attributed to (1) stochastic variation in projected values derived from a 10% sample of deaths; and (2) a major epidemic of influenza, which had hastened the deaths of people seriously ill with cancer. When the full data became available, the age-adjusted death rate for cancer in 1975 was actually lower than in the preceding year.

24.5.3. *Applying Standardizations*

Because heterodemic data are based on rates of events for ecologic populations having major denominator differences in age, gender, and race, the data can regularly be standardized to avoid susceptibility bias arising from disproportions in these demographic attributes. The demographic standardizations may be direct or indirect (see Section 20.3.6.1) according to the type of information that is available. The indirect method is particularly popular because it is more easily applied. If we have the census data and the crude event rates for a particular region, we can do an indirect standardization without having to know the stratum-specific event rates for that region. The convenience of the indirect standardization is responsible for the frequency with which its products, such as *standardized mortality ratios,* appear in epidemiologic literature.

Although satisfactory for public health maneuvers applied to a presumably healthy general population, this type of standardization is obviously inadequate for therapeutic maneuvers. Because the main determinants of prognosis for therapeutic maneuvers are the clinical baseline state and indications for treatment, a standardization based on demography alone may be mathematically impressive but scientifically useless.

A separate hazard of the standardizing process is the possibly distorting impact of the particular population used for the standardization. As noted earlier (Section 20.3.6.1.3), the standardization process can produce misleading results for comparisons of different ecologic regions and particularly for analysis of secular trends. Ecologically, the single adjusted result that is produced for each region may fail to reflect important distinctions that can be noted only from inspection of the rates in individual strata. Secularly, the trend in the adjusted results can be substantially altered according to the composition of the population in the particular year chosen for the standardization. For example, because the United States population is progressively getting older, the adjusted rates will fall below the crude rate whenever an earlier secular population (such as 1970) is used to standardize mortality rates for a later secular year (such as 1983). Conversely, if standardized according to the population for 1980, the adjusted rate for any year in an earlier era (such as anything that preceded 1980) will rise above the corresponding crude rate.

Although the standardization process has the virtues previously described, the standardized rates are merely adjustments. The crude rates tell what is really happening; and the best way to make precise comparisons is to analyze the crude results within individual strata rather than in the standardized conglomerate. Despite various scientific complaints[10–12] about the possible distortions produced by the adjustment process, its epidemiologic popularity remains unabated.

24.5.4. *Substituting Indexes*

In some instances, the main information available for certain outcome phenomena may consist of an enumeration rather than a rate of events. For example, we might know the number of deaths that have been ascribed in a particular region to disease A, disease B, disease C, and all other diseases, but we may not have an accurate count of the denominators needed to convert these numbers into rates of death for each disease. Alternatively, although we know the rates of death, we may worry about the possible distortions imposed by the choice of a particular standardizing population. Either one of these problems can be avoided if we abandon the rates of death and substitute a different index, called the *proportionate mortality ratio,* for each disease. Despite its impressive name, this ratio is merely a proportion. If we take the number of deaths ascribed to disease A and divide by the total number of deaths, we get the proportionate mortality ratio (PMR) for disease A.

Although easy to calculate, the PMR can be a highly deceptive index because it represents a proportion among a spectrum of deaths, not an occurrence rate of deaths in a population. The PMR for a particular disease can show wide fluctuations, unrelated to its true impact in the population, according to what is happening to all the other diseases. For example, suppose the actual occurrence rates of death per thousand people in a region are 20 for disease A, 15 for disease B, 30 for disease C, and 125 for all others. The total death rate for the population will be 190 per thousand, and the proportionate mortality ratio for disease A will be 10.5% (= 20/190). Now suppose that the population has major improvements in mortality rates so that the individual rates per thousand drop to 18 for disease A, 5 for disease B, 15 for disease C, and 87 for all others. The total mortality rate will fall to 125 per thousand, but the proportionate mortality for disease A will rise to 14.4% (= 18/125). Someone who examines proportionate mortality ratios alone may wonder why disease A has had so striking a rise in its mortality, although in fact, the disease is causing fewer deaths than before. Because of the propensity for these fallacies, the best use of the proportionate mortality ratio is to indicate the relative magnitude of a problem in a particular region at a particular time. Although the PMR has inspired some ingenious mathematical models for its application, the index seems too unstable to warrant serious scientific attention.

24.5.5. *Multivariate Explorations*

Heterodemic data can receive a great many multivariate explorations, some of which were outlined in Chapter 22. The stratified clusters that would directly display the observed evidence are seldom used, however. Instead, the analyses generally depend on various statistical indexes of association, determined with mathematical models based on diverse forms of linear regression. The models are often expanded for two types of analyses that seldom appear in other forms of epidemiologic research.

One type of analysis makes use of the secular features of the data. Instead of being processed with the linear model employed for most types of multivariate associations, the data at different secular points are fitted with polynomial models that are called *time series*. The mathematical activity is used for finding factors that explain the secular trends and for predicting future trends. Although a fertile source of biomathematical publications, the time series analyses are seldom validated, and their pragmatic scientific contributions are uncertain.

An additional type of multivariate mathematical analysis has been fashionable in using heterodemic data to explore the public health impact of various socioeconomic phenomena. The procedure, called *path analysis*, relies on a type of recursive regression strategy. The outcome event is first regressed to find the first-order variables that best explain it. These variables then become used as the outcomes of a new set of second-order regressions, searching for the second-order variables that best explain the first-order variables. The procedure can continue into third-order and higher-order steps until nothing more can be explained. The result of the recursive regressions is a set of *path coefficients*, which allegedly indicate the important factors and stages in the causal sequence. This mathematical method of demonstrating a chain of causation has often been used by social scientists, but has not yet become popular in epidemiology.

With or without path analysis, the mathematical associations found between mortality rates and socioeconomic data have led to strong but instructive controversy. According to certain sociologists[13] and economists,[14] secular changes in mortality from heart disease can be attributed to economic changes. According to epidemiologists,[15] medical statisticians,[16] and other economists,[17] the socioeconomic analyses are based on "tenuous associations or highly dubious bioassays"; and the results, produced "in splendid statistical isolation," are "opaque, unhelpful, potentially misleading" and should be viewed with "profound skepticism." (The excerpted quotations show the flavor of the published controversy. Readers who want to see more should check the cited references and the other publications to which the citations will lead.)

24.6. THE SCIENTIFIC PATHOLOGY OF HETERODEMIC RESEARCH

Heterodemic research contains so many potential fallacies and so few scientific safeguards against those fallacies that many clinical readers may be tempted to dismiss the research as totally worthless. Although this temptation is sometimes difficult to resist, oases can be found in the scientific desert. Just as the ailments noted in human pathology are not all lethal, the many impairments that constitute the scientific pathology of heterodemic research are not all fatal flaws. At selected levels of data and analyses, certain types of questions can receive answers that might warrant scientific credibility. This section and Section 24.7 are concerned with the many types of pathology that prevent heterodemic research from being scientifically useful for more than the few roles cited in Section 24.8. Because not all epidemiologists will agree with these appraisals, readers should have a look at the spirited defense offered in D. D. Reid's discussion[18] of the "long and respectable history" of heterodemic research.

24.6.1. *Problems in Communication*

Aside from the difficulties of understanding the mysteries of standardized rates and proportionate ratios, medical readers are often confused by the vocabulary of heterodemic expressions. When a clinician and a public health epidemiologist think about a rate of death, each person has a different denominator in mind. The clinician is thinking about a group of diseased patients; the epidemiologist, about a general population. Because of these different denominators, the phrase "death rate for myocardial infarction" can mean dramatically different things to a public health epidemiologist and to a clinical investigator. In public health, the denominator of this rate is a general population and the numerator is the deaths ascribed to myocardial infarction; but clinically, the denominator is a group of patients with myocardial infarction and the numerator is the members of that group who have died. Similarly, a clinical epidemiologist contemplating a rate of mortality for cancer of the pancreas thinks about deaths occurring in a group of people with pancreatic cancer; a public health epidemiologist thinks about deaths attributed to pancreatic cancer in a general population. Having been able to set the standards of nomenclature, the public health epidemiologist usually calls the general population death rate a *mortality rate* and the clinical group death rate a *case-fatality rate*.

When not adequately recognized, these conceptual distinctions can lead to fruitless controversy about the merits of diagnostic and therapeutic procedures. In evaluating cervical Pap smears for uterine cancer, clinicians may assert that death rates for cancer of the cervix have declined since introduction of the Pap test, whereas public health epidemiologists may claim that the rates have not changed and may even have increased. The controversy is fruitless because the two groups are talking about different things and because both groups may be right and wrong. Clinically, the case fatality rate may have declined only because widespread use of the Pap smear enables more patients to be treated in a more favorable prognostic stage or at an earlier serial time for the disease. In public health, the general mortality rate may show no change only because a true decline in the old general rate has been counterbalanced by an increase in previously undetected cervical cancer deaths that would have escaped diagnosis in the absence of the Pap smear test.

24.6.2. *Problems in Quantification*

The denominators of heterodemic rates depend on census enumerations that may be either grossly inaccurate (particularly in underdeveloped countries) or substantially distorted by inadequate estimations of either the numbers or composition of migrant populations and other intercensal populational changes. For example, suppose that unhealthy people leave Maine for Arizona and are replaced by equal numbers of healthy people moving from Arizona to Maine. If the exchanged populations are demographically similar, the enumerated values of strata in the two populations will be unaffected, but their prognostic composition will be greatly altered.

The numerators of heterodemic data are reasonably trustworthy if they refer merely to deaths (and if all deaths become enumerated), but the data for *causes* of death contain the many inaccurate, bizarre, and sometimes farcical diagnoses that will be discussed further in Section 24.7.

Heterodemic data for external maneuvers may or may not be accurate; but even when accurate, the data may not be suitable. A pharmaceutical manufacturer may be able to supply reasonably accurate information on the sales of a particular drug as it leaves the factory, but the manufacturer may not know how much of the drug is purchased at retail outlets or what kinds of people are buying (or using) it. The frequent dissociation between the magnitude of sales or production for a particular maneuver and the actual imposition of that maneuver on the presumed recipients is responsible for the ecologic fallacy described in Section 24.6.4.3 and for several other major errors in cause-effect reasoning.

24.6.3. *Problems in Comparison*

The difficulties just cited in quantitative accuracy of data for an individual ecologic group can create important biases when comparisons are performed among different groups. The methods of enumerating census and deaths may differ in time, place, and demographic groups; the identification of events, such as causes of death, may be grossly different; and the data about external maneuvers may also have major differences in quality. For reasons cited previously, these problems are seldom solved by attempts to standardize rates. The wrong variables may have been used for the standardization; the selected standardizing population may have produced its own distortions; or the data may have been too inaccurate to be helped by mathematical manipulations.

24.6.4. *Problems in Causal Reasoning*

Perhaps the greatest problem of all, however, is that the causal reasoning of heterodemic surveys is based on indirect associations. In homodemic data, we at least know that the involved people were or were not exposed to the alleged causal agents and we know each person's outcome. The outcome may or may not be due to the alleged cause, but we can form a direct association between an alleged cause and its putative effect. In heterodemic data, however, the suspected causal agent occurs in the milieu of the exposed populations, but we do not know who was exposed and who was not.

24.6.4.1. SELECTING CAUSAL CANDIDATES

The problem of indirect exposure produces three major hazards. The first is that we can select anything we want to examine as a maneuver for causal relationships: sales of television sets, membership in churches, attendance at basketball games, introduction (or recall) of a new type of candy, or phases of the moon. If we are particularly lucky, we may be right in choosing the suspected maneuver, but the methods contain no safeguards to keep us from being badly wrong.

24.6.4.2. ESTABLISHING A CAUSE-EFFECT SEQUENCE

The second main hazard is the difficulty of establishing a cause-effect sequence when the suspected causal maneuver is a therapeutic agent. If a public health maneuver—such as an atmospheric agent or a change in water—is introduced into an ecologic environment, the maneuver will not be specifically prescribed for sick people; and changes in outcome rates can be referred to the secular date of the maneuver's introduction. If the new maneuver is used for clinical therapy, however, the cause-effect sequence for a therapeutic agent cannot be properly evaluated without considering the baseline state of people receiving the agent. For example, if an epidemic of a serious and potentially lethal disease strikes an ecologic region, a newly introduced therapeutic agent for that disease may be given mainly to the moribund people who have failed to improve with standard treatment. Even if the new treatment is highly efficacious, it may not save all of the moribund patients. Because the rise that occurs in the ecologic death rate for the disease will be associated with the ecologic introduction and usage of the new treatment, a clinically naive investigator, who examines the temporal sequence in the heterodemic data and who overlooks the reverse therapeutic sequence in the clinical events, may then conclude that the new therapeutic agent was a cause of the deaths.

This type of problem may have occurred in the still unresolved controversy about a powerful bronchodilator aerosol whose allegedly lethal effects in the treatment of asthma were demonstrated only with heterodemic data. (Exercise 24.4 at the end of the chapter asks you to evaluate the available evidence and form your own opinion.)

24.6.4.3. **DEMONSTRATING A DIRECT RELATIONSHIP: THE ECOLOGIC FALLACY**

Because maneuvers and outcomes are not noted in individual people, there is no way to determine directly that an ecologic maneuver was received by the same people who had the outcome events. Dealing with data for the *entire* ecologic region, the investigator has no way to check the possibility that the maneuver was applied mainly in one part of the region, whereas the outcome events occurred mainly in a different part of the region. The rise in occurrence for the maneuver and for the outcome event, although not directly related, will coexist and become related in the indirect data for the entire region.

This type of error—in which incorrect conclusions about individual people are drawn from associations in group data—has occurred often enough to have received a specific name: *ecologic fallacy*.[19] Although often suspected, this fallacy is hard to demonstrate with good medical examples because so few homodemic studies have been done to check the conclusions of heterodemic research. In one noteworthy investigation,[20] the authors found no significant correlation when the data of individual patients were examined for the relationship between prematurity and adequate prenatal care. Relatively high correlations occurred, however, when the data were examined heterodemically in ecologic aggregates of townships or census tracts.

24.6.4.4. **REQUIREMENTS OF SCIENTIFIC INFERENCE**

Because of all the cited difficulties, almost none of the requirements of a scientific causal inference can regularly be attained in heterodemic research. We have no evidence that the people allegedly exposed to causal maneuvers were indeed exposed and no evidence that the target event was absent before the exposure took place. We can try to classify baseline states according to overt demographic data, but we seldom have information about clinical, behavioral, familial, or other cogent attributes that must be checked to avoid comparisons distorted by susceptibility bias.

Because we examine a temporal-spatial concurrence of events rather than an imposed principal maneuver and comparative maneuver, we cannot check directly for performance bias. We seldom, in fact, have a defined maneuver whose performance can be examined. Instead, we analyze different levels of exposure and look for an appropriate pattern of dose response in the statistical associations. If additional co-maneuvers have contaminated the responses, we will be unaware of the contamination unless separate efforts are made to obtain the sales curves, patterns of usage, or other suitable information about those co-maneuvers.

Because we are not collecting data about individual people, we may not have any major problems in transfer bias, but the unresolved difficulties of detection bias are formidable. When data are contrasted for different ecologic regions or for different secular intervals, we have no assurance that the outcome events were identified with similar methods of surveillance and identification. For clinical readers, the inaccurate or biased detection of the diseases used as outcome events is perhaps the most obvious scientific weakness of heterodemic research. Every clinician who has prepared a discharge summary for a patient is aware of the vicissitudes of nomenclature for diagnosing disease; and anyone who has filled out a death certificate knows about the further inconsistencies with which diagnoses are recorded in the stipulated format. Because these summaries and forms are filled out as an administrative requirement, not as an act of science, clinicians are well aware of the gross inadequacies with which different diseases are cited. These gross inadequacies, however, may be accepted and tabulated to become the fundamental data used for outcome events in heterodemic research.

24.6.4.5. DELUSIONS ABOUT CAUSE-SPECIFIC MORTALITY AND OCCURRENCE OF DISEASES

For the general goals of heterodemic research, certain parts of the second-hand data can be regarded as reasonably trustworthy. In well-developed countries, the census information about denominator populations may have no major inaccuracies; the number of total deaths reported in the numerators is close to a complete count; and the information from sales or other data about magnitude of maneuvers is unlikely to be falsified.

A major delusion does occur, however, when the occurrence rate of diseases is determined from cause-specific mortality rates. This delusion has two contributing components, each of which is a prime source of error. The first error is the assumption that the multiple diagnoses listed on death certificates can be effectively sorted to choose a single entity, which is then called *the* cause of death and counted as the patient's sole disease. The second error is the assumption that the cause-specific mortality rates, determined from counts of those isolated causes of death, can be used to represent the occurrence rates of the cited diseases.

The medical historians who review the epidemiologic events of the 20th century will doubtlessly have great difficulty interpreting the persistence of these two conceptual errors. How could this astonishing *nosologic fallacy* have managed to endure and prevail for so long in the same scientific medical era that gave rise to molecular biology, precise diagnosis, and potent therapy? No knowledgeable clinician or pathologist in the second half of the 20th century believes that single choices of death certificate diagnoses can indicate disease-specific causes of death and that those choices can represent the actual occurrence of the specified diseases. Nevertheless, the deluded beliefs continue to produce the nosologic fallacy that has been established as a basic, standard, operating paradigm in heterodemic research.

24.7. THE SCIENTIFIC PATHOLOGY OF DEATH CERTIFICATE DATA

The epidemiologic analysis of death certificate data is said to have begun in 1662, when John Graunt initiated[21] *Bills of Mortality* in the city of London. The "bills" contained a systematic recording of each dead person's name, date of death, gender, and type of illness. Figure 24–4 shows Graunt's list of identities and frequencies for lethal illnesses in

The Diseases, and Casualties this year being 1632.

A Bortive, and Stilborn ..	445	Grief	11
Affrighted	1	Jaundies	43
Aged	628	Jawfaln	8
Ague	43	Impostume	74
Apoplex, and Meagrom	17	Kil'd by several accidents..	46
Bit with a mad dog.......	1	King's Evil..............	38
Bleeding	3	Lethargie	2
Bloody flux, scowring, and flux	348	Livergrown	87
		Lunatique	5
Brused, Issues, sores, and ulcers, ...	28	Made away themselves.....	15
		Measles	80
Burnt, and Scalded.......	5	Murthered	7
Burst, and Rupture.......	9	Over-laid, and starved at nurse	7
Cancer, and Wolf.........	10		
Canker	1	Palsie	25
Childbed	171	Piles.....................	1
Chrisomes, and Infants.....	2268	Plague...................	8
Cold, and Cough..........	55	Planet	13
Colick, Stone, and Strangury	56	Pleurisie, and Spleen......	36
Consumption	1797	Purples, and spotted Feaver	38
Convulsion	241	Quinsie	7
Cut of the Stone..........	5	Rising of the Lights......	98
Dead in the street, and starved	6	Sciatica	1
		Scurvey, and Itch........	9
Dropsie, and Swelling......	267	Suddenly	62
Drowned	34	Surfet	86
Executed, and prest to death	18	Swine Pox	6
Falling Sickness..........	7	Teeth	470
Fever	1108	Thrush, and Sore mouth...	40
Fistula	13	Tympany	13
Flocks, and small Pox.....	531	Tissick	34
French Pox..............	12	Vomiting	1
Gangrene	5	Worms	27
Gout	4		

Christened { Males .... 4994 / Females .. 4590 / In all ... 9584 } Buried { Males .... 4932 / Females .. 4603 / In all ... 9535 } Whereof, of the Plague. 8

Increased in the Burials in the 122 Parishes, and at the Pest-house this year.. 993

Decreased of the Plague in the 122 Parishes, and at the Pest-house this year................................ 266

Figure 24–4. Excerpts from "Natural and Political Observations Mentioned in a Following Index, and Made Upon the Bills of Mortality," John Graunt, London, 1662. (From Wilcox WF, ed. Natural and Political Observations Made Upon the Bills of Mortality by John Graunt [a reprint of the first edition, 1662]. Baltimore: Johns Hopkins Press, 1937.)

1662. A modern enumeration of this old nosologic taxonomy was prepared when Thomas Forbes tabulated the burial records maintained by sextons in the 17th century at a London parish.[22] The diagnoses found by Forbes for 15,856 deaths at that parish are shown in Figure 24–5.

A modern reader will have difficulty recognizing most of the diseases shown in Figures 24–4 and 24–5, and even the ones whose names endure today may be diagnosed with substantially different criteria. Graunt paid little attention to the diagnostic names, but he saw the potential value of the demographic data. He used the demographic information to evaluate infant mortality rates and to introduce the first form of life-table analysis for estimating life expectancy.

About 200 years later, when the preparation of death certificates had become universal in Great Britain, William Farr, who was then the Registrar-General, wanted to make better statistical use of the diagnostic data. Thomas Forbes has also given us a modern look at the diagnoses recorded for deaths in that era. Figure 24–6 shows his enumeration of the causes of death entered in a London parish's mortality books[23] from 1820 to 1849. Although more familiar to modern readers than the nosography of two centuries earlier, the diagnostic nomenclature is still strikingly different from what would be used today. The diagnostic terms include many ailments that are too vague to be acceptable in modern nomenclature (e.g., debility, chest diseases, fevers), that are diagnosed with different

	No.	Percent		
Consumption, tissick	2636	16.6	Worms	59
Flux, gripes, colic	2112	13.3	French pox	45
Teeth	1643	10.4	Gangrene	44
Convulsions	1637	10.3	Jaundice	40
Fever, ague	1511	9.5	Palsy	37
Aged	863	5.4	Pleurisy	37
Smallpox	843	5.3	Rupture	36
Stillborn	513	3.2	Strangury	30
Rising lights,	447	2.8	Lunatic	27
Stoppage	438	2.8	Fistula	24
Dropsy	340	2.1	Suddenly	23
Rickets	337	2.1	Stone	17
Abortive	280	1.8	Measles	14
Thrush	271	1.7	Rheumatism	13
Surfeit	267	1.7	Quinsy	10
[Not stated]	250	1.6	Gout	7
Accidents, violence	217	1.4	Tympany	7
Childbed	203	1.3	Decay, decline, lethargy	6
Ulcer	167	1.1	Scald head	4
Apoplexy	97	0.6	Cough	2
Evil	87		Asthma	1
Impostume	87		Cholera	1
Cancer	63		Falling sickness	1
Scurvy	60		Spotted fever	1
Total				15,856

Figure 24–5. Causes of death in order of frequency in the 17th century. (From Forbes TR. Yale J Biol Med 1973; Chapter reference 22.)

'Causes'	Number	Percent M	F	'Causes'	Number	Percent M	F
Debility, decay, decline	770	47.1	52.9	Scarlet fever	69	55.1	44.9
Consumption	432	56.9	43.1	Cholera	59	37.3	62.7
Convulsions	253	62.5	37.5	Paralysis, palsy	59	52.5	47.5
Age	252	41.3	58.7	Teeth	56	57.1	42.9
Inflammation	246	53.3	46.7	Heart diseases	55	47.3	52.7
Asthma	221	61.1	38.9	Childbirth	48		100.0
[Not stated]	208	54.8	45.2	Liver diseases	45	55.6	44.4
Brain, water on	183	61.2	38.8	Typhus, putrid fever	42	40.5	59.5
Dropsy	173	38.2	61.8	Insane, lunatic	36	47.2	52.8
Whooping cough	148	41.2	58.8	Croup	30	66.7	33.3
Chest diseases	108	57.4	42.6	Mortification (gangrene)	28	53.6	46.3
Measles	104	51.9	48.1	Cancer	26	11.5	88.5
Accidents and violence	84	72.6	27.4	Coroner's warrant	24	79.2	20.8
Smallpox	84	46.4	53.6	Epilepsy	24	45.8	54.2
Apoplexy	81	55.6	44.4	Throat diseases	14	64.3	35.7
Bowel diseases	80	53.8	46.2	Influenza	10	30.0	70.0
Lung diseases	79	51.9	48.1	Rheumatic fever	10	50.0	50.0
Brain diseases, injuries	74	64.9	35.1	Spasms	10	50.0	50.0
Fevers	73	39.7	60.3	Tumor	10	50.0	50.0

Figure 24–6. Most frequent causes of death, with proportions by gender, in 4513 parish deaths during 1820–1849. (From Forbes TR. J Hist Med 1972; Chapter reference 23.)

standards and criteria (e.g., whooping cough, asthma, rheumatic fever), or that have disappeared because they receive different names (e.g., dropsy, consumption).

In trying to analyze the death certificates of the early 19th century, Farr[24] complained that "each disease has in many instances been denoted by three or four terms, and each term has been applied to as many different diseases; vague, inconvenient names have been employed, and complications have been registered instead of primary diseases." Trying to improve the situation, Farr and Marc D'Espine of Geneva, working under the aegis of the "First Statistical Congress," in 1853 drew up a nosologic classification for international use with death certificate data.[24]

The Farr-D'Espine classification attempted to standardize the diagnostic labels that might be used on death certificates, but no attention was given to the things being labeled. A standard list of names was developed for diagnosis of disease, but no criteria were established for applying the names diagnostically. This criterion-free tradition has been maintained during the many subsequent revisions of the original taxonomy. In its current status, the taxonomy is called *International Classification of Diseases, Clinical Modification* (ICD-CM).[25] It is issued every 10 years as a document that provides names, coding digits, and groupings for the diseases that can be recorded as death certificate data.

The achievement of international agreement on names of diseases is alone so difficult a task that our admiration of the accomplishment should not be mitigated by how much more remains to be done before the ICD taxonomy can be used as a scientific instrument.

24.7.1. *Problems in Classification of Death*

In contemporary patterns of application, the ICD taxonomy for diagnoses in death certificate data contains the following major problems: no standard criteria for making diagnoses; no provision for the impact of secular changes in diagnostic technology and in nosologic concepts of disease; no standard criteria for clinically deciding which of several diagnoses is *the* cause of death; no instruction to clinicians in preparing death certificates; arbitrary instructions for coding clerks to alter the causal sequences recorded by clinicians; arbitrary rearrangements of groupings for diseases; and acceptance of incidence of diagnoses on death certificates as a surrogate for incidence of disease.

These manifold problems are so extensive that they will be discussed here only briefly. Interested readers should consult a thorough critique,[26] written in 1968, and a more recent annotated bibliography[27] of cause-of-death validation studies during 1958–1980.

24.7.1.1. INCONSISTENCIES IN DIAGNOSES BY CLINICIANS

In the absence of diagnostic criteria that are distinctly specified, widely disseminated, and universally applied, two clinicians observing the same clinical condition may give it different names. For example, clinicians in the United Kingdom often use the name *chronic bronchitis* for an ailment that might be called *pulmonary emphysema* or *chronic obstructive lung disease* in the United States. Two clinicians who both use the name *pulmonary emphysema* might apply the diagnosis differently according to their individual requirements in the clinical, radiographic, and laboratory standards for emphysema.

24.7.1.2. CHANGES PRODUCED BY AVAILABILITY AND DISSEMINATION OF TECHNOLOGY

A different source of variation is the availability and applicability of diagnostic technology. If a disease requires specific morphologic or other paraclinical evidence to be diagnosed, its diagnosis will not be made in locations where the technology is not available or not used. For example, many lung tumors and other internal neoplasms will be detected or undetected according to the application of appropriate methods of imaging, endoscopy, biopsy, cytology, and surgical exploration.

The availability of diagnostic technology may also change the occurrence rate of certain diseases by changing the criteria required for diagnosis. Thus, many clinical conditions that formerly received a diagnosis of pulmonary tuberculosis or gastric cancer could no longer receive that diagnosis when it began to require specific radiographic and microscopic evidence.

24.7.1.3. CHANGES PRODUCED BY ALTERED NOSOLOGIC CONCEPTS AND METHODS

The rise or fall in rates of certain diseases may reflect changes in clinical concepts of nosology rather than variability in clinical decisions or improvements in technology. For example, the disappearance of dropsy, one of the great killer diseases of the 19th century, was not accompanied by any claims that the triumph was produced by the concomitant activities of the sanitary movement, which had improved the supply of water and disposition of sewage. Most analysts of the data recognized that dropsy was being called by another name (such as congestive heart failure or venous insufficiency).

During the past half century, many other ailments have been extirpated by changes in nosologic identification, increased by altered technologic tests and concepts, or "newly" discovered. Beeson[28] has described a series of diseases that seem to have vanished between the 1927 and the 1977 editions of a major textbook of medicine. Other ailments such as systemic lupus erythematosus, Kaposi's sarcoma, and end-stage renal disease have become far more common than before, and yet other diseases, such as Legionnaire's disease, clear cell adenocarcinoma of the vagina, toxic shock syndrome, and graft-vs.-host disease, seem to have been newly discovered.

In all these circumstances, the contributions of nosologic and technologic identification are difficult to separate from real changes in the occurrence of the disease. When chlorosis and Banti's syndrome "disappeared," the ailments probably received other names. The modern rise in lupus erythematosus is readily ascribed to better knowledge about the disease and better methods of detection. The rise in end-stage renal disease can be attributed to the increased data and statistics produced by federally sponsored methods of paying for treatment. The rise in Kaposi's sarcoma, however, is probably real, occurring as a consequence of certain homosexual patterns of behavior.

Graft-vs.-host disease is obviously new, because it could not have occurred (in its current nosologic concept) before the frequent use of transplanted tissue and cells. Legionnaire's disease, however, is newly identified but probably not really new, because it has been retrospectively detected in many previous circumstances in which sera were preserved and available for testing. Clear cell vaginal adenocarcinoma also occurred long before it was associated with in-utero exposure to stilbestrol, although it formerly often received different diagnostic names and was much less likely to be discovered because young women did not receive gynecologic examinations as frequently as today. The newness of toxic shock syndrome is also uncertain. Most older clinicians today can recall seeing patients years ago who were diagnosed as having something else but who, in retrospect, probably had toxic shock syndrome. The occurrence rate of toxic shock syndrome is also uncertain. It seemed to decline after a particular brand of tampons was removed from the market, but the decline seems to have occurred mainly because the monitoring federal agency reduced its surveillance. At state health agencies that continued active surveillance, the incidence of toxic shock syndrome seems unchanged.

The distinctive roles of nosology, technology, and surveillance seldom receive adequate attention when data analysts become excited about patterns of rise or fall for a particular disease. The pattern is regularly ascribed to an external maneuver, which is then credited for the fall or indicted for the rise. The causal implications are almost never accompanied by evidence to rule out the possibility that the entire statistical pattern is an artefact.

24.7.1.4. INACCURACIES IN CLINICAL DIAGNOSES OF CAUSE OF DEATH

The advances of modern technology have provided a precise identification of many diseases, but have not solved the problem of determining which disease was the actual cause of death. Clinicians may often disagree about this choice; and the choices may often disagree with what is found when necropsy yields a clear-cut answer.[29] The problem is dramatically evident in adults with sudden unexpected deaths. Although usually ascribed to coronary artery disease, these deaths are commonly due to other causes, which remain unidentified if necropsy is not performed.[30]

24.7.1.5. INCONSISTENCIES IN CHOOSING A CAUSE OF DEATH

In filling out a death certificate, a clinician is asked to record two fundamental sets of decisions in causality. The first decision involves choosing a sequential chain of diseases that led to death. Thus, the death certificate asks the clinician to cite:

Part I. Death was caused by
Immediate cause (a) _____
Due to (b) _____
Due to (c) _____

The (a), (b), (c) elements chosen for this trio should give the sequence of events that led to death, specifying last the underlying cause that initiated the train of events.

The second decision asks for the following:

Part II: Other significant conditions contributing to death but not related to the terminal disease condition given in Part Ia.

These requests do not allow a clinician to supply information that involves straightforward observation and direct evidence. There is no room to state what diseases were known to be present in the dead patient; and the clinician is specifically asked *not* to report symptoms or mode of dying. Instead, the assignment is to prepare a sequence of inferences that will seem suitably plausible to someone who reviews the death certificate. This request for a sequential chain of inference, rather than an account of observed evidence, is one of the fundamental scientific flaws of the death certificate process.

A clinician frequently cannot be sure of which disease among several was the prime cause of death, and he often has great difficulty in deciding how to arrange the order of contributory and unrelated diseases. Because each decision can be made only from knowledge of the patient's clinical course, and because no clinical criteria currently exist for evaluating the sequential causes of fatality, two different clinicians observing the same clinical situation and reaching the same diagnostic conclusions about diseases may nevertheless differ in the choice of which disease has caused death. The problem is magnified by the absence of systematic training or even discussion in most medical schools today to provide students with concepts of clinical principles to use in preparing death certificates.

What makes the problem of multiple diseases particularly treacherous in vital statistics is that only a single disease—the one listed as the main cause of death—is chosen for the tabulations. For example, if a patient depressed by an incurable chronic disease commits suicide, the suicide may be listed as the cause of death, and the chronic disease may not appear in the mortality statistics; if a patient with a stroke develops a fatal aspiration pneumonia, the death may be recorded as due to the stroke, and the pneumonia may be omitted from the tabulation of lethal diseases.

A separate problem in the sequential listing of cases arises from nosologic concepts about relationships of disease. For patients who have both cardiovascular disease and diabetes mellitus, the diabetes may be listed as an associated disorder by some clinicians and as an underlying cause by others. The frequency of occurrence of diabetes can rise or fall according to this decision about nosologic co-morbidity.

24.7.1.6. ABSENCE OF NECROPSY CONFIRMATION

Because necropsy is often performed for deaths at academic medical centers, the assumption is sometimes made that most death certificate diagnoses have been confirmed by necropsy. This assumption is wrong for at least four reasons: (1) necropsies are now performed much less frequently than before at academic institutions; (2) the ecologic data that receive statistical analyses come from all deaths, not just from those at academic centers, and fewer than 20% of all deaths (in the United States) have received necropsy; (3) most death certificates are prepared and submitted to state health agencies before necropsy and are seldom altered after necropsy; and (4) the pathologist may be just as inconsistent as the clinician in choosing a single cause of death from the diverse diseases noted at necropsy.

24.7.1.7. PROBLEMS IN HEALTH AGENCY GUIDELINES FOR CODING

The death certificates prepared by clinicians do not become statistical data until appropriately processed by the health agencies to which the certificates are submitted.

Although the clinician who prepared the certificate may list a sequence of causes leading to death, these agencies use their own criteria for reviewing the list of cited diseases to choose one of them as *the* cause of death. The clinician's statements on the death certificate thus become a list of possibilities to be organized into a correct rank and sequence, as determined by the data coder at the agency. The criteria for these ranking or re-ranking decisions are contained in documents having such names as *Manual of Joint Causes of Death* or *Nosology Guidelines*. In these documents, diseases are arranged into hierarchical orders and sequences of lethality that determine the single disease to be designated as *the* cause of death.

Most clinicians do not realize that their conscientious attempts to allocate diagnoses in the format of the death certificate can be greatly altered by these arbitrary systems of coding and hierarchical ranking. Although the systems are intended to be reasonable, their application may sometimes produce capricious or shocking changes in what really happened to the patient. Because the existence of these subsequent coding activities is generally unknown, their effects on statistical tabulations have seldom been investigated. To appreciate these effects would require reading the extensive details of the coding instructions, envisioning what would be done to the information listed in diverse death certificates, and checking what actually occurs.

For example, one of the coding rules says that "If there is more than one sequence (terminating in the condition first entered on the certificate), select the underlying cause of the first mentioned sequence." With this principle, when the patient dies of an anesthetic or surgical "therapeutic misadventure," the underlying disease may be cited as a cause of death. In this way, the statistical tabulations may include fatalities ascribed to such lethal ailments as *hemorrhoids, cataract, dental caries, strabismus,* or *bunion.*

In an investigation of death certificates coded for coal miners in the United Kingdom, Cochrane and Moore[31] found that deaths due to pneumoconiosis were substantially undercounted because pneumoconiosis, although cited on a death certificate, would often be supplanted by chronic bronchitis, which has a higher priority in the coding system.

My own favorite among the peculiarities of arbitrary coding is the following death certificate, which has been used as an illustration for the coding clerks:

Male, 75 years

I (a) Chronic congestive heart failure 2 yr.
  (b) Arteriosclerotic heart and cardiovascular disease 4 yr.
  (c) Carcinoma of lung (pneumonectomy) 8 yr.

A clinical reader of this death certificate would recognize that it has been filled out improperly. The lung cancer should have been omitted or perhaps cited under Section II, as an associated disease. Nevertheless, because the diagnosis was placed in I(c), it becomes regarded as an underlying cause of the ailments listed in I(a) and I(b). The therapeutic triumph of the pneumonectomy becomes lost, and the occurrence of cardiac disease falls, as the death is ascribed to the cancer because of coding instructions that say the following: "The fact that surgery had been performed for a malignant neoplasm is not evidence that malignancy did not exist at the time of death."[32]

24.7.1.8. INCONSISTENCIES IN HEALTH AGENCY GUIDELINES FOR CODING

Because the hierarchical rankings have been changed at regular intervals, the occurrence rate of certain diseases can rise or fall according to the arbitrary positions they are assigned in the nosologic rankings. For example, for a patient diagnosed as having both *nephritis* and *cardiac disease,* the selected cause of death would have been nephritis during 1900 to 1912 and cardiac disease during 1913 to 1924. If the clinician had used a somewhat different nomenclature to list these two joint diagnoses as *uremia* and *cardiac insufficiency,* the cause of death would have been reversed. It would have been cited as cardiac during 1900 to 1912 and renal during 1913 to 1924.

Beyond these obvious caprices, the listed rankings can be applied with substantial observer variability. In one of the few studies of this problem, the statistical offices of several different countries were asked to choose the primary cause of death from the diseases cited on the same large series of death certificates. According to the investigators, "the results showed a disagreement great enough to largely nullify the comparability of national mortality statistics."[33]

24.7.1.9. PROBLEMS IN GROUPS AND RUBRICS

When the international classification of diseases is revised every 10 years, the numerical codes and rubrics are altered, and certain diseases may be rearranged, consolidated, or shifted from the group of one coding rubric to another. For example, in one recent arrangement, the number 527 was used for *emphysema, atelectasis, hernia of lung, mediastinitis,* and *acute pulmonary edema.* If acutely decompensated cardiac patients without lung disease are included in this rubric, the occurrence of cardiac disease can fall fallaciously while pulmonary disease appears to rise.

Another problem in the international classification schemes is the difficulty of assigning a *single* category of classification to diseases containing different etiologic and morphologic components. Should *bacterial endocarditis* be listed as an infectious or cardiac disease? Is *cerebral arteriosclerosis* to be counted as a neurologic or degenerative disorder? As Harold Dorn pointed out,[34] "Substantial changes in the number of deaths assigned to specific causes of death can be brought about by changes in coding rules, even though the basic classification of disease remains unchanged."

24.7.1.10. DECISIONS REGARDING INCIDENCE OF DISEASES

The foregoing difficulties produce substantial obstacles for the scientific credibility of any of the diverse trends, associations, or other mathematical manipulations derived from vital statistics data about individual diseases. Nevertheless, the information exists and, like any other statistical data, it becomes used in diverse ways.

Perhaps the most scientifically peculiar aspect of this usage is the decision to let the death certificate codings represent the *incidence* of different diseases. This strategy grossly underestimates the occurrence and importance of the many arthritic, gastroenterologic, metabolic, genetic, neurologic, and psychiatric ailments that can be major sources of human morbidity, although they are seldom directly lethal. Furthermore, because death certificates may not be kept confidential, clinicians are often reluctant to list alcoholism, sexually transmitted diseases, suicide, or other ailments that may be embarrassing to the deceased patient or to the family.

24.7.1.11. PROBLEMS IN DEMOGRAPHIC DATA

Aside from the occurrence and date of death itself, the only generally trustworthy information on a death certificate is demographic information about the person's gender, age, and place of death.

Other types of demographic data are difficult to analyze because of their variability within the patient. For example, in a highly mobile society, should a person's *place of residence* be cited as the site of the most recent home or the site where most of life was lived? If a person has had several different occupations, including a job held after retirement, which one should be cited as *usual occupation*? Will a citation as *steel-mill worker* include someone who was a watchman at the factory as well as someone exposed directly to the furnaces?

Finally, the problem of race is no more solved in vital statistics than in social relations. In current classifications, someone with eight black great-grandparents will emerge looking black and be cited as *black*. Someone with eight white great-grandparents will emerge looking white and be cited as *white*. Someone who had one black and seven white great-grandparents, however, is more white than black but may still be listed as *black*. Thus, in a racially mixed society, the term *black* may often be more indicative of socioeconomic status, which is not entered on death certificates, than of the recorded race.

24.7.2. *Evaluations of Death Certificate Data*

Whenever the quality of death certificate diagnoses has been evaluated, the res· ˌˌs have been scientifically dismal. Aside from the major inconsistencies previously noted among international agencies, the few tests of observer variability in clinicians preparing diagnostic citations have shown discrepancies so great that the investigators raised serious doubts about the use of present death certificate data for research purposes. In a recent study[35] of about 48,000 cancer deaths in hospitalized patients, the underlying cause coded on the death certificate was found to be accurate for only 65%. In a separate review[36] of data sustaining the diagnoses on 1362 certificates on which death was attributed to cardiovascular disease, 12% of the major diagnoses were regarded as well established and 41% seemed reasonable. The remaining 47% of diagnoses were regarded as inadequately supported or incorrect. The investigators concluded that "there should be another basis for the compilation of mortality statistics."

These distressing results come only from investigations of *false-positive* diagnoses. The rates of error would be substantially raised if they included the many *false-negative* diagnoses for diseases that are undetected during life and first found—if found at all—at necropsy. In addition, a huge number of diseases such as diabetes mellitus or lupus erythematosus, which are not demonstrable by histopathology, may never be recognized if not adequately sought during life.

About 15 years ago, I showed a simple mathematical formula for demonstrating the difference between the true occurrence of a disease, T, and its diagnosis, D, on death certificates.[26] The formula is $D = T - A - U - G + F$. In this formula, the F group consists of people with false-positive diagnoses, and the false-negative group contains people in the A, U, and G categories. The A group has not received appropriate medical surveillance; the U group, although clinically examined, was not suspected of having the disease; and the G group had negative results when tested for the disease. With changes in medical care and technology, changing values of A, U, G, and F can lead to substantial changes in D, although the true value, T, is unaltered.

24.7.3. *Attempts to Improve Statistics for Occurrence of Disease*

To avoid relying on death certificate data, epidemiologists have established special registries to collect data about diseases identified in living people rather than at death. The main diseases under scrutiny have been cancers; and the denominator data for occurrence rates depend on census estimations for a particular region. The numerator data for these morbidity rates have been obtained in two different ways. In one approach, a regional tumor registry that has been effective in eliciting voluntary cooperation from the clinicians (and other nosocomial sources) in the region becomes the central source of data. In the second approach, the investigators create an *ad hoc* registry by arranging to receive data from hospitals, laboratories, and other regional sites where the diagnostic tests are performed.

By improving the thoroughness with which identified cancers appear as statistical data, these new techniques can be expected to raise the occurrence rates for many cancers. Because of problems cited previously, however, the investigators will have great difficulty in determining whether changes in the occurrence rates represent a changing incidence of cancer, the effects of screening campaigns, or the impact of improved diagnostic technology.

24.8. THE SCIENTIFIC ROLE OF HETERODEMIC RESEARCH

Because of all the foregoing problems, the important societal and legal roles of death certificates are accompanied by relatively few data that are satisfactory for scientific purposes. As Raymond Pearl[24] pointed out, the scientifically trustworthy information is confined to age, gender, total deaths (i.e., from *all* causes), and deaths ascribed to a few obvious individual causes, such as trauma and homicide. Using this type of information, demographers, sociologists, and actuaries of life insurance companies have been able to make valuable and important analyses of data based on all deaths.

The analyses that are much more difficult to accept scientifically are appraisals based on cancer, cardiac disease, and other individual causes of death. The elaborate analyses, maps, and statistical correlations drawn from these investigations often seem as incongruous in medical science as the methods of alchemy would be if applied in molecular biology.

The fundamental scientific improvements needed in death certificates have been discussed elsewhere[26] and are too extensive to be repeated here. The point to be considered now is whether heterodemic analyses for any individual diseases—beyond trauma and homicide—are trustworthy enough to warrant scientific credibility. Because several such circumstances may occur, their conditions and criteria will be cited here.

24.8.1. *Standards for Acceptable Relationships*

The discussion in this section contains specifications for conditions in which scientific credibility might be given to heterodemic data for a proposed cause-effect relationship. The suggestions are not intended to be complete or definitive. They can be regarded as a first draft for improvement in future research.

24.8.1.1. ACCEPTABLE NUMERATORS

An individual disease can be accepted for numerator data if it is clinically overt and routinely reported when present, and if the reporting system enables all or most instances of the disease to be detected. For example, fracture of the hip may not always be cited on death certificates but is clinically overt and routinely recorded. If an active registry is maintained for these reports, the registry data can be used to denote incidence.

24.8.1.2. ACCEPTABLE CANCERS

A well-run cancer registry, which maintains active surveillance in a particular ecologic region, can be used to supply data about the occurrence of *certain* cancers in that region. The acceptable cancers, however, are relatively few. Because they must be clinically overt, they would be confined to solid tumors involving the skin, limbs, or appendages of the body. For example, osteosarcomas and chondrosarcomas of the arm or leg are unlikely to escape detection when they occur. Malignant melanoma, breast cancer, cancer of the vulva (not vagina), and testicular cancer are also easy to detect, but their diagnostic rate will often depend on the screening techniques with which patients examine themselves. Results for all other cancers in internal organs are relatively untrustworthy because they vary too greatly with both screening procedures and diagnostic technology.

24.8.1.3. OTHER CLINICAL EVENTS

Dramatic, non-oncologic clinically overt events—such as ruptured ectopic pregnancy, the classic presentation of acute myocardial infarction, and stroke—are likely to be cited accurately when they are causes of death, provided the citation is a *clinical* observation rather than a morphologic inference. Thus, unless specific morphologic evidence is available (from appropriate imaging or other techniques) to show bleeding and an anatomic location, the diagnosis of *stroke* is much more trustworthy than the diagnosis of *hemorrhage from lenticulostriate artery*.

24.8.1.4. SURVEILLANCE AND DETECTION

A rise or fall in a heterodemic rate of occurrence for a disease cannot be related to any particular maneuver unless the mechanism used for surveillance and detection of the disease has been unchanged. For example, recent changes in death rates for coronary disease have produced rejoicing in the United States and the United Kingdom, where the rates have declined, and concern or chagrin in Switzerland and Sweden, where the rates have increased.[37-39] The decline in rates has usually been attributed to improvements in such maneuvers as diet, smoking, or other aspects of life style—but inadequate attention has been given to the effect of nosographic customs, national systems of ranking and coding death certificate data, and changes in the ICD rubrics of classification.

24.8.1.5. CREDIBILITY OF NEGATIVE ETIOLOGIC ASSOCIATIONS

If a disease meets the identification criteria noted in points 1 to 3, a negative or negligible heterodemic association with changes in a proposed etiologic agent can be reasonable evidence to exonerate the agent as a cause of the disease. Thus, if a rising sales curve for agent X is *not* accompanied by a rise in the occurrence rate of disease D, or if disease D shows a steady rise in occurrence while the sales curve of X remains flat, it seems unlikely that X is a cause of D.

24.8.1.6. CREDIBILITY OF POSITIVE THERAPEUTIC ASSOCIATIONS

Positive heterodemic associations between diseases and therapeutic agents leave so much to be desired that they cannot be regarded as scientific evidence of etiologic causation. If suspicions arise that a therapeutic agent is noxious, homodemic research (even if only a retrospective case-control study) can easily be performed. If an investigator will not make the effort to do a suitable homodemic study, the heterodemic analyses may often be regarded as statistical acrobatics rather than scientific investigation.

24.8.2. *Examples of Useful and Harmful Heterodemic Studies*

In 1974, Hadden and McDevitt[40] employed heterodemic data to investigate the popular belief that stress is in some way implicated in the pathogenesis of thyrotoxicosis. Using a technique of therapeutic auditing, in which the occurrence of a disease is determined from National Health Service prescriptions, the investigators noted the incidence of treated thyrotoxicosis during two 3-year periods, 1966 to 1968 and 1969 to 1971, before and after the beginning of the civil unrest in Northern Ireland in 1969. The occurrence of thyrotoxicosis was noted not from death certificates but from reports of patients treated with antithyroid drug therapy, radioiodine, or thyroid surgery. Using careful methods to distinguish courses of treatment and treated patients, and applying cautious clinical reasoning to account for possible sources of bias, the authors found no difference in the incidence rates of thyrotoxicosis for the two secular periods. The conclusion was that no evidence had been found to support the concept that environmental stress causes thyrotoxicosis.

In 1978, after research in mice had raised the specter that injection-site sarcomas might be caused by alum-adsorbed allergenic extracts, Jekel, Freeman, and Meigs[41] performed a heterodemic study of data in the Connecticut Tumor Registry. Because the allergenic extract for humans is injected almost exclusively in the upper arm, the investigators looked for the ratio of occurrence of upper to lower extremity sarcomas before and after the introduction of the alum-absorbed extract in 1963. No changes were found that could be related to the introduction of the new treatment. Because sarcomas of the extremity seldom escape diagnostic detection and because the Connecticut Tumor Registry maintains excellent surveillance, the results seem scientifically credible in demonstrating no apparent effect for the suspected agent.

During 1975 to 1977, a public furor about industrial carcinogens was raised when data-dredging activities produced heterodemic associations between cancer mortality in U.S. counties and the industries located in those counties. Excess mortality from diverse cancers was ascribed to residence near the petrochemical industry and various other industries. In 1980, however, Hearey and coworkers[42] checked these heterodemic alarms by doing a cohort study, examining medical and domiciliary records for a 10% sample of 1.2 million people receiving medical care in the Kaiser Foundation Health Plan. The results indicated that place of residence near petrochemical industries is not associated with increased cancer risk. In accordance with general custom for these matters, no publicity was given to the cohort refutation of the heterodemic contentions.

24.9. SYNOPSIS

In heterodemic research, the basic biologic unit is a group of people rather than the individual persons examined in all other forms of clinical and epidemiologic investigation. Information about these groups is collected and supplied by civil and commercial agencies working with methods, criteria, and standards that were not determined by the investigator.

The second-hand information is usually arranged as statistical associations between occurrence of an alleged maneuver and the rate of an outcome event in a general population. The link for these occurrences can be their concomitant values in different ecologic regions or in different points of secular time in the same region. The data under association usually come from three different sources. The maneuver variable depends on information about sales, usage, or exposure to a particular agent. The outcome is a rate whose denominators come from census estimations and whose numerators come from disease registries or, more commonly, from death certificates.

Although particularly easy to do, the research contains almost none of the safeguards used to improve accuracy and eliminate bias in other forms of scientific investigation. The numbers that are calculated or estimated may often be misleading despite (and sometimes because of) efforts to standardize the results. The indirectness of the associations and the ecologic fallacies that can occur in large groups will often provide evidence to support erroneous causal hypotheses.

The demographic data recorded on death certificates can be used scientifically for various actuarial and public health purposes, but the diseases listed as causes of death are usually too untrustworthy for serious analysis. Although changes in the death certificate occurrence of individual diseases are often ascribed to various maneuvers in public health or clinical therapy, many other sources are seldom adequately excluded as possible causes of the changes. The sources include alterations in the names and concepts of disease, altered methods of technologic identification, changes in the hierarchical nosologic system used by public health agencies to rank the importance of the diseases listed on a death certificate, and changes in the categories established and revised in the international system of disease classification.

Because of these problems, analyses of death certificate diagnoses have relatively little scientific credibility, although heterodemic data about disease may be trustworthy in certain special circumstances in which careful criteria are fulfilled for the information or the proposed association.

EXERCISES

Exercises 24.1. Write a brief critique of the way the results are presented in Figures 24–2 and 24–3. Do you regard these presentations as an adequate way of displaying evidence? If not, what features of the data are ambiguous or unsatisfactory, and what corrections would you suggest?

Exercise 24.2. The four subexercises here refer to claims that have been made in heterodemic studies. The sources are cited with reference numbers, in case you want to review them, although the questions that follow can be answered without such a review:

    24.2.1. The rate of occurrence of colon cancer increases as average income rises. (Data come from an association between identified cases of colon cancer in a Nebraska county and income status of people in census tracts in which the cases live.[43])

    24.2.2. Ventricular septal defects may be caused by an environmental agent that is particularly prevalent in winter and in cities. (Data come from an association between VSD cases found in a New England regional cardiac program and their months of birth, county of residence, and population counts in that county.[4])

    24.2.3. "Excessive consumption of animal protein may . . . encourage malignant changes."[2] (Data come from an ecologic association between lymphoma deaths and per capita bovine protein consumption in different countries.)

    24.2.4. An etiologic link exists between cancer of the penis and cancer of the cervix.[44] (Data come from a high correlation found in China for mortality rates between cancer of the penis and cancer of the cervix.)

If we assume that none of these relationships is actually true, what types of innate bias might account for the data that led to each of the four claims?

Exercise 24.3. During the past decade, the state of New Jersey has received the unenviable reputation of being a "cancer alley." The occurrence rate of cancer is higher in New Jersey than in any of the 49 other states in the U.S. Because the cancer rates also seem to be highest in parts of New Jersey that are heavily industrialized, the toxic effects and exposures of industry have generally been accused of causing the high carcinogenesis. The new governor of the state of New Jersey has appointed you to be a one-person committee charged with performing a thorough scientific review of the evidence and with making recommendations. What would be your first steps in dealing with this assignment?

Exercise 24.4. The references listed below, in their order of chronologic appearance, contain reports of a prominent unresolved controversy arising from heterodemic data about the role of bronchodilators in producing deaths due to asthma. The reports can be assigned to different members of a class and can lead to an interesting debate about the dispute, which can be divided into three chronologic periods. References 1, 2, and 4 to 7 represent the original case for the "prosecution" in the U.K.; and reference 3 gives the "defense" in Australia. The claims on behalf of the prosecution are then extended in reference 8 and counterattacked in references 9 to 11. Finally, references 12 to 15 represent the later resolution of clinical opinion, counterattacked by prosecution epidemiologists in reference 16.

1. Speizer FE, Doll R, Heaf P. Observations on recent increase in mortality from asthma. Br Med J 1968;1:335–9 (Feb 10).
2. Speizer FE, Doll R, Heaf P, Strang LB. Investigation into use of drugs preceding death from asthma. Br Med J 1968;1:339–43 (Feb 10).
3. Gandevia B. The changing pattern of mortality from asthma in Australia: 2. Mortality and modern therapy. Med J Aust 1968;1:884–91 (May 25).
4. Speizer FE, Doll R. A century of asthma deaths in young people. Br Med J 1968;1:245–6 (July 27).
5. Inman WHW, Adelstein AM. Rise and fall of asthma mortality in England and Wales in relation to use of pressurised aerosols. Lancet 1969;2:280–5 (Aug 9).
6. Editorial. Aerosol bronchodilators and asthma mortality. Lancet 1969;2:305–7 (Aug 9).
7. Fraser PM, Speizer FE, Waters DM, et al. The circumstances preceding death from asthma in young people in 1968 to 1969. Br J Dis Chest 1971;65:71–84.
8. Stolley PD. Asthma mortality: Why the United States was spared an epidemic of deaths due to asthma. Am Rev Respir Dis 1972;105:883–90.
9. Gandevia B. Changing patterns of morbidity and mortality in relation to isoproterenol therapy of asthma. In: Isoproterenol therapy symposium. Ann Allergy 1973;31:30–4 (Jan).
10. Herxheimer H. (Letter to Editor) Asthma mortality. Am Rev Resp Dis 1973;107:306.
11. Gandevia B. (Letter to Editor) Asthma mortality. Am Rev Resp Dis 1973;107:307.
12. Spilker B. (Letter to Editor) Increase in asthma mortality. Br Med J 1973;2:171–2 (Oct 20).
13. Crompton GK. (Letter to Editor) Deaths in asthma. Br Med J 1975;2:458 (Nov 22).
14. Lewis HE. (Letter to Editor) Deaths in asthma. Br Med J 1975;2:650 (Dec 13).
15. Editorial. Fatal asthma. Lancet 1979;2:337–8 (Aug 18).
16. Stolley PD, Schinnon R. (Letter to Editor) Fatal asthma. Lancet 1979;2:897 (Oct 27).

Exercise 24.5. Using any suitable collection of data, such as the Statistical Abstract of the United States or publications issued by the National Center for Health Statistics, please assemble heterodemic collections of data to perform the following two research projects.

24.5.1. Demonstrate the most bizarre relationship you can construct from the data.

24.5.2. Demonstrate a plausible relationship that has not hitherto been shown, and explain why the relationship is plausible.

Exercise 24.6. Which, if any, of the diseases and casualties noted in Figures 24–4 and 24–5 as causes of death in 1632 or in the later 17th century might still be accepted and used as causes of death today?

Exercise 24.7. Which, if any, of the causes of death noted in Figure 24–6 for 1820 to 1849 would serve as nonspecific ailments that could be diagnosed more precisely today, thus raising the rates of the associated diagnosis?

Exercise 24.8. What instruction did you receive in medical school about the existence of an international classification of disease? What instruction did you receive about how to complete a death certificate? Do you believe such instruction should be given to students? If so, how would you arrange it?

Exercise 24.9. Each of the 22 examples in the death certificate entries that follow has been employed as a teaching case in material issued by the U.S. National Center for Health Statistics. The statements below are verbatim copies of material issued by the NCHS. In each case, which entry would you code as the main cause of death? (The object here is to determine what seems clinically sensible, not necessarily for you to employ the rules or decision tables of the NCHS. Your answers will later be compared with the official answers issued by the NCHS.)

(1) I   (a) Fatty degeneration of liver   1 yr.
         (b) Cerebral hemorrhage   2 days
         (c) Chronic alcoholism
     II Large bowel obstruction

(2) I   (a) Esophageal varices and congestive heart failure
         (b) Cirrhosis of liver and chronic rheumatic heart disease

(3) I   (a) Rheumatic and arteriosclerotic heart disease

(4) I   (a) Diabetes
         (b) Arteriosclerosis

(5) I   (a) Renal failure
         (b) Heart failure

(6) I   (a) Pneumonia
         (b) Cleft palate

(7) I   (a) Heart failure
         (b) Curvature of spine
         (c) Rickets in childhood

(8) I   (a) Parkinsonism
         (b) Arteriosclerosis

(9) I   (a) Arteriosclerosis
     II Parkinsonism

(10) Female, 70 years
     I   (a) Pneumonia
         (b) Aspiration of food
         (c) Cerebral arteriosclerosis

(11) Male, 83 years
     I   (a) Arteriosclerosis, generalized   10 yr.
         (b) Myocardial and renal failure   1 yr.
         (c) Chronic interstitial nephritis   12 yr.

(12) Male, 56 years
     I   (a) Cardiac arrest   1 min.
         (b) Coronary embolism   3 mo.
         (c) Cholelithiasis

(13) Male, 84 years
     I   (a) Cirrhosis of liver with congestive failure   4 yr.
         (b) Generalized arteriosclerosis   3 yr.
         (c) Diabetes   15 yr.

(14) Male, 65 years
I   (a) Bronchopneumonia, right lung   4 days
    (b) Chronic pyelonephritis and emphysema, right 10 yr.
    (c) Hemiplegia, right side   45 yr.

(15) Female, 87 years
I   (a) Acute myocardial infarction   2 wk.
    (b) Fracture of left hip   8 mo.
    (c) Congestive failure, flu   2 wk.

(16) Male, 3 years
I   (a) Infection
    (b) Treatment delayed of
    (c) Small cut on shoulder
        Accident: Yard—child stumbled and fell on electric lawn-
        mower his mother was using

(17) Female, 65 years
I   (a) Pulmonary edema
    (b) Uremia, chronic renal disease
    (c) Hypertensive vascular disease

(18) Male, 58 years
I   (a) Confluent bronchopneumonia
    (b) Bacterial endocarditis aortic valve
    (c) Rheumatic heart disease

(19) Male, 16 years
I (a) Aspiration of vomitus   momentary
   (b) Gastroenteritis and pneumonitis
   (c) Influenza
II Muscular dystrophy—severe deformity

(20) Male, 47 years
I   (a) Dehydration severe   hours
    (b) Vomiting
II Mental deficiency

(21) Female, 74 years
I   (a) Congestive heart disease   2 days
    (b) Arteriosclerotic heart disease and
    (c) Splenectomy 5 days before death
II Reticulum cell sarcoma—spleen

(22) Female, 63 years
I (a) Pulmonary embolism—coronary artery disease
   (b) Knee surgery—3 weeks prior
II Paranoia—arteriosclerotic heart vascular disease

CHAPTER REFERENCES

1. Armstrong, 1975; 2. Cunningham, 1976; 3. Beral, 1976; 4. Rothman, 1974; 5. Mancuso, 1974; 6. Keys, 1953; 7. Yerushalmy, 1957; 8. Anonymous, 1977; 9. "Minerva," 1977; 10. Yerushalmy, 1951; 11. Hickey, 1980; 12. Fleiss, 1981; 13. Brenner, 1979; 14. Bunn, 1979; 15. Kasl, 1979; 16. Lew, 1979; 17. Gravelle, 1981; 18. Reid, 1975; 19. Selvin, 1958; 20. Oreglia, 1977; 21. Graunt, 1662; 22. Forbes, 1973; 23. Forbes, 1972; 24. Pearl, 1940; 25. International Classification of Diseases, 1978; 26. Feinstein, 1968; 27. Gittlesohn, 1982; 28. Beeson, 1980; 29. Medical Services Study Group, 1978; 30. Lundberg, 1979; 31. Cochrane, 1981; 32. National Center for Health Statistics, 1968; 33. Dorn, 1964; 34. Dorn, 1961; 35. Percy, 1981; 36. Moriyama, 1966; 37. Levy, 1982; 38. Heller, 1983; 39. Welin, 1983; 40. Hadden, 1974; 41. Jekel, 1978; 42. Hearey, 1980; 43. Lynch, 1975; 44. Rogan, 1983.

PART SIX

EVALUATION OF PROCESSES

The domain of *health services research* was developed to deal with issues in the distribution, delivery, costs, and quality of medical care. After determining the frequency with which people receive optimum forms of medical care, health services investigators try to develop methods of raising that frequency while lowering its expense.

An immediate problem in such research is to define *optimum care*. When several competing tactics are available to manage a particular clinical condition, which one is best? Although a randomized trial is the preferred method of answering this question, relatively few tactics have been studied with randomized trials. The number of clinical conditions and managerial strategies that require evaluation is much greater than our ability to conduct an experimentally designed test for each condition and strategy. Furthermore, even when randomized trials are done, they do not always produce unequivocal answers to the questions.

Accordingly, health services researchers have been forced to rely on nonexperimental evidence. Because this evidence contains all the pitfalls described in previous chapters, investigators who want to study the delivery of optimum care would be stymied by the problems of obtaining suitable data to show that the care is optimum. To avoid these problems and to focus on questions of delivery rather than efficacy, the investigators often establish arbitrary standards for optimum management of clinical conditions. The standards are chosen as sensibly as possible; and conformity with those standards is used to denote satisfactory performance in giving care.

When the standards are unaccompanied by direct evidence of their value in producing optimum results, the appraisals are directed at the process rather than the outcome of patient care. To distinguish this difference in goals, the name *process research* has often been used for audits and other appraisals of management strategies in which the focus has been a clinician's performance rather than a patient's change.

Many other evaluations in medical research, however, are also concerned with a process rather than with a cause-effect impact. We evaluate a process when we check the accuracy of a diagnostic test; when we compare the variability of radiologists or pathologists in interpreting images and tissues; when we determine a patient's compliance in maintaining a prescribed pharmaceutical regimen; and when we test a candidate's decisions in an examination given to check clinical competence for purposes of academic grading, medical licensure, or specialty board certification.

If each of these topics in process research received extensive discussion, this text would become too great a burden to read (as well as to write). Consequently, readers who are particularly interested in the study of compliance[1, 2] or in the psychometric methods[3, 4] used for clinical competence are urged to seek other sources of discussion. The three chapters presented here on process research are concerned with marker procedures, observer variability, and audits of quality of care.

REFERENCES

1. Haynes, 1979; 2. DiMatteo, 1982; 3. Barro, 1973; 4. Levine, 1978.

Chapter 25

Diagnostic and Spectral Markers

Although the name *diagnostic test* is commonly applied to the phantasmagoria of laboratory, radiographic, electrographic, and other paraclinical procedures that are ordered in modern medical practice, the results are often used for many clinical decisions beyond diagnosis alone. Some of the decisions deal with prognostic estimations or therapeutic choices; others relate to the evaluation of post-therapeutic change or the provision of reassurance for clinicians and patients.

For example, a radionuclide scan of bones is used for the staging with which prognosis is predicted in patients with cancer; a test of bacterial sensitivity to antibiotics is used to choose treatment; an alteration of erythrocyte sedimentation rate or of blood glucose will indicate the regulatory control achieved in the treatment of a patient with rheumatoid arthritis or diabetes mellitus; a computerized tomographic scan of the brain can reassure clinicians and patients that a stroke is not caused by a lesion that can be surgically cured.

Even when used for purely diagnostic purposes, the test can play diverse roles in the diagnostic process. One of these roles is derived from the strength of the evidence provided by the test. Certain procedures, such as a glucose tolerance test for diabetes mellitus or a liver biopsy for hepatitis, produce *definitive* diagnostic evidence. The diagnosis depends directly on the result found in the test. Other procedures, such as a measurement of creatine phosphokinase (CPK) in a patient with suspected myocardial infarction, produce *contributory* diagnostic evidence. When combined with other results, such as the clinical history and the electrocardiographic data, the contributory test can lead to a diagnostic decision; but it is not used alone for making the decision. A third type of procedure acts as a *surrogate* test, which substitutes for a definitive test. The results are used directly as a diagnostic marker. Thus, the alpha fetoprotein (AFP) test is used as a surrogate for the diagnosis of fetal abnormality; and the VDRL test is a surrogate for the diagnosis of syphilis. Because the surrogate tests are intended to be easy and inexpensive, they are often used for screening purposes in people who are not overtly diseased. A positive result is then checked by confirmation with the definitive test, which is more powerful but less easy to do and more expensive.

A different aspect of the tests is in the type of discrimination that they perform. Thus, a *diagnostic marker* test is expected to demarcate a particular disease from other entities contained in the spectrum of human diseases and states of health. A *spectral marker* test is expected to demarcate a particular condition within the spectrum of an established disease. For a spectral marker, the discrimination is between one stage of the disease and other stages of the same disease. For example, the carcinoembryonic antigen (CEA) test was first introduced as a diagnostic marker that would discriminate cancer of the colon from other clinical conditions. When the CEA test was found to have low discrimination for this purpose, it became employed as a spectral marker, separating localized from metastatic cancer of the colon. The CEA test receives its main usage today as a spectral marker, not as a diagnostic marker.

This chapter is concerned mainly with evaluating the discrimination of diagnostic and spectral marker procedures, particularly when applied for surrogate purposes. Because many of the issues in evaluation are similar for diagnostic and spectral markers, most of the discussion will emphasize diagnostic markers. The variations introduced by spectral marker goals will then be described briefly, and the chapter will conclude with an outline of the strategies that can be used to evaluate definitive and contributory tests.

25.1. **STATISTICAL ISSUES IN EXPRESSING RESULTS**

Unlike a cause-effect maneuver, whose accomplishments can be expressed in means, proportions, rates, or some other measured level of an outcome event, a surrogate marker test is judged by its agreement with the results of a definitive standard. The method of measuring and expressing this agreement has been a source of fertile mathematical creativity (and extensive clinical confusion) for several decades. Although the fundamental scientific issues in choosing and using the tests all depend on clinical goals that are often overlooked during the mathematical enchantment, published literature has concentrated on statistical strategies for expressing results.

These strategies will be the first main topic of discussion here, so that we can get them out of the way and then turn to the fundamental scientific principles that underlie the mathematics. A reader who wants to avoid the mathematics can skip directly to Section 25.2.

25.1.1. *Indexes of Efficacy*

In Chapter 20, we considered the diverse mathematical tactics that have been developed for expressing the efficacy of a diagnostic marker test. Its *diagnostic sensitivity* and *diagnostic specificity* refer to the predictive accuracy of the results when the test is positive or negative. Although these "batting averages" are what a clinician really wants to know in using the test, the most commonly cited indexes of efficacy for diagnostic marker tests refer to *nosologic sensitivity* and *nosologic specificity*. The nosologic index of sensitivity shows the proportion of people correctly identified by the test in a collection of cases who have the disease; and nosologic specificity shows the correctly identified proportion of people in the control group, without the disease. The complex manipulations of *Bayes theorem* can then be applied to convert these vertical nosologic indexes into the desired horizontal indexes of diagnostic prediction.

A more recently developed set of indexes, called *likelihood ratios,* has the advantage of expressing results in the horizontal direction of diagnosis, but the ratios refer to odds rather than probabilities, and the indexes must receive a complex reconstruction to produce the probability values desired by a clinician as "batting averages" for diagnostic efficacy.

25.1.2. *Problems in Dichotomous Indexes*

In all of the foregoing mathematical structures, the tabulations are arranged in a dichotomous manner. Nosologically, the tested people are divided into two groups, with or without the disease. Diagnostically, the results of the test are cited as positive or negative. Although the fourfold tables produced by this double dichotomy are not required to calculate likelihood ratios, each likelihood ratio is nevertheless formed from four numbers and thus resembles a doubly dichotomous arrangement.

The difficulty with all these dichotomous strategies is that the patient's true condition as well as the results of the test may not always be easily cited in two sharply separated categories. The patient's true condition may be *equivocal* rather than *diseased* or *nondiseased;* and the results of the test may be regarded as *uncertain* rather than definitely *positive* or *negative*. In some instances, more than three categories may be needed to demarcate either the patient's condition, the results of the test, or both.

A simple example of the demarcation problem occurred in a study[1] in which the investigators wanted to determine whether the fever discerned with a thermometer could be detected equally well by a nurse's palpation of the child's forehead or chest. The results of that study are shown in Table 25-1. In this situation the actual temperature (obtained with a thermometer) indicated the definitive state of disease. The diagnostic test was the temperature estimated by palpation of the forehead. To simplify the analyses, the results

Table 25–1. RESULTS OF PALPATION VERSUS THERMOMETRY FOR DIAGNOSING FEVERS*

Temperature Estimated by Palpation	≥39°C (Major Fever)	Actual Temperature 38.0–38.9°C (Minor Fever)	No Fever	Total
≥39°C (major fever)	15	3	3	21
38.0–38.9°C (minor fever)	19	43	15	77
No fever	3	55	993	1051
Total	37	101	1011	1149

*Table rearranged from data reported by Bergeson PS, Steinfeld HJ. How dependable is palpation as a screening method for fever? Clin Pediatr (Phila) 1974; 13:350–1.

were presented in three categories for each variable, thus forming the nine cells shown in Table 25–1.

To summarize the results, the investigators decided to cite the palpation test as being *correct, too high,* or *too low.* Thus, the test was correct in the three downward left-to-right diagonal cells of the table, yielding a correct result in $15 + 43 + 993 = 1051$ cases. The palpation method gave a falsely high result in 21 instances ($= 15 + 3 + 3$) and gave a falsely low result in 77 instances ($= 55 + 3 + 19$). When these results are expressed as proportions of the total of 1149 challenges, the palpation method was correct in 91% ($= 1051/1149$), too high in 2%, and too low in 7%.

The investigators did not attempt to dichotomize their trichotomous categories, but if the customary indexes of efficacy were used, dichotomies would be necessary. One arrangement would be to compare *fever* versus *no fever.* With this demarcation, Table 25–1 would reduce to

Result of Palpation Test	Fever	Definitive State of Disease No Fever	Total
Fever	80	18	98
No Fever	58	993	1051
Total	138	1011	1149

The nosologic sensitivity of the palpation test would become $80/138 = 0.58$ and nosologic specificity would be $993/1011 = 0.98$. The diagnostic sensitivity would be $80/98 = 0.82$ and diagnostic specificity would be $993/1051 = 0.94$.

An alternative demarcation is to compare *major fever* versus *not major fever.* With this arrangement, Table 25–1 becomes

Result of Palpation Test	Definitive State of Disease Major Fever	Not Major Fever	Total
Major fever	15	6	21
Not major fever	22	1106	1128
Total	37	1112	1149

The nosologic sensitivity is now reduced to $15/37 = 0.41$, but nosologic specificity has increased to $1106/1112 = 0.99$. Diagnostic sensitivity is lowered to $15/21 = 0.71$, but diagnostic specificity is raised to $1106/1128 = 0.98$.

These results show that we can obtain at least two different sets of nosologic indexes according to arbitrary decisions in partitioning the same set of data. The mathematical problems of choosing this arbitrary mechanism of partition will be discussed shortly in Section 25.1.3, but before we reach that section, we might note a clinical (rather than mathematical) method of eliminating the problem.

Suppose we decide that we are really uninterested in whether palpation of the forehead is good for detecting minor fevers. Our main interest is in determining the efficacy of palpation in separating the distinctively sick children from those who are distinctively well (at least in temperature). With this focus, we would eliminate all patients with minor fever from the vertical columns of the challenges contained in Table 25–1. We would also eliminate all palpations in which the diagnosis was minor fever. The nine cells of Table 25–1 would then be reduced to the following fourfold table:

	Definitive State of Disease	
Result of Palpation Test	*Major Fever*	*No Fever*
Major fever	15	3
No fever	3	993

The nosologic sensitivity would now climb to $15/18 = 0.83$ and nosologic specificity would be $993/996 = 0.996$. The values for diagnostic sensitivity and specificity would also be 0.83 and 0.996. Our conclusion would be that palpation of the forehead—which might be called the *cutaneous thermometric surrogate test*—is quite effective in performing the assigned clinical task. We shall return later to the way in which *clinical* decisions about the desired goal of a test can enormously simplify the mathematical expression of results. A reader who wants to get to those clinical decisions, which are the main "meat" of this chapter, can skip the next few sections and go directly to Section 25.2. Readers who want a guide to the mathematical maneuvers that commonly appear in published literature about diagnostic tests can peruse the next few sections.

25.1.3. *Mathematical Choices and Consequences of Demarcation Boundaries*

The data shown in Table 25–1 could yield two different sets of index values because we could choose different boundaries for converting a 3×3 table to a 2×2 table. A more common dichotomous problem in clinical literature occurs when the cases and controls are cleanly divided into two groups, but the diagnostic test produces a dimensional result, such as level of serum calcium or depression of electrocardiographic ST segment. A statistical problem then arises from the need to choose a boundary that will split the dimensional range into two parts, with one part being regarded as *high, abnormal,* or *positive* and the other part regarded as *low, normal,* or *negative.* The challenge of choosing this boundary line has led to a mathematical strategy that is usually labeled as *ROC analysis.*

25.1.3.1. **RECEIVER-OPERATING-CHARACTERISTIC (ROC) CURVES**

The receiver-operating-characteristic (ROC) curves that have become so popular in medical literature were originally developed as a statistical contribution[2] in engineering. When an apparatus yields an output product, the occurrence or quality of that product will vary with the operating characteristics of the apparatus. The effects produced by different operating characteristics—in voltage, position, or other attributes of the apparatus—can be noted in relation to the occurrence of an all-or-none response or to the quality of the image, film, or other output of the apparatus. By displaying what emerges from different operating characteristics, the ROC curve has been a splendid aid for the engineering decisions needed to choose the particular operating arrangement that yields the best image, film, or other output.

The strategy became particularly valuable when radiologists started working with new apparatus that produced nuclide scintigrams, computerized tomographic scans, and other new media in modern imaging.[3-5] In trying to decide which voltages, chemical concentrations, object positions, and other engineering characteristics to use in operating the apparatus, radiologists have been greatly aided by the ROC technique.

This engineering application of ROC strategy in an apparatus/product relationship is very different from the subsequent application of the strategy for choosing the cutting points that demarcate dimensional data in a diagnostic marker/disease relationship.[6-8] To yield a product, an apparatus must receive a definite set of operating instructions; and a definite decision must be made about which set of instructions to give. When an item of data is interpreted diagnostically, however, a definitive **yes/no** decision is not necessary. The decision may be expressed as **uncertain** or with different degrees of certainty about **yes** or **no**. Nevertheless, when applied in diagnostic reasoning, the ROC technique demands that an intellectual decision be expressed with the same sharp dichotomous separation that would be used in the engineering operation of an inanimate apparatus.

The advantages (and disadvantages) of the ROC strategy for diagnostic marker tests are best demonstrated with an example. Let us consider the problem of choosing an abnormal boundary value for ST segment depression in an electrocardiographic stress test. We have assembled a series of 150 cases and 150 controls who have been shown with coronary arteriography to either have or not have definitive evidence of coronary disease. As we correlate the ST segment results with the arteriographic diagnoses, we find the data shown in Table 25–2.

25.1.3.2. **PATTERN OF DISTRIBUTION FOR TEST RESULTS**

Perhaps the best way to understand the problems of obtaining suitable statistical indexes for the data in Table 25–2 is to convert the data into the frequency distributions shown in Table 25–3. In Table 25–3, the test results have been moved to the center column, which is surrounded on its left and right with the relative individual frequency and cumulative frequency of results for the cases and controls. The results of Table 25–3 can be depicted with the horizontal bar graph shown in Figure 25–1. In that bar graph, the individual relative frequencies at each value of the test are shown as solid bars, with a line

Table 25–2. RESULTS IN A DIAGNOSTIC MARKER STUDY OF CORONARY ARTERY DISEASE AND LEVEL OF S-T DEPRESSION IN EXERCISE STRESS TEST

Patients with ST Segment Depression of	Definitive State of Disease	
	Cases of Coronary Disease	*Controls Without Coronary Disease*
≥3.0 mm.	31	0
≥2.5 mm. but <3.0 mm.	15	0
≥2.0 mm. but <2.5 mm.	27	7
≥1.5 mm. but <2.0 mm.	30	8
≥1.0 mm. but <1.5 mm.	32	39
≥0.5 mm. but <1.0 mm.	12	43
≤0.5 mm.	3	53
Total	150	150

Table 25-3. FREQUENCY DISTRIBUTIONS FOR RESULTS OF TABLE 25-2

Cases of Coronary Disease		Results of Test, Showing S-T Segment Depressions of	Controls Without Coronary Disease	
Cumulative Relative Frequency	Individual Relative Frequency		Individual Relative Frequency	Cumulative Relative Frequency
0.21	0.21	≥3.0	0	0
0.31	0.10	≥2.5–<3.0	0	0
0.49	0.18	≥2.0–<2.5	0.05	0.05
0.69	0.20	≥1.5–<2.0	0.05	0.10
0.90	0.21	≥1.0–<1.5	0.26	0.36
0.98	0.08	0.5–<1.0	0.29	0.65
1.00	0.02	<0.5	0.35	1.00

connecting them to form a frequency polygon for the distribution of values in the cases and controls. The cumulative relative frequencies are shown with the speckled bars.

The cumulative frequencies for the diseased cases will represent the nosologic sensitivity of the test at any level of demarcation. The cumulative frequencies for the nondiseased controls represent the inverse of the nosologic specificity at the selected demarcation point. Because this inverse value is shown as $1 -$ specificity, the specificity is obtained by subtracting each displayed value from 1. The concomitant rise in the two sets of cumulative frequencies indicates the problem of trying to pick a suitable cutting point. As we lower this cutting point to try to increase sensitivity, we will inevitably reduce the specificity of the test—and vice versa.

For example, because seven different levels of S-T depression are represented in Table 25–2, we have six possible choices of demarcation points for the abnormal versus normal boundaries. The results obtained with those choices are summarized in Table 25–4. If we let our first boundary, designated as A, be placed so that ≥3.0 mm. is defined as *abnormal*, the fourfold table becomes $\begin{Bmatrix} 31 & 0 \\ 119 & 150 \end{Bmatrix}$. The sensitivity of the test becomes quite

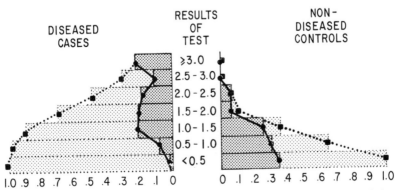

Figure 25–1. Horizontal bar graph showing relative individual (solid line) and cumulative (dotted line) frequencies for data in Table 25–3.

Table 25–4. SUMMARY OF NOSOLOGIC SENSITIVITY AND SPECIFICITY OBTAINED FOR DEMARCATIONS OF TABLE 25–2

Identification	Location of Boundary for Abnormal	Number of Cases Included	Sensitivity	Number of Controls Included	Specificity	1 – Specificity
A	≥3.0 mm.	31	0.21	0	1	0
B	≥2.5 mm.	46	0.31	0	1	0
C	≥2.0 mm.	73	0.49	7	0.95	0.05
D	≥1.5 mm.	103	0.69	15	0.90	0.10
E	≥1.0 mm.	135	0.90	54	0.64	0.36
F	≥0.5 mm.	147	0.98	97	0.35	0.65

low (0.21 = 31/150), but its specificity is the perfect value of 1 (= 150/150). At demarcation point B, where any ST depression of ≥**2.5 mm.** is defined as *abnormal,* sensitivity rises to 0.31 (= 46/150), whereas specificity still remains perfect. At demarcation point C, with a depression of ≥**2.0 mm.** defined as *abnormal,* sensitivity rises to 0.49, but we begin to get some false-positive results. Specificity falls to 143/150 = 0.95. At point D, with ≥**1.5 mm.** demarcated as *abnormal,* the fourfold table becomes $\begin{bmatrix} 103 & 15 \\ 47 & 135 \end{bmatrix}$; sensitivity rises to 0.67, but specificity falls to 0.90. At point E, sensitivity becomes 0.90, but specificity drops to 0.64. At point F, sensitivity is a splendid 0.96, but specificity is a dismal 0.35.

This inverse relationship between sensitivity and specificity is an inevitable feature of any diagnostic marker test. As we lower (or raise) the boundary of demarcation, trying to "catch" all the cases, we will inevitably increase the false-positive trapping of controls. The inverse attribute of the relationship could readily be shown on a graph, but makers of ROC curves prefer to have things look more positive. Accordingly, the value of 1 – specificity is plotted on the graph, thereby providing an internal inversion before the values are drawn on the curve. (The values of 1 – specificity are presented in the far right–hand column of Table 25–4.)

Figure 25–2 shows the conventional format of an ROC curve used for depicting results of a diagnostic marker test, with sensitivity plotted against 1 – specificity. The curve has its lowest sensitivity at the A and B points where specificity is highest. As the curve ascends, it gains sensitivity at the cost of specificity. At its highest point, F, sensitivity is at a peak value of 0.96, but 1 – specificity has also increased to 0.65, so that specificity is down to 0.35.

25.1.3.3. **FREQUENCY DISTRIBUTIONS AND ROC CURVES**

An ROC curve can be drawn for any diagnostic test that has an ordinal or dimensional scale of results. When the scale is partitioned at different locations, the changing values of nosologic sensitivity and specificity will generate the points of the ROC curve. Because of these distinctions, ROC curves will have a relatively similar shape and location, ranging between the shape found with a useless test and the shape found for a perfect test.

The top part of Figure 25–3 shows the relative individual and cumulative frequency distributions of results for a useless test. The distributions are identical for both the cases and controls. The middle part of Figure 25–3 shows corresponding distributions for a perfect test. All of the cases occur in the upper three levels of the test result, and all of the controls occur in the lower three levels. If we draw the demarcation boundary between

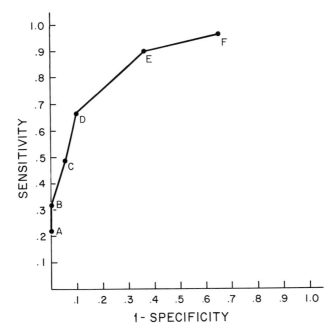

Figure 25–2. Format of a receiver-operating characteristic (ROC) curve. (For further details, see text.)

the 3rd and 4th levels, we will have a perfect separation of the groups, with 100% sensitivity and 100% specificity for the test.

The bottom part of Figure 25–3 shows what is usually encountered with the ordinary tests performed in clinical reality. There is a substantial overlap of the two distributions of cases and controls. Except for the very top zone, which contains only diseased cases, and the very bottom zone, which contains only nondiseased controls, any other demarcations will produce a mixture of cases and controls.

Figure 25–4 shows the ROC curves that correspond to the three tests whose distributions are shown in Figure 25–3. The diagonal line drawn at a 45-degree angle in Figure 25–4 shows the ROC performance of the useless test. The values of sensitivity and 1−specificity are identical at each point. The right-angle line in Figure 25–4 shows the ROC curve for the perfect test. Its value of 1−specificity is 0 at different levels of sensitivity. Its sensitivity remains 1 for different levels of 1−specificity. The upper triangle formed between the useless and perfect ROC curves is what becomes available for the location of ordinary ROC curves. The line drawn in this zone displays the ROC curve for the ordinary test shown at the bottom of Figure 25–3.

25.1.3.4. ROC CURVES FOR COMPARING TESTS

As new technologic procedures are developed and proposed, clinicians will often want to see whether a new test has more or less efficacy than an old one. Although a proper comparison of the tests will require suitable attention to the architectural features discussed later, some type of statistical index will be needed to express the numerical results.

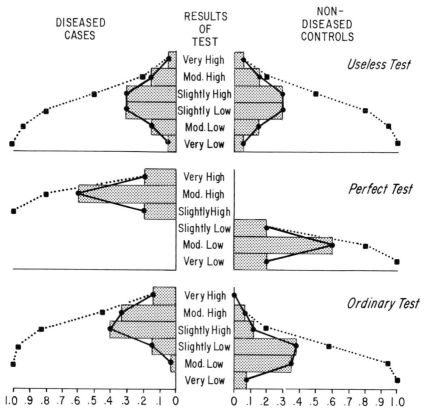

Figure 25–3. Distributions of relative individual and cumulative frequencies for a useless, perfect, and ordinary diagnostic test.

If the results are originally cited in a dichotomous scale as *positive* or *negative*, the indexes of sensitivity and specificity can be compared directly. Because these indexes should be calculated and compared only when the two tests are performed on the same group of people, the statistical expressions can follow either a nosologic or diagnostic direction for sensitivity and specificity.

If the test results are cited in ordinal or dimensional scales, however, a problem will occur because direct comparisons will be difficult to achieve for the dichotomous indexes of sensitivity and specificity. Perhaps the greatest value of ROC curves is their role in solving this problem. An ROC curve can be plotted for each test; and the two curves can be compared. The curve that has the higher location on the graph, i.e., closest to the inverted-L shape of a perfect performance, will denote the test that has the better overall performance.

25.1.3.5. **ROC CURVES AND CHOICE OF AN OPTIMAL DICHOTOMOUS DEMARCATION**

A different role of ROC curves has been their proposed application in choosing a single optimum boundary for dichotomous demarcation of a diagnostic test. Before we

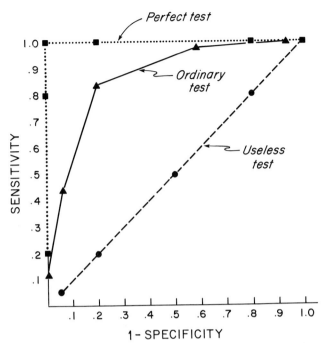

Figure 25–4. ROC curves for the three sets of distributions shown in Figure 25–3.

discuss this choice, you might wonder why it is necessary. Why could we not use two (or more) cutting points? Thus, above a boundary of ⩾**2.5 mm.** in Table 25–2, we have excellent *diagnostic sensitivity* for the test. Everyone in this zone has coronary artery disease and there are no false-positives. Our positive predictive accuracy in this zone would be 46/46 = 100 %. Conversely, below a lower boundary of ⩾**0.5 mm.** (point F), we would have excellent *diagnostic specificity*. A false-negative diagnosis would occur in only 3/56 = 0.05 of the instances in which we classified such patients as *normal*. Why could we not use these two boundaries for demarcating three zones? We could make positive and negative diagnoses for people in the upper and lower zones and then say we are diagnostically uncertain about the people in between. After all, the zone that extends from above 0.5 mm. to just below 2.5 mm. of ST depression contains 101 cases and 97 controls. Although segments of this zone have a distinct diagnostic gradient, our predictive accuracy for the total zone will only be about 50%.

These are important questions; and their implications will be discussed later when we finally reach the clinical interpretation of diagnostic marker tests. For the moment, however, because we remain temporarily enthralled by the mathematical activities, they call for a single demarcation point to be chosen. Accordingly, we shall continue pursuing the mathematical strategy, if only to understand what it does before we later find a possible way of rejecting it.

One way to choose the desired cutoff point is to try to minimize the sum of false-positive and false-negative test results. (The tactic is analogous to maximizing the index of validity.) Using mathematical calculus, it can be shown that this point occurs when the slope of the ROC curve is equal to n_2/n_1, where n_2 represents the number of controls, and n_1 represents the number of cases. Because calculations of slope are a nuisance, a simpler way to find this point is to note that it occurs when the number of false-positive values begins to exceed the number of false-negative values. Thus, for the data of Table 25–2, we would have the following:

Cutting Point	Number of False-Negatives	Number of False-Positives	Total Number of False Results
A	119	0	119
B	104	0	104
C	77	7	84
D	47	15	62
E	15	54	69
F	3	97	100

At point D there are 47 false-negatives and 15 false-positives. At point E, this ratio is reversed, with 15 false-negatives and 54 false-positives. Therefore, point D (with $\geq$**1.5 mm.** elevation) would minimize the total numbers of false results in the test. Its choice as a demarcation boundary would give the test a nosologic sensitivity of 0.67 and a nosologic specificity of 0.90.

A different goal in choosing a cutoff point is to maximize the predictive accuracy of the test with respect to its performance in *diagnostic* sensitivity and specificity. For this decision, the likelihood ratio can be a helpful guide. For any horizontal row in Table 25–2, the likelihood ratio for a positive result in that row will be [no. of cases in row/150]/[no. of controls in row/150]. Thus, for the fourth row in Table 25–2, the likelihood ratio is (30/150)/(8/150) = 3.75 for a positive result. Because the values of 150 = n_1 and 150 = n_2 are fixed in the table, the likelihood ratios can be compared for each row simply as (no. of cases in row)/(no. of controls in row). Because L_{pos} for a fourfold table is determined from the nosologic indexes as sensitivity/(1 – specificity), we can examine the values of L_{pos} at various cutting points by using the appropriate data in Table 25–4. If we were interested in minimizing L_{neg}, we could also use those data to calculate the consequent L_{neg} values as (1 – sensitivity)/specificity. The results would be as follows:

Cutting Point	Value of L_{pos}	Value of L_{neg}
A	∞	0.79
B	∞	0.69
C	9.8	0.48
D	6.7	0.26
E	2.5	0.16
F	1.5	0.11

Because the goal in overall prediction is to maximize L_{pos} while simultaneously minimizing L_{neg}, the results show that we cannot achieve the desired goal with a single cutting point. These likelihood ratios also confirm what we noted before when nosologic indexes were examined in Section 25.1.3.2. The best value of L_{pos} is obtained at cutting points A or B. The best value of L_{neg} is obtained at cutting point F. In between, what we gain in L_{neg} is lost in L_{pos}, and vice versa.

Several other strategies[4, 6] are available for choosing a single cutting point. One strategy involves efforts to maximize the information content of the test by noting the pretest and post-test certainties of diagnosis. The information content is calculated as a logarithmic function of sensitivity, specificity, and prevalence. Because no provision is made for the different diagnostic goals with which marker tests are ordered, this procedure has the same disadvantages as the two that preceded.

Some ingenious mathematical dexterity[7] has been used to propose a combined index that includes the costs as well as the efficacy of diagnostic tests. With various forms of economic sorcery, estimates are made for the direct and indirect costs and benefits of each of the four results in the diagnostic marker table: false-negatives, false-positives, true-negatives, and true-positives. For this estimate, monetary values are assigned to the costs of the tests, costs of caring for complications, and fiscal benefits of the enhanced survival or improved quality of life made possible by the test results. Using the C symbol to represent the net value of costs minus the benefit for each type of result, the expression $C_{FP} - C_{TN}$ is calculated for the increment of false-positive and true-negative results in the control group. A corresponding expression, $C_{FN} - C_{TP}$, is calculated for the net values of false-negative and true-positive results in the diseased case group. The ratio of these two expressions is then multiplied by $(1-P)/P$, where P = the prevalence of the disease. After all these things are done, it can be shown mathematically that the costs attributable to diagnostic error will be minimized if the cutoff value for the ROC curve is set at the point on the curve where its slope is

$$\frac{1 - P}{P} \times \frac{[C_{FP} - C_{TN}]}{[C_{FN} - C_{TP}]}$$

The intricate ingenuity of computations and estimations in this strategy is exceeded only by the unlikelihood of the strategy ever being applied in practical clinical reality.

25.1.3.6. CLINICAL INADEQUACY OF DICHOTOMOUS DEMARCATIONS

Although the choice of a cutting point has evoked the described acts of mathematical creativity, dichotomous demarcations are really inadequate for the diverse clinical goals with which diagnostic tests are ordered. In diagnosis, clinicians begin with different degrees of suspicion about the possible presence of the disease. According to these suspicions, which are further described in Section 25.2.1, the test may be used to rule in or rule out the disease during such activities as screening, differential diagnosis, or confirmation.

For these activities, a clinician usually wants the test to have either high *diagnostic* sensitivity or high *diagnostic* specificity rather than a compromise that lowers accuracy for both. Consequently, the clinician will really look for three zones of operation rather than two. The upper and lower zones will be the sites of high diagnostic accuracy. The middle zones, as places of diagnostic uncertainty, will require the performance of additional diagnostic procedures. Furthermore, when the tests are used for purposes other than diagnosis, the dimensional values of the test result will usually be arranged quite differently from a mere separation into high or low zones.

25.2. CLINICAL OBJECTIVES IN USING DIAGNOSTIC TESTS

The main reason for learning about the preceding statistical strategies is prophylactic: to keep them from obscuring the more fundamental underlying clinical and scientific issues. These issues may be neglected or left unexamined by a reader who is confused (or by an investigator who is infatuated) by likelihood ratios, indexes of validity, Bayesian conditional probabilities, and other mathematical elegances; or by someone whose head is rolling with ROC curves.

Once we begin to think about the reasons why clinicians order diagnostic tests, we can promptly begin to discern the scientific inadequacy of all the mathematical folderol.

25.2.1. *The Functional Roles of Diagnostic Tests*

Diagnostic tests are usually ordered for at least three different purposes: discovery, exclusion, and confirmation. Each of these activities is performed under different circumstances and with different goals.

25.2.1.1. DISCOVERY TESTS

A discovery test is ordered to find a particular disease that currently exists in a silent or lanthanic form, having produced no prominent clinical manifestations to suggest its presence. Although the testing process is properly called *screening* when applied to members of a general population in a community survey and *case-finding* when applied to patients in a medical setting, the word *screening* is now commonly used for both types of activity. The main difference between the discovery procedures of community screening and of clinical case-finding is in the prevalence of the diagnosed diseases. Because the diseases are more likely to be found in clinical than in community groups, the *nosologic* and *diagnostic* indexes of sensitivity and specificity will not be as dramatically different in clinical groups as in community groups. (An example of this distinction is shown in Exercise 25.1 at the end of the chapter.)

Examples of discovery tests are the examination of urine glucose in a search for diabetes mellitus, the measurement of serum calcium for hyperparathyroidism, palpation of the breast to find breast cancer, or palpation of the rectum to find rectal cancer. When a clinician routinely does a complete physical examination, an act of screening is conducted with most of the questions asked in the *review of systems* and with all parts of the physical examination that are directed at sites unassociated with pertinent symptoms. Many of the laboratory tests ordered in ordinary clinical practice and many (if not most) of the tests ordered when patients are admitted to the hospital are also performed as acts of screening.

25.2.1.2. EXCLUSION TESTS

An exclusion test is an act of differential diagnosis, done to rule out the presence of a disease that is suspected because of a particular clinical or paraclinical manifestation. Exclusion tests are usually too expensive or inconvenient to be employed merely for discovery purposes during routine screening. For example, a chemical test of blood in the stool might be used to screen for gastrointestinal lesions, but a more elaborate roentgenographic or endoscopic examination would be needed if a particular disease is suspected because of clinical symptoms or because the stool has a positive test for blood. Certain exclusion tests are sufficiently cheap and convenient to be used for screening purposes. Thus, in healthy people, an appropriate skin test for tuberculosis will signal the need for further examination if positive and can exclude the presence of active disease if negative.

25.2.1.3. CONFIRMATION TESTS

A confirmation test is used in differential diagnosis when the disease is strongly suspected of being present. The suspicions may have been induced or supported by a particular set of manifestations or by the results found in an exclusion test. For example, if upper GI endoscopy and colonoscopy are negative in demonstrating the source of GI bleeding, and if small bowel imaging shows a potential lesion, a special small bowel biopsy procedure may be performed as a confirmation test. In more ordinary clinical circumstances, confirmation tests are the ones that provide the definitive or "gold standard" diagnostic results. A glucose tolerance test provides confirmation for the diagnosis of diabetes mellitus, and diverse types of biopsy provide confirmation for the diagnosis of cancer. (The use of Pap smears in sputum, gynecologic, and other examinations can be regarded as a screening test.)

25.2.2. *Clinical Requirements for Efficacy*

Some tests can be used for all three purposes of discovery, exclusion, and confirmation. Some are good for two purposes, and some for only one. For example, sigmoidoscopy (together with biopsy as needed) can usually be employed to discover, exclude, and confirm cancer of the rectum. A glucose tolerance test can be used to exclude or to confirm diabetes mellitus but is too inconvenient for use in screening. Histologic examination of tissues from a bronchoscopic biopsy is an excellent way to confirm lung cancer, but the procedure cannot be used alone (without chest films) as an exclusion test, and it is too expensive and inconvenient for screening purposes.

These different roles for diagnostic tests will create different demands when the desired indexes of efficacy[8] are calculated from data arranged as shown in Table 25–5.

25.2.2.1. REQUIREMENTS FOR DISCOVERY TESTS

Because a discovery test should be able to detect the disease whenever it is present, we would want the test to have high nosologic sensitivity. This goal can be undesirable, however, if the test also has a very low nosologic specificity. The high sensitivity will give us a proportionately high value for the a cell in Table 25–5, but the low specificity will produce a high value for the b cell. Consequently, the test will yield a large number of false-positive results when it is used in screening, and the calculation of *diagnostic* sensitivity as $a/(a+b)$ will produce a low value. For example, if we diagnose lung cancer in everyone who has a nose, we will miss very few cases of lung cancer, and nosologic (the pun is not bad but was not intended) sensitivity will be quite high. The huge number of false-positive diagnoses, however, will give terrible results for nosologic specificity and diagnostic sensitivity.

We might be willing to perform a confirmation test when a discovery test is positive, but if the rate of false-positive diagnoses is too high, the advantages of a low-cost screening test will be ruined by the disadvantages of the high-cost confirmation tests. Accordingly, we would be willing to sacrifice some nosologic sensitivity (or convenience) in a screening test if it can be made to have higher nosologic specificity.

This is the reason why a fasting blood sugar (FBS), rather than a urinalysis, is often used clinically as a case-finding test for diabetes mellitus. The FBS value will have better nosologic specificity than the test of urinary sugar. Besides, when other tests are being done simultaneously on the same specimen of blood, the incremental cost and inconvenience of the FBS test is minor. On the other hand, in community screening procedures, the urinary test is much easier to do and is therefore preferred over the blood test, despite lower nosologic indexes of efficacy.

25.2.2.2. REQUIREMENTS FOR EXCLUSION TESTS

We want an exclusion test to have high *diagnostic specificity,* because the goal is to be confident that a negative result has excluded the disease. This goal requires a very low

Table 25–5. BASIC ARRANGEMENT OF DATA IN A DIAGNOSTIC MARKER STUDY

Result of Diagnostic Test	Definitive State of Disease	
	Positive	*Negative*
Positive	a (True-positive)	b (False-positive)
Negative	c (False-negative)	d (True-negative)

value for the c cell and a reasonably high value for the d cell in Table 25–5. To obtain a low value of c, we would want *nosologic sensitivity* to be as high as possible, preferably very close to 1, whereas nosologic specificity is reasonably high. (Alternatively, we would want a very low value for L_{neg}.)

25.2.2.3. **REQUIREMENTS FOR CONFIRMATION TESTS**

A confirmation test should have high *diagnostic sensitivity*, which requires a low value for the b cell in Table 25–5. To obtain this low value for b, we would want *nosologic specificity* to be as high as possible.

Because we want to be sure that the disease is present when the test is positive, we would have no major objection to occasional false-negative results, because the confirmation test would probably be ordered after an exclusion test was used to find any cases that might otherwise be missed as false-negatives.

25.2.2.4. **THE PROBLEMS OF NOMENCLATURE**

The foregoing requirements indicate the confusion that can be produced by the terms *sensitivity* and *specificity*. The original names and nosologic values of these terms are produced by "vertical" information about diseased cases and nondiseased controls; but the clinical goals and diagnostic (or predictive) values require "horizontal" thoughts about positive and negative test results. Consequently, the requirements for clinical goals produce an apparent reversal of the nosologic terminology: high diagnostic sensitivity requires high nosologic specificity; and high diagnostic specificity requires high nosologic sensitivity.

Perhaps the greatest virtue of the likelihood ratios is that they eliminate this ambiguity. An even simpler way to achieve clarity, for readers who are not repulsed by additional neologisms, might be to replace *diagnostic sensitivity* with *diagnostic inclusivity* for the value of $a/(a+b)$, which currently is usually called *accuracy for positive prediction*. *Diagnostic specificity* can then be replaced with *diagnostic exclusivity* for the value of $d/(c+d)$, which is usually called *accuracy for negative prediction*. Because an exclusion test is intended to rule out and an inclusion (or confirmation) test is intended to rule in, the words *inclusivity* and *exclusivity* would communicate both the form and the function of the statistical indexes used in making diagnostic decisions.

25.2.2.5. **COMBINATIONS OF TESTS**

A single test can seldom be excellent for the goals of both discovery and confirmation. With rare exception, the same procedure cannot be sensitive enough to find all cases of the disease while simultaneously being specific enough to avoid false-positive identifications.

For example, the chest x-ray is a quite sensitive but nonspecific way of finding lung cancer. Almost all patients with lung cancer have abnormal roentgenograms, but not all people with abnormal roentgenograms have lung cancer. Conversely, a positive result in tissue obtained at bronchoscopic biopsy is a quite specific but often nonsensitive way of identifying lung cancer. The bronchoscopic biopsy seldom gives false-positive results but regularly fails to capture tissue from lung cancers located at inaccessible sites.

For these reasons, many diagnostic tests are regularly used in combinations that are ordered in tandem or sometimes concomitantly as part of a work-up. When employed in deliberate combinations, the individual procedures become contributory rather than surrogate tests. The appropriate indexes of efficacy should then focus either on the accomplishments of the patterns found in the combined results or on the contributions made by an additional single test when a particular pattern already exists in the results of previous tests. Unfortunately, the Bayesian models and dichotomous strategies of the currently popular mathematical approaches are unsuitable (or have not yet been suitably applied) for these requirements. If diagnostic procedures are to be properly evaluated for the combinations with which they are constantly used in clinical practice, an additional set of statistical strategies and indexes will be required.

25.3. THE SPECTRUM OF GROUPS USED FOR EVALUATING TESTS

With all of the arithmetic behind us, we can now turn to the fundamental scientific and clinical issues that have been neglected during the mathematical quantophrenia of the past two decades. Although randomized trials and carefully selected criteria have been established to give suitable attention to issues in spectrum, bias, and reliability for the statistical evaluation of *therapeutic* agents, no counterpart activity has occurred for the statistical evaluation of *diagnostic* agents.

Because randomized trials and double-blind procedures have seldom been used for diagnostic evaluations, the compared groups and data can often be distorted by many innate biases that occur when the tests are obtained in ordinary clinical activities. These innate biases in groups and data will be discussed in Section 25.5. Our main concern now is with a different problem that is particularly cogent but commonly neglected in the evaluation of diagnostic tests: the choice of a suitably challenging spectrum.[9]

25.3.1. *The Concept and Role of Spectrum*

When therapeutic agents are compared, we can usually learn what kinds of patients were treated by inspecting the admission criteria for the study. Even if the criteria are somewhat vague and the comparison biased, we can still draw certain conclusions merely by knowing about the agents of therapy. For example, we can generally assume that surgically treated patients fulfilled criteria for operability, even if those criteria were unstated in the published report; and that patients treated with anticoagulants had no evidence of gastrointestinal or other bleeding before treatment began.

In studies of diagnostic agents, however, criteria for admission to the study seldom receive extensive attention; and the types of patients under scrutiny cannot always be deduced from the types of tests. Thus, when exercise stress tests are compared with coronary arteriography in the diagnosis of coronary artery disease, we can assume that the patients were well enough to undergo both procedures, but we have little or no idea about the particular kinds and proportions of patients who composed the spectrum of the tested groups.

The fourfold statistical table will have one axis showing the arteriographic results that identified people as diseased cases and nondiseased controls, and another axis showing positive or negative results in the exercise stress test. The published report may contain no information, however, about the different anatomic types of coronary disease that are included as cases, about the main sources and diseases of the controls, and about the presenting clinical manifestations of the patients in either the case or control groups. Did the patients have classic angina pectoris, atypical angina pectoris, or no angina pectoris? Were the exercise stress test and the arteriograms done to confirm the diagnosis of coronary disease, to exclude it, to check post-therapeutic status, or to predict prognosis after myocardial infarction?

Although diagnostic marker tests are used to discriminate between a particular disease and all other entities in the spectrum of human health and disease, the composition of that spectrum receives relatively little attention when a control group is chosen; and careful thought is seldom given either to the internal spectrum of the disease itself or to the spectrum of clinical manifestations that evoke the diagnostic tests. Nevertheless, these different issues in spectrum are crucial determinants of the efficacy of a diagnostic test. If we want to use the test as a screening procedure for discovering disease in *asymptomatic ambulatory* patients, can we rely on indexes of sensitivity, specificity, or likelihood that were calculated from results found in *symptomatic hospitalized* patients? If we want to use the test in differential diagnosis to exclude or confirm the disease in patients with a distinctive pattern of manifestations, can we rely on statistical indexes obtained in patients who did not have that pattern of manifestations?

If you answered "No" to both of the two foregoing questions, you have just discovered a useful mechanism for evaluating the medical literature on screening and other diagnostic tests. As you examine the published literature, do not be impressed or awed by the superficial grandeur of the mathematical expressions. Look at the clinical science that was used in assembling the groups under study. Did the investigators choose a suitable spectrum of cases and controls, and were the results analyzed separately *within different parts of the spectrum*? The scientific importance of these clinical questions will be discussed in the next few sections.

25.3.2. *The Role of Component Evaluations*

When nosologic indexes, Bayes theorem, and ROC curves are used to evaluate a test's diagnostic performance, the crucial underlying assumption is that the nosologic indexes remain constant for either the presence or absence of the disease under study. Thus, when we calculate the nosologic indexes of sensitivity and specificity for the coronary disease identified with an exercise stress test, we expect the indexes to retain the same values thereafter when applied to patients with or without coronary disease. Despite the many mathematical models that have been based on this assumption, no pragmatic evidence has been obtained to demonstrate that the assumption is indeed correct. On the contrary, in the few situations in which it has been checked, the assumption has been found to be erroneous. Exercise stress and radionuclide tests have shown[10-14] different nosologic sensitivities for patients with different forms of coronary disease. The carcinoembryonic antigen (CEA) test has shown different nosologic specificities in different groups of patients without cancer of the colon[15-17]; and the nosologic sensitivity of the CEA test has been so varied in patients with different forms of colon cancer that the test has been converted from a diagnostic to a spectral marker. Two other well-established procedures that have now been shown to vary in nosologic specificity are the VDRL slide test for syphilis[18] and the fluorescent antinuclear antibody test.[19]

If this type of variability is confirmed for the nosologic indexes of other tests, the entire mathematical industry currently developed for diagnostic marker procedures will have been built on an erroneous foundation. The nosologic indexes and the Bayesian and ROC models that have become so popular in contemporary iatromathematics will have to be replaced by a new set of indexes that are more correctly suited to clinical reality. To determine the suitability of the existing models or to create new ones will require specific attention to the different components of diseased cases and nondiseased controls who enter the spectrum of people under evaluation.

For example, suppose we consider a group of asymptomatic, presumably healthy people who would receive the diagnostic test during screening as a detection test. When this group is assembled in a fourfold table, the results would be as follows:

Result of Screening Test	Presence of Disease	
	Yes	*No*
Positive	a′	b′
Negative	c′	d′

The nosologic indexes of sensitivity and specificity would be, respectively, $a'/(a'+c')$ and $d'/(b'+d')$.

Now suppose we consider a group of people with medical manifestations arousing suspicions that make us want to exclude or confirm the disease in differential diagnosis. When this group is assembled in a fourfold table, the results would be:

| Result of Diagnostic | Presence of Disease | |
Suspicion Test	Yes	No
Positive	a''	b''
Negative.	c''	d''

The nosologic indexes of sensitivity and specificity for this group of people would be $a''/(a''+c'')$ and $d''/(b''+d'')$.

If the two sets of indexes give similar results in the screened group and suspected group, we can conclude that the test is constant in its nosologic indexes (or likelihood ratios). If the results are not similar, the indexes will yield different values in different studies in which screened and suspected patients have been combined without regard to the stratification that would permit an effective evaluation of clinical components.

25.3.3. *The Use of Spectral Distinctions*

In the evaluation just described, the groups under study were assembled from a single framework of people who were being either screened or differentially diagnosed for presence or absence of the disease. In that single-framework approach, the investigator works prospectively to find the outcome of the disease associated with the results of the test. This uni-group approach is quite different from the customary two-group framework in which the investigator chooses a group of diseased cases, then chooses another group of controls, and then retrospectively finds the test results that were associated with these outcomes.

The retrospective framework is commonly used because—like other case-control methods—it is easier, cheaper, and quicker than the prospective technique. On the other hand, because the scientific and clinical attributes of the prospective approach make it much more desirable than the case-control technique, we might try to identify and use the virtues of the prospective strategy as a basis for improving the case-control technique. The main virtues of the prospective uni-group technique arise from its capacity to show a complete spectrum of consecutive challenges to which the test is exposed. If we think about the constituent elements of that spectrum, we might be able to use the information for better plans in case-control diagnostic marker studies.

The sections that follow contain a discussion of the three main components of spectrum, together with some illustrative examples of problems created when spectral distinctions were ignored or inadequately managed.

25.3.3.1. CLINICAL SPECTRUM

The clinical component of a disease's spectrum refers to the particular clinical reasons why the test was ordered or to other clinical distinctions that may affect its results. For example, a test that becomes positive when patients are symptomatic or severely ill may be negative when they are asymptomatic. Unless this distinction is noted "horizontally" as a feature of clinical spectrum rather than "vertically" as a feature of nosologic disease, the nosologic indexes may be obtained and interpreted erroneously. A test that is excellent in differential diagnosis may be dismissed as useless because it had low nosologic indexes in an evaluated group that contained many asymptomatic people. Conversely, a test with high indexes in a group of hospitalized patients may give unexpectedly poor results when used for screening in the general community.

For example, the high sensitivity reported for the limulus lysate test in diagnosing gram-negative meningitis may be an artefact that arose because the evaluated group was not stratified for clinical severity. The test may have been positive only in patients with the most severe forms of meningitis.[9, 20]

25.3.3.2. CO-MORBIDITY SPECTRUM

The spectrum of co-morbidity refers to coexisting ailments, which may or may not be related to the disease under study, that can alter the test results in several different ways. In one alteration, the co-morbid ailment produces chemical abnormalities that interfere with a chemical reaction used in the test. A different alteration occurs if the co-morbid ailment has led to an associated clinical phenomenon—such as malnutrition or cachexia—that indirectly affects the results of the test. Another attribute to be considered under co-morbidity is the chemical or other impact of concomitant pharmaceutical therapy.[21] If the case and control groups are chosen without regard to concomitant pharmacologic effects, the sources of unexpectedly erroneous results in the test may be impossible to identify.

With any of the cited effects, a co-morbid phenomenon may be responsible for false-positive or false-negative results or even for the main distinction attributed to the test. For example, diagnostic marker tests for cancer are commonly first evaluated in patients hospitalized with advanced cancer. Because many of these patients may also have malnutrition or cachexia, a positive result in the test may be due to these manifestations rather than the cancer. To avoid this diagnostic error, the test should be checked in a control group component of patients with ailments that have produced the same manifestations.

An example of inadequate checking for related co-morbid sources of false-positive results occurred when e antigen was studied as a diagnostic marker for chronic liver disease.[22] Although a false-positive result might be due to severe cachexia rather than the liver disease, patients with other sources of severe cachexia were not deliberately checked in the control group. Another example of the same problem occurred when a radiolabeled dye marker was studied for diagnosing the patency of the cystic duct in cholecystitis.[23] Although patients with severe liver disease might have false-positive results if the liver does not adequately excrete the dye, such patients were not examined in the control group. The converse phenomenon—inadequate checking for co-morbid sources of false-*negative* results—occurred when coexisting pulmonary disease, which might produce a falsely negative breath test for lactose deficiency, was not specifically cited in the reported evaluation of the test.[24]

25.3.3.3. PATHOLOGIC SPECTRUM

In cancers, infarctions, and other diseases that are identified morphologically, the pathologic spectrum of the disease refers to its location, anatomic extensiveness, and microscopic features. In inflammatory or infectious diseases, the pathologic spectrum includes consideration of the etiologic agent as well as the morphology of the disease.

An adequate pathologic spectrum of morphology in a *control* group would contain people with other diseases in the same location or with the same microscopic features in other locations. For example, in a diagnostic marker test for cancer of the prostate, the control group could include patients with cancers in other organs and with non-neoplastic diseases of the prostate. In the *case* group of diseased people, the pathologic spectrum will be inadequate if it is confined to patients with disease that is topographically too extensive or too localized. For example, a test that has a nosologic sensitivity of 100% in patients with a widespread cancer may later be found useless for diagnosing the same cancer when it is localized.

An inadequate pathologic spectrum of diseased cases occurred when the anatomic size of the tumors was not reported in an evaluation of ultrasound as an exclusion test for renal cancer.[25] The pathologic spectrum of cases was also inadequate when the size of the investigated infarctions was not cited in an evaluation of efficacy for radionuclide scanning in ruling out myocardial infarction.[26] An inadequate pathologic spectrum occurred in the control group when patients with severe staphylococcal infections in bone and other noncardiac sites were omitted from a diagnostic marker study of the teichoic acid test for staphylococcal endocarditis.[27]

25.3.4. *Consequences of Inadequate Spectrums*

When two therapeutic agents have received an inadequate comparison, we may still be able to learn something worthwhile from the biased results. If each treatment was suitably tested, we might be able to use what was learned about each treatment individually while withholding a decision about which treatment is superior. This type of compensatory knowledge is almost never obtainable from an inadequate diagnostic marker study. When we find major inadequacies in either the case group or the control group or both, nothing can be done with the information except to lament its inadequacy.

The reason for this problem is that the diagnostic use of the information requires a "horizontal" application of results from the "vertically" collected cases and controls. As noted earlier (Section 25.2.2.4), the nosologic data from the two vertical columns are combined and then divided horizontally when the information is used to make positive or negative diagnoses. If gross inadequacies have occurred in the vertical spectrum of either the cases or the controls, almost nothing can be salvaged diagnostically when the groups are rearranged in horizontal layers.

Consequently, the main flaw of inadequate spectrums in diagnostic marker studies is the production of results that are erroneous, misleading, or inconsistent. Tests that are hazardous or expensive (or both) may become accepted, disseminated, and installed as standard procedures before their inadequacies become recognized, often after many false results are noted in pragmatic clinical experience. Different evaluations of the same diagnostic test for the same disease may yield huge ranges of variation in the values of nosologic sensitivity and specificity.[28] When these inconsistencies occur, the subsequent controversy about the diagnostic value of the test may involve an intense scrutiny of the mathematical models, the cutting points in ROC curves, or the equipment used in performing the test, with little or no attention given to the main source of difficulty: the inadequate scope and stratification of the spectrum of people under study.

Because sufficiently detailed results are seldom published for subgroups of the spectrum, relatively few examples can be cited to demonstrate sources and solutions for the problem. In one recent appraisal,[9] however, an inadequate scope of spectrum in both cases and controls was shown to be the source of the erroneous belief that CEA was an efficacious diagnostic marker test for cancer of the colon. A similar problem in the scope and stratification of spectrum has been shown[28] to be the source of the extensive variability found in nosologic indexes for exercise stress testing as a diagnostic marker for coronary artery disease. Because the exercise stress test has now been shown[10, 11, 14] to have variable nosologic indexes that violate the fundamental assumptions of all the mathematical models, and because this type of spectral variability probably occurs in most other diagnostic tests, a suitable scope, demarcation, and appraisal of spectrum will be essential to avoid misleading results in the future.

During a recent demonstration of spectral inadequacies in evaluations of the dexamethasone suppression test for diagnosis of endogenous depression, the authors[29] proposed three new names for the problems that were cited previously and in this section. *Prevalence bias* was suggested as a title for the difficulty that makes nosologic indexes inadequate for diagnostic predictions: the predictive results of a test will change when it is applied to a group in which the prevalence of disease is different from the group in which the test was originally studied. *Sensitivity bias* and *specificity bias* were proposed as labels for the instabilities of nosologic indexes in varying with different types of patients in the spectrum of disease or in the spectrum of various types of control groups.

25.3.5. *The Role of Spectrum in Pathodynamic Studies*

In some instances, such as a streptococcal antibody measurement in patients with rheumatic fever, the entity that is tested diagnostically is regarded as an etiologic factor for the disease. In most circumstances, however, the disease is usually regarded as having produced the marker, with which the disease is then associated pathodynamically (or pathoconsortively). Because of this distinction, the main difference between the outcome entity in a pathodynamic study and the marker entity in many diagnostic studies is the statistical rate of occurrence or the convenience of measuring the entity. If a particular entity is easy to measure, with high prevalence in the cases and low prevalence in the controls, it is likely to be proposed as a marker test.

For these reasons, the selection of suitable spectrum for a pathodynamic study (or for a pathoconsortive study) contains the same challenges as in a diagnostic marker study. The spectrum of cases and controls in a well-designed pathodynamic study should be chosen to deal with the same problems noted for spectrums in a diagnostic marker study.

25.4. **PROBLEMS IN BIAS**

All of the difficulties just discussed can be avoided with adequate attention to choosing suitable spectrums and analyzing results in spectral components. A separate set of problems is more difficult to avoid, because they arise as innate biases that are produced when the tests are ordered, performed, and interpreted. Because the biases are innate, they may not always be found, remedied, or eliminated in studies that are conducted in retrospect, using routinely collected information available in archival sources such as medical records or diagnostic rosters. Beyond the innate biases that can be expected in any form of observational research, certain additional biases can be created by the investigator's decisions during the research.

These diverse biases can be divided into those that affect the comparison of groups and those that affect the accuracy of the basic data.

25.4.1. *Bias in Comparison of Groups*

Two sources of bias can occur when groups are chosen for comparison in diagnostic marker tests. One bias is innate, produced by the circumstances in which tests are ordered as part of an ordinary diagnostic work-up. The other bias is produced by the investigator's decisions about what to do with equivocal data or uncertain results.

25.4.1.1. **SEQUENTIAL-ORDERING (WORK-UP) BIAS**

If the results of a diagnostic test affect the decision to order the test that provides the definitive result about the disease, a work-up or sequential-ordering bias can greatly distort the indexes calculated for nosologic sensitivity and specificity.[9] For example, if the diagnostic marker test is positive, the clinician may look intensely for the disease, thereby ordering the definitive diagnostic procedure, which is solicited much less often if the diagnostic test is negative. These selective decisions in ordering definitive procedures are particularly likely to occur if the diagnostic test (such as exercise stress testing or a liver function test) is noninvasive, whereas the definitive procedure (such as coronary arteriography or a liver biopsy) is invasive.

If the statistical evaluation employs data only from people who have had both the diagnostic marker and the definitive diagnostic procedure, many people with negative test results will be omitted from the fourfold diagnostic table. The result will be an excess proportion of people in the two upper horizontal cells (the *a* and *b* cells of Table 25–5), where the marker test results are positive. The consequence in nosologic indexes for the test will be a relative false elevation in sensitivity and false reduction in specificity. The horizontal predictive results—particularly if determined directly from the fourfold table—may be relatively accurate for diagnostic sensitivity but may be excessively high for diagnostic specificity because many falsely negative results of the marker test will not be detected.

A noncardiac example of this problem occurred when a radiolabeled dye scan was studied as a diagnostic marker for cholecystitis. The surgical exploration that provided the definitive evidence of cholecystitis was often performed in patients with a positive gallbladder scan test, but not in those whose scan results were negative.[23]

The problem of sequential-ordering bias is not easy to solve. It can be avoided in a preplanned (i.e., prospective) diagnostic marker study by insisting that the sequence of diagnostic work-up be established *before* the results are known for the diagnostic test, i.e., the definitive procedure would be ordered without regard to the results of the diagnostic test. Because this strategy may be refused by many clinicians and patients, an alternative approach is to ask the clinician to indicate, when ordering the diagnostic marker test, whether the definitive test is also planned. Patients in whom the definitive test is ordered (or not ordered) only in response to the results of the marker test would be excluded from the statistical tabulations. This approach would provide unbiased data for the compared groups, but it might be difficult to carry out because relatively few clinicians might be willing to state their pre-test work-up plans, and the data available for analysis might be drastically curtailed.

An alternative approach is to abandon the calculation of the vertical nosologic indexes. What the clinician wants to know, after all, are the horizontal indexes of diagnostic sensitivity and diagnostic specificity. These indexes—particularly if calculated for a *consecutive* rather than a case-control series of patients receiving both the marker and the definitive tests—would directly indicate what is likely to happen when the definitive test is ordered. Without the benefit of Bayes' theorem, ROC curves, or other mathematical tactics, the horizontal results in a consecutive series of patients would indicate exactly what has transpired in the prospective use of the test. This "radical" approach will be further discussed in Section 25.6.2.

25.4.1.2. **BIAS DUE TO EXCLUSION OF EQUIVOCAL RESULTS**

When choosing whom to include or exclude in a retrospective case-control study, an investigator can create the transfer bias noted in previous chapters. An analogous bias can arise when analogous decisions are made for the cases and controls to be admitted to a diagnostic marker evaluation.

In the customary two-group framework of selection, the investigator finds the diseased cases from people who had positive results in the definitive diagnostic procedure. The control group is then chosen from a framework of people regarded as free of that disease. The controls are usually healthy normals, patients with other diseases, or people with negative results in the definitive diagnostic procedure. Regardless of which framework (or combination of frameworks) is used for obtaining the controls, the investigator's next step is to find the results of diagnostic marker tests that were performed concomitantly in the cases and controls. The statistical tabulations are then formed from data for the two variables: result of marker test and result of definitive diagnostic procedure.

During this process, the investigator will encounter diagnostic marker results that cannot be clearly classified as positive or negative because they were cited as *equivocal, uncertain, indeterminate, inconclusive,* or some other term indicating that the test had not provided a distinctive decision. What should be done with these results? If the statistical tabulations are examined horizontally, the predictive diagnostic efficacy of these equivocal results can be readily determined. The investigator forms a sixfold table as $\begin{Bmatrix} a & b \\ x & y \\ c & d \end{Bmatrix}$, where the x and y would represent the equivocal findings. The predictive accuracy can promptly be determined horizontally for the positive $(a+b)$, equivocal $(x+y)$, and negative $(c+d)$ results of the test.

In the customary tabulations, however, the statistics are calculated vertically to provide the nosologic indexes. Because these nosologic calculations contain no mechanism for including the equivocal results, they are usually omitted from the data. Thus, the investigator creates a fourfold table as $\begin{Bmatrix} a & b \\ c & d \end{Bmatrix}$. The consequence is a substantial distortion in the nosologic indexes. The true nosologic sensitivity, which should be $a/(a+x+c)$, becomes inflated to $a/(a+c)$. The true nosologic specificity, which should be $d/(b+y+d)$, becomes inflated to $d/(b+d)$. Furthermore, when these inflated indexes are published to show the efficacy of the test, the investigator may not mention the number of equivocal results that were excluded from the calculations. Consequently, a test that often makes no diagnostic contribution, because its equivocal result cannot be interpreted, may be reported as having a relatively high nosologic sensitivity and specificity.

The prevalence of this problem is difficult to discern because reports of diagnostic marker tests seldom include an indication of the excluded patients. In one recent study,[30] in which observations were made in a uni-group prospective consecutive series of tests rather than in a two-group collection of cases and controls, the investigators noted a remarkable phenomenon. After the removal of patients with equivocal results and a series of other reasons for exclusion, only about 3% of the patients who received exercise stress tests would have been retained for calculating the test's nosologic indexes in diagnosis of coronary disease. Because the "tip of the iceberg" seldom represents the true state of events, this iceberg phenomenon is obviously a prominent source of distortion in the conventional determination of nosologic indexes.

The phenomenon can occur, in the manner just cited, if equivocal results are excluded for the diagnostic marker test. A different source of the phenomenon is the exclusion of equivocal results for the definitive-diagnostic procedure. In fact, when equivocal results can occur in both the marker and the definitive procedures, the true state of the statistical data is a ninefold table, containing positive, equivocal, and negative results for each of the two main variables. Opportunities for biased demarcations become abundant when this ninefold table is reduced to the fourfold table used for calculating the nosologic indexes. The kinds of variations that can occur with these reductions were illustrated earlier with the fever measurements of Section 25.1.2.

25.4.2. *Bias in Acquisition of Data*

In ordinary clinical practice, the person who interprets a diagnostic procedure is usually told about the patient's clinical condition and the results of previous tests. Although regarded as desirable by radiologists, pathologists, electrocardiographers, and other consultants who interpret diagnostic procedures, the background information can regularly cause biased interpretations.

25.4.2.1. BIAS IN MAKING A DEFINITIVE DIAGNOSIS (DIAGNOSTIC REVIEW BIAS)

The results found in a diagnostic marker test can readily affect the decision made by the person interpreting the definitive diagnostic procedure. A strongly positive exercise stress test may influence a radiologist who is deciding about a possibly inconclusive coronary arteriogram; a Class V Pap smear may influence a pathologist deciding whether the associated biopsy shows malignant tissue. Unless objectivity is maintained by the interpreter, the definitive procedure may have a falsely high rate of agreement with the diagnostic marker procedure. For example, in an evaluation of the Doppler ultrasound test as a diagnostic marker for venous thrombosis, the investigators provided no assurance that the definitive venograms had been examined independently by interpreters who were unaware of the Doppler results.[31]

This type of problem can be easily remedied. Although consultants can be given all the data they want in ordinary clinical practice, a scientific evaluation of procedures requires assurance of objectivity. Therefore, when the results are to be used as research data, the specimens or other material should be reviewed and re-interpreted by someone who is objectively "blind," i.e., unaware of the findings of other pertinent tests. The "blind" review may not be necessary for laboratory measurements that are performed with inanimate equipment, but is essential whenever a human observer produces a subjective interpretation that becomes the research data.

25.4.2.2. BIAS IN INTERPRETING THE MARKER TEST (TEST REVIEW BIAS)

The reverse type of bias can occur if the diagnostic marker test is performed or interpreted after the definitive results are known. If the marker requires a subjective decision, the decision can readily be affected to yield interpretations that agree with the definitive findings.

For example, about 15 years ago, the nitroblue tetrazolium (NBT) test was optimistically introduced to the medical community as a surrogate marker for the diagnosis of bacterial infection. The test required a subjective interpretation for certain microscopic features of chemically treated white blood cells, but the early evaluations did not include double-blind interpretations for both the marker test and the definitive diagnosis. When these precautions were eventually employed, the high values originally found for the test's sensitivity and specificity began to plummet.[9] The test lost its popularity and is seldom used today.

25.4.2.3. INCORPORATION BIAS

In this type of bias, the investigator works out a "sure bet" arrangement. The results of the marker test are incorporated into the evidence used to make the definitive diagnosis; and the marker then appears to be a good surrogate test for a diagnosis to which it has already contributed. An example of this problem occurred in the previously cited evaluation[23] of a radiolabeled dye scan in diagnosing acute cholecystitis. The results of the scan were included in the data used to establish the definitive diagnosis of the disease. The problem can easily be eliminated. The definitive diagnostic result should depend on information that excludes whatever was found in the diagnostic marker test.

25.5. **PROBLEMS IN CHOOSING A DEFINITIVE STANDARD**

Most of the discussion so far has been concerned with "horizontal" issues in stipulating what is *normal* or *abnormal* for a marker test and with obtaining an undistorted calculation of the test's diagnostic accuracy. We can now turn to the "vertical" problems of choosing and demarcating the definitive result on which everything else depends.

25.5.1. *Issues in Observer Variability*

Some of the main difficulties in diagnostic marker studies are never identified because they arise from observer variability in performance of the *definitive* diagnostic procedure. Unlike a marker test, which can be refuted or confirmed by the definitive procedure, the definitive procedure usually has no independent standard against which to be checked. If a urine sugar test suggests diabetes mellitus, it can be checked with a glucose tolerance test, but the glucose tolerance test is the end of the line. No separate diagnostic procedure is used to verify its results. The same type of decision occurs when a liver biopsy is the definitive standard for a diagnosis of acute hepatitis. The biopsy specimen can be re-interpreted by the same or another observer, but there is no further additional test that checks the results of the biopsy.

In these situations, an important scientific safeguard in the research is to be sure that the definitive procedure was properly performed (e.g., with administration of the appropriate amount of glucose and with appropriate timing of blood specimens); and that the results were interpreted with standard criteria (e.g., checking that the sum of the five blood glucose values exceeds a stipulated boundary). Because the operational performance and interpretive criteria may change from one era to the next or from one institution to another, the efficacy of a diagnostic marker test may sometimes be inconsistent because of variations in the definitive standard rather than in the marker itself.

This variability is particularly likely to occur, as noted in Chapter 26, when the definitive standard depends on subjective interpretations by a pathologist or radiologist. For example, coronary arteriography is customarily used as the definitive standard for appraising the diagnostic results of exercise stress tests—yet the same arteriograms can be interpreted with substantial variability by different observers or even in repeated independent examinations by the same observer.[32]

25.5.2. *The Absence of a Definitive Standard*

The greatest problem in choosing a definitive standard, however, occurs when definitive evidence cannot always be obtained. For example, the results of serum amylase tests are often used to make a diagnosis of pancreatitis, but direct histologic tissue is seldom acquired as definitive evidence that pancreatitis is present or absent. In many instances, definitive evidence may not be obtained because of sequential-ordering bias. For example, when a child is suspected of having appendicitis, a barium enema may be performed as a marker test. If the marker is positive, surgery may be performed, thereby allowing a direct inspection of the appendix to confirm or refute the results of the test. If the marker test is negative, however, surgery is seldom performed, so that definitive diagnostic evidence will not be available. The absence of definitive evidence for most of the patients with negative results may then create a major impediment in evaluating the marker test.

25.5.2.1. **ALTERNATIVE DIAGNOSTIC STANDARDS**

One escape from the dilemma just described is to use a different type of procedure for the definitive diagnosis. For example, instead of requiring surgery and histopathologic inspection of the appendix, we might assemble a panel of appropriate experts and use their consensus as the definitive standard for concluding that the patients did or did not have appendicitis. Another approach is to let the patient's diagnosis be confirmed or refuted by the subsequent clinical course. Thus, such diagnoses as appendicitis or deep vein thrombosis[33] could be accepted or rejected according to the events that take place during a suitable interval after diagnosis.

25.5.2.2. **CHANGE TO MANAGERIAL GOALS**

A more clinically cogent approach to some of these diagnostic dilemmas is to recognize that clinicians often aim at a managerial rather than diagnostic decision. For a patient with suspected appendicitis, pancreatitis, or deep vein thrombosis, the clinician's main goal is what to do about the ailment, not just what to call it. If used for a managerial rather than diagnostic decision, a marker test might be appraised quite differently. The definitive results would be cited according to the successful (or unsuccessful) outcomes that followed different plans of management. The marker tests would be appraised not for their contributions to the often intellectually sterile diagnostic labels of disease, but for their roles in the main clinical decisions—in prognosis and therapy—that are of prime concern in patient care. This strategy was used several years ago for evaluating the contributions that upper gastrointestinal endoscopy had made to choices of treatment rather than names of diseases alone.[34] An analogous approach was proposed for examining the exercise stress test as a prognostic rather than diagnostic marker in patients with suspected coronary disease.[35]

The development of appropriate methods for converting diagnostic process research into clinical management research is a major challenge for future investigators.

25.6. IMPROVEMENTS OF ARCHITECTURE IN DIAGNOSTIC MARKER RESEARCH

Until the new forms of research are developed, we can use what was learned in the foregoing sections to arrive at methods of improving the architectural quality of diagnostic marker research.

25.6.1. *Sequential Phases of Research*

As noted in Chapter 18, a new drug undergoes different phases of development in its pathway from laboratory inception to widespread human usage. The initial animal experiments are usually followed by Phase I and Phase II studies in people, followed by Phase III randomized trials. The next step may be Phase IV studies for post-marketing surveillance before the drug receives unqualified approval and usage.

An analogous set of phases can be contemplated for the development of diagnostic marker tests. In Phase I, the test would be compared for cases of substantially diseased people and for healthy controls. If good discrimination is shown in Phase I, the test can advance to Phase II, in which the spectrum of comparison is extended. The test would now be challenged with different types of diseased cases and controls, covering a suitably wide spectrum of disease and health. If discrimination remains good, the challenge spectrum would be enlarged in Phase III so that the selected cases and controls encompass the clinical, co-morbid, and pathologic issues discussed throughout Section 25.3.3.

If the test passes the challenges of Phase III, the architecture of Phase IV can become prospective rather than case-control. The results of the marker test would be noted, reported, and analyzed for a large *consecutive* series of clinically suitable patients. If the definitive standard results are not known for many of these patients, their data would be analyzed separately, using the alternative standards cited in Section 25.5.2.1.

25.6.2. *Development of Horizontal Diagnostic Indexes*

Because the Phase IV marker study would be prospective, its results need not be cited in the clinically awkward expressions of nosologic indexes and likelihood ratios. In a consecutive series of patients, the efficacy of the test can be cited horizontally as a direct index of its "batting average" for positive and negative values.

Furthermore, if the Phase IV series of patients is suitably stratified for the manifestations that evoked the tests and also for the diagnostic conclusions reached in each patient, the horizontal indexes will show exactly how the test performs in diverse clinical, co-morbid, and pathologic situations. Because these indexes will come from a direct series of patients for whom the test would be applied in pragmatic clinical reality, there will be no need to use Bayes theorem or other mathematical esoterica to compensate for prevalence of disease while converting nosologic indexes or likelihood ratios. The prevalence of disease will be an inherent component of the consecutive series, and no special adjustments will be required for the direct, immediate clinical predictions provided by the horizontal indexes of diagnostic accuracy.

25.6.3. *Management of Uncommon Phenomena*

Although a consecutive series has the major advantage of offering a single rather than double framework for evaluating marker procedures, the approach also has a major disadvantage. The consecutive series may not be large enough to include certain uncommon phenomena that produce some of the most intriguing sources of false-positive or false-negative results in the marker test. For example, if the co-morbid presence of acute monocytic leukemia produces a false result in a marker test, but if acute monocytic leukemia occurs in only 1 of 1000 hospital admissions, a consecutive series of 750 patients may fail to include anyone with this co-morbid disease. The impact of the leukemia would be left unrecognized.

This disadvantage is more apparent than real, however, because the false results produced by leukemia should have been detected when the spectrum of cases and controls was assembled for the Phase III evaluations of the marker. If we recall that the Phase III case-control series is intended to find sources of false-positive and false-negative results, the spectrum can be made broad enough to include diverse sources of suspicious phenomena. With these sources identified in Phase III, their impact can be suitably evaluated and adjusted when the Phase IV indexes are calculated for the test's diagnostic performance in a consecutive series.

25.6.4. *Maintenance of Other Scientific Principles*

Because all results of the marker test will be examined and accounted for, the consecutive series studied in Phase IV will avoid the two forms of group bias noted in Section 25.4.1. The only other biases to worry about may occur in acquisition of data. Because the procedure will be conducted prospectively, the marker test will be interpreted before the results of the definitive procedure are known. Consequently, the main problems to be avoided are the diagnostic review or incorporation biases that can arise if the results of the marker test are known or used in making the definitive diagnosis. These problems can be eliminated by having a separate blinded review of the definitive diagnostic data for each patient included in the evaluation study.

25.7. STUDIES OF CONTRIBUTORY AND DEFINITIVE DIAGNOSTIC TESTS

All of the foregoing discussion has been devoted to the evaluation of surrogate tests whose diagnostic accuracy is the main focus of the evaluation. The evaluation processes will differ, however, when applied to contributory and to definitive diagnostic tests.

25.7.1. *Contributory Tests*

Because a contributory test does not get used alone and cannot have specific statistical indexes calculated for its isolated achievement, it cannot be evaluated in the same way as a surrogate test. A contributory test can receive a quasi-surrogate evaluation, however, if the accompanying clinical and paraclinical data are suitably demarcated to produce component parts of a spectrum in which the contributory test is ordered. For example, a measurement of creatine phosphokinase (CPK) is often employed as a contributory test in the diagnosis of acute myocardial infarction. The distinctive contributions of CPK can be determined by noting its diagnostic performance (i.e., the predictive accuracy for positive and negative results) in a spectrum of appropriate patients demarcated into subgroups with and without different types of chest pain, electrocardiographic abnormalities, and so on. The definitive diagnosis of myocardial infarction, of course, should not include data from the CPK test. If other laboratory measurements are included in the definitive diagnosis, they should be omitted from the spectrum of subgroup challenges given to the CPK tests. Laboratory tests that are *not* included in the definitive diagnosis can be used, however, for further demarcation of the spectrum.

25.7.2. *Definitive Tests*

Because a definitive test is the procedure that gives the correct standard diagnosis, it cannot be evaluated for diagnostic accuracy. The test can be checked for its hazards, costs, observer variability, or clinical value in nondiagnostic decisions but not for its diagnostic accuracy.

The inability to perform such evaluations creates a problem when the definitive test consists of a set of arbitrary diagnostic criteria rather than a single pathognomonic test. For example, fulfillment of the Modified Jones Diagnostic Criteria[36] is currently the definitive test for a diagnosis of acute rheumatic fever. How can we evaluate the accuracy of the criteria, particularly if we want to determine whether the most recent modification of the criteria is better than the previous modifications[37, 38] or better than the original version?[39]

There is no easy answer to this question, particularly because relatively few specific studies have been done to evaluate the accuracy of these (or any other) criteria. A set of diagnostic criteria can regularly be checked for false-positive results by determining the performance in patients who have been demonstrated (by other methods) to have other diseases. For example, we could see how often the Jones criteria would lead to a false-positive diagnosis of rheumatic fever in patients known to have lupus erythematosus, rheumatoid arthritis, congenital heart disease, or other ailments that might be initially suspected as being rheumatic fever. This type of false-positive appraisal was used several years ago to evaluate a new set of diagnostic criteria for systemic lupus erythematosus.[40]

A method for appraising the false-negative aspects of diagnostic criteria remains available for creation by the fertile ingenuity of young readers. The main problem to be solved arises because whatever procedure demonstrates the false-negative results would probably either replace the existing diagnostic criteria or be incorporated into them. A new or modified set of criteria would then have to be evaluated for false-negative results.

25.8. SPECTRAL MARKERS

The distinction between a diagnostic and spectral marker is shown in Figure 25–5. The strategy of forming and using spectral markers is still so relatively new that many investigators who have done such research may not recognize that they were studying *spectral markers.*

Perhaps the main impetus for the recent growth and development of this field was disappointment in the performance of the CEA test as a diagnostic marker in screening presumably healthy people for cancer of the colon. When the results of the CEA test were often negative for localized colon cancer but positive for disseminated colon cancer, investigators began thinking of CEA as a spectral marker that could discriminate localized from advanced or metastatic disease. When used as an index of the patient's clinical course, a conversion from a positive to a negative value of the CEA test would suggest that the treatment had extirpated the cancer. A change from a negative to a positive value of the CEA test might then signal that the cancer had recurred or spread.

Almost all the clinical principles discussed for diagnostic marker evaluations also pertain to the evaluation of spectral markers. There are the same problems in obtaining a suitably broad spectrum of challenges, an unbiased comparison of groups, and objective interpretations for both the marker and the definitive test. The main differences between spectral and diagnostic markers arise in patterns of demarcation for disease, choice of statistical indexes, and an expanded set of clinical applications.

25.8.1. *Patterns of Demarcation*

Unlike the diagnosis of a disease, which is present or absent, the spectrum of an existing disease can be demarcated into many different parts. Because spectral markers are

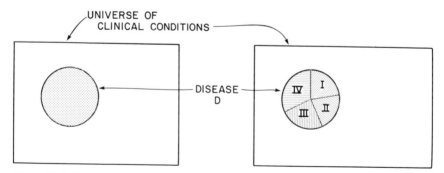

Figure 25–5. Diagnostic and spectral markers. In the figure on the left, a *diagnostic marker test* is intended to discriminate between disease D and all other conditions in the clinical universe. In the figure on the right, a *spectral marker test* is intended to discriminate among different portions (such as stages I, II, III, and IV) of the spectrum of disease D.

used to identify these different parts of the disease's spectrum, the evaluations cannot be readily expressed with the simple fourfold tables that are often possible for diagnostic marker tests.

In most studies, the spectrum is divided nosologically, according to the results of the definitive diagnostic procedure used to identify that part of the spectrum. The spectral marker is then checked for its performance in each of those nosologic components. For example, the CEA test might be checked for its relative frequency of positive and negative results in patients with Stage I, Stage II, or Stage III of a particular cancer. Examples of well-known spectral marker tests are the use of glycosylated hemoglobin to assess the control of blood glucose in patients with diabetes mellitus and the correlation of creatine kinase levels with the size of an acute myocardial infarction.

If the spectral marker is expressed as a dimensional value, the dimensional results may be cited for their direct correlation with the different parts of the spectrum. In some circumstances, a dimensionally measured spectral marker may be directly correlated with the dimensional value of a more definitive test that is more expensive or less convenient to do.

25.8.2. *Choice of Statistical Indexes*

Because of multiple components in the spectrum, the accomplishments of spectral markers would best be cited with a horizontal index of predictive accuracy. Nevertheless, as noted in Section 20.2.3, this index is sometimes calculated in a confusing vertical manner because the denominator is the nosologic condition rather than the results of the spectral marker test. Thus, a spectral marker may be reported as having a mean value of 6.3 in Stage I and 9.2 in Stage II of the disease. This type of post-spective index may demonstrate the discriminatory distinction of the spectral marker test, but the distinction may not be useful for clinical predictions or other identifications. Confronted with a patient who has a spectral marker value of 7.1, the clinician needs to know whether the patient is more likely to be in Stage I or Stage II. These probabilities could be determined only if the results of the spectral index markers were partitioned horizontally to form the denominators of rates of accuracy, for which the numerators would consist of the appropriate nosologic stages. The reversed statistical index, which cites a mean spectral value per stage, uses a nosologic denominator and does not provide an expression applicable to clinical predictions.

25.8.3. *Other Clinical Applications*

Although a spectral marker is commonly used to identify the single state of a particular clinical condition, the marker can also be used for other clinical purposes. Successive values of the marker can be compared to form a transition variable, indicating changes in state from one point in time to another. The marker can also be used in forecasting, to make prognostic estimations. For example, a patient with cancer of the colon may be told that prognosis has improved because the CEA test has changed from positive to negative.

25.9. MARKER TESTS AND THE EVALUATION OF TECHNOLOGY

The explosion of new technologic tests has created enormous problems in clinical medicine. The tests can make an appealing contribution to patient care, but many of them are hazardous or expensive. The people who bear the costs (and the risks) of the technology have increasingly insisted that the tests be evaluated for their cost/benefit or risk/benefit ratios.

These demands are based on the assumption that satisfactory methods exist for doing the evaluations. The assumption, however, is incorrect. The strategies described in this chapter can show the *diagnostic* efficacy of technologic tests but not the many contributions the tests make to all the nondiagnostic decisions that occur when clinicians estimate prognosis, choose therapy, appraise post-therapeutic changes, and provide reassurance.

Because statistical indexes have been relatively well developed (or at least relatively well publicized) for diagnostic efficacy, the diagnostic indexes are commonly used to assess the value of new technologic procedures.[8] If the diagnostic indexes are unimpressive, the evaluators may conclude that the new procedures have little or no merit. The major merits of the procedures may occur, however, in clinical activities that were not suitably evaluated with statistical indexes of diagnosis.

An excellent example of this problem appeared when computerized tomography (CT) first became available. In an elderly patient with an acute stroke, a CT scan of the head did not greatly improve the accuracy of a clinical diagnosis of *cerebrovascular accident*. The result of the CT scan also seemed to add relatively little when prognosis was estimated or suitable rehabilitation therapy was chosen for a patient with stroke. Accordingly, many medical economists regarded the CT scan as a costly, wasteful technologic extravagance.

What the economists overlooked, however, was the magnificent contribution of the CT scan in reassuring clinicians, patients, and patients' families that the diagnosis was indeed *cerebrovascular accident* and that efforts at rehabilitation should proceed as planned. Perhaps 1 of 100 patients with stroke may have a surgically remediable lesion, such as a benign meningioma or a subdural hematoma. An occurrence rate of 0.01 may seem small to economic analysts, but it is critically important for patients and clinicians. Clinicians want to find that one patient in a hundred so that a curable stroke can be cured rather than consigned to slow deterioration. Accordingly, clinicians will regularly try to rule out the presence of a curable lesion in a patient with stroke. In the days before the CT scan, the additional diagnostic procedures used for this rule-out function produced the painful horrors of pneumoencephalography or the invasive hazards of cerebral arteriography. Today, however, both of these unpleasant diagnostic procedures can be replaced by a pain-free, risk-free, noninvasive CT scan of the head.

If evaluated merely for a role in verifying the clinical diagnosis of cerebrovascular accident, the CT scan will seem to make a negligible contribution to diagnosis, prognosis, or therapy in about 99 of 100 patients with stroke. Consequently, the CT scan will have a low statistical score for incrementing diagnostic efficacy; and the high costs of the equipment will not be balanced by positive data for clinical benefits. On the other hand, the statistically low index of efficacy will completely omit the major contributions that the CT scan makes to patient care by providing the desired reassurance so easily and safely.

These distinctions should be kept in mind when new technology is evaluated from mathematical models and statistical indexes that focus only on diagnosis. For properly appraising and mastering new technology, clinicians will need a new, expanded set of models and indexes. The new strategies, which have not yet been fully developed, will have to include attention to many clinical activities beyond diagnosis alone; and the methods of measurement, which also remain to be developed, will have to include new clinimetric scales for reassurance and other benefits that are now omitted from the constrained scope of risk/benefit and cost/benefit computations.

25.10. SYNOPSIS

To use current mathematical strategies for indexing the efficacy of diagnostic marker tests, the results must be divided into a double dichotomy, with the test demarcated sharply as positive or negative, and the disease as present or absent. These demarcations often misrepresent the nondichotomous events of clinical reality, in which many tests yield equivocal results and many tested patients receive inconclusive diagnostic decisions. For receiver-operator-characteristic (ROC) curve analysis, the dichotomous demarcation of dimensional or ordinal values also creates a clinical artefact. The dichotomy provides vertical indexes of nosologic sensitivity and specificity, but because clinical diagnostic reasoning proceeds in a horizontal direction, a better approach would be to divide the test results into three (or more) horizontal zones rather than two. The upper and lower zones would have high accuracy for positive and negative diagnoses; and the middle zone would be too uncertain for diagnostic conclusions.

Aside from these problems, cogent clinical issues in diagnosis cannot be adequately managed if the analysis depends exclusively on mathematical strategies. The requirements for success will differ according to the test's purpose in discovery, exclusion, or confirmation of disease and according to the test's application alone or in combination. A particularly important but commonly neglected problem is the spectrum of the groups under evaluation. Many indexes are inaccurate or misleading because they were calculated from diseased and nondiseased groups that had an inadequate scope in their clinical, co-morbid, or pathologic spectrum. The groups under study may have a biased composition because the definitive test is often not ordered when the marker test is negative, or because equivocal results are excluded from the analysis. The data may be biased if the results of the marker test are incorporated into the definitive diagnostic evidence, or if the tests are not interpreted objectively, so that decisions about the marker test are made with knowledge of results in the definitive test, or vice versa. The most distressing problem of all, however, is that all the mathematical computations depend on the assumption that each test has a constant value for its nosologic sensitivity and specificity. In the few instances in which this assumption has been checked, it was found to be erroneous, thus raising doubt about all subsequent mathematical derivations.

The definitive diagnostic evidence needed for evaluating marker tests may be uncertain because of observer variability, or may be unobtainable because a definitive result does not exist or requires inappropriate invasion. When a definitive result is not routinely available, the marker process may be better evaluated if aimed at managerial rather than diagnostic decisions.

The architectural quality of diagnostic marker research can be improved if conducted in a sequence of phases analogous to those used for testing new drugs. The spectrum of tested cases and controls would be progressively extended as the appraisal proceeds from Phases I through III, but the final premarketing evaluations, during Phase IV, would occur in a uni-group, consecutive series of suitable patients, whose results could be cited in the directly observed horizontal indexes of diagnostic accuracy, with no need for indirect mathematical processes.

The evaluation of spectral marker tests, which are used to indicate different parts of a disease's spectrum, contains many of the same problems and solutions as those just cited for diagnostic markers. The use of inappropriate vertical indexes is particularly common for spectral marker tests, producing mean (or median) values that cannot be used for horizontal predictions.

Perhaps the greatest clinical difficulty in all of the cited diagnostic and spectral approaches, however, is that they are too intellectually restricted to be satisfactory for evaluating modern informational technology. The information supplied by the technology is constantly used for estimating prognosis, choosing therapy, appraising post-therapeutic status, providing reassurance, and making many clinical decisions other than diagnosis alone. Whatever strategies are used for diagnostic evaluation cannot be adequate for appraising the role of the technology in all of the other nondiagnostic clinical decisions. The solution to this problem will require development of a new set of architectural models and clinical indexes.

EXERCISES

Exercise 25.1. About 4% of school-aged children in Megalopolis are believed to be physically abused by their parents. The schools in the city might be able to screen all children for evidence of abuse (e.g., scars, bruises, and burns), with the intent of follow-up by contacting the suspected parents. A great deal of potential damage can be caused either by letting an abused child go undetected or by erroneously suspecting a parent. To avoid the latter problem, school and health officials should be very confident of their suspicions before approaching the parents. School health officials assert that the physical examination they use is very reliable: 96% of the abused children will be detected by a positive physical examination, whereas only 8% of nonabused children will be falsely positive.

    a. What is the nosologic sensitivity of the physical examination?

    b. What is the nosologic specificity of the physical examination?

    c. If the screening program is indeed implemented in Megalopolis schools, what will be the diagnostic sensitivity, i.e., the positive predictive accuracy, of the physical examination?

Exercise 25.2. From the literature at your disposal, select a study of a diagnostic marker test and in one or two sentences, outline its basic arrangement. Comment on the selection of case and control groups. If you do not fully approve of the selections, what alternatives would you suggest? Make any other critical comments or architectural suggestions that occur to you as you review the study.

Exercise 25.3. The ratio of the renal clearance of amylase relative to creatinine has been proposed as a possible test for acute pancreatitis, which is usually diagnosed when a patient with abdominal pain has an elevated serum and/or urinary amylase. Two problems in the evaluation are that amylase activity may be elevated in conditions other than pancreatitis and may be normal with proved pancreatitis; and that the clinical impression of acute pancreatitis is seldom documented by pathologic examination of tissue or by some other unequivocal "gold standard" technique. These two problems create a virtually insoluble dilemma: How can you prove that the new amylase clearance ratio is better than amylase measurements when amylase values are the usual yardstick to diagnose pancreatitis? Please solve the dilemma of the gold standard and suggest a method for confirming the existence of the diseased state (pancreatitis). What kinds of patients would you assemble as a suitable challenge for checking the diagnostic value of the test?

Exercise 25.4. Assume that Roth spots (of retinal hemorrhage) provide a perfectly specific sign for bacterial endocarditis; their presence confirms endocarditis beyond doubt. The sign, however, is rarely present. For this assignment, assume that the probability of endocarditis is 0.2 for a particular patient under consideration. Also assume that the probability of Roth spots in endocarditis is 0.005 but that the spots never occur unless endocarditis is present.

    a. Given that the patient has endocarditis, what is the probability that the patient shows Roth spots?

b. Given that a patient does not have endocarditis, what is the probability that the patient shows Roth spots?

c. Given that a patient shows Roth spots, what is the probability that the patient has endocarditis?

d. Given that a patient does not show Roth spots, what is the probability that the patient has endocarditis?

Exercise 25.5. Screening for disease is technically defined as the application of diagnostic testing to a healthy population in order to separate the population into groups with high and low probabilities for a given disorder. What circumstances and test characteristics would you cite as justifying efforts to screen for disease?

Exercise 25.6. Find a set of diagnostic criteria for any disease in which you are interested. If the criteria were tested for their diagnostic efficacy, please comment on how well the test was done. If the criteria have not been tested, please outline the procedure you would suggest for this purpose.

CHAPTER REFERENCES

1. Bergeson, 1974; 2. Statistical Research Group, Columbia University, 1948; 3. Ackerman, 1972; 4. Metz, 1973; 5. Johnstone, 1979; 6. McNeil, 1975; 7. Weinstein, 1980; 8. Griner, 1981; 9. Ransohoff, 1978; 10. Goldschlager, 1976; 11. Weintraub, 1983; 12. Rozanski, 1983; 13. Osbakken, 1984; 14. Hlatky, 1984; 15. Moertel, 1978; 16. Goslin, 1981; 17. National Institutes of Health, 1981; 18. Hart, 1983; 19. Richardson, 1981; 20. Ross, 1975; 21. Anonymous, 1978; 22. Sheikh, 1975; 23. Eikman, 1975; 24. Newcomer, 1975; 25. Sherwood, 1975; 26. Ennis, 1975; 27. Nagel, 1975; 28. Philbrick, 1980; 29. Shapiro, 1983; 30. Philbrick, 1982; 31. Meadway, 1975; 32. Detre, 1975; 33. Hull, 1983; 34. Lichtenstein, 1980; 35. Harrell, 1982; 36. American Heart Association, 1984; 37. American Heart Association, 1955; 38. American Heart Association, 1965; 39. Jones, 1944; 40. Fries, 1973.

Chapter 26

Observer Variability

When I was in high school, a science instructor taught me an important lesson about observer variability. "If you want to know the length of this board," he said, "measure it once and quit. If you measure it again, you may get confused."

The lesson was valuable for its application in determining the length of something as simple as a flat board, using a well-calibrated tape measure or ruler, and getting a dimension that would probably serve as an approximation. The minor differences of intraobserver variability in repeated measurements of the board might not be worth discovering. They would probably produce uncertainty about which measurement was correct, doubt about which one to choose, and delay in making use of the information.

Many phenomena of clinical medicine, however, are not as easily measured as the length of a board; and the consequences of variability may be much greater. The value obtained for blood pressure can make a patient be regarded as healthy or unhealthy; a measurement of serum cholesterol may produce major changes in diet; a radiologist's interpretation of a thoracic image may lead to a surgical operation; a pathologist's reading of a tissue slide may determine whether a woman keeps her breast or loses it; and a clinician's auscultatory decision that a heart murmur is new may evoke an intensive course of costly, risky antibiotic therapy.

Because clinicians must make so many measurements while acquiring the data of routine patient care, an attention to observer variability has often been regarded as undesirable. To learn and check the different types of variability that can occur in each of the measurements might simply produce uncertainty and doubt. The resultant confusion might impede the promptness, prudence, and efficiency with which clinical decisions must be made from the data. On the other hand, as clinicians have become increasingly aware of their inconsistencies, and as patients increasingly seek second opinions for many of the decisions, the problem of observer variability has gained major medical importance and a vital scientific role. Clinicians may not need to worry about measurements that have little or no impact on major decisions, but the validity of clinical science and practice depends on certain items of crucial information. If that information affects the main results of a research project, or if it leads to surgical operations, courses of medical therapy, and changes in life style, we need to know whether the information is trustworthy.

One way of checking the trustworthiness of information was described in Chapter 25. When a definitive or reference standard is available, the data can be checked against that standard. In many (if not most) medical circumstances, however, a definitive standard is not available, or there may be problems in the standard itself. When we want to license a commercial laboratory that measures chemical constituents of blood, who or what is to be used as the source of the "correct" answers? When two radiologists disagree about whether a chest film shows a cancer, we can use the pathologist's examination of tissue as the standard, but what do we do if no tissue is removed or if a second pathologist disagrees with the first pathologist's interpretation? And what does a patient do when surgery is vigorously urged by one board-certified internist and vigorously opposed by another?

The foregoing questions set the stage for the topics to be discussed in this chapter. They deal with variability in observations for which a definitive standard does not exist; with the different observational and decisional sources of the variability; and with efforts to reduce the variability or to draw conclusions amid the uncertainty.

26.1. OBJECTIVES OF THE RESEARCH

As in any other form of research, a study of observer variability should have a clearly specified goal that has both overt and latent components. The *overt* objective is usually easy to state. A particular entity or set of entities is chosen to be appraised; the results are to be reported by observers who have been chosen to do the appraisal and who are willing to do it; and their degree of agreement will be noted and summarized. This overt objective can usually be easily converted into an architectural plan for the research.

The *latent* objective of the research is seldom clearly stated, however, and its choice is particularly important. Is the study being done to demonstrate observer variability or to remove it? If the goal is to remove variability, the work may need a set of plans quite different from those used merely to demonstrate variability. To remove variability (as noted later), many more details of the observations may have to be specified, and the investigator may have to arrange confrontations that do not occur and are not required if the only objective is merely to quantify the presence or absence of major inconsistencies.

The distinction between descriptive documentation and remedial improvement becomes particularly striking when we compare the way that observer variability is studied in clinical epidemiologic research and in laboratory medicine. The people who run medical laboratories study variability so they can determine what went wrong, try to fix it, and check that it is fixed. Because of this objective, the name *observer variability* is almost never used for this type of laboratory research. It produces, and it is called, *quality control.*

In contrast, when *observer variability* is studied and reported in the activities of pathologists, radiologists, clinicians, and other medical personnel, the investigators usually arrange merely to demonstrate the variability. Few or no efforts are made to dissect or probe the sources of variability, to remove it, or even to suggest methods of possible removal. The work is quite properly called a study of *observer variability,* because it neither improves nor controls quality. Having added a bit of quantified sagacity to their bibliography, the investigators usually depart in an aura of wisdom, but the *status* is left as *quo.* (I was guilty of exactly this type of activity in a study of observer variability among histopathologists conducted almost 15 years ago.[1])

The methods and standards used to achieve quality control in laboratory medicine are well developed, well established, and reported extensively in several publications[2-4] to which interested readers are referred. The rest of this chapter will be devoted to the underdeveloped territory of observer variability and to the efforts that can be made for improving quality control among pathologists, radiologists, and clinicians.

26.2. SCALES AND STATISTICAL INDEXES OF EXPRESSION

The principle of "begin at the end" is particularly valuable in planning studies of observer variability. Because the variability will be judged from disparities in expressing the results, a prime feature of the research will be the scales available for the expressions.

26.2.1. *Use of Commensurate Scales*

If two observers use exactly the same scale for reporting their results, the data will be relatively easy to analyze because the variability will arise from the observational process, not from the scales. For example, suppose we want to check for observer variability in obstetricians' or pediatricians' ratings for the condition of newborn babies. If we ask that the ratings for each baby be expressed as an *Apgar score*—a well-known, well-accepted, standard scale—any differences in the ratings can be attributed to differences in the observers. If we ask the observers to express the babies' conditions as **excellent, good, fair,** or **poor,** the observers would all use the same scale, but considerable variability might occur because no criteria have been specified for each of the ratings. If no rating scale were stipulated, however, and if a standard scale did not exist, each observer might use a different set of categories of expression. One person might rate the babies as **healthy** or **unhealthy;** another observer might use a scale such as **perfect, splendid, very good, no major problems, alarming,** or **moribund.** The use of different scales would make it difficult to decide whether the varying results arise from the observational process itself or from the choice of terms that expressed the results.

This type of problem constantly occurs when observer variability is studied for the many medical phenomena that lack a standardized scale of expression. Because of different taxonomies of classification, the scales of expression may differ substantially for two pathologists designating the cellular type of a cancer, for two radiologists expressing degree of cardiac enlargement, or for two clinicians citing the magnitude of pitting peripheral edema.

Because the sources of variability will be difficult to analyze if the observers use different scales, an investigator should arrange (if possible) for the observers to use the same scale, containing the same available categories of expression. If one radiologist rates pulmonary embolism as **present** or **absent** and another rates it as **present, uncertain,** or

absent, the results can be used to examine the trend of the two sets of observations but not their actual agreement or disagreement.

In choosing a scale that will make the observations commensurate, the investigator may immediately remove a prime source of variability. This removal may be undesirable if the research is intended to show differences in the actual categories of expression. For such a goal, the observers should be left to their own devices. If the research has some other goal—such as studying sources of variability in the observational process or reducing the variability—the establishment of a commensurate scale of expression for all observers is highly desirable before the research begins.

When the scale is chosen, however, the investigator should negotiate with the observers to be sure that the scale is both acceptable and suitable for its purpose. For example, several years ago I helped a radiologist design a study of observer variability among his colleagues in making the diagnosis of pulmonary embolism from a plain chest film in a series of patients for whom pulmonary arteriograms were available to provide the definitive result. To keep his colleagues from "sitting on the fence," the investigator originally wanted each plain chest film to be cited as **yes** or **no** for the diagnosis of pulmonary embolism. Although this binary scale would prevent equivocation in diagnosis, the participating radiologists might complain that it was unfair. A radiologist could contend that when she was sure about the presence or absence of an embolism, she would happily record the result as **yes** or **no.** When she was unsure, however, she wanted to be able to express the uncertainty and not be forced into an unequivocal **yes** or **no** decision. The rating scale was therefore changed to **yes, uncertain,** or **no.** This choice satisfied the participating radiologists and was also acceptable to the investigator after he became persuaded that enough data would probably be available for demonstrating substantial inaccuracies even in the unequivocal **yes** or **no** categories of diagnosis.[5]

26.2.2. *Choice of a Scale*

After deciding to have the observers use commensurate scales, the investigator must often establish the categorical contents of the scale. If the scale is already well established, no choice is necessary because the observers can use the standard categories; but if the scale is being created for the research (as in the foregoing study of pulmonary embolism), a decision must be made about the number of categories. Should the scale have three categories, such as **yes, uncertain,** or **no**? Or should there be five categories: **definitely yes, probably yes, uncertain, probably no,** or **definitely no**?

An increased richness of categories will allow the observers greater freedom to express all their nuances of observation but will also increase the opportunity for variability. A smaller number of categories may reduce the variability, but if the number becomes too small, variability may be increased (as noted earlier) because of the truncated opportunity to express important distinctions.

I am not aware of any effective, medically oriented research about the optimum number of categories to be used in a categorical rating scale. If the scale is nominal, as in the histologic types of a cancer, the choice seems to depend more on scientific progress than on statistical principles. Thus, with new staining or microscopic techniques, the taxonomy of a histologic classification is often changed not for quantitative distinctions in number of categories in a rating scale, but for new scientific discoveries that lead to new schemes of classification. The main decisions about number of categories usually arise in scales concerned with the presence or absence of a particular entity (as in the example of pulmonary embolism) or in scales that provide an ordinal grade of relative magnitude.

Ordinal rating scales are constantly used by clinicians and radiologists to rate the relative magnitude of such entities as severity of illness, degree of physical incapacitation, enlargement of heart, congestion of pulmonary vessels, and so on—but the scales are often informal and unstandardized. For studies of observer variability in these phenomena, the investigator must then choose the contents of the scale. In general, very few scales seem to exceed 10 categories; and the idea of a graded rating is impaired if the scale has less than three categories. Scales with four or five categories seem quite popular, but many have only three. In one test of observer variability[6] in use of the Karnofsky scale of performance status,[7] which can be cited in either 10 or three categories, the amount of variability was substantially reduced when the observers were compared for their three-category rather than 10-category ratings.

26.2.3. *Expressions of Disagreement*

Regardless of what scale was used to express the observations, a prime focus of the research is the magnitude of disagreement. Two observers obviously disagree if they use different categories in the selected rating scale, but the magnitude of disagreement may be trivial, minor, or major. For example, a difference of 10 points may be relatively unimportant if the diastolic blood pressure is cited as 150 mm. Hg by one observer and 160 by another, but this same increment may make the difference between untreated health and treated hypertension if the respective readings are 85 and 95.

26.2.3.1. DIMENSIONAL SCALES

Because dimensional data offer an almost unlimited number of categories, disagreements in results will be quite common, but many of the disagreements will be trivial. For example, if two measurements of the same fasting blood glucose are reported as 86 and 87 by a hospital laboratory, the distinction would probably be ignored. If they were cited as 76 and 86, we might begin to worry. If the two values were 86 and 126, we might stop using the laboratory for that measurement.

The foregoing example demonstrates that dimensional data, despite their mensurational advantages, are often converted into ordinal grades for assessing magnitude disagreement. The boundaries used for these grades of disagreement will vary according to the scale and the criteria used by the boundary maker, but what usually emerges is a rating scheme such as **identical, very close, reasonably close, far apart,** and **distressingly far apart.** The boundaries would establish a central zone of **very close** agreement, with subsequent zones demarcated above and below the central region.

26.2.3.2. ORDINAL SCALES

Because disagreements in ordinal data are easily cited according to the number of categories of disparity, the main decisions are to choose how many categories create a real disparity and whether all disparities have equal importance.

In many instances, we might decide that a difference of one category is relatively unimportant and that a true disagreement (or change) requires a two-category difference. For example, despite the dimensional expression of results, streptococcal antibody titers are cited in an ordinal scale that depends on a finite number of dilutions in the tubes used for the measurement process. The dilutions may create a scale based on reciprocal values of 8, 16, 32, 64, 128, 256, 512, and so on. Such a scale is essentially ordinal rather than dimensional because a particular measurement must occupy one of these categories and cannot lie between them. Consequently, a patient whose antibody titer was cited as **128** on one occasion and **256** on another occasion may actually have had the same intermediate value on both occasions. To avoid this type of problem, clinicians will insist on a change of at least two tube dilutions as evidence of a recent streptococcal infection.

Analogously, if cardiac size is reported as **slightly enlarged** by one radiologist and **moderately enlarged** by another, we may not want to regard the one-category disparity as a real disagreement. If the respective categorizations, however, are **slightly enlarged** and **massively enlarged,** the disparity of two (or more) categories will obviously be impressive.

A separate problem in rating disagreements for ordinal data occurs when the same scale is used to indicate both existence and magnitude. For example, when cardiac enlargement exists, we can use a scale such as **slight, moderate,** or **massive** to characterize the degree of enlargement. Alternatively, we can use a single scale, such as **none, slight, moderate,** or **massive** to indicate that the heart has either normal size or various grades of enlargement. In the first scale, a difference of one category between **slight** and **moderate** might be regarded as essentially equivalent to the one-category disagreement between **moderate** and **massive.** In the second scale, a one-category disagreement between **none** and **slight** might create the difference between a diagnosis of health or disease, and might therefore be accorded more importance than the other one-category differences, each of which occurs within the spectrum of disease.

Analogously, in the three categories of a TNM staging for cancer, a one-category difference between **localized** and **regionally disseminated** might have much greater therapeutic implications and might be accorded more importance as a disparity than a one-category difference between **regional** and **distant dissemination.**

Cicchetti[8] has provided a detailed account of the impact of these distinctions in scoring and summarizing disagreements in ordinal scales.

26.2.3.3. BINARY SCALES

When observations are reported in binary scales, the disagreements are especially easy to express. Because the individual results can be cited in only two categories, such as **yes** or **no**, the observers will either agree or disagree on any pair of observations. When the two responses are **yes-yes** or **no-no**, the observers agree; but a distinctive pattern can occur in the disagreements. Are they equally divided among **yes-no** and **no-yes** responses, or does one pattern of disagreement occur substantially more often than the other?

For example, a series of 50 disagreements may occur as 26 instances of **yes-no** and 24 instances of **no-yes**; or as 45 instances of one and 5 of the other. If b and c are used to represent the number of instances of these two types of disagreement, their pattern can be summarized with the McNemar bias index of $(b-c)/(b+c)$. In the first example, this index would be $(26-24)/50 = 0.04$. In the second example, the index would be $(45-5)/50 = 0.80$. At values near 0, the index shows no distinctive pattern of disagreement; at values near $+1$ or -1, the index shows that one of the observers is much more likely to say **yes** (or **no**) than the other. The stochastic significance of the bias can be interpreted, at one degree of freedom, with the McNemar chi-square test, which is calculated as $X_M^2 = (b-c)^2/(b+c)$.

When an investigator plans to use a binary scale for investigating observer variability, the most challenging decision is whether, in fact, to use only the two categories, or to expand the binary scale into some additional categories as noted earlier in Section 26.2.1. An analogous set of problems in using binary scales to evaluate diagnostic marker tests rather than observer variability was discussed in Chapter 25.

26.2.3.4. NOMINAL SCALES

Studies of observer variability become particularly interesting when the observations are expressed in nominal scales. Although the observations themselves cannot be ranked, a rating scale can often be established for ranking the observed disagreements. For example, the rating scale for *birthplace in United States* contains 50 states as a set of nominal, unranked categories. For observer variability in citing geographic location, however, a disagreement of **Maine** versus **Vermont** is substantially less striking than a disagreement between **Maine** versus **California.**

Because of various attributes associated with the nominal categories, a scale of ranked disagreements can often be established so that the disparities can be analyzed as ordinal rather than nominal data. An arrangement of this type was used to evaluate the observer variability of pathologists in diagnosing the histologic type of lung cancer.[1] In other circumstances, however, the investigators may prefer to avoid a scale of ranked disagreements.[9] Two observations will then be rated simply as **agree** or **disagree** if they are stated in the same category of the nominal scale.

26.2.4. *Statistical Indexes for Summarizing Disagreement*

In Chapter 10, we saw that agreements or disagreements should be summarized with statistical indexes of concordance, not with the customarily used indexes of trend (or correlation).

The inappropriate indexes are actually used more often for the dimensional data of quality control studies than for the nondimensional data investigated in most studies of observer variability. Knowing that the customary statistical coefficients of dimensional correlation (such as Pearson's r) cannot be readily applied to nondimensional data, investigators of observer variability have had to search for alternative indexes to summarize the results. For nondimensional data, the investigators have then used such appropriate statistical indexes as percentage agreement, kappa (for binary or nominal data), and weighted kappa (for ordinal data).

In quality control studies, however, the Pearson r coefficient is readily applicable, and has often been applied, to index the associations of the compared dimensional data. The summaries are often unsatisfactory because r is an index of trend, not of agreement. Two sets of measurements can be strikingly different and yet have a strikingly high coefficient of correlation if they show the same trend. Thus, an r value of 1 could be found if method A always yields a result that is 20 units higher or three times higher than the corresponding result of method B. To avoid this problem, the appropriate index of concordance in dimensional data is the *intraclass correlation coefficient,* not the conventional correlation coefficient.

Readers who want more detailed accounts of these statistical indexes can consult several appropriate reference sources.[10-12] The textbook by Fleiss[12] contains a particularly lucid discussion and good illustrations of the statistical issues. Readers should also be warned that all of the discussion thus far pertains to comparison of disagreement for *two* observers. When more than two observers are being evaluated simultaneously, the indexes must be modified appropriately. Although a generalized index of concordance can encompass the variations in all observers simultaneously, the multiple-observer results are often hard to understand. Most investigators therefore prefer to calculate standard indexes for the disagreements of each pair of observers. The overall index for the multiple observers is then calculated as the average of values for the paired disagreements.

26.3. **THE INPUT CHALLENGE**

The choice of specimens (or other objects) for the input challenge is as important in studying observer variability as in evaluating marker procedures. If the study is intended to demonstrate observer variability in the real world, the input spectrum should have a proportionate distribution that will adequately represent the real world. If the spectrum is chosen mainly to contain a set of challenging cases, or if the difficult cases occur in a much higher proportion than in customary circumstances, the observers may seem to have a distressingly high rate of disagreement. This type of problem has often occurred in studies of observer variability. When a collection of such studies is reviewed[13] without attention to the problem, the results may unfairly suggest the nihilistic conclusion that clinical observations are too unreliable to receive serious attention.

On the other hand, if the selected spectrum of specimens merely reflects the proportions encountered in reality, there may be too few cases to provide any difficult challenges for the observers. They may then seem to have results that are falsely high when assessed by percentage of agreement and perhaps punitively low when assessed by the kappa index. The reason for the latter distinction is that the kappa index, like the indexes used for diagnostic prediction, is affected by the prevalence of the disease (or condition) that serves as the main challenge in the group used for evaluation.[14]

For example, consider the challenge given to two ophthalmologists who are asked to diagnose the retina of the eye as being normal or abnormal in a group of 300 people. Let us assume, from previous studies using ophthalmologist C as the definitive standard, that ophthalmologist A has a nosologic sensitivity of 95% for diagnosing abnormality in people with abnormalities, and a specificity of 90% for diagnosing normality in people who are normal. For ophthalmologist B, the corresponding values are 85% for nosologic sensitivity and 80% for specificity.

When ophthalmologists A and B are tested for observer variability, however, these underlying aspects of their accuracy are obscured. What is appraised is their variability, not their accuracy, in the group of people who are used as the input spectrum. Let us first give the observers a group of 300 predominantly normal people—10 with abnormal retinas and 290 with normal retinas. With some algebra that is not shown here, the marginal totals for the table of observer variability can be determined. If we then fill in the four cells to give the observers excellent agreement, we might find the following results:

| | Observer B | | |
Observer A	Abnormal	Normal	Total
Abnormal	38	29	67
Normal	1	232	233
Total	39	261	300

For this table, the percentage agreement is 90% $[= (38 + 232)/300]$, but kappa is substantially lower. The expected number of agreements is $[(39 \times 67)/300] + [(261 \times 233)/300] = 211.42$ and the observed agreement is 270, so kappa is $(270 - 211.42)/(300 - 211.42) = 0.66$, which is good but less impressive than the 90% value for agreement.

On the other hand, if we challenge observers A and B with a different group of 300 people with 150 abnormal and 150 normal retinas, and if we make the same assumptions about the underlying sensitivity and specificity for each observer, we can determine the marginal values of their agreement matrix. We can then fill in the cells to get the following table:

| | Observer B | | |
Observer A	Abnormal	Normal	Total
Abnormal	138	20	158
Normal	20	122	142
Total	158	142	300

The two observers now seem to have a relatively worse performance because their percentage index of agreement has dropped to 87% $[= (138 + 122)/300]$. Their value of kappa, however, will show a rise to 0.73, because the expected number of agreements would be $[(158 \times 158)/300 + (142 \times 142)/300] = 150.42$ and kappa would be $(260 - 150.42)/(300 - 150.42) = 0.73$.

Perhaps the best way to obtain an adequate and relatively unbiased challenge spectrum is to begin with a consecutive series of patients who are (or were) candidates for the examination under scrutiny. This consecutive series will have the advantages both of coming from a uni-group framework and of showing the actual reality of the procedure's application in routine practice. The contents of this consecutive series, however, would be supplemented by additional patients, chosen from the infrequently occurring extremes of the spectrum, who will expand the total challenge to include phenomena seldom found in routine practice. The number of these unusual cases should be adequate to provide a good idea of how they are appraised by the observers, without becoming so large that the unusual patients either cannot be obtained or become the dominant feature of the total spectrum.

26.4. PERFORMANCE OF PROCEDURE

The main items to be considered under *procedure* are the choice of a suitable focus in the procedure and the arrangement of objectivity in performance.

26.4.1. *Choice of Focus of Variability*

As noted in Chapter 5, the research objective should be clearly aimed at checking the instrumental methods, the performing observers, or a combination of both. Thus, if we want to compare different types of ophthalmoscopes, we would want the instruments to be used by ophthalmologists of equal competence, and preferably the same ophthalmologist would check each instrument. If the goal is to investigate mainly the observational process of the ophthalmologists, and if we think the quality of the ophthalmoscope will affect the observations, we would want the different observers to use the same (or same type of) ophthalmoscope.

Finally, if our main concern is the output of the total process, consisting of a combination of instrument plus observer, we might let the observers use whatever type of ophthalmoscope they employ routinely. For example, when the detection of diabetic retinopathy was compared among ophthalmologists and nonophthalmologists,[15] the investigators were interested mainly in determining whether the nonophthalmologists were equally skillful in detecting the retinal lesions. No attempt was made to standardize the work of the two sets of observers in such procedures as type of ophthalmoscope and techniques of pupil dilatation. The results, which showed that the nonophthalmologists were not as adept as the ophthalmologists, provided a satisfactory answer to the research question, but not an explanation for the distinction. Had the nonophthalmologists dilated the pupils, used the same instruments, and taken the same amount of procedural time as the ophthalmologists, the agreement of the two sets of observers might have been substantially higher.

26.4.2. *Objectivity in Performance*

Because observer variability is seldom evaluated without a specifically designed plan for the research, the investigators almost always recognize the need for objectivity in the compared performances. The investigators can then plan to "blind" the observers appropriately. When intraobserver variability is being checked by having the observers reexamine the same specimens, the "mask" used for the blinding may be "perforated" if an observer can regularly recall individual specimens and remember the previous interpretations. To avoid this problem, studies of intraobserver variability are usually planned to contain a large number of specimens, with a reasonably long interval between the two sets of examinations.

As noted in Chapter 25, this attention to objectivity is often overlooked in diagnostic or spectral marker research. Because the results of the marker test and the definitive test are readily available in patients' medical records, the research can be often conducted retrolectively, using the available archival data. The recorded results for one procedure, however, may have been biased by the examiner's awareness of what had already been found in the other procedure. Because observer variability studies are almost always conducted prolectively, this type of bias can easily be avoided if the investigators make the necessary efforts.

26.4.3. *Cooperation of Participants*

A separate challenge for the investigators of observer variability is to acquire the necessary observers and persuade them to participate in the research. Many people may refuse to participate because they do not like the idea of submitting their authoritative status to objective verification. Consequently, the spectrum of participating observers may not include some of the persons whose opinions most need to be checked. Other observers, who are willing to participate, may not be able to give the work the necessary time and effort. This difficulty can usually be reduced by making the activities as easy as possible for the observers (the investigator obtains the specimens, provides the formats for recording data, etc.) and by keeping the sample size small enough to be manageable while still being large enough to yield statistically and clinically cogent distinctions.

One unique problem that I encountered in a study of observer variability was the distress of a renowned participating pathologist after he learned the results of the research. Claiming that the demonstration of high variability was a disservice to pathologists, he wanted to have the study suppressed and left unpublished. Fortunately, he was overruled by the four other participating pathologists; and the results were eventually reported in scientific literature,[1] although the name of the dissenter was omitted from the list of authors.

26.5. FORMATION OF OUTPUT

Probably the main reason that variability can arise and persist in subjective medical observations is the common neglect—during both instruction and investigation—of the two different phases of the observational process. In the first phase, the observational procedure transforms the observed phenomena into certain raw elements of descriptive data. Thus, a cardiac auscultator hears a set of noises that may be descriptively converted into such raw data as **systolic murmur, Grade 3/6, loudest at apex, high-pitched, blowing**, and so on. In the second phase, these raw descriptive elements are converted into a category of final expression, such as **murmur of mitral regurgitation.** Analogously, a series of lesions on the skin may first be transformed descriptively from visual to verbal entity with phrases such as **erythematous, flat, peripheral blanching with pressure, small darker red central zones that do not blanch.** In the second step, these descriptive elements are converted to a final expression, such as **petechiae.**

This two-step process often receives inadequate attention during medical education because it would take too much time both for the instructor to concentrate on specific identification of all the basic descriptive elements, and for clinicians to try to use all the elements during communication. Consequently, the second-step expressions became the major elements of primary communication. Patients are described as having a **mitral regurgitation murmur, petechiae**, or some of the other nondescriptive attributes that were cited earlier in Exercise 6.5. The use of second-step expressions is prudent and economical in saving everyone's time and energy, but it leads to major difficulties in observer variability. When a disagreement occurs in the second-step expression, the source of the disagreement may be difficult to discover and correct. Do the observers vary mainly in the first phase of the observational process, transforming the observed entities into primary data; or in the second phase, transforming the primary data into categories of final citation?

The problem is perpetuated by observer variability investigations in which the main or only focus is the categories of output citation. This focus is quite reasonable, because these citations represent the bottom line of the variability that is being scrutinized. When the scrutiny is finished, however, the variability cannot be improved unless its component sources are identified. In trying to make the improvements, the investigator may then discover that the observers have difficulty dissecting the observational process into its two phases. When asked to cite the constituent elements of the basic descriptive data, an observer who has become habituated to using second-phase expressions may no longer be able to recall the primary ingredients. The observer may simply say it "sounds that way" or "looks like that," without being able to identify the fundamental acoustic or visual constituents.

This problem seldom occurs during quality control research in laboratory measurements, because the measurements usually produce a first-phase element of descriptive data. In quality control research, the investigators can therefore concentrate exclusively on the procedural activities that transform an observed specimen into raw data. When the raw data are produced, the process is finished. In clinical, radiologic, and microscopic observations, however, the final expressions emerge from a two-stage process; and different types of problems can occur in each stage. When the laboratory tells us that the serum calcium is 11.3 mg./dl., we receive a primary item of elemental description. We can wonder about the accuracy of the measurement, but we can use our own separate criteria for the interpretations that decide whether this measurement represents hypercalcemia or hyperparathyroidism. When a cardiac auscultator says the patient has the murmur of mitral regurgitation, however, we receive a secondary item of interpretation, and we do not know what criteria were used either for the descriptive observations or the interpretive conclusions.

26.5.1. *Procedural Criteria*

For the reason just cited, a fully satisfactory study of observer variability will contain attention to two separate sets of criteria. One set refers to the events involved in acquiring and preparing the specimen for observation, doing the observations, and expressing the primary elements of descriptive data.

In laboratory measurements, these procedural criteria often occupy many pages of instruction for such work as acquiring specimens, preparing reagents, and calibrating equipment. When medical data are obtained with a questionnaire, an analogous set of instructions is (or should be) provided for directions about the way in which each question is to be asked and answered. In many studies of observer variability, however, the procedural criteria or details of the first-phase observations may be omitted. The observer may be asked only to state the second-phase interpretations.

26.5.2. *Conversion (Interpretation) Criteria*

The second set of criteria refers to the second phase of the observational process, which converts the elemental data into categories of interpretation. These interpretive categories can be designations, such as **hypercalcemia** for a serum calcium level of 11.3 mg./dl., or inferences such as **hyperparathyroidism**, which can be proved with information obtained by some other mode of examination.

A *designation* reflects a category that is assigned as an arbitrary appraisal. The assignment cannot be proved right or wrong. Thus, if someone decides that any persons above age 40 will be categorized as **old age**, we can disagree with the decision, but we cannot prove that it is right or wrong. It is an arbitrary designation. On the other hand, if a decision is made to classify anyone with gray hair as being **old**, we can prove that the inference is right or wrong for individual persons by finding the person's actual age. If we accept >40 as being **old**, we could prove that the decision is wrong for a gray-haired person who is 35.

Many clinical observations are expressed in ranked ordinal grades that represent designations, such as **excellent response, moderate dyspnea,** or **4+ sick.** Many other clinical observations are inferences, such as **mitral regurgitation, petechiae,** or **moribund**, that can be proved with additional data obtained via radiography, histopathology, or observation of subsequent clinical course. Observations made by radiologists can also be designations or inferences—according to the available mechanism for proving the accuracy of the interpretation. Ordinarily, when a radiologist says a heart is slightly enlarged or that pulmonary vessels are engorged, the interpretation is a designation for which direct proof will not be available. Most radiographic decisions, however, are anatomic inferences that can be proved right or wrong if the actual anatomy can be inspected via biopsy, surgery, or necropsy.

A cytopathologist's interpretations are usually inferences that can be proved with histopathologic examination, but almost all of a histopathologist's interpretations are designations. The histopathologist is often used as the final word to decide about the accuracy of the inference made by a clinician or radiologist, but there is no external standard against which we can check the accuracy of the histopathologist. Thus, the clinical diagnosis of *mitral stenosis*—using the data of auscultation, radiography, and echocardiography—is an inference. The pathologist's diagnosis of *mitral stenosis*—examining the opened heart—is a designation.

Although the distinctions between designations and inferences have major importance for testing "accuracy" in clinical decisions,[16] the main point to be noted now is that we can study observer variability for both designations and inferences, but we can study accuracy only for inferences. Consequently, the scientific quality of designations can be easily improved, without the need for checking accuracy, if we can get the observers to specify both sets of criteria and become *consistent* in the observational process.

26.6. SUBSEQUENT ANALYSIS

After the results are obtained and summarized in a study of observer variability, the subsequent analyses depend on the four types of objectives that can be chosen as direct or latent goals of the research. The objectives and subsequent analyses are discussed in the next four subsections.

26.6.1. *Demonstrating Consistency of a New Index*

When a new clinical index or rating scale has been developed, a study of observer variability is often included in the original publication to demonstrate that the new technique produces consistent results. The investigators usually conduct the formal research after various pilot studies have been done to improve the procedure during its developmental activities. Because the pilot studies were used to find and remove sources of variability, and because the formal research is done to show the consistency of the fully developed technique, the results are usually presented without further analysis.

When a new technique or index is presented without studies of observer variability, the procedure can become accepted, disseminated, and widely used before its variability is formally investigated. After the study is done, everyone may be shocked to discover the inconsistencies it demonstrated. Aware of the frequent disagreements that occur in the clinical examination process, most medical readers are seldom surprised to learn about observer variability in signs, symptoms, and composite clinical indexes (such as the Apgar score), but clinical readers may often be crestfallen to discover the discrepancies found in studies of observer variability among histopathologists or radiologists.

26.6.2. *Demonstrating Unreliability or Bias*

Certain studies of observer variability may be done to show that a particular procedure is (or has been) unreliable or biased. The investigators may have the latent goal of discrediting the procedure or raising doubt about the results of research using the procedure.

For example, as described in Section 26.2.1, the radiologists' variability was studied to discredit the idea that pulmonary embolism could be accurately diagnosed from a plain chest film. In some instances, observer variability may be studied as an experiment with the goal of demonstrating the bias produced by concomitant information. Thus, in Exercise 2.2.9, the decisions made about pulmonary status in each film of a sequential series of chest roentgenograms were altered when the radiologists received the series of films in a random sequence rather than in the expected natural sequence.[17] In another experimental study of observer variability, the investigators found that exactly the same set of medical data received the diagnosis of toxic shock syndrome much more often when the accompanying information indicated that the patient was a tampon-using woman rather than a man or a non–tampon user.[18]

Studies of this type may be necessary to alert the scientific community to substantial problems that may have been overlooked or complacently regarded as nonexistent. Public health epidemiologists have been much luckier than clinicians in having their research data generally accepted, despite relatively little attention to issues of variability and bias. When a clinician wants to claim a cause-effect benefit for a particular agent, the scientific community is aware of the potential for biased observations. Rigorous standards of evidence are often imposed, usually containing the demand for double-blind procedures whenever the agent and outcome are related with subjectively obtained data. If these precautions were not used, the results of a therapeutic trial may be summarily rejected. On the other hand, when a public health epidemiologist wants to claim a cause-effect risk, these scientific standards are often abandoned.[19] Although the data were obtained subjectively with procedures containing few scientific precautions against diverse innate biases that can readily be expected in the research, the results are often received without qualm or skepticism.

Even when several studies have demonstrated an unreliability so great as to destroy any scientific credence in the basic data, epidemiologic investigators can continue using the unreliable data and having the results accepted. For example, most clinicians recognize that the diagnoses listed on death certificates have little or no scientific value; and many studies of death certificate diagnoses have shown that they are grossly unreliable. Nevertheless, as noted in Chapter 24, the diagnostic information continues to be used for diverse investigative tabulations and analyses that receive serious scientific attention and that sometimes affect major decisions in national health policy.

26.6.3. *Demarcating a Spectrum of Variability*

Although many studies of observer variability seem to be done for no other reason than to demonstrate and quantify its existence, some studies may include further analyses of the spectrum of variability. In such analyses, the investigators may show that major variability is particularly likely to be present or absent in certain subgroups of the spectrum of observations.

For example, in diagnosing the histologic types of lung cancer, pathologists were shown to have less intra- and interobserver variability for well-differentiated cancers than for cancers that were not well differentiated.[1] Similar types of distinctions may be noted when the spectrum of challenges is demarcated for appropriately stratified analyses of age, gender, and clinical or morphologic attributes associated with the observational process.

26.6.4. *Reducing Variability and Improving Quality*

Ultimately, the most useful feature of a study of observer variability is its role in reducing variability and improving quality. For this purpose, the investigator would try to determine the criteria used in the two phases of the observational process. The distinctions noted in these criteria will reveal the sources of variability and will allow suitable attention to be given to each disparity. If the observers discuss the disparities and then develop agreement about each criterion that produced a disparity, the criteria can be used subsequently with high consistency.

To achieve this type of consensus, the investigator will often need to arrange a confrontation in which the two observers repeat the observation that produced disagreement and then try to identify the elements of their phase-one descriptions and phase-two interpretations. As the observers conduct this discussion, they will usually find where they disagree and can usually resolve the disagreement fairly easily. The elements of observation and interpretation that are revealed during this discussion will indicate the particular attributes to be noted in the new, improved criteria.

This type of strategy can sometimes be used to improve the quality of an observational process, without any formal studies of observer variability and without any formal publication of the results. For example, many years ago, when my colleagues and I began doing "blind" auscultation (i.e., without first looking at the patient's medical record) in a special research clinic, we discovered our own capacities for intraobserver and interobserver variability.[16] At the time, we did not know that the phenomenon was called *observer variability* and that we could try to quantify it. Instead, we described some of its clinical consequences in creating a spurious new appearance (or disappearance) of rheumatic heart disease;[20] and we began efforts to remove the variability by standardizing ourselves as a group of collaborating auscultators.

The first step in this procedure was to develop our skills in vocalizing a set of cardiac "bird calls" so that we could reproduce the acoustic noises[21] and agree that we all heard the same thing. After this agreement was achieved, we then asked anyone who dissented about the final diagnostic category to cite the reasons for the dissent. These citations would usually indicate an element of observation that was being ignored by the other observers. Thus, everyone might agree that a murmur was holosystolic, loud, high-pitched, and blowing, but one observer might state that the murmur was also loudest at the left sternal border rather than at the apex. After everyone agreed that *site of maximum loudness* was an important criterion, we then discovered that another element of observation was used by some observers but neglected by others. Thus, *response of loudness to changes in position* was discerned and became accepted as another important criterion. In this way, we progressively discovered all our elements of observation and interpretation, and we eventually became a highly standardized, consistent group in our individual and collective auscultatory decisions. Unfortunately, the process was accomplished before I realized that it should be documented, and so it has remained unpublished, although the results of the team auscultators have been used in several major investigations of the clinical course of rheumatic fever and rheumatic heart disease.[22, 23]

I know of several circumstances in which similar activities have been used, also without publication of results, to reduce variability among radiologists and pathologists. In a formally published study[24] of methods for improving clinical skills, individual instructions based on videotapes of personal interviews were used in a residency program to help family physicians raise their accuracy in rating patients' psychiatric disturbances. In another interesting analysis, the investigators[25] studied sources of disagreement among observers making decisions about adverse drug reactions. Because the adverse reactions were diagnosed with a formal algorithm that had 56 possible questions, the investigators could check the performance of the observers at each step in the sequence of questions. This retraceability tactic showed that disagreement occurred more commonly when the questions involved judgmental rather than factual answers. The authors concluded that improvements in consistency among observers would require an effective method for dealing with difficult issues in judgment.

26.6.5. *Management of Uncertainties*

Avoiding bias and eliminating inconsistencies are a necessity of scientific research, but the necessary efforts are often omitted, particularly if the investigator begins with a preconceived hypothesis about the risks or benefits of a particular agent. Although scientific precautions are an obligation of the investigator, not of the reviewer, some investigators become outraged if a reviewer is reluctant to accept results of research conducted without such precautions. A clinical investigator may become incensed if his trial of therapy is rejected because of inadequate double-blinding; and an epidemiologist who took no scientific precautions to avoid biased data or decisions may demand that a reviewer produce direct evidence to support the suspicion of bias. Because the reviewer has no way of obtaining evidence that the investigator failed to examine, the suspicion can be documented only with separate studies of the type described in Section 26.6.2.

Problems of unresolved variability (or bias) frequently occur in the daily activities of clinical practice. Whenever these activities are studied, and particularly when a set of studies is collectively reviewed, the results can be dismaying. They usually show a variability so rampant and massive as to suggest that clinicians are too inconsistent to be trusted about anything. (Because the variability of epidemiologists has not been frequently examined,[26] analogous suggestions have not been prominent for epidemiologic research.)

The impact of biased or inconsistent data is substantially different in epidemiologic research and in clinical practice. In many forms of epidemiologic research, the main conclusions usually depend on the relationships found for two variables, representing the maneuvers and the outcomes. If the data for either one (or both) of those two crucial variables are grossly unreliable, the conclusions of the research cannot be scientifically acceptable. In clinical practice, however, decisions about patient care usually involve data from scores of different variables. Because the decisions often rely on patterns or clusters of information from the different types of data, a single item of data may have relatively little impact on the decisive pattern.

Furthermore, different items of data describing the same clinical phenomenon can be expected to show a distinctive biologic coherence. The presence of this coherence tends to suggest that the phenomenon is correctly described; and its absence will lead either to dismissal of the outlyer data or to reappraisal of the results. For example, a patient's cardiac size can be estimated from physical examination, electrocardiography, echocardiography, routine roentgenograms of the chest, other forms of imaging, or cardiac catheterization. An inconsistency between the results of physical palpation and certain paraclinical data may make the clinician decide to reject the physical findings or to preserve them, leading to the discovery that the transmitted x-ray interpretation referred to the wrong patient. For these reasons, clinicians may disagree about many individual observations while often agreeing on the main conclusions and management recommendations in patient care. Studies of observer variability in patient care can therefore be particularly cogent if devoted to the final conclusions and recommendations rather than to individual items of observational data.

Although patients are often justified in seeking second opinions about many clinical decisions, the extensiveness and ramifications of the problems have not been well studied. Substantial challenges exist for future investigators who want to check the impact of observer variability or bias in clinical practice as well as in epidemiologic research.

26.7. **SYNOPSIS**

Studies of observer variability can have at least four different goals. The first three are documentary. The objective is to demonstrate consistency for a new index, unreliability or bias in an existing procedure, or the particular circumstances in which variability is likely to be high or low. The fourth goal is remedial: to reduce variability and improve the quality of the observational process.

To document the variability of the total process, observers can be allowed to use whatever scale they wish for expressing results; but to find and remove sources of variability, a suitable scale should be negotiated beforehand and used by all observers participating in the study. The existence and magnitudes of disagreement will be rated according to disparities in cited categories of the scale. The decisions about what constitutes an important disparity will affect the choice of analytic statistical tests as well as their results.

The spectrum of challenges given to the observers should represent commonly encountered phenomena, particularly in a consecutive series of cases, but should be enriched to include unusual cases from extreme parts of the spectrum in which variability may be important and otherwise undetected. The plans for the study should be suitably aimed to distinguish variability among observers, instrumental methods, or both; and the observers should be suitably "blinded" to results obtained previously.

To reduce variability and improve quality, the observational process must be divided into its two phases. Procedural criteria should be developed for the first-phase activities that transform phenomena or specimens into primary raw descriptive data; interpretational criteria are needed for the second-phase activities that convert raw descriptions into categories of interpretation in the final scale of expression. By discussing disagreements and noting their sources in the first or second phases of the process, the participating observers can work with the investigator to identify, improve, and standardize the criteria used in both phases. The results can help convert studies of observer variability into the kind of quality control research needed for the fundamental data of clinical science.

EXERCISES

Exercise 26.1. The assignment here is to select and critique a study of observer variability. (In classroom activities, students can be divided into teams to share assignments and make reports.) You may choose the study from any source at your disposal. You should first outline the basic structure and results found in the research. Although you can discuss as many things as you wish within the scope of reasonable brevity, your critique should cover at least the following attributes of the study:

1. *Purpose*: Was the goal of the research clearly specified? Was it to demonstrate or to remove observer variability?

2. *Input challenge*: Was the group of specimens or subjects suitably representative of both the customary group and the scope of entities exposed to this procedure?

3. *Procedural components*: Was the research aimed at the instrumental methods, the performing observers, or both? If the research was aimed at only one of these components, was the other component suitably standardized?

4. *Observations*: Were they made independently or, if necessary, "blindly"?

5. *Observers*: Were they appropriately competent and suitably chosen for performing the procedure?

6. *Scale of reporting output*: Was the scale expressed in a satisfactory manner? Was it chosen and agreed upon before the research began? Should it have been chosen beforehand?

7. *Scale of disagreement*: Was a suitable scale desirable or necessary for describing the disagreement between any two readings? If so, was such a scale developed and was it satisfactory? If each specimen received more than two readings (i.e., multiple observers), how did the investigators deal with an index of multiple disagreement?

8. *Index of concordance*: Were the results expressed in a suitable statistical index of concordance? Did it make provision for agreement that might have occurred by chance alone?

9. *Procedural criteria*: Were criteria stated or developed for the first-phase process of converting observations into raw data?

10. *Interpretation criteria*: Were criteria stated or developed for the second-phase process of converting the raw data into the output scale of interpretation?

11. *Analysis*: Was the source (or sources) of variability identified by evaluating disagreements in basic raw data as well as in categories of interpretation?

12. *Improvements*: Were attempts made to have the observers confront their disagreements and try to determine (or remove) the sources of dissent?

13. *Recommendations*: Were any suggestions made about how to improve the defects that were noted?

CHAPTER REFERENCES

1. Feinstein, 1970; 2. Benson, 1969; 3. Whitehead, 1977; 4. Barnett, 1979; 5. Greenspan, 1982; 6. Hutchinson, 1979; 7. Karnofsky, 1949; 8. Cicchetti, 1976; 9. Fleiss, 1975; 10. Kramer, 1981; 11. Cochrane, 1968; 12. Fleiss, 1981; 13. Koran, 1975; 14. Kraemer, 1979; 15. Sussman, 1982; 16. Feinstein, 1974; 17. Reger, 1974; 18. Harvey, 1984; 19. Feinstein, 1982; 20. Feinstein, 1959; 21. Feinstein, 1968; 22. Feinstein, 1964; 23. Feinstein, 1967; 24. Goldberg, 1980; 25. Hutchinson, 1983; 26. Gordis, 1979.

Quality-of-Care Evaluations

Of all the different forms of research discussed in this text, perhaps the most difficult is the evaluation of quality of care. There are multiple factors to be considered individually, interactively, and collectively. There are multiple targets that can be selected as the focal goals of the research. And there are multiple opinions and conflicting beliefs about what those goals should be.

In studying cause-effect maneuvers or the processes involved in marker tests and observer variability, we might have had problems in choosing a suitable research structure, finding an appropriate comparison, obtaining credible data, and achieving an effective analysis of results, but there was usually no difficulty in stipulating the basic goal of the research and no controversy about whether the research was worth doing. In quality-of-care investigations, however, problems begin in the very title of the research, because major disagreements exist about what is meant by "quality" and by "care." Furthermore, according to the way those concepts are specified, there may be substantial dissent about the goals of the research and whether its performance is worthwhile.

Because work in quality of care has received so much discussion and attention, this chapter can present only a relatively brief outline of the activities. Readers who want more information are urged to check various sources[1-9] that contain more extensive details and that provide examples of particularly successful accomplishments.

27.1. OBJECTIVES OF THE RESEARCH

In all of our previous discussions, the objectives of the research were relatively easy to specify. Once those objectives were clearly stated, the main challenges in the research were to choose and carry out suitable methods for answering the basic questions. In quality-of-care research, the choice and execution of methods creates many formidable problems, but the most difficult obstacle is the selection of a research objective. This task is particularly difficult not because objectives are so hard to find and specify, but because whatever choice is made may later be regarded as unsatisfactory. The conduct and subsequent appraisal of the research involves so many people who hold different views about quality of care that the results may be downgraded or rejected, no matter how well the research was done, because of conflicts in value judgments rather than flaws in scientific methods.

The largest part of this chapter, therefore, is devoted to these issues in choosing the objectives. Because the objectives differ, and because all of them cannot be achieved in a single study (if at all), the necessary distinctions should be recognized by both investigators and reviewers. Without this recognition, an excellent study may be dismissed as poor research because the reviewer disagrees with the objectives; conversely, a relatively poor study may be regarded as splendid because its results coincide with the reviewer's prejudices. In quality-of-care research, the quality of the research itself may therefore depend on what the investigator has chosen and defined as quality of care.

27.1.1. *The Latent Goals*

The latent objective discussed earlier in Section 14.1.2 is one of the most important features of the goals of quality of care research. The overt objective is usually easy to specify; but the latent objective, which denotes what is to be done with the overt results, will often determine how well the original (stated) objective was chosen and how successfully the results will accomplish their ultimate mission.

27.1.1.1. ELEVATING PERFORMANCE VERSUS REMOVING INCOMPETENCE

One fundamental distinction in the latent goals of the research is similar to the problem noted in the previous chapter for studies of observer variability: Are we trying to demonstrate or to remove the variability? In quality-of-care research, a similar decision must be made, but the decision is more complex. Because very few investigators would want merely to provide documentation for variations in quality, the research often has some type of improvement as a direct or latent goal. The problem, however, is to decide what type of improvement is desired. Is the research intended to elevate the general quality of clinical care or to discern (and remove) incompetence? Are we trying to protect the public by "getting the dangerous driver off the road"—a tactic that would elevate the general level of performance without changing any individual performers—or are we trying to improve individual performances regardless of their high or low original levels?

Either one of these goals is quite desirable, but the methods chosen for the research can differ substantially according to whether we want to find the unsatisfactory "dangerous drivers" or provide ratings for different levels of satisfactory performance.

27.1.1.2. EDUCATING PERFORMERS VERSUS IMPROVING PERFORMANCE

Regardless of whether the latent goal is to demarcate incompetence or to provide general ratings, a separate decision involves the use of the results. Are they intended to rate the performers, educate them, or produce changes in performance? In Chapter 26, we noted that a study of observer variability can be clinically useless, despite its intellectual interest, if no subsequent efforts are made to reduce the variability of the observers. If such efforts are to be made, however, the original plans of the study may need a redesign that will allow better detection of the constituents of variability.

Analogously, if the latent goal is to improve performance in quality of care rather than merely to rate or educate the performers, different methods may be needed in planning the investigations. Occasionally, the improvement may be better achieved by authoritative edict than by analytic research. Thus, although various tactics can be studied for their efficacy in getting the house staff to stop ordering needless tests, nothing may work as well as a ban issued (and enforced) by the chief of the clinical service.

27.1.1.3. WHAT IS TO BE RATED AND/OR CHANGED?

Regardless of whether the latent goal is to rate or to change performance, the performer that is the target of the research must be clearly specified. Are we aiming at individual clinicians; at the health care providers formed by a consortium of clinicians, nurses, and allied personnel; at a particular institution, such as a hospital; at a particular mechanism for delivering health care, such as prepaid or fee-for-service arrangements; or at a national system of health care, such as autonomous private practice, national heath insurance, or socialized medicine?

Here, too, the methods of doing the research and the value judgments with which results are appraised will differ dramatically according to what is chosen as the main target of the evaluated performance.

27.1.1.4. WHO CHOOSES THE GOALS?

Finally, beyond the inevitable disagreements about how to answer the foregoing questions, there will be other disagreements about *who* answers them. Should these choices be made by society, i.e., government officials or legislators, or by individual clinicians and patients? Should there be a strict set of guidelines or should they be flexibly adapted for the many *ad hoc* vicissitudes that occur in patient care? Should economic goals in cost containment be the main priority or should we try to achieve high-quality care for everyone, regardless of cost? If we cannot provide high-quality care for everyone, who chooses the persons to whom it will be given or denied?

These questions are particularly difficult to answer because of the inevitable conflict between the goals of lowering costs and raising quality. As noted earlier, statistical data can be particularly treacherous when used to answer these questions, because the benefits of high-quality care may sometimes have a low rate of occurrence. Even worse, the benefits may be left undelineated and unquantified. For example, in Section 25.9, we noted that a CT scan of the head would detect a remediable lesion in perhaps 1 of 100 elderly patients with stroke. Is something that has an occurrence rate of only 0.01 worth trying to find? In a society concerned mainly with economics, this question would probably receive a negative answer, but individual patients and their families almost always regard the search as worthwhile.

Would the efforts still be worthwhile if the occurrence rate were 0.001 rather than 0.01? Economically, the costs of preventing or treating such phenomena may be excessive, yet in certain circumstances, the efforts may be regarded as worthwhile by both individuals and society. For example, the attack rate of paralytic poliomyelitis was about 0.001 in the days before polio vaccine, but society was willing to invest the research funds for developing a vaccine and to pay the costs of administering the vaccine to everyone.

Even if the risk of a particular entity were as low as 0.0001, so that its prevention or remedy would seem to have particularly small merit, how could we measure the benefits of the reassurance given to the remaining 0.9999 of people who could feel secure in knowing they would avoid the risk or could cure the problem if it occurred? Because the statistical data needed to answer these and other questions about cost/benefit and cost/effectiveness ratios are either unsuitable or unavailable, the questions must be answered with value judgments—and the decisions will usually depend on the values held by the individual judges.

27.1.2. *The Delineation of Quality of Care*

Assuming that the latent goals have been selected in a manner that will at least satisfy the investigator, we can now turn to the direct goals of the research itself. The next few sections will be concerned with research aimed at evaluating or rating the performance of care. In Section 27.5, we shall turn to research aimed at improving performance. The terms *quality assessment* and *quality assurance* are often used, respectively, to distinguish these two different goals.

27.1.2.1. **PROCESS VERSUS OUTCOME**

As noted earlier, the phrase *process research* was created to indicate that quality-of-care assessments would usually depend on what went on during the care, not on its ultimate accomplishments. At least three reasons can be cited for this decision.

27.1.2.1.1. *Absence of Adequate Comparative Data in Outcomes*

Unequivocal proof of superiority does not exist for many (perhaps most) of the patterns of care that come under evaluation in modern medicine. To rate pattern A as optimum because it achieves better outcomes than any other regimen would require impeccable evidence of the achievement—but the evidence is seldom available. The only available data may come from observational studies that may be regarded as unacceptable because the treatments were not assigned with randomization. If randomized trials have been conducted, they may have compared pattern A versus B and C, but not versus D or E; or the trials may have included somewhat different patients examined for somewhat different outcomes than what are desired.

27.1.2.1.2. *Absence of Correlations Between Process and Outcome*

Health care also has the distinction of being one of the main technologic activities in which interventional processes do not always closely correlate with their outcomes. The work of a plumber, a television repairman, an automobile mechanic, or an airplane pilot can usually be evaluated directly by the product that emerges from their use of the associated technology. The water pipe did or did not stop leaking; the image on the TV screen did or did not become clear; the automobile engine did or did not stop sputtering; the airplane did or did not reach its intended destination safely.

In medical activities, however, the human body and the diverse forces of nature can often pursue pathways that have good outcomes despite poor care or poor outcomes despite good care. Someone may live a long, healthy (and happy) life while continuing to smoke and drink heavily, exercise negligibly, eat imprudently, drive a car carelessly, and dwell in a polluted environment. Someone else may die young of acute myocardial infarction despite vigorous attempts at a health-promoting life style and the best efforts of an intensive care unit. An unexpected pulmonary embolus may bring sudden postoperative death to a patient whose disease has just been removed by masterful surgery; another patient may be cured while believing that an unnecessary colonoscopy was a therapeutic procedure.

A separate problem is that the outcome may occur too long after the process to allow the acquisition of satisfactory evidence proving that the two events are associated. For example, we generally believe that good parenting enables children to become good adults, but very little documentary evidence is available to prove this belief. The long interval between childhood and adulthood would make a suitable investigation logistically difficult; and even if the logistic difficulties could be overcome, the analytic problems would be formidable. Because an enormous number of nonparental co-maneuvers would intervene between a person's childhood and adult status, how well could we identify all those co-maneuvers and adjust for their effects to arrive at a confident conclusion about the individual impact of the good parenting many years earlier?

These and other difficulties that keep process and outcome from being directly associated in individual people have given statistics so prominent a role in medical research. Because we can seldom be sure of exactly what will happen in individual people, we have to look at groups and make decisions by comparing results in groups. These decisions may allow therapeutic choices to be made as prudently as possible, but clinicians cannot guarantee that optimum care will always produce an optimum outcome or that poor outcomes are due to poor care.

27.1.2.2. THE CHOICE OF OUTCOME

A third problem that makes quality of care often focus on process rather than outcome is the difficulty of choosing and evaluating outcomes. As noted in Section 27.1.1.4, different people may use different value systems in weighing the diverse benefits, hazards, and costs that occur as the outcomes of care; and there may be major disagreements about which outcomes are most important. If we cannot do both, is it more important to prolong duration of life or to improve quality of life? If a disease can be prevented or cured by making a person miserable, is the effort worthwhile? For example, the performance of a bilateral mastectomy at or before puberty would probably eliminate breast cancer in women, but no one has seriously proposed that this doubtlessly effective process be regularly used to achieve the outcome of preventing a major disease.

27.1.2.3. THE COMPONENTS OF PROCESS

Finally, even if we decide to focus on process rather than outcome, there are problems in choosing and evaluating the constituent components of the process. The totality of care can readily be divided into at least four distinct components: the activities used to determine what is wrong, i.e., the diagnostic process; the principal therapeutic interventions that are aimed at the main target, e.g., eliminating a cancer; the interventions aimed at ancillary targets, e.g., relieving symptoms or raising hematocrit; and the communication, consideration, compassion, or bedside manner that a clinician contributes uniquely as iatrotherapy.

Different people may disagree about the relative merits of the first three technologic components. Should the right treatment be given full credit if the preceding diagnostic work-up was incomplete? Should the right work-up be given full credit if followed by the wrong treatment? How much credit should be given to a splendidly conceived and executed plan for the principal treatment, while the patient's ancillary problems of pain and nausea are neglected? And how do we assess iatrotherapy—a nontechnologic activity that is often of prime importance to patients, but that is seldom described in medical records and seldom included in evaluations of care?

27.1.2.3.1. *Ambiguities in Classification*

Because iatrotherapy is so generally neglected as an important component of care, there may also be disagreements on how to classify another important entity: the patient's *satisfaction*. Is satisfaction to be regarded as an *outcome* that is worth achieving even if other desired outcomes are not attained; or is it part of the *process* as something contributing to the goals but not requiring identification as a separate goal?

Another phenomenon that is also difficult to classify as process or outcome is the patient's *compliance* with the clinician's recommendations. Suppose the clinician does an optimum job in making a diagnosis, formulating therapy, communicating the results and plans, and understanding the patient's psychic needs—but suppose the patient ignores the recommendations or forgets to carry them out properly. Is the defective compliance a flaw in the process or in the outcome?

A third entity that creates ambiguity in classification is the patient's *education*. With modern media of communication, many patients are much better informed about medical activities than they used to be. The patients usually ask for (or demand) more explanation from their clinicians, and today's clinicians are more willing to provide the additional information. In fact, arguments are regularly offered (although not always supported by data[10]) that compliance depends on how well the patient has been educated about his clinical condition and its recommended management. If the patient's education is an important component of care, should we try to evaluate it, and if so, is it part of process or outcome?

27.1.2.3.2. *Measuring What Is Available to Be Measured*

Regardless of how the foregoing questions are answered, the people who do quality-of-care research will usually behave like all other clinical investigators. They will rely on what *can* be done with the available data rather than what *should* be done. Accordingly, the investigators will usually do the best they can, working with what can be found retrolectively in medical records or with information that can be attained prolectively without loss of cooperation and interest from the clinicians whose work is being appraised. The components of process are usually chosen as entities that are readily identified in medical records: the tests that were ordered, the treatments that were given, the lengths of stay in the hospital, and the statement of instructions given at time of discharge. Although the clinician's iatrotherapy and the patient's psychic comfort, education, and satisfaction with care are all important (and sometimes crucial) components of the process, they are often omitted from analysis.

This separation of components is inevitable if any research is to be accomplished, but it often leaves the research open to the legitimate complaint that a focus has been placed on cure rather than care, and on the technology of medical practice rather than on the clinician's total role as a healer.

27.1.3. *Choosing the Standard Agent of Comparison*

The last main item to be considered in formulating the basic plan of quality-of-care research is to choose the comparative agent. Regardless of what (or who) is to be rated for performance and what components of the process are to be examined, a decision must be made about the definitive standard to be used in the comparison.

Are we looking for conformity with optimum standards of care (whatever they may be) or with the ordinary standards used in the community (whatever it may be)? And who decides what is *optimum* or *ordinary*? The choice of a standard-setting mechanism is one of the most important decisions in the research, and it often evokes considerable dispute. If we let the standard be set by a group of academic professors, the practitioners who are to be rated may complain that the academicians often have unrealistic goals and expectations, and that academic standards may call for an excessive amount of technologic testing. The practitioners can also cite examples, such as the "academic epidemic" of retrolental fibroplasia about 30 years ago (see Exercise 4.4.4 at the end of Chapter 4), in which the highest academic standards of care were actively harmful rather than just passively wrong. On the other hand, if we let the standards be set by the practitioners themselves, society may have no reassurance that the community's practitioners have kept up to date, that they are as judicious as practitioners elsewhere, and that the quality of care is as high as it can or should be.

An increasingly successful approach to this problem is to let the standards be set by a group of practitioners who are generally accepted as leaders in the community and who have maintained enough liaison with medical progress to be able to incorporate its worthwhile features into the standards. This mechanism of standard-setting usually works quite well. It allows the practitioners to be judged by a group of peers; the judges will usually discuss things with the practitioners when the standards are set, thus producing education as well as cooperation; and the standards that emerge are usually readily accepted by academic experts. The result may be neither a theoretical *optimum* nor an inferior *ordinary* but a set of goals for *optimum reality*.

27.2. THE SPECTRUM OF INPUT

If all of the cited decisions about the basic plans of the research have been satisfactory, the rest of the work, although still difficult, becomes comparatively easy. As in any type of process research, the investigator must make suitable choices of input, procedures, and output, and must arrange appropriate similarity in the comparison. The rest of this section is concerned with issues in choosing and comparing the input.

The input in quality-of-care research consists of the patients whose care is being evaluated and the particular setting in which the main performance of care takes place.

27.2.1. *The Setting or Structure of Medical Care*

The word *structure* was introduced by Donabedian[1] to denote the setting in which the procedures of health care occur. In this concept, the structure includes the technical capacity and geographic location of the health care facility; the arrangements used to finance and deliver the care; and the availability and qualifications of the ancillary personnel, beyond the particular personnel whose performance is being evaluated. The decision to regard these structural components as *input* is arbitrary. They could also be regarded as a type of co-maneuver, occurring during the procedures of health care.

The structural components of health care have two important roles. First, these components must be considered when comparative standards are established for the evaluations. If an intensive care unit or computerized tomography (CT) is not available for usage in a particular setting, the practitioner should not be faulted for having failed to use them. The latter comment indicates the second role of structural components. They can sometimes be chosen, instead of personal performances, as the main focus of the quality-of-care research. For example, we might decide to rate the quality of care at a particular institution as inferior if the institution does not have an intensive care unit or a CT apparatus. If these components of the total care process become the focus of evaluation, the personnel and other concomitants of health care would become part of the structure rather than primary targets in the research.

Because the structural components can have a wide spectrum of facilities, ancillary personnel, fiscal systems, and administrative mechanisms, these distinctions must be borne in mind when performances of health care are compared for evaluation. Distinctions that are attributed to the particular performers may arise from overlooked differences in the associated structural setting in which the care occurs.

27.2.2. *The Choice of Patients*

If a structural component is used as the main focus of evaluation, the research can often be done without studying *any* patients. Thus, we might decide that good care at a hospital requires an intensive care unit, a CT apparatus, an appropriate number of nurses, suitable arrangements for social work, an occupational therapist, and the availability of consultants in certain clinical specialties. With a check list for these components, we could rate the hospital's capacity for quality of care without having to appraise any individual performances.

In general, however, quality of care is evaluated by observing what is done for individual patients, who become the main input for the process. As in the other process activities described in Chapters 25 and 26, this spectrum should be carefully chosen. Its components, i.e., the different types of patients, should be proportionately distributed in a way that suitably represents the realities of clinical care for the particular clinical condition(s) under evaluation. On the other hand, the spectrum should be broad enough to contain the uncommon phenomena that constitute major challenges in clinical practice.

For example, because human beings were having babies quite successfully for millennia before the invention of midwives and obstetricians, it is clear that most pregnancies can be successfully delivered without any form of professional assistance. If a live baby and a healthy mother form the main criterion of successful care, a quite high rate of success can be attained in deliveries that are unattended or in those performed by husbands, policemen, or taxi drivers as well as in the work of midwives and obstetricians. The main reason for having a routine delivery performed by a skilled professional is to deal with the uncommon, unanticipated complications in which the professional's talents can make a real difference between disaster or a healthy baby and mother.

If the quality of obstetric care is to be appraised merely from a consecutive series of routine deliveries, however, the series may not contain enough complicated cases to provide the challenges that will distinguish a skilled professional from a collaborating unskilled bystander. If the success rates are 99% for the professional and 98% for the nonprofessional, the erroneous conclusion may be that the added increment of skill is quite small.

For this reason, when the comparison involves performers with different levels of skill, the spectrum of challenges must be suitably chosen. To provide a suitable scope of challenges, the contents of a consecutive series of cases may need deliberate augmentation with cases that contain the appropriate distinctions. Furthermore, unless the challenges are suitably classified and analyzed, a retrospective review of cases may produce statistics in which a highly skilled professional seems worse than someone who is unskilled.

For example, a home delivery may be planned for a woman who appears to be in excellent health, with no risk factors. If no complications occur during labor, the delivery may be successfully consummated at home, thus incrementing the percentage of successful home deliveries. If the pregnant woman has risk factors, however, or if complications become evident during labor, an obstetrician may be called for a hospital delivery. Because these pregnancies may end unsuccessfully, despite exceptionally skillful obstetric management, the obstetrician's percentage of in-hospital success will be lowered. If we then simply compare the success rates, ignoring the types of challenges, the obstetrician's results for hospital deliveries may be lower than what is attained at home.

27.3. THE DELINEATION OF PROCEDURE

In the obstetric vignette just described, we were really examining an outcome—a healthy baby and mother—rather than the procedures involved in supervising the gestation, monitoring the labor, and delivering the baby. In the strictest sense of *process* research, these procedural activities would be the prime foci of assessment. As noted earlier, we would have to decide which and how many procedures are to be examined; how to examine their performance; and how to rate the performance.

27.3.1. *Choice of Procedures*

Examples of obstetric care are good illustrations because the events of a pregnancy are well known and relatively easy to anticipate. Even for this relatively simple common clinical condition, however, we might have difficulty deciding what procedural components to include for evaluating quality of care. Should we focus mainly on the management of labor and delivery, omitting the care given earlier in the pregnancy? Do we concentrate on technologic issues in ordering diagnostic tests, recommending proper diets, prescribing suitable medications, monitoring the labor adequately, and performing the appropriate manipulations during parturition—or do we also include the obstetrician's pattern of iatrotherapy in communication, compassion, and attention to psychic needs?

Ideally, we might want to look at everything, but pragmatically, there are many constraints. The more attributes we examine, the greater is the difficulty of obtaining suitable data and the problems of appraising the contributions of each of a series of multiple variables. Even if we could acquire all the data we wanted and could manage the multivariate analysis, there would still be problems in obtaining *suitable* data because no satisfactory mechanisms may exist for observing and recording the basic raw information. The difficulties are increased by the current absence of well-established, generally accepted indexes or scales for rating communication, compassion, attention to psychic needs, or other aspects of iatrotherapy.

If we leave the work of an obstetrician and consider what is done by other clinicians, things become much more difficult because so many diverse clinical conditions must be considered. If we had major problems trying to decide what to appraise as quality of care in a routine pregnancy, the problems become huge if we consider all the different clinical conditions encountered by nonobstetric practitioners. To evaluate the practitioner's work, we would need to examine and to be able to rate all the procedural distinctions used in the care of all those different maladies. Even if we wanted and were able to develop all these rating schemes, we might have difficulty applying them effectively to individual practitioners with a varied clinical clientele, because there might not be enough patients with each of the diverse conditions to allow statistically distinctive results for each condition.

27.3.2. *Use of Tracer or Indicator Conditions*

To simplify the evaluation technique, Kessner[11] proposed the use of a selected set of tracer or indicator conditions. These conditions are chosen to be clinical challenges that commonly occur in the practice under appraisal and that receive straightforward, generally accepted methods of care. The tracer conditions might include management of a common complaint—such as sore throat or ear ache in children, low back pain in adults, or urinary tract infection in women. The tracer conditions might also include justifications for the ordering of certain diagnostic tests, such as ultrasonography, or for prescribing therapeutic agents, such as antibiotics or tranquilizers. In some instances, the practitioner's tactics might be scrutinized for the complete approach to a particular tracer condition, such as the screening, diagnostic testing, management, and follow-up of hypertension.

The tracer procedure has been effective and relatively easy to use—even in retrolective reviews of medical records—because the conditions can be readily identified and because relatively uncontroversial standards can be established for the management decisions. The disadvantages are that the tracer conditions do not include iatrotherapy and other important aspects of care; the individual rating systems are often crude; and aggregates of scores for individual tracer conditions are difficult to interpret.

27.3.3. *Duration of Episodes*

A separate issue in choice of procedures is the decision about when a particular episode of care has ended. In many quality-of-care studies, the episode is the set of events that took place while the patient was hospitalized, but many (perhaps most) important issues in quality of care occur outside a hospital. The relative brevity of inpatient episodes of care may make them easier to evaluate than longer-term encounters, but a focus on hospital activities alone may miss many of the most important events. For example, in patients hospitalized with stroke, the use (or avoidance) of steroids to treat cerebral edema can be examined as a tactic in care, but some of the most important elements of care for a patient with stroke occur after discharge from the hospital, when the patient receives blood pressure control, physical therapy, occupational adaptation, and other rehabilitative efforts.

27.3.4. *Formulation of Criteria for Evaluation*

As noted in Chapters 5 and 26, the evaluation of a process often requires two separate sets of criteria. The *procedural* criteria deal with basic activities in performing the task; the *interpretation* criteria transform the results of the procedural criteria into the output rating. Thus, we might have procedural criteria to rate a clinician's performance in managing sore throat, back pain, and urinary tract infection. The interpretation criteria would combine those three individual ratings into the final score given to the overall performance.

27.3.4.1. CONSENSUAL VERSUS EMPIRIC CRITERIA

Criteria are created *consensually* when they represent the opinion of a selected group of judges who may be academicians, community practitioners, or some other designated source of authority. The criteria are created *empirically* when they are justified with specific evidence. The evidence is usually a documentary demonstration of the outcome value of the process. For example, prophylactic administration of lidocaine to a patient with acute myocardial infarction can be justified with evidence showing that ventricular arrhythmias are prevented. Alternatively, the documentation may consist of evidence (obtained from questionnaires or surveys) showing that the process is generally accepted as valuable and generally employed in care, even though its outcome benefits have not been formally proved.

The consensual approach is often preferred in quality-of-care research because the criteria can be established more easily and promptly, because empiric evidence may not be available, and because the existing empiric evidence is usually carefully considered when the judges form their consensual standards.

27.3.4.2. **IDEAL VERSUS MINIMAL STANDARDS**

According to the purpose of the evaluation, as noted in Section 27.1.1.1, the pass/fail standards might be set at relatively low levels, to detect gross errors in management, or at relatively high levels, to instruct practitioners and to elevate general quality. The minimal standards will usually be easier to apply and will help screen out the "dangerous drivers." The ideal standards, although generally preferred, are more difficult to establish and apply; and they will often detect unimportant errors.

27.3.4.3. **EXPLICIT VERSUS IMPLICIT CRITERIA**

Explicit criteria contain a set of stipulated directions, created before the audit, about each topic to be checked, each decision to be made during the checking, and each rating to be assigned during the decisions. Because of all these specifications, the criteria will usually be clear and consistent. On the other hand, the specifications are often difficult to create. The makers of the criteria may not be able to anticipate all the events that will be encountered and may not reach agreement on how to specify and rate the management of each event. To develop the specifications and consensus ratings, the criteria may therefore emphasize overt events—such as duration of hospitalization or ordering of tests—that are easy to stipulate but that do not indicate cogent distinctions or important subtle nuances in care.

In contrast, implicit criteria are not overtly stipulated and are applied as a set of subjective decisions by the individual judge who performs the audit. The judge can evaluate all the events occurring during the entire episode of clinical care and can reach an overall rating of the performance, but may have no specific guidelines or reproducible mechanisms for making the decisions. The distinction between explicit and implicit criteria thus resembles the difference between a multiple-choice, machine-scored written examination and an individual oral examination in evaluating a clinician's competence for specialty board certification. The implicit criteria are more likely to be aimed at the important things but will often be applied inconsistently. The explicit criteria will be consistent but aimed at less important phenomena.

27.3.5. *Sources of Data*

The most direct way of obtaining data about performance is with a preplanned study that is arranged to observe, monitor, and record the audited events. Such research is seldom conducted because it is so difficult to do, although it has been achieved in special circumstances, such as a randomized trial in which quality of care was compared between nurse practitioners and family physicians.[12] The audited events can be standardized if presented as simulated patients or as written case vignettes, but the scope of the simulations is often limited by the range of physical findings; and the written case vignettes, despite their intellectual challenges, cannot simulate many important attributes of a real patient.

Because of these problems, most studies of quality of care are conducted retrolectively from information available in archival sources. For audits of individual clinicians, these sources are the medical records maintained by the clinicians. Other sources can be insurance claim forms and information assembled by diverse agencies concerned with health care. These sources have the advantage of being readily available for the research, but the data are often of dubious scientific quality, and many important phenomena, as noted earlier, are not recorded.

27.4. ASSESSMENT OF OUTPUT

The output of the study will have been determined by the choices of goals for the study, the performers under evaluation, and the procedures to be rated. The main decisions that remain to be made as *output* will be the scoring systems used for rating performance. If the criteria are implicit, the judges may agree to use the same rating scale, such as pass/fail, but no further specifications may be cited for each rating. With explicit criteria, however, the scoring system and its ingredients will be fully specified. Three basic strategies can be used for this activity.

27.4.1. *Uniform Linear Scoring*

In uniform linear scoring, a listed series of individual phenomena are each rated as *yes* or *no* according to the performer's conformity with the stipulated standard. The positive scores are then added together to form the final result. This was the tactic used by Nobrega and coworkers[13] in a recent study of management of patients with hypertension.

27.4.2. *Weighted Linear Scoring*

The same basic activity takes place in weighted linear scoring, except that the phenomena receive individual scores that are weighted according to the postulated importance of each phenomenon. As illustrated by Mates and Sidel[14] in an evaluation of emergency room care for asthma, the weighting allows clinical judgment to be more closely approximated in the rating system, but both of the linear scoring techniques have major disadvantages. They demarcate a set of phenomena to be scored, but not all of the phenomena are pertinent for each patient. Neither of the two linear rating systems is flexibly adapted to the individual distinctions of individual patients.

27.4.3. *Criteria Mapping*

In the technique called *criteria mapping,* Greenfield and coworkers[15] developed a scoring system that follows a stipulated algorithm or flow chart, which reaches different decision points according to the clinical distinctions of each patient. This type of scoring strategy, which was illustrated in an evaluation of the emergency room management of chest pain,[15] follows the pattern of sequential logic used in clinical decision making and provides ratings for only those events that are appropriate in each pattern of the sequence.

The strategy has the major advantage of approximating the flexible logic used in clinical decisions. The disadvantage is that the criteria maps are difficult to create, and they will be unsatisfactory or incomplete unless the map makers have been able to develop an algorithm that anticipates all of the diverse pathways of events and decisions occurring in clinical phenomena.

27.5. QUALITY ASSURANCE

For all the reasons cited in Sections 27.1 to 27.4, no clinical or scientific agreement has been set for the best way to assess quality of care, and there are often major disputes about its definition. Nevertheless, as the containment of health care costs became a major issue in the United States, political considerations led to the legislatively mandated development of methods for assuring quality of care. These assignments were legally delegated to Professional Standards Review Organizations (PSRO) and to federally supported Health Maintenance Organizations (HMO); and the challenge was spontaneously taken on by the Joint Commission on the Accreditation of Hospitals (JCAH). These groups have generated various requirements for the medical profession to use in evaluating and improving health care.

27.5.1. *Medical Audits*

The main focus of the requirements has been the use of medical audits to assess (and alter) performance by individual practitioners. The audits are usually based on medical records, most commonly for inpatients (although ambulatory care is checked by HMOs), with an emphasis on the process rather than outcome of care. The topics to be studied and the corresponding criteria and standards of assessment are chosen locally. The criteria are usually explicit and are concerned exclusively with technical aspects of management, omitting iatrotherapeutic and other personal aspects of the art of care.

In the PSRO activities, which have been most prominently publicized, one main focus of review was hospital *utilization.* Justifications were reviewed for elective admissions, nonelective (emergency) admissions, and hospitalizations having protracted durations (which exceeded a threshold for length of stay). The utilization reviews were often performed concurrently rather than retrospectively from medical records, and were relatively easy to do because the standards for admission and duration of hospitalization could be relatively simple. This simplicity, however, meant that the reviews were concerned more with cost containment than with actual quality of care.

Another type of review, called *profile analysis,* compared the pattern of an aggregate of patient care data against the corresponding pattern in regional or national standards. The main type of review instituted by PSRO groups consisted of Medical Care Evaluation (MCE) studies. They involved the *feedback loop* technique of performing audits for a selected set of tracer conditions, applying corrective procedures for any deficiencies that were noted, and then conducting repeated audits to check that the deficiencies were corrected.

In view of the enormous number of problems, it is not surprising that these quality assurance activities have not been particularly successful. Nelson[16] has described the difficulties of applying the feedback loop technique; and the entire quality assurance process was viewed with strong skepticism by a committee of the Institute of Medicine.[17] The committee concluded that "existing information does not substantiate the effectiveness of Medical Care Evaluations (audits). . . . There is no reliable data to reflect the numbers, topics, and associated costs (of the audits), the identified deficiencies in patient care, the remedial actions proposed and taken, or the extent and duration of improvement in patient care."

27.5.2. *Other Activities*

An alternative or supplemental approach to quality-of-care assurance is to monitor the process that educates clinicians rather than their actual performance of care. This process includes the selection of applicants, curriculum of instruction, and methods of pedagogy used in the education of medical students, house staff, and specialty fellows. One obvious component of the total process is the examination system given for medical licensure, specialty board certification, and recertification. Another component is the clinicians' postgraduate continuing medical education.

All of these activities are frequently discussed, but no agreement has been achieved about how they should be conducted and what contributions are most valuable and important. A strong argument is often made that all of the activities contain an inappropriate focus. The instructional and examination processes tend to emphasize technologic aspects of care, although most malpractice suits and other manifestations of public discontent seem to arise from failures in iatrotherapy, not in use of technology. The content of postgraduate education tends to emphasize sophisticated new information, although most of the identified problems in health care seem to arise from defective habits in the application of mundane knowledge.

For example, various studies have demonstrated substantial inadequacies in the immunization of healthy children, in the unnecessary prescription of iron for anemic children, in the use of antibiotics for nonbacterial ailments, and in the detection and management of hypertension. These deficits represent flaws in the clinician's pattern of routine practice rather than a lack of sophisticated knowledge or technologic information—but the prevention and remedy of these flaws has not yet been effectively achieved in either the educational process or the quality assurance process.

If the health care system is unwilling or unable to develop the necessary methods, perhaps the most effective (and inevitable) technique will be the evaluations and decisions made by individual members of the public, using the informal methods, implicit criteria, and unquantified results of personal judgment. Patients will choose clinicians and hospitals according to their own perceptions of good care. This traditional method of evaluating quality of care may have nothing to recommend it except tradition, but it will often be less costly, more readily applicable, and more universally available than all the other procedures whose merits are currently also unsubstantiated.

27.6. SYNOPSIS

The quality of medical care is difficult to assess and affect. Different evaluators often disagree about whether the main goals are to elevate general quality or remove isolated incompetence; to rate or improve performance; and to focus on individual performers or on the total system of care. Other major disputes are whether these goals should be chosen by patients, clinicians, legislators, or society and whether high quality and low costs are compatible.

The evaluations have often emphasized the process rather than outcomes of care because of disagreements about the choice of outcomes, because good process and good outcome are often dissociated, and because satisfactory data may not be available for the process/outcome relationship. The evaluation of process, however, involves controversial decisions about technologic versus personal components of care, problems in obtaining suitable data, and difficulties in choosing the people who set comparative standards of care.

The input for the evaluation process consists of both the people receiving the care and the setting (or *structure*) in which the care is delivered. The performance of clinicians or other individual care-givers should be evaluated with standards appropriate for the setting; and the spectrum of patients should have suitable proportions of customary events and an adequate scope of challenges.

Because of difficulties in trying to evaluate all of a clinician's activities, the appraisal may be confined to certain *tracer* (or *indicator*) conditions, which often consist of relatively brief episodes of care. The criteria used in the evaluation can be created by consensus or derived empirically, aimed at ideal or minimal standards, and applied with implicit judgments or explicit citations. The performances can be rated uniformly with a linear or weighted scoring system, or with a criteria-mapping technique that is adapted to different clinical challenges.

The diverse efforts made to improve (or assure) quality of care have had little direct evidence of success. The efforts have included reviews of hospital utilization, comparisons of profiles of patterns in patient care, and a feedback loop of audit, followed by correction of deficiencies, followed by re-audit to check the corrections. The roles and contributions of medical schools, primary postgraduate education, licensure examinations, specialty board certification, and continuing postgraduate education have also not been explicitly investigated and convincingly documented. One of the most effective although unquantified methods of evaluating and assuring quality of care may be the traditional approach in which patients make up their own minds about what they like. When they don't like it, they can choose other doctors or aid from lawyers.

EXERCISES

Note: The exercises that follow are derived from five published reports in medical literature. Because the reports are too long to be reproduced here, replicated copies should be made available for classroom or seminar instruction.

Exercise 27.1. After reading the paper by Nobrega and coworkers,[13] please answer the following questions:

27.1.1. If process and outcome are really related in the treatment of hypertension, how could the relationship have been missed in the architecture of this study?
27.1.2. Does Table 4 provide a satisfactory descriptive account of the process/outcome relationship? If not, why not?
27.1.3. The patients in Table 4 are stratified according to initial diagnosis of hypertension. What is the purpose of this stratification? How does it help or impair the analysis of the data?

Exercise 27.2. The paper by Mates and Sidel[14] is particularly interesting because it shows a positive correlation between process and outcome in the emergency room care of asthma. Please read the paper and answer the following questions:

27.2.1. What are the main units of analysis in this study? Are you happy with this choice? If not, why not?
27.2.2. Were the comprehensive outcome criteria appropriate for the process criteria?
27.2.3. What was the rate of follow-up for the assessment of outcomes? Was this rate satisfactory? If not, why not?
27.2.4. How impressive are the coefficients shown for the correlation of process and 24-hour outcome in Table 2? Why did the correlation diminish for the 7-day outcome score?

Exercise 27.3. Please read the paper on criteria mapping by Greenfield and coworkers,[15] and answer the following questions:

27.3.1. Does the branching logic used in this technique correspond to the type of branching logic used in clinical decision making?

27.3.2. What are the relative advantages (and disadvantages) of this technique versus the type of process auditing used by Nobrega and coworkers in Exercise 27.1?

27.3.3. Why did the authors study the correlation between process and outcome mainly in patients discharged from the emergency room? Was this a reasonable strategy and did it really measure the correlation between the process and outcome of care?

Exercise 27.4. Mushlin and coworkers[18] made an interesting attempt to achieve quality assurance by measuring outcome and then determining the reasons for poor outcome. Please read that paper and answer the following questions:

27.4.1. Are you satisfied with the way the authors defined and ascertained health care outcomes? If not, why?

27.4.2. What are the limitations of this outcome-based type of audit?

Exercise 27.5. In the previously cited paper by Nelson,[16] Figure 1 shows the success of quality assurance efforts in improving blood transfusion practices in Utah. Do you regard this information as convincing evidence of success? (Please state the reasons for your decision.)

CHAPTER REFERENCES

1. Donabedian, 1980; 2. Donabedian, 1982; 3. Brook, 1977; 4. Brook, 1979; 5. Lewis, 1974; 6. McLachlan, 1976; 7. Payne, 1976; 8. Sanazaro, 1980; 9. Smits, 1981; 10. Haynes, 1979; 11. Kessner, 1973; 12. Spitzer, 1974; 13. Nobrega, 1977; 14. Mates, 1981; 15. Greenfield, 1977; 16. Nelson, 1976; 17. Institute of Medicine, 1976; 18. Mushlin, 1978.

PART SEVEN

ADDITIONAL TOPICS

The last three chapters of the book contain several topics that have not yet received specific formal attention. Chapter 28, which refers to descriptive research, is concerned with quantitative studies that set boundaries for the customary contents, or "range of normal," of a spectrum of group data. Chapter 29, on randomized clinical trials, has been saved for near the end of the book so that the discussion can refer to various scientific principles that have been thoroughly described earlier in the text. Chapter 30 contains an inventory of other epidemiologic topics that are traditionally discussed in conventional courses in public health. Those topics are outlined here so that clinical epidemiologists can recognize and acknowledge their predecessor kinfolk in the epidemiologic family.

The Range of Normal

When a univariate spectrum is examined in most types of research, the immediate goal is usually to demonstrate, quantify, and summarize the contents of the spectrum. In descriptive research, spectral surveys commonly appear in medical literature as a report of a collected series of cases of people with a particular disease or clinical condition. The spectrum is usually partitioned cross-sectionally according to the demographic, clinical, and paraclinical characteristics of the diseased patients at the time the disease was encountered.

In many instances, however, the cross-sectional spectrum may be partitioned in a way that shows correlations with subsequent treatment and future outcomes. Such reports will therefore contain a combination of a single-state spectral description and a cohort study of clinical course for the members of the spectrum. The components of the two research structures are often used for many internal correlations and contrasts. Thus, after describing the univariate spectrum of gender and cholesterol in patients with disease D, the investigator may see whether the average cholesterol values are higher in men than in women. Separate comparisons may then be done to see whether prognosis is affected by different levels of the initial cholesterol values. These reports are invaluable for the detailed portraits they provide of a particular clinical condition; and the reports often serve as a basis for articles in textbooks and discussions at educational conferences.

In one special circumstance, however, the descriptive research is not intended to show the contents and associated events of a spectrum. Instead, the goal is to establish boundaries that circumscribe the scope of the spectrum. The circumscribed spectrum is usually called a *range of normal*.

Although ranges of normal are constantly published as the results of specific research or as boundaries suggested for the measurements issued by medical laboratories, the arbitrarily chosen *range* is often unsuitable for the stated goals, and the basic concept of *normal* is often applied ambiguously or inconsistently. The problems of establishing the concept and demarcating the range are the subject of this chapter.

28.1. THE MEANING OF NORMAL

To help clarify the associated confusion, E. A. Murphy[1] has pointed out that the word *normal* can be used for at least seven different meanings. They can be divided into two main categories of definition: isolated and correlated.

28.1.1. *Isolated Meanings*

In the isolated definitions, *normal* is a strictly univariate concept, emerging from boundaries set on values of the spectrum of a single variable, such as height, weight, or serum cholesterol level.

The boundaries demarcate a zone that is chosen to represent the conventional, customary, habitual, or average values found in the spectrum. With this approach, we might use such expressions as "he normally begins work at 9 A.M." or "families these days normally have two children." The spectral boundaries are usually demarcated as a purely statistical act, based on a particular mathematical principle that has been chosen for the purpose.

28.1.2. *Correlated Meanings*

In the correlated approaches, the idea of normal is medically associated with an innocuous, harmless, or ideal feature of health. If an item of data implies a current state of ill health, it is called *abnormal;* if it implies the hazard of some future ailment, it may be called a *risk factor.* For example, a person who seems to be in excellent health and who has a series of otherwise unremarkable results in a battery of laboratory tests might be regarded as having an abnormal serum cholesterol level if it seems high enough to be a risk factor for future coronary disease. A person with sickle cell trait could go through a medically uneventful lifetime but might be thought to have an abnormality because the trait is a potential genetic hazard for future offspring.

Many medical concepts of normal were established with this type of clinically correlated rather than statistically univariate approach. For example, long before any formal cohort studies were done, the clinical decision that 90 or 95 mm. Hg was the boundary for a normal diastolic blood pressure depended on the relationships noted between blood pressure values and subsequent vascular complications. Today, after cohort studies have provided data for arguments that the boundary should be lowered, the justifications also rest on observed correlations. Clinical decisions for the normal range of blood pressure have never depended on a purely statistical univariate demarcation of values found in a large population.

Decisions about abnormalities in temperature have also been made in a correlated manner. When someone with a temperature of 39° C. is regarded as having the abnormality of *fever*, the designation is based on the associated clinical phenomena, not on a range demarcated from a univariate distribution of temperature frequencies.

Because correlated approaches have been the traditional method for making clinical decisions about *normal* or *abnormal*, the terms have implied a direct relationship to a past, present, or future state of health. The relationships have been particularly easy to perceive for the many states of deranged health that are diagnosed categorically by observation and verbal description, not by dimensional measurement. Such categories include the many diseases that are identified morphologically (as *cancers, infarctions, degenerative changes,* and so on) or as clusters receiving psychiatric or clinical designations (such as *schizophrenia* or *lupus erythematosus*). The association between one of these categorical ailments and a univariate spectrum of data would be analyzed with the diagnostic marker technique discussed in Chapter 25. With this technique, zones of normality or abnormality could be delineated for a particular variable according to its direct relationship to the diagnosed ailment.

28.1.3. *Therapeutic Correlations*

A different clinical approach to correlation depends on making an action decision about treatment rather than an intellectual decision about diagnosis. For example, Cochrane and Elwood[2] have suggested that the upper limit of normal for a screening test be chosen as the point below which treatment does more harm than good. In proposing guidelines for decisions about levels of inorganic lead and mercury in urine, Elkins and coworkers[3] divided the values into three zones in which the managerial action was to be *none*, a *periodic check*, or *active medical surveillance*.

28.1.4. *Problems of Correlated Approaches*

Despite an appealing medical sensibility, the correlated approaches have often been difficult to use in an era of burgeoning technology. The correlational technique may not be applicable if the correlation is not unique, if the necessary data are not available, or if the data require multivariate analysis.

28.1.4.1. **NONUNIQUE CORRELATIONS**

In many circumstances, the same item of data (such as a value of alkaline phosphatase or creatine phosphokinase) may be pertinent for several different diagnoses, as either a surrogate or contributory test. For variables of this type, zones of abnormality cannot be demarcated uniquely. A different zone might be required for each of the diagnoses in which the variable participates. An array of different zones can be established and used appropriately for each situation, but the results will seldom yield a *single* set of boundaries for the range of normal of that variable.

28.1.4.2. **UNAVAILABLE OUTCOME DATA**

To be used for future prediction rather than current diagnosis, a variable must be correlated with data indicating a subsequent outcome rather than a concomitant state. Relatively few long-term cohort studies are available to provide the data needed for such analyses. In clinical research, many groups of diseased patients have been followed as cohorts, but the results often become obsolete as new technologic advances produce data and treatments that were not formerly available or incorporated in the analyses. In epidemiologic research, risk factors are difficult to study in cohorts; and the few suitable studies may not include information about the impact of all the variables whose consequences might be chosen for examination.

28.1.4.3. **MULTIVARIATE ANALYSES**

Perhaps the greatest problem in forming correlations, however, is the many types of data that must often be considered simultaneously. Clinical decisions about normality frequently involve a multivariate rather than bivariate analysis. For example, before deciding that a particular measurement is abnormal, a clinician may want to consider its mensurational variability, duration, previous levels, and association with other abnormalities as well as the therapeutic or other consequences for the patient. Thus, from various considerations, we might decide that a diastolic blood pressure of 96 is desirable in an octogenarian or not alarming if it appears only sporadically in a middle-aged adult. A temperature of 38° C. could be greeted happily if the patient's previous temperature was 39.5° C. The occurrence of asymptomatic sickle cell trait might be a welcome genetic event in a family in which most members have suffered from sickle cell disease.

Although the multivariate appraisals might be expressed with a suitable statistical model or clinical algorithm, the complexity of the expression would offer a cumbersome approach. Besides, when new types of measurements become available, they will not be initially accompanied by all the additional data needed for the multivariate model.

28.2. **CHOICE OF A ZONE**

For all these reasons, decisions about a range of normal are usually made as isolated univariate demarcations. The basic assumptions are that the technique can be easily standardized and that the demarcated zone will serve as a type of screening test. Values that fall inside the zone can often be safely accepted as normal; and values that fall outside the zone will be called to the clinician's attention and appraised accordingly, often with the additional correlations just discussed.

Having made the basic decision to demarcate normality in a univariate manner, the investigator must now choose a suitable mathematical method to define the numerical boundaries, and a suitable group of people to provide the demarcated data. The selected boundaries for the data will have to account for three different sources of variability: the epidemiologic spectrum of characteristics in the people under study, the intrapersonal physiologic fluctuations within each of the studied people, and the intrinsic mensurational variations within the system of measurement. Because each of these three sources of variability can affect what is found in the collected data, several zones of demarcation could be constructed to cover the epidemiologic, intrapersonal, and mensurational spectrums of variation.

These separate sources of variability are generally disregarded, however, when a range of normal is demarcated statistically. Instead, the main focus of attention is the choice of an appropriate mathematical process.

28.2.1. *Statistical Decisions*

A statistical choice of a demarcated zone requires decisions about its relative size, location, and symmetry.

28.2.1.1. SIZE OF THE ZONE

What proportion of the values in an array of univariate data should be regarded as common or uncommon? And how uncommon must something be to be called *abnormal*?

Because these questions have no standard biologic or clinical answers, they are usually approached with the statistical strategy proposed by Sir Ronald Fisher, who regarded 95% of the inner values as common and the remaining 5% as significantly uncommon. Although the strategy is regularly used to designate the outer 5% of values as *abnormal*, Murphy[1] has pointed out that "contrary to popular opinion," this demarcation of abnormality "is *not* a recommendation of statisticians and . . . has no support from statistical theory." Fisher's proposed boundary of uncommon occurrences was intended for inferential decisions about P values, not for descriptive decisions about normality. Nevertheless, after years of exposure to 0.05 as the magic level of stochastic significance, many clinicians have become thoroughly conditioned to accept the same boundary marker for abnormality.

28.2.1.2. LOCATION OF THE ZONE

Having decided that 5% of the values would be *abnormal*, the investigator must now choose their location. Do they lie only at one or the other end of the spectrum, or are they located at both ends? Is there a single boundary, above or below which everything is normal; or are there two boundaries, forming an inner zone of normality and two outer zones in which the abnormalities are too high and too low?

In pragmatic reality, many laboratory measurements have a single boundary; and the normal zone is located beyond or below this boundary. These single-boundary demarcations, however, are usually derived from diagnostic correlations, not from univariate statistical models. When a statistical model is used, the usual mathematical strategy is to split the zone of abnormality and to choose two boundary markers. The array of data is thus divided into three parts: an interior normal zone, surrounded by upper and lower zones of abnormality.

This decision creates an intriguing mathematical irony. When abnormality is demarcated with a purely statistical model, using no clinical correlations, clinicians are regularly willing to have two boundaries and three zones. On the other hand, when boundaries can be established using direct clinical correlations for diagnostic marker tests, as noted in Chapter 25, clinicians regularly accept a single boundary, forming two zones. Although the diagnostic precision of the diagnostic marker tests could be sharply improved with the three-zone pattern discussed in Section 25.1.3.6, clinicians have retained the logical inconsistency of using two zones for decisions about diagnosis, but three zones for decisions about abnormality. The awkward mathematical mechanisms currently used in statistical indexes of diagnosis can be attributed to this two-zone rather than three-zone system of demarcation.

28.2.1.3. SYMMETRY OF THE ZONE

Having decided that the 5% zone of abnormality is to be divided into an upper and a lower zone, we must now apportion the size of each zone. Should the two zones be split symmetrically, with 2.5% at either end; or should the two parts be unequal, with perhaps 1% at one end and 4% at the other?

In the absence of a correlational mechanism for making this decision, we have no clinical or biologic reason for assuming that abnormality is asymmetric. Therefore, on a purely esthetic basis, we split it evenly, putting 2.5% at each end.

28.2.1.4. CHOICE OF THE GAUSSIAN MODEL

With all of these basic decisions completed, the last step is to choose the particular mathematical model that would do the desired job. For the cited specifications, the choice is obvious: the Gaussian curve. In a Gaussian curve, a zone calculated from the mean ± 2 (actually, 1.96) standard deviations around the mean contains 95% of the values of data. This inner zone is centrally located, with the remaining 5% of data symmetrically distributed in the lower and upper 2.5% zones of abnormality.

The choice of a Gaussian curve is compelling not so much because it fits the desired strategy, but because the strategy was actually derived from the Gaussian model. Ronald Fisher's concept of a symmetrically centered 95% zone of common data, surrounded by two 2.5% zones of uncommon data, was derived from mathematical attributes of the Gaussian curve. In fact, through an interesting quirk in cross-disciplinary jargon, mathematicians have traditionally used the term *normal distribution* to refer to the shape of a Gaussian curve. Having already been sanctified by the mathematical title of *normal*, the Gaussian model could be immediately transplanted for its medical role in determining a range of normal.

With all these decisions completed, the range of normal became easily determined in a simple sequence: Find the mean. Add 2 standard deviations on either side. Proclaim the boundaries.

28.2.2. *Biologic Peculiarities*

When biologic problems receive so simple a solution, we can expect to find many instances in which the solution either does not work or creates strange phenomena. The most striking peculiarities produced by this method of demarcating the range of normal are the implications of the nomenclature, the factitious designations of abnormality, and the impossible ranges that can be formed with the Gaussian procedure.

28.2.2.1. IMPLICATIONS OF NOMENCLATURE

For univariate calculations of a range of normal, the data are often obtained from a group of people who were deliberately chosen to be medically healthy or normal. Having been selected for their normality, these people might be expected to remain normal after having their mathematical adventures in the data processing. Nevertheless, the statistical strategy is relentless. No matter how healthy those people may have been, 5% of them must emerge as abnormal after the statistical partitions.

This problem can be eliminated in two ways. The first is to recognize that the range of values found in those healthy people is indeed the range of normal. It can be designated directly, without any calculations, as spanning the zone from the lowest to highest observed value. Although appealing, this tactic may be inaccurate if some of the apparently healthy people have a latent disease; and it may be misleading if some of the truly healthy people have peculiar outlyer values.

A second solution, which seems more attractive and more universally applicable than the first, is to avoid using the word *normal* for the demarcated zone. The term is inappropriate if the zone is calculated (as it often is) from laboratory data that include diseased as well as healthy people; and the word constantly acts as a source of mischief when it is misinterpreted or misunderstood by patients. Instead of being called a *range of normal,* the zone can be called the *customary range* or *customary zone.* Although this zone need not occupy 95% of the distribution, the 95% tradition may be desirable and can be preserved if clinicians and patients understand that the 95% zone demarcates what is customary rather than what is normal.

28.2.2.2. FACTITIOUS ABNORMALITIES

When normality is defined exclusively according to a 95% statistical boundary, a healthy person who receives a large series of screening tests is quite likely to emerge by chance as abnormal in something. Suppose the person is tested for hematocrit, white blood count, and serum values of cholesterol, sodium, and alkaline phosphatase. Because the person has a 95% chance of being normal in any one of these tests, the chance of being normal in all five, if they vary independently, is $0.95 \times 0.95 \times 0.95 \times 0.95 \times 0.95 = 0.77$. Instead of having a 5% chance of being abnormal in a single test, a healthy person receiving five tests would have a 23% chance of abnormality.

In the batteries of tests now applied routinely with modern technology, in which 30 different measurements may be done with a single specimen of serum, a person receiving the 30 tests has a chance of only $(0.95)^{30} = 0.21$ of being normal in all of them. The likelihood of finding an abnormality by chance somewhere in the screening battery will be 79%.

Alternative tactics of adjusting for multivariate normality have been proposed[4] to deal with this issue. Because the adjustment still depends on the idea that 5% of medically normal people will arbitrarily be called abnormal, the adjustment would reduce the frequency of the peculiarities without altering the source of the basic defect, which arises from an inappropriate use of the word *normal.*

28.2.2.3. IMPOSSIBLE RANGES

The two problems just cited can easily be solved with a simple change in nomenclature, and with greater awareness of the chance likelihood that a barrage of multiple tests will produce at least one value falling outside the customary range. A much more substantial and statistical problem is produced by the Gaussian strategy for demarcating the central 95% zone.

Most medical data do not have a Gaussian spectrum. The patterns of frequency distribution are often significantly skewed; or the curve may have a leptokurtic (too tall), platykurtic (too short), bi-modal (two humps), or other shape that deforms the classic "bell-shaped" pattern of the Gaussian model. When the distribution of data contains these aberrations, a central 95% zone cannot be determined from the $\bar{X} \pm 2s$ tactic used for a Gaussian curve.

Aside from the basic mathematical theory that is violated by the Gaussian calculations, the results are often biologically bizarre. For example, in 265 children and adolescents, the duration of activity in an episode of acute rheumatic fever was found to have a mean of 109 days, with a standard deviation of 57 days.[5] Adding and subtracting $2 \times 57 = 114$ for the mean value of 109, the normal range for a rheumatic episode would therefore be 223 days at the upper end and -5 days at the lower end. An imaginative data analyst might claim some profound undiscovered meaning for those negative five days, but a biologic scientist would recognize the result as silly. Similarly, the range of normal values for fasting blood sugar would take on a negative lower boundary if the range were based on Gaussian calculations from the widely skewed curve usually found in a hospital population.

28.2.3. *Transformations and Modifications*

The problems produced by the inappropriate Gaussian model can be managed by preserving the model and changing the data, or by using a different model.

28.2.3.1. TRANSFORMATION OF DATA

With careful choice of a mathematical method of transformation, we can often convert the original data into a new set of values that have a Gaussian distribution. Instead of working with the original measurements, we may work with their logarithms, square roots, arc sines, or some other derived value that transforms the spectrum of data into a Gaussian pattern. The mean, standard deviation, and customary range are then determined by applying the Gaussian formula to the transformed data. The results are then reconverted for final expression in the original units of measurement.

The justification for these arbitrary transformations is that the original data were themselves measured with an arbitrarily chosen scale. For example, it is a purely arbitrary act to measure height on a scale that is linear, with intervals of equal length between any two adjacent points on the scale. We could just as arbitrarily have decided to express height in logarithmic rather than linear units. The value of pH is an instance of a common biologic measurement that is actually logarithmic, but that is expressed as though it were linear. Another widely employed transformation is our method of expressing biologic antibody titers as the reciprocal of values: we often talk about an antistreptolysin O titer of 250, but the actual value is 1/250.

Because there is nothing mathematically sacred about the arbitrary units of biologic measurement, we should presumably have no reluctance to transform the units into a new scale that will provide a Gaussian pattern for the data. The difficulty with many of the transformations, however, is that they are alien to the basic units with which a biologist has learned to think. In dealing with logarithms, cube roots, or other conversions that make the data attain a Gaussian distribution, the investigator may lose track of whatever biologic meaning is under scrutiny. After the arc sine of the data is used to find a Gaussian mean and standard deviation, and after the appropriate arc sine values are converted back to the original units, the customary range of the results may become statistically acceptable, but the investigator may then be somewhat bewildered in trying to explain them.

Several types of tactics have been proposed to avoid transforming the data while still adjusting for non-Gaussian distributions.[6,7] These indirect methods for estimating a range of normal include such procedures as using truncated distributions; replacing the mean by the mode; taking averages of normals; and preparing composite distributions. After performing a pragmatic evaluation of the indirect methods, Amador and Hsi[6] concluded that they were "quite inaccurate, because the estimated means were shifted significantly toward pathologic values and the estimated standard deviations were unacceptably wide."

28.2.3.2. USE OF PERCENTILES

At this point in the discussion, an intelligent person bereft of statistical education might ask a simple, common-sense question: "If you want to know the zone that contains the inner 95% of the data, why not find it directly?"

The direct approach would require no transformations and no calculations of means and standard deviations. We would rank the observed values of data in ascending order from lowest to highest. To find the inner 95% of the data, we would locate the 2.5 percentile point, which demarcates the lower 2.5% of data, and the 97.5 percentile point, which demarcates the upper 2.5%. We would then have the ipr_{95} range, discussed in

Chapter 7, as a symmetrically placed inner 95% zone for the data. The procedure would be quite simple with no muss, no fuss, and no unreasonable or impossible ranges.

28.2.3.2.1. *Advantages of Percentiles*

The percentile technique for determining the central 95% of a distribution has existed for many years and has impeccable credentials in both statistics and biology. The technique was statistically proposed by Thompson[8] and developed by Wilks.[9] It was biologically explored further by Herrera[10] and has been particularly well described by Mainland.[11] The procedure is simple, realistic, and direct, requiring no transformations of data and no assumptions about the distribution of frequencies or Gaussian parameters. For Gaussian data, the percentile technique produces the same 95% range that would emerge from the Gaussian calculations; and for non-Gaussian data, the technique produces a result that is biologically sensible and easily comprehended.

Nevertheless, the percentile technique is not mentioned in many standard textbooks used for teaching statistics to medical people, and when mentioned in the books, the technique is usually quickly traversed en route to a more extensive discussion of the Gaussian models. Because clinicians do not receive adequate instruction in using the percentile procedure, it seldom appears in general medical literature[12] and it has not been used for calculating the range of normal in most of the tests reported in the past few decades. Consequently, prominent general medical journals have begun to publish papers calling the profession's attention to the defects of Gaussian strategies and urging adoption of a better "modern" method that has existed for more than 45 years. One of the best papers on this topic was by Elveback, Guillier, and Keating.[13]

28.2.3.2.2. *Resistance to Percentiles*

Because the percentile technique is so obviously superior to its Gaussian predecessor, another common-sense question to ask would be why the Gaussian procedure has endured so long and remained so popular. Although a simple explanation is that the scientific community has always resisted a change in paradigms,[14] the reasons for such behavior are usually much more complex. In this instance, at least two main sources of resistance can easily be identified.

The first type of resistance arises from statistical misconceptions about the scientific role of descriptive summaries. Clinicians examine a spectrum of data to determine purely descriptive boundaries for a customary range, but many statisticians regard description only as a primitive appetizer for the main course, which is estimation of a parameter. To estimate a confidence interval for a parametric mean, we need the standard error that is calculated from the standard deviation. The Gaussian formulas are appealing because they offer this parametric bonus. We can use the standard deviation descriptively to obtain a zone for the data, and inferentially to find a confidence interval for the parametric mean. Thus, although a clinician demarcating a customary zone may have no interest in estimating a parametric mean and would have no use for the confidence interval produced by the calculations, the Gaussian procedure may be maintained because it allows the parameters to be inferentially estimated, even when they are biologically unnecessary, unrealistic, or absurd.

A more substantial resistance, however, has come from the work involved in determining the percentiles. For many years, a mean and standard deviation could readily be obtained for a set of data if the appropriate keys were pushed on a conventional desk calculator, but the percentile procedure does not involve classic acts of statistical calculation. Because the observed values must be ranked in ascending order of magnitude, and because an ordinary calculator does not perform rankings, a data analyst who wanted to use the percentile technique had to do the rankings himself. For large amounts of data, the manual ranking procedure was too oppressive to be appealing, no matter how receptive the analyst might have been to new and improved paradigms.

Modern techniques of computation, however, have ended all this calculational oppression. With a suitably programmed calculator or a terminal connected to a computer, we can now obtain the percentile values just as easily as we formerly calculated the mean and standard deviation. In fact, if we make the right plans, we can obtain both sets of results simultaneously from a single run of the data.

As these new computational devices become increasingly available and increasingly used by a new generation of data analysts, the old excuse about difficulty in calculating will no longer be tenable. The failure to use percentile techniques will then be attributable only to professional recalcitrance and intellectual inertia.

28.2.3.3. STANDARDIZED UNITS OF DEVIATION

A quite different approach to the range-of-normal problem is to determine the customary ranges (by whatever method is desired) and then to convert the original data into expressions cited as standardized units of normality or deviations from normal. The strategy is analogous to the principle used for the Z-scores described in Chapter 7.

The avowed goal of these transformations is to free the clinician's mind from the "conversion drudgery" that occurs when different numerical boundaries must be examined for the customary range of each test. In current pragmatic approaches to this problem, clinicians often carry a card that lists all the boundaries of the customary ranges, or the laboratory publishes appropriate boundaries adjacent to the result of each test. In the new proposals, however, all of the customary scales of expression would be abandoned. The value of any test would be cited only according to the relative magnitude of its deviation from a central reference point. The proposed systems of citation have received such names as *probits, normal quotient units, standard deviation units, statens, stanines, clinical units,* and *physician liberation units.* The systems differ mainly in the choice of the central reference point (mean or median) and the tactic used for expressing deviations.

Despite the appeal of the "liberation," these systems have several major flaws. Because they are inapplicable whenever a laboratory result is expressed in nondimensional scales, the systems are not suitable for morphologic data or for quantitative data (such as antibody titers) that are expressed in arbitrary ordinal categories. More importantly, for those clinicians who prefer to correlate the results with judgmental interpretations, the systems create unfamiliar new units that impair usage of the background of experience on which the judgments depend. The new systems may actually increase rather than reduce clinicians' mnemonic difficulty by forcing them to remember how the standard units were calculated so that they can be reconverted for purposes of clinical correlation. Most importantly, however, the standard units are population dependent. They will vary according to the group of people and the particular set of data chosen as the reference population. If the standard units are determined without regard to any of the epidemiologic, intrapersonal, or mensurational variations to be discussed shortly, a clinician may have no direct way of considering the effect of these variations on the result of the test.

28.3. CHOICE OF A REFERENCE GROUP

The main focus thus far in this chapter has been the statistical strategies used for determining a customary range or perhaps for transforming the basic data. These strategies are the usual and often the only topics considered in most discussions of the range of normal. A quite different issue, which is commonly overlooked in the discussions, is the source of the greatest problem in most studies of the customary range. The problem is epidemiologic, and it arises from the lack of suitable attention to the choice and contents of the reference group whose data will be analyzed.[15]

In many instances, a customary range is reported with no information about the people whose data were used for the calculations. Were these people all medically normal, and how was their normality determined? Were they a group of hospital inpatients or outpatients? If so, how might their clinical abnormalities affect the results? Were their age, gender, and other biologic features similar to those of the person to whom the results will be applied? Is the customary range for certain tests in young women different from that of elderly men? If so, were the data listed separately for each biologic category? Were there enough people in each biologic category for the results to be numerically cogent?

28.3.1. *Components of the Epidemiologic Spectrum*

Almost none of these questions receives a satisfactory answer in most current approaches to the range of normal. The zone is calculated or published as an accomplished fact, and the reader is left to divine the constituents with which the fact was obtained. The epidemiologic spectrum of the group is ignored and the different mixtures of demographic and clinical components in the spectrum are neither identified nor quantitatively partitioned.

Nevertheless, as Files, van Peenen, and Lindberg[16] have noted, "different subpopulations vary enough in mean values and breadth of frequency distribution so that age and sex differences are sometimes reversed." Furthermore, in addition to age and gender, important subgroups may be delineated by dietary habits, medication, and other clinical attributes. For example, Hamburger[17] has pointed out that the customary ranges noted for tests of thyroid function have "no meaning without defining the patient population in terms of thyroid abnormality, medications, and quantitative data on iodine ingestion." In assessing laboratory values for a pregnant patient, obstetricians might want to use a range based on healthy women who have not only the same age and race but also the same trimester of pregnancy.

28.3.2. *Suitability of Hospital Groups*

Another important but generally ignored epidemiologic issue is the suitability of demarcating a customary range by using data assembled in a hospital laboratory. The data are easy to collect, particularly if stored in a computer system; the analyses are easy to do; and the results will properly characterize the customary range found in that laboratory's measurements—but the range cannot be used as a surrogate for normal because the reference group contained many diseased people.

If the investigators try to edit the collection of data so that only healthy people are included in the reference group, the research can become quite difficult. The investigators would have to check each person's medical record, not just the stored laboratory data, and would have to choose and apply criteria for the diagnosis of *healthy*. The latter problem can be disregarded only if the investigators are willing to use certain statistical theories,[18] which have been elegantly demolished by Elveback,[19, 20] that propose to distinguish between good and ill health by mathematical analysis alone.

An alternative and easily justified argument is that the laboratory's results should not be edited. They are derived from the clinical population observed at that laboratory and they will be applied to other people tested there. If this approach is used, however, the demarcated zone must be regarded as a *customary range* and should not receive the medically misleading title of *normal.*

28.3.3. *Suitability of Healthy Controls*

A different approach, having much less epidemiologic desirability than the mixed population just described, has been used for many years by clinical investigators who devise a new test. After developing a new method to measure substance X in the serum, the investigator who wants to determine its range of normal obtains blood from some apparently healthy people. The people usually consist of himself and his laboratory technicians, some itinerant house officers, several cooperative secretaries, a few indentured medical students, and an orderly who happened to pass the lab that morning. From the mean and standard deviation of the values found in this haphazardly assembled group, the investigator calculates, publishes, and disseminates the range of normal for substance X.

After this range becomes applied in general usage, many people are unexpectedly found to be suffering from a deficit or surplus of X. They then receive elaborate, expensive further tests that produce no useful explanation for the apparent abnormality. Eventually someone looks up the original publication and discovers the unsatisfactory epidemiologic scope of the healthy control group used for establishing the customary range. A new group—including people much older and younger than the original convenience sample—is assembled and tested. Suddenly the normal range becomes considerably expanded and the previous abnormalities vanish.

Although a defective scope of the reference spectrum is a recurrent source of flawed data both for evaluating diagnostic marker tests (as noted in Chapter 25) and for establishing customary ranges of normal, the strategy is still often used and the results are often accepted for publication. A striking recent variation on this theme has occurred during the contemporary development of chromosome studies. For several years, genetic investigators performed such analyses only on people with obvious clinical abnormalities. The correlations between the chromosomal and clinical abnormalities were excellent until someone had the idea of testing some healthy people and determining a range of normal. To the surprise of the genetic fraternity, a relatively high frequency of chromosomal abnormalities was found[21] in babies with no congenital malformations or other clinical defects.

28.3.4. *Specifications in Reporting Results*

Regardless of how the reference group is chosen, it need not be viewed as a single homogeneous mixture. In an era in which most laboratories use computers to store and analyze data, the customary ranges can regularly be partitioned and reported for groups of similar age, gender, and (when pertinent) clinical attributes. If a particular subgroup is too small to warrant calculating its customary range, the results can be combined with an adjacent group, and the laboratory can warn the reader appropriately.

Epidemiologists have traditionally used stratifications by age, gender, and other pertinent attributes to produce precise data for mortality and morbidity. Similar stratifications could be employed for improving precision in data issued about the customary ranges of laboratory tests. The appropriate computer programs are easy to develop; and Elveback[19, 20] has presented some excellent illustrations of the appearance of the reports.

28.4. ADDITIONAL SOURCES OF VARIABILITY

Beyond the statistical and epidemiologic features just cited, certain additional sources of variability can greatly affect the customary range of normal, although their contributions are often overlooked. They arise from physiologic variations within a particular person, and from mensurational variations in the procedure of measurement.

28.4.1. *Intrapersonal Variations*

Certain phenomena can maintain a basic level in individual people while varying within each person according to a daily, weekly, monthly, or other cycle of periodicity. Other phenomena can change their basic level as people grow older. The fluctuations can be due to circadian rhythms,[22] seasonal patterns, or such imposed features[23] as eating, emotion, exercise, pain, and posture.

If not recognized, the effects of these intrapersonal variations will not be suitably included in the mathematical procedures used to determine a customary range. More importantly, when successive measurements are obtained in the same person, the recipient of the data may falsely conclude that a significant change has occurred, even though the distinctions lie within the intrapersonal range of normal. For example, within the same person the electrocardiogram[24] may show substantial daily variation; major diurnal fluctuations[23] can occur in serum albumin and in volume of urinary excretion; serum iron[23] can vary both diurnally and menstrually; uric acid may show both diurnal and hebdomadal patterns;[25] the neutrophil count may have long-term cyclic oscillation;[26] and serum cholesterol levels may be affected by exercise[27] and by posture.[28]

Fortunately, healthy people have been found[29] to be generally more chemically stable than the mensurational variability of the chemical tests themselves. Nevertheless, certain individual people might have wide intrapersonal fluctuations that must be considered when decisions are made about whether a single value lies in the customary range. These fluctuations become particularly important when the decision deals not with the normality of a single value but with the magnitude and possible causes of a change observed in serial values. Without such awareness, a therapeutic agent may be credited or blamed for having produced a change that was entirely within the customary range of variation for that patient.

28.4.2. *Mensurational Variation*

The physiologic variation that occurs within a single person can often be distinguished mathematically[30] from the mensurational (or analytic) variation in a laboratory's system of measurement, but the main point for clinicians to remember is that the laboratory results can be inconsistent when the same test is applied repeatedly to the same specimen in the same or different laboratories.

Experts in laboratory medicine are well aware of these variations and have developed many techniques to improve quality control by increasing the stability of mensuration.[31-35] The process is relatively easy to study because the work can be done within the confines of the laboratory, concentrating on specimens whose epidemiologic and clinical origins are relatively unimportant for the chemical and other technologic activities of the analytic system.

Although laboratory experts usually know which tests are highly consistent and which ones are not, clinical clients are generally much less sophisticated. To help improve the clinicians' interpretations of test results, the laboratory experts could report the range of mensurational variability for each test, along with the usually reported range of normal values. When clinicians learn (and think about) the effect of a test's own range of mensurational variability, certain results that seem abnormal or changed from previous values may lose their distinctions and become either borderline or unimpressive.

28.5. THE RANGE OF SERIAL CHANGE

Until we reached the intrapersonal and mensurational variability discussed in Section 28.4, the data under consideration were all cross-sectional. The demarcated spectrum consisted of individual values of data obtained at a single point in time for each member of the spectrum. In that cross-sectional spectrum, the additional sources of variability were important because their effects could make a particular person's result lie inside or outside the circumscribed zone of normal. The additional variability was also important, however, for a phenomenon that is not cross-sectional: a person's serial change from one measurement to the next, or during a series of measurements.

Serial changes have sometimes been studied mainly to discern the types of intrapersonal variation described in Section 28.4.1, but most serial investigations are aimed at finding change rather than variability. In cause-effect research, serial changes may be examined from a pair of before-and-after values or from a series of longitudinal results that follow the imposition of a maneuver. Before-and-after patterns are commonly checked in studies of remedial therapy. Longitudinal patterns are commonly examined when long-term efforts are made to lower the magnitude of risk factors or to examine new therapeutic agents for unexpected side effects. Serial changes can also be investigated to determine patterns of growth and development in normal children, in aging adults, and in the course of specific diseases.

The evaluation of serial changes and the demarcation of a customary or normal range of change produce many challenging issues in statistics and in research architecture. To keep this chapter from becoming excessively long, only four of those issues will be briefly outlined here. Readers who want additional details can consult other sources.[36-39]

28.5.1. *When Is a Change a Change?*

One of the most common errors in clinical practice and medical research is the assumption that a newly reported finding is new or that a change is indeed a change. The error occurs when this assumption is made without checking the results of a previous examination or without considering the intrapersonal or mensurational sources of variability. A lump in the breast, a shadow in the chest roentgenogram, or a carcinoma in tissue removed during an endometrial dilatation and curettage may all be regarded as recent new events even though the pertinent sites had never been previously examined in the same way. Alternatively, a patient may be regarded as having newly developed hypertension when previous but unexamined records would show it has existed in labile form for many years. Another patient may be deemed to have a new heart murmur that was previously present without being recognized by the auscultators.

Epidemiologists regularly calculate rates of incidence for various cancers by tabulating the cases that have been newly reported to tumor registries. Such cases may be newly detected and newly reported, but they are not necessarily new incidences, because most of the patients were not previously checked and found free of the cancer. As discussed previously (Chapter 24), the rates of incidence can rise or fall spuriously in relation to screening campaigns, effects of publicity, improvements in technology, dissemination of technology, and changes in diagnostic criteria.

In laboratory measurements, spurious changes can be produced by alterations in the system of measurement (a common problem in such data as serum cholesterol and alkaline phosphatase) and by errors in the collection of specimens, processing of specimens, and transformation of observed result to reported result.

All of these distinctions require careful consideration before decisions are made that a change is a change or that the change is new or recent.

28.5.2. *Regression to the Mean*

When Francis Galton[40] introduced the word *regression,* he was using it in its original meaning. Studying the corresponding heights in a series of fathers and sons, he found that the values were generally well correlated in the middle ranges of height. At the extremes of height, however, the correlation was not as good. The tallest fathers tended to have somewhat shorter sons and the shortest fathers had somewhat taller sons. Galton explained this phenomenon by saying that in successive generations the extremes of height tended to regress toward the mean values, with the high values becoming lower and the low values becoming higher.

Because the regression relationship was shown with a line depicting trend in the two sets of heights, that same word—*regression*—later became applied for any linear pattern of statistical association between two variables. In Galton's original usage, *regression to the mean* implied a pattern in which both ends were moving centripetally toward the middle, but *regression* is now applied for any statistical relationship in which one variable appears to depend on some other variable. In the classic pattern, $Y = a + bX$ expresses a *simple linear regression* of y on x. In more complex patterns, $Y = b_0 + b_1X_1 + b_2X_2 + b_3X_3 + b_4X_4 + \ldots$ expresses a *multiple linear regression* of Y on the variables $X_1, X_2, X_3, X_4, \ldots$. In a tactic called *time series*, $y = a + bt + ct^2 + dt^3 + ct^4 + \ldots$ expresses a *polynomial regression* of y on the variable t (for time).

Nevertheless, Galton's original concept of regression to the mean is still encountered for the serial changes noted in cohort studies. The centripetal movement of data is particularly common when people are enrolled in an interventional study designed to lower the level of some risk factor, such as elevated blood pressure, blood lipids, or blood glucose. The enrollees are often recruited after a screening process demonstrated their higher-than-normal values of the target factor. Because some of these above-normal values may have been due to random fluctuations of intrapersonal or mensurational variability, the values can be expected to return toward normal levels in subsequent measurements, even if no real changes have occurred in the individual persons. Consequently, during the serial follow-up of a cohort, some of the initially high values can be expected to decline because they regress to the mean. Because the interventional maneuver is being used to make high values fall, the observed changes in the group must be carefully analyzed to separate the effects of the maneuver from those attributable to regression to the mean. A variety of mathematical strategies have been proposed for performing this analytic dissection.[41, 42]

28.5.3. *Longitudinal Cross-Sections*

Because of the logistic difficulties of cohort research, certain studies that imply long-term changes are conducted with longitudinal cross-sections, not with cohorts. As noted in Section 18.4.3.3.2, the charts used by practicing pediatricians to monitor the growth and development of children were determined from cross-sections of children at different ages. The charts are admirable because they express the data in percentiles rather than standard-deviation units; but the results do not show the tracking of individual children.

During a particular age period, if the speed of growth increases in some children and decreases in others, the frequency of these individual occurrences might be important to know for future application in clinical practice; but the individual rises and falls would not be detected in the collection of cross-sectional spectrums. Because of this distinction, longitudinal cross-sections can be used effectively for demonstrating each child's relative location in a particular age group, and the data can also be used as a crude index of change, but precise analyses of change would require the tracking of a cohort.

In adults, when longitudinal cross-sections are used instead of cohort studies to determine the effects of aging or disease, many errors or biases can occur, as discussed earlier, because of the attrition of the cohort.

28.5.4. *Serial Normality*

An interesting problem has been produced in recent years by the many laboratory tests used as screening monitors in Phase III randomized trials of new therapeutic agents. In ordinary clinical practice, these tests would not be repeated at frequent intervals; but when new agents are investigated, the tests may be done each week or every two weeks in search of an unexpected adverse reaction.

The location of any individual result can be identified in relation to the customary range, but the collection of longitudinal data poses a new problem. What is the customary range of serial change, and how should it be determined? Should we find the scope of variability for each person, regard each scope as a univariate index, and then establish boundaries for the range of scopes? Should we note each serial value merely as being inside or outside the customary cross-sectional range, with concerns being raised if a particular patient's values become and remain outside this range? Should a coefficient of linear trend be calculated for each person's serial values, with a customary range being developed from these coefficients?

These questions currently have no established or standard answers; and the issues are available as topics for future research. In the meantime, the serial laboratory data of Phase III randomized trials continue to produce oddities that require judgmental rather than purely statistical interpretations. These oddities arise because the trials often have a large sample size that was chosen to demonstrate stochastically significant distinctions for discrete outcome events, such as relief of symptoms. The large sample size, however, may then produce stochastically significant results for trivial distinctions in the serial values of such dimensional measurements as white blood counts, serum sodium, and uric acid. A data analyst who concentrates on the P values rather than on the quantitative or clinical importance of the observed distinctions may then reach the erroneous or misleading conclusion that something significant has happened in the serial variations of the laboratory test.

28.6. SYNOPSIS

When a spectrum of data for a single variable is demarcated with boundaries that form a *range of normal,* the word *normal* can be used in two basically different meanings. In an isolated definition, *normal* refers to the customary, common, or average values found in the spectrum. In a correlated definition, *normal* depends on external information about medical features of current or future health.

Although desirable for clinical activities, a correlated demarcation is often difficult to achieve. The same spectrum may need different boundaries for different clinical phenomena; the data needed for correlations with health may not be available; and a correlated demarcation may require complex multivariate considerations. Consequently, a *range of normal* is usually formed in an isolated manner, according to the contents of a spectrum of univariate data.

In the customary procedure, the range is chosen to be a zone occupying the central 95% of the spectrum. The upper 2.5% and lower 2.5% of values in the spectrum become the abnormal results that are regarded as too high or too low. For a Gaussian spectrum of data, the central range is readily demarcated with two standard deviations around the mean and is expressed as $\bar{X} \pm 2s$. Because most medical data are not Gaussian, this tactic often creates peculiar or distorted ranges. Although various types of transformations (such as logarithms) can be used to convert non-Gaussian data into Gaussian patterns, the inner 95-percentile range is a simple, preferable approach for demarcating the desired central zone. Because the central 95% zone is not directly correlated with health and may often be determined from a group of people who were all chosen as medically normal, the name *customary zone* or *customary range* is a better title than the *range of normal*.

Although demarcated from a univariate collection of data, the customary range can have three other sources of substantial variation: the epidemiologic and clinical characteristics of the people who form the reference group; the individual physiologic status of each person; and the mensurational fluctuations of the analytic method used for measurement. Unless suitable attention is given to these additional epidemiologic, intrapersonal, and mensurational sources of variation, erroneous decisions may be made about changes and abnormalities for individual persons.

To avoid misleading conclusions about longitudinal changes within members of a cohort, a separate range of change may be needed for the customary patterns of serial data, and the phenomenon of *regression to the mean* should be considered when values that are initially extreme later become more centrally located.

EXERCISES

Exercise 28.1. From publications in the medical literature, find a reported survey of the spectrum of a disease. In one or two sentences, briefly outline the topic and apparent purpose of the research. Prepare a list of all the variables whose univariate spectrum was presented or summarized in the report. Are you content with the way these spectrums were shown? If not, what improvements would you suggest? If any bivariate associations were presented, give one illustration. If any comparative contrasts were presented, give one illustration. Are you content with the way the selected association and contrast were presented? If not, what changes would you propose?

Exercise 28.2. From publications in the medical literature, find a report that describes the demarcation of a range of normal for a particular type of data. If the report does not contain enough quantitative or qualitative information, use its references to find the (or an) appropriate source. After choosing an appropriate publication, prepare a critique of the work. The critique should give the reader a reasonably good outline of what the investigators actually did and found (so that the reader need not review the original publication). The critique should include your own favorable (or unfavorable) comments on the statistical, epidemiologic, or other methods that were used in the research.

CHAPTER REFERENCES

1. Murphy, 1972; 2. Cochrane, 1969; 3. Elkins, 1972; 4. Grams, 1972b; 5. Feinstein, 1961; 6. Amador, 1969; 7. Keyser, 1965; 8. Thompson, 1938; 9. Wilks, 1942; 10. Herrera, 1958; 11. Mainland, 1971; 12. Feinstein, 1974; 13. Elveback, 1970; 14. Feinstein, 1971; 15. McCall, 1966; 16. Files, 1968; 17. Hamburger, 1969; 18. Hoffman, 1963; 19. Elveback, 1972; 20. Elveback, 1973; 21. Ratcliffe, 1970; 22. Tedeschi, 1973; 23. Anonymous, 1967; 24. Willems, 1972; 25. Rubin, 1969; 26. Morley, 1966; 27. Mirkin, 1968; 28. Reece, 1973; 29. Cotlove, 1970; 30. Harris, 1970; 31. Benson, 1978; 32. Whitehead, 1977; 33. Barnett, 1979; 34. Mefferd, 1967; 35. Grams, 1972a; 36. Goldstein, 1979; 37. Healy, 1958; 38. Rosner, 1979; 39. Harris, 1980; 40. Galton, 1885–1886; 41. Davis, 1976; 42. Healy, 1978.

Chapter 29

Randomized Clinical Trials

Historians will surely regard randomized clinical trials as one of the main scientific advances in methods of clinical research during the 20th century. The widespread adoption of randomized trials and their required use as a standard for demonstrating therapeutic efficacy have led to an extraordinary clinical event. For the first time in the long history of medicine, unequivocal evidence of efficacy is now usually provided when new pharmaceutical agents are introduced. The efficacy is not always transferrable from one goal to another. We may not know whether an agent that relieves pain also improves physical function and satisfaction with life, or whether the lowering of blood glucose also prevents the vascular complications of diabetes mellitus—but at least we can be assured that the agents do indeed relieve pain or lower blood glucose.

29.1 HISTORICAL EVOLUTION OF CONTROLLED TRIALS

A brief historical review of the evolution of controlled trials is valuable to indicate the way in which the components of modern randomized trials were developed, and to enlighten readers who may mistakenly believe that controlled comparisons of therapy suddenly began when a table of random numbers was first generated. In preparing this summary, I have relied mainly on four excellent historical reviews,[1-4] which should be consulted for further details.

The idea of doing controlled trials is not at all recent or new. In the Bible,[5] to avoid the religious problem of eating food supplied by a conquering king, Daniel proposed a trial of culinary contrast. He arranged for the state of health to be compared in two groups of youths who for 10 days would eat either the royal cuisine or a "kosher" collection of leguminous plants and water. Although obviously applicable for evaluating therapeutic agents, Daniel's strategy of comparison was either disregarded or rejected by practicing clinicians. For many centuries, the clinical paradigm in choosing treatment was to rely not on documented observations and comparisons but on the pathophysiologic rationales provided by authoritative experts. This paradigm was used in ancient times when blood-letting was employed to let out bad humors but is also used today when special diets are planned to lower blood glucose.

Throughout the centuries, the clinicians' obsession with reasoned theory rather than pragmatic evidence aroused many complaints from laymen who had not been educated to ignore what they observed. In a letter to Boccacio in the 14th century, Petrarch said he had "no doubt as to which half would escape" if a clinical trial were conducted to compare "the prescriptions of the doctors" versus "Nature's instincts" in the treatment of "a hundred or a thousand men of the same age, same temperament and habits, together with the same surroundings, (who) were attacked at the same time by the same disease."[4]

By the middle of the 19th century, the situation had not greatly improved. Although Pierre Louis in 1835 had performed comparisons using the numerical method to demonstrate the relative lack of efficacy of blood-letting, and had urged that all future treatments be evaluated with quantified comparisons,[6] clinicians remained generally refractory to the idea. Observing the consequences of this refractoriness, Oliver Wendell Holmes—a physician best known for his nonmedical writings—delivered his celebrated indictment[7] in 1860: "If the whole materia medica as now used could be sunk to the bottom of the sea, it would be all the better for mankind and all the worse for the fishes."

According to what is defined as a controlled comparison of treatment, several candidates can be suggested[1-4] as the first recorded clinical trial. They include: a comparative study by Ambroise Paré done inadvertently in 1537 when he ran out of boiling oil and had to treat battle wounds with a "bland digestive"; a 17th-century cross-over trial in which Wiseman tested the mechanical treatment of peripheral edema by placing, removing, and replacing laced stockings; and several 18th-century events. Among these events were: experiments on prisoners or "charity children" to test smallpox inoculation; Jenner's observational studies of vaccination with cowpox; Withering's evaluation of foxglove (digitalis) as a remedy for dropsy; John Pearson's appraisal of different treatments for syphilis; and Robertson's statistical comparisons of case fatality rates for the use of bark in the treatment of continuous fever.

Perhaps the best known and most dramatic of the "ancient" clinical trials was James Lind's famous experiment[8] in 1747. He used a balanced allocation in which 12 sailors with scurvy were divided into groups of two for a comparison of six regimens: cyder, elixir vitriol, vinegar, sea water, purgatives, and citrus fruits (oranges and lemons). Fortunately, Lind had no advisors to tell him that his sample sizes were statistically inadequate. The prompt and striking improvement in the two sailors receiving the citrus fruits provided convincing evidence of efficacy. (In classic bureaucratic tradition, Lind's evidence was not promptly converted into policy action. Almost 50 years elapsed before the British navy began to supply lemon juice routinely to its ships, thus eliminating scurvy and producing the sobriquet of "limey" for British sailors.)

29.1.1. *The Rise of Documentary Evidence*

In the 19th century, mainly prompted by the impact of Pierre Louis, a larger series of historical landmarks can be identified, although the events and evidence generally had little immediate effect on the contemporaneous clinical practice and medical research. In 1844, Elisha Bartlett,[9] an American student of Louis, established a set of requirements that are still pertinent today as criteria for a satisfactory clinical trial. Among the additional treatments subjected to direct evaluation in the 19th century were tartar emetic for pneumonia, mint water for rheumatic fever, and a nutritious diet for beri-beri. Clinical comparisons were also used to show efficacy for new therapeutic maneuvers, such as Lister's techniques of antisepsis, thyroid extract, serum treatment of diphtheria, and prophylactic inoculation for typhoid fever. John Snow, best known for his work in the public health epidemiology of cholera, engaged in a clinical epidemiologic comparison of chloroform and other new anesthetic agents. Probably the most dramatic clinical comparison of the 19th century—Semmelweis' demonstration of the iatrogenic sources of puerperal fever—was discussed in Chapter 19.

During the first half of the 20th century, clinicians became accustomed to seeing documentary evidence for the value of therapeutic agents. The documentary studies conducted before World War II included the following evaluations: digitalis, vitamin supplements and irradiation for rickets, the nutritional prevention of pellagra, various agents used to prevent or remedy infectious diseases before the advent of sulfonamides, the various types of sulfonamides, insulin for diabetes mellitus, liver for pernicious anemia, ergotamine for migraine, plasma treatment for burns, methionine for hepatitis, stilbestrol for diverse gynecologic conditions, and penicillin.

29.1.2. *The Rise of Concurrent Controls*

Although evidence was now being produced and often reported with quantified statistical expressions, the merits of therapeutic agents were seldom compared directly and concurrently. Almost all the comparisons of a new agent were with historical controls: patients with the same disease who had been treated before the arrival of the new agent. Lind had used concurrent controls as early as 1747, but the principle of concurrent comparison had not yet become established. It was deliberately employed in 1898, when

Fibiger[10] gave an antidiphtheria serum to patients alternatingly (one received it; the next did not; the next received it, and so on), but the principle did not take hold.

The use of serum treatment—this time for pneumonia—led to another revival of the concurrent control principle a generation later. In a series of studies[11] at Boston City Hospital in the 1920s, the concurrent untreated controls were sometimes alternating patients on the same ward and sometimes groups of patients in other wards. In the United Kingdom in 1934, serum treatment of pneumonia was also studied with alternating patients as concurrent controls.[12] This trial was probably the first cooperative study involving multiple collaborating institutions.[4]

In 1930, the concurrent control principle was used in a different manner. Instead of alternating treatment in a direct sequence of patients, Wycoff and coworkers[13] studied the danger of routine digitalis therapy for pneumonia by using a sophisticated arrangement of concurrent assignments to four treatment groups, based on the date and hour of admission to Bellevue Hospital in New York.

29.1.3. *The Introduction of Randomization*

The idea of assigning treatment by randomization was proposed by R. A. Fisher[14] (with W. A. Mackenzie) in 1923 for application in agricultural research. Like most innovations, Fisher's idea was not initially received with enthusiasm by colleagues in the two domains he spanned. His coworkers at the agricultural experimental station did not accept and use randomization in an actual experiment until 3 years after he first proposed it.[15] Among Fisher's fellow statisticians, several prominent leaders in the field—including W. S. Gossett (the "student" creator of the t test) and F. W. Yates (the corrector of chi square)—feared that randomization would increase the error variance in the statistical data. They preferred the balance achieved by assigning treatments within homogeneous strata.

In addition to producing concurrent controls, randomization offered a novel concept in experimental research: unpredictability. When treatment is assigned in an alternating manner or given in any other preset plan (such as time of admission), a clinician who wants his patient to receive a particular treatment can learn the plan and can then arrange to admit the patient at a propitious moment. With randomization, however, each patient's treatment is assigned according to the luck of the draw. This unpredictability, unless subverted by clinicians who peek at the randomization schedule, should prevent the susceptibility bias that can arise when treatments are assigned according to clinicians' preferences.

Fisher's idea seems to have been first used clinically, without being called *randomization*, in the same year (1926) that it entered agricultural experimentation. To test the value of sanocrysin (a gold compound) in treating tuberculosis, Amberson and coworkers[16] arranged two closely matched groups containing 12 patients each. A flip of a coin was then used to assign one group to receive the sanocrysin and the other to act as controls. This trial, reported in 1931, was also the first study (according to Lilienfeld[4]) in which patients were kept unaware of the treatment they received.

A random assignment by group rather than by individual person was not exactly what Fisher had in mind, however. Beyond the scientific merits of concurrent comparison and unpredictable assignments, randomization had a desirable statistical virtue. When stochastic calculations are done to show the role of chance in statistical data, each person is assumed to have a distinctive probability of appearing in a particular group. The variance, standard errors, and other calculations customarily used in stochastic tests all depend on random probabilities for individual persons, not for groups.

This stochastic virtue of randomization, however, is honored much more in statistical theory than in actual practice. Tests of statistical significance are constantly calculated for situations in which the people under study were neither selected randomly from a larger group nor individually assigned the compared maneuvers by randomization. In fact, if either randomized selection or randomized allocation of individual persons were demanded as a prerequisite for conducting tests of statistical significance, an enormous amount of clinical and epidemiologic literature would have to be expunged of all the P values, confidence intervals, and other stochastic calculations used for data collected in nonrandomized studies.

Randomization of individuals rather than groups soon became the preferred investigative procedure, however, not because it was stochastically compelling, but because it was pragmatically necessary. In most clinical trials, the compared groups of patients are not assembled at a single point in time to be assigned treatment and have the trial begin. Instead, the patients are accrued in a successive series as they are sequentially found by the investigator, evaluated for admission, and persuaded to join the study. In this customary situation, there are no initial groups; and the sequential randomized assignment of individual people actually creates the groups that become compared. Group randomization is still sometimes used today, however, particularly in modern trials of interventions administered en masse to communities or to hospital units.

Fisher's idea of randomizing individual people appears to have been first used in studies of immunization against acute respiratory disease. In 1938, Diehl and coworkers[17] reported that students at the University of Minnesota were assigned at random to the experimental or control groups. In 1944, Hinshaw and Feldman[18] at the Mayo Clinic used the toss of a coin to choose actively treated and control patients for evaluating antituberculosis therapy.

29.1.4. *The Rise of Randomization*

The evaluation of treatment for tuberculosis set the stage for the entrance of the modern era of randomized trials. When streptomycin became available shortly after World War II, prompt evaluation was necessary. Clinicians wanted to know if the drug was efficacious; and manufacturers wanted to know if it worked well enough to warrant major industrial efforts to produce it. In the United Kingdom in 1946, the Medical Research Council's Therapeutic Trials Committee initiated a study[19] in which the toss of a coin was replaced by random sampling numbers to assign patients to experimental and control groups. A. B. Hill, a statistician involved in that study, later became an outstanding authority on randomized trials and an eloquent spokesman for their sensible usage. (In the United States in 1946, the Veterans Administration network of hospitals also began a study of streptomycin,[20] but the investigators did not use an untreated control group. This collaboration of investigators at multiple hospitals later evolved into the V.A. Cooperative Studies program, which has subsequently been responsible for so many excellent, successful, and relatively inexpensive randomized trials.)

Because streptomycin was in short supply for the U.K. trial, the investigators designed their study with several adaptations that turned out to be quite lucky. Instead of giving streptomycin to a general group of patients with active pulmonary tuberculosis, the investigators confined the study to a subgroup of severely ill patients with rapidly advancing bilateral pulmonary tuberculosis unsuitable for collapse therapy. By selecting this stratified subgroup, the investigators worked with a relatively homogeneous clinical condition and avoided all the problems that would later arise when randomized trials were used in heterogeneous clinical mixtures of patients having the same disease. The U.K. investigators could also, with a clear conscience, arrange to study an untreated group, because the additional streptomycin was not available for usage. Finally, because of the paucity of streptomycin and because the post-therapeutic improvements were prompt and dramatic, the trial had a short duration. The long-term adverse side effects of streptomycin did not appear.

The spectacular success of the U.K. streptomycin trial is usually regarded as the landmark event in the development of modern randomized trials—but the success had occurred without providing any anticipations or warnings of major problems that would later arise. These problems in randomized trials involved the ethics of placebo therapy, the complexities of heterogeneous clinical groups, and the detection of adverse long-term side effects.

29.1.5. *Placebo and Double-Blind Therapy*

During the examination of concurrently treated control groups, clinicians began to recognize the value of administering inert preparations to the control patients to exclude the factor of mental suggestion. In the Amberson trial[16] of sanocrysin, the control patients received intravenous injections of distilled water. In the Diehl study[17] of prophylactic vaccination against colds, the word *placebo* was reportedly first applied in reference to the saline solution given to the controls.

The Amberson trial also seems to have pioneered the use of a blind procedure, and the MRC streptomycin study was probably the first to use a double-observer technique, because blinding was employed not for the patients or clinicians, but for the radiologists who interpreted the x-ray films.

Although the double-blind procedure is often used mainly to prevent biased observation of the outcome of treatment after a trial is under way, the procedure can have two other advantages when patients are admitted. If a particular treatment is strongly desired for an individual patient, the randomization process can be thwarted if the patient decides to withdraw from the trial after discovering that the undesired agent was allocated. This problem is prevented if neither patient nor clinician knows which agent was assigned.

The other main virtue of double-blind allocation is its avoidance of individual ethical qualms when a potentially effective agent is being compared with placebo. For example, when a vaccine was prepared against poliomyelitis, efficacy had to be demonstrated in a controlled trial[21] before major efforts could be justified to manufacture and disseminate the vaccine. If the vaccine was indeed efficacious, however, the person administering an open placebo to an individual patient would know that the patient was being denied active treatment and exposed to the preventable risk of paralysis. Because this knowledge could jeopardize the vaccinator's willingness to inject placebo, particularly for patients who might be personal acquaintances, the double-blind technique eliminated the problem.

29.1.6. *The 1950s Decade*

In the decade that followed the landmark streptomycin trials, all the ingredients of the modern randomized clinical trial became well established. The structure offered a concurrent comparison of agents that were assigned unpredictably, often with double-blinding and often with placebo controls. The stratifications that provided increased homogeneity were also introduced so that randomization could be scheduled in block fashion, within subgroups of similar patients, rather than given in a complete schedule that did not differentiate among clinical components of a heterogeneous spectrum of disease.

By 1960, enough activity had occurred to be summarized[22-30] in symposia and books devoted to randomized trials, but the trials themselves were still not a commonplace event. They were established, accepted, and respected as a scientific procedure, but they were generally regarded as somewhat recondite clinical enterprises, conducted by academicians who had probably not found ways of being creative or productive in laboratory research.

29.1.7. *Stimulus and Consequences of Thalidomide*

The seminal event that led to the increased popularity of clinical trials and that helped make them a household word was a major therapeutic catastrophe: the phocomelia produced by thalidomide in the early 1960s. The egregious deformities were dramatic; the publicity was extensive; and appropriate action to prevent similar future disasters became an obvious necessity in both medical and public policy.

In the United States, the Food and Drug Administration became required, by legislation passed in 1962, to require proof of efficacy before new drugs were approved for marketing. Because proof of efficacy was usually construed to mean evidence from randomized trials, they promptly became a hallmark of research in the pharmaceutical industry. A similar impetus to greater use of randomized trials occurred in other countries, where regulatory agencies also increased the intensity and scope of their pharmaceutical supervision and demands.

Required for getting new drugs on the market, randomized trials became ubiquitously used by individual practitioners who were directly commissioned to do pharmaceutical studies, by commercial research groups formed to meet the industry's needs, and by clinical academicians whose main rewards often consisted of special equipment or additional research funded by the industry. Results from randomized trials also became extensively used in advertising, thus bringing the concept and the evidence to wide public attention.

In medical research policy, large-scale trials funded by federal agencies or by other noncommercial organizations became increasingly applied to study phenomena that often would not be investigated in ordinary pharmaceutical research for new drugs. These phenomena included studies of nonpharmaceutical agents (such as surgery), comparisons of relative efficacy for well-established old drugs, or investigations of long-term prophylactic efficacy (such as prevention of vascular complications) for drugs whose Phase III trials had proved short-term remedial efficacy in such actions as lowering blood glucose, blood pressure, or blood lipids, but whose long-term accomplishments were uncertain.

One interesting irony in the current regulatory demands is that none of them would prevent recurrence of the thalidomide disaster today. The adverse effects of thalidomide could have been shown in appropriate experiments with animals, but demands for animal experiments are not included in the new regulations concerned with human therapy; and besides, a suitable animal model is often hard to find. In the current regulatory policies for human research, pregnant women, particularly in the first trimester of gestation, would be excluded from admission to randomized trials of new therapy. Consequently, a thalidomide-like substance would be tested in Phase III trials of nonpregnant people who might show no adverse side effects and an efficacious relief of symptoms. Thus, another thalidomide could be developed tomorrow, tested in animals without untoward reactions, shown to be highly efficacious in Phase III randomized trials, and extensively marketed before it becomes received by any vulnerable fetuses. Under the current policy, the only way to prevent another thalidomide disaster is to forbid pregnant women from taking any but the most essential medications—but this mode of prevention was well known and readily applicable *before* the new regulations were instituted.

29.1.8. *Current Status of Randomized Trials*

During the past 15 years, randomized trials have undergone the customary evolution of any major new paradigmatic advance in science. They have become thoroughly established, universally admired, sometimes revered, and frequently criticized.

The establishment of randomized trials as an important branch of medical research is demonstrated by the many additional major summaries or books on the subject,[31-41] by the creation of a special professional journal[42] concerned exclusively with controlled trials, and by the development of a new academic "industry": the biostatistical coordinating center for multi-institutional trials.

The universal admiration for randomized trials arises from the many obvious benefits they have brought to medical research and clinical practice. The list of therapeutic advances mediated and of ineffectual treatments eliminated through randomized trials is too extensive to be cited here. It can be found in the cited books and other appropriate reference sources. Even the most antagonistic critics of randomized trials today will usually focus on specific problems, rigidities, or other inadequacies, and do not seek abandonment of the basic policy or a retrogression to the pretrial era.

The reverence for randomized trials is manifested by quasi-religious devotion[43] in the zeal of enthusiasts who would want any new treatment to be evaluated with immediate randomization, starting with the first patient;[44] who urge readers to accept no evidence about therapeutic efficacy unless the evidence comes from randomized trials;[45] and who would even invoke an editorial censorship that prohibits publication of therapeutic comparisons conducted without randomization.[46] This type of reverence has developed despite A. B. Hill's warning:[47] "Any belief that the controlled trial is the only way (to study therapeutic efficacy) would mean not that the pendulum had swung too far but that it had come right off its hook."

The criticism has come from multiple sources and for multiple reasons, which include conflicts in the design and analysis of the trials, unhappiness about controversies in which the trials have raised more questions than they answered, complaints about their costliness and potential stifling of creativity, and concerns about every aspect of their ethics, ranging from recruitment to long-term follow-up of the treated patients.

Because this discussion is intended to have limited length and scope, I shall focus on the discontent, rather than the enthusiasm, and shall try to note some of the reasons for the problems.

29.2. POLICY CONFLICTS IN DESIGN AND ANALYSIS

A randomized trial is designed and analyzed according to strategic policies about what questions the trial is intended to ask, what answers are to be obtained, what is to be done with the data, and who is to be convinced by the results. These decisions will depend on one of two basic policies, each of which is reasonable and readily justifiable. The approaches that emerge from the choice of basic policies, however, will often be conflicting, so that a trial carried out with one of these policies will often be regarded as unsatisfactory and unacceptable by a proponent of the other policy. The resultant problems are reminiscent of the definition of tragedy as a destructive collision of two opposing protagonists, both of whom are right.

29.2.1. *Pragmatic Versus Fastidious Policies*

The opposing policies arise from different views about the latent objectives of a clinical trial. The overt goal of a clinical trial is readily apparent: it demonstrates the outcomes of a principal maneuver and its comparative maneuver(s) in groups of people with a selected baseline state. The latent goals of a trial, however, reflect the underlying purpose and the standards to be used in interpreting its results. The two different philosophic views about these latent objectives are the source of the current difficulties. In one set of views, a trial is intended to ask questions and obtain answers that are directly pertinent for decisions in clinical practice. In the other viewpoint, a trial must be an explicitly scientific activity. Its results should provide accurate, unbiased answers to the proposed questions; and it should help increase our understanding of the action of the investigated regimens. Both viewpoints are entirely reasonable and defensible, but they often produce conflicts for the many circumstances in which a single trial cannot satisfy both sets of requirements.

The conflict in clinical trials seems to have been first described in 1958 by Modell and Houde,[48] who stated that "there are two fundamentally different goals . . . (1) to predict the value of a drug in the treatment of a particular disease, i.e., a therapeutic evaluation (and) (2) to define the action of a drug in man, i.e., a pharmacological examination." The cited contrast referred mainly to the different goals of a biodynamic explicatory experiment and a remedial (or prophylactic) therapeutic experiment. These disparate objectives in evaluating pharmaceutical substances now often receive numerical labels, with *Phase I* or *II* applied to the explicatory trials of a new drug and *Phase III* or *IV* applied to the therapeutic studies.

In 1967, Schwartz and Lellouch,[49] recognizing that the conflict extended well beyond the goal of studying new drugs and could affect the design of many other trials as well, used the terms *pragmatic* and *explanatory* for the contrasting attitudes with which a trial can be designed. In the Schwartz-Lellouch concepts, the *explanatory* approach is aimed at scientific understanding. The treatments are chosen and compared in a way that facilitates a biologic explanation of their distinctive actions. The goal is to explain how a treatment works or to show that it does work. The *pragmatic* approach, on the other hand, is aimed at the empiric decisions made by clinical practitioners in preferring one treatment rather than another. Thus, when a new active treatment is to be evaluated, the explanatory goal would use a placebo comparison to test for efficacy. The pragmatic goal would compare the new treatment against a standard active agent. In choosing a baseline state for the patients, the explanatory goal is to obtain a cleanly delineated answer. The admitted group might be restricted to a limited spectrum of patients who are particularly likely to cooperate and to respond to the treatment. The pragmatic goal would be to determine what happens in the realities of clinical practice. The admitted group might be a relatively unrestricted collection of diverse patients to whom the new treatment could be given. According to which of these policies is pursued in the initial design, the trial will contain a different comparison in a different spectrum of patients. The results may be able to satisfy the pragmatic goal or the explanatory goal but not both.

More than a decade later, Sackett and Gent[50] pointed out that this conflict in policy for designing a trial was often followed by a different but analogous conflict in the analysis of results. After a trial has been completed, many decisions must be made about how to attribute the events and count the people under observation. Some of the people may have dropped out of the trial for diverse reasons. Other people may have failed to comply with the prescribed regimen or may have taken contaminating regimens. Some of the events may have occurred before a treatment had a chance to exert its action, or the events may have been phenomena that are not amenable to the treatment.

These problems can be analyzed with two opposing viewpoints, which Sackett and Gent called *management* and *explanatory*. In the management approach, which has also been called the *intention-to-treat* approach, all events that occur after randomization are attributed to the treatment assigned by randomization, regardless of when they occurred and how well the treatment was maintained. This policy depends on the principle that avoidance of bias is a prime goal in the trial, that randomization is the prime mechanism for avoiding bias, and that bias can arise from any postrandomization decisions made by patients in maintaining treatment or by investigators in attributing events. To avoid these potential sources of bias, everything that happens after someone has been randomly assigned to a treatment is ascribed to that treatment. The approach is designated as a *management* policy because the results of a decision to follow a given course of therapy can be assessed. In the alternative *explanatory* policy, the investigators want to analyze what happened rather than what was initially decided. The investigators may not want to count events that seem inappropriate for the treatment or to evaluate results for treatments that were not properly maintained.

Although the two sets of policies in design and analysis can be sharply delineated, the associated nomenclature is confusing. The *explanatory/pragmatic* titles clearly denote the contrasting goals in design, but the *explanatory/management* terms are ambiguous for the conflict in analysis, particularly because many of the explanatory goals in analysis seem pragmatic, and some of the management goals are not pragmatic. For example, most pragmatic clinicians would pay relatively little attention to statistics in which the results are summarized for everyone assigned to a treatment, regardless of whether the treatment was actually received or maintained. Yet this type of intention-to-treat analysis is called a *management* policy. Conversely, most pragmatic clinicians would want to see the results of a trial analyzed according to different degrees of compliance or intermediate regulation for the treatments; but this approach is designated as *explanatory*.

The problems in nomenclature arise because three different objectives are being covered with two words. One set of objectives refers to policies aimed directly at answering the questions raised by practicing clinicians in both design and analysis. The second set of objectives refers to *designing* a trial that will provide clear explanations of a treatment's action. The third set of objectives refers to *analyzing* the data in a manner that will yield unbiased results. The word *pragmatic* offers a quite satisfactory title for the first set of objectives, but the *explanatory* and *management* titles create confusion. Thus, an intention-to-treat analysis may be called a *management* policy, but it is not pragmatic; an analysis according to compliance and intermediate regulation may be called *explanatory* but it is also pragmatic.

Because the second and third objectives are often combined in a single policy, we can eliminate the confusion by giving a different name to the two nonpragmatic, scientific goals of understanding mechanisms and obtaining unbiased results. The word *scientific* does not seem right for this purpose because of its inappropriate connotation that the opposite (pragmatic) approach is unscientific. Consequently, to encompass the two aims of the nonpragmatic approach in obtaining knowledge and avoiding bias, I shall use the word *fastidious*. All of the policy conflicts described by Modell and Houde, by Schwartz and Lellouch, by Sackett and Gent, and by other investigators from biometry divisions of national agencies in the U.S. or U.K.[51–53] can be unambiguously catalogued under the rubrics of *pragmatic* versus *fastidious*.

The conflicting goals of pragmatic or fastidious policies can affect every aspect of the design, analysis, and interpretation of a randomized clinical trial. The diverse conflicts, which are discussed in the sections that follow, can be particularly well illustrated with examples from what is probably the most controversial randomized trial ever conducted: the famous UGDP study of hypoglycemic agents.

Begun in the early 1960s and reported in publications that began to appear almost a decade later,[54–57] the UGDP randomized trial evoked a furious dispute[58–66] that has still not been fully resolved.[67] At the peak of the battle, the assaults from both sides contained emotional accusations, self-righteous fervor, and hyperbolic invective of a degree that has probably not occurred clinically since Pierre Louis more than a century earlier[68] used statistical data to impugn the therapeutic value of blood-letting. Now, as the basic flames have subsided with only uncleared smoke remaining, it becomes apparent that both sides in the UGDP controversy could effectively justify their positions with a defensible argument. The opposing arguments, however, could not be reconciled because of their conflicting basic sources in the pragmatic goals of the clinical reviewers and in the fastidious policies used for the trial's design and analysis.

29.2.2. *Conflicts in Basic Design*

When a trial is first being planned, the conflicts in pragmatic versus fastidious policies can affect each aspect of suitability in choice of the baseline state, the outcome, the individual maneuvers, and the strategy of comparison.

29.2.2.1. CHOICE OF BASELINE STATE

Seeking a "clean" answer to the research question, a fastidious designer will want the baseline state to contain a relatively homogeneous group of patients. The admission criteria may therefore arrange to purify the baseline state, by including people of only one gender and race, within a limited age span, with no coexisting other diseases or medications, who have been checked for their willingness to cooperate well with the requirements of the experimental protocol. These restrictions will simplify the conduct of the trial and sharpen the statistical precision of the results. A pragmatic designer, however, may complain that the pure results are not pertinent and may be inapplicable for the impure heterogeneous spectrum of patients in clinical reality.

In the UGDP controversy, pragmatic clinicians were interested in knowing the value of strict versus relaxed regulation of blood glucose—an issue that is particularly cogent for diabetic patients who require insulin to remain free of ketosis. Because the UGDP group wanted fastidiously to investigate oral hypoglycemic agents and placebo as well as insulin, patients who required insulin were not allowed into the trial. The elimination of insulin-dependent diabetes made the study immediately unacceptable to many practicing clinicians. The value of regulating blood glucose in patients with diabetes would be tested only in the restricted subset of patients who could stay free of acidosis with placebo treatment alone.

29.2.2.2. CHOICE OF OUTCOME EVENTS

Because precise decisions about sample size and stochastic significance will depend on the entity chosen as the outcome event, fastidious designers will try to avoid using phenomena described in soft data. Consequently, death—the hardest of all events—is often chosen as the index of outcome. If deaths do not occur frequently, the sample size needed for stochastic significance may be greatly inflated, and the trial may require the cumbersome logistics of multiple collaborating institutions, but the results will be statistically trustworthy.

The absence of suitable soft data, however, may evoke complaints from pragmatic clinicians who want to honor their ancient obligation "to cure occasionally, to relieve often, to comfort always." The clinical pertinence of therapeutic accomplishments cannot be evaluated when suitable data have not been analyzed (or collected) to indicate relief, comfort, or other personal reactions that are of prime interest to patients and patients' families.

The UGDP trial was originally intended to measure the prevention of such vascular complications as retinopathy, neuropathy, nephropathy, and arterial lesions in the extremities. The fastidious design did not include attention to the patients' convenience in using oral rather than injectable agents, to the frequency or distress of insulin-provoked hypoglycemic reactions, or to the infections that may have been prevented or reduced by good control of blood glucose. In measuring the target of vascular complications, the investigators sought "hard data," but the results were often uninterpretable (such as photographs of retinal fundi) or clinically useless (such as the biothesiometric measurements of neuropathy). Consequently, the hard mortality data for deaths—an unanticipated finding—became the main outcome event, and the original question about vascular complications has never received a satisfactory answer.

29.2.2.3. **CHOICE OF INDIVIDUAL REGIMENS**

If a pharmaceutical agent must be regulated with the flexibility used in clinical practice, a fastidious designer may have two sources of distress. The flexible dosage schedules may have too many variations to allow the drug to be analyzed as a single regimen; and, more importantly, the adjustment of dosage may unmask the double-blind procedure. Accordingly, a particular agent (such as anticoagulants or anti-inflammatory doses of aspirin), which practicing clinicians usually titrate for each patient, may be given fastidiously in an invariant fixed dosage or in an arbitrary escalating pattern that may miss the optimal schedule. This type of regimen will usually be unacceptable to a pragmatist, who may complain that the treatment was given in a nonproficient or perhaps unethical manner.

In the UGDP trial, the oral hypoglycemic agents were assigned fastidiously in a fixed, invariant dosage, which represented the customary regimen used by most practitioners, but which was not adjusted for the needs of individual patients. Even if blood glucose was poorly regulated, the fixed dosage remained unchanged. Another of the compared treatments was chosen with an explanatory goal: one group of patients received a fixed, invariant dosage of insulin—a regimen that would be avoided in clinical practice.

29.2.2.4. **STRATEGY OF COMPARISON**

The conflict in fastidious versus pragmatic viewpoints can produce many problems in the strategy of comparison. The ones to be cited here arise from the choice of a comparative agent, the format of comparison, and the applicability of cross-over arrangements.

29.2.2.4.1. *Choice of Comparative Agent*

Although a pragmatic designer would want to compare a new agent against an existing active agent, the choice of a single active agent may be difficult if too many are available. Besides, if the outcome event has an unexpectedly low attack rate in the groups under study, the compared active agents may have similar results because neither agent has been adequately challenged. Accordingly, a fastidious designer will usually choose placebo for a comparison that is both standardized and unequivocally indicative of efficacy.

A pragmatist may then object that a placebo comparison is useless for demonstrating the relative merits of alternative active regimens and may also suggest that the use of placebos is unethical. The pragmatist may even argue, using an explanatory attitude, that the use of a placebo alone, without a concomitant comparison of no treatment, prevents discernment of the major contributions made by iatrotherapy.[69]

29.2.2.4.2. *Format of Comparison*

A different issue in the strategy of comparison refers to the format in which it is arranged. Schwartz and Lellouch[49] give an example of this issue in evaluating the merits of preoperative radiotherapy for patients with operable cancer. A pragmatic designer, answering the practical clinical question, would compare immediate surgery versus surgery that follows a course of radiotherapy. A fastidious designer, trying to achieve a balanced physiologic effect, would give the control patients a course of sham radiotherapy before the surgery is performed.

The format of comparison also creates a conflict in trials of medical versus surgical therapy for patients with unstable angina pectoris. In pragmatic clinical reality, a patient who will be treated medically may not receive a coronary arteriogram while the angina is unstable. A pragmatic comparison, therefore, would randomize one group to be medically treated and the other group to receive surgery preceded by coronary arteriography. In a fastidious comparison, everyone would receive arteriography first; and the anatomically eligible patients would then be randomized to medical or surgical therapy.

29.2.2.4.3. *Applicability of Cross-over Arrangements*

A cross-over design has the universal appeal of reducing the costs of a trial, because fewer patients will be needed if the same people can be tested with each (or most) of the compared agents. The cross-over arrangement also appeals to fastidious designers, because statistical variance is reduced (as noted in Section 9.4.2.7) when the same agents are contrasted within each patient.

During the 1960s, these attractions led to the frequent use of cross-over designs in circumstances that were clinically inappropriate. While the study was in progress, a secular trend might change the general conditions accompanying the first and last agents tested in any individual sequence, and a serial trend might alter the clinical state of individual patients between earlier and later treatments. A carry-over effect might extend either the pharmacologic or psychologic impact of a drug beyond the time frame of that drug and into the action of the next drug.

When these problems were recognized, data obtained in cross-over trials were often rejected by regulatory agencies. The agents received as the *first* treatment for patients in the trial could be compared in a parallel contrast—but the subsequent cross-over information was deemed unacceptable. The washout period that is now often used between successive agents has eliminated the carry-over problem of extended pharmacologic action, but not the possible carry-over of psychic effects.[70, 71] By lengthening the duration of the total trial for each patient, the washout period also increases the costs of the study and the chances of problems due to secular or serial trends.

Although various statistical tactics[71–74] can be used to adjust for trends and carry-over effects, cross-over studies are generally shunned today by both the pragmatic and fastidious camps. Clinical pragmatists are put off by the problems of understanding the intricate mathematical analyses, and fastidious designers fear that the analyses may not adequately cope with the diverse clinical possibilities for bias. Cross-over investigations are now in such disrepute that they may be avoided even in situations in which they can be used effectively and well—such as studying the bioavailability of drugs and testing short-term treatment of chronic or recurrent stable conditions in which the selected outcome variables are not profoundly influenced by psychic effects.

The UGDP study was not planned as a cross-over trial, although many patients changed their originally assigned treatments. The main problems in the strategy and format of comparison arose from the decision to use an oral placebo. It created the previously cited restriction in the scope of admitted patients and it was given in a double-blind manner for comparison with the two oral hypoglycemic agents. Because attempts to titrate the individual dosages might unmask those agents, they were given in fixed dosages. The consequences of these decisions then evoked the pragmatists' objections to the clinical unsuitabilities of both the baseline state and the proficiency of maneuvers.

29.2.3. *Conflicts in Analysis of Results*

After the planned trial has begun, a much more complex set of problems arises in decisions about when to end or extend it, and whom or what to include in the analysis of results.

29.2.3.1. ANALYSIS OF BASELINE STATE

Although randomization creates the groups whose baseline state is scheduled to be treated in the trial, the contents of the analyzed groups can be affected by many things that happen after the randomization. The retrograde effects of outcome events and of treatment itself will be discussed in separate sections later. This section is concerned with events in the baseline state that preceded randomization.

29.2.3.1.1. *Ineligible Admissions*

Patients who do not fit the criteria for admission may be entered into a trial inadvertently or deliberately. The inadvertencies occur when someone failed to check the patients' credentials closely enough and the error is discovered afterward. The deliberate admissions occur when active treatment must be started promptly, without the delay required for the results of tests that confirm the diagnosis. If it is not confirmed, the treatment is stopped.

The pragmatic approach to these problems is simple. The ineligible patients are de-admitted from the trial and replaced by new patients. The replacements can receive whatever treatment is next in the randomization schedule; or the coordinating center (or pharmacist) can arrange, if necessary, for the new patients to receive the same agents that were assigned to the de-admitted patients.

The fastidious approach to the problems has varying levels of intensity. At one extreme, many fastidious analysts are willing to use the same de-admission strategy employed by the pragmatists. In the middle levels, the ineligible patients are allowed to stop treatment, but their data are maintained and analyzed (for whatever duration they are available) in the therapeutic group to which each patient was assigned. At the other extreme, the act of randomized admission to a trial is regarded almost as a permanent statistical sanctification. Not only the data, but the patients themselves must be maintained in the trial, continuing to receive the treatments for which they were ineligible.

The UGDP group used this last approach. Although the results were analyzed with and without inclusion of the ineligible patients, the investigators continued treatment and repeated follow-up visits at regular intervals for 69 patients whose glucose tolerance tests did not fulfill the original quantitative criteria for diabetes mellitus. In justification of the policy, the investigators noted that many of the originally ineligible patients eventually *did* fulfill the glucose tolerance test criteria.

29.2.3.1.2. *Clinical Pertinence of Prognostic Analyses*

Although randomization is intended to produce an unbiased distribution of prognostic factors that affect susceptibility to outcome events, the randomization (as noted earlier) may not always succeed in this goal. The treatment schedule may have received unauthorized modifications at the research sites, or the luck of the draw may have produced major imbalances. To check for this problem, the baseline distribution of prognostic factors is regularly compared in the treated groups.

This baseline state comparison, however, does not indicate the effects of the treatments in those different groups. As noted in earlier chapters, the therapeutic differences may have been confined only to patients with good or poor prognoses, rather than occurring across the board in all of the prognostic groups under study. In certain circumstances, the total results may show no difference between disparate treatments because therapy had opposite effects in different prognostic subgroups. To check for these possibilities, the results of the treatments are prognostically analyzed, usually by comparing results in prognostically similar strata of patients.

Beyond the statistical goal of checking for distorted therapeutic comparisons, however, a suitable prognostic stratification has a crucial role in making the trial clinically pertinent. When clinicians choose treatment for a particular new patient, they want to know what was achieved by the candidate treatments not merely in previous patients with the same disease, but in patients who were clinically similar to the current patient. In the taxonomy that demarcates a suitably similar resemblance, clinicians often classify patients according to severity of illness, duration, auxometry, co-morbidity, and other clinical characteristics that affect prognosis as well as judgments about therapy.

Although a vital feature of analysis in a clinical trial, the choice and arrangement of variables for prognostic stratification has been another important source of conflict in the pragmatic and fastidious approaches. In choosing variables, fastidious planners seek the reliability of hard data and may not analyze or even collect information for the many soft phenomena to which clinical pragmatists often give paramount attention. In arranging variables, fastidious analysts tend to prefer the complex scores that emerge from multivariate mathematical models, and to avoid the stratified clusters or simple scores formed with clinical judgment. When the fastidious prognostic analyses are completed, pragmatic clinicians may then complain that the results are either inscrutable, because of the incomprehensible mathematical tactics, or inadequate, because so many important soft clinical variables have been omitted from consideration.

This problem was an important persistent source of dispute in the UGDP controversy. The defenders of the trial insisted that their many multivariate mathematical analyses provided satisfactory evidence of an equitable prognostic distribution in the treated groups. The opponents insisted that important clinical distinctions had been omitted and that statistically significant differences and inconsistencies had been ignored. This aspect of the controversy has never been resolved.

29.2.3.2. **ANALYSIS OF OUTCOME EVENTS**

The analysis of outcome events may determine how and when a trial is ended, and may have retrograde effects on the choice of patients to be included in the analysis.

29.2.3.2.1. *Premature Termination or Postmature Extension*

While a trial is in progress, the investigators may find significant differences that suggest ending the trial prematurely before it has accrued the planned number of patients or reached the intended duration of follow-up. Conversely, the differences found at or near the end of the trial may have borderline significance, suggesting the need for either more patients or an extended duration.

The pragmatic approach to these problems is to give priority to *clinical* concepts of significance. If the trial shows a distinction that has quantitative clinical significance, the trial can be ended early if the difference is also stochastically significant, or extended if stochastic significance has not yet been achieved.

The fastidious approach to this decision has been to give priority to stochastic concepts of significance, regardless of the quantitative clinical distinctions. With this approach, the fastidious analyst will worry about the stochastic adjustments[75-77] needed to compensate for the significance that can arise by chance when accumulating data are repeatedly checked with "multiple peeks." If the trial is planned with the fastidious technique of *sequential analysis*,[78] the sample size and ending of the trial are all determined by a stochastic decision rule for the distinctions noted in a *single* outcome variable in sequentially admitted pairs of patients.

In the UGDP study, the trial was terminated prematurely when the cardiovascular death rate for tolbutamide was found to be impressively higher than the rate for placebo. Because the finding was unexpected, the investigators used several different stochastic methods for testing statistical significance before becoming persuaded that the tolbutamide-placebo difference was not an artefact of chance. Neither the pragmatic attackers nor the fastidious supporters of the trial commented on the multiple-comparison problem in the stochastic contrasts. The tolbutamide-placebo decisions were made with an unadjusted α level of 0.05, although five regimens had been tested simultaneously, thus permitting 10 pairs of contrasts, for which other fastidious analysts might have dropped α to 0.005.

The main controversy about premature termination of the trial was produced not by the stochastic procedures, however, but by the associated publicity for implications that tolbutamide was a lethal substance. As noted later, statistical significance was initially present only for deaths ascribed to cardiovascular disease, not for the rates of total deaths. Furthermore, in longer-term follow-up, the tolbutamide group was found to have a significantly *lower* death rate for cancer.

29.2.3.2.2. *Patients with Inappropriate Vulnerability*

The vulnerability problem described in Section 15.5.2.3 occurs if a treatment is started too late (or sometimes too early) to exert its anticipated effects. For example, antibiotic therapy is usually regarded as able to prevent rheumatic fever if the treatment is started at satisfactory dosage at any time within nine days after streptococcal pharyngitis is overtly manifested. (This period of vulnerability is what allows practicing clinicians to wait for the result of a throat culture before starting therapy.) In a patient with acute myocardial infarction, the period of vulnerability for lidocaine prophylaxis is the first two days. If started on the fourth day, lidocaine could not be given credit for preventing arrhythmias that do not appear. Conversely, if a patient receives a penicillin injection for a sore throat that was first noted today, and if manifestations of rheumatic fever appear tomorrow, we would not regard the penicillin as a failure. We would decide that it had not been given at the right time to do its job.

The issue of vulnerability arises most often in circumstances in which a patient fulfills the eligibility criteria for admission, starts treatment, and then promptly has an undesirable event before the treatment has had a suitable chance to exert its action in preventing (or producing) that event. How should these events of inappropriate vulnerability be counted and attributed in a randomized trial? This question is easily answered by a fastidious analyst. The events are counted and ascribed to whatever treatment the patient received. A pragmatic analyst, however, will not want to associate the event and the treatment, and will exclude such patients from the analysis. Although some fastidious analysts may be willing to accept this approach, the criteria for inappropriate vulnerability may not evoke universal clinical agreement; and the approach may be outrightly rejected if the criteria seem to have been developed after, rather than before, the data were analyzed.

This type of difficulty did not occur in the UGDP trial, but it has been a major source of controversy in another much-disputed randomized trial, in which sulfinpyrazone therapy was used for the goal of preventing recurrent myocardial infarction.

In the sulfinpyrazone trial,[79, 80] the investigators evaluated their results as rates of analyzable deaths in eligible patients. Eligibility was defined both for admission to the study and for continuing maintenance in the denominator of the life-table type of cohort analysis. Although 71 of the 1629 originally admitted patients were immediately excluded because they did not meet the admission criteria, many other patients were later withdrawn as ineligible because of unacceptable concomitant medication or a variety of medical and nonmedical reasons. As these withdrawals occurred, the follow-up denominators were progressively decremented so that the total eligible denominator of 1558 patients at zero time dropped to about 1100 patients 1 year later and to 204 patients at the 2-year outcome date.

Analyzable deaths were defined, according to a pharmacologic rationale about appropriate vulnerability for the action of sulfinpyrazone, as deaths that occurred more than 7 days after initiation of trial therapy or less than 7 days after withdrawal of therapy. Deaths that occurred outside this therapeutic window or that could be attributed to unrelated surgery were regarded as nonanalyzable. Of the observed 149 deaths in the study, 43 were nonanalyzable and about equally distributed among sulfinpyrazone and placebo. The 106 analyzable deaths, when examined either as a direct proportion of the initial denominators or in the life-table analyses, formed rates that were significantly in favor of sulfinpyrazone.

In the FDA's critique[81] of the trial, the reviewers contended that the conclusions were unreliable and that there was insufficient evidence of sulfinpyrazone's efficacy. The FDA reviewers had a few major disagreements about some of the diagnosed causes of death, but the main complaints arose from possible biases caused by the after-the-fact exclusion of the many ineligible patients and nonanalyzed deaths. The reviewers argued that many of these exclusions had been unplanned because they were not "clearly stated in the ... protocol ... (of) predetermined guidelines and principles" for the trial.

The investigators responded by convening an external, independent "blue-ribbon" committee, which performed a blinded classification of all deaths and the associated analyses. The results[82] were regarded as supporting the investigators' original results and conclusions. The FDA has neither replied to this response nor approved the additional claim for sulfinpyrazone, although a subsequent randomized trial[83] in a somewhat different clinical population showed apparently unequivocal evidence that sulfinpyrazone had reduced thromboembolic events and prevented recurrent myocardial infarction.

29.2.3.2.3. *Patients with Inappropriate Outcome Events*

In the vulnerability problem just described, the outcome event and the treatment can be reasonably related to one another, but the timing is wrong. A different type of problem involves decisions about how to analyze an outcome event that seems unrelated to the treatment.

The pragmatic and fastidious camps often approach this issue in two different ways, according to whether the event is lethal. If the patient survives the event, fastidious analysts usually insist on counting it as part of a tally of potential adverse reactions; pragmatic analysts usually dismiss it as an incidental, unrelated phenomenon. On the other hand, if the event is death, the policies become reversed. Fastidious analysts will usually count only the deaths ascribed to causes that the principal treatment was intended to prevent, whereas clinical pragmatists, troubled by inaccuracies and inconsistencies in the selection of causes of death, want to count all deaths. Thus, in a trial of agents intended to prevent cardiovascular complications, deaths due to myocardial infarction or other atherosclerotic phenomena would be the main focus of a fastidious analysis, whereas all deaths—including those caused by cancer, trauma, or infection—would be counted in a pragmatic approach.

The differences in these two approaches to death can greatly affect statistical distinctions in a trial's results. For example, in a randomized trial of the efficacy of screening for breast cancer,[84] the screened and unscreened groups had significant differences only in deaths ascribed to breast cancer, not in total deaths. Conversely, in a trial of clofibrate primary prophylaxis of coronary disease in healthy patients with relatively high lipid levels,[85] the mortality rates showed a significant difference for all causes but not for myocardial infarction.

Because death itself is hard data, but cause of death is a subjective judgment, a fastidious analysis of causes of death should be preceded by rigorous efforts to ensure that each cause is decided by someone who has suitable data and is suitably blinded to therapy. These efforts would require that each patient's medical record be excerpted objectively, with a procedure such as the differential xeroxing described earlier. Unless the judge works with the original but blinded data rather than with a summary prepared by someone who was aware of treatment, the objectivity of the final decisions will be dubious.

In the UGDP study, the death rates in the tolbutamide versus placebo comparisons were significantly higher for cardiovascular causes but not for all deaths. The causes of death, however, were determined by a special committee who worked not with the original, blinded medical record data, but with summaries prepared by people who knew which treatment had been used when the text of the summary was arranged.

In the sulfinpyrazone controversy, the main statistical significance in favor of the active treatment arose from an unanticipated finding. The drug had been expected to prevent recurrent myocardial infarction, but the most striking distinction in outcome events was a lower rate of sudden death. The causes of death that were originally diagnosed during the double-blind phase of the trial were later reconfirmed by two different committees[82] in blinded reviews, using material that had been differentially xeroxed from the patients' medical records. Although many of the original diagnostic decisions were disputed in the FDA critique, the FDA reviewers did not work blindly and made cause-of-death diagnoses while aware of the treatment each patient had received. The regulatory agency had thus used a fastidious policy for analyzing eligibility and vulnerability, but not for interpreting outcome events.

29.2.3.2.4. *Other Withdrawals from a Trial*

Living patients can withdraw from a trial because they become lost to follow-up or because they have had a prematurely successful or unsuccessful outcome event.

In a long-term trial, the pragmatic and fastidious camps both agree that the losses should be managed with suitable methods of cohort analysis, as discussed in Chapter 17. In a short-term trial (lasting several weeks or months), however, patients are seldom lost. They usually withdraw because they either have been cured or dislike the treatment. The management of these causal losses can create another source of pragmatic versus fastidious disputes.

The pragmatic analyst may want to appraise categorical data for success or failure, regardless of when these events occurred and regardless of whether the decisions were made by patients or clinicians. The fastidious analyst may insist on analyzing the final results of the dimensional or ordinal data of a preestablished outcome variable. Because these data will be available only for patients who completed the trial, a good drug may look bad if its successful patients dropped out, and a bad drug may look good if it lost its failures.

29.2.3.3. ANALYSIS OF THERAPEUTIC PROFICIENCY

Because no planned protocol is ever carried out perfectly by either patients or clinicians, free-living people will regularly violate their instructions. The data analysts will thus find many situations in which some patients never received the assigned regimen; others complied so poorly that the regimen was hardly used; some may have complied well but never achieved the desired degree of intermediate regulation; others may have been well regulated despite poor compliance; yet others may have transferred to a competing regimen in the trial; and everyone may have used various additional treatments beyond the ones that were authorized.

For a fastidious analyst, the paramount role of randomization is to eliminate an unbiased comparison, and the prevention of bias is the prime goal in the analysis of data. Because bias can be created by any personal or clinical decisions that are made *after* randomization, the goal of avoiding bias requires that priority in the analysis of data be given to the randomized intention to treat, rather than to whatever treatment the patient actually received. With this approach, all patients randomly assigned to a particular regimen are included thereafter in the analysis of results for that regimen, regardless of how the original assignment may have been violated or altered.

Despite its defensibility as the only apparent standard mechanism for preventing a biased analysis, this policy evokes sharp disagreement from pragmatic clinicians. They say it is irrational to make decisions about the clinical value of a regimen by evaluating it in patients who were untreated by that regimen, poorly treated, or possibly even treated by the competing regimen. The dissenters can even conjure up a scenario in which all patients receiving an ineffectual regimen become transferred during the trial to a new effective treatment—and then have their successful outcomes ascribed to the original useless treatment.

29.2.3.3.1. *Unplanned Additional Treatment*

No one has a good solution for the problems of unplanned additional treatment, and everyone wishes it would go away. In one study in which I was involved, we tried to avoid the problem by dealing with it in the *design,* rather than the *analysis,* of the trial. Because we were testing the long-term efficacy of antistreptococcal prophylaxis, we wanted the patients (whenever possible) to avoid receiving antibiotic treatment for nonstreptococcal intercurrent upper respiratory infections. With the consent of the referring clinicians, our group of investigators became the primary care physicians for the patients in the study.[86] We were thus able to prevent many of the problems of contamination that would occur if the patients often received additional unscheduled antibiotics.

In other trials, particularly when one group of patients is assigned to a routine care that is not conducted under the auspices of the investigators, a major degree of contamination of the control group is an ominous possibility. It obviously occurred and it remains an unresolved source of dispute in the MRFIT trial,[87, 88] in which the patients receiving routine care nevertheless used many of the tactics and achieved many of the intermediate regulations that were ·desired for the special interventions group.

The problem of contamination is not confined to untreated control groups, however, because any type of additional treatment can have effects that arise as supplements or interactions for the assigned treatment. The intention-to-treat analysis of data is based on the rational hope that the additional treatments will have been randomly distributed among the compared groups, but because the additional treatments are given for clinical indications (which are not considered in the fastidious analyses), the events of reality may not always coincide with the rational hopes. Clinical pragmatists would want to analyze results according to all the reasons why the additional treatments were given, but no one has worked out a satisfactory method for dealing with the attendant complexities of small numbers in diverse groups. The development of a suitable method for analyzing contaminated treatment is another challenge available for future research.

Contamination of treatment was a major problem in the UGDP study. Most of the placebo group had transferred to other treatments before the trial was completed, and large proportions of patients in other groups had also changed to regimens different from their original assignments. Neither the original fastidious analyses, in which everyone was counted according to the initial assignment of treatment, nor the subsequent mathematical models,[64] which allegedly adjusted for changes in treatment, were acceptable to the pragmatic clinical viewpoint.

29.2.3.3.2. *Compliance and Intermediate Regulation*

For analyzing compliance and intermediate regulation, the pragmatic-fastidious conflict has two component problems. The first problem occurs as a simple misunderstanding. Certain fastidious analysts may not realize that the two phenomena are different, and may present results for compliance instead of regulation, or vice versa. The second problem occurs when a fastidious analyst, contending that differences in compliance and regulation may produce biased results because they occur *after* randomization, is reluctant to appraise therapy separately in groups of patients who have had different degrees of compliance or different levels of success in regulating such intermediate targets as blood pressure, blood glucose, or serum lipids.

A dramatic argument in favor of the fastidious approach was demonstrated in the Coronary Drug Project,[89] a randomized trial of several regimens intended to prevent recurrent myocardial infarction. When the initial results, analyzed only according to randomized regimen, showed no favorable impact for any of the active treatments, many clinicians wanted to see what the outcomes were for patients with different degrees of lipid lowering. The results of the trial have never been presented for degrees of intermediate regulation, but an analysis was later reported according to degrees of compliance.[90] The results showed that patients who complied well with clofibrate had significantly higher survival rates than those who complied poorly. This distinction would suggest that clofibrate was highly efficacious. However, when the same analysis was also conducted for the placebo group, the results were similar. Patients who faithfully maintained the placebo regimen had significantly higher survival rates than those who neglected taking the placebo.

The decision to avoid analyzing therapy in subgroups of compliant or well-regulated patients can therefore be well justified, because a patient's *ability* to comply or to be well-regulated can be a nonrandomized prognostic determinant that leads to the distortions of susceptibility bias. The avoidance of such an analysis, however, leaves pragmatic clinicians in a major predicament, unable to determine the value of either faithfully maintaining a fixed dose of treatment or carefully adjusting the dosage of agents that require suitable intermediate regulation. To determine these values with a strictly fastidious approach would require an unethical study in which patients are randomly assigned to clinically unsatisfactory degrees of compliance or regulation, and are then urged (or coerced) to maintain the unsatisfactory regimen.

An alternative but acceptable fastidious approach, used in the VA cooperative trial of treatment for hypertension,[91] is to precede the trial with a protracted qualification period in which patients are appraised for their ability to comply or to be regulated. In the VA study, the qualification period was actually aimed at a different goal. The investigators wanted to screen and eliminate noncompliant patients from admission, so that the research efforts were not inefficient. In more general application, however, the qualification period would be used for characterization rather than for screening. After the eligible people are appropriately characterized according to their capacities for intermediate regulation or compliance, they could be stratified into different levels of these capacities, with separate randomization schedules used for each level.

In the UGDP trial, the analysis of blood glucose regulation was another focus of sharp dispute. Because superior survival results were not found in patients receiving the flexible insulin regimen, the investigators concluded that careful regulation of blood glucose had little value. Pragmatic clinical reviewers then contended that the regulation had not been particularly good, and besides, from informal analyses of the published early results, a distinct survival gradient could be shown in favor of good regulation. In the formal mathematical analyses eventually reported by the investigators, however, such a gradient was not identified.

29.2.4. *Reconciliation of the Conflicts*

Because the opposing policies can affect every aspect of design and analysis in a clinical trial, many of the controversies that have occurred in the past decade are inevitable. A trial conducted with one set of policies cannot please the proponents of the other policy.

The two policies are also difficult to reconcile. After the trial is finished, the analyses can be conducted in both ways, but the conflict will then be transferred to decisions about which set of analyses to accept if the two sets do not agree. If the conflict occurred—as it often does—in the original design, a reconciliation may be impossible, because the designers may not have arranged the appropriate comparisons, chosen suitable patients, or collected the necessary information.

Certain types of reconciliation are easily possible if both sides are willing to make reasonable compromises. In baseline state, a realistically heterogeneous clinical population can be studied if the necessary clinimetric procedures have been developed to improve the quality of soft data.[91a] The data can then be used for suitable prognostic stratifications before or after the randomization. A suitable collection of clinimetrically improved data can also be used to develop better measures of outcome events, to reduce sample sizes, and to allow prerandomization characterizations of compliance and regulation.

Regimens that would not be used in clinical practice should be avoided in clinical trials, unless the trial is specifically intended to answer nonpragmatic questions. The pragmatic view can be given greater attention in decisions about ending or extending trials; and the fastidious view can be given greater attention in decisions for definding eligibility, vulnerability, and inappropriate outcomes *before* the trial begins or under suitably blinded conditions afterward. The analysis of unplanned additional treatment can receive new creative attention, with fastidious models developed to meet pragmatic goals.

29.2.5. *Role of Remedial Versus Prophylactic Objectives*

The most magnificent and generally unchallenged successes of randomized trials have occurred in situations in which the therapy had a remedial purpose. In these circumstances, the baseline state is relatively homogeneous, because everyone has the same target at which treatment is aimed. The sample sizes can be relatively small, because the main outcome events are transitions in the target, rather than appearance of the events that were to be prevented. The remedial trials can also have relatively short durations, because changes in the target phenomenon can be directly and promptly observed.

With relatively homogeneous groups, easy-to-observe outcomes, small sample sizes, and brief durations, trials of remedial therapy can often avoid the expense and cumbersome logistics of cooperative studies, and can also avoid the protracted observational period that allows so many other problems to arise in therapy and outcome events. Randomized trials have also been successful in short-term prophylactic studies, such as surgical trials of the prevention of postoperative infection by antibiotics or prevention of bedsores by steroids.

Most of the main controversies or disappointments in randomized trials have arisen in studies of long-term prophylactic therapy. The prophylaxis may have been used in primary prevention (as in the cited clofibrate trial) or in secondary prevention (with such agents as anticoagulants, hypoglycemics, or antithrombotics). In these circumstances, the low attack rate of the event to be prevented will necessitate large sample sizes. If the incubation period is long, protracted durations of follow-up will be required. During a long period of follow-up, diverse difficulties can arise in proficiency of therapy and in evaluating causes of unexpected outcomes. If the trial is used in studying secondary prevention (and even sometimes in primary prevention), the baseline state will contain a heterogeneous spectrum of patients whose clinical distinctions will create problems in acquiring and analyzing suitable prognostic data.

These problems have not made all prophylactically oriented trials unsuccessful. Successful studies have occurred, for example, in primary prevention of poliomyelitis,[21] "needlestick" hepatitis,[92] and homosexually transmitted hepatitis[93] and in such secondary prevention activities as recurrent rheumatic fever, antihypertensive treatment, chemotherapy for cancer, and beta blocker therapy after myocardial infarction. In many other prophylactic circumstances, however, the trials have been disappointing. The results may not have given unequivocal answers to the original questions, or the answers may not have justified their costs. The results have been particularly distressing when apparently similar studies yielded contradictory findings or when the findings evoked major disputes and controversy.

29.3. **INTERPRETATION OF CONFLICTING RESULTS**

The diverse sources of conflicting options in planning or analyzing a trial can also produce conflicts in the results of two trials that seemed similar in their objectives and methods. In these situations, the investigators seem to have obtained opposite results in trials in which the same therapeutic agents were tested for apparently the same clinical conditions. When the components of the trials are carefully examined, however, the conflict can usually be traced to substantial differences in baseline states, outcome events, or proficiency of treatment.

The differences in results can usually be reconciled when these other differences are discovered, but some clinicians may then unfairly condemn randomized trials as having failed again. Because there is no good clinical reason to believe that a single therapeutic agent will have the same effect in all of the patients exposed to it, there is no good reason to expect all trials of that agent to give the same results. The sources of disparity can usually be found with a careful inspection of all the many components, beyond the therapeutic agents themselves, that are involed in a therapeutic comparison. This information will be found in the *methods* section, rather than the *results,* of the published report. Sometimes, however, particularly in large-scale studies, the crucial methodologic details are not published and can be found (if at all) only in administrative documents prepared by the coordinating center.

Things are much more difficult to interpret when only one trial has been performed, when additional trials of the same topic are unlikely to occur for a long time (if ever), and when the results are disputed. During the disputes, arguments will be brought forth from either the fastidious or pragmatic viewpoints, but the way in which the arguments are used will often depend on underlying unstated policies that depend on the passion of human beliefs rather than dispassionate scientific reasoning. Like the goals of therapy, the goals of these beliefs can be either remedial, in attacking something regarded as evil, or prophylactic, in preventing a pet ox from being gored. The designated evils can be profit-making organizations, costly technology, bureaucratic rigidity, or anything that disturbs the status quo of an established paradigm. The oxen to be defended include academic reputations and the fruits of an investigator's labor, as well as investments in a comfortable status quo, drugs, or technology.

When different disputes produce different targets as the evil to be attacked or the ox to be defended, the disputing protagonists will often choose (or reverse) whatever pragmatic or fastidious policies can support their arguments. For example, according to the fastidious orientation, the intention-to-treat analyses in a randomized trial of an active versus control intervention should provide final conclusions, regardless of what has been found in nonrandomized observational studies of the same relationship. With this policy orientation, tolbutamide would be regarded as a dangerous cardiac agent after the UGDP trial, and multiple risk factor intervention would be regarded as a usefuless activity after the MRFIT trial. Nevertheless, many people who will fastidiously accept the UGDP's conclusion for tolbutamide will argue that the results of the MRFIT trial should be disregarded because of the contaminated control group and that conclusions about multiple risk factor interventions should depend on previous nonrandomized observations.

Although scientific methods and standards can be used for obtaining evidence and evaluating its credibility, the editorial interpretation of results is a human activity, affected by all of the rational mechanisms, foibles, and prejudices of human judgment.

29.4. ADDITIONAL PROBLEMS AND CHALLENGES

Of the many additional problems and challenges that might be discussed for randomized trials, only seven will be briefly cited here. They involve complex issues in ethics, generalization of results, double-blind procedures, nonrandomized controls, coordination of multi-institutional collaborative studies, pooling of studies, and unconventional applications.

29.4.1. *Ethical Issues*

Almost every aspect of randomized trials—ranging from broad ideas about their basic goals to minute details of their implementation—has been the subject of ethical scrutiny and controversy. Like the basic policy conflicts discussed throughout Section 29.2, these disputes arise from two sets of viewpoints that also can each be readily justified individually but that often cannot be reconciled. The fundamental distinctions in the two policy viewpoints might be labeled as *societal* versus *samaritan*. In the societal viewpoint, clinicians are obligated to find and demonstrate worthwhile agents of therapy. In the samaritan viewpoint, clinicians are obligated to do their best for individual patients.

Both viewpoints are entirely ethical, but they will regularly collide during decisions about whether, when, and how to do a randomized trial. In the samaritan viewpoint, randomization itself is an often unacceptable method of choosing therapy, because it removes clinical judgment from choices tailored to the nuances of a patient's personal needs. Because these individualized samaritan judgments have led to the many past delusions about therapeutic merits, randomization is welcomed in the societal viewpoint as a prime mechanism for avoiding the delusions. Although proponents of the samaritan approach may claim that certain treatments are too well established to warrant randomized trials, a societal response can cite a long list of well-established treatments that were eventually shown, often with randomized trials, to be useless or harmful. The two policies will also collide in the attitude toward placebos, which will often be rejected in the samaritan viewpoint, but accepted for societal needs in evaluating therapy.

The societal-samaritan conflict also occurs when informed consent is sought from patients solicited to enter a trial. Because randomized trials are almost always conducted with the suspicion that one treatment is superior to another, and because sample sizes are calculated on the basis of that suspicion, clinicians seeking a patient's informed consent will not be fully truthful, according to the samaritan viewpoint, in stating that the trial is intended merely to see whether a difference exists in the two treatments. The societal viewpoint, however, can ethically justify a statement that the trial is intended to provide convincing evidence of a difference and to detect unsuspected complications.

Several publications contain extensive bibliographies[94-100] that can be used as starting points for readers who want further information about these and other ethical dilemmas.

29.4.2. *Generalization of Results*

The filtration process described in Chapter 15 creates two major problems in randomized trials. One problem is the difficulty of obtaining enough patients for the trial. When investigators estimate the number of patients who might be available for a particular trial at a particular medical setting, the estimate is almost always much too high. The investigator usually makes the estimate by counting the number of people at that setting who were diagnosed during a selected time interval as having the disease under investigation. Many (and often most) of those people, however, may fulfill the main diagnostic criteria without satisfying the other strict qualifications established for admission to the trial. Beyond the patients who are unqualified, a second overlooked source of losses is the need for both the patients and their individual clinicians to consent to participation. Even if qualified for admission, many patients may refuse. The result of all these losses is that the trial may not be able to enroll enough patients.

This problem was strikingly illustrated in a review of a randomized trial of psychotropic therapy for depressive illness. In more than 4½ years, 95 investigators working in nine centers had recruited only 136 patients; and in two large cities, only three patients had been admitted. After wondering what went wrong in the trial, the editorial writer[101] also wanted to know what made those three patients so uniquely suitable.

Aside from difficulties in recruiting patients, however, the filtration process creates a second major problem: the difficulties in generalizing results. Regardless of how well the comparison is conducted within the trial, the relatively small proportion of eligible patients under investigation may not suitably represent the population for whom the results are intended. In an enumeration of the losses produced at each stage of filtration in a randomized trial, Hampton[102] has shown the steps in which the large numbers of patients originally considered for acceptance were eventually winnowed down to the small proportions who were actually admitted. In some trials, the investigated remnant may still be sufficiently large and general to allow easy extrapolation of results; but in others, the trial may yield a horticultural rather than clinical product. The result may resemble a type of hothouse flower, which cannot bloom or be successfully removed beyond its special greenery.

29.4.3. *Double-Blind Procedures*

Although randomization is intended to prevent delusions in clinical judgment, double-blind procedures may create delusions in randomized results. The main problems arise, as discussed earlier, because the efforts to preserve a double-blind design may lead to a peculiar or unproficient regimen; the double-blind masks may be perforated by diverse associated phenomena; or the attending clinicians may be discouraged by their inability to augment clinical experience by immediately observed correlations between treatments and outcomes.

A problem that seldom receives much attention is the need to check whether patients and clinicians did indeed remain ignorant of the treatment under study. When remedial therapy involves subjectively observed transitions in outcome events, double-blind observations may be more of a safeguard against bias than a randomized assignment of treatment. Investigators in the randomized Aspirin Myocardial Infarction Study (AMIS)[103] have published an account of how the double-blind process can be checked, some of the startling results it revealed, and a good review of the pertinent literature.

Although double-blinding (or an appropriate form of single-blinding) is an obvious necessity in many studies, the use and abuse of the procedure can be substantially reduced when suitable clinimetric improvements have been developed for obtaining data. The main incentive for the double-blind technique has often been the hope of avoiding bias and having an equal distribution of imprecision for ratings that were made without standardized specifications or criteria. If standardized methods are developed for making the observations, however, the double-blind process could be reserved for situations in which it is most necessary, and it need not be used as a surrogate for obtaining satisfactory scientific data.

29.4.4. *Nonrandomized Controls*

Arguing that new treatments must be tested in controlled clinical trials but that the control groups need not be randomized or even concurrent, Gehan and Freireich[104] have thoughtfully presented the case for choosing nonrandomized controls, particularly in studies of new chemotherapy for cancer. The nonrandomized controls can be either concurrent, selected from other patients treated at the same institution (or elsewhere), or historical, selected from published literature, preceding trials, or preceding patients.

The subsequent disputes about the acceptability of this technique have contained contributions from both the pragmatic/fastidious and societal/samaritan policy conflicts. The proponents of nonrandomized trials have contended, at the samaritan level, that patients and clinicians will be reluctant to participate in trials testing an "inferior" conventional treatment and, at the pragmatic level, that randomized trials are too expensive and difficult to be used for every new treatment that comes along. The opponents have usually responded that the new treatment may actually be inferior to the old one and that the nonrandomized comparisons, although inexpensive, may be worthless because of the potential for distorted results.

As is customary in these policy disputes, both sides can be right and wrong. A prominent focus of dispute is the role of randomization in reducing susceptibility bias. Supporters of nonrandomized comparisons claim that this bias can be eliminated by choosing patients with similar prognoses. As noted earlier and elsewhere,[105] however, some of the important clinical prognostic distinctions are not managed well either in randomized or nonrandomized comparisons. As long as cogent prognostic distinctions continue to be overlooked, a nonrandomized comparison will often have problems, but neither type of comparison can be confidently assured—particularly with the relatively small sample sizes used to test cancer chemotherapy—of having avoided susceptibility bias.

An important problem often ignored in this dispute is the role of ancillary supportive therapy. If the supportive treatment is different from one span of time to the next, historical controls may be unacceptable not because of the feared prognostic differences, but because of performance bias introduced by changes in the concomitant therapy. This problem can usually be avoided if the controls are concurrent in both secular time and institutional site of treatment, but the best approach will require development of suitable clinimetric methods to identify and analyze concomitant therapy.

A different problem in historical versus concurrent comparisons of cancer therapy is produced by improved methods of diagnostic imaging. In a phenomenon analogous to lead-time bias, the stage migration produced by the detection of clinically silent metastases can improve prognosis in a metastatic stage identified with recent diagnostic techniques, although actual survival is unaffected.[106] If the distinction is not recognized in the baseline state of the compared groups, the recent therapy will fallaciously be credited with improving survival.

29.4.5. *Multi-Institutional Collaborative Studies*

When multiple institutions collaborate in a randomized trial, the multicentric aspects of the study produce a series of problems that do not arise for work done at a single medical setting.

The most obvious problem is the need to standardize variability among the diverse investigators in all aspects of performance of the trial, ranging from compliance with the planned protocol to completion of the requested formats for data. Special arrangements may be required for a central pharmacy to prepare drugs, a central laboratory to do special measurements, and a central committee (or reader) to provide interpretation for roentgenograms or other specimens that require visual review. The collaborators will have to hold regular meetings; a steering committee will be needed to coordinate routine operations; and an external policy committee will have to review the results periodically for making decisions about the progress or termination of the study. The opportunities and tribulations created by these activities have received detailed descriptions elsewhere.[107–112]

An issue that is seldom discussed is the problem of ego gratification and rugged individualism in the self-selected group of people who have become medical clinicians. For ego gratification, most clinical investigators like to see their names attached to published papers, and most practitioners like the satisfaction of a job well done in the samaritan function of patient care. As rugged individualists, both the academicians and the practitioners like to be in charge of what they are doing.

The desire for gratification and individualism in both groups may be sacrificed, however, when a rigid protocol must be followed to maintain standardization in a multicenter trial, when samaritan or pragmatic compromises must be made for the societal or fastidious consensus of the group, and when results are reported with only the "group" cited as author, leaving the participating collaborators' names buried in a telephone-book array of small type. Analogous problems involving the ego can arise when the granting agency maintains a separate monitoring committee that has power to suspend support of the study if the collaborators "misbehave," and when individual collaborators want to present their own results separately in a manner not authorized by the steering committee.

Multicenter collaborative studies are a splendid mechanism for answering questions that require such studies—but they are not easy to do, and they usually involve special approaches not only in design, conduct, and analysis, but also in the choice of temperament and other personal attributes for the participating investigators.

29.4.6. *Pooled Results*

In a multi-institutional collaborative trial, deliberate plans are made for the results of the individual institutions to be combined in a single pooled analysis. According to those plans, the individual centers all use the same research protocol, admit the same kinds of patients, administer the same kinds of treatments, follow the patients in the same way, and look for the same outcome events. Because of problems in observer variability or the types of patients found at different institutions, this similarity is not always achieved; but the efforts to attain it provide the justification for the subsequent pooling.

As noted in Section 22.4.4.1, however, data analysts may sometimes want to pool data from studies that were not conducted with the same common protocol and with maneuvers that were not assigned with randomization. For example, in the era before the MRFIT trial produced a randomized evaluation of public health interventions, a special pooling project was conducted.[113] The results of diverse observational studies were combined for estimates of the risk of coronary heart disease in relation to levels of smoking, blood pressure, and serum cholesterol. In more recent years, the results of randomized trials performed with different protocols have been pooled to evaluate the effects of anticoagulant[114] or intravenous streptokinase therapy[115] in acute myocardial infarction, the role of antibiotic prophylaxis in colon surgery,[116] and the association of adrenocorticosteroid therapy with subsequent peptic ulcer disease.[117]

The dispute[118, 119] about the scientific merits of heterogeneous pooling has elements of the fastidious/pragmatic policy problems noted earlier. A fastidious analyst would contend that because randomization eliminates bias, randomized trials of similar agents can justifiably be pooled and analyzed without bias. A pragmatic analyst would respond that the results may be too heterogeneous and vague to be cogently applied in clinical practice. A pragmatist might argue that when no other answers are available, the results of the pooled analyses are better than nothing; a fastidious reviewer might insist that no answer is better than one that is probably misleading.

Regardless of scientific issues in the intellectual dispute, the main problems arise in deciding what to do about the results. If the concomitant or major treatments have sufficiently changed, the comparisons of therapy given in an earlier era may no longer be pertinent for the subsequent era in which the pooled analysis is presented. Practitioners may then regard the results as an interesting historical relic, inapplicable to current medical practice. If the results of treatment compared in the pooled analysis are to be pertinent for current medical practice, the comparison should refer to current therapeutic conditions, employing the many additional diagnostic procedures and treatments that were not available in the earlier era. This type of evaluation may be difficult to do, however, particularly if conclusions from the pooled analyses are accompanied by claims that subsequent evaluations would be unethical.

29.5. UNCONVENTIONAL APPLICATIONS

This section describes some valuable but unorthodox ways in which randomized trials have been used. Most clinicians think of a randomized trial as a comparison of pharmaceutical or other specific therapeutic agents used in clinical treatment. During the past few decades, however, randomized trials have been used in various unconventional ways, some of which are listed in the subsections that follow.

29.5.1. *Randomized Cessation of Active Therapy*

Although the efficacy of a treatment is usually tested by seeing what happens when it is newly imposed on a patient, an alternative approach is to discontinue an allegedly efficacious agent. My colleagues and I used this strategy about two decades ago to determine whether long-term antistreptococcal prophylaxis might be successfully stopped in adolescent children, without heart disease, who had gone for many years without an episode of rheumatic fever.[120] In a randomized trial, half the patients had their active prophylactic agent discontinued and replaced by a placebo. The patients receiving placebo thus became the experimental group, and the patients continuing active prophylaxis were the controls. An analogous design was used by Rimland and coworkers[121] to show the efficacy that was lost when high doses of vitamin B_6 were replaced by placebo in autistic children.

The randomized cessation technique might be particularly useful for showing the efficacy of nonprescription drugs. Instead of testing for efficacy by giving the drugs *de novo* to unselected patients, the investigators can check the results of double-blind randomized discontinuation of the drug in patients who claim to be benefited by it.

29.5.2. *Tests of Etiology*

By exposing patients to an agent that provokes episodes of clinical illness, a clinical trial can be used for etiologic rather than therapeutic purposes. This technique, which is particularly applicable for investigating dietary pathogens, has been used to study the etiologic role of cow's milk in infantile colic[122] and various foods in migraine headaches.

29.5.3. *Tests of Screening*

The virtues of screening for lanthanic disease are often preached and practiced but seldom documented. The main problem in documentation is to show that the patient was actually benefited, rather than merely diagnosed early, by the screening procedure. If the only outcome under investigation is diagnosis of the disease, the research activity is really a study of process and becomes a direct demonstration of how detection bias operates: People who receive appropriate diagnostic tests have disease detected more frequently than people who do not receive the tests.

This type of result was noted in a randomized trial of testing feces for occult blood to detect colorectal cancer.[123] The patients of a collaborating group of general practitioners in the United Kingdom were randomly assigned to receive or not receive the screening tests. During the year after onset of the trial, colorectal carcinomas were found at rates 3.6 times higher in the screened group than in the control group, and, as might be expected from lead-time bias, the cancers detected by screening had more favorable pathologic stages. The investigators noted, however, that a larger study is necessary to determine whether mortality rates in the long term are altered.

The investigation of a screening procedure can become a cause-effect study, and patient's benefits can be demonstrated, if the outcome is a morbid or mortal event that was presumaby altered by the early diagnostic detection. Because of the difficult problems in logistics and in evaluating the contributing co-maneuvers of intervening therapy, this type of long-term cohort screening study is seldom done (or reported). In several well-known instances, however, the outcome efficacy of screening has been evaluated with randomized trials. In one study, described earlier, patients who were screened for breast cancer had lower rates of breast cancer mortality but not of total mortality than the unscreened control group.[84] In several randomized trials of multiphasic screening procedures, no striking advantages were noted in the outcomes of people who were screened.[124–126]

29.5.4. *Comparison of Diagnostic Procedures*

Randomized trials have been used to appraise the diagnostic value of new technologic procedures, such as flexible endoscopy in upper gastrointestinal bleeding. In this type of acute, serious clinical condition, the trial can readily focus on outcome rather than process, because only two major forms of treatment (medical or surgical therapy) will follow the diagnosis and because the outcome of the acute condition can be noted soon after onset of treatment.

If the post-therapeutic outcome does not occur until long after the diagnosis, however, and if many different therapeutic regimens can intervene between diagnosis and outcome, the results of randomized diagnostic procedures will be more difficult to interpret.

29.5.5. *Comparison of Technologic Processes or Devices*

Although technologic processes were discussed in Chapter 25, the compared agents were seldom randomized and they were usually studied for diagnostic identifications rather than clinical impacts. Randomized trials have been used, however, for evaluating technologic processes or devices in studies done to see the impact of different barium sulfate suspensions on the quality of gastrointestinal roentgenograms,[127] to determine whether daily versus weekly monitoring of glucose would affect perinatal morbidity in the pregnancies of diabetic women,[128] and to compare the risk of infusion-associated bacteremia when the intravenous sets were changed at 24-hour or 48-hour intervals.[129]

29.5.6. *Tests of Purveyant Maneuvers*

Readers who have worked their way through the text may recall that back in Section 11.5.3.3, a purveyant maneuver was defined as a cause-effect intervention involving specifically human activities associated with health care delivery, rather than the usual agents considered in etiology or therapy of disease. Among the things that can be purveyant maneuvers are distinctions in health care personnel, patterns of communication, educational programs, or administrative and fiscal mechanisms. The recipients of the maneuvers can be a general population, groups of patients, or the personnel who provide health care. When the maneuvers consist of health care personnel, they can be different types of practitioners or practitioners trained in different ways. The patterns of communication can include instructions given by written documents, telephone calls, outlined protocols, audiovisual presentations, or computer displays. The educational programs can involve presentations that are given individually or to groups, in tailored or routine manners, or with other variations. Aside from conventional outcome events in health, the goals of the trials may be patients' compliance with maneuvers, understanding of disease, or attendance at clinics. Clinicians rather than patients have been the subjects of trials done to evaluate methods of postgraduate medical education, to alter patterns of prescribing, and to reduce the costs (and risks) of ordering excessive diagnostic tests.

The foregoing remarks appear without reference citations because the individual listings would add about 50 additional numbers to the already huge list that appears at the end of this chapter. If only one reference could be cited, however, I would list the landmark study in randomized trials of purveyant maneuvers: the classic Burlington comparison of family physicians versus nurse practitioners in delivering primary care.[130] I also cannot resist mentioning my own personal favorite among randomized trials: a double-blind experimental test, by Joyce and Welldon, of the objective efficacy of prayer.[131] (Because I don't want to ruin your guesses about what happened in that trial, you should check the report to learn the results.)

29.6. LIMITATIONS OF RANDOMIZED TRIALS

Despite their many splendid and admirable accomplishments, randomized trials have some substantial limitations, which arise not from anything inherent in the trials themselves, but from the limited spectrum of scientific challenges to which the trials can be successfully applied. Although invaluable for appraising many issues in therapy, the trials cannot be used effectively for answering all the questions that occur in patient care.

The many nonexperimental structures discussed in previous chapters were developed because of scientific necessity, not because of creative inertia or intellectual resistance to the trials. The observational structures were needed as substitutes for randomized trials in the many research circumstances for which the trials cannot be used because they are unethical, unfeasible, or ineffectual.

29.6.1. *Studies of Etiologic Agents*

One prominent type of research to which randomized trials cannot be applied is in answering the many cause-effect questions about the etiologic role of presumably noxious agents. As soon as an agent is suspected of being noxious, the opportunity to test it in a randomized trial has passed. For this reason, almost all of the environmental, occupational, nutritional, behavioral, and other public health agents that become suspected of causing disease will have to be investigated with nonexperimental epidemiologic studies. We can do randomized trials to see whether cessation of an allegedly noxious maneuver (such as stopping smoking or changing to a "prudent" diet from a high-fat diet) can be used in a positive way to prevent disease, but we cannot experimentally assign people to begin using the noxious maneuvers (such as starting smoking or converting to a high-fat diet) to demonstrate that the maneuvers will indeed cause disease.

29.6.2. *Studies of Distant or Rare Adverse Reactions to Therapy*

Another entity that is not amenable to study with randomized trials is the distant or rare occurrence of adverse effects from therapeutic agents. We cannot assemble enough people and follow them long enough under a rigorous experimental protocol to compare the occurrence rates for hazards that may not appear until decades later; and when the hazards do appear, we may not be able to separate the long-term effect of a single therapeutic agent from the impact of all the other maneuvers that will have intervened. Thus, we can use randomized trials to demonstrate the short-term remedial action of hypoglycemic agents in lowering blood glucose and to appraise their longer-term prophylactic impact in preventing vascular complications. We would not be able, however, to follow huge groups of diabetic patients long enough, well enough, and strictly enough to obtain suitable experimental proof that a distant effect of hypoglycemic agents is to cause (or prevent) cancers.

For certain short-term therapeutic quesions—such as the possible adverse effects of aspirin in the treatment of acute childhood illness—the occurrence rate of outcome events such as Reye's syndrome is too low. We could not assemble the huge sample sizes that would be required for convincing randomized trials of the aspirin/Reye's syndrome relationship.

29.6.3. *Studies of Diagnostic Technology*

The agents of diagnostic technology can sometimes be compared with randomized trials, but the spectrum of potential clinical application is very narrow. As discussed in Section 29.5.4, randomized trials can be successfully used in certain acute clinical conditions, such as an episode of gastrointestinal bleeding, in which a distinctive outcome promptly follows the tested diagnostic agent and the ensuing treatment. In all other circumstances, in which the outcome event is delayed, the effects of diverse intervening events in the patient's management will be impossible to separate from the preceding contribution of the diagnostic agent itself.

29.6.4. *Evaluation of Proliferating New Therapeutic Alternatives*

Although seemingly well suited for evaluating most therapeutic agents, randomized trials will be difficult to use in an economical manner as a burgeoning technology constantly produces distinctively new agents, different alternatives for old agents, and variations in established agents.

29.6.4.1. **PREMATURE OBSOLESCENCE OF RESULTS**

The proliferation and development of distinctively new agents creates the threat that the results of a long-term trial will be obsolete before the trial is finished. By the time the data are assembled and analyzed to compare the respective merits of agents A and B, one or both agents may have been replaced by newly developed treatments that seem preferable.

For example, about 15 years ago, a randomized trial of medical therapy versus tunnel-implant surgery for coronary disease was abandoned after almost 2 years of work because bypass grafting had become the preferred surgical procedure. Today, before all the results have been thoroughly evaluated for randomized trials of bypass grafts, another new type of treatment has arrived: transluminal coronary angioplasty. Even in the unlikely possibility that angioplasty can be successfully studied with randomized trials, some other new (and presumably better) surgical procedure may be developed before the trials are completed.

Furthermore, most of the trials of surgical versus medical therapy for coronary disease were conducted before antithrombotic agents, beta blockers, calcium-channel blockers, and other powerful new weapons were regularly being used in the medical armamentarium. Even if the surgical procedures had not changed, the medical therapy used in the randomized comparisons would have been substantially altered before the trials were finished. Another example of this problem is shown by the large-scale, multi-institutional randomized trial called the Coronary Drug Project, which was previously discussed in several places in the text. Although the trial showed that none of the tested agents—estrogen, thyroid, and clofibrate—seemed more effective than placebo in preventing recurrent myocardial infarction, the subsequent development of better pharmacologic agents would have made them the leading choices in medical therapy today regardless of what had been found in the trial.

A similar type of problem has occurred in a multi-institutional randomized trial of hemodialysis versus intermittent peritoneal dialysis for patients with advanced renal disease. The results of the trial were obsolete before it was completed, because the continuous form of peritoneal dialysis had replaced the intermittent treatment.

29.6.4.2. COMPARISON OF MULTIPLE ALTERNATIVE AGENTS

A different type of problem arises when many alternative active agents are available for comparison with a particular new (or old) agent. Because the new agent cannot be compared against each of the many available alternatives, what agent(s) should the investigator choose for the comparison?

This type of difficulty regularly places the investigator in a no-win situation. No matter which agents (or combinations of agents) are selected for comparison in the trial, someone will complain that other choices would have been better. Furthermore, if the investigator decides to use a placebo, which is the only standard agent of comparison, the results may be acceptable to a regulatory agency, but the trial may be denounced as undesirable (or possibly unethical) by patients and their physicians.

29.6.4.3. MINOR VARIATIONS IN ESTABLISHED AGENTS

A quite different problem arises if regulatory agencies or other societal groups insist on having randomized clinical trials as evidence of efficacy when minor variations are produced in the physical formulation of an established therapeutic agent. Can society afford to use precious resources of time, effort, and money for conducting randomized clinical trials of these minor variations? For example, are randomized clinical trials necessary to demonstrate that a chemically similar but physically different form of a particular drug has the same clinical effects as the original product, or can we be satisfied with suitable laboratory evidence and pharmacologic demonstrations of bioavailability? Are randomized trials needed to compare long-acting versus short-acting aspirin, or company A's aspirin versus company B's aspirin, or one brand of cephalosporin versus another, or type X versus type Y surgical sutures?

To save the diversion of research funds that might be better used for more creative purposes, and to spare society the costs of expensive trials devoted to minor issues, can acceptable answers to these questions be obtained with other forms of suitable research?

29.6.5. *The Problem of Inevitable Controversies*

In all the circumstances just cited, the limitations of randomized trials become apparent as soon as we consider the question that is proposed and the architectural arrangement needed to find the answer. The most vexing difficulties of all, however, occur when an important question having an obtainable answer gets caught in the fastidious/pragmatic conflict discussed throughout Section 29.2. In this circumstance, a randomized trial may be ethical, possible, feasible, and valuable, but its results will inevitably create major controversy because the trial cannot be designed and analyzed in a way that will satisfy proponents of the opposing policies.

Because a single trial can seldom simultaneously placate both the fastidious and pragmatic viewpoints, the desired answer to the research question may require several trials, each designed and analyzed according to the different policies employed for approaching the pertinent issues. Because even a single trial may be extremely costly for certain topics, an unacceptable burden may be placed on resources allocated for research if several trials must be done to obtain a noncontroversial mosaic of results. On the other hand, the expense may also be uncomfortable or unacceptable if only a single trial is conducted, and if the fastidious/pragmatic conflict inevitably makes the results produce confusion and controversy rather than clarification.

29.6.6. *The Role of Randomized Trials in Basic Clinical Science*

The diverse limitations that have just been cited do not in any way affect the status of randomized trials as the methodologic gold standard in scientific comparison. The stature of William Osler is unaffected if we point out that he was not a competent statistician, and Ronald Fisher's achievements are not demeaned by his failure to become a board-certified internist. The limitations do indicate, however, that randomized trials often cannot be used as a practical research structure for answering all the questions that arise as basic issues in scientific clinical medicine. Furthermore, just as a surgeon's activities inside the operating room are ultimately more important than his immaculate washing of hands before he enters, the crucial scientific issues depend on what is asked and how it is answered in the basic architecture of the research, not on the particular mechanism used to allocate the compared maneuvers.

If we want to find credible answers to important fundamental questions in clinical science, we shall often have to use research structures other than randomized trials. For this reason, the main discussions in this text have emphasized the architectural components of scientific comparison, and the principles that make the results acceptable as scientific evidence. When randomized trials can be done, they are obviously desirable because the scientific demands are easier to fulfill than with other research structures. The rigidity of a randomized trial protocol or a policy choice in the pragmatic/fastidious conflict, however, may sometimes alter the architectural components that were most desired for the trial. The results may then be satisfactory statistically but unsatisfactory as clinical science. Alternatively, when randomized trials are not or cannot be done, the desired architectural components can be chosen without inhibition, but the scientific demands for accurate data and unbiased comparison may be difficult to fulfill. The results may then be satisfactory clinically but unsatisfactory as statistical science.

Perhaps the most important ultimate role of randomized trials in basic clinical science is as intellectual models rather than as practical structures. By using the randomized trial as an architectural model for planning and analyzing both experimental and nonexperimental research, we can improve the scientific quality of observational studies while expanding the nonexperimental application of basic experimental principles. The approaches that can be used for these activities have been discussed throughout this book, and further details have been presented in a recent set of essays[132] on "An Additional Basic Science for Clinical Medicine."

29.7. **SYNOPSIS**

The Book of Daniel in the Bible describes a controlled trial of diets, and therapeutic agents were compared for many centuries thereafter, but the idea of quantitative documentation for concurrent comparisons did not take firm hold until the 20th century; and the allocation of treatment by statistically designed randomization was not proposed until 1923. With the frequent use of placebo agents for comparison and double-blind methods for observation, and with the incentives provided by the thalidomide disaster in the early 1960s, the randomized controlled trial became established as the modern experimental gold standard for evaluating therapeutic agents.

Although extraordinarily successful for demonstrating the remedial effects of pharmaceutical and other agents in altering or removing an existing target, randomized trials have not always been successful in clarifying issues in prophylactic therapy, which is intended to prevent the primary development of a disease or to thwart the secondary adverse effects of an existing disease. Problems in prophylactic trials have often been inevitable because of an irreconcilable conflict in two opposing policies for the design and analysis of a trial. In the pragmatic policy, a trial is intended to answer direct questions about the use of treatment in clinical practice. The answers should be immediately pertinent for the heterogeneous "messiness" of clinical practice, even if the answers are sometimes "messy." In the fastidious policy, a trial is intended to satisfy rigorous scientific standards for explaining therapeutic mechanisms and for avoiding biased comparisons. The main goal is to obtain scientifically "clean" results, even if the answers are not always cogent for practitioners' questions.

Both sets of policies are reasonable, justifiable, and defensible, but they often lead to conflicting choices in every aspect of architecture used for planning the components of a trial and for analyzing the results. Consequently, a trial that was conducted and interpreted with one set of policies will often be unsatisfactory or unacceptable to the other set of viewpoints. Until the opposing features of these viewpoints are mediated into compromises that can satisfy both sides, major controversies will continue to occur as a distressing sequel of devoted efforts and enormous expense.

Successful randomized trials have made many contributions to clinical science and to effective knowledge about therapy, but the trials have also led to many other important problems. An ethical conflict often occurs between the societal need for comparing therapeutic effectiveness and the clinician's samaritan obligations to individual patients. The filtration process that precedes admission to a trial may impair its conduct because of difficulties in enrolling enough patients; and the patients who are admitted may not suitably represent the external population to which the results are to be generalized. The need for double-blind procedures may produce undesirable modifications in the research architecture; the process is not always checked for the effectiveness of the blinding; and the reliance on blinding may inhibit the development of improved clinimetric indexes. The attempt to replace randomization with historical controls may lead to comparisons that are distorted by susceptibility bias in baseline states and, more importantly, by differences in the ancillary supportive treatment used in the two eras under contrast.

Multi-institutional collaborations are often necessary to obtain adequate numbers of patients; and the cooperative trials require special efforts to coordinate the protocol, to standardize variability among the institutions, and to satisfy the diverse goals and gratifications of the participating investigators. Although the pooling of results is a basic principle in cooperative studies, no generally accepted principles have been developed for the standards under which results can be pooled, outside the cooperative study framework, for heterogeneous patients, treatments, and protocols.

Randomized clinical trials have been effectively applied in several unconventional situations. Therapy has sometimes been evaluated by stopping rather than starting treatment; etiologic (rather than therapeutic) agents have sometimes been tested, particularly for dietary pathogens; and the investigated agents have included screening procedures, diagnostic tests, and the purveyant action of clinical or other medical personnel in delivering clinical services or educational programs.

Despite their many splendid accomplishments, randomized trials have the practical limitation of not being applicable for many important questions in clinical science. Randomized trials cannot be used successfully to investigate the etiologic role of many suspected noxious agents, to determine adverse therapeutic reactions that occur too long or too rarely after treatment, or to evaluate diagnostic agents used in circumstances in which the patient's outcome is delayed and preceded by diverse therapeutic interventions. The continuing proliferation of new technologic agents makes the trials unappealing if the compared agents may be obsolete before the trial is completed, if the comparative agent must be chosen from many available active candidates, or if the expensive effort of a trial is demanded to test minor new variations in existing old agents. Even when a randomized trial is feasible and desirable, its results may be inevitably controversial because the trial could not be designed and analyzed in a way that would satisfy both the pragmatic and fastidious viewpoints. For all these reasons, nonexperimental research will continue to be a basic necessity in clinical science, and an additional prime scientific contribution of randomized trials will be their role not as a practical research structure, but as an architectural model for improving the scientific quality of observational studies.

EXERCISES

This chapter contains many opportunities for readers and instructors to evaluate individual randomized trials, to consider trials that have produced conflicting results in studies of the same relationship, and to debate the merits of certain trials (such as the UGDP, sulfinpyrazone, and MRFIT studies) that have evoked major public controversies. Beyond these individual opportunities, the following exercises can be useful.

Exercise 29.1. Find a report of a randomized trial concerned with *remedial* therapy. Using the classification of policy options presented throughout Section 29.2, please identify and comment on the options used for each issue in that trial. Do you agree with what was done?

Exercise 29.2. Find a report of a randomized trial concerned with *prophylactic* (primary or secondary prevention) therapy and do the same things requested in Exercise 29.1.

Exercise 29.3. The Hypertension Detection and Follow-up Program (HDFP)[133] was a community-based, nonblinded, randomized controlled trial designed to compare the effects of two programs on 5-year mortality in patients with hypertension. The active program was systematic antihypertensive treatment, given by the investigative team in a pattern called Stepped Care, which consisted of a free program, in special HDFP centers, in which medication was increased stepwise according to a standard protocol to achieve the desired diastolic blood pressure. The control program, designated as Referred Care, consisted of whatever treatment the patients received from their customary sources of care in the community.

To recruit participants for the trial, community surveys encouraged people aged 30 to 69 years to report for sequential blood pressure measurements. Persons with mean diastolic blood pressures of ≥ 90 mm. Hg were invited to enter the trial and participants were randomized to receive either Referred Care or Stepped Care. Referred Care participants were seen once a year to measure blood pressure and to obtain interval medical histories. Stepped Care patients were seen at least every 4 months for blood pressure checks and for evaluation and management of risk factors such as overweight, increased cholesterol, and smoking.

After 5 years of follow-up, mortality from all causes was significantly lower in the total Stepped Care group than in the Referred Care group. This outcome was particularly distinct for patients who had mild hypertension (diastolic BP 90 to 104) on admission to the trial. Preliminary analysis of the data also suggests a lower cause-specific mortality (for cardiovascular deaths and for noncardiovascular deaths) for the Stepped Care group.

Please answer the following questions:

29.3.1. What aspects of the design of this trial may complicate the interpretation of morbidity data and the cause-specific mortality data?

29.3.2. How could the protocol be changed to avoid these problems?

Exercise 29.4. During 1972 to 1977, a randomized, controlled clinical trial[134] was done to determine whether vigorous antacid therapy would prevent the development of acute gastrointestinal bleeding in 100 critically ill patients hospitalized in a respiratory-surgical intensive care unit. The actively treated patients received antacids, through a specially placed nasogastric tube, to maintain gastric pH above 3.5. The control group also had a nasogastric tube inserted, but no antacid was given, and the tube was connected to intermittent suction. All patients received a stool guaiac test daily to monitor gastrointestinal bleeding. The results of the study were as follows:

Treatment Group	Development of G.I. Bleeding	No Bleeding	Total
Antacids	2	49	51
No antacids	12	37	49
Total	14	86	100

Because the attack rates for GI bleeding were 4% in the antacid group and 25% in the control group, with $X^2 = 8.8$ and $P<0.005$, the investigators concluded that antacids reduce the occurrence of gastrointestinal bleeding among critically ill patients. Please answer the following questions:

29.4.1. What problems do you perceive in the compared maneuvers? How do these problems affect your interpretation of the results?

29.4.2. What alternative design would you propose to avoid the problems, if any, that you noted in 29.4.1?

29.4.3. From the information provided, do you perceive any other problems in the design or analysis of this study?

CHAPTER REFERENCES

1. Gaddum, 1954; 2. Green, 1954; 3. Bull, 1959; 4. Lilienfeld, 1982; 5. Book of Daniel; 6. Louis, 1836; 7. Holmes, 1860; 8. Lind, 1753; 9. Bartlett, 1844; 10. Fibiger, 1898; 11. Finland, 1930; 12. Therapeutic Trials Committee, 1934; 13. Wycoff, 1930; 14. Fisher, 1923; 15. Box, 1980; 16. Amberson, 1931; 17. Diehl, 1938; 18. Hinshaw, 1944; 19. Medical Research Council, 1948; 20. Streptomycin Committee, 1947; 21. Francis, 1957; 22. Underwood, 1951; 23. Reid, 1954; 24. Lasagna, 1955; 25. Dodds, 1958; 26. Greenberg, 1959; 27. Waife, 1959; 28. D'Arcy, 1960; 29. Hill, 1960; 29. Mainland, 1960; 31. Cox, 1968; 32. Harris, 1970; 33. Good, 1976; 34. Johnson, 1977; 35. Peto, 1978; 36. Schwartz, 1980; 37. Friedman, 1981; 38. Friedewald, 1982; 39. Tygstrup, 1982; 40. Bulpitt, 1983; 41. Shapiro, 1983; 42. Controlled Clinical Trials (Journal); 43. Rimm, 1978; 44. Chalmers, 1977; 45. Department of Clinical Epidemiology, 1981; 46. Spodick, 1980; 47. Hill, 1966; 48. Modell, 1958; 49. Schwartz, 1967; 50. Sackett, 1979; 51. Byar, 1976; 52. Peto, 1976–1977; 53. May, 1981; 54. University Group Diabetes Program, 1970; 55. University Group Diabetes Program, 1971a; 56. University Group Diabetes Program, 1971b; 57. University Group Diabetes Program, 1975; 58.

Cornfield, 1971; 59. Schwartz, 1971; 60. Feinstein, 1971; 61. Schor, 1971; 62. Schor, 1973; 63. O'Sullivan, 1975; 64. Report of the Committee, 1975; 65. Feinstein, 1976a; 66. Feinstein, 1976b; 67. Kilata, 1979; 68. Feinstein, 1967; 69. Feinstein, 1972; 70. Lasagna, 1962; 71. Barsky, 1983; 72. Grizzle, 1965; 73. Hills, 1979; 74. Brown, 1980; 75. McPherson, 1982; 76. Pocock, 1978; 77. Freedman, 1983; 78. Armitage, 1975; 79. Anturane, 1978; 80. Anturane, 1980; 81. in Temple, 1980; 82. Anturane Reinfarction Trial Policy Committee, 1982; 83. Anturane Reinfarction Italian Study, 1982; 84. Shapiro, 1982; 85. Oliver, 1978; 86. Gavrin, 1964; 87. MRFIT, 1982; 88. Stallones, 1983; 89. Coronary Drug Project, 1973; 90. Coronary Drug Project Research Group, 1980; 91. VA Cooperative Study Group on Antihypertensive Agents, 1970; 91a. Feinstein, 1983; 92. Seef, 1978; 93. Szmuness, 1980; 94. Hill, 1963; 95. Feinstein, 1974; 96. Burkhardt, 1978; 97. Levine, 1979; 98. Howard, 1981; 99. Brewin, 1982; 100. Jonsen, 1982; 101. Anonymous, 1981; 102. Hampton, 1981; 103. Howard, 1982; 104. Gehan, 1974; 105. Feinstein, 1977; 106. Feinstein, 1984; 107. Gorringe, 1970; 108. Ramshaw, 1973; 109. Chan, 1981; 110. Meinert, 1981; 111. Cancer Research Campaign Working Party, 1980; 112. Sullivan, 1981; 113. Inter-society Commission for Heart Disease Resources, 1970; 114. Chalmers, 1977; 115. Stampfer, 1982; 116. Baum, 1981; 117. Messer, 1983; 118. Elashoff, 1978; 119. Goldman, 1979; 120. Feinstein, 1966; 121. Rimland, 1978; 122. Jakobsson, 1978; 123. Hardcastle, 1983; 124. Olsen, 1976; 125. Southeast London Screening Study Group, 1977; 126. Dales, 1979; 127. Bircher, 1971; 128. Varner, 1983; 129. Buxton, 1979; 130. Spitzer, 1974; 131. Joyce, 1965; 132. Feinstein, 1983; 133. Hypertension Detection and Follow-up Program, 1979; 134. Hastings, 1978.

Chapter 30

Other Epidemiologic Topics

When John R. Paul (1893–1971) introduced *clinical epidemiology*[1-3] as a name for the "application of a new philosophy to old diseases," he wanted to expand both the methods and topics of epidemiology.

In methods, Paul advocated homodemic research, based on careful studies of individual people, rather than heterodemic investigations, which he called "statistical epidemiology." In the statistical approach, epidemiology was defined as a heterodemic activity. It consisted of "the study of diseases as a mass phenomenon. . . . The unit of observation is a group, not an individual."[4] Paul wanted to escape from this methodologic boundary. He stated that

> . . . the role of the clinical epidemiologist is like that of a detective visiting the scene of the crime. He starts with the examination of a sick individual and cautiously branches out into the setting where that individual became ill and where the patient may also become ill again. In this respect the *clinical* epidemiologist stands in relation to the *statistical* epidemiologist perhaps as a physician does to a health officer. The statistician may validate his analyses by increasing the number of observations, whereas the clinician has the opportunity of improving the accuracy of a limited number of observations by intimate study and exacting measurements.[2]

In topics, Paul wanted to expand beyond another set of constraints: "the fallacies of the orthodox concepts that epidemiology is the study of epidemics and belongs wholly in the public health field."[2] Paul believed that "epidemiology is concerned with the ecology of disease and deals, therefore, with the general circumstances under which people get sick—an approach which may involve a great variety of factors: immunologic, toxicologic, social, climatic, even political or religious."[2] The topics for which Paul wanted to open the epidemiologic door had sometimes "been presented by others as examples of *social medicine, community medicine, population pathology,* and *social pathology*" and also as "*geographical medicine* or *geographical pathology.*"[3] To illustrate the scope of these ecologic topics, Paul cited the examples of Henry Sigerist's contention[5] "that medicine is a social science," John Ryle's emphasis[6] on "environmental, domestic, occupational, economic, habitual, and nutritional factors" in human illness, and James Spence's concern[7] that "the full picture of disease" will require clinical investigators "to carry observations beyond hospitals."

Paul's original proposal for this expansion of epidemiologic research was first delivered in 1938 as his Presidential Address to the American Society for Clinical Investigation.[1] His clinical investigative colleagues at that time, however, were unpersuaded. They were moving their research inward, toward the pathophysiology and molecular biology of disease, rather than outward, toward ecology and environmental factors. Not until 34 years later, in 1972, did *clinical epidemiology* become a specified title for research presented at the Society's annual meeting.[8]

In the meantime, however, the broadened scope that Paul wanted as a *clinical* expansion of epidemiology was achieved by investigators who were based in nonclinical departments (having such names as *epidemiology, hygiene, public health,* and *community medicine*) and who gave their work titles different from what Paul had suggested. His methodologic distinction between the homodemic *clinical* study of individuals and the heterodemic *statistical* study of group data became cited with the respective terms "shoe-leather" and "armchair" epidemiology. His methodologic goal of "intimate study and exacting measurements" became realized as epidemiologists turned increasingly from heterodemic investigations to the homodemic research structures of randomized trials, observational cohorts, cross-sectional surveys, case-control studies, and detective work with one or several cases.

Despite the pertinence of Paul's *clinical/statistical* distinctions, they were too nonspecific to provide precise labels for the many different topics into which epidemiologic research evolved. With the same type of disease-oriented taxonomy used in clinical investigation, epidemiologic investigators began to demarcate their research topics as *infectious* or *chronic disease*. (Yet another disease-oriented partition today is reflected in the progressive development of *genetic epidemiology*.) Later on, with increased attention to the many etiologic factors that Paul had described, specialized foci of research were given such names as *occupational, environmental,* and *social epidemiology*.

Because these topics had not received the *clinical* title that Paul envisioned, the word was left available as a name for the new form of *clinical epidemiology* that I proposed[9-11] in 1968, as the study of groups of patients to evaluate the diagnostic, prognostic, and therapeutic decisions made in patient care. I do not know what Paul, if alive today, would think about the altered modern contents of *clinical epidemiology,* but I am sure he would be pleased that it now receives what he sought as "recognition and study by university departments of clinical medicine";[2] and he would doubtlessly be delighted that the "child" he christened at the American Society for Clinical Investigation is reborn, well, and thriving at the Society's annual meetings.

The new form of clinical epidemiology, together with some of its ramifications in other aspects of epidemiology, has been emphasized throughout this book. This last chapter, therefore, is intended to acknowledge some of the many other topics that John Paul might have regarded as *clinical epidemiology* but that today are given other names. I shall briefly outline the contents of these additional forms of epidemiology, note some of their main scientific challenges and problems, and cite a few references where interested readers can look for further details.

30.1. DETECTIVE-WORK EPIDEMIOLOGY

The view of epidemiologists as "disease detectives" was also proposed by Paul when he described the research function of "visiting the scene of the crime." He presented a series of epidemiologic case reports[2] in which good detective work helped reveal the cause of small-scale outbreaks or individual episodes of trichinosis, tuberculosis, rheumatic fever, poliomyelitis, psittacosis, and carbon tetrachloride hepatotoxicity.

The type of detective work described by Paul in 1958 was already becoming well known to the public, through the efforts of a nonscientist writer, Berton Roueché. In 1947, under the title *Annals of Medicine* in The New Yorker magazine, Roueché began writing a series of articles about epidemiologic (and other medical) exploits in tracking down diverse etiologic culprits. Roueché's stories continued over many years and have now been collected in several books, of which the latest is called *The Medical Detectives*.[12] The stories, which can be read as a fascinating informal textbook of medicine, contain accounts of the presentation and eventual etiologic solution of diverse medical detective problems. Some of the problems were infectious diseases, often transmitted by unusual mechanisms, such as anthrax, hepatitis, histoplasmosis, pseudomonas, rabies, salmonellosis, schistosomiasis, rickettsial pox, tetanus, trichinosis, tularemia, and typhoid fever. Other problems were poisonings, toxicities, or skin reactions caused by botulism, carbon tetrachloride, carotenes and lycopenes, clothing dye, metallic copper, jimson weed, organic mercury, organic phosphate, salicylate, and sodium nitrite. Roueché has also dramatically described some of the diagnostic puzzles that were met in instances of mass hysteria in schoolchildren, hypogeusia, labyrinthitis, and Wilson's disease.

Probably the most outstanding recent example of detective work in Paul-style clinical epidemiology occurred when a group of academic-based rheumatologists and epidemiologists at Yale, after being alerted by a physician in the Connecticut State Health Department, began with the examination of several sick patients and then branched out into the setting in which the patients had become ill. The research led to the identification of Lyme arthritis as a "new" ailment, to the extension of its clinical spectrum as Lyme disease, to effective therapy with antibiotics, and to the eventual demonstration of a spirochete as the etiologic agent.[13]

30.2. INFECTIOUS DISEASE EPIDEMIOLOGY

Because epidemiology started to become a scientific discipline about a century ago, and because the outbreaks of that era were usually infectious diseases, modern epidemiology began with studies of infectious disease in the community. Some of the most dramatic accomplishments of epidemiologic research a century ago—including Snow's work with cholera and the development of effective sanitation for water and sewage—and some of the most striking modern successes—including the unraveling of etiologic mechanisms that led to a poliomyelitis vaccine and the detection and vaccination process that recently eradicated smallpox—are all rooted in public health concerns with infectious disease. Probably the most dramatic episode of public health detective work in epidemiology was the pursuit of the last known person with smallpox and the vaccination activities that halted its further spread.[14] The story is unique in citing the name of the person with the *last* case of one of the world's major diseases.

From a public health base in the community, infectious disease epidemiology was brought to a clinical location when Ignaz Semmelweis in the 19th century studied puerperal sepsis in hospitalized patients. Although the work was not yet recognized as infectious disease, microbial organisms were the thwarted etiologic agents when Semmelweis[15] identified the iatrogenic carriers and (eventually) persuaded doctors to prevent the disease by washing their hands. This research gave Semmelweis two pioneering roles in epidemiology. He can be regarded as the founder of the hospital-based infectious disease activity that is now called *nosocomial epidemiology*. Together with Pierre Louis,[16] who studied therapy rather than transmission of disease in hospitalized patients, Semmelweis also helped create the *clinical epidemiology* discussed in the preceding chapters of this book.

The outstanding sources of information today about the bacterial and viral domains of infectious disease epidemiology are two textbooks edited by Evans[17] and by Evans and Feldman.[18] The books contain a bounty of well-organized and well-presented information about historical background, methodologic principles, and analytic techniques in the general field of infectious disease as well as specific discussions of the epidemiology of individual infections.

The investigation of outbreaks of food poisoning, hepatitis, Legionnaire's disease, and other acute illnesses has been a prime activity (in the U.S.) of the Centers for Disease Control, and the work has helped enhance the image of epidemiologists as disease detectives.[19] Although *ad hoc* outbreaks evoke remedial action to determine immediate etiology, an ongoing prophylactic activity for the CDC is the surveillance of infectious disease.[20] From the data obtained with four different systems of disease surveillance, epidemiologists can determine the status of diverse infectious diseases and can develop special efforts for disease control and prevention.

Although most surveillance procedures involve efforts to learn about clinically overt morbidity and mortality, a special type of community surveillance with homodemic research is called *seroepidemiology*. Through laboratory examination of blood components indicative of past or current infection, serologic surveys in a community can cover the lanthanic as well as the overt part of a disease spectrum and can thereby discern total infection rates rather than rates for clinically apparent infections alone. Two other major advantages of seroepidemiology are the detection of community responses to a vaccination campaign, and the development of banks in which sera are stored for later testing that can reveal important secular trends or new infectious agents.

30.2.1. *Infectious/Chronic Distinctions*

Although every other branch of science has been suitably labeled to denote the specialized domains created by modern progress (e.g., inorganic chemistry, organic chemistry, physical chemistry, biochemistry, etc.), epidemiologists are sometimes distressed by analogous developments in the nomenclature of epidemiology. The distress is often stated in objections to the separation of epidemiology into the specialties of infectious disease and chronic disease.[21]

Because epidemiology can be classified in one way according to methodologic strategies and in another way according to topical contents, the infectious/chronic distinction can be lamented for both reasons. Methodologically, the argument is that methods that worked well in infectious disease could be successfully applied to chronic disease[21] and that both domains use similar research structures involving cohorts, ecologic cross-sections, case-control studies, and heterodemic associations. Topically, the argument is that the contents of the two domains are often difficult to separate. Like chronic diseases, many infectious diseases have long latent intervals, are not transmitted from person to person, have multiple contributory causes, and involve characteristics of personal behavior.[21]

Despite the shared research structures and etiologic concepts, however, epidemiologic investigations of infectious and noninfectious disease have profound differences in the scientific quality of the basic raw data. Infectious disease researchers have had the good scientific fortune to work with ailments in which the disease itself and the main etiologic agent are often both identified with the same relatively simple laboratory test. For noninfectious ailments, however, two different types of information are required. The suspected etiologic agent (smoking, diet, occupation, etc.) is identified with one set of data; the disease (cancer, infarction, stones, etc.) is identified with a different set of data; and both sets of data are often difficult to obtain, verify, and standardize. By contrast, an appropriate measurement of a blood component or microbial culture can often be used to demonstrate both the existence and the etiologic agent of an infectious disease.

This concomitance of a relatively simple identification for both maneuver and outcome creates three major scientific advantages for the basic raw data of infectious disease research. The investigators can concentrate on attaining high quality in a reduced scope of data; the measurement process can be carried out in a single laboratory and can be given an accuracy and consistency that is impossible to achieve for the diverse sources and types of information needed in noninfectious disease; and the specimens of blood (or cultures) that are measured are usually much easier to obtain than x-ray films, tissues, electrographic tracings, detailed archival data, and extensive interviews.

An additional scientific advantage for infectious disease has come from seroepidemiologic surveys showing that each disease has a large lanthanic or subclinical spectrum. This realization has helped the investigators avoid the problems of detection bias that arise when an analogous spectral distribution is not adequately recognized for noninfectious diseases. These modern scientific advantages, however, cannot always prevent problems when concepts of infectious disease are applied in the retrospective interpretation of past events, in the investigation of current ailments, and in the prediction of future epidemics.

30.2.2. *Historical Identification of Infectious Disease*

In past events, many scholars have written about the scientific history of individual infectious diseases and also about the impact of infectious diseases on political, military, and other aspects of human history. The main scientific difficulty in these historical accounts is uncertainty about whether the diseases of long ago were the same entities that receive those names today. In the absence of microscopic or serologic evidence, how many of the ancient episodes of malaria, typhoid fever, and other infectious diseases would be given those same diagnoses today?

An excellent illustration of the problems is provided by tuberculosis. For many centuries, the term *consumption* was used for an ailment clinically characterized by anorexia and weight loss, often associated with fever, dyspnea, and hemoptysis. With the advent of frequent necropsy in the 19th century, the lungs of people with consumption were often found to have the histologic abnormality of *tubercles*. After the tubercle bacillus was identified in many of these lesions, evidence of the bacillus (and also of appropriate roentgenographic abnormalities) became required for a clinical diagnosis of *pulmonary tuberculosis*. In the era before routine microbial cultures and x-rays, however, the clinical diagnosis of tuberculosis depended mainly on symptoms and auscultatory patterns of rales. With these symptoms and physical signs as the sole diagnostic requirement, the label of *tuberculosis* could easily have been given to many entities that today would be identified more precisely as primary pulmonary cancer, metastatic pulmonary cancer, noninfectious pulmonary disease, or even pneumonia.[10]

Similar problems occur in evaluating the many plagues of past history. Were they really due to plague bacilli or were they similar to some of the severe viral epidemics encountered today? For example, in a dramatic modern recollection of patients and events in the influenza epidemic of 1918, Isaac Starr[22] described the high case-fatality rate and the intense cyanosis that led to the contemporary rumor that the "black death" of plague had returned. Without modern diagnostic and therapeutic methods, we have no way of knowing how many old epidemics of "plague" might have been outbreaks of influenza.

30.2.3. *Modern Problems in Infectious Etiology and Prediction*

In the investigation of current ailments, research methods that rely on a concomitant demonstration of infectious agent and disease may get into difficulty if the ailment is a syndrome (rather than a disease) produced by either a toxin or by an as-yet-unidentified microbial organism. For example, the etiologic riddle of Legionnaire's disease was eventually solved when suitable culture media were used to grow and demonstrate the infectious organism. In the syndrome of rheumatic fever, however, the ubiquitous etiologic role of the group A streptococcus was not accepted for many years until the organism, which often escaped growth on culture media, could be demonstrated with newly developed antibody measurements. In Stevens-Johnson syndrome, for which an infectious organism has still not been demonstrated, inappropriate investigations and an error in protopathic bias led to a false accusation of a causal role for a then-new antibiotic agent.[23] Analogous problems may exist today[24] in causal indictments that have been proposed for aspirin in Reye's syndrome and for tampons in toxic shock syndrome.

In the prediction of future epidemics, infectious disease scientists have ruefully discovered that prognostication can be as difficult in public health as in clinical medicine. Less than a decade ago, a distinguished group of epidemiologists concluded that the probability of an epidemic of swine flu influenza was high enough to warrant massive public health efforts in vaccination. When the expected epidemic did not occur, the attendant political fall-out was unpleasant, but a worse set of problems arose when the prophylactic vaccine was associated with many adverse reactions and a few deaths.[25, 26]

30.3. NOSOCOMIAL EPIDEMIOLOGY

The old saying that hospitals can be dangerous places for sick people is supported by the modern development and need for nosocomial epidemiology.[27, 28] Most large hospitals in the U.S. now contain special teams[29] whose job is to prevent or control the infections transmitted intra-institutionally. In the most recently published survey data,[30, 31] about 5% to 10% of patients admitted to acute care hospitals will develop nosocomially related infections, of which about 40% are in the urinary tract and about 20% are in the lungs or bloodstream.

Nosocomial infections have been provoked by almost every inanimate or human object that enters or remains in a hospital.[32] The inanimate items have been the equipment used in hospital rooms (air conditioners, bedding, furniture, flower vases, sinks, and bathtubs), in personal care (shaving brushes, urinals), in minor technology (stethoscopes, sphygmomanometers), and in major technology (x-ray cassettes, respiratory apparatus, prostheses, dialysis machines). Contamination has also occurred within the hand creams, ingested food, and injected fluids used in therapy; and infections have been facilitated by indwelling catheters placed in bladders, veins, and arteries. Perhaps the greatest treacheries have been bacterial contamination of the agents used in cleansing: floor mops and antiseptic or disinfectant solutions.

The human sources of infection include patients' visitors and patients themselves, particularly when transferred from nursing homes. In an irony that Semmelweis probably would have savored, however, the greatest human sources of intrahospital infectious transmission today are the members of the hospital staff: doctors, nurses, and technicians.[33, 34] The decline of conscientious cleansing by hospital staff is probably attributable, paradoxically, to the antibiotics that have brought so many clinical triumphs in the treatment of infectious disease. As many infections became conquered by antibiotics, the special precautions formerly used by hospital personnel seemed to become unnecessary. Masks, gowns, gloves, and isolation procedures gradually disappeared from the standard routines of hospital practice, and other sanitary precautions also became less frequent. To confirm the old maxim of *plus ça change, plus c'est la même chose,* hospital staff members today are being once again entreated, a century after Semmelweis, to wash their hands more often and more carefully.

The most interesting methodologic challenges for nosocomial epidemiologists are the problems of getting hospital staff to comply with appropriate precautions, choosing suitable models in statistical analysis,[35] evaluating cost/benefit ratios for different strategies in controlling infections,[36] and coping with the false accusations that occur as pseudoepidemics produced by laboratory errors or by artefactual clustering of infections.[37]

Although infectious diseases are currently the main focus of nosocomial epidemiology, not all of the ailments produced in hospitals have infectious origins. Many ailments can arise as complications of devices used in diagnosis or therapy, as fears or anxieties produced during miscommunication, and as adverse reactions to drugs. Because these events can also occur outside hospitals, they are often called *iatrogenic* rather than *nosocomial.* A special new form of epidemiologic research[37a] has been developed for the collection and analysis of group data in studying adverse drug reactions.

30.4. NUTRITIONAL EPIDEMIOLOGY

From a traditional public health base in community locations, epidemiology has expanded its etiologic topics to include noninfectious causes of disease. Probably the most dramatic early event in this expansion was a heroic set of investigations in which Joseph Goldberger,[38] ignoring entrenched beliefs about an infectious etiology and working with substantial opposition from leaders of the "establishment," demonstrated that pellagra was due to a dietary deficiency.

Although James Lind[39] almost two centuries earlier had shown that nutritional inadequacy could cause scurvy, Lind's work and the principle it should have taught had been forgotten. Goldberger's discovery helped initiate better clinical attention to nutrition and eventually led to the modern era of vitamin supplementation. His demonstration of a nutritional etiology in disease also helped set the stage for the modern era of epidemiologic concern for dietary risk factors.

Despite the frequency with which these risk factors are studied today, however, nutritional epidemiology is seldom regarded as a separate specialty. It is usually subsumed as part of chronic disease epidemiology or within the social epidemiology described in the next section. The most pressing scientific problem in nutritional epidemiology is the difficulty of obtaining accurate data about nutritional intake.

30.5. SOCIAL EPIDEMIOLOGY

The role of social factors in disease has been a concern of epidemiologists ever since statistical data were first collected and made available to relate deaths to occupation, education, and social class. Because the investigations usually depended on heterodemic data, however, a prime contribution of Paul, Ryle, Spence, and other social-minded clinical epidemiologists was to urge and institute research that was directly homodemic.

In more modern times, the outstanding advocate of scientific homodemic research in social epidemiology has been the late John Cassel.[40-42] Having been an active medical practitioner before he became a professor, Cassel brought an intimate knowledge of sick people to the research, and—together with such epidemiologic colleagues as Graham,[43] Syme,[44] and Tyroler[45]—he helped produce a strong foundation for scientific research in social epidemiology. Interested readers can learn more about this field by reviewing the references just cited, other publications by Cobb,[46] Kasl,[47, 48] and Berkman,[49] and the books by Freeman, Levine, and Reeder[50] and by Eisenberg and Kleinman.[51]

Social epidemiologists focus on a variety of factors that have long been regarded as the basic staples of demography: age, gender, race, ethnicity, education, housing, smoking and drinking habits, physical activity, and socioeconomic status. In recent years, however, the traditional demographic variables have been expanded to include factors that are more specifically cultural and behavioral. Among these factors are household composition, family structure and function, social networks and bonds, social support systems, health practices, and use of health services. Certain behavioral variables, which are also part of a growing domain called *psychiatric epidemiology,* include cognitive function, personality traits,[52, 53] and the effects of special life events such as relocation, changes in employment, retirement, and bereavement. Although the direct effects of industrial agents are usually studied in occupational epidemiology (as noted in the next section), social epidemiologists are often concerned with work-induced personal stress.

The cultural and behavioral variables of social epidemiology have two unique distinctions that give the investigators a particularly difficult scientific job. The first distinction is that the variables refer to intangible entities, such as a social network or personality pattern, rather than more tangible phenomena, such as cigarettes, food, or severity of pain. Because of this problem, the investigators trying to measure a social factor must often justify not merely the structure of the scale of measurement but also the basic validity of the measurement process. In other types of epidemiology, we may have trouble obtaining accurate measurements of cigarette smoking, food intake, or severity of pain, but there are few disputes about what is meant by smoking, food, or pain. Considerable dissension may arise, however, about what is meant and who or what is to be included when social variables are created to measure a social network, a support system, or behavioral reactions.

The second difficult problem for social epidemiologists is that social factors may appear in all three major locations of the architectural structure for a cause-effect relationship. Social factors can identify baseline states, maneuvers, and outcome events. For example, when we do research to see whether a type A personality makes healthy people more or less likely to develop coronary disease, the type A personality is regarded as a maneuver. When we see whether coronary disease occurs more commonly in cigarette smokers than in nonsmokers, and when the results are stratified for people with type A and type B personalities, the social factor demarcates a baseline state. When we see whether group therapy, family support, or other interventions alter a person's behavior from type A to type B, the change in the social variable is an outcome event.

These three different architectural roles for social factors make the research particularly complicated. In other epidemiologic investigations, we can easily define the architectural role of such factors as cigarette smoking, antibiotic therapy, severity of illness, and relief of pain. The scales used to express those factors can then be easily chosen for their assigned location in the causal pathway. With social variables, however, a scale that is satisfactory for demarcating their role as maneuvers may not work well for their role in baseline states or in outcome events. A scale that works well for outcome events may not be suitable for describing the same factor's role as a maneuver or baseline state. Consequently, three different indexes or scales may be needed to describe the same social factor in its different architectural roles. Furthermore, unless the investigator is particularly careful about where the social factor appears in the architectural model, statistical analyses of covariance or other multivariate tactics may yield a confusing pastiche of baseline states, maneuvers, and outcomes.

In the cross-disciplinary interchange between clinical and social epidemiologists, clinicians do not often seek or receive some of the best quantitative tools of social science. These tools are the mathematical models developed by social scientists for analyzing multivariate data with targeted-cluster strategies rather than additive scores. Because the strategies are generally unknown to the biostatisticians who consult in the research, clinicians and nonsocial epidemiologists seldom become aware of the targeted-cluster procedures and may then spend a great deal of analytic effort in "re-inventing the wheel" and giving it new names, such as *recursive partitioning*.

Instead of learning these distinctive social science strengths in obtaining and analyzing data, clinical investigators may rely on social science consultants for help mainly in a different type of research challenge: the construction of clinimetric indexes and scales. Although quite suitable for preparing scales of attitudes or opinions, the sociometric approach may differ greatly from the strategy needed to describe overt clinical phenomena, such as pain or severity of illness. The resulting product may then be grossly unsuitable for qualitative sensibility in the clinical goals, despite all the statistical accolades offered in the quantitative appraisal of reliability and validity. An important challenge in future research by both clinical and social epidemiologists will be the development of an improved collaborative approach for the suitable measurement of clinimetric phenomena.

30.6. OCCUPATIONAL AND ENVIRONMENTAL EPIDEMIOLOGY

After establishment of the etiologic principle that disease could be caused by microbial contamination, the obvious next step was to expand the principle to include other types of contaminants—particularly the chemical agents produced in an increasingly technologic and industrialized society. Direct high-dose exposure to chemicals could readily be identified as sources of individual ailments in the "detective stories" described by Paul and by Roueché, but the effects of indirect and low-dose exposures have become a major problem in health and in scientific research. The effects on exposed industrial workers are explored in *occupational epidemiology*, and the community effects of polluted air, water, food, radiation, or other substances have led to the development of *environmental epidemiology*.

Both types of epidemiology are beset with many scientific, statistical, and political difficulties. The political problems are evident in the intense publicity that is given to almost any type of accusation, regardless of the accompanying evidence, and in the ideologic beliefs that often preclude a dispassionate evaluation of whatever evidence is available. The scientific problems arise because occupations and the environment have been generally neglected as a focus of careful scientific investigation during the past century. In the absence of a suitably extensive background in either laboratory or clinical research, these two forms of epidemiology do not have a strong basic foundation to provide rigorous scientific principles and investigative standards.

Because the era of computers readily allows etiologic vacuums to be filled with statistical data, a great deal of heterodemic information has been processed in search of adverse associations between diseases and either environmental agents or employment in different occupations. Heterodemic research has been particularly prominent in occupational epidemiology, as noted in Chapter 24.

A major statistical problem in this type of research is the difficulty of distinguishing between a real clue to a cause-effect relationship and a stochastic artefact of the computerized number crunching. With many occupations and many diseases recorded in huge amounts of data, an enormous number of positive associations can be expected to emerge by chance alone as the computer spews out its barrage of myriads of cross-tabulations, maps, or other quantitative displays. For example, a computerized search of data for as few as 50 occupations and 50 diseases can lead to 2500 associations that are examined for stochastic significance. At an α level of 0.05, about 125 of these associations can be expected to have a significance that arises spuriously as a random act of chance even if the occupations and diseases have no real relationships.

The examination of 2500 associations is actually much smaller than the numerical scope of some of the data-dredging expositions. Thus, in one typical study,[54] the investigators constructed 2×2 tables and determined odds ratios for the 5858 associations of 202 employment categories with 29 cancer sites. Although 293 ($= 0.05 \times 5858$) of these odds ratios could be stochastically significant by chance alone, the investigators added a series of stratifications that gave chance a greatly increased opportunity to act. Within each of the basic 5858 tables, odds ratios were further calculated for each of 768 cross-tabulations derived from two categories of gender, four categories of age, three categories of education, four categories of alcohol intake, and eight geographic locations. Within each occupation/disease association, therefore, an additional opportunity was given for chance alone to produce 38 ($= 0.05 \times 768$) odds ratios that could be significant solely by stochastic variation. In a tabulation reported by the investigators for one of these occupation/disease stratifications, only 26 odds ratios were marked as "P<0.05." Because α levels were not altered for the mammoth numbers of comparisons, the occurrence of only 26 positive relationships, instead of the 38 expected by chance alone, might be optimistically interpreted as showing that the cited occupation was highly protective for the cited cancer.

For investigators who want to avoid these heterodemic acts of statistical epidemiology, the problems of doing scientific homodemic research are formidable. With environmental agents, the assembly of a homodemic group is difficult because the exposure occurs heterodemically in the environment, and its direct magnitude may be impossible to measure in individual people. With occupational agents, problems of accuracy and bias can occur in each component of the cause-effect architecture for baseline states, principal occupational maneuvers, comparative maneuvers, and outcome events. In baseline state, the people employed in a particular occupation will be affected by criteria used in hiring, thus leading to the healthy worker effect described earlier and to the problems of finding suitable comparison groups. Although commonly used to contrive a simulated control group, a general population (for reasons cited earlier in the text) is not really suitable for this purpose; and no standard criteria have been developed for choosing comparison groups from workers in the same or other occupations. The proportions and scope of spectrum in occupational cohorts may be uncertain because of the vagaries of data and completeness in the employment records from which the cohorts are constructed.

In maneuvers, occupational exposure is usually difficult to demarcate because it is seldom accurately recorded in industrial archives. When exposure is ascertained in retrospect, the workers' recollections may be biased by the outcome events. For example, during the period of roughly 1950 to 1965, almost every elderly man admitted to a U.S. Veterans Administration Hospital with a diagnosis of chronic pulmonary disease said he had been "gassed" during World War I. The number of men retrospectively reporting this exposure to poison gas in Europe was probably more than the total number of U.S. troops actually sent there.

In detection of outcome events, many tricky problems have arisen as workers' health care benefits have increased. Because of better medical care and more extensive testing with modern diagnostic technology, a worker whose death years ago might have been ascribed to pneumonia is now identified as having cancer or a more precise pulmonary diagnosis. The occurrence rate of the neoplastic and chronic diseases may thus rise merely because of better detection, not because of more or new industrial exposure. Analogous problems in detection bias arise when the rates of diseases found during screening procedures in an industrial population are compared with the rates found in a general population, which did not receive screening. Although the same era of technologic advances that produced the new chemical substances has also produced the new diagnostic identifications, the phenomena have not yet been adequately disentangled to distinguish cause-effect relationships from those that are merely concomitant markers.

In collection of enumerated outcome events, transfer bias has been rampant in occupational epidemiology. In his thoughtful textbook, Monson[55] has given several excellent examples of transfer bias produced when outcome events in a group of selected coworkers were reported by other workers holding a distinct hypothesis about a particular exposure-disease relationship. The rates calculated in the selected group differed substantially from the rates found when the same outcome was sought in an unbiased cohort.

Because of the intense political, social, and economic conflicts that develop in the workplace and in the environment, and because these conflicts affect the diverse vested interests of management, labor, government, academia, and the public, it is not surprising that science is often the first casualty in the controversies. Although methods that might help reduce the magnitude of some of these problems have been discussed by Monson,[55] Morris,[56] and Hinkle et al.,[57] the methods are not always employed; and the research often becomes public without passing through the customary evaluative processes used in scientific investigation. The results may appear in lay media long before any formal documents are issued, and the formal documents may be published privately or by governmental agencies, without having been scrutinized according to the standards that might be used by referees for a cautious scientific journal.

The consequence of the activities is the current epidemic of apprehension that Lewis Thomas[58] has described so eloquently. For example, the Love Canal region was branded as dangerous and its residents were badly frightened by the results of a single study in which an abnormally high frequency of chromosome damage was found in residents of the region. The research was done without a control group, and the investigator (who had previously developed a causal hypothesis) examined the chromosome slides without blinding or any other precautions for objectivity. When the work was later repeated with a control group and with objective readings of the slides, no difference was found between the Love Canal residents and a suitable control group.[59] By then, however, it was too late to fix things. The correction did not receive the publicity given to the original erroneous accusation, and *Love Canal* has already entered the vernacular as a synonym for deadly chemical pollution.

If industrial workers and the public are to receive suitable protection against occupational and environmental hazards, and if everyone is to be protected against irrational fears that may lead to a needless loss of income, jobs, and homes, the first step in the process is to obtain accurate, unbiased information about what the hazards are, where they occur, and how relatively great they may be. The task of acquiring credible information is difficult but not impossible. Until this task is approached with rigorous scientific methods, workers and the public may be victimized far more often by the products of defective research than by the toxins of occupation or the pollutions of environment.

30.7. SYNOPSIS

The *clinical epidemiology* advocated in John R. Paul's introduction of that term was intended to expand the methods and contents of traditional epidemiologic activities in public health. In methods, Paul wanted the investigators to do homodemic research, with "intimate study and exacting measurements" of individual people rather than the hetero-demic analyses conducted in what he called *statistical epidemiology*. In contents, Paul advocated attention to the total ecology of disease, not just a focus on outbreaks of infectious disease.

Paul's goals have now been generally achieved but under titles different from what he proposed. Intimate studies of individual people are now frequently conducted as detective-work activities; and homodemic studies have become a standard activity in many branches of epidemiology. Infectious disease investigators have had particular success with seroepidemiologic community surveys; and the research methods of both infectious disease and the detective-work approach have been applied to hospital infection studies in nosocomial epidemiology.

The ability to demonstrate both etiologic agent and outcome disease with a single simple laboratory test has been a scientific boon for the quality of data in infectious disease epidemiology; and the study of community spectrums has helped the investigators avoid the problems of detection bias that are so prominent in the epidemiology of noninfectious disease. These scientific advantages, unfortunately, cannot be applied in retrospective evaluations of ancient ailments and epidemics, in current studies of presumably infectious syndromes that are ill defined in etiology or manifestations, and in predictions about future epidemics.

After Goldberger's demonstration that pellagra was caused by a nutritional deficiency, epidemiologists began to examine many noninfectious factors as etiologic agents for disease. Social epidemiologists have developed excellent homodemic methods for the research, but major scientific difficulties arise in developing and applying appropriate instruments to measure social, cultural, and behavioral factors. The difficulties are increased by the potential role of these factors in all three basic locations of cause-effect architecture: baseline state, maneuvers, and outcome.

Occupational and environmental epidemiology are hampered by the absence of a scientific tradition and by the presence of conflicting political beliefs or other prejudices that may impair rational appraisals for almost any topic under discussion. Aside from the basic difficulties of obtaining scientifically suitable groups, data, and comparisons in homodemic research, the results are often published without careful scientific review, and the agent/disease relationships are often determined from heterodemic data dredgings conducted without suitable statistical adjustments for the massive number of positive associations that can arise by stochastic chance alone. Clinically trained investigators who want to work in the particular type of clinical epidemiology proposed by John Paul can find abundant opportunities in the scientific investigation of occupational and environmental pathogens.

EXERCISES

If you have come this far in the text, you deserve thanks from the author, congratulations for your perseverance, and a reward. Here is the reward: There are no exercises for this chapter. (Instead, you are urged to read some of the many pertinent references.)

CHAPTER REFERENCES

1. Paul, 1938; 2. Paul, 1958; 3. Paul, 1966; 4. Greenwood, 1932; 5. Sigerist, 1946; 6. Ryle, 1948; 7. Spence, 1950; 8. Feinstein, 1972; 9. Feinstein, 1968 (Ann Intern Med, a); 10. Feinstein, 1968 (Ann

Intern Med, b); 11. Feinstein, 1968 (Ann Intern Med, c); 12. Roueché, 1947; 13. Malawista, 1984; 14. Henderson, 1980; 15. Semmelweis, 1861; 16. Louis, 1836; 17. Evans, 1982 (Viral infections of humans); 18. Evans, 1982 (Bacterial infections of humans); 19. Astor, 1983; 20. Thacker, 1983; 21. Barrett-Connor, 1979; 22. Starr, 1976; 23. Bianchine, 1968; 24. Horwitz, 1984; 25. Neustadt, 1978; 26. Silverstein, 1981; 27. Thoburn, 1968; 28. Bennett, 1979; 29. Emori, 1981; 30. Brachman, 1981; 31. Haley, 1981; 32. Bagshawe, 1978; 30. Schaffner, 1977; 34. Albert, 1981; 35. Freeman, 1981; 36. Eickhoff, 1981; 37. Maki, 1980; 37a. Cluff, 1964; 38. Terris, 1964; 39. Lind, 1753; 40. Cassel, 1960; 41. Cassel, 1974; 42. Cassel, 1976; 43. Graham, 1974; 44. Syme, 1974; 45. Tyroler, 1964; 46. Cobb, 1976; 47. Kasl, 1977; 48. Kasl, 1981; 49. Berkman, 1980; 50. Freeman, 1979; 51. Eisenberg, 1980; 52. Jenkins, 1967; 53. Review panel on coronary-prone behavior and coronary heart disease, 1981; 54. Williams, 1977; 55. Monson, 1980; 56. Morris, 1964; 57. Hinkle, 1976; 58. Thomas, 1983; 59. Kolata, 1980.

REFERENCES

[Numbers in brackets at the end of each reference indicate the chapter(s) where the reference is cited. References at the end of each chapter are made by senior author and year of publication, with name of journal added for multiple references by a senior author in one year, and letters (a, b, c, etc.) used for multiple annual references in a single journal.]

Ackerman LV, Gose EE. Breast lesion classification by computer and xeroradiograph. Cancer 1972;30:1025–35. [25]

Adar R, Papa MZ, Halpern Z, et al. Cellular sensitivity to collagen in thromboangiitis obliterans. N Engl J Med 1983;308:1113–6. [23]

Advisory Committee to the Surgeon General of the Public Health Service. Smoking and health. Washington DC: US Dept of HEW, 1964. (Public Health Service Publication No. 1103) [23]

Agrez MV, Valente RM, Pierce W, et al. Surgical history of Crohn's disease in a well-defined population. Mayo Clin Proc 1982;57:747–52. [15]

Albert RK, Condie F. Hand-washing patterns in medical intensive-care units. N Engl J Med 1981;304:1465–6. [30]

Amador E, Hsi BP. Indirect methods for estimating the normal range. Am J Clin Pathol 1969;52:538–46. [28]

Amberson JB, McMahon BT, Pinner M. A clinical trial of sanocrysin in pulmonary tuberculosis. Am Rev Tuberculosis 1931;24:401–35. [29]

American Heart Association Committee on Standards and Criteria for Programs of Care. Jones criteria (modified) for guidance in the diagnosis of rheumatic fever. Mod Concepts Cardiovasc Dis 1955;24:291. [13, 25]

American Heart Association Ad Hoc Committee to Revise the Jones Criteria (modified) of the Council on Rheumatic Fever and Congenital Heart Disease. Jones criteria (revised) for guidance in the diagnosis of rheumatic fever. Circulation 1965;32:664. [13, 25]

American Heart Association Committee on Rheumatic Fever and Bacterial Endocarditis. Jones criteria (revised) for guidance in the diagnosis of rheumatic fever. Circulation 1984;69:203A–8A. [13, 25]

American Joint Committee for Cancer Staging and End-Results Reporting. Manual for staging of cancer 1978. Chicago, 1978. [15]

Anonymous. Annotation. Interpretation of laboratory tests. Lancet 1967;1:1091–2. [28]

Anonymous. Apparent rise in cancer death rate fades on closer study of figures. JAMA 1977;237:2173–4. [24]

Anonymous. Serum enzymes and myocardial infarct size: The effect of drugs. Lancet 1978;2:1082–3. [25]

Anonymous. Editorial. Multicentre depression. Lancet 1981;2:563–4. [29]

Anturane Reinfarction Trial Research Group. Sulfinpyrazone in the prevention of cardiac death after myocardial infarction. N Engl J Med 1978;298:289–95. [15, 22, 29]

Anturane Reinfarction Trial Research Group. Sulfinpyrazone in the prevention of sudden death after myocardial infarction. N Engl J Med 1980;302:250–6. [17, 29]

Anturane Reinfarction Italian Study. Sulphinpyrazone in post-myocardial infarction. Lancet 1982;1:237–42. [29]

Anturane Reinfarction Trial Policy Committee. The Anturane Reinfarction Trial: Reevaluation of outcome. N Engl J Med 1982;306:1005–8. [17, 29]

Armitage P. Sequential Medical Trials. 2nd ed. New York: Wiley, 1975. [29]

Armstrong B, Stevens N, Doll R. Retrospective study of the association between use of rauwolfia derivatives and breast cancer in English women. Lancet 1974;2:672–5. [19, 21]

Armstrong BK, Mann JI, Adelstein AM, et al. Commodity consumption and ischemic heart disease mortality, with special reference to dietary practices. J Chron Dis 1975;28:455–69. [24]

Astor G. The Disease Detectives: Deadly Medical Mysteries and the People Who Solved Them. New York: New American Library, 1983. [30]

Austin MA, Criqui MH, Barrett-Connor E, et al. The effect of response bias on the odds ratio. Am J Epidemiol 1981;114:137–43. [22]

Axelsson G, Rylander R. Exposure to anaesthetic gases and spontaneous abortion: Response bias in a postal questionnaire study. Int J Epidemiol 1982;11:250–6. [15]

Bagshawe KD, Blowers R, Lidwell OM. Isolating patients in hospital to control infection. Part I. Sources and routes of infection. Br Med J 1978;2:609–12. [30]

Baird PJ. Serological evidence for the association of papillomavirus and cervical neoplasia. Lancet 1983;2:17–8. [23]

Barnett RN. Clinical Laboratory Statistics. 2nd ed. Boston: Little, Brown, 1979. [26, 28]

Barrett-Connor E. Infectious and chronic disease epidemiology: Separate and unequal? Am J Epidemiol 1979;109:245–9. [30]

Barro A. Survey and evaluation of approaches to physician performance measures. J Med Educ 1973;48:1048–93. [Part Six]

Barsky AJ. Nonpharmacologic aspects of medicine. Arch Intern Med 1983;143:1544–8. [29]

Bartlett E. An essay on the Philosophy of Medical Science. Philadelphia: Lea and Blanchard, 1844. [30]

Batuman V, Landy E, Maesaka JK, et al. Contribution of lead to hypertension with renal impairment. N Engl J Med 1983;309:17–21. [23]

Bauer FW, Robbins SL. An autopsy study of cancer patients. JAMA 1972;221:1471–4. [21]

Baum ML, Anish DS, Chalmers TC, et al. A survey of clinical trials of antibiotic prophylaxis in colon surgery: Evidence against further use of no-treatment controls. N Engl J Med 1981;305:795–9. [29]

Beadenkopf WG, Abrams M, Daoud A, et al. An assessment of certain medical aspects of death certificate data for epidemiologic study of arteriosclerotic heart disease. J Chron Dis 1963;16:249. [21]

Beeson PB. Changes in medical therapy during the past half century. Medicine 1980;59:79–99. [24]

Bennett JV, Brachman PS, eds. Hospital Infections. Boston: Little, Brown, 1979. [30]

Benson ES, Strandjord PE, eds. Multiple Laboratory Screening. New York: Academic Press, 1969. [26]

Benson ES, Rubin M, eds. Logic and Economics of Clinical Laboratory Use: Proceedings of a Conference at Cancun, Mexico, March 1978. New York: Elsevier, 1978. [28]

Beral V. Cardiovascular-disease mortality trends and oral-contraceptive use in young women. Lancet 1976;2:1047–51. [24]

Bergeson PS, Steinfeld HJ. How dependable is palpation as a screening method for fever? Clin Pediatr (Phila) 1974;13:350–1. [25]

Bergstrand R, Vedin A, Wilhelmsson C, et al. Bias due to non-participation and heterogeneous sub-groups in population surveys. J Chron Dis 1983;36:725–8. [17]

Berkman LF. Physical health and the social environment: A social epidemiological perspective. In: Eisenberg L, Kleinman A, eds. The Relevance of Social Science for Medicine. New York: Reidel, 1980:51–75. [30]

Berkson J. Limitations of the application of fourfold table analysis to hospital data. Biomet Bull 1946;2:47–53. [21]

Best EWR, Josie GH, Walker CB. A Canadian study of mortality in relation to smoking habits. A preliminary report. Can J Public Health 1961;52:99–106. [23]

Bianchine JR, Macaraeg PVS, Lasagna L. Drugs as etiologic factors in the Stevens-Johnson syndrome. Am J Med 1968;44:390–405. [22, 30]

Bibbo M, Gill WB, Azizi F, et al. Follow-up study of male and female offspring of DES-exposed mothers. Obstet Gynecol 1977;49:1–8. [18, 23]

Bibbo M, Haenszel WM, Wied GL, et al. A twenty-five year follow-up study of women exposed to diethylstilbestrol during pregnancy. N Engl J Med 1978;298:763–7. [15, 18, 23]

Bircher J, Bourquin J, Wirth W, et al. Controlled clinical trial of barium sulfate suspensions for upper gastrointestinal x-ray examinations. Eur J Clin Pharmacol 1971;4:38–45. [29]

Blot WJ, Winn DM, Fraumeni JF Jr. Oral cancer and mouthwash. J Natl Cancer Inst 1983;70:251–3. [23]

Boice JD Jr. Follow-up methods to trace women treated for pulmonary tuberculosis, 1930–1954. Am J Epidemiol 1978;107:127–39. [17]

Book of Daniel. I:v 1–15. [29]

Boston Collaborative Drug Surveillance Program. Oral contraceptives and venous thromboembolic disease, surgically confirmed gallbladder disease, and breast tumours. Lancet 1973;1:1399–1404. [22]

Boston Collaborative Drug Surveillance Program. Reserpine and breast cancer. Lancet 1974;2:669–71. [19, 22, 23]

Box GP. Science and statistics. J Am Statist Assoc 1976;71:791–9. [19]

Box JF. RA Fisher and the design of experiments, 1922–1926. Amer Stat 1980;34:1–7. [29]

Brachman PS. Nosocomial infection control: An overview. Rev Infect Dis 1981;3:640–8. [30]

Bradley JV. Distribution-free Statistical Tests. Englewood Cliffs: Prentice-Hall, 1968. [9, 10]

Brenner MH. Mortality and the national economy: A review, and the experience of England and Wales 1936–1976. Lancet 1979;2:568–73. [24]

Brewin TB. Consent to randomised treatment. Lancet 1982;2:919–21. [29]

Brook RH, Avery AD, Greenfield S, et al. Quality of medical care assessment using outcome measures: An overview of the method. Med Care 1977;15(12):Supplement. [27]

Brook RH, Ware JE, Davies-Avery A, et al. Conceptualization and measurement of health for adults in the Health Insurance Study: Overview. Med Care 1979;17(7):Supplement. [27]

Brown BW Jr. The crossover experiment for clinical trials. Biometrics 1980;36:69–79. [29]

Bull JP. The historical development of clinical therapeutic trials. J Chron Dis 1959;10:218–48. [29]

Bulpitt CJ. Randomized Controlled Clinical Trials. Boston: Martinus Nijhoff, 1983. [29]

Bunn AR. Ischaemic heart disease mortality and the business cycle in Australia. Am J Public Health 1979;69:772–81. [24]

Burch PRJ. Smoking and lung cancer. Tests of a causal hypothesis. J Chron Dis 1980;33:221–38. [18]

Burkhardt R, Kienle G. Controlled clinical trials and medical ethics. Lancet 1978;2:1356–59. [29]

Buxton AE, Highsmith AK, Garner JS, et al. Contamination of intravenous infusion fluid: Effects of changing administration sets. Ann Intern Med 1979;90:764–8. [29]

Byar DP, Simm RM, Friedenwald WT, et al. Randomized clinical trials: Perspectives on some recent ideas. N Engl J Med 1976;295:74. [29]

Cancer Research Campaign Working Party. Trials and tribulations: Thoughts on the organisation of multicentre clinical studies. Br Med J 1980;281:918–20. [29]

Cassel J, Patrick R, Jenkins D. Epidemiological analysis of culture change: A conceptual model. Ann NY Acad Sci 1960;84:938–49. [30]

Cassel JC, ed. Evans County cardiovascular and cerebrovascular epidemiologic study. Arch Intern Med 1971; 128:883–986. [23]

Cassel J. An epidemiological perspective of psychosocial factors in disease etiology. Am J Public Health 1974;64:1040–3. [30]

Cassel J. The contribution of the social environment to host resistance. Am J Epidemiol 1976;104:107–23. [30]

Centers for Disease Control Cancer and Steroid Hormone Study. JAMA 1983;249:Long-term oral contraceptive use and the risk of breast cancer: 1591–5. Oral contraceptive use and the risk of ovarian cancer: 1596–9. Oral contraceptive use and the risk of endometrial cancer: 1600–4. [22]

Chalmers TC. Randomize the first patient. N Engl J Med 1977;296:107. [29]

Chalmers TC, Matta RJ, Smith H Jr, et al. Evidence favoring the use of anticoagulants in the hospital phase of acute myocardial infarction. N Engl J Med 1977;297:1091–6. [15, 16, 22, 23, 29]

Chalmers TC. In defense of the VA randomized control trial of coronary artery surgery. Clin Res 1978;26:230–5. [16]

Chambers LW, Spitzer WO. A method of estimating risk for occupational factors using multiple data sources: The Newfoundland lip cancer study. Am J Public Health 1977;67:176–9. [22]

Chan YK, Collins D. Some aspects of data management in multi-center clinical trials. Trends Pharmacol Sci 1981;2:29–31. [29]

Chaput de Saintonge DM. Aide-mémoire for preparing clinical trial protocols. Br Med J 1977;1:1323–4. [23]

Charlson ME, Feinstein AR. The auxometric dimension. A new method for using rate of growth in prognostic staging of breast cancer. JAMA 1974;228:180–5. [15]

Charlson ME, Feinstein AR. A new clinical index of growth rate in the staging of breast cancer. Am J Med 1980;69:527–36. [21]

Chiang CL. A stochastic model of competing risks of illness and competing risks of death. In: Gurland J, ed. Stochastic Models in Medicine and Biology. Madison: Univ Wisconsin Press, 1964. [17]

Chu J, Schweid AI, Weiss NS. Survival among women with endometrial cancer: A comparison of estrogen users and nonusers. Am J Obstet Gynecol 1982;143:569–73. [17, 22]

Chuong J, Fisher RL, Spiro HM, et al. Plasma pepsinogen as predictive marker for the development of duodenal ulcer: A long-term follow-up questionnaire study. Clin Res 1981;29:667A. [15]

Cicchetti DV. Assessing inter-rater reliability for rating scales: Resolving some basic issues. Br J Psychiatry 1976;129:452–6. [26]

Clemens JD, Chuong JJH, Feinstein AR. The BCG controversy. A methodological and statistical reappraisal. JAMA 1983;249:2362–9. [17]

Cluff LE, Thornton GF, Seidl LG. Studies on the epidemiology of adverse drug reactions. I. Methods of surveillance. JAMA 1964;188:976–83. [30]

Cobb LA, Thomas GI, Dillard DH, et al. An evaluation of internal-mammary-artery ligation by a double-blind technic. N Engl J Med 1959;260:1115–8. [12, 17]

Cobb S. Social support as a moderator of life stress. J Psychosom Med 1976;38:300. [30]

Cochran WG. Errors of measurement in statistics. Technometrics 1968;10:637–66. [26]

Cochrane AL, Elwood PC. Laboratory data and diagnosis. Lancet 1969;1:420. [28]

Cochrane AL. Effectiveness and Efficiency: Random Reflections on Health Services. London: Nuffield Provincial Hospitals Trust, 1972. [12]

Cochrane AL, Moore F. Death certification from the epidemiological point of view. Lancet 1981;2:742–3. [24]

Cole P. The evolving case control study. J Chron Dis 1979;32:15–27. [18, 20, 23]

Colin-Jones DG, Langman MJS, Lawson DH, et al. Cimetidine and gastric cancer: Preliminary report from post-marketing surveillance study. Br Med J 1982;285:1311–3. [23]

Conn HO, Snyder N, Atterbury CE. The Berkson bias in action. Yale J Biol Med 1979;2:141–7. [21]

Controlled Clinical Trials: Design and Methods. Official Journal of the Society for Clinical Trials. New York: Elsevier Science Publishing. [29]

Cornfield J. A method of estimating comparative rates from clinical data. Applications to cancer of the lung, breast and cervix. J Natl Cancer Inst 1951;11:1269–75. [20]

Cornfield J. A statistical problem arising from retrospective studies. In: Neyman J, ed. Proceedings of the Third Berkeley Symposium, Volume IV. Berkeley: Univ California Press, 1956;135–48. [20]

Cornfield J. The University Group Diabetes Program. A further statistical analysis of the mortality findings. JAMA 1971;217:1676–87. [29]

Coronary Drug Project Research Group. The Coronary Drug Project: Design, methods, and baseline results. Circulation, 1973;47:I-1–44. [16, 29]

Coronary Drug Project Research Group. Influence of adherence to treatment and response of cholesterol on mortality in the Coronary Drug Project. N Engl J Med 1980;303:1038. [16, 29]

Cotlove E, Harris EK, Williams GZ. Biological and analytic components of variation in long term studies of serum constituents in normal subjects. Clin Chem 1970;16:1028–32. [28]

Cox DR. Regression models and life tables (with discussion). J R Stat Soc 1972;B34:187–200. [17]

Cox KR. Planning Clinical Experiments. Springfield: Charles C Thomas, 1968. [29]

Cullen K, Stenhouse NS, Wearne KL, et al. Multiple regression analysis of risk factors for cardiovascular disease and cancer mortality in Busselton, Eastern Australia—13 year study. J Chron Dis 1983;36:371–7. [23]

Cunningham AS. Lymphomas and animal-protein consumption. Lancet 1976;2:1184–6. [24]

Cutler SJ, Ederer F. Maximum utilization of the life table method in analyzing survival. J Chron Dis 1958;8:699–713. [17]

Dales LG, Friedman GD, Collen MF. Evaluating periodic multiphasic health checkups: A controlled trial. J Chron Dis 1979;32:385–404. [29]

Daniels J, Goodman AD. Hypertension and hyperparathyroidism. Inverse relation of serum phosphate level and blood pressure. Am J Med 1983;75:17–23. [23]

D'Arcy HR. Controlled Clinical Trials. Springfield: Charles C Thomas, 1960. [29]

Davis CE. The effect of regression to the mean in epidemiologic and clinical studies. Am J Epidemiol 1976;104:493–8. [28]

Davis JP, Vergeront JM. The effect of publicity on the reporting of toxic-shock syndrome in Wisconsin. J Infect Dis 1982;145:449–57. [22]

Dawber TR. The Framingham Study. The Epidemiology of Atherosclerotic Disease. Cambridge: Harvard Univ Press, 1980. [23]

Day TK, Powell-Jackson PR. Fluoride, water hardness, and endemic goitre. Lancet 1972;1:1135–8. [18]

Department of Clinical Epidemiology and Biostatistics, McMaster University Health Sciences Center. Clinical epidemiology rounds: How to read clinical journals. V. To distinguish useful from useless or even harmful therapy. Can Med Assoc J 1981;124:1156–62. [19, 29]

Department of Clinical Epidemiology and Biostatistics, McMaster University Health Sciences Center. Clinical epidemiology rounds: The interpretation of diagnostic data. V. How to do it with simple maths. Can Med Assoc J 1983;129:947–54. [20]

Detre KM, Wright E, Murphy ML, et al. Observer agreement in evaluating coronary angiography. Circulation 1975;52:979–86. [25]

Diamond GA, Forrester JS. Clinical trials and statistical verdicts: Probable grounds for appeal. Ann Intern Med 1983;98:358–94. [19]

Dieckmann WJ, Davis ME, Rynkiewicz LM, et al. Does the administration of diethylstilbestrol during pregnancy have therapeutic value? Am J Obstet Gynecol 1953;66:1062–81. [15, 18, 23]

Diehl AK. Gallstone size and the risk of gallbladder cancer. JAMA 1983;250:2323–6. [23]

Diehl HS, Baker AB, Cowan DW. Cold vaccines: An evaluation based on a controlled study. JAMA 1938;111:1168. [29]

DiMatteo MR, DiNicola DD. Achieving Patient Compliance: The Psychology of the Medical Practitioner's Role. Elmsford: Pergamon Press, 1982. [Part Six]

Dimond EG, Kittle CF, Crockett JE. Comparison of internal mammary artery ligation and sham operation for angina pectoris. Am J Cardiol 1960;5:483–6. [12, 17]

Dodd C. Report of a symposium on clinical trials held at the Royal Society of Medicine. London: Pfizer Ltd, 1958. [29]

Doll R, Hill AB. A study of the aetiology of carcinoma of the lung. Br Med J 1952;2:1271–86. [23]

Doll R, Hill AB. Mortality in relation to smoking: Ten years' observations of British doctors. Br Med J 1964;1:1399–1410, 1460–7. [15, 23, 29]

Donabedian A. Explorations in Quality Assessment and Monitoring. I. Definition of Quality and Approaches to Its Assessment. Ann Arbor: Health Administration Press, 1980. [27]

Donabedian A. Explorations in Quality Assessment and Monitoring. II. The Criteria and Standards of Quality. Ann Arbor: Health Administration Press, 1982. [27]

Dorn H. Some applications of biometry in the collection and evaluation of medical data. J Chron Dis 1955;1:638–64. [19]

Dorn HF. The mortality of smokers and non-smokers. Am Stat Assoc Proc Soc Stat Sec 1958;33–71. [23]

Dorn HF. Tobacco consumption and mortality from cancer and other diseases. Public Health Rep 1959;74:581–93. [23]

Dorn HF. The increasing mortality from chronic respiratory diseases. Am Stat Soc Proc 1961;148–52. [24]

Dorn HF, Moriyama IM. Uses and significance of multiple cause tabulations for mortality statistics. Am J Public Health 1964;54:400. [24]

Dunn JE Jr, Linden G, Breslow L. Lung cancer mortality experience of men in certain occupations in California. Am J Public Health 1960;50:1475–87. [23]

Eickhoff TC. Nosocomial infections—a 1980 view: Progress, priorities and prognosis. Am J Med 1981;70:381–8. [30]

Eikman EA, Cameron JL, Colman M, et al. A test for patency of the cystic duct in acute cholecystitis. Ann Intern Med 1975;82:318–22. [25]

Eisenberg L, Kleinman A, eds. The Relevance of Social Science for Medicine. New York: Reidel, 1980. [30]

Elashoff JD. Combining results of clinical trials. Gastroenterology 1978;75:1170–2. [29]

Elkins HB, Pagnotto LD, Brugsch HG. Confusion concerning "normal" values in biologic analysis. N Engl J Med 1972;286:1268–9. [28]

Elveback LR, Guillier CL, Keating FR. Health, normality, and the ghost of Gauss. JAMA 1970;211:69–75. [28]

Elveback LR. How high is high? A proposed alternative to the normal range. Mayo Clin Proc 1972;47:93–7. [28]

Elveback LR. The population of healthy persons as a source of reference information. Hum Pathol 1973;4:9–16. [28]

Emori TG, Haley RW, Garner JS. Techniques and uses of nosocomial infection surveillance in U.S. hospitals, 1976–1977. Am J Med 1981;70:933–40. [30]

Ennis JT, Walsh MJ, Mahon JM. Value of infarct-specific isotope (99m Tc-labeled stannous pyrophosphate) in myocardial scanning. Br J Med 1975;3:517–20. [25]

Evans AS. Viral Infections of Humans. Epidemiology and Control. 2nd ed. New York: Plenum Medical Book Co, 1982. [30]

Evans AS, Feldman HA, eds. Bacterial Infections of Humans. Epidemiology and Control. New York: Plenum Medical Book Co, 1982. [30]

Eyler JM. William Farr on the cholera: The sanitarian's disease theory and the statistician's method. J Hist Med Allied Sci 1973; 28:79–100. [19]

Farr W. Influence of elevation on the fatality of cholera. J Stat Society 1852;15:155–83. [19]

Feinstein AR, DiMassa R. The unheard diastolic murmur in acute rheumatic fever. N Engl J Med 1959;260:1331–3. [26]

Feinstein AR, Spagnuolo M. The duration of activity in acute rheumatic fever. JAMA 1961;175:1117–9. [28]

Feinstein AR, Wood HF, Spagnuolo M, et al. Rheumatic fever in children and adolescents: A long-term epidemiologic study of subsequent prophylaxis, streptococcal infections, and clinical sequelae. Ann Intern Med 1964;60:87–123 (Suppl 5). [26]

Feinstein AR, Spagnuolo M, Jonas S, et al. Discontinuation of antistreptococcal prophylaxis. A double-blind study in rheumatic patients free of heart disease. JAMA 1966;197:949–52. [29]

Feinstein AR, Stern E. Clinical effects of recurrent attacks of acute rheumatic fever: A prospective epidemiologic study of 105 episodes. J Chron Dis 1967;20:13–27. [26]

Feinstein AR. Clinical epidemiology. I. The populational experiments of nature and of man in human illness. Ann Intern Med 1968;69:807–20. (a) [30]

Feinstein AR. Clinical epidemiology. II. The identification rates of disease. Ann Intern Med 1968;69:1037–61. (b) [24, 30]

Feinstein AR. Clinical epidemiology. III. The clinical design of statistics in therapy. Ann Intern Med 1968;69:1287–1312. (c) [30]

Feinstein AR. Acoustic distinctions in cardiac auscultation. With emphasis on cardiophonetics, synecphonesis, the analysis of cadence, and the problems of hydraulic distortion. Arch Intern Med 1968;121:209–24. [26]

Feinstein AR. A new staging system for cancer and a reappraisal of "early" treatment and "cure" by radical surgery. N Engl J Med 1968;279:747–53. [15]

Feinstein AR, Gelfman NA, Yesner R, et al. Observer variability in histopathologic diagnosis of lung cancer. Am Rev Respir Dis 1970;101:671–84. [26]

Feinstein AR. The pre-therapeutic classification of co-morbidity in chronic disease. J Chron Dis 1970;23:455–69. [21]

Feinstein AR. Clinical biostatistics. VIII. An analytic appraisal of the University Group Diabetes Program (UGDP) study. Clin Pharmacol Ther 1971;12:167–91. [29]

Feinstein AR. Clinical biostatistics. XII. On exorcising the ghost of Gauss and the curse of Kelvin. Clin Pharmacol Ther 1971;12:1003–16. [28]

Feinstein AR. Clinical biostatistics. XV. The process of prognostic stratification. Clin Pharmacol Ther 1972;13:442–57 and 609–24. [20]

Feinstein AR. Clinical biostatistics. XVII. Synchronous partition and bivariate evaluation in predictive stratification. Clin Pharmacol Ther 1972;13:755–68. (e) [13]

Feinstein AR. Why clinical epidemiology? Clin Res 1972;20:821–5. [30]

Feinstein AR. The need for humanised science in evaluating medication. Lancet 1972;2:421–3. [29]

Feinstein AR. Clinical biostatistics XX. The epidemiologic trohoc, the ablative risk ratio, and "retrospective" research. Clin Pharmacol Ther 1973;14:291–307. [18]

Feinstein AR. Clinical Judgment. Huntington: Robert E Krieger, 1974. (Reprinting of original edition published in 1967 by Williams and Wilkins Co, Baltimore) [15, 19, 21, 26, 29]

Feinstein AR. Clinical biostatistics. XXV. A survey of the statistical procedures in general medical journals. Clin Pharmacol Ther 1974;15:97–107. [28]

Feinstein AR. Clinical biostatistics. XXVI. Medical ethics and the architecture of clinical research. Clin Pharmacol Ther 1974;15:316–34. [29]

Feinstein AR. Clinical biostatistics. XXVII. The biostatistical problems of pharmaceutical surveillance. Clin Pharmacol Ther 1974;16:110–23. [17]

Feinstein AR. Clinical biostatistics. XXXIV. The other side of "statistical significance": Alpha, beta, delta, and the calculation of sample size. Clin Pharmacol Ther 1975;18:491–505. [9]

Feinstein AR. Clinical biostatistics. XXXV. The persistent clinical failures and fallacies of the UGDP study. Clin Pharmacol Ther 1976;19:78–93. (a) [15, 29]

Feinstein AR. Clinical biostatistics. XXXVI. The persistent biometric problems of the UGDP study. Clin Pharmacol Ther 1976;19:472–85. (b) [29]

Feinstein AR, Schimpff CR, Andrews JF Jr, et al. Cancer of the larynx: A new staging system and a re-appraisal of prognosis and treatment. J Chron Dis 1977;30:277–305. [17]

Feinstein AR, Wells CK. Randomized trials vs. historical controls: The scientific plagues of both houses. Trans Assoc Am Physicians 1977;90:239–247. [29]

Feinstein AR. Clinical biostatistics. XLVII. Scientific standards vs. statistical associations and biologic logic in the analysis of causation; and XLVIII. Efficacy of different research structures in preventing bias in the analysis of causation. Clin Pharmacol Ther 1979;25:481–92 and 26:129–41. [19]

Feinstein AR, Kramer MS. Clinical biostatistics. LII. A primer on quantitative indexes of association. Clin Pharmacol Ther 1980;28:130–45. [10]

Feinstein AR. Clinical biostatistics. LVI. The t test and the basic ethos of parametric statistical inference (conclusion). Clin Pharmacol Ther 1981;30:133–146. [9]

Feinstein AR. Clinical biostatistics. LVII. A glossary of neologisms in quantitative clinical science. Clin Pharmacol Ther 1981;30:564–77. [18]

Feinstein AR, Horwitz RI, Spitzer WO, et al. Coffee and pancreatic cancer. The problems of etiologic science and epidemiologic case-control research. JAMA 1981;246:957–61. [16, 20]

Feinstein AR, Horwitz RI. An algebraic analysis of biases due to exclusion, susceptibility, and protopathic prescription in case-control research. J Chron Dis 1981;34:393–403. [22]

Feinstein AR, Horwitz RI. Double standards, scientific methods, and epidemiologic research. N Engl J Med 1982; 307:1611–7 [19].

Feinstein AR. Wells CK. Lung cancer staging: A critical evaluation. Clin Chest Med 1982;3:291–305. [15]

Feinstein AR. The Jones criteria and the challenges of clinimetrics. Circulation 1982;66:1–5. [13]

Feinstein, AR. An additional basic science for clinical medicine. Parts I–III. Ann Intern Med 1983; 99:393–397, 544–550, and 705–712. [29]

Feinstein AR. An additional basic science for clinical medicine: IV. The development of clinimetrics. Ann Intern Med 1983;99:843–8. [6,13,29]

738   REFERENCES

Feinstein AR, Sosin DM, Wells CK. The Will Rogers phenomenon: Improved technologic diagnosis and stage migration as a source of non-therapeutic improvement in cancer prognosis. Clin Res 1984;32:543A. [29]

Ferencz C, Matanoski GM, Wilson PD, et al. Maternal hormone therapy and congenital heart disease. Teratology 1980;21:225–39. [22, 23]

Fibiger J. Om serum behandling of difteri. Hospitalshdende 1898;6:309–25. [29]

Files JB, van Peenan HJ, Lindberg DAB. Use of "normal range" in multiphasic testing. JAMA 1968;205:94–8. [28]

Finland M. The serum treatment of lobar pneumonia. N Engl J Med 1930;202:1244–47. [29]

Finney DJ. Systematic signalling of adverse reactions to drugs. Methods Inf Med 1974;13:1–10. [17]

Fisher RA, Mackenzie WA. Studies in crop variation: II. The manurial response to different potato varieties. J Agric Sci 1923;13:315. [29]

Fisher RA. Statistical Methods for Research Workers. 5th ed. Edinburgh: Oliver and Boyd, 1934. [9]

Fisher RA. The Design of Experiments. Edinburgh: Oliver and Boyd, 1935. [16]

Fisher RA. Smoking. The Cancer Controversy. Some Attempts to Assess the Evidence. Edinburgh: Oliver and Boyd, 1959. [18]

Fisher RA. Statistical Methods and Scientific Inference. 2nd ed. Edinburgh: Oliver and Boyd, 1959:42. [19]

Fleiss JL. Measuring agreement between two judges on the presence or absence of a trait. Biometrics 1975;31:651–9. [26]

Fleiss JL. Confidence intervals for the odds ratio in case-control studies: The state of the art. J Chron Dis 1979;32:69–82. [20]

Fleiss JL. Statistical Methods for Rates and Proportions. 2nd ed. New York: Wiley, 1981. [9, 10, 20, 24, 26]

Forbes TR. Mortality books for 1820 to 1849 from the parish of St. Bride, Fleet St., London. J Hist Med Allied Sci 1972;27:15–29. [24]

Forbes TR. Sextons' day books for 1685–1687 and 1694–1703 from the parish of St. Martin-in-the-fields, London. Yale J Biol Med 1973;46:142–150. [24]

Francis T Jr, Napier JA, Voight RB, et al. Evaluation of the 1954 Field Trial of Poliomyelitis Vaccine: Final report. Ann Arbor: Edwards Brothers, 1957. [29]

Francis T Jr, Epstein FH. Survey methods in general populations. Studies of a total community. Tecumseh, Michigan. Milbank Mem Fund Q 1965;43:333–42. [23]

Franks LM. Latent carcinoma of the prostate. J Pathol Bacteriol 1954;68:603–21. [21]

Freedman LS, Spiegelhalter DJ. The assessment of subjective opinion and its use in relation to stopping rules for clinical trials. The Statistician 1983;32:153–60. [29]

Freeman HE, Levine S, Reeder LG, eds. Handbook of Medical Sociology. 3rd ed. Englewood Cliffs: Prentice-Hall, 1979. [30]

Freeman J, McGowan JE. Methodologic issues in hospital epidemiology. I. Rates, case-finding, and interpretation. Rev Infect Dis 1981;3:658–67, 668–77. [30]

Freeman LC. Elementary Applied Statistics. New York: Wiley, 1965. [9, 10]

Freiman JA, Chalmers TC, Smith H, et al. The importance of beta, the type II error and sample size in the design and interpretation of the randomized control trial. N Engl J Med 1978;299:690–4. [9, 19]

Frerichs RR, Webber LS, Voors AW, et al. Cardiovascular disease risk factor variables in children at two successive years—the Bogalusa Heart Study. J Chron Dis 1979;32:251–62. [23]

Friedewald WT, Furberg CD. Clinical trials: Key references. Circulation 1982;65:213–5. [29]

Friedman GD, Klatsky AL, Siegelaub AB, McCarthy N. Kaiser-Permanente epidemiologic study of myocardial infarction. Study design and results for standard risk factors. Am J Epidemiol 1974;99:101–6. [18]

Friedman LM, Furberg CD, DeMets DL. Fundamentals of clinical trials. Boston: John Wright, PSG Inc, 1981. [29]

Fries JF, Siegel RC. Testing the "Preliminary Criteria for Classification of SLE." Ann Rheum Dis 1973;32:171–7. [25]

Frost WH. The age selection of mortality from tuberculosis in successive decades. Am J Hygiene 1939;30:91–6. [2, 17]

Gaddum JH. Discoveries in therapeutics. J Pharm Pharmacol 1954;6:497–512. [29]

Galton F. Regression towards mediocrity in hereditary stature. J Anthropol Inst 1885–86;15:246–63. [28]

Garceau AJ, Donaldson RM, Ottara ET, et al. A controlled trial of prophylactic portal caval shunt surgery. N Engl J Med 1964;270:496–500. [15]

Gavrin JB, Tursky E, Albam B, et al. Rheumatic fever in children and adolescents: A long-term epidemiologic study of subsequent prophylaxis, streptococcal infections, and clinical sequelae. II. Maintenance and preservation of the population. Ann Intern Med 1964;60:18–30. [17, 29]

Gehan EA, Freireich EJ. Non-randomised controls in cancer clinical trials. N Engl J Med 1974;290:198–203. [29]

Gerber L, Wolf A, Braham RS, et al. Effects of sample selection on the co-incidence of hypertension and diabetes. JAMA 1982;247:43–6. [21]

Gillum RF, Feinleib M, Margolis JR, et al. Community surveillance for cardiovascular disease: The Framingham Cardiovascular Disease Survey. J Chron Dis 1976;29:289–99. [23]

Gittlesohn A, Royston PN. Annotated bibliography of cause-of-death validation studies 1958–80. Washington DC: US Government Printing Office, 1982. (Vital and health statistics. Series 2: no. 89) (DHHS publication no. [PHS] 82–1363). [24]

Glindmeyer HW, Diem JE, Jones RN, et al. Noncomparability of longitudinally and cross-sectionally determined annual change in spirometry. Am Rev Respir Dis 1982;125:544–8. [20]

Goldacre MJ, Holford TR, Vessey MP. Cardiovascular disease and vasectomy: Findings from two epidemiologic studies. N Engl J Med 1983;308:805–8. [20]

Goldberg DP, Steele JJ, Smith C, et al. Training family doctors to recognise psychiatric illness with increased accuracy. Lancet 1980;2:521–3. [26]

Goldman L, Feinstein AR. Anticoagulants and myocardial infarction. The problems of pooling, drowning, and floating. Ann Intern Med 1979;90:92–4. [22, 29]

Goldschlager N, Selzer A, Cohn K. Treadmill stress tests as indicators of presence and severity of coronary artery disease. Ann Intern Med 1976;85:277–86. [25]

Goldstein H. The Design and Analysis of Longitudinal Studies: Their Role in the Measurement of Change. London: Academic Press, 1979. [28]

Goldstein HR. No association found between coffee and cancer of the pancreas. N Engl J Med 1982;306:997. [22]

Good CS, ed. Principles and Practice of Clinical Trials. Edinburgh: Churchill-Livingstone, 1976. [29]

Gordis L. Assuring the quality of questionnaire data in epidemiologic research. Am J Epidemiol 1979;109:21–4. [22, 26]

Gorringe JAL. Initial preparation for clinical trials. In: Harris EL, Fitzgerald JD, eds. Principles and Practice of Clinical Trials. Edinburgh: E & S Livingstone, 1970:41–6. [29]

Goslin R, O'Brien MJ, Steele G, et al. Correlation of plasma CEA and CEA tissue staining in poorly differentiated colorectal cancer. Am J Med 1981;71:246–53. [25]

Graham S. The sociological approach to epidemiology. Am J Public Health 1974;64:1046–9. [30]

Grams RR, Johnson EA, Benson ES. Laboratory data analysis system. II. Analytic error limits. Am J Clin Pathol 1972;58:182–7. (a) [28]

Grams RR, Johnson EA, Benson ES. Laboratory data analysis system: III. Multivariate normality. Am J Clin Pathol 1972;58:188–200. (b) [28]

Graunt J. Natural and political observations mentioned in a following index, and made upon the bills of mortality. London, 1662. (Reprinted Baltimore: Johns Hopkins Press, 1939). [24]

Gravelle HSE, Hutchinson G, Stern J. Mortality and unemployment: A critique of Brenner's time-series analysis. Lancet 1981;2:675–9. [24]

Green FHK. The clinical evaluation of remedies. Lancet 1954;267:1085–91. [29]

Greenberg BG. Conduct of cooperative field and clinical trials. Am Stat 1959;13:13. [29]

Greenfield S, Nadler MA, Morgan MT, et al. The clinical investigation and management of chest pain in an emergency department. Quality assessment by criteria mapping. Med Care 1977;15:898–905. [27]

Greenspan RH, Ravin CE, Polansky SM, et al. Accuracy of the chest radiograph in diagnosis of pulmonary embolism. Invest Radiol 1982;17:539–43. [26]

Greenwald P, Barlow JJ, Nasca PC, et al. Vaginal cancer after maternal treatment with synthetic estrogens. N Engl J Med 1971;285:390–2. [20]

Greenwood M. Epidemiology. Historical and experimental. Baltimore: Johns Hopkins, 1932. [30]

Griner PF, Mayewski RJ, Mushlin AI, et al. Selection and interpretation of diagnostic tests and procedures: Principles and applications. Ann Intern Med 1981;94:553–600. [25]

Grizzle JE. The two-period change-over design and its use in clinical trials. Biometrics 1965;21:467–80. [29]

Hadden DR, McDevitt DG. Environmental stress and thyrotoxicosis: Absence of association. Lancet 1974;2:577–8. [24]

Haley RW, Hooton TM, Culver DH, et al. Nosocomial infections in U.S. hospitals, 1975–1976. Estimated frequency by selected characteristics of patients. Am J Med 1981;70:947–59. [30]

Hamburger JI. Normal ranges de-emphasized. N Engl J Med 1969;281:331. [28]

Hammond EC, Horn D. Smoking and death rates—report on forty-four months of follow-up of

187,783 men. JAMA 1958; I. Total mortality 166:1159–72. II. Death rates by cause. 166:1294–1308. [23]

Hampton JR. Presentation and analysis of the results of clinical trials in cardiovascular disease. Br Med J 1981;282:1371–3. [29]

Hardcastle JD, Farrands PA, Balfour TW, et al. Controlled trial of faecal occult blood testing in the detection of colorectal cancer. Lancet 1983;2:1–4. [29]

Hardyck C, Goldman R, Petrinovich L. Handedness and sex, race, and age. Human Biol 1975;47:369–75. [10]

Harrell FE, Califf RM, Pryor DB, et al. Evaluating the yield of medical tests. JAMA 1982;247:2543–6. [25]

Harris EK. Distinguishing physiologic variation from analytic variation. J Chron Dis 1970;23:469–80. [28]

Harris EK, Cooil BK, Shakarji G, et al. On the use of statistical models of within-person variation in long-term studies of healthy individuals. Clin Chem 1980;26:383–91. [28]

Harris EL, Fitzgerald JD, eds. The Principles and Practice of Clinical Trials. Edinburgh: Livingstone, 1970. [29]

Hart G. Predictive value of serologic tests. Am J Public Health 1983;73:1288–92. [25]

Harvey M, Horwitz RI, Feinstein AR. Toxic shock and tampons: Evaluation of the epidemiologic evidence. JAMA 1982;248:840–6. [21, 22]

Harvey M, Horwitz RI, Feinstein AR. Diagnostic bias and toxic shock syndrome. Am J Med 1984;76:351–60. [21, 26]

Hastings PR, Skillman JJ, Bushnell LS, et al. Antacid titration in the prevention of acute gastrointestinal bleeding. N Engl J Med 1978;298:1041–5. [29]

Haybittle JL, Freedman LS. Some comments on the logrank test statistic in clinical trial applications. Statistician 1979;28:199–208. [17]

Haynes RB, Taylor DW, Sackett DL, eds. Compliance in Health Care. Baltimore: Johns Hopkins Univ Press, 1979. [16, Part Six, 27]

Healy MJR. Variation within individuals in human biology. Hum Biol 1958;30:210–8. [28]

Healy MJR, Goldstein H. Regression to the mean. Ann Hum Biol 1978;5:277–80. [28]

Hearey CD, Ury H, Sieglaub A, et al. Lack of association between cancer incidence and residence near petrochemical industry in the San Francisco Bay area. J Natl Cancer Inst 1980;64:1295–9. [24]

Heasman MA, Lipworth L. Accuracy of certification of causes of death. General Register Office, Studies on Medical and Population Subjects No. 20, H. M. Stationery Office, London, 1966. [21]

Heinonen OP, Shapiro S, Tuominen L, et al. Reserpine use in relation to breast cancer. Lancet 1974;2:675–7. [19]

Heller RF, Hayward D, Hobbs MST. Decline in rate of death from ischemic heart disease in the United Kingtom. Br Med J 1983;286:260–2. [24]

Henderson DA. The history of smallpox eradication. In: Lilienfeld AM, ed. Times, Places, and Persons. Baltimore: Johns Hopkins, 1980:99–108. [30]

Henderson M, Reinke WA. Analytical bias in studies of pregnancy outcome. Am J Obstet Gynecol 1966;96:735–40. [20]

Herbst AL, Ulfelder H, Poskanzer DC. Adenocarcinoma of the vagina. Association of maternal stilbestrol therapy with tumor appearance in young women. N Engl J Med 1971;284:878–81. [20]

Herbst AL, Kurman RJ, Scully RE, et al. Clear-cell adenocarcinoma of the genital tract in young females: Registry report. N Engl J Med 1972;287:1259–64. [23]

Herrera L. The precision of percentiles in establishing normal limits in medicine. J Lab Clin Med 1958;52:34. [28]

Hickey RJ, Clelland RC, Clelland AB. Epidemiological studies of chronic disease: Maladjustment of observed mortality rates. Am J Public Health 1980;70:142–50. [24]

Hill AB. Observation and experiment. N Engl J Med 1953;248:995–1001.[23]

Hill AB, ed. Controlled Clinical Trials. Oxford: Blackwell, 1960. [29]

Hill AB. Medical ethics and controlled trials. Br Med J 1963;1:1457. [29]

Hill AB. Reflections on the controlled trial. Ann Rheum Dis 1966;25:107–113. [29]

Hills M, Armitage P. The two-period cross-over clinical trial. Br J Clin Pharmacol 1979;8:7–20. [29]

Hinkle LE Jr, Dohrenwend BP, Elinson J, et al. Social determinants of human health. In: Preventive Medicine USA: Task Force Reports. New York: Prodist, 1976:617–74. [30]

Hinshaw HC, Feldman WH. Evaluation of chemotherapeutic agents in clinical trials: A suggested procedure. Am Rev Tuberculosis 1944;50:202–13. [29]

Hlatky MA, Pryor DB, Harrell FE Jr, et al. Factors affecting the sensitivity and specificity of the exercise electrocardiogram: A multivariable analysis. Am J Med 1984; 77:64–71. [25]

Hoffman RG. Statistics in the practice of medicine. JAMA 1963;185:864. [28]

Holmes OW. Currents and counter-currents in medical science. Annual meeting of the Massachusetts Medical Society. Boston, 1860. [29]

Hoover R, Gray LA Sr, Cole P, et al. Menopausal estrogens and breast cancer. N Engl J Med 1976;295:401–5. [11, 12]

Hoover RN, Strasser PH. Artificial sweeteners and human bladder cancer: Preliminary results. Lancet 1980;1:837–40. [22]

Horwitz RI, Feinstein AR. Alternative analytic methods for case-control studies of estrogens and endometrial cancer. N Engl J Med 1978;299:1089–94. [22]

Horwitz RI, Feinstein AR. Methodologic standards and contradictory results in case-control research. Am J Med 1979;66:556–64. [23]

Horwitz RI, Feinstein AR. Advantages and drawbacks of Zelen design for randomized clinical trials. J Clin Pharmacol 1980;20:425–7. [16]

Horwitz RI, Feinstein AR, Stremlau JR. Alternative data sources and discrepant results in case control studies of estrogens and endometrial cancer. Am J Epidemiol 1980;111:389–94. [22]

Horwitz RI, Feinstein AR. An improved observational method for studying therapeutic efficacy, with evidence suggesting that lidocaine prophylaxis prevents death in acute myocardial infarction. JAMA 1981;246:2455–9. [21, 23]

Horwitz RI, Feinstein AR. The application of therapeutic-trial principles to improve the design of epidemiologic research: A case-control study suggesting that anticoagulants reduce mortality in patients with myocardial infarction. J Chron Dis 1981;34:575–83. [16, 21, 23]

Horwitz RI, Feinstein AR, Horwitz SM, et al. Necropsy diagnosis of endometrial cancer and detection bias in case/control studies. Lancet 1981;2:66–8. [21]

Horwitz RI, Feinstein AR, Stewart KR. Exclusion bias and the false relationship of reserpine and breast cancer. Circulation 1981;64 (Suppl IV):42. [21]

Horwitz RI, Stewart KR. Effect of clinical features on the association of estrogens and breast cancer. Am J Med 1984;76:192–8. [22]

Horwitz RI, Feinstein AR, Harvey MR. Temporal precedence and other problems of the exposure-disease relationship in case-control research. Arch Intern Med 1984;144:1257–9. [22, 30]

Howard J, Friedman L. Protecting the scientific integrity of a clinical trial: Some ethical dilemmas. Clin Pharmacol Ther 1981;29:561–70. [29]

Howard J, Whittemore AS, Hoover J, et al. How blind was the patient blind in AMIS? Clin Pharmacol Ther 1982;32:543–53. [17, 29]

Huggins C. Endocrine-induced regression of cancer. Nobel lecture, December 13th 1966. In : Nobel lectures: Physiology or medicine. 1963–1970. New York: Elsevier, 1973:235–47. [11]

Hull RD, Carter CJ, Jay RM, et al. The diagnosis of acute, recurrent, deep-vein thrombosis: A diagnostic challenge. Circulation 1983;67:901–6. [25]

Hutchinson TA, Boyd NF, Feinstein AR. Scientific problems in clinical scales, as demonstrated in the Karnofsky index of performance status. J Chron Dis 1979;32:661–6. [26]

Hutchinson TA, Polansky SM, Feinstein AR. Post-menopausal oestrogens protect against fractures of hip and distal radius: A case-control study. Lancet 1979;2:705–9. [17, 23]

Hutchinson TA, Flegel KM, HoPingKong H, et al. Reasons for disagreement in the standardized assessment of suspected adverse drug reactions. Clin Pharmacol Ther 1983;34:421–6. [26]

Hylen JC, Kloster FE, Herr RH, et al. Phonocardiographic diagnosis of aortic ball variance. Circulation 1968;38:90–102. [19]

Hypertension Detection and Follow-up Program Cooperative Group. Five-year findings of the Hypertension Detection and Follow-up Program. I. Reduction in mortality of persons with high blood pressure, including mild hypertension. JAMA 1979;242:2562–71. [29]

Ingelfinger FJ. Significance of significant. N Engl J Med 1968:278; 1232–3. [19]

Institute of Medicine. Assessing quality in health care: An evaluation. Washington DC: National Academy of Sciences, 1976. [27]

The International Classification of Diseases, 9th Revision, Clinical Modification, ICD-9-CM. Ann Arbor: Commission on Professional and Hospital Activities, 1978. [13, 24]

Inter-society Commission for Heart Disease Resources. Primary prevention of the atherosclerotic diseases. Circulation 1970;42:A55–95. [29]

Irey NS. Diagnostic problems and methods in drug-induced diseases. Parts I, II, and III. Washington DC: American Registry of Pathology, Armed Forces Institute of Pathology, 1966, 1967, 1968. [17]

Jakobsson I, Lindberg T. Cow's milk as a cause of infantile colic in breast-fed infants. Lancet 1978;2:437–9. [29]

Jason J, Anderek N, Marks J, et al. Child abuse in Georgia: A method to evaluate risk factors and reporting bias. Am J Public Health 1982;72:1353–8. [21]

Jekel JF, Freeman DH, Meigs W. A study of trends in upper arm soft tissue sarcomas in the state of Connecticut following the introduction of alum-adsorbed allergenic extract. Ann Allergy 1978;40:28–31. [24]

Jenkins CD, Rosenman RH, Friedman M. Development of an objective psychological test for the determination of the coronary-prone behavior pattern in employed men. J Chron Dis 1967;20:371–9. [30]

Jick H, Vessey MP. Case-control studies in the evaluation of drug-induced illness. Am J Epidemiol 1978;107:1–7. [23]

Johnson FN, Johnson S, eds. Clinical Trials. Oxford: Blackwell Scientific, 1977. [29]

Johnstone DE, Wackers FJT, Berger HJ, et al. Effect of patient positioning on left lateral thallium-201 myocardial images. J Nucl Med 1979;20:183–8. [25]

Jones TD. The diagnosis of rheumatic fever. JAMA 1944;126:481. [13, 25]

Jonsen AR, Siegler M, Winslade WJ. Clinical Ethics. New York: Macmillan, 1982. [29]

Joyce CRB, Welldon RMC. The objective efficacy of prayer: A double-blind clinical trial. J Chron Dis 1965;18:367–77. [29]

Karch FE, Lasagna L. Adverse drug reactions: A critical review. JAMA 1975;234:1236–41. [17]

Karnofsky DA, Burchenal JH. The clinical evaluation of chemotherapeutic agents in cancer. In: MacLeod CM, ed. Evaluation of Chemotherapeutic Agents. New York: Columbia Univ Press, 1949:191–205. [26]

Kasl SV. Contributions of social epidemiology to studies in psychosomatic medicine. In: Kasl SV, Reichsman F, eds. Advances in Psychosomatic Medicine: Epidemiologic Studies in Psychosomatic Medicine. Basel: S Karger, 1977:160–223. [30]

Kasl SV. Mortality and the business cycle: Some questions about research strategies when utilizing macro-social and ecological data. Am J Public Health 1979;69:784–8. [24]

Kasl SV, Berkman LF. Some psychosocial influences on the health status of the elderly: The perspective of social epidemiology. In: McGaugh JL, Kiesler SB, eds. Aging: Biology and Behavior. New York: Academic Press, 1981:345–85. [30]

Kendall MG, Stuart A. The Advanced Theory of Statistics. New York: Hafner Press. Vol 1. Distribution theory. 4th ed. 1977. Vol 2. Inference and relationship. 4th ed. 1979. Vol 3. Design and analysis, and time series. 4th ed. 1983. [19]

Kessler II, Levin ML. The Community as an Epidemiologic Laboratory. A Casebook of Community Studies. Baltimore: Johns Hopkins, 1970. [15, 23]

Kessner DM, Kalk CE, Singer J. Assessing health quality—a case for tracers. N Engl J Med 1973;288:189–94. [27]

Keys A. Atherosclerosis: a problem in newer public health. J. Mt. Sinai Hosp. 1953;20:118–139. [24]

Keyser JW. The concept of the normal range in clinical chemistry. Postgrad Med J 1965;41:443–7. [28]

Killip T, Kimball JT. Treatment of myocardial infarction in a coronary care unit. Am J Cardiol 1967;20:457–64. [23]

Kish L. Survey Sampling. New York: Wiley, 1965. [18]

Kleinbaum DG, Kupper LL, Morgenstern H. Epidemiologic Research. Principles and Quantitative Methods. Belmont: Lifetime Learning Publications, 1982. [20, 23]

Klemetti A, Saxén L. Prospective versus retrospective approach in the search for environmental causes of malformations. Am J Public Health 1967;57:2071–5. [16, 22]

Kolata GB. Controversy over study of diabetes drugs continues for nearly a decade. Science 1979;203:986–90. [29]

Kolata GB. Love Canal: False alarm caused by botched study. Science 1980;208:1239–42. [30]

Koran LM. The reliability of clinical methods, data and judgments. N Engl J Med 1975;293:642–6, 695–701. [26]

Kraemer HC. Ramifications of a population model for κ as a coefficient of reliability. Psychometrika 1979;44:461–72. [26]

Kramer MS, Rooks Y, Pearson HA. Growth and development in children with sickle-cell trait. A prospective study of matched pairs. N Engl J Med 1978;299:686–9. [15]

Kramer MS, Leventhal JM, Hutchinson TA, et al. An algorithm for the operational assessment of adverse drug reactions. 1. Background, description, and instructions for use. JAMA 1979;242:623–32. [5, 17]

Kramer MS, Hutchinson TA, Rudnick SA, et al. Operational criteria for adverse drug reactions in evaluating suspected toxicity of a popular scabicide. Clin Pharmacol Ther 1980;27:149–55. [17]

Kramer MS, Feinstein AR. Clinical biostatistics: LIV. The biostatistics of concordance. Clin Pharmacol Ther 1981;29:111–23. [10, 26]

Kuhn TS. The Structure of Scientific Revolutions. 2nd ed. Chicago: Univ Chicago Press, 1970. [14, 16]

Labarthe D, Reed D, Brody J, et al. Health effects of modernization in Palau. Am J Epidemiol 1973;98:161–74. [18]

Labarthe D, Adam E, Noller K, et al. Design and preliminary observations of National Co-operative Diethylstilbestrol Adenosis (DESAD) Project. Obstet Gynecol 1978;51:453–8. [21, 22, 23]

Labarthe DR. Methodologic variation in case-control studies of reserpine and breast cancer. J Chron Dis 1979;32:95–104. [19, 21, 22]

Landis RJ, Koch GG. The measurement of observer agreement for categorical data. Biometrics 1977;33:159–74. [10]

Lanier AP. Cancer and stilbestrol: A follow-up of 1,719 persons exposed to estrogens in utero and born 1943–1959. Mayo Clinic Proc 1973;48:793–9. [23]

Lasagna L. The controlled clinical trial: Theory and practice. J Chron Dis 1955;1:353. [29]

Lasagna L. Some unexplored psychological variables in therapeutics. Proc R Soc Med 1962;55:773–6. [29]

Lee ET. Statistical Methods for Survival Data Analysis. Belmont: Lifetime Learning Publications, 1980. [17]

Levine A, Mandel SPH, Santamaria A. Pattern signalling in health information monitoring systems. Methods Inf Med 1977;16:138–44. [17]

Levine HG. Selecting and evaluating instruments. In: Morgan MK, Irby DM, eds. Evaluating Clinical Competence in the Health Professions. St. Louis: CV Mosby, 1978:33–51. [Part VI]

Levine RJ, Lebacqz K. Some ethical considerations in clinical trials. Clin Pharmacol Ther 1979;25:728–41. [29]

Levy RI, Moskowitz J. Cardiovascular research: Decades of progress, a decade of promise. Science 1982;217:121–9. [24]

Lew EA. Mortality and the business cycle: How far can we push an association? Am J Public Health 1979;69:782–3. [24]

Lewis CE. State of the art of quality assessment. Med Care 1974;12:799–806. [27]

Lichtenstein JL, Feinstein AR, Suzio KD, et al. The effectiveness of panendoscopy on diagnostic and therapeutic decisions about chronic abdominal pain. J Clin Gastroenterol 1980;27:567–78. [25]

Lilienfeld AM. Ceteris paribus: The evolution of the clinical trial. Bull Hist Med 1982;56:1–18. [29]

Lin KS, Kessler II. A multifactorial model for pancreatic cancer in man. JAMA 1981;245:147–52. [16]

Lind J. A Treatise of the Scurvy, in Three Parts. London: A. Millar, 1753. Reprinted in: Stewart CP, Gutherie D. Lind's Treatise on Scurvy. Edinburgh: University Press, 1953. [19, 29, 30]

Lionel NDW, Herxheimer A. Assessing reports of therapeutic trials. Br Med J 1970;3:637–40. [23]

Loeb HS, Pifarre R, Sullivan H, et al. Improved survival after surgical therapy for chronic angina pectoris. One hospital's experience in a randomized trial. Circulation 1979;60:I-22–30. [22]

Louis PCA. Researches on the effects of bloodletting in some inflammatory diseases and on the influence of tartarized antimony and vesication in pneumonitis. (Trans. Putnam CG). Boston: Hillard, Gray, 1836. [19, 29, 30]

Lundberg GD, Voigt GE. Reliability of a presumptive diagnosis in sudden unexpected death in adults. JAMA 1979;242:2328–30. [24]

Lynch HT, Guirgus H, Lynch J, et al. Cancer of the colon: Socioeconomic variables in a community. Am J Epidemiol 1975;102:119–27. [24]

McBride WG. Thalidomide and congenital abnormalities. Lancet 1961;2:1358. [12]

McCall MG. Normality. J Chron Dis 1966;19:1127–32. [28]

McDermott W, Rogers DE. Technology's consort. Am J Med 1983;74:353–8. [18]

McDonald TW, Annegers JF, O'Fallon WM, et al. Exogenous estrogen and endometrial carcinoma: Case control and incidence study. Am J Obstet Gynecol 1977;127:572–9. [16, 22]

McLachlan G, ed. A Question of Quality? Roads to Assurance in Medical Care. London: Oxford Univ Press, 1976. [27]

MacMahon B. Prenatal X-ray exposure and childhood cancer. J Natl Cancer Inst 1962;28:1173–91. [18]

MacMahon B, Yen S, Trichopoulos D, et al. Coffee and cancer of the pancreas. N Engl J Med 1981;304:630–3. [16, 20, 22]

McMichael AJ, Haynes SG, Tyroler HA. Observations on the evaluation of occupational mortality data. J Occup Med 1975;17:128–31. [17]

McNeil BJ, Keeler E, Adelstein SJ. Primer on certain elements of medical decision making. N Engl J Med 1975;293:211–5. [25]

McNemar Q. Note on the sampling error of the difference between correlated proportions or percentages. Psychometrika 1947;12:153–7. [9]

McPherson CK. On choosing the number of interim analyses in clinical trials. Statistics in Medicine 1982;1:25–36. [16, 30]

Mack TM, Pike MC, Henderson BE, et al. Estrogens and endometrial cancer in a retirement community. N Engl J Med 1976;294:1262–7. [22]

Mahon WA, Daniel EE. A method for assessment of reports of drug trials. Can Med Assoc J 1964;90:565–9. [23]

Mainland D. The clinical trial: Some difficulties and suggestions. J Chron Dis 1960;11:484. [29]

Mainland D. Elementary Medical Statistics. Philadelphia: WB Saunders, 1963. [Reprinted, 1978. Ann Arbor: Biometry Imprint Series Press] [9]

Mainland D. Remarks on clinical "norms." Clin Chem 1971;17:267–74. [28]

Maki DG. Through a glass darkly: Nosocomial pseudoepidemics and pseudobacteremias. Arch Inter Med 1980;140:26–8. [30]

Malawista SE, Steere AC, Hardin JA. Lyme disease: A unique human model for an infectious etiology of rheumatic disease. Yale J Biol Med 1984; (in press). [30]

Mancuso TF, Sterling TD. Relation of place of birth and migration in cancer mortality in the U.S.—a study of Ohio residents (1959–1967). J Chron Dis 1974;27:459–74. [24]

Mantel N, Haenszel W. Statistical aspects of the analysis of data from retropsective studies of disease. J Natl Cancer Inst 1959;22:719–48. [20]

Marks SH, Barnett M, Calin A. Ankylosing spondylitis in women and men: A case-control study. J Rheumatol 1983;10:624–8. [18]

Mates S, Sidel VW. Quality assessment by process and outcome methods: Evaluation of emergency room care of asthmatic adults. Am J Public Health 1981;71:687–93. [27]

May GS, DeMets DL, Friedman LM, et al. The randomized clinical trial: Bias in analysis. Circulation 1981;64:669–73. [29]

Mayes LC, Horwitz RI. Personal communication. 1984. [23]

Meadway J, Nicolaides AN, Walker CJ, et al. Value of Doppler ultrasound in diagnosis of clinically suspected deep vein thrombosis. Br Med J 1975;552–4. [25]

Medical Research Council. Streptomycin treatment of pulmonary tuberculosis. Br Med J 1948;2:769–82. [29]

Medical Services Study Group of the Royal College of Physicians of London. Death certification and epidemiological research. Br Med J 1978;2:1063–5. [24]

Mefferd RB, Pokorny AD. Individual variability reexamined with standard clinical measures. Am J Clin Pathol 1967;48:325–31. [28]

Meinert CL. Organization of multicenter clinical trials. Controlled Clin Trials 1981;1:305–13. [29]

Melton AW. Editorial. J Exp Psychol 1962;64:553–7. [19]

Messer J, Reitman D, Sacks HS, et al. Association of adrenocorticosteroid therapy and peptic-ulcer disease. N Engl J Med 1983;309:21–4. [29]

Metz CE, Goodenough DJ, Rossman K. Evaluation of receiver operating characteristic curve data in terms of information theory, with applications in radiography. Radiology 1973;109:297–303. [25]

Miettinen OS. Estimability and estimation in case-referent studies. Am J Epidemiol 1976; 103:226–35. [20]

Miettinen OS, Cook EF. Confounding: Essence and detection. Am J Epidemiol 1981; 114:593–603. [23]

Miller RG Jr. Simultaneous Statistical Inference. New York: McGraw-Hill, 1966. [9]

Miller RG Jr. Survival Analysis. New York: Wiley, 1981. [17]

"Minerva." News and notes. Br Med J 1977;1:1476. [24]

Mirkin G. Labile serum cholesterol values. N Engl J Med 1968;279:1001. [28]

Modell W, Houde RW. Factors influencing clinical evaluation of drugs with special reference to the double-blind technique. JAMA 1958;167:2190–9. [29]

Moertel CG, Schutt AJ, Go VLW. Carcinoembryonic antigen test for recurrent colorectal carcinoma. Inadequacy for early detection. JAMA 1978;239:1065–6. [25]

Monson RR. Occupational epidemiology. Boca Raton: CRC Press, 1980. [30]

Moriyama IM, Dawber TR, Kannel WB. Evaluation of diagnostic information supporting medical certification of deaths from cardiovascular disease. Natl Cancer Inst Monogr 1966;19:405–19. [24]

Morley AA. A neutrophil cycle in healthy individuals. Lancet 1966;2:1220–2. [28]

Morris JN. Uses of Epidemiology. 2nd ed. Edinburgh: E & S Livingstone, 1964. [30]

Moses LE, Oakford RV. Tables of Random Permutations. Stanford: Stanford Univ Press, 1963. [16]

Moss AJ, Davis HT, Odoroff CL, et al. Digitalis-associated mortality in postinfarction patients. Circulation 1983;68:III 368. [23]

Moussa MAA. Statistical problems in monitoring adverse drug reactions. Methods Inf Med 1978;17:106–112. [17]

MRFIT Research Group. Multiple Risk Factor Intervention Trial. JAMA 1982;248:1465–77. [11, 16, 21, 22, 29]

Murphy EA. The normal, and perils of the sylleptic argument. Perspect Biol Med 1972;15:566–82. [28]

Murphy ML, Hultgren HN, Detre K, et al. Treatment of chronic stable angina. N Engl J Med 1977;297:621–7. [16, 22, 29]

Mushlin AI, Appel FA, Barr DM. Quality assurance in primary care: A strategy based on outcome assessment. J Community Health 1978;3:292–305. [27]

Nagel JG, Tuazon CU, Cardella TA, et al. Teichoic acid serologic diagnosis of staphylococcal endocarditis: Use of gel diffusion and counterimmunoelectrophoretic methods. Ann Intern Med 1975;82:13–7. [25]

National Center for Health Statistics. Vital statistics instruction manual. Part 2. Cause-of-death coding for deaths occurring in 1968. Washington: US Government Printing Office, 1968. [24]

National Center for Health Statistics. Plan and operation of the Health and Nutrition Examination Survey, United States, 1971–1973. Washington: US Government Printing Office, 1973. (Vital and health statistics. Series 1, 10a, 10b) (DHEW Publication No. (HSM) 73-1310). [15]

National Institutes of Health. CEA as a cancer marker: National Institutes of Health Consensus Development Conference Summary. Vol 3. No. 7, 1981. [25]

Nelson AR. Orphan data and the unclosed loop: A dilemma in PSRO and medical audit. N Engl J Med 1976;295:617–9. [27]

Neustadt RE, Fineberg HV. The swine flu affair: Decision-making on a slippery disease. Washington DC: US Dept of Health, Education, and Welfare, 1978. [30]

New York Heart Association Criteria Committee. Diseases of the heart and blood vessels. Nomenclature and criteria for diagnosis. Boston: Little, Brown, 1964. [15]

Newcomer AD, McGill DB, Thomas PJ, et al. Prospective comparison of indirect methods for detecting lactase deficiency. N Engl J Med 1975;293:1232–5. [25]

Neyman J. Statistics—servant of all sciences. Science 1955;122:401. [17]

Nobrega FT, Morrow GW, Smoldt RK, et al. Quality assessment in hypertension: Analysis of process and outcome methods. N Engl J Med 1977;296:145–8. [27]

Nuland SB. The enigma of Semmelweis—an interpretation. J Hist Med Allied Sci 1979;34:255–72. [19]

O'Neill R, Wetherill GB. The present state of multiple comparison methods. J R Stat Soc (Meth) 1971;33:218–50. [9]

O'Sullivan JB, D'Agostino RB. Decisive factors in the tolbutamide controversy. JAMA 1975;232:825–9. [29]

Oliver MF, Heady JA, Morris JN, et al. A co-operative trial in the primary prevention of ischemic heart disease using clofibrate: Report from the Committee of Principal Investigators. Br Heart J 1978;40:1069–1118. [29]

Olsen DM, Kane RL, Proctor PH. A controlled trial of multiphasic screening. N Engl J Med 1976;294:925–30. [29]

Oreglia A, Duncan P. Health planning and the problem of the ecological fallacy. Am J Health Planning 1977;2(2):1–6. [24]

Osbakkan MD, Okada RD, Boucher CA, et al. Comparison of exercise perfusion and ventricular function imaging: An analysis of factors affecting the diagnostic accuracy of each technique. J Am Coll Cardiol 1984;3:272–83. [25]

Paradise JL, Bluestone CD, Bachman RZ, et al. Efficacy of tonsillectomy for recurrent throat infection in severely affected children: results of parallel randomized and nonrandomized clinical trials. N Engl J Med 1984;310:674–83. [15]

Paul JR. Clinical epidemiology. J Clin Invest 1938;17:539. [1, 30]

Paul JR. Clinical Epidemiology. Chicago: Univ Chicago Press, 1958. [1, 30]

Paul JR. Clinical Epidemiology. Revised edition. Chicago: Univ Chicago Press, 1966. [30]

Payne BC. The Quality of Medical Care: Evaluation and Development. Chicago: Hospital Research and Educational Trust, 1976. [27]

Pearl R. Introduction to Medical Biometry and Statistics. Philadelphia: Saunders, 1940. [24]

Percy C, Stanck E III, Gloeckler L. Accuracy of cancer death certificates and its effect on cancer mortality statistics. Am J Public Health 1981;71:242–50. [24]

Peto R, Pike MG, Armitage P, et al. Design and analysis of randomised clinical trials requiring prolonged observation of each patient. Br J Cancer I. Introduction and design. 1976;34:585–612 and II. Analysis and examples. 1977;35:1–39. [15, 17, 29]

Peto R. Clinical trial methodology. Biomedicine 1978;28:24–36. [29]

Philbrick JT, Horwitz RI, Feinstein AR. Methodologic problems of exercise testing for coronary artery disease: Groups, analysis and bias. Am J Cardiol 1980;46:807–12. [25]

Philbrick JT, Horwitz RI, Feinstein AR, et al. The limited spectrum of patients studied in exercise test research. JAMA 1982;248-2467–70. [5, 25]

Pitman EJG. Significance tests which may be applied to samples from any population. J R Stat Soc (Series B) 1937;4:119–30. [9]

Pocock SJ. Size of cancer trials and stopping rules. Br J Cancer 1978;38:757–66. [29]

Pocock SJ. Clinical Trials. New York: Wiley, 1984. [29]

Proudfit WL. Criticisms of the VA randomized study of coronary bypass surgery. Clin Res 1978;26:236–40. [16]

Pryor JP, Castle WM, Dukes DC, et al. Do beta-adrenoceptor blocking drugs cause retroperitoneal fibrosis? Br Med J 1983;287:639–41. [23]

Ramcharan S, ed. The Walnut Creek Contraceptive Drug Study: A prospective study of the side effects of oral contraceptives. Vol III. Washington: US Government Printing Office, 1981. [23]

Ramshaw WA, Latvis VF, Collins DD, et al. The use of a computer for data management in large-scale long-term cooperative studies. J Chron Dis 1973;26:201–17. [17, 29]

Ransohoff DF, Feinstein AR. Problems of spectrum and bias in evaluating the efficacy of diagnostic tests. N Engl J Med 1978;299:926–30. [5, 25]

Ratcliffe SG, Stewart AL, Melville MM, et al. Chromosome studies on 3500 newborn male infants. Lancet 1970;1:121–2. [28]

Reece RL. Effect of posture on laboratory values. N Engl J Med 1973;289:1374. [28]

Reger RB, Petersen MR, Morgan WKC. Variation in the interpretation of radiographic change in pulmonary disease. Lancet 1974;1:111–3. [26]

Reid DD. The design of clinical experiments. Lancet 1954;2:1293. [29]

Reid DD. International studies in epidemiology. Am J Epidemiol 1975;102:469–76. [24]

Report of the Committee for the Assessment of Biometric Aspects of Controlled Trials of Hypoglycemic Agents. JAMA 1975;231:583–608. [29]

Review Panel on Coronary-prone Behavior and Coronary Heart Disease. Coronary-prone behavior and coronary heart disease: A critical review. Circulation 1981;63:1199–1215. [30]

Richardson B, Epstein WV. Utility of the fluorescent antinuclear antibody test in a single patient. Ann Intern Med 1981;95:333–8. [25]

Rimland B, Callaway E, Dreyfus P. The effect of high doses of vitamin B_6 on autistic children: A double-blind crossover study. Am J Psychiatry 1978;135:472–5. [29]

Rimm AA, Bortin M. Clinical trials as a religion. Biomedicine 1978;28:60–3. [29]

Robboy SJ, Szyfelbein WM, Goellner JR, et al. Dysplasia and cytologic findings in 4,589 young women enrolled in Diethylstibestrol-Adenosis (DESAD) Project. Am J Obstet Gynecol 1981;140:579–86. [17]

Roberts RS, Spitzer WO, Delmore T, et al. An empirical demonstration of Berkson's bias. J Chron Dis 1978;31:119–28. [21]

Robinson WS. Ecological correlations and the behavior of individuals. Am Sociol Rev 1950;15:351–7. [24]

Rogan WJ, Milne KL. Correlation between cancers of the cervix and penis. J Natl Cancer Inst 1983;71:427. [24]

Rosner B. The analysis of longitudinal data in epidemiologic studies. J Chron Dis 1979;32:163–73. [28]

Ross S, Rodriguez W, Controni G, et al. Limulus lysate test for Gram-negative bacterial meningitis: Bedside application. JAMA 1975;233:1366–9. [25]

Rothman KJ, Fryler DC. Seasonal occurrence of complex ventricular septal defect. Lancet 1974; 2:193–7. [24]

Roueché B. The Medical Detectives. New York: Times Books, 1947. [30]

Royal College of General Practitioners. Oral Contraceptives and Health: An Interim Report from the Oral Contraception Study. London: Pitman Medical, 1974. [20]

Royal College of General Practitioners' Oral Contraception Study. Further analyses of mortality in oral contraceptive users. Lancet 1981;1:541–6. [23]

Rozanski A, Diamond GA, Berman D, et al. The declining specificity of exercise radionuclide ventriculography. N Engl J Med 1983;309:518–22. [25]

Rubin RT, Plag JA, Arthur RJ, et al. Serum uric acid levels: Diurnal and hebdomadal variability in normoactive subjects. JAMA 1969;208:1184–6. [28]

Rudnick SA, Feinstein AR. An analysis of the reporting of results in lung cancer drug trials. J Natl Cancer Inst 1980;64:1337–43. [13]

Ryle JA. Changing disciplines. Lectures on the History, Methods, and Motives of Social Pathology. London: Oxford Univ Press, 1948. [30]

Sackett DL, Gent M. Controversy in counting and attributing events in clinical trials. N Engl J Med 1979;301:1410–12. [15, 17, 29]

Sackett DL, Macdonald L, Haynes RB, et al. Labeling of hypertensive patients. N Engl J Med 1983;309:1253. [22]

Sanazaro PJ. Quality assessment and quality assurance in medical care. Annual Rev Public Health 1980;2:37–68. [27]

Sandler M, Ruthven CRJ, Goodwin BL, et al. Phenylethylamine overproduction in aggressive psychopaths. Lancet 1978;2:1269–70. [21]

Santen RJ, Worgul TJ, Samojlik E, et al. A randomized trial comparing surgical adrenalectomy with aminoglutethimide plus hydrocortisone in women with advanced breast cancer. N Engl J Med 1981;305:545–51. [16]

Sartwell PE, Masi AT, Arthes FG, et al. Thromboembolism and oral contraceptives, an epidemiologic case-control study. Am J Epidemiol 1969;90:365–80. [22]

Sartwell PE. Retrospective studies: A review for the clinician. Ann Intern Med. 1974;81:381–6. [23]

Schaffner W. Humans: The animate reservoir of nosocomial pathogens. In: Cundy KR, Ball W, eds. Infection Control in Health Care Facilities: Microbiological Surveillance. Baltimore: Univ Park Press, 1977:57–70. [30]

Scheaffer RL, Mendenhall W, Ott L. Elementary survey sampling. North Scituate: Duxbury Press, 1979. [18]

Schlesselman JJ. Case-control studies: Design, conduct, analysis. New York: Oxford Univ Press, 1982. [20]

Schor SS. The University Group Diabetes Program. A statistician looks at the mortality results. JAMA 1971;217:1671–5. [29]

Schor SS. Statistical problems in clinical trials. The UGDP study revisited. Am J Med 1973;55:727–32. [29]

Schwartz D, Lellouch J. Explanatory and pragmatic attitudes in therapeutic trials. J Chron Dis 1967;20:637–48. [29]

Schwartz D, Flamant R, Lellouch J. Clinical Trials. (Trans. Healy MJR). London: Academic Press, 1980. [29]

Schwartz TB. The tolbutamide controversy: A personal perspective. Ann Intern Med 1971;75:303–6. [29]

Seeff LB, Wright EC, Zimmerman HJ, et al. Type B hepatitis after needle-stick exposure: Prevention with hepatitis B immune globulin: Final report of the Veterans Administration Cooperative Study. Ann Intern Med 1978;88:285–93. [29]

Semmelweis IP. The Etiology, the Concept, and the Prophylaxis of Childbed Fever. 1861. Translated by FP Murphy. Birmingham: Classics of Medicine Library, 1981. [19, 30]

Severson RK, Davis S, Polissar L. Smoking, coffee, and cancer of the pancreas. Br Med J 1982;285:214. [22]

Shands KN, Schmid GP, Dan BB, et al. Toxic shock syndrome in menstruating women. N Engl J Med 1980;303:1436–42. [22]

Shapiro MF, Lehman AF, Greenfield S. Biases in the laboratory diagnosis of depression in medical practice. Arch Intern Med 1983;143:2085–8. [25]

Shapiro S, Venet W, Strax P, et al. Ten–fourteen year effect of screening on breast cancer mortality. J Natl Cancer Inst 1982;69:349–55. [17, 29]

Shapiro SH, Louis TA, eds. Clinical trials: Issues and approaches. New York: Marcel Dekker, 1983. [29]

Sheikh NE, Woolf IL, Galbraith RM, et al. e Antigen-antibody system as indicator of liver damage in patients with hepatitis-B antigen. Br Med J 1975;4:252–3. [25]

Sherwood T. Renal masses and ultrasound. Br Med J 1975;4:682–3. [25]

Siegel S. Nonparametric Statistics for the Behavioral Sciences. New York: McGraw-Hill, 1956. [9, 10]

Sigerist HS. The University at the Crossroads. New York: H Shuman, 1946. [30]

Siler JF, Garrison PE, MacNeal WJ. A statistical study of the relation of pellagra to use of certain foods and to location of domicile in six selected industrial communities. Arch Intern Med 1914;14:293–373. [19]

Silverstein AM. Pure politics and impure science: The swine flu affair. Baltimore: Johns Hopkins, 1981. [30]

Siscovick DS, Weiss NS, Hallstrom AP, et al. Physical activity and primary cardiac arrest. JAMA 1982;248:3113–7. [21]

Smits HL. The PSRO in perspective. N Engl J Med 1981;305:253–9. [27]

Snedecor GW. The statistical part of the scientific method. Ann NY Acad Sci 1950;52:792–9. [19]

Snow J. On the Mode of Communication of Cholera. London: John Churchill, 1855. Reprinted: New York: Commonwealth Fund, 1936. [19]

South-east London Screening Study Group. A controlled trial of multiphasic screening in middle-age: Results of the South-east London Screening Study. Int J Epidemiol 1977;6:357–63. [29]

Spence JC. Family studies in preventive pediatrics. N Engl J Med 1950;243:205. [30]

748   REFERENCES

Spitzer WO, Sackett DL, Sibley JC, et al. The Burlington randomized trial of the nurse practitioner. N Engl J Med 1974;290:251-6. [17, 27, 29]

Spitzer WO, Feinstein AR, Sackett DL. What is a health care trial? JAMA 1975;233:161-3. [13]

Spitzer WO, Hill GB, Chambers LW, et al. The occupation of fishing as a risk factor in cancer of the lip. N Engl J Med 1975;293:419-42. [22]

Spodick DH, Aronow W, Barber B, et al. Letter to the editor. J Chron Dis 1980;33:127-8. [29]

Stallones RA. Mortality and the Multiple Risk Factor Intervention Trial. Am J Epidemiol 1983;117:647-50. [22, 29]

Stampfer MJ, Goldhaber SZ, Yusuf S, et al. Effect of intravenous streptokinase on acute myocardial infarction. N Engl J Med 1982;307:1180-2. [29]

Starr I. Influenza in 1918. Recollections of the epidemic in Philadelphia. Ann Intern Med 1976;85:516-B. [30]

Statistical Research Group, Columbia University. Sampling Inspection. New York: McGraw-Hill, 1948, Chapter 17. [25]

Stravraky KM, Clarke EA. Hospital or population controls? An unanswered question. J Chron Dis 1983;36:301-7. [21]

Stern E, Clark VA, Coffelt CF. Contraceptive methods: Selective factors in a study of dysplasia of the cervix. Am J Public Health 1971;61:553-8. [15]

Streptomycin Committee, Central Office, Veterans Administration. The effect of streptomycin upon pulmonary tuberculosis. Am Rev Tuberculosis 1947;56:485-507. [29]

Stuart MJ. Aspirin and maternal or neonatal hemostasis. N Engl J Med 1983;308:281. [18]

Student (WS Gossett). The probable error of a mean. Biometrika 1908;6:1-25. [9]

Sullivan SN. Tribulations of a clinical trial. Can Med Assoc J 1981;125:1325-7. [29]

Sussman EJ, Tsiaras WG, Soper KA. Diagnosis of diabetic eye disease. JAMA 1982;247:3231-4. [26]

Syme SL. Behavioral factors associated with the etiology of physical disease. A social epidemiological approach. Am J Public Health 1974;64:1043-5. [30]

Szmuness W, Stevens CE, Harley EJ, et al. Hepatis B vaccine: Demonstration of efficacy in a controlled clinical trial in a high-risk population in the United States. N Engl J Med 1980;303:833-41. [29]

Taves DR. Minimization: A new method of assigning patients to treatment and control groups. Clin Pharmacol Ther 1971;15:443-53. [16]

Taylor KG. Hypocholesterolaemia and cancer? Br Med J 1983;286:1598-9. [23]

Tedeschi CG. Circadian challenges in "Quality control." Biochemical rhythms and spacial phenomena. Hum Pathol 1973;4:281-7. [28]

Temple R, Pledger GW. The FDA's critique of the Anturane Reinfarction Trial. N Engl J Med 1980;303:1488-92. [17, 29]

Terris M, ed. Goldberger on Pellagra. Baton Rouge: Louisiana State Univ Press, 1964. [19, 30]

Thacker SB, Choi K, Brachman PS. The surveillance of infectious diseases. JAMA 1983;249:1181-5. [30]

Therapeutic Trials Committee of the Medical Research Council. The serum treatment of lobar pneumonia. Lancet 1934;1:290-5. [29]

Thoburn R, Fekety FR, Cluff LE, et al. Infections acquired by hospitalized patients. Arch Intern Med 1968;121:1-10. [30]

Thomas L. An epidemic of apprehension. Discover 1983;4(11):78-80. [30]

Thompson WR. Biological applications of normal range and associated significance tests in ignorance of original distribution forms. Ann Math Stat 1938;9:281. [28]

Tukey JW. Some thoughts on clinical trials, especially problems of multiplicity. Science 1977;198:679-84. [9]

Turnbull LW, Turnbull LS, Crofton J, et al. Variation in chemical mediators of hypersensitivity in the sputum of chronic bronchitics: Correlation with peak expiratory flow. Lancet 1978;2:184-6. [10]

Tygstrup N, Lachin JM, Juhl E. The Randomized Clinical Trial and Therapeutic Decisions. New York: Marcel Dekker, 1982. [29]

Tyroler HA, Cassel J. Health consequences of culture change. II. The effect of urbanization of CHD mortality in rural residents. J Chron Dis 1964;17:167-77. [30]

Underwood EA. The history of the quantitative approach in medicine. Br Med Bull 1951;7:265. [29]

University Group Diabetes Program. A study of the effects of hypoglycemic agents on vascular complications in patients with adult-onset diabetes. Part I. Design, methods, and baseline characteristics. Part II. Mortality results. Diabetes 1970;19:747-830 (suppl 2). [12, 13, 15, 16, 22, 29]

Ibid. Part III. Clinical implications of the UGDP results. JAMA 1971;218:1400-8. (a) [29]

Ibid. Part IV. A preliminary report on phenformin results. JAMA 1971;217:777–84. (b) [29]

Ibid. Part V. Evaluation of phenformin therapy. Diabetes 1975;24:65–84. [29]

Varner MW. Efficacy of home glucose monitoring in diabetic pregnancy. Am J Med 1983;75:592–6. [29]

Vessey MP, Doll R. Investigation of relation between use of oral contraceptives and thromboembolic disease. Br Med J 1968;2:199–205. [22]

Vessey MP, McPherson K, Yeates D. Mortality in oral contraceptive users. Lancet 1981;1:549–50. [23]

Veterans Administration Cooperative Study Group on Antihypertensive Agents. Effects of treatment of morbidity in hypertension. II. Results in patients with diastolic blood pressure averaging 90 through 114 mm Hg. JAMA 1970;213:1143–52. [15, 29]

Veterans Administration Cooperative Urological Research Group. Carcinoma of the prostate: Analysis of patient morbidity at the 6-month, 12-month and 18-month follow-up examinations. J Chron Dis 1964;17:207–223. [17]

Veterans Administration Cooperative Urological Research Group. Treatment and survival of patients with cancer of the prostate. Surg Gynecol Obstet 1967;124:1011–17. [11]

Waife SO, Shapiro AP, eds. The Clinical Evaluation of Drugs. New York: Harper, 1959. [29]

Weinstein MC, Fineberg HV. Clinical Decision Analysis. Philadelphia: Saunders, 1980, [25]

Weintraub WS, Madeira SW, Bodenheimer MM, et al. A critical analysis of the application of Bayes' theorem to sequential testing. Circulation 1983;68:III-413. [25]

Weiss W. Heterogeneity in historical cohort studies: A source of bias in assessing lung cancer risk. J Occupational Med 1983;25:290–4. [20]

Welch BL. On the z test in randomized blocks and latin squares. Biometrika 1937;29:21–52. [9]

Welin L, Larsson B, Svärdsudd K, et al. Why is the incidence of ischaemic heart disease in Sweden increasing? Study of men born in 1913 and 1923. Lancet 1983;1:1087–9. [24]

Wells CK, Feinstein AR. Routine radiographic measurement and prognostic importance of rate of growth (auxometry) in patients with lung cancer. Clin Res 1977;25:266A. [15]

Wells CK, Stoller JK, Horwitz RI, et al. The prognostic impact of symptoms and comorbidity in the staging of endometrial cancer. Arch Intern Med 1984;144:2004–009. [17, 22]

Werf SDJ van der, Nagengast FM, Berge Henegouwen GP van, et al. Colonic adsorption of secondary bile-acids in patients with adenomatous polyps and in matched controls. Lancet 1982;1:759–62. [23]

Whitehead TP. Quality Control in Clinical Chemistry. New York: Wiley, 1977. [26, 28]

Whittemore S, Paffenbarger RS Jr, Anderson K, et al. Early precursors of pancreatic cancer in college men. J Chron Dis 1983;36:251–6. [16]

Wilcoxon F, Wilcox RA. Some Rapid Approximate Statistical Procedures. Pearl River: Lederle Laboratories, 1964. [9]

Wilks SS. Statistical prediction with special reference to the problem of tolerance limits. Ann Math Stat 1942;13:400. [28]

Willems JL, Poblete PF, Pipberger HV. Day-to-day variation of the normal orthogonal electrocardiogram and vectorcardiogram. Circulation 1972;45:1057–64. [28]

Williams RR, Stegens NL, Goldsmith JR. Associations of cancer risk and type with occupation and industry from the Third National Cancer Survey Interview. J Natl Cancer Inst 1977;59:1147–85. [30]

Wood HF, Stollerman GH, Feinstein AR, et al. A controlled study of three methods of prophylaxis against streptococcal infection in a population of rheumatic children. 1. Streptococcal infections and recurrences of acute rheumatic fever in the first two years of the study. N Engl J Med 1957;257:394–8. [16]

Wood HF, Feinstein AR, Taranta A, et al. Rheumatic fever in children and adolescents: A long-term epidemiologic study of subsequent prophylaxis, streptococcal infections, and clinical sequelae. III. Comparative effectiveness of three prophylaxis regimens in preventing streptococcal infections and rheumatic recurrences. Ann Intern Med 1964;60 (suppl 5): 31–46. [17]

Woolf B. On estimating the relation between blood group and disease. Ann Hum Genet 1955;19:251–3. [20]

World Health Organization. Arterial hypertension and ischaemic heart diseases. Preventive aspects. Technical report series 1962;231:3–28. [15]

Wright IS, Marple CD, Beck DF. Report of Committee for Evaluation of Anticoagulants in Treatment of Coronary Thrombosis with Myocardial Infarction: Progress report on statistical analysis of first 800 cases studied by this committee. Am Heart J 1948;36:301–15. [16]

Wulff HR. Rational Diagnosis and Treatment. Oxford: Blackwell Scientific Publications, 1976. [7]

Wyckoff J, Dubois EF, Woodniff IO. The therapeutic value of digitalis in pneumonia. JAMA 1930;95:1243–9. [29]

Wynder EL, Kabat G, Rosenberg S, et al. Oral cancer and mouthwash use. J Natl Cancer Inst 1983;70:255–60. [23]

Yano K, McGee D, Red DM. The impact of elevated blood pressure upon 10-year mortality among Japanese men in Hawaii—the Honolulu Heart Program. J Chron Dis 1983;36:569–79. [23]

·Yates F. Contingency tables involving small numbers and the χ^2 test. Supplement, J R Stat Soc 1934;1:217–35. [9]

Yates F. Theory and practice in statistics. J R Statist Soc (Series A) 1968;131:463–75. [19]

Yates F. Sampling Methods for Censuses and Surveys. 4th ed. New York: Macmillan, 1980. [18]

Yerushalmy J. A mortality index for use in place of the age-adjusted death rate. Am J Public Health 1951;41:907–22. [24]

Yerushalmy J, Hilleboe HE. Fat in the diet and mortality from heart disease. A methodologic note. NY State Med J 1957;57:2343–54. [24]

Yerushalmy J. On inferring causality from observed associations. In: Ingelfinger FJ, Relman AS, Finland M, eds. Controversy in Internal Medicine. Philadelphia: Saunders, 1966:659–88. [13]

Youden WJ. Index for rating diagnostic tests. Cancer 1950;3:32–5. [20]

Zelen M. The education of biometricians. Am Statist 1969;23:14–5. [19]

Zelen M. Play the winner rule and the controlled clinical trial. J Am Stat Assn 1969;64:131–46. [16]

Zelen M. A new design for randomized clinical trials. N Engl J Med 1979;300:1242–5. [16]

ANSWERS TO EXERCISES

Chapter 1

Answer 1.1. Because at least one of the denominators (the cases) is clinical and because the controls are commonly chosen from patients in the same medical setting as the cases, a strong argument can be made that this type of study really belongs to clinical epidemiology. Even when the controls come from healthy nonclinical persons, at least half of the study still has a clinical denominator.

On the other hand, the basic question here is really rhetorical and has no definite answer. As will be noted later, during detailed discussion of the retrospective case-control method, the technique seems to have been first used in the 19th century by epidemiologic clinicians studying causes of infectious disease and trying to test the Henle-Koch postulates of causation. Later on, the same approach was used in etiologic studies of chronic disease by public health epidemiologists who, with the help of statistical consultants, developed a complex set of mathematical indexes and analyses for the results.

Not understanding the mathematical strategies, clinical investigators have used the retrospective case-control technique only rarely and have generally regarded it as a classical public health epidemiologic activity. In recent years, however, clinical investigators have begun using case-control studies for answers to diverse questions beyond etiology alone and have also tried to reduce or eliminate some of the scientific defects contained in the classical approaches. Because the research today is being conducted by both types of investigators, the retrospective case-control study currently occurs in the domains of both classical and clinical epidemiology.

Answer 1.2. These questions are also intended to provide stimulating thought, rather than a divisive taxonomy. Almost any plausible answers can be satisfactory. The official answers are as follows:

1.2.1. Because the sites of the occupations are in the community, studies based on exposure or nonexposure are classical. Studies that follow the subsequent course of the diseased patients are clinical.

1.2.2. This is a classic activity of infectious disease epidemiologists.

1.2.3. Either answer or both can be correct. The patient denominators are clinical, but studies of infectious disease transmission are classical.

1.2.4. Because the community environment is studied for possible sources of exposure, the activity is classical. (If the research is concerned with the clinical spectrum, therapy, and subsequent course of the diseased people, the activity is clinical.)

Chapter 2

Answer 2.1. The studies described in Exercises 2.1.1. to 2.1.5 are all homodemic, because data for the same people will be directly related. Study 2.1.6 is heterodemic, because gross national product is not an entity observed in the individual people under study. The temporal arrangements are as follows:

2.1.1. Cross-sectional
2.1.2. Longitudinal
2.1.3. First part is cross-sectional; second is longitudinal
2.1.4. Longitudinal
2.1.5. First part is cross-sectional; second is longitudinal
2.1.6. Cross-sectional for each year.

Answer 2.2. Each of the projects is homodemic except for 2.2.5, in which two different groups of data were combined to form the numerators and denominators of the heterodemic death rates. Because of the implication that death followed the prescriptions, Project 2.2.5 is cited as longitudinal. The remaining citations are as follows:

	Brief Title	Purpose	Allocation	Temporal Status
2.2.1	Placental lactogen	Process	Survey	Cross-sectional for dysmaturity. ?Longitudinal for fetal distress. Longitudinal for neonatal asphyxia
2.2.2	Trigeminal neuralgia	Impact	Survey	Cross-sectional
2.2.3	Postoperative thrombosis	Impact	Experiment	Longitudinal
2.2.4	Leukocyte electrolytes	Impact	Survey	Cross-sectional
2.2.5	Safety of barbiturates	Impact	Survey	Longitudinal
2.2.6	Antenatal diagnosis	Process	Survey	Cross-sectional*
2.2.7	Urea treatment	Impact	Survey	Longitudinal
2.2.8	Mortality and anemia	Impact	Survey	Longitudinal
2.2.9	Radiographic interpretation	Impact†	Experiment	Cross-sectional
2.2.10	Liver scans	Process	Survey	Cross-sectional
2.2.11	Plasma prolactin	Impact††	Survey	Cross-sectional

*This study is cross-sectional rather than longitudinal because although the anencephaly may not be actually observed until later, it exists when the test is done.

†This is an impact experiment, in which the reversed chronology of films was a maneuver intended to make the radiologists change their minds. Because this type of maneuver differs from the usual causal intervention, the classification of temporal status is moot. It is here classified as cross-sectional, but a reasonable argument can be made for longitudinal.

††The assumption is that prolactin is a risk factor contributing to the etiologic development of breast cancer.

Answer 2.3. *Longitudinal experiment:* Controlled clinical trial comparing subsequent appearance of schizophrenia in children of mothers randomized to give either breast feeding or bottle feeding.

Longitudinal survey: Arrange to do long-term follow-up observations for appearance of schizophrenia in children of mothers who made their own decision about whether to breast feed. Compare rate of occurrence of schizophrenia in the breast-fed or non–breast-fed infants.

Cross-sectional survey: Assemble a case group of schizophrenics and a control group of nonschizophrenics, matched for age, race, and gender. Determine whether each of the people was or was not breast-fed. Compare the exposure rate in the two groups for the risk factor of non–breast feeding.

Heterodemic study: Assemble data on annual frequency rates of mothers who did breast feeding during a defined calendar period such as 1945 to 1965. Assemble data on annual occurrence rates of schizophrenia during a calendar period 20 years later, such as 1965 to 1985. See whether changes in rate of schizophrenia correlate with changes in rate of breast feeding.

Answer 2.4. The research is an impact study, because the causal action of sulfate is being contrasted against saline. The study is also experimental, because the compared agents are assigned randomly. The temporal status, however, is cross-sectional rather than longitudinal, because the effect under assessment is brief and transient. At the end of the experiment, each patient returns (or so the investigators hope) to the baseline state. This type of research is commonly conducted by clinical investigators whose major concern is a pathophysiologic explanation of biologic mechanisms rather than a therapeutic intervention in the course of health or disease. This type of pathophysiologic research is one of the few types of cause-effect experiment in which the temporal status is cross-sectional rather than longitudinal. Another type, cited in Exercise 2.2.9, is an experiment in which the impact is produced by an intervention intended to create temporary alteration in a physician's diagnostic reasoning.

Answer 2.5. This is a tricky issue, with complexities creating distinctions that have made various authors contend that every act of clinical therapy is analogous to an experiment. In the situation described here, the physician can assign the treatments that are carried out; he assigns them according to a predesigned plan; and he compares the treatments concurrently. He has thus fulfilled all the requirements of an experiment, according to Section 2.2.3. On the other hand, the plan does not call for comparing the treatments in similar groups of patients. Thus, patients in group A may receive diet; and a different kind of patient, belonging to group B, may receive oral agents, and so on. You could argue that the clinician's work would be a designed experiment if each group (A, B, C, and so on) had its members exposed to each form of treatment. If you make this argument, however, you are demanding *similarity of baseline state* as another criterion for regarding the comparison of maneuvers as an experiment. This demand seems reasonable, but it would deprive the word *experiment* from being used for randomized clinical trials in which (as we shall see later) the randomization, as an act of chance, did *not* produce similar baseline states for the compared groups.

Your best advice here might be to tell the physician that if the results are indeed worth reporting for each treatment, he should present them reportorially without any editorial implications that one treatment is superior to another. Because the treated patients were different at baseline, he cannot justify a claim of therapeutic superiority. If presented without such contentions, the results may be of considerable descriptive interest to other diabetologists and clinicians, even though the *J. Prest. Med.* may not want to accept the work for publication. The physician can then try submitting the paper to another journal that is willing to publish worthwhile reportorial data obtained without randomization.

Chapter 3

Answer 3.1.

The following problems occur when we try to set up a diagram that specifies a distinctive initial state, principal maneuver, and subsequent state for each of the cited research goals:

3.1.1. What is meant by "unusual family background"? Is the background regarded as an etiologic maneuver for a healthy initial state, or an outcome (subsequent) effect of schizophrenia?

3.1.2. What subsequent state will be noted as "superior"? (Survival time; medical complications; psychic comfort; esthetic appearance)

3.1.3. The basic objective here seems reasonably well specified. (We would need to know later, during implementation of the objective, about the kinds of patients, with and without colon cancer, who will be used for comparison.)

3.1.4. What is meant by "peculiar"? (That is, what constituents of serum do you plan to examine?) Do you regard these changes as a cause or effect of diabetes?

3.1.5. If baseline state is health and marijuana is the maneuver, what outcome will be assessed as "harm"? (Soma versus psyche; long-term versus short-term effects)

3.1.6. This is a policy decision, about which you might want to take a public opinion poll, but the question as such is not susceptible to scientific research.

3.1.7. If initial state contains different clinical conditions and if NMR is the procedure, what subsequent events will be assessed as benefits?

3.1.8. This objective seems well specified. During the subsequent implementation of the research, each constituent will require detailed definition.

3.1.9. The model we have discussed for comparative research is not pertinent for this stated objective, which is an issue in descriptive mensuration. If a "better" index is to be developed, its evaluation will depend on the mensurational goals.

3.1.10. Despite the vague statement, the main objective is clear. Input will be surgical specimens; procedure is the pathologist's examination; output is the pathologist's reading. (Main problem here is that the comparative agent is not known. Will the pathologist be tested for intra-observer variability, inter-observer variability, or conformity with a "gold-standard" pathologist's readings?)

3.1.11. The maneuvers will be different doses of Excellitol, but what kinds of clinical conditions and outcomes will be the inititial and subsequent states?

3.1.12. Are menstrual cramps an initial state to be treated with the Excellitol maneuver, or an outcome event to be prevented?

3.1.13. The research structure has problems similar to those of Exercise 3.1.7: What is to be regarded as the benefits? The main issue, however, becomes a matter of policy, rather than research, when we make a value judgment about "worth."

Answer 3.2.

3.2.1. This proposal has one problem in suitability and two problems in similarity. The problem of suitability arises in the initial state. Because surgery and radiotherapy were used to treat patients with cancer 20 years ago and also today, we shall need some careful thought about what kinds of patients will be entered into this study, which seems concerned only with chemotherapy. Assuming this problem is solved, we must deal with two problems in similarity. Were the patients of 20 years ago found and treated in the same stages of cancer as those treated today? (The comparison of survival rates can be greatly distorted if the patients 20 years ago were sicker or in later stages of cancer than the modern patients.) There is also a problem in similarity for the proficiency of therapy. Today's patients receive many types of supportive treatment (with blood products, antibiotics, steroids, and so on) that were not available years ago. How will the role of these ancillary agents be disentangled from the effect of the direct agents under comparison?

3.2.2. The main problem here is in suitability of the subsequent event. By choosing *survival* as the subsequent event, we may fail to detect many valuable contributions of CT scans to such important aspects of care as reassurance, comfort, and avoidance of hazardous invasive procedures. There is also a problem in similarity of initial states. Are the types of stroke admitted to hospital A similar to those admitted to hospital B?

3.2.3. The main problem here is in suitability of the initial state. Chicken soup is commonly employed at home for people who do not seek medical attention for the stated symptoms. The people who come to the doctor's office may be sicker than the stay-at-homes and less amenable to the chicken soup's beneficial impact. Consequently, by doing the study in doctors' offices, we may aim our research at the wrong group of people. You may also want to complain about the vagueness of the proposed comparative agent. What will be used as alternative forms of treatment?

Chapter 4

Answer 4.1
    4.1.1.

HEALTHY PERSONS ⟨ SMOKING / NO SMOKING → ⟩ BLADDER CANCER

    4.1.2.

NEWBORN BABIES ⟨ BREAST FEEDING / BOTTLE FEEDING → ⟩ INFECTIONS IN FIRST TWO YEARS OF LIFE

    4.1.3.

FERTILE — VASECTOMY → ⟩ STERILE OR NONSTERILE, (i.e., MOTILE SPERM)

(No control group is needed because the question refers to quantity in the outcome, not comparative efficacy of the maneuver.)
    4.1.4.

POPULATION RECEIVING MEDICAL CARE ⟨ PREPAID PRACTICE / FEE-FOR-SERVICE PRACTICE → ⟩ COSTS

    4.1.5. The diagram is difficult to draw because the question does not indicate what outcome is to be regarded as "useful." Is it a reduction in costs of therapy, in the patient's time away from work, in level of serum bilirubin, or in development of hepatic cirrhosis? Without specification of that outcome, all we can draw is

$$\text{CHRONIC ACTIVE HEPATITIS} \left\{ \begin{array}{c} \xrightarrow{\text{STEROID THERAPY}} \\ \xrightarrow{\text{NO STEROID THERAPY}} \end{array} \right\} \text{OUTCOME}$$

4.1.6. Because no comparison is sought, this is an issue in descriptive rather than comparative research. If any diagram is pertinent, it would be

$$\text{ELDERLY PEOPLE} \xrightarrow{\begin{array}{c}\text{MAINTENANCE IN}\\\text{NURSING HOME}\end{array}} \text{COSTS}$$

Answer 4.2.

4.2.1. The main form of susceptibility bias that might be considered here is the possibility that people who decide to smoke (or continue smoking) are also constitutionally more likely than nonsmokers to develop bladder cancer. The possibility seems far-fetched here, but it is still offered, sometimes with plausible arguments, as an explanation for some of the other diseases associated with smoking.

4.2.2. If the less healthy babies are more likely to develop infections than perfectly healthy babies, but are also more likely to have troubles in maintaining breast-feeding (or in bottle-feeding), a susceptibility bias will occur in data for the feeding group to which the less healthy babies are transferred.

4.2.3. Not pertinent.

4.2.4. Susceptibility bias will occur if people with an increased degree of sickness, who will require increased care and costs, deliberately seek treatment in a prepaid practice, or conversely, if such people are deliberately rejected from admission to such a practice.

4.2.5. Susceptibility bias will occur, regardless of the selected outcome, if the steroid treatment is given mainly to people with a particularly high (or low) degree of clinical severity in the chronic active hepatitis.

4.2.6. Not pertinent.

Answer 4.3. The BUN change before and after administration of agent A is merely a transition for each person. Without a control maneuver, we would have no idea of the transitions in BUN that can occur with other anesthetics or as a response to whatever surgery is done during the anesthesia.

Answer 4.4.

4.4.1. Because of referral patterns to hospitals in NYC, Bellevue receives a flotsam and jetsam "skid row" population, whereas New York–Cornell gets a more "elite" group. The derelicts with pneumococcal meningitis are usually comatose—a subgroup for which the mortality rate is about 50%. The "beautiful people" with pneumococcal meningitis are usually noncomatose—a subgroup for which the mortality rate is about 10%. The different hospital rates of death can thus readily arise from susceptibility bias in the disproportionate distribution of these two prognostic subgroups.

4.4.2. The complaint is based on an issue in performance bias for the principal maneuver. Because a high postoperative mortality rate was noted in the surgically treated patients, a conclusion was drawn that the V.A. surgeons were either still learning how to do the operation or were otherwise not as skillful as surgeons at other institutions. For this reason, the efficacy of the operation was regarded as not suitably tested in the V.A. study.

4.4.3. Perhaps the main problem among the many that could be noted here is the attitude of the students who take the National Board examination. The students who were previously exam-free, knowing that everything rides on their performance in the Board examinations, will study vigorously for it and may therefore do much better than the students from other institutions, who approach the "Boards" in a more relaxed manner, hoping only to pass. (The situation described here pertains at the Yale University School of Medicine, where the high performance of the exam-free students on their "Boards" has regularly been used as evidence of [a] the value of the exam-free program and [b] the good teaching done by the faculty.) If the diagram is drawn as follows,

$$\text{MEDICAL STUDENTS TAKING EXAM} \left\{ \begin{array}{c} \xrightarrow{\text{NO-EXAM SYSTEM}} \\ \xrightarrow{\text{OTHER SYSTEMS}} \end{array} \right\} \begin{array}{l}\text{SCORE ON}\\\text{PART I OF}\\\text{NATIONAL}\\\text{BOARDS}\end{array}$$

the problem can be catalogued as *performance bias,* due to an unrecognized co-maneuver: the extra studying and other preparations made by the no-exam students before taking the National Board examinations.

4.4.4. A problem in proficiency of the maneuver. The incubators used at the Charity Hospital were found to have had a faulty construction so that the oxygen leaked out and did not reach its destination. Thus, although prescribed, the high-dose oxygen was not really administered at that institution.

4.4.5. This particular trial—the University Group Diabetes Program (UGDP)—has been a fertile source of many controversies for almost 15 years. For the instance cited here, the main complaint is an issue of distorted assembly. By restricting the admitted population to adult-onset nonketotic diabetic patients, the investigators excluded the particular kinds of diabetes mellitus that many clinicians believe are most benefited from tight control of blood glucose. Thus, even if the comparisons conducted during the trial were valid (another dispute that is not under discussion here), the opponents argue that the results still cannot be extrapolated beyond the particular kinds of diabetic patients under study.

Chapter 5

Answer 5.1.

5.1.1. Let a panel of experts, using other data that exclude the radionuclide scan, decide by consensus whether the patient has acute cholecystitis. Better yet, because the main issue in suspected acute cholecystitis is whether to operate surgically, change the goal of the project to evaluate a management decision. Did the result of the radionuclide scan lead to surgical decisions whose outcomes were good or bad for each patient?

5.1.2. Without data from the invasive test of cardiac catheterization, no standard is available. A panel of experts can provide a consensus about the result of the scan but not an external reference standard. To achieve a standard here, the goal of the project would have to be aimed at the contribution the scan makes to some other decision, such as diagnosis, prognosis, or therapy.

5.1.3. Choose a single standard diagnosis for each specimen from the consensus of the participant pathologists (or from some other group of pathologists). Then see how each observer deviates from the consensus reading.

5.1.4. Use the same tactic as in 5.1.1. Let a panel of experts decide the diagnosis, without using the amylase test; or correlate the amylase result with the patient's outcome.

Answer 5.2. Choose a small set of conditions (sometimes called *indicator conditions* or *tracer conditions*) that can be the focus of evaluation. The conditions can represent the diagnostic management of certain ailments, such as urinary tract infections or head trauma, or the appropriate prescription of certain pharmaceutical substances, such as antibiotics or tranquilizers. Set up explicit criteria for management of these indicator challenges. Then see how they were managed by the audited clinicians.

Answer 5.3. Medical record data almost never include an account of the personal interchange between patient and clinician, although this interchange is one of the most important constituents of clinical care.

Answer 5.4.

5.4.1. Cause-effect.

5.4.2. The answer is disputable. If we regard cost as a consequence created by the intervention of care, it is an outcome; and the research is a cause-effect study. If cost is regarded as a concomitant aspect of care and if the patients' subsequent condition is the main outcome, then cost is part of the process of care.

5.4.3. Process.

5.4.4. Also disputable. If we regard patients' compliance as the outcome of the communicative process, the research is cause-effect; but if the patients' clinical conditions are the outcome of care, compliance is merely a contributory process.

5.4.5. Most clinicians would regard patient satisfaction as an important outcome event (thus making the evaluation a cause-effect study), but some might argue that patient satisfaction is merely part of the process.

5.4.6. Again, satisfaction of clinicians can be regarded as an outcome event in a suitably aimed cause-effect study—but such an outcome does not focus on the superiority of clinical care for the patients and is part of the process.

5.4.7. Same issue as in 5.4.6.

5.4.8. Another debatable subject. If outcome is what eventually happens to the patient, the detection of early disease is an activity in the process of care, not its outcome. For a true cause-effect study of the consequences of care, we would need to know the eventual results in the patients treated early.

Answer 5.5.

5.5.1. "Similar clinical conditions" would have to be clearly stipulated as *similar* in prognostic and therapeutic categories, not merely in general diagnostic categories, such as *coronary disease.* Criteria for "getting better" would have to be defined suitably and applied similarly in both groups.

5.5.2. Methods of determining cost must be similar in both groups; and the patients should present similar clinical conditions for which costs of care are being calculated.

5.5.3. Decisions about agreement with guidelines should be made blindly by someone unfamiliar with the patients' health care plan.

5.5.4. Decisions about degree of compliance should also be made blindly.

5.5.5. Index of satisfaction should be suitably defined and should be made as objective as possible. Blinding the investigator will not help avoid bias here, because the patients will know what form of care they received.

5.5.6. Same problem as in 5.5.5. Find an index of professional satisfaction that can be applied as objectively as possible but also usefully.

5.5.7. Aside from a problem in measuring "up-to-date," there is a problem analogous to susceptibility bias. Have clinicians who have an easy time keeping up-to-date, or who are particularly eager to do so, deliberately chosen to practice in one of the two compared health care plans?

5.5.8. No problem here as long as the patients are similar clinically and "early stage" is defined and categorized the same way in both groups.

Chapter 6

Answer 6.1. The observational characteristics create the basic difficulties encountered by an automaton in observing an image and converting it into data. In the case of an electrocardiogram, the automaton receives a voltage and does not view an image. The pattern of voltage is axially oriented (up-and-down), contains only two variables (height and time), has no distinctions of color or shading, and (unlike an electroencephalogram) has distinctively demarcated, usually repetitive patterns.

Answer 6.2. Automated recognition of patterns is difficult for major arrhythmias because of the complexity of the algorithms needed to describe places at which to start and stop in the succession of voltage segments that are to be converted into data. Successive tracings are difficult to automate because transition criteria for interpreting change have not been created as counterparts of the diagnostic criteria for interpreting a single tracing.

Answer 6.3. Let us assume that the two auscultators hear the same noise and call it a *systolic murmur,* and let us assume they agree on the various characteristics of loudness, quality, transmission, site of maximal intensity, changes of intensity in response to positional changes of chest, and so on. If so, the source of disagreement is different criteria for converting this set of designated elements into a diagnosis of *mitral regurgitation* versus *physiologic systolic murmur.* If the auscultators use the same diagnostic criteria for the conversion, then the difficulty lies in the basic observation and designation of the characteristics that are elements of the criteria. The disagreement over aortic regurgitation can involve both these problems (in designation and interpretation) but often arises from two others: (1) some physicians fail to "tune in" and may not hear a faint AR murmur; (2) the physician may be incorrect in the timing of a faint regurgitant murmur and call it systolic (and therefore physiologic) rather than diastolic. A further problem in interpretation is that both M.D.'s may hear and describe the same thing, but one regards the diastolic noise as so faint that he calls it an echo effect rather than a murmur.

Answer 6.4. Specimen mislabeled (wrong patient); specimen put into wrong type of tube (e.g., containing anticoagulant or other proscribed substance); specimen taken at wrong time (e.g., not fasting); reagents used in lab were improperly standardized; equipment used in lab was not correctly calibrated; lab technician did not add reagents in correct manner; error made in transcribing results by technician or by subsequent clerk (or key puncher).

Answer 6.5. All of the cited terms are conclusions or inferences about the evidence rather than descriptions of what was observed. Better replacements for the terms in parenthesis would be the following: pale (anemic); ammoniacal (uremic); Grade 4/6, blowing, holosystolic, etc. (mitral regurgitation); inspiratory (pleuritic); dry (dehydrated); 8 cm. below costal margin in midclavicular line (enlarged).

Answer 6.6.

6.6.1. An inmate of a state mental institution, when asked his identity, repeatedly answers, "I am Napoleon, Man of LaMancha, born on February 30, 1776." Another example, for dimensional data, is the following: The 0 point on a scale has been improperly placed at 100 gm. The scale is precise enough to read to 0.1 mg. and the skillful technician uses it consistently so that an object actually weighing 10 gm. is recorded as 110.0 gm., 109.9 gm., and 110.1 gm.

6.6.2. You want to know a patient's place of birth. He repeatedly says "Africa" and he has documents verifying that location, but he does not know the particular place or country.

6.6.3. This is a somewhat tricky question. Does "consistent" mean that the observational process yields the same results when it is repeated? If so, consistency cannot be determined if the entity under observation has been altered so that it is not the same when the second set of observations occurs. One example of this situation is the problem that would occur if we tried to measure the size of a melting ice cube. Another example would be the following scenario: At the conclusion of a particular patient's operation, a surgeon has dictated an operative note that contains an extensive description of everything that occurred. All of the personnel who were present at the operation concur that the description is entirely correct. The precise and presumably accurate data can not be checked for consistency because the operation will not be performed again for this patient.

If consistency refers to achieving the same result on a substance that *can* be measured repeatedly, we can cite the problem created by an alcoholic pathologist. When sober, he provides a magnificent description of the details noted in a specimen of tissue; and he is so highly respected by colleagues that his diagnostic conclusions are accepted as the authoritative standard in the field. These two attributes make him precise and accurate. Unfortunately, he is often drunk; and on such occasions he may disagree with the interpretations he previously gave to the same tissue.

Answer 6.7.

6.7.1. One main problem, as suggested in the text, is the thoroughness of the enumeration of blacks (or whites) in regions where census takers may be greeted with suspicion or hostility, so that people fail to register. A more likely possibility is that census takers may not want to spend protracted time in "unpleasant" regions (such as ghettos or barrios) and may thereby take incomplete counts. Another problem, in comparing annual enumerations, is whether the enumerating techniques have changed so that certain kinds of people are more (or less) likely to be counted. Finally, there is the fundamental problem of what is *black*. Is it a social, ethnic, pigmentary, or genetic condition? According to social customs, someone with seven pure-white great-grandparents and one pure-black great-grandparent is obviously more white than black but may regularly be categorized as black.

6.7.2. The problems are manifold and immense. The prime source of all the difficulty is that the information tabulated here is *not* the occurrence of these diseases. It is the occurrence of the diagnoses listed on death certificates. (For further details, see Chapter 24.)

6.7.3. The most overt problems here seem to be (1) do the cities have similar systems of surveillance for noting and recording serious crimes and (2) what is included as a serious crime? Is New Britain relatively free of crime, or are many crimes unreported or unrecorded? Also, because the cited list does not include arson, embezzlement, serious injuries caused by drunken driving, or child abuse, many people may wonder whether motor vehicle theft is a more serious crime than those that have been omitted.

Answer 6.8. The following answers are official, but many others might also be acceptable:

6.8.1. Diagnostic and therapeutic warning.

6.8.2. Etiologic suspicion.

6.8.3. Therapeutic warning.

    6.8.4. Diagnostic hint.
    6.8.5. Diagnostic hint.
    6.8.6. Diagnostic hint.
    6.8.7. Diagnostic hint and pathologic curiosity.
    6.8.8. New therapeutic procedure.
    6.8.9. Diagnostic hint.
    6.8.10. Diagnostic hint and etiologic suspicion.
Answer 6.9. Not all knowledge comes from experiments and control groups. Most of these 10 reports make immediate, important contributions to medical knowledge and to clinical practice by virtue of the various hints and warnings that are offered. The other papers act as clues for future research and as general intellectual stimulants. To insist that all studies be controlled is counterproductive pedantry; and to prevent such papers from being published would deprive clinicians and the public of valuable information.

Chapter 7

Answer 7.1.

Name of Variable	Type of Scale	Value for This Patient	Summary Indexes
Gender	Binary (or nominal)	Male	Proportions
Occupation	Nominal	Farmer	Proportions
Marital status	Nominal	Married	Proportions
Number of children	Dimensional	2	Median and ipr_{95} (or range)
Chief complaint	Nominal	Fever	Proportions
Duration of illness (mos.)	Dimensional	3	Median and ipr_{95} (or mean and s.d.)
White blood count	Dimensional	8700	Median and ipr_{95} (or mean and s.d.)
Urinalysis	Binary	Normal	Proportions

Answer 7.2. Mean $= \bar{X} = 129.14$; median $=$ 11th value $= 96$; geometric mean $= (9.916753488 \times 10^{42})^{1/21} = 111.54$; range $= 62$ to 400; standard deviation $= 88.72$ (calculated with $N-1$). The coefficient of variation is $s/\bar{X} = 88.72/129.14 = 0.69$. The inner 90-percentile range spans the distance between the 5th and 95th percentiles. Each data point here occupies 1/21 or 0.0476 of the distribution. The 5th percentile therefore occurs within the 2nd ranked value, and the 95th percentile occurs within the 20th ranked value. Thus, the ipr_{90} is from 78 to 310. The standard error is $88.72/\sqrt{21} = 19.36$. The 95% confidence interval is $129.14 \pm (1.96)(19.36)$ and runs from 91.19 to 167.09.

Answer 7.3. These data are obviously not Gaussian. In particular, if we used the Gaussian formula to get an inner 95% range, we would have $\bar{X} \pm 2s = 129.14 \pm (2 \times 88.72) = 129.14 \pm 177.44$. The span would go from an impossible -48.30 at the lower end to a high of 306.58, which does not include the two highest numbers (almost 10% of the data) at the upper end. The median of 96 is therefore the best choice for central tendency, although the geometric mean of 112 could also be suitable. For spread, because the ipr_{95} here is the same as the range, we could simply show the range.

Answer 7.4.
    7.4.1. Outcome is binary; therapy is nominal.
    7.4.2. $360/1055 = 0.34$.
    7.4.3. $50/345 = 0.14$.
    7.4.4. The overall total success rate is $160/1055 = .15$.

Answer 7.5. We want a 97.5% confidence interval around 0.55, and the lower limit should exceed 0.50. Let us assume the lower limit is 0.501. Then half of the confidence interval is $0.55 - 0.501 = 0.049$. Because this half of the interval equals Z_α times the standard error, and because $Z_{0.025} = 2.24$ (in Table 7–2), we can calculate standard error $= 0.049/2.24 = 0.021875$. Because standard error $= \sqrt{pq/N}$, we can calculate

$$(s.e.)^2 = \frac{pq}{N} , \text{ and}$$

$$N = \frac{pq}{(s.e.)^2} = \frac{(0.55)(0.445)}{(0.021875)^2} = 517.22$$

The political poll would require a sample of at least 518 people to achieve the desired results.
Answer 7.6. Let each candidate's raw score be X_i. From the array of candidate scores calculate $\bar{X}$ and s and then calculate $Z_i = (X_i - \bar{X})/s$ for each candidate. These results will have a mean of zero and s.d. of 1. To make the s.d. 100, multiply each Z_i by 100, to get $100Z_i$. The results will have a mean of zero and s.d. of 100. Then add 500 to each $100Z_i$. The results will have a mean of 500 and s.d. of 100. Thus the formula is: Final score = $[100(X_i - \bar{X})/s] + 500$.
Practical demonstration of the formula:
Three candidates get 75, 83, and 92 in the raw scores. For these data, $\bar{X} = 83.33$ and s = 8.50. The original Z_i scores for the three candidates will be $(75 - 83.33)/8.50 = -0.98$, $(83 - 83.33)/8.50 = -0.04$, and $(92 - 83.33)/8.50 = 1.02$. Multiplied by 100, these scores become -98, -4, and 102. When 500 is added, the scores become 402, 496, and 602. For these three values, a check on your calculator will confirm that $\bar{X} = 500$ and s = 100.
Answer 7.7.
   7.7.1. Z = $(114 - 101.6)/5.2 = 2.38$. According to Table 7–2, the one-tailed exterior proportion is 0.0125 for Z = 2.24 and 0.006 for Z = 2.5. For Z = 2.38, the proportion lies between 0.0125 and 0.006. The probability is between 0.6% and 1.25%.
   7.7.2. For an interior zone of 90%, Table 7–2 shows that Z_α is 1.645. Therefore, the inner zone is $101.6 \pm (1.645)(5.2) = 101.6 \pm 8.55$. It extends from 93.0 to 110.2.
   7.7.3. Z = $(88.6 - 101.6)/5.2 = -2.5$. From Table 7–2, we see that 0.006 of patients would have even smaller values of Z. (Because the table refers to positive values of Z, things have to be reversed for negative values.)
Answer 7.8. The laboratory is trying to indicate a 95% interval for the range of the observed data, but the phrase "95% confidence interval" refers to dispersion around an estimate of the mean, not to dispersion of the data. The correct phrase should be simply "range of normal" or "customary inner 95% range." The word *confidence* should be used only in reference to the location of a *mean* (or proportion).

Chapter 8

Answer 8.1. Different people will offer different arguments for these answers, and, assuming that the argument is rational and reasonable, everyone can be correct. One set of responses is as follows:
   8.1.1. The criterion is a ratio of at least 1.20 and an increment of at least 10%. Because 55% success offers an increment of 10% and a ratio of 55/45 = 1.22, it can be the boundary.
   8.1.2. Because mortality is already low, much of the decision will depend on the risks and inconvenience of the active treatment. Assuming that reduction in mortality (rather than increase in survival) is the point here, a purely quantitative approach is to seek a proportionate incremental reduction of at least 25%. This would lower the 12% to 9% or less.
   8.1.3. Assuming that we are not denied permission to calculate a dimensional mean for these ordinal grades, at least a 50% proportionate increment (i.e., a ratio of 1.5) could be sought for the active group. Because $1.3 \times 1.5 = 1.95$, the treated group should have a mean of about 2.0 or higher.
   8.1.4. The answer to this question ought to produce a rousing discussion in class. Suppose you choose a risk ratio of 2. The rate in the treated group will be 0.002, and the incremental risk will be $0.002 - 0.001 = 0.001$. For a risk ratio of 10, the incremental risk will be only $0.01 - 0.001 = 0.09$. Are these incremental risks scary enough to make you want to let the distressing menopausal symptoms return? Besides, who should make that decision: you or the patient? Many clinicians would tell a woman about the ratios and incremental risks, and then let her make the choice.

Answer 8.2. Death rates for cardiovascular causes are 3.5% (= 10/205) for placebo and 12.7% (= 26/204) for tolbutamide. The corresponding death rates for noncardiovascular causes are 5.3% for placebo and 2.0% for tolbutamide. Probably the best expression is to give *total* death rates, which are 10.2% (= 21/205) for placebo and 14.7% (= 30/204) for tolbutamide. These data do not lend themselves to expression in a single index of contrast, and most clinicians would want to know the individual death rates for each treatment.

Answer 8.3. This was a trap question. If you fell in the trap, please use it as a learning experience. Because the research is a case-control study, with the groups assembled according to outcomes, not maneuvers, the risk of breast cancer cannot be determined for users and nonusers. Thus, you cannot calculate an incremental risk or a risk ratio from these results. If you tried to do this inappropriate calculation, you would find the rate of breast cancer in nonusers to be 139/1313 = 11%. If true, this would represent an extraordinary and almost overwhelming epidemic of breast cancer in the general population. A more suitable thing to do with these data is to compare the prevalence of reserpine usage in cases and controls. The results would be, respectively, 7.3% (= 11/150) in cases and 2.2% (= 26/1200) in controls. Actually, the best thing to do here is to calculate an odds ratio as $(11 \times 1174)/(26 \times 139) = 3.57$. For reasons mentioned briefly in the text and discussed later in Chapter 20, the odds ratio—if no distortions have occurred—would approximate the risk ratio for breast cancer in reserpine users. If you calculated the incremental risk as 19% $[= 30\% - 11\% = (11/37) - (139/1313)]$, the arithmetic was right, but the science was wrong.

Answer 8.4.

    8.4.1. Prevalence.

    8.4.2. Incidence.

    8.4.3. Because 350 people received B and 705 did not, the odds in favor of B are 350/705 or about 1:2.

    8.4.4. Because odds cannot be construed as a rate, the result is neither prevalence nor incidence. Of the two alternatives, however, *prevalence* is the better idea.

    8.4.5. Failure rates are 320/360 = 0.89 for A and 280/350 = 0.80 for B. Risk ratio for failure with B is 0.80/0.89 = 0.90. Success rates are 40/360 = 0.11 for A and 50/345 = 0.14 for C. Risk ratio for success with C is 0.14/0.11 = 1.30.

    8.4.6. Failure odds are 280/70 for B and 320/40 for A. Odds ratio is $(280/70) \div (320/40) = 0.5$. Success odds are 50/295 for C and 40/320 for A. Odds ratio is $(50/295) \div (40/320) = 1.36$.

Answer 8.5. The percentages show the proportionate distribution of age groups in the spectrum of omphalosis at the medical center. The composition of this spectrum may be greatly affected by referral patterns to that center. The actual occurrence rates of omphalosis in the various age groups of the general population are not shown by these results.

Chapter 9

Answer 9.1. The correct statement is 9.1.3. Statement 9.1.1 is close to correct, but it is based on the impossible idea that we could actually repeat this trial 1000 times. Statement 9.1.2 is overtly wrong because it describes a quantitative magnitude or frequency, not a stochastic probability. Statement 9.1.4 has erroneously converted a stochastic probability into odds for an undefined outcome as "effective"; but even if this conversion were justified, the odds were calculated improperly. For a probability of 1/1000, the odds are 999 to 1, not 1000 to 1. Statement 9.1.5 is presumptuous in claiming that the stochastic test allows a scientific conclusion about efficacy. The stochastic test merely validates the numerical distinction as being a nonchance event; we would need to know more about the scientific structure of the trial before forming the scientific conclusion. Statement 9.1.6 is a perversion of the statistical concept of *power*. The idea of *power* applies to tests for Type-II error under an alternative hypothesis and is not pertinent for the cited distinction.

Answer 9.2. The one-tailed argument would be that we ordinarily expect a placebo to have a lower rate of *adverse* reactions than an active agent. The two-tailed argument is that this expectation, although customary, may not be pertinent for this particular clinical situation. Unless more information is provided to allow a more specific hypothesis here, the test should be two-tailed.

Answer 9.3. The observed difference in pain relief scores is -0.6, which is a proportionate reduction of $-0.6/2.3 = -26\%$. This quantity cannot readily be dismissed as trivial. For the t test, the respective standard errors are $0.8/\sqrt{6} = 2.449$ and $0.9/\sqrt{7} = 2.646$. The pooled variance is $s_p^2 = [5(0.8)^2 + 6(0.9)^2]/(6+7-2) = 1.073$, and the variance of the difference in means is $s_C^2 = [(1/6)+(1/7)](1.073) = 0.332$. Since the value of t is $-0.6/\sqrt{0.332} = 1.04$, the distinction is not stochastically significant. Nevertheless, if we put a 95% confidence interval around the difference, we get $-0.6 \pm (t_{11,.05})(\sqrt{0.332}) = -0.6 \pm (2.20)(0.576)$. The interval goes from -1.87 to $+0.67$. At its lower end, the difference of -1.87 would give the new agent a mean pain relief score of only $2.3 - 1.87 = 0.43$. The claim of "similar efficacy" would be hard to sustain.

A quicker but coarse way of examining this same issue is to put crude 95% confidence intervals around each mean and then to compare the two extreme values. For the new agent, the standard error of the mean is $0.8/\sqrt{6} = 0.327$, and its 95% confidence interval can be found crudely, using $Z_{0.05} = 1.96$, from $(1.96)(0.327) = 0.640$. The lower boundary would be $1.7 - 0.640 = 1.06$. For the standard agent, the s.e. is $0.9/\sqrt{7} = 0.340$; and $(1.96)(0.340) = 0.667$. The upper boundary would be $2.3 + 0.667 = 2.97$. The difference of $2.97 - 1.06 = 1.91$ is impressive (and not far off the -1.87 found with the t values).

Either approach would make us reluctant to accept the contention that similar efficacy has been demonstrated.

Answer 9.4. $X^2 = 3.4 = [(12^2/43) + (5^2/42) - (17^2/85)] \times [85^2/(17)(68)]$ with Equation 9.15, and $[(12)(37) - (5)(31)]^2 85/[(42)(43)(17)(68)]$ with Equation 9.14. Because a value of 3.84 is required for stochastic significance, the two-tailed P value is <0.1 but not <0.05. If you insist on a one-tailed interpretation, however, this value of X^2 will be <0.05.

Answer 9.5. The distinction in the fractured femur group is 26% versus 19% and is not particularly impressive quantitatively. Stochastically, it is not significant, because X^2 for 7/27 versus 5/26 is 0.34. The distinction in the hip replacement group is striking, however, as 31% versus 0%. These small numbers are best tested with the Fisher test; and the calculation is easy because we start with the extreme table and have only that one to consider. Using Equation 9.1, we have $P = (16! \times 16! \times 5! \times 27!)/(5! \times 11! \times 0! \times 16! \times 32!) = 0.02$. This is a one-tailed value. Because each group has 16 members, we can double the result and have 0.04 as the two-tailed value. The stratified results are entirely consistent with the basic conclusion formed in Answer 9.4, and they help fortify it—although they suggest that the preoperative corticotrophin gel is probably worthwhile only in the patients having hip replacement.

Chapter 10

Answer 10.1.

   10.1.1. First determine the median value for each of the three variables. It is 33.8 for peak expiratory flow rate (PEFR), 0.51 for histamine, and 3.8 for eosinophils. Next, after classifying each patient's values as being above or below the median for that variable, arrange a 2×2 table for the relationship of PEFR and the other two variables. (You can put the median in with the low or the high group. In the first set of results here, the medians are in the low group.) The two tables are as follows:

PEFR	Histamine Low	High	Eosinophils Low	High
Low	5	1	3	3
High	1	4	3	2

If the medians are put in the high group, the tables show the following:

PEFR	Histamine Low	High	Eosinophils Low	High
Low	3	2	2	3
High	2	4	3	3

With either pair of arrangements, no correlation is apparent between PEFR and eosinophils. In the first arrangement, however, and somewhat in the second, histamine and PEFR seem to have a positive rather than negative correlation. This would not contradict the authors' claims, but might make us suspicious enough to check the calculations carefully in Answer 10.1.2.

10.1.2. We can directly check the claims by determining the correlation coefficient for the relationships. If we let PEFR be represented by Y, histamine by X, and eosinophils by W, the basic information is as follows:

$$\begin{aligned}
\Sigma Y &= 407.1 & ; & & S_{yy} &= 2956.0491 \\
\Sigma X &= 7.9 & ; & & S_{xx} &= 3.011164 \\
\Sigma W &= 126.5 & ; & & S_{ww} &= 2168.98 \\
\Sigma XY &= 351.77 & ; & & \Sigma WY &= 4144.54 \\
S_{xy} &= 59.398 & ; & & S_{wy} &= -537.11
\end{aligned}$$

The correlation coefficient for PEFR and histamine is

$$r_{xy} = \frac{S_{xy}}{\sqrt{S_{xx}S_{yy}}} = 0.630$$

The correlation coefficient for PEFR and eosinophils is

$$r_{wy} = \frac{S_{wy}}{\sqrt{S_{ww}S_{yy}}} = -0.212$$

Consistent with what we found in Answer 10.1.1, the detailed calculations show a high positive correlation (0.63) between PEFR and histamine and a small negative correlation (-0.212) between PEFR and eosinophils. The authors' claims do not seem substantiated by these calculations.

10.1.3. The main problem here is that the relationships have been examined separately for each variable with PEFR. If histamine and eosinophils are highly correlated, however, the univariate tests may be misleading. We do not yet know how to test PEFR versus the other two variables simultaneously, but we can see if they correlate with one another. The correlation coefficient for histamine and eosinophils is $r_{wx} = S_{wx}/\sqrt{S_{ww}S_{xx}}$. The value of ΣWX is 62.838 and so S_{wx} turns out to be -28.012. Therefore $r_{wx} = -0.347$, and a modest negative correlation exists between histamine and eosinophils.

Answer 10.2. Perhaps the simplest approach here is to compare the proportion of left-handers among boys and girls. It is 10.5% ($= 417/3960$) for boys and 8.7% ($= 324/3728$) for girls. The increment is 1.8%; and the ratio is 1.21. You may or may not want to regard this as a quantitatively significant distinction. Regardless of its quantitative importance, the result is stochastically significant because $X^2 = [(3543 \times 324) - (417 \times 3404)]^2 \times 7688/(6947)(741)(3728)(3960)] = 7.46$; and so P<0.01. You could calculate ϕ^2 as $X^2/N = 7.46/7688 = 0.00097$ and $\phi = 0.03$, thus indicating a very weak association. You can then decide whether you want to draw your final conclusion from the stochastic value of P<0.01, from the correlation coefficient of 0.03, or from the ratio of 1.21. It's dealer's choice. The original investigators stated that "even though this association is significant, it seems of little importance."

Answer 10.3. This problem, which does not involve statistical association, is put here to remind you of descriptive issues that can occur under various disguises.

You can approach this problem in two different but basically similar ways. The first way is to assign arbitrary numbers to grades expressed in categories or letters. For example, the A, B, C, D, E grades could be called 5, 4, 3, 2, 1. The high honors, honors, pass, fail grades could be called 4, 3, 2, 1. Using these numerical values for each clerkship, transform the grades of each clerkship into standardized Z-scores. These Z-scores are commensurate and can be added for the results of each clerkship. The class can then be ranked according to each person's total for the five Z-scores.

The second way is even simpler and requires little or no calculation. Instead of computing the Z-scores for each clerkship, rank the students for their grades in that clerkship. If several people have the same grade, give them the appropriate value of the tied rank, as discussed in Section 7.2.3.3. For example, suppose the class contains 20 students. In Psychiatry, five of the students were rated *superior*, 11 were *satisfactory*, and four *failed*. The first five students, who are tied for the ranks of *1* through *5*, are all given the rank of *3*. The next 11 students, who are tied for the ranks of *6* through *16*, are each ranked as *11*. The last four students, tied for the ranks of *17* through *20*, are each ranked as *18.5*. (To check the accuracy of these assigned ranks, we would expect the sum of ranks to be $(20 \times 21)/2 = 210$. In our assignments here, the sum is $(5 \times 3) + (11 \times 11) + (4 \times 18.5) = 210$.) After the rankings are determined for each of the five clerkships, the students' scores will be the sum of the rankings. These total scores can then be ranked to provide the class standing.

Answer 10.4.

10.4.1. In the first table, the results are tied in 80 patients. For the 12 patients where the results differ, we can compute the McNemar Bias Index as a way of indicating that drug B seemed more likely to be associated with no pain than drug A. If the two drugs are equal, this ratio should be close to zero. Its value here is $(10 - 2)/12 = 8/12 = 0.67$. The result is difficult to interpret, however, because it ignores the 80 patients in whom the two drugs gave equal results.

To obtain an overall result for each drug, we can turn to the second table and see that the success rate for "no pain" was 54% ($= 50/92$) with drug A and 46% ($= 42/92$) for drug B. This result is easier to understand, but it does not make use of the cross-over matching design.

An intriguing way to use this design is to eliminate the patients who had pain with both drugs. In patients capable of achieving pain relief with either drug, the rates of success would then be 96% ($= 50/52$) with drug B and 81% ($= 42/52$) with drug A. This arrangement might be disdained by many statisticians, because it was not part of the original design, but it might be the most clinically meaningful expression of the results.

Measures of association, such as ϕ, would not be a particularly informative way of citing these results.

10.4.2. The stochastic test here depends on which arrangement we used for expressing the results. In the first expression cited in Exercise 10.4.1, the appropriate test would be McNemar's Chi-Square, as described in Section 9.4.2.7.2. Using the formula $X_M^2 = (b - c)^2/(b + c)$, we would get $(10 - 2)^2/12 = 5.3$ for X_M^2. (Some statisticians prefer a Yates-like correction here, and calculate X_M^2 as $(|b - c| - 1)^2/(b + c)$. With this calculational formula, X_M^2 is $(|10 - 2| - 1)^2/12 = 49/12 = 4.1$. With either calculation, the associated P value is <0.05.

For the comparison of 50/92 versus 42/92, the standard X^2 turns out to be $[(50 \times 50) - (42 \times 42)]^2 \times 184/92^4 = 1.4$. This result is *not* stochastically significant.

For the comparison of 50/52 versus 42/52, X^2 turns out to be 6.0, and the result *is* stochastically significant. (If you decide to use the Yates correction, X_c^2 is 4.6, and the result is still stochastically significant.)

We thus have three different ways of approaching the calculation, and the results disagree. You might argue that the third approach is unsatisfactory because it involves *post hoc* classifications; and that the second approach is unsatisfactory because it counts each patient twice, making it seem as though 184 people were tested rather than 92. On the other hand, the first approach seems unsatisfactory because it is based on the 12 people who remain after we throw out the 80 patients whose results were similar for both drugs.

The main point is that there is no *ideal* analysis for this problem. The McNemar procedure, i.e., the first approach, is generally recommended by statisticians, but the *scientific* interpretation of the results is uncertain. My own preference would be to use the third approach, but many statisticians would reject it as a *post hoc* activity, although the removal of the 80 tied patients in the statistical format of the McNemar calculations is also a *post hoc* activity.

If you are troubled by all this ambiguity, you may regard it as a useful lesson in the realities of data analysis. When we say "there is more than one way to skin a cat," we assume that the same cat emerges underneath the removed skin. In many types of data analysis, however, a different cat comes out with each type of dissection, and you then have to decide which one you like most. We shall meet many more of these ambiguities later in other aspects of policy or formulas for data analysis.

Answer 10.5. The percentage agreement is $80/92 = 0.87$. A better expression would be kappa, calculated as $2(ad - bc)/[n_1f_2 + n_2f_1] = 2[(40 \times 40) - (2 \times 10)]/[(50 \times 50) + (42 \times 42)] = 0.74$. If calculated as $[N(a + bd) - (n_1f_1 + n_2f_2)]/[N^2 - (n_1f_1 + n_2f_2)]$, we get $K = [92(80) - \{(42 \times 50) + (42 \times 50)\}]/[92^2 - \{(42 \times 50) + (42 \times 50)\}] = 0.74$. With either result, the agreement seems quite good.

Chapter 11

Answer 11.1

Original Designation of Exercise	Principal Maneuver	Function	Reality of Maneuver
2.2.2	Religion, drinking, smoking	Etiologic	Virtual
2.2.3	Phenformin and ethylestrenol	Contrapathic	Actual
2.2.4	Heart disease	Pathodynamic	Virtual
2.2.5	Barbiturate	Etiologic, i.e., adverse effect	Virtual
2.2.7	Urea	Remedial	Actual
2.2.8	Anemia	Pathodynamic	Actual
2.2.9	Reversed sequence of films	Purveyant	Actual
2.2.11	Prolactin	Etiologic	Virtual

Answer 11.2.

11.2.1. The costs of *hospitalization* may be reduced, but the costs of the rest of total medical care may be increased. [Information process]

11.2.2. If the examination is voluntary, incompetent specialists may refuse to take it. [Susceptibility factor]

11.2.3. The mothers who want to bond [susceptibility] may be the ones who decide to breast-feed. Besides, is bonding measured [information process] in a way that is wholly independent of breast-feeding?

11.2.4. Assuming that adequate data exist, the statement itself is a descriptive observation and creates no problem, because a causal claim is not made. The results would usually be very good, of course, if time merely passed with no therapy given. If a causal claim is inferred, other arguments could be offered. For example, in ancillary maneuvers, a parent or spouse who is devoted enough to make chicken soup may have other salubrious attributes. Lest the sanctified efficacy of chicken soup come under a cloud, however, this answer will stop here.

11.2.5. All three types of bias can occur here. In susceptibility, the Ivy League graduates can come from families that have higher socioeconomic status, and the graduates may simply maintain that status thereafter. In ancillary maneuvers, the prestige of the Ivy League (rather than the actual education) may help its graduates obtain better jobs. In information processes, the rating of socioeconomic status will be biased if it includes a prestige factor for the college attended.

Answer 11.3.

Original Designation of Exercise	Baseline State	Outcome	Function of Maneuver
3.1.1	Healthy child	Schizophrenic	Etiologic
3.1.2	Breast cancer	Appearance of breast	Remedial
		Death	Contratrophic
3.1.4	Healthy	Serum manganese	Pathodynamic
3.1.5	Healthy	Homicidal or suicidal impulses	Etiologic
3.1.8	Healthy infants	Death of infants	Etiologic
3.1.11	Chronic arthritic pain	Relief of pain	Remedial
		Blood level of drug	Pharmacologic
3.1.12	Patients who get menstrual cramps	Relieve cramps on occurrence	Remedial
		Prevent cramps	Contrapathic
3.1.13	Patients receiving renal dialysis	Lowered BUN	Remedial
		Prolonged life (prevention of death)	Contratrophic

Answer 11.4.

11.4.1. Is the chemotherapy being used as a solo maneuver or in conjunction with other maneuvers, such as radiotherapy or surgery? If used in conjunction with other maneuvers, is the chemotherapy a conjugate or conditional maneuver; and does it come before or after the others?

11.4.2. The main issue here is susceptibility. Was aspirin treatment given for a clinical illness that was actually the early first manifestation of the Reye's syndrome?

11.4.3. Was the hormone treatment given during the vulnerable first trimester of pregnancy?

11.4.4. Was the hormone treatment started at an appropriate time in the pregnancy and maintained long enough?

11.4.5. Has the operation been carried out in exactly the manner in which it was proposed?

11.4.6. Assuming that the diet is maintained as proposed, there is no problem in proficiency.

11.4.7. At what age should the diet have been used and how long should it have been maintained to regard a patient as exposed to it?

11.4.8. How soon after the previous acute myocardial infarction will the beta blocker treatment be started?

Chapter 12

Answer 12.1.

12.1.1. Some other maneuver that is currently regarded as the best way to prevent hangovers, e.g., reduced alcohol intake, increased sleep, maintenance of hydration, or some combination of these. The existing best maneuver might also be used additively in combination with Excellitol.

12.1.2. No comparative maneuver needed. If it works, it works. (If need be, invoke historical controls.)

12.1.3. Continuing and stopping smoking are the compared maneuvers. (Main issue in comparison here is not the maneuvers but whether the people who persist or stop smoking have similar characteristics and susceptibility to the diseases.)

12.1.4. Pump warm air (same temperature as the cigarette smoke) into the trachea of beagle dogs.

12.1.5. The principal maneuver is not clearly stated in the objective of the research. Is the main cause of the respiratory distress syndrome believed to be prematurity? If so, the comparison is with nonpremature children delivered by cesarean section. If the main cause of RDS is believed to be cesarean section, then the comparison is with premature children who were delivered by customary vaginal route. The comparative maneuver cannot be chosen here until the principal maneuver is stipulated.

12.1.6. Eating a non–high-fat (or a low-fat) diet.

12.1.7. Gargling with a placebo that looks and tastes like Xanadine but that lacks its active ingredient.

12.1.8. No comparison group needed. This is a descriptive study, because no comparison is implied, although the term "very expensive" requires definition. If you insist on a comparative maneuver, it is probably living in locations other than an old-age home. A really argumentative person might want to contend, however, that "elderly people" is the principal maneuver and that the comparison should be with non–elderly people.

12.1.9. The question is difficult to answer because "beneficial" is not defined and because the Pap smear is a diagnostic agent, not a cause-effect intervention. If benefit refers to convenience in mass diagnostic screening, the comparative agent is presumably something like biopsy of the cervix or endometrium, but this comparison is not logistically possible. If benefit refers to the therapeutic consequences in patients with Pap smear–detected cancers, the comparison is against cancers that were not so detected. (Major biases would have to be considered in the baseline states and serial-time outcomes of the compared patients.)

12.1.10 Treatment of congestive failure with either digitalis or diuretics (or bed rest) alone.

12.1.11. This is one of those projects in which a control group would be almost impossible to assemble. The virtues of prosthetic hip replacement are now so generally accepted that it would not be denied to an appropriate candidate. Its efficacy would have to be compared either in historical controls or in people who refused the offered operation.

Answer 12.2. Exercises 12.1.1 and 12.1.7 could be done as cross-overs if each person's hangovers or sore throats occurred with consistent severity each time. Conditional maneuver is a risk in Exercise 12.1.10 if digitalis (or diuretic) is added to the regimen after diuretic (or digitalis) alone has been tried and failed.

Answer 12.3. If data were assembled regarding compliance of patients with therapy, classify each patient as having had *good* or *not good* compliance. If attack rates of the infections are lower in the *good* than in the *not good* group for a particular antistreptococcal prophylactic agent, the agent was probably efficacious (unless you can think of some good reasons why compliance was related to the patient's susceptibility to infections).

Answer 12.4. *Argument by Bayer*: (a) It is impossible to do randomized therapeutic trials comparing 223 agents. The sample sizes, which would need to be enormous just to cover all the agents, would have to be even larger to show the relatively small therapeutic distinctions that would be involved in relieving headache or other symptoms. (b) The claim of "better" does not require a huge difference or even a statistically significant difference. Thus, the baseball batting championship may be won by someone whose average is only 0.001 higher than the next contender, with the difference not being statistically significant. Nevertheless, this batter is the winner. (c) The adverse reactions to aspirin may be caused by impurities, and Bayer has the least impurities. Because clinical data are extremely difficult to obtain to prove that impurities cause adverse reactions, clinicians or patients may want to use the chemical data for choosing the aspirin with the least impurities.

Argument by FTC: (a) The issue is therapeutic, not pharmacologic, superiority. At suitable dosage of salicylate, the pharmacokinetic superiorities of Bayer vanish, and all aspirins can have similar results. Why should the public pay more for Bayer when *therapeutic* efficacy is unproved? (b) If 223 therapeutic trials are impossible, why not do comparative trials against the 3, 4, or 5 leading contenders?

Decision by ARF as Judge: The decision here is largely a matter of ideologic viewpoint with respect to the role of individuals, industry, and government in a free society. As long as reasonable evidence can be offered, Bayer has the right to advertise that it is "better," and the evidence here is not unreasonable (although many readers may disagree with this appraisal). Members of the public have the right and the responsibility to be skeptical about advertising claims and also have the right to buy the aspirin that is cheapest as long as the aspirin is efficacious. (Analogously, a Rolls Royce can advertise that it is better than a Chevelle, but more people will buy the Chevelle for its advantages in price.) Besides, doesn't the FTC have more important crooks to catch or deceptions to correct than a *possible* deception that ended more than a decade previously?

Answer 12.5. What the investigator found was an example of the susceptibility bias called the "healthy worker effect," which was discussed in Section 4.2.1. The occurrence of the bias was facilitated by the use of a contrived control group rather than people who were in similar good health but not exposed to the occupational hazard.

Answer 12.6.

    12.6.1. Condition of mother and child at onset of the serious labor that was followed by delivery.

    12.6.2. (a) Status on admission to unit. (b) Status on discharge from unit.

    12.6.3. Time of *first* antineoplastic therapy, with surgery or nonsurgery.

    12.6.4. For surgical patients, date of surgery. For nonsurgical patients, date on which surgery was considered and rejected (or refused). If surgery was never considered, use the date (probably soon after first overt diagnosis of angina) when surgery might have been considered.

    12.6.5. Date of discharge from hospital.

    12.6.6. Date of diagnosis of diabetes.

    12.6.7. Date (or year) of pepsinogen test.

    12.6.8. Date of birth.

    12.6.9. Time of decision re management of sore throat.

    12.6.10. Date of onset of psychotropic treatment (or of decision not to use it).

Answer 12.7. Because randomization at each center may produce prognostic inequalities, use a central randomization stratified according to prognosis. Each new patient who enters the trial, regardless of medical site, is phoned in to the central source, designated in fair or poor prognostic category, and randomized to receive either X or old treatment.

Answer 12.8. The basic virtues of the two regimens could be adequately determined with a comparison of four groups, as follows: Excellitol plus whiskey placebo; whiskey plus Excellitol placebo; Excellitol plus whiskey; and Excellitol placebo plus whiskey placebo.

Chapter 13

The individual choices of research projects preclude any official answers to these questions. A comment can be offered, however, about the difficulty in answering questions about the outcome variables in Exercise 13.3 if the etiologic study was conducted with a case-control structure. (In a casual search of the literature, readers are much more likely to encounter a case-control than a cohort study of an alleged etiologic agent.) In a case-control study of etiology, the main groups under investigation are selected on the basis of the postmaneuver outcome events that made each person become either a diseased *case* or a nondiseased *control*. After these selections are completed, the subsequent variables and analyses all refer to the baseline state (age, race, gender, and so on) for each person or to the performance of maneuvers (exposure to suspected etiologic agents). Because no further attention is given to any of the other outcome events that may have followed the investigated maneuvers, there are no outcome variables to be classified as ancillary or incidental.

In a case-control study, however, the investigator's main outcome activity (in contrast to the actual outcome of the maneuvers) is obtaining information for each case and control about the antecedent exposure to maneuvers. Thus, the actual performance (or proficiency) of the maneuvers is often more likely to have been carefully investigated in a case-control study of etiology than in an experimental or observational cohort study of therapy. Other distinctions of the case-control architecture will be discussed in Chapters 18 and 21–23.

Chapter 14

Answer 14.1.

14.1.1. *Value:* important. *Feasibility:* Can patients be followed long enough for intellectual capacity to be noted? How will effects of postuterine events and environment be disentangled from the impact of nutrition during pregnancy? *Stipulations:* What will be measured as nutrition during pregnancy? What will be measured as intellectual capacity? When will it be measured?

14.1.2. *Value:* Uncertain. You may want to argue that the behavior of clinical personnel (in attitudes toward patients, not keeping them waiting long before being seen, explaining what is proposed, and so on) is more important for patient satisfaction than the physical setting of the clinic and should be studied instead. On the other hand, changing the physical setting may be much more feasible to accomplish than changing the behavior of the staff. *Feasibility:* Within the confines and space restrictions of most hospitals, how will this trial be conducted? Will the old clinic be maintained and a new attractive facility established elsewhere? If two different facilities are not envisioned, how will the randomized assignment be carried out? *Stipulations:* OK.

14.1.3. *Value:* Important. *Feasibility:* OK, except for problem of deciding whether outcome events are attributable to intervening co-maneuvers rather than contraception. *Stipulations:* OK. (Adverse side effects will presumably be defined in a satisfactory manner.)

14.1.4. *Value:* Important. *Feasibility:* OK, except for two problems. Will the patients who consent to enter such a trial represent suitable clinical challenges for the clinical practitioners? Will the period of follow-up observation be long enough to provide those challenges? *Stipulations:* How long is the period of follow-up observation?

14.1.5. *Value:* Important. *Feasibility:* Has a pilot study been done to demonstrate that hard-core unemployed people can be suitably trained and can function effectively in this role? *Stipulations:* OK.

14.1.6. *Value:* Important. *Feasibility:* Will enough women be willing to volunteer for randomization in this trial? Will enough clinicians be willing to encourage their patients to be randomized? *Stipulations:* Will women with any type of breast cancer be admitted or will the study be confined to a certain subgroup, such as apparently localized breast cancer?

14.1.7. *Value:* Seems like a trivial question to be subjected to a randomized trial. Why not investigate what is done *after* the blinded veterans get to the clinic? *Feasibility:* OK, assuming that the mailed letters can be read and that the tape-recorded announcements can be played. *Stipulations:* OK.

14.1.8. *Value:* Important. *Feasibility:* What mechanism will be used for assigning patients to be treated by the nonpsychotherapists? What biases will be introduced by a nonrandomized assignment of the compared maneuvers? Can the maneuvers be maintained long enough to appraise their individual outcomes? *Stipulations:* What kinds of "disturbed patients"? What will be measured to decide if they have been helped?

14.1.9. *Value:* Important. *Feasibility:* Dubious. Can enough patients be obtained and followed long enough to observe the outcome of the proposed maneuvers? Can the effects of different susceptibility factors, intervening maneuvers, and detection procedures be separated from those of the compared maneuvers? *Stipulations:* OK.

Answer 14.2. Individual choices to be made. Here is one example of a published retrolective cohort study:

$$
\text{UNSTABLE ANGINA PECTORIS} \left\{ \begin{array}{c} \text{SURGICAL} \\ \text{BY-PASS GRAFT} \\ \longrightarrow \\ \text{MEDICAL} \\ \longrightarrow \\ \text{THERAPY} \end{array} \right\} \text{SURVIVAL AT 2 YEARS}
$$

This study would have two major advantages as an experiment. The randomized allocation of treatment would prevent the susceptibility bias that can arise if surgical treatment is given to good prognostic risks and medical treatment to inoperable patients with poor prognoses. The improved data obtained in a planned experiment would also allow a suitable stratification of prognostic expectations for patients with unstable angina pectoris. Treatment could be analyzed with such a stratification in an effort to adjust for the potential bias in an observational study, but the data assembled retrolectively from patients' medical records may not be satisfactory to demarcate the strata effectively. This project, which has now been conducted as an experimental trial, was long resisted as an experiment because of doctors' dilemmas about ethics and because of vigorous opposition by advocates of each of the compared maneuvers.

Answer 14.3. Individual choices to be made. Here are two examples:

14.3.1. *Clinical trial*

$$
\text{PATIENTS WITH METASTATIC CANCER} \left\{ \begin{array}{c} \text{OLD CHEMOTHERAPY AGENT} \\ \longrightarrow \\ \text{NEW CHEMOTHERAPY AGENT} \end{array} \right\} \text{SURVIVAL TIME}
$$

Latent objective: Palliative therapy
    Problem: Survival time, as an index of palliation, does not include the palliated comfort of patient and family

14.3.2. *Case-control study*

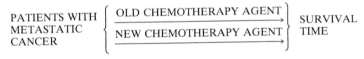

PATIENTS WITH   PATIENTS WITHOUT
THROMBOPHLEBITIS   THROMBOPHLEBITIS

Antecedent use of oral contraceptive pills

Stated objective: Do oral contraceptive pills predispose to thrombophlebitis?
Latent objective: Should oral contraceptive pills be withdrawn from the market?
        Problem: The use of drugs, or their authorization for availability, requires careful appraisal of all risks *and benefits*. This study contains no data regarding benefits of oral contraceptive preparations, and only one type of risk is cited.

Chapter 15

Answer 15.1. (The answers are identified according to the previous citation of the study.)
    2.2.3. Because no particular thrombotic potential is associated with most of the

conditions that receive gynecologic operations, the main prognostic feature here is the vulnerability imposed by the extensiveness, duration, and other stress of the operation itself. A complete hysterectomy and bilateral salpingo-oophorectomy may be much more likely to predispose a patient to postoperative thrombosis than the repair of a cystocele.

2.2.5. The main prognostic point to be noted here is the goal of the persons who selected (or received) the maneuvers. Were barbiturates preferred by people who intended to commit suicide?

2.2.7. Extensiveness or anatomic severity of the treated carcinomas.

2.2.8. Prognostic severity of the co-morbid ailments associated with the reduced or elevated levels of hematocrit.

3.1.2. Anatomic extensiveness and clinical severity of the breast cancers.

4.1.2. Clinical status (healthy or different degrees of unhealthiness) of the infants. (The socioeconomic status and nutritional patterns of the family and the infant's exposure to infections are not features of the baseline state; they all occur while the maneuvers are in progress.)

4.1.4. Clinical status and needs of the people who choose to use either form of practice.

4.1.5. Clinical severity of the chronic active hepatitis and reasons why steroid therapy was chosen (or rejected).

Answer 15.2.

15.2.1. *Cancer of lung:* A demand for histologic evidence of cancer will severely restrict the trial's patient population because of omission of patients whose histologic evidence of lung cancer cannot be obtained until after thoracotomy (or necropsy) is performed. Patients with lesions that are inaccessible to biopsy will also be excluded. The admitted population will overemphasize patients with metastatic lesions that were amenable to easy biopsy, e.g., scalene nodes and liver.

15.2.2. *Acute myocardial infarction:* Because ECG evidence of infarct is not always present on admission, criteria I will exclude patients from entering the trial immediately. By the time the ECG evidence develops, some of the most important issues in therapy may already have been resolved.

15.2.3. *Relief of sore throat symptoms:* Because the target is to be relief of symptoms and because no antibiotic has been mentioned, the goal may be to test an analgesic or anti-inflammatory agent. The demand for evidence of streptococcal infection may be unnecessary.

15.2.4. *Prevention of post-streptococcal inflammation:* Unless arrangements are made for special facilities to provide immediate laboratory answers (e.g., fluorescent antibody tests), admission to the trial will be delayed if criteria I are used. If ordinary (overnight) facilities are used for identifying the streptococcus, the patients will have to be recalled or otherwise retrieved from home before admission to the study. This delay may lead to many refusals. With criteria II, patients can be admitted immediately and then later de-admitted if the laboratory tests are negative.

15.2.5. *Low back pain:* The agent to be tested for relief of symptoms is presumably a pharmaceutical or physical form of therapy that would be applied in regular clinical practice, where x-rays are often not taken unless such therapy fails to provide relief. Accordingly, criteria II would be more realistic.

15.2.6. *Psychiatric depression:* Neither set of criteria seems optimal. A combination of both sets, particularly with careful specifications for clinical diagnosis, might allow a better identification of depressed patients.

Answer 15.3. Suppose that the docile compliant hypertensive patients are also particularly likely to have blood pressures that can be easily lowered by the tested drugs; whereas the nondocile, hostile group, who are unwilling to comply, are also relatively refractory to the drugs (even if the drugs were faithfully maintained). The results of the trial would thus make the drugs look especially effective because the refractory patients have been excluded. Consequently, the true rate of effectiveness, when the drugs are given to the general population of hypertensives, may be substantially lower than what was found in the trial.

Answer 15.4. The heretic here was Joseph Berkson, one of America's foremost clinical biostatisticians. Although the proposed scenario seems far-fetched, it has never (to my knowledge) been convincingly excluded as a possible source of falsely elevated death rates in the smokers. Berkson's proposal[28] was as follows:

Assume that the population of doctors contains two strata: s_1—the proportion of sick doctors, who are likely to die in the next few years with death rate d_1; and s_2—the proportion of healthy doctors, who are likely to die with a much lower death rate, d_2. Assume that the death rates, d_1 and d_2, are unaffected by smoking. Now assume that sick doctors return their questionnaires with the same frequency, f_1, regardless of whether they smoke or do not smoke. Assume that healthy smoking doctors, annoyed by having to answer all the details of questions about their smoking habits, return their questionnaires at a rate f_2, that is much lower than the return rate, f_3, of the non-smoking doctors, who have very few questions to answer after having indicated that they do not smoke.

The rate of returned questionnaires will be as follows:

$$\text{Smokers: } s_1f_1 + s_2f_2$$
$$\text{Nonsmokers: } s_1f_1 + s_2f_3$$

The rate of deaths encountered in the next few years among doctors who returned the questionnaires will be as follows:

$$\text{Smokers: } s_1f_1d_1 + s_2f_2d_2$$
$$\text{Nonsmokers: } s_1f_1d_1 + s_2f_3d_2$$

Since d_2 (the death rate in the healthy doctors) is substantially smaller than d_1, the occurrence of deaths in the numerator of the smoking and nonsmoking cohorts will be essentially similar, because it depends mainly on $s_1f_1d_1$. But the denominator of the nonsmoking population will be relatively larger than that of the smokers (because $f_3 > f_2$). Therefore, the death rate calculated for the nonsmokers may be spuriously lower than that for the smokers.

Answer 15.5. Because no cogent prognostic factors are known for susceptiblity to mesothelioma, cancer of the bladder, cancer of the pancreas,or toxic shock syndrome, there are no susceptibility biases to be considered in Exercises 15.5.1, 15.5.3, 15.5.4, 15.5.7, or 15.5.8. (There may be other biases to worry about in these studies, but susceptibility bias is not one of them.) The other potential problems are as follows:

15.5.2. If people with particularly tense type AAAA personalities are especially likely to develop coronary disease and also to smoke cigarettes, the smoking may be a predictive marker rather than a cause of the disease. If suitable tests of personality were available, the cohorts should be appropriately restricted or stratified for those factors.

15.5.5. and 15.5.6. The bleeding or other manifestations of a threatened abortion, or the habitual occurrence of spontaneous abortions in the past, can signal the likelihood of an overt or subtle deformity in the fetus. Women with habitual previous abortions may be particularly likely to seek a diagnostic test in a new pregnancy; and those with a currently threatened abortion were usually the ones who received treatment with DES. For the pregnancy-test study, stratify the cohorts according to the patient's previous pregnancy history and the reason why the test was ordered. For the DES study, restrict the compared cohorts to women who have a suitable therapeutic indication for receiving DES.

15.5.9. Although hypertension is not known to be a risk factor for breast cancer, the cohorts should be restricted to people with hypertension, because it is the therapeutic indication for use of reserpine. (If the breast cancer is to be appraised only in women, the cohort should also be restricted to women.)

15.5.10. If we really believe the old clinical aphorism that gallstones are most likely to appear in women who are "fair, fat, and 40," and if such women (for some unknown reason) are particularly likely to be tea drinkers, we might try to use this aphorism in choosing the cohort. Because the cohort would be selected before the women reach age 40 and before some of them have later become fat, the admission criteria would be tricky to establish. Probably the best bet here is to let an unrestricted cohort enter the study and then stratify the data later for features of gender, complexion, and weight.

Answer 15.6. Individual answers to be submitted.

Chapter 16

Answer 16.1.

16.1.1. You can start with any number you want in Table 16–1. This answer starts with the first number in the third horizontal block of digits. The first strategy is to assign the letters A, B, C in recurrent succession to each number and then to rank the sequence of random numbers. The results will be 70-A; 45-B; 100-C; 28-A; 42-B; 78-C; 62-A; 75-B; 87-C; 11-A; 46-B; 9-C; 20-A; 69-B; 6-C; 16-A; 18-B; 27-C; 100-A; 98-B; 62-C; 16-A; 27-B; 86-C; 56-A; 100-B; 70-C; 44-A; 73-B; 21-C.

When we rank this sequence, we get 6-C; 9-C; 11-A; 16-A; 16-A; 18-B; 20-A; 21-C; 27-C; 27-B; 28-A; 42-B; 44-A; 45-B; 46-B; 56-A; 62-A; 62-C; 69-B; 70-A; 70-C; 73-B; 75-B; 78-C; 86-C; 87-C; 98-B; 100-C; 100-A; and 100-B. We have problems with 16-A, 27-B, 70-C, 100-A, and 100-B, because each of these ranks has already been chosen. We therefore use the next digits after the *21* that we stopped with in Table 16–1 and reassign these "tied" treatments. Thus 16-A becomes 7-A; 27-B becomes 67-B; 70-C becomes 22-C; 100-A would again be 100-A, so we skip that number and go to the next one, which is 42-A. Because we already have a 42, we go to the next, which is 14. Thus 100-A becomes 14-A. Finally, 100-B becomes 17-B.

When these new ranked numbers are inserted appropriately, the final sequence would be 6-C; 7-A; 9-C; 11-A; 14-A; 16-A; 17-B; 18-B; 20-A; 21-C; 22-C; 27-C; 28-A; 42-B; 44-A; 45-B; 46-B; 56-A; 62-A; 62-C; 67-B; 69-B; 70-A; 73-B; 75-B; 78-C; 86-C; 87-C; 98-B, and 100-C. In batches of six, the final sequence would be:

    CACAAA   BBACCC   ABABBA   ACBBAB   BCCCBC

Although the total group of 30 assignments is balanced, with 10 members for each treatment (because we planned things that way), the early sequence is substantially unbalanced. The first six patients contain no B's and four A's. The first 12 patients contain only two B's.

A different and easier approach is to divide each random number by 3. If the result is even, assign treatment A. If the result has a remainder of 1, assign treatment B. If the remainder is 2, assign treatment C. To make things fair, use only the digits from 1 to 99. Thus, if we start with the random number 97 in the fourth main block, $97/3 = 32$ with 1 left over. We assign B. 67/3 also has 1 left over. Assign B. The rest of the sequence is 3-A; 60-A; 62-C; 6-A; 32-C; 55-B; 65-C; 6-A; 12-A; 2-C; 74-C; 79-B; 55-B; 46-B; 62-C; 4-B; 7-B; 4-B; 39-A; 45-A; 46-B; 50-C; 48-A; 92-C; 81-A; 83-C; 48-A; 16-B. This tactic is easier because we do not have to deal with ties. However, when we examine the sequence in batches of six, we see the following:

    BBAACA   CBCAAC   CBBBCB   BBAABC   ACACAB

There are 10 A treatments, 11 B treatments, and nine C treatments and so the group of 30 assignments still contains a slight imbalance.

16.1.2. Starting with the fifth block of the table, we assign A-100, A-49, B-82, B-2, C-24, C-98. In ranked sequence of these random numbers, the first batch of six would be BCABCA. The next batch would come from A-22, A-2, B-78, B-23, C-41, and C-81 (skipping the two that already occurred in this block). The sequence for the second batch would be AABCBC. The third batch would come from A-38, A-54, B-11, B-75, C-64, C-18, and the sequence would be BCAACB. Continue this way for two more batches to determine a schedule for 30 patients, balanced at every six cases.

16.1.3. Basic strategy is to prepare a randomization for the first agent to be taken. The cross-over will always go to the other agent. Letting even numbers go to A and odd numbers go to B, and starting with the first number in the sixth block of Table 16–1, we get 78-A, 67-B; 52-A; 32-B; 83-A; 27-B; 43-B; 40-A; 85-B; and 22-A. The sequence of assignments for the first treatment would be ABABABBABA. The corresponding sequence for the crossed-over second treatment would be BABABAABAB.

Diagram of conventional design:

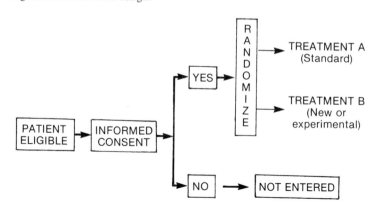

Answer 16.2. Diagram of randomized consent design:

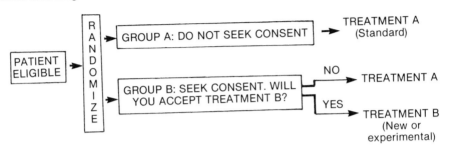

The randomized consent design has the following main advantages: First, the patient knows which therapy will be offered before consenting to participate in the trial. Second, because the patient decides to enter the trial only if the experimental treatment seems desirable, the decision-making process is greatly simplified. Third, the physician need not discuss with the patient the process of randomized allocation of treatment.

The randomized consent design has the following major limitations: First, because the proper statistical comparison is between all patients randomized to group A versus all patients randomized to group B, the effectiveness of the new treatment may be masked if many patients in group B elect to use standard therapy. Second, because both the patient and the physician know which treatment is being used, double-blinding will be impossible. Third, many clinical trials require frequent follow-up visits for data collection. This increased surveillance creates no problem for group B, but the follow-up may be troublesome in group A, because informed consent has not been obtained.

Answer 16.3. The investigators are being reasonable, but their high hopes depend on the ability to maintain a perfect double-blind mask throughout the trial. If the true identity of treatment becomes revealed for even a single patient, the identity of treatment may become known for everyone. Because a patient's treatment is usually deliberately revealed when an adverse reaction occurs (so that the reaction can be properly managed), the investigators would also have to hope either that no one develops an adverse reaction or that each such reaction will be managed by a separate clinician who can successfully hide what she or he discovered about the treatment. Because these additional hopes seem unlikely to be attained, the double-blinding will probably be destroyed at some point during the trial.

Answer 16.4. Consider the following three choices: (1) In a parallel design, randomize each psychiatrist's patients so that the psychiatrist uses each of the two treatments on different patients. (2) In a parallel design, randomize the psychiatrists so that each one uses only one of the two treatments for whatever patients come to see him. (3) In a cross-over design, randomize each psychiatrist's patients to be treated for a period of time with one type of treatment and then later with the other. These designs have various advantages and disadvantages, but none of the designs deals with the problem of prejudice/skill among the psychiatrists, i.e., that some really prefer Freudian or behavioral therapy and are better at it.

To avoid this problem, try doing the following. Before the trial begins, devise some method for determining which type of treatment each psychiatrist prefers or does better. Classify the psychiatrists as type F or type B, according to whether they prefer Freudian or behavioral therapy. Prepare a random sequence of the psychiatrists so that they are arranged as B-1, B-2, . . . and F-1, F-2, F-3, and so on. When patients appear, they are asked to consent to a central randomization, which assigns them to treatment B or F. The first patient randomized to treatment B goes to psychiatrist B-1. The second patient randomized to treatment F goes to psychiatrist F-2, and so on.

(You may think this scheme is wild and impractical, but if so, why did you realistically accept the premise that a group of psychiatrists actually wanted to do this study and that it was feasible?)

Answer 16.5. The answer to this question is debatable. In one view, if we assume that patients with mandatory indications or contraindications for anticoagulants were excluded from the trial, there would be no reason for suspecting a regulation-determined susceptibility bias, and the proposed procedure would therefore seem fair. The opposing view might hold that patients who were well regulated also received special clinical attention, which evoked ancillary therapy. This ancillary treatment, rather than the anticoagulants alone, may have produced superior results in this group. If the well-regulated group, on the other hand, failed to show better results than placebo, this argument is untenable.

Answer 16.6. Unless you have reason to think the clinician is a liar, you can believe his statement. The main issue here is not the accuracy of the statement but its potential extrapolation. Can this diet be applied successfully to other people? Suppose the diet, although offered to 100 people, was successfully maintained by only three, who respectively lost 51, 42, and 27 pounds to provide the average loss of 40 pounds per person?

Answer 16.7.

16.7.1. The best way of rehabilitating the patients may be an additive combination of mechanical plus psychosocial therapy. Hence it is not good design to test the two maneuvers as alternatives unless the intention is to determine which is better.

16.7.2. Aspirin should be tested not at fixed dosage, but at whatever titrated dose is optimal for each patient who receives it.

16.7.3. The comparison is nonconcurrent. The patients treated in the later secular group may be initially in milder or more severe stages of disease than the group of 1983 to 1984. Possible reasons are changes in inter-iatric referral patterns for that hospital or changes in diagnostic standards for myocardial infarction. Also, other aspects of therapy may have changed since January 1, 1985.

16.7.4. There are many historical controls for the conduct and results of a routine abortion. Assuming that the gynecologist is a careful observer and honest reporter, we can accept his statement.

16.7.5. The problem is that of a conditional maneuver. Suppose there are two types of cancer: rapid-growing and slow-growing. The patients who receive surgery immediately will be a mixture of the two types. For those assigned to the combined regimen, patients who have rapid-growing tumors may no longer be operable after a two-month delay, so that the radiotherapy + surgery group will contain mainly patients with slow-growing tumors and will probably have better outcomes because of this biologic distinction, regardless of therapy.

16.7.6. In the absence of a special diet for the control group, this design has a strong potential for compliance-determined susceptibility bias. Suppose psychically tense people are likely to develop coronary artery disease but are unable to comply with a special diet. The compliers will then consist of nontense people who are not likely to develop coronary disease but whose success, compared with the controls, may then be attributed to the diet.

16.7.7. Because DES was used for pregnant women with a threatened abortion or with a history of previous repeated abortions, this therapeutic indication should be a qualification for admission to the study. Therefore, the control group should not be casually chosen; it should consist of women who had the same indication but who were not treated with DES.

16.7.8. There are at least three main problems here. First, the women who choose to use estrogen replacement therapy may be more conscious of physical appearance because they initially are more attractive than other women. The persistence of this greater attractiveness may then be falsely ascribed to the therapy. Second, the women who continue using estrogens may be those who continue to remain attractive (i.e., the women who stop using estrogen may be those who feel they have lost their good looks or who have not had their good looks restored). Third, the esthetics of current physiognomy may affect a woman's decision to volunteer to participate in the study.

Chapter 17

Answer 17.1. The policy has the major statistical advantage of avoiding answers to questions such as "How high is up?" Because dimensional or ordinal changes must be categorized to be tabulated as transition events, we would have to confront such categorical decisions as whether a reduction of 5 pounds represents a *small, large,* or *good* loss of weight and whether the transition event should be rated differently if the person's initial weight is 250 or 120 pounds.

The expression of an average transition allows an escape from these decisions. On the other hand, in choosing treatment for individual patients, clinicians usually are interested in the likelihood of transition events. Thus, a clinician wants to know not the average change in blood pressure after treatment, but the chances that a patient's elevated blood pressure will become normal. A statistical analysis that omits this type of outcome information may not be useful in clinical practice.

Answer 17.2. Did the nausea and vomiting (N & V) occur long enough after receipt of the medication to be regarded as an adverse drug reaction rather than as a local dysfunction of the esophageal-gastric transmission mechanism? Had any N & V occurred before the medication was given? Was it given for a condition that could readily produce N & V at about the same time the N & V occurred? Was the medication given in a manner, e.g., swallowed with whiskey or sour milk, that could lead to N & V? Was the patient exposed to any concomitant phenomena (other medication, bad news, the sight of other people having N & V, etc.) that might provoke the reaction? A particularly desirable set of additional data would be information about the past history of this medication. Was it followed by N & V in other people? If only one tactic is available, perhaps the best procedure would be the rechallenge conducted by seeing what happens when the patient is given the medication again at a later date, after the acute events have subsided and preferably with the patient blind to the medication's identity.

Answer 17.3. Calculate an average duration (mean or median) for the interval between randomization and performance of surgery in the surgical cohort. Any deaths that occur in the medical group during that interval are managed in the same way as the preoperative surgical deaths. The average survival in the medical group is then calculated, beginning at that point, for the medically treated patients who were alive at that point. (Alternatively, you might delay the onset of medical treatment until completion of the preoperative interval, but this tactic is less appealing clinically and is unfeasible unless you have advance knowledge of the average length of the preoperative interval.)

Answer 17.4. If the observations used to judge the outcome state are made by the recipient of the maneuver, a direct comparison with a highly mimetic placebo is needed. If someone else makes the judgments, the judge should be suitably blinded, but the placebo itself need not be highly mimetic. For this reason, we need highly mimetic placebos in Exercises 17.4.1 and 17.4.2, but only suitably blinded judges in the rest of the studies. Accordingly, you can propose the following:

    17.4.1. Double-blind trial with a placebo that has the peppermint-like flavor of Rolaids and a somewhat chalky texture but no antacid constituent.

    17.4.2. Double-blind gargling with a placebo that has a strong medicinal taste and flavor but no ingredients that are believed efficacious. The placebo's taste and flavor need not be identical to Listerine but should convey the idea of a medicinal effect.

    17.4.3. The control infants should have ordinary petrolatum (or Vaseline) applied to the chest. The petrolatum should resemble Vicks Vapo-Rub in visual appearance. The judges should be kept unaware of each infant's treatment when inspecting the nasal passages, and each judge, before the inspection, should have Vapo-Rub spread on her/his upper lip to prevent the smell of the thoracic Vapo-Rub from revealing its identity.

    17.4.4. For the control treatment, use some other lotion that contains no active ingredients. Wash the patients' faces before they are inspected by a judge who is kept unaware of treatment.

    17.4.5. Let a panel of judges, unaware of the culinary ingredients, rate the taste of batches of chicken prepared with and without mustard in the gravy.

    17.4.6. Let a panel of judges, unaware of preceding skin care, rate the "loveliness" of skins treated with Lux and with whatever comparative agent is under consideration. If the skins were recently washed, so that the faint residual smell of Lux might reveal its identity, let the judges wear clips that keep their nostrils tightly closed.

Answer 17.5. This exercise is intended to provoke a discussion of ethical issues in double-blinding. Because many ethical issues do not have correct or incorrect answers, none will be offered here. The societal versus samaritan approaches to ethics in randomized trials are discussed further in Chapter 29.

Answer 17.6. Without considering any ethical issues, the argument seems justified purely on clinical and scientific grounds. We would be testing regimens constructed in a manner that may impair their actual efficacy and that cannot be used for direct extrapolation to clinical practice. Because the trial cannot be suitably designed in a double-blind manner, we would have to drop the double-blind requirement, administer the regimens in a manner that is suitably proficient for each treatment, and arrange for the outcome events, 5 years later, to be evaluated as objectively as possible, perhaps by separate observers who are kept blind to the treatments.

Answer 17.7.

17.7.1. Women receiving oral contraceptive agents had to see their physicians for renewal of prescriptions to supply "the pill." At those times, the women could report minor episodes of leg pain that might receive attention and a thromboembolic diagnosis. In women using mechanical barriers and not receiving medical surveillance, similar episodes could be overlooked and undiagnosed.

17.7.2. A woman taking oral agents is in constant control of her contraception and also need not interrupt sexual foreplay for the insertion of *ad hoc* mechanical barriers. The resultant sexual freedom may lead to greater exposure to gonorrhea.

17.7.3. The technology needed to diagnose lung cancer is more likely to be available and employed in urban than in rural regions.

17.7.4. Estrogens commonly produce the side effect of vaginal bleeding, which then evokes diagnostic testing with dilation and curettage (D & C) or other intra-endometrial procedures. The diagnostic tests will reveal the presence of many silent endometrial cancers that will escape detection in women who did not have bleeding evoked by estrogens.

17.7.5. Anticipating that estrogen replacement therapy may restore youthful beauty and sex appeal, women who begin the treatment with those hopes may be more vocal in expressing their later disappointment (if the hopes are not realized) than women whose sex life is equally unsatisfactory but who have not taken estrogen and raised their hopes.

17.7.6. Believing that someone with coronary disease would not be jogging, the person who fills out the death certificate may ascribe sudden death in a nonjogger to a stroke.

17.7.7. The diagnostic methods used to detect cancer may be better in the municipalities that also fluoridate water.

17.7.8. Many otherwise silent colon cancers become detected by the increased medical surveillance that begins at or after the appendectomy.

17.7.9. A malignant gastric ulcer that was mistakenly regarded as benign in the era before easy and frequent endoscopy may be revealed today when the ulcer receives endoscopic biopsy only after the treatment is initiated.

Answer 17.8.

17.8.1. Because the statement is an assertion and no causal comparison is being made, there is no comparative bias. For generalization to "elderly people," however, the studied group has a distorted assembly, because people living in an old-age home may not get along with their children.

17.8.2. Susceptibility bias. If psychic tension causes high death rates and also causes the "drive" that makes people migrate from their homeland, the U.S. Irish may be people with higher tension and shorter longevity.

17.8.3. Transfer bias in a residue group. Patients who do not have cardiac damage do not die during an acute attack of rheumatic fever and will not be available for autopsy.

17.8.4. Transfer bias in a residue group. The discontent patients may have stopped coming to the clinic, leaving behind only a small and imperceptible but happy group. This study also contains a problem in substitution of variables. Does patient satisfaction alone denote good quality of primary health care?

Answer 17.9.

17.9.1. *Calculations for actuarial method:*

Interval	Alive at Beginning	Died During Interval	Lost to Follow-up	With-drawn Alive	Adjusted Denomi-nator	Proportion Dying	Proportion Surviving	Cumulative Survival Rate
0–1	126	47	4	15	116.5	0.403	0.597	0.597
1–2	60	5	6	11	51.5	0.097	0.903	0.539
2–3	38	2	0	15	30.5	0.066	0.934	0.503
3–4	21	2	2	7	16.5	0.121	0.879	0.443
4–5	10	0	0	6	7.0	0.000	1.000	0.443

17.9.2. *Calculations for direct method:*

Interval	Censored People Removed	Cumulative Mortality Rate	Cumulative Survival Rate
0–1	19	47/107 = 0.439	0.561
1–2	17	52/90 = 0.578	0.422
2–3	15	54/75 = 0.720	0.280
3–4	9	56/66 = 0.848	0.151
4–5	6	56/60 = 0.933	0.067

17.9.3. The distinctions clearly illustrate the differences between analyses in which the censored people do or do not contribute to the intervening denominators. At the end of the fifth year of follow-up in this cohort of 126 people, we clinically know only two things for sure: 56 people have died and 60 people have actually been followed for at least 5 years. Everyone else in the cohort is either lost or in the stage of censored suspended animation called *withdrawn alive.* Assuming that the 12 (= 4+6+0+2) lost people are irretrievably lost, we still have 54 people (= 15+11+15+7+6) who are percolating through the follow-up process at various stages of continuing observation before 5 years. The cumulative survival rate of 0.067 in the direct method is based on the two clearly known items of clinical information at 5 years. The cumulative survival rate of 0.443 in the actuarial method is based on the interval contributions made by all the censored people. In fact, if you take 33 as half the number of the 66 (= 12+54) censored people and add 33 to the *direct* denominator at 5 years, the cumulative mortality at 5 years becomes 56/(60+33) = 56/93 = 0.602; the direct cumulative survival becomes 0.398; and the two methods agree more closely.

Rather than dispute the merits of the two methods, we might focus our intellectual energy on the basic scientific policy here. Why are 5-year survival rates being reported at all when the 5-year status is yet to be determined for almost as many (54) people as the 60 for whom the status is known? Why not restrict the results to what was known at a 1-year or at most 2-year interval, for which the fate of the unknown group has much less of an impact? A clinician predicting a patient's 5-year chances of survival from these data might be excessively cautious in giving the direct estimate of 0.067. On the other hand, the clinician would have a hard time pragmatically defending an actuarial estimate of 0.443, when the only real facts are that four people of a potential 60 have actually survived for 5 years.

Answer 17.10.

Number of Interval	Cumulative Survival Rate Before Death	Time of Deaths That End Interval	Number Alive Before Deaths	Number of Deaths	Number of Survivors	Interval Survival Rate	Censored Before Next Death
1	1.00	0.5 yr.	126	32	94	0.746	8
2	0.746	1.0 yr.	86	15	71	0.826	11
3	0.616	1.5 yr.	60	3	57	0.950	10
4	0.585	2.0 yr.	47	2	45	0.957	7
5	0.560	2.5 yr.	38	2	36	0.947	19
6	0.531	4.0 yr.	17	2	15	0.882	5
7	0.468	—	10	—	—	—	(6)

Answer 17.11. See Figure 17.4.
Answer 17.12. The variable-interval results are more like the actuarial than the direct method. The main reason is that the censored people, although not augmenting the variable-interval denominators, make distinctive contributions before they are removed. When many people have been censored, the direct method leads to an underestimation of cumulative survival time.
Answer 17.13. When there are no losses due to censoring or competing risks, the denominator for the cumulative survival rate at each interval in the direct method is simply N, the total number of people in the cohort. The numerator of the cumulative mortality rate is the sum of deaths = Σd_i that have accrued at that point. The cumulative mortality rate will be $\Sigma d_i/N$ and the cumulative survival rate will be $1-(\Sigma d_i/N)$.

In the actuarial method, the mortality rate for the first interval will be d_i/N, and the survival

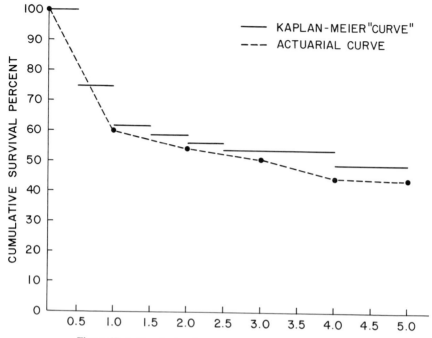

Figure 17–4. Graph showing answer to Exercise 17.11.

rate will be $(N-d_1)/N$. For the second interval, $N-d_1$ will be the denominator; d_2 deaths will occur; the interval mortality rate will be $d_2/(N-d_1)$; and the interval survival rate will be $(N-d_1-d_2)/(N-d_1)$. For a denominator of $N-d_1-d_2$ people and for d_3 deaths in the third interval, the interval survival rate will be $(N-d_1-d_2-d_3)/(N-d_1-d_2)$. At the end of the third interval, the cumulative survival rate will be

$$\frac{N-d_1}{N} \times \frac{N-d_1-d_2}{N-d_1} \times \frac{N-d_1-d_2-d_3}{N-d_1-d_2}$$

With suitable cancellation of numerators and denominators, this expression becomes $(N-d_1-d_2-d_3)/N$, which is $1-[(d_1-d_2-d_3)/N]$. At this interval (and for all successive intervals), the actuarial result is the same as $1-[\Sigma d_i/N]$.

In the Kaplan-Meier method, the individual interval and cumulative for survival rates are calculated according to the same algebraic formulas used in the actuarial method. The lengths of the intervals may vary, but the mathematical principles are the same. If there are no losses due to censoring or competing risks, the algebra and the results will be identical in the two methods, and both will yield the same value of $1-(\Sigma d_i/N)$ produced by the direct method. Q.E.D.

Chapter 18

Answer 18.1. (The answers are cited according to the original number of the exercise.)
   2.2.1. A diagnostic marker study for dysmaturity or for concomitant fetal distress; a prognostic marker study for neonatal asphyxia. The basic structure is V versus W, where W is the level of human placental lactogen and V is the result for dysmaturity, fetal distress, or neonatal asphyxia. If the categories are partitioned suitably, we can use T for

a positive result in the test and D for the abnormal clinical condition. The structure would then be T/D versus $\bar{T}/\bar{D}$.

2.2.2. A retrospective case-control study. The outcome variable, F, can be shown as F_1 for cases with lower-face trigeminal neuralgia; F_2 for cases with upper-face trigeminal neuralgia; and $\bar{F}$ for the healthy control group. Several different factors were examined as the maneuver, M. These were religion, smoking, drinking, and age. The comparisons seem to have been M/F_1 versus M/F_2 versus $M/\bar{F}$.

2.2.4. This is a complicated pathodynamic study examining leucocyte-electrolyte abnormalities as the outcome of two maneuvers (heart disease and diuretic therapy). The cases with heart disease and the controls without it can be shown as M and $\bar{M}$. Each of these groups could be stratified, according to the use or nonuse of diuretics, as M_D and $M_{\bar{D}}$; and as $\bar{M}_D$ and $\bar{M}_{\bar{D}}$. With leucocyte-electrolyte values marked as F, the structure of the research was F/M_D versus $F/M_{\bar{D}}$; F/M_D versus $F/\bar{M}_D$; and so on.

2.2.6. Diagnostic marker study. It can be portrayed with a pathodynamic structure if we let M = anencephalic fetus and F = level of the selected protein in amniotic fluid. The structure is then F/M versus F/$\bar{M}$. Otherwise, let V = protein measurement and W = state of fetus. The study is then V versus W. If the fetal state is marked D for anencephaly and $\bar{D}$ for its absence, and if the protein measurement is demarcated for a positive result, T, the structure is T/D versus $\bar{T}/\bar{D}$.

2.2.9. This is a cross-sectional experiment in observer variability research. The compared maneuvers are the presentation of films in a reversed and correct chronologic sequence. The outcomes are the readings given by the radiologists. We could show the structures as F/M versus F/$\bar{M}$, but because we would want to compare agreement, we could use V_M and $V_{\bar{M}}$ to represent readings given in response to the active and control maneuvers. The comparison would then be structured as $V_M \leftrightarrow V_{\bar{M}}$.

2.2.10. A diagnostic marker study, analogous to Exercise 2.2.6 and cited the same way if you let M (or W or D) represent presence of cancer and F (or V or T) represent result of the liver scan.

2.2.11. You can offer several acceptable interpretations for this study, according to whether prolactin is regarded as a marker factor or (as in the approach offered here) as an etiologic factor. Etiologically, this is a retrospective case-control study, with F and $\bar{F}$ representing presence or absence of breast cancer and M representing level of prolactin. The structure is M/F versus M/$\bar{F}$. In a separate analysis, the case group was stratified into a high–family-risk group, F_1, and a low–family-risk group, F_2. The comparison was then M/F_1 versus M/F_2.

Answer 18.2. Answers depend on individual reports.

Chapter 19

Because individual reports were selected for each of the exercises, there are no official answers.

Chapter 20

Answer 20.1.

      20.1.1. $81/2943 = 0.0275$

      20.1.2. $36/1476 = 0.0244$

      20.1.3. $0.0244/0.0275 = 0.89$ or $(36 \times 2943)/(81 \times 1476) = 0.89$

      20.1.4. We have three ways of calculating the confidence interval.

      With the simple method, we find $\sqrt{(1/36)+(1/2943)+(1/81)+(1/1476)} = \sqrt{.0411} = 0.203$. The s.e. of o is $(0.203)(0.89) = 0.180$; and 1.96 times this s.e. is 0.35. The 95% confidence interval will be 0.89 ± 0.35 and extends from 0.54 to 1.24.

      With the Wolff method, we take the square root of $[(1/36.5)+(1/2943.5)+(1/81.5)+(1/1476.5)]$. This is $\sqrt{0.0407} = 0.202$. Multiplied by 1.96, 0.202 becomes 0.395.

The ln of o is -0.1165, and the 95% interval for the ln is -0.1165 ± 0.395. These values will be -0.5115 and 0.2785. Taking e to those powers, we get the interval of 0.60 to 1.32.

With the Miettinen method, we first find $X^2 = 0.355$ and $X = 0.596$. With Z_a set at 1.96, we calculate $1.96/0.596 = 3.288$. The values of 1 ± 3.288 extend from -2.288 to 4.288. When the latter two values are multiplied by the ln of o, which is -0.1165, we get a zone from $+0.2666$ to -0.4996. When raised to the appropriate powers of e, these values give a 95% confidence interval that goes from 0.61 to 1.31.

The three sets of results seem reasonably similar. Because all three confidence intervals include the neutral value of 1, and because the upper limits of the confidence intervals go no higher than the relatively benign value of 1.31, we can conclude (at least at the 0.05 stochastic level) that vasectomy has no distinctive relationship to cardiovascular disease.

20.1.5. This is a trap question. This cohort risk cannot be determined from these noncohort data. Because we did *not* assemble our basic groups as exposed and nonexposed people, you should *not* calculate the risk as $36/(36+81) = 0.31$. If you calculated the value as $36/81 = 0.44$, you have found an odds, not a risk.

20.1.6. Same problem as in Exercise 20.1.5. If you calculated $1476/4419 = 0.33$, the proportion is correct, but the concept of risk is wrong. If you calculated $1476/2943 = 0.50$, you are doubly wrong. This result is an odds, not a risk, and the risk (if that is what you were looking for) cannot be determined from these data.

20.1.7. Having neither risk value available from Exercises 20.1.5 or 20.1.6, we cannot calculate a risk ratio. The best we can do is to say that the risk ratio is approximated by the odds ratio of 0.89. Because cardiovascular disease may occur at a rate larger than 0.1, this approximation may not be totally correct.

Answer 20.2. Because of the small numbers, stochastic significance for these data is best calculated with the Fisher Exact Test. Because one of the cells already contains a zero, we have only one table to examine in the same direction as the observed difference. Its p value is $(7!)(33!)(8!)(32!)/(7!)(1!)(0!)(32!)(40!) = 0.0000004$. Because this is a one-tail hypothesis, we can accept this single table as the only one to be checked. The P value is thus 0.0000004.

If you want to do stochastic significance with a chi-square test (which we will need for the Miettinen confidence interval), it is $X_c^2 = [(7 \times 32)-(1 \times 0)-(40/2)]^2 \times 40/[7 \times 33 \times 8 \times 32] = 28.15$, and $X = 5.31$. This result also has an extremely small P value.

The odds ratio here will be $(7.5 \times 32.5)/(0.5)(1.5) = 325$ and $\ln(o) = 5.78$. For the Miettinen confidence interval, $1.96/5.31 = 0.369$, and 1 ± 0.369 extends from 0.631 to 1.369. Multiplied by 5.78, this zone runs from 3.65 to 7.91. When each number is raised to the appropriate power of e, the 95% confidence interval extends from 38.4 to 2732.1. Although the result is stochastically impressive, this wide confidence interval is very imprecise. We cannot be sure what the correct odds ratio really is, other than to say it is quite highly elevated above 1.

For the Wolff confidence interval, we first take the square root of $(1/7.5)+(1/32.5)+(1/0.05)+(1/1.5) = \sqrt{2.83} = 1.68$. The 95% confidence interval around $\ln(o)$ will be 5.78 $(1.96)(1.68)$, which is 5.78 ± 3.30. This will go from 2.48 to 9.08. When these numbers are raised to the powers of e, the 95% confidence interval is seen to extend from 11.9 to 8777.9. Again, the interval is extremely wide; and this one does not closely agree with what was found with the Miettinen technique.

The simple technique is probably inappropriate for these small numbers. If you tried it anyhow, you presumably used the results obtained with 0.5 added to each number. The s.e. of o will be $(325)(1.68) = 546$, which, when multiplied by 1.96, becomes 1070. The confidence interval would then become 325 ± 1070 and would extend from -745 to 1395. Because this zone includes the neutral value of 1, someone might want to claim that the result is *not* stochastically significant, despite the impressive P values.

The decision you make here depends on your preconceptions about the relationship, your beliefs about the confidence you can have in small numbers, your tolerance of results that disagree when calculated with different methods, and your faith about which method is correct. Any rational argument can be accepted.

Answer 20.3.

20.3.1. The fourfold table becomes

215	16	231
15	114	129
230	130	360

For this table,

$$
\begin{aligned}
\text{Nosologic sensitivity} &= 215/230 = 0.93 = & P(T|D)\\
\text{Nosologic specificity} &= 114/130 = 0.88 = & P(\bar{T}|\bar{D})\\
\text{Diagnostic sensitivity} &= 215/231 = 0.93 = & P(D|T)\\
\text{Diagnostic specificity} &= 114/129 = 0.88 = & P(\bar{D}|\bar{T})\\
\text{Positive likelihood ratio} &= (215/16)/(230/130) = 7.6\\
\text{Negative likelihood ratio} &= (15/114)/(230/130) = 0.07
\end{aligned}
$$

20.3.2. $P(D) = 230/360 = 0.64$, $P(D|T) = 215/231 = 0.93$, and $P(T|\bar{D}) = 16/130 = 0.12$. $P(\bar{D}|\bar{T}) = 114/129 = 0.88$.

$$
P(D|T) = \frac{(215/230) \times 0.64}{[(215/230) \times 0.64] + (1-0.88)(1-0.64)} = \frac{0.596}{0.596 + 0.043} = 0.93
$$

20.3.3. The fourfold table becomes

97	1	98
133	129	262
230	130	360

$$
\begin{aligned}
\text{Nosologic sensitivity} &= 97/230 = .42\\
\text{Nosologic specificity} &= 129/130 = .99\\
\text{Diagnostic sensitivity} &= 97/98 = .99\\
\text{Diagnostic specificity} &= 129/262 = .49\\
\text{Positive likelihood ratio} &= (97/1)/(230/130) = 54.8\\
\text{Negative likelihood ratio} &= (133/129)/(230/130) = .58
\end{aligned}
$$

The results become substantially different from what was noted previously.

20.3.4. The easiest approach is to cite the likelihood ratio for each of the three levels at which CPK is partitioned. At the level of ≥ 280, L_{pos} is $(97/1)/(230/130) = 54.8$. At the level of $80-279$, L_{pos} is $(118/15)/(230/130) = 4.4$. At <80, L_{pos} is what we found previously in Exercise 20.3.1 for L_{neg}. It is $(15/114)/(230/130) = 0.07$.

20.3.5. Without going through the complexities of converting the likelihood ratios into probability values, there does not seem to be a simple way of explaining this information. (If you have found a simple way, please let me know.) The best I could do would be to say that with lower levels of CPK, the chance of myocardial infarction is reduced. This remark does not say much, because the point is evident from the original table.

Answer 20.4.

20.4.1. Because the numbers are reasonably large, we can do a Z-test for stochastic significance, using the formula $Z = (\bar{X}_1 - \bar{X}_2)/\sqrt{(s_1^2/n_1) + (s_2^2/n_2)}$. The result is $(9265 - 8130)/\sqrt{(487^2/100) + (640^2/100)} = 1135/\sqrt{6467.69} = 14.1$. The P value associated with this value of Z is well below 0.05.

20.4.2. The results are presented in a postspective rather than prospective manner. To use the information clinically, we would want to know the throat culture results that are found at different levels of WBC. The statistical evidence should be structured as culture per WBC, but the data are presented as WBC per culture.

20.4.3. In the absence of a better presentation of data, we cannot tell how well the WBC does its diagnostic job. If the data have a Gaussian distribution, we can assume that the 95% interval range is roughly $9265 \pm (2)(487)$ for the cases and $8130 \pm (2)(640)$ for the controls. This range is from 8291 to 10,239 in the cases and from 6850 to 9410 in the controls. The two ranges will obviously have a great deal of nondiscriminating overlap. It is possible that very low values of WBC and very high values have relatively good discrimination at the two ends of the spectrum, but we would need to see the stratified results to examine this possibility.

Answer 20.5. The expected success rate in hospital A would be

$$
\left(\frac{98}{198} \times \frac{40}{49}\right) + \left(\frac{48}{198} \times \frac{88}{151}\right) + \left(\frac{52}{198} \times \frac{94}{302}\right) = 0.63
$$

Because the observed rate is 0.63, the ratio of observed and expected rates is $0.63/0.63 = 1$. This standardized ratio multiplies the standard rate to give the indirect standardized rate. In this instance, because 0.44 is the success rate at the standardizing hospital, we would have $1 \times 0.44 = 0.44$ as the standardized value for hospital A.

Answer 20.6. Taking the stratum death rates for Houston and the stratum proportion rates from Tampa–St. Petersburg, we would get $(5.2 \times 0.067) + (0.8 \times 0.308) + (2.6 \times 0.201) + (11.9 \times 0.222) + (54.9 \times 0.203) = 14.9$. As might be expected from a comparison of the stratified rates, the standardized result is similar to the death rate of 14.1 in the standardizing population.

Answer 20.7.

20.7.1. The standardizing year was 1940, when the two rates are identical.

20.7.2. Because the U.S. population is progressively aging, the proportion of elderly people will increase with secular time. If a later population is used to standardize an earlier population, the larger proportion of older people in the standardizing population will elevate the crude rate. Conversely, if an earlier population standardizes a later population, the crude rate of the later population will be lowered when standardized. With method A, the rate is above method B before the standardizing year, and the rates of method A are below method B after the standardizing year. The elevation followed by the fall indicates that method A produced the standardized rate and method B gave the crude rate.

Answer 20.8.

20.8.1. There are seven subgroups each for age and social class and six subgroups each for parity and cigarette smoking. The result of $7 \times 7 \times 6 \times 6 = 1764$.

20.8.2. Excluding the 13 unknown people, find the morbidity events and calculate their rates in each of the 1764 total subgroups, regardless of treatment. These calculations will produce the standard morbidity rates, R_i, for each subgroup, where $i = 1, 2, \ldots,$ 1764. Now suppose a particular treatment group with a crude morbidity rate, r, contains n_1 people in subgroup 1, n_2 people in subgroup 2, and so on. If n is the total number of people receiving that treatment, the subgroup proportions will be $p_1 = n_1/n$, $p_2 = n_2/n$, $\ldots$, and $P_{1764} = n_{1764}/n$. The standardized expected morbidity in each subgroup will be $p_i R_i$; and the expected morbidity rate for the treatment will be $\Sigma p_i R_i$. (An easier way to obtain this value is to multiply each $n_i \times R_i$ directly, find $\Sigma n_i R_i$, and then divide it by n.) The standardized morbidity ratio will be $r/\Sigma p_i R_i$, and it will become an indirectly standardized rate when multiplied by the total morbidity rate, R, for the entire cohort.

20.8.3. If the morbid events were relatively infrequent, many of the 1764 cells for each treatment would contain no morbid events and would have an attack rate of zero. If these rates were used in a direct standardization, the adjustment would depend on the positive results found in relatively few cells. The indirect standardization allows all of the cells to contribute, even if they contaned no morbid events.

20.8.4. The standardization process seems mathematically quite reasonable, although we can wonder whether its complexity was understood by the general practitioners who performed the research. The main problem is that the process, despite its elaborate statistics, does not account for the susceptibility and detection biases that can readily be suspected as prime sources of distortion in the results. Why did the takers and ex-takers decide to use or to discontinue the use of oral contraceptives? If these reasons were related to health, there might be major susceptibility biases present at baseline. Did the three groups receive similar surveillance and diagnostic procedures for the outcome events? If the takers were under more intense medical surveillance (as the investigators acknowledged), the surveillance alone could elevate the detection of many morbid events that might be unrecognized or uncounted in the other two groups.

Answer 20.9.

20.9.1. The odds ratios become $(5 \times 104)/(13 \times 6) = 6.67$ for old men, $(4 \times 80)/(10 \times 7) = 4.57$ for young men, $(7 \times 40)/(5 \times 12) = 4.67$ for old women, and $(5 \times 72)/(6 \times 24) = 2.50$ for young women. These new values do not change any previous conclusions, but they suggest that age has a distinct effect that should be adjusted if we want to express everything as a single odds ratio.

20.9.2. If we recombine the data, irrespective of gender, we get the following two tables:

Presence of Hypercholesterolemia	Presence of Diabetes in:			
	Old People		Young People	
	Yes	No	Yes	No
Yes	12	11	9	13
No	25	144	34	152

The overall odds ratios will be $(12 \times 144)/(11 \times 25) = 6.28$ for old people and $(9 \times 152)/(13 \times 34) = 3.10$ for young people.

20.9.3. We want to get a Mantel-Haenszel adjusted odds ratio across the four tables having the respective group sizes of 128, 101, 64, and 107. The adjusted numerator will be $(5 \times 104/128) + (4 \times 80/101) + (7 \times 40/64) + (5 \times 72/107) = 14.97$. The adjusted denominator will be $(13 \times 6/128) + (10 \times 7/101) + (12 \times 5/64) + (24 \times 6/107) = 3.59$. The adjusted odds ratio will be $14.97/3.59 = 4.17$.

Answer 20.10. Cancer cases in the hospital may be there because of later development of malnutrition or other complications. These complications, rather than the cancer alone, may raise the level of neoplasmognome. Alternatively, the level of neoplasmognome may be low or high early in the disease but may then change to normal levels later by the time the patient is found in the hospital group.

Answer 20.11. Status of cohort is shown at the two ages. Abbreviations are A = alive; D = dead; R = retinopathy; N = no retinopathy; O = old retinopathy. For combinations of symbols, AR = alive with retinopathy; DO = dead with old retinopathy, and so on.

Age 35

AR:(0.75)(0.20) = 0.15
DR:(0.75)(0.15) = 0.1125
DN:(0.75)(0.10) = 0.075
AN:(0.75)(0.55) = 0.4125

Age 55

AO:(0.15)(0.60) = 0.09
DO:(0.15)(0.40) = 0.06
AR: × (0.25) = 0.103125
DR: × (0.30) = 0.12375
DN: × (0.18) = 0.07425
AN: × (0.27) = 0.111375

AR:(0.25)(0.08) = 0.02
DR:(0.25)(0.06) = 0.015
DN:(0.25)(0.02) = 0.005
AN:(0.25)(0.84) = 0.21

× 0.82 = 0.0164:AO
× 0.18 = 0.0036:DO
× 0.12 = 0.0252:AR
× 0.14 = 0.0294:DR
× 0.06 = 0.0126:DN
× 0.68 = 0.1428:AN

Rates of Retinopathy

Incidence

= 0.15 + 0.1125 + 0.02 + 0.015 = 0.2975 ≈ 30%

= 0.2975 + 0.103125 + 0.12375 + 0.0252 + 0.0294 = 0.5789 ≈ 58%

Prevalence

= (0.15 + 0.02) ÷ (0.15 + 0.02 + 0.4125 + 0.21) = (0.17)/(0.7925) = 0.2145 ≈ 21%

= (0.09 + 0.103125 + 0.0164 + 0.0252) ÷ (0.09 + 0.103125 + 0.0164 + 0.0252 + 0.111375 + 0.1428) = 0.234725/0.4889 = 0.4801 ≈ 48%

Conclusions: The longitudinal prevalence rates produce an underestimate of incidence rates of retinopathy. At age 35, incidence is 30%, but longitudinal prevalence is 21%. At age 55, incidence is 58%, but longitudinal prevalence is 48%.

Chapter 21

Answers 21.1 and 21.2. No official answers, because studies are to be chosen individually.
Answer 21.3.
21.3.1. This is a population-based retrospective case-control study.
21.3.2. Three main problems come to mind. Because the authors discuss all three of

the potential problems in the published report, you can decide for yourself whether the problems were suitably managed. The problems are as follows:

(1) How accurately can the interview technique and the special rating discern the candidate's customary expenditure of energy in physical activities?

(2) Were the interviewers blinded to the research hypothesis or to the identity of spouses as cases or controls when the interview was conducted? (If not, how was objectivity maintained?)

(3) Protopathic bias can occur if people with angina pectoris (or other appropriate symptoms) had not sought medical attention and had not told their spouses about the symptoms, but had gradually reduced their level of physical activities. If such people later died of sudden cardiac arrest, they would not be excluded from the case group but would be cited as having a reduced level of physical activities.

Answer 21.4. The compared results are based on longitudinal cross-sections. Because patients with recurrences of rheumatic fever must emerge from those who have had first attacks, the following circumstances might exist for a cohort:

	Status in First Attack	Patients with: No Recurrence	Patients with: Recurrent Attacks	Rate of Recurrence
No Cardiac Damage	116 ———→	100 ———→	16	16/116 = 14%
Cardiac Damage	84 ———→	20 ———→	64	64/84 = 76%
TOTAL	200	120	80	
Prevalence of Cardiac Damage	84/200 = 42%		64/80 = 80%	

This chart shows how, without a change in the cardiac status of individual patients, the prevalence of cardiac damage can rise from 42% to 80%. To check whether this possible interpretation is correct, perform a cohort study and check stratified rates of recurrence and cardiac outcome.

Answer 21.5. This is a pathoconsortive study. The high phenylacetic acid coexists with the aggressive behavior, but we cannot tell whether it is cause or effect. Both the case and control groups are unsatisfactory because of the prisoners used as the framework for the study. The outcomes of the research hypothesis are aggressive and nonaggressive behavior, not imprisonment for violent and nonviolent crimes. Why not classify a group of *nonprisoners* for aggressive characteristics and then correlate their levels of phenylacetic acid?

Answer 21.6. None of the suggested groups is very good. Detection bias, a prominent issue in patients with colon cancer, would be neglected if the control groups were chosen from neighbors or siblings. Unless the patients with anemia had been suitably tested for colonic sources of the anemia, they would also not compensate for detection bias. The patients receiving elective surgery would be unsuitable because of the unilateral exclusions applied to that group. Because alpha-methyldopa is used to treat hypertension, the elimination of patients with cerebrovascular, kidney, and cardiac disease from the control group would factitiously lower the antecedent prevalence of alpha-methyldopa usage in that group. The colonoscopy patients would be a good choice if they came from County General rather than Suburban Hospital, whose source population may be quite different in its susceptibility to colon cancer and antecedent usage of alpha-methyldopa. A better control group, therefore, would be chosen from patients receiving barium enemas or colonoscopy at County General Hospital during the past 5 years. After the cases are identified in these diagnostic rosters, the remaining controls (with diagnostic findings that are negative for cancer) could be matched to the cases by age, gender, and year of diagnosis.

Answer 21.7. Without regard to the effects of Excellitol, the rates of hospitalization for each disease will produce the following table, arranged in the same manner as Table 21–2:

$$\begin{Bmatrix} 40 & 39 & 746 \\ 120 & 462 & 2218 \end{Bmatrix}$$

The remaining people receiving Excellitol in the community will be arranged as 10, 38, and 24,127. If hospitalized at a rate of 0.1, the Excellitol patients will augment the upper row of the foregoing table by the following numbers: 1, 4, and 2413. Consequently, the hospital data will show the following sixfold table:

$$\begin{Bmatrix} 41 & 43 & 3159 \\ 120 & 462 & 2218 \end{Bmatrix}$$

With other cancers as controls, the odds ratio will be $(41 \times 462)/(43 \times 120) = 3.7$. Although having no effect on lung cancer, Excellitol would still be falsely indicted as a possible cause, according to this odds ratio. With noncancers as controls, the odds ratio will be $(41 \times 2218)/(120 \times 3159) = 0.24$. Excellitol may now be regarded as a protective agent that prevents lung cancer. With all other patients as controls, the odds ratio will be $[41 \times (462 + 2218)]/[120 \times (42 + 3159)] = 0.29$ and would still suggest a fallacious protective role for Excellitol.

Answer 21.8. Using the formula $(b-c)^2/(b+c)$, the matched value of X_M^2 is $(16-4)^2/20 = 7.2$. If you use $(|b-c|-1)^2/(b+c)$ as the formula, X_M^2 is $(|16-4|-1)^2/20 = 6.05$. With either value of X_M^2, $P<0.05$. For the unmatched arrangement, the basic table would be as follows:

	CASES	CONTROLS
EXPOSED	56	44
NONEXPOSED	44	56

The odds ratio here is $(56 \times 56)/(44 \times 44) = 1.6$. The regular X^2 calculation could be simplified to $[56^2 - 44^2]^2 \cdot 200/100^4 = 2.88$; and $P>0.05$.

Answer 21.9. As shown in the text, the matched odds ratio is b/c and the unmatched ratio is $(a+b)(b+d)/(a+c)(c+d)$. If we expand the latter expression, we get $(b^2 + ab + bd + ad)/(c^2 + ac + cd + ad) = [b(a+b+d)+ad]/[c(a+c+d)+ad]$. Because $N = a+b+c+d$, we can substitute $N-c = a+b+d$, and $N-b = a+c+d$. The unmatched ratio then becomes $[b(N-c)+ad]/[c(N-b)+ad] = [bN+ad-bc]/[cN+ad-bc] = \{b+[(ad-bc)/N]\}/\{c+[(ad-bc)/N]\}$. The value of the unmatched ratio will equal b/c when $ad-bc = 0$, i.e., when $ad = bc$. The unmatched odds ratio can substantially depart from b/c when the term $(ad-bc)/N$ is relatively large compared with the individual values of b or c.

Chapter 22

Answer 22.1.

22.1.1. Because the cases are no longer alive, the surviving informants's comments will depend on second-hand data, which may be affected by the responder's beliefs about efficacy of jogging.

22.1.2. Parents may not remember the particular antibiotics that were given to the children. If the study were being done today, the already established association between stained teeth and tetracycline may make the parent of a stained-teeth child assume that a preceding antibiotic must have been tetracycline.

22.1.3. Not all people can recall the particular type of antibiotic they received in previous treatment. Patients with chronic pulmonary disease are particularly likely to have received (and to recall having received) a cephalosporin antibiotic for a pulmonary episode (such as pneumonia) that preceded the formal diagnosis of chronic pulmonary disease.

22.1.4. Because of publicity about a possible fluoride-cancer relationship, recollections of amount and schedule of antecedent fluoride usage may be approached more avidly by people with cancer than by control patients without cancer.

22.1.5. No particular problem, except for the general difficulty of identifying tranquilizers among the many prescribed and nonprescribed drugs to which people are exposed.

22.1.6. Same problem as in Exercise 22.1.3. In addition, people with Alzheimer's disease may not be able to remember possible exposures, whereas people without Alzheimer's disease may forget them.

22.1.7. Most people should know whether they have ever been to Eastern Connecticut. If the interview is conducted long after development of Lyme disease, however, knowledge of the time relationship may be compromised. Did the visit occur at an appropriate preceding time in relation to the subsequent development of Lyme disease?

Answer 22.2.

22.2.1. Check with friends, colleagues, or fellow joggers to obtain confirmation from people other than the surviving informant.

22.2.2. Check with records of prescribing physicians or pharmacists.

22.2.3. Same as Exercise 22.2.2.

22.2.4. Difficult to check, unless people who lived with patient (parents, siblings, and so on) are available and reliable.

22.2.5. Difficult to check, unless you can find reliable people who lived with patient throughout life and who were initimately familiar with patient's medication patterns.

22.2.6. Same problem as in Exercise 22.2.5, except physician's *and dentist's* records might be checked for episodes at which general anesthesia might have occurred.

22.2.7. Check with physicians re timing of Lyme disease. Check with fellow travelers or hosts re timing of visit to Eastern Connecticut.

Answer 22.3.

22.3.1. Protopathic bias. People with poor health may have avoided or discontinued jogging.

22.3.2. Anamnestic bias if tetracycline is believed to cause stained teeth.

22.3.3. Protopathic bias. The infection that evoked cephalosporin treatment may have been an early manifestation of chronic pulmonary disease.

22.3.4. Anamnestic bias if fluoride is believed to cause cancer.

22.3.5. Protopathic bias. Was tranquilizer used to treat nonspecific abdominal pain that was an unrecognized early manifestation of pancreatic cancer?

22.3.6. No particular bias seems evident to me. What did you suggest?

22.3.7. Anamnestic bias that may produce a false temporal sequence.

Answer 22.4.

22.4.1. Because jogging is widely regarded as health-promoting, results suggesting it is harmful might not be welcomed or accepted.

22.4.2. Results suggesting tetracycline does *not* stain teeth might be rejected because they are contrary to prevailing opinion.

22.4.3. Because chronic pulmonary disease was abundant before cephalosporins became available, they are not a plausible etiologic agent. Results showing they contribute to chronic pulmonary disease might be more acceptable than those suggesting direct causality.

22.4.4. Acceptance of hypothesis depends on prior beliefs about carcinogencity of fluorides.

22.4.5. There is no explicatory mechanism for the biologic hypothesis, although heterodemic data might show a rising occurrence of pancreatic cancer in association with increased sales of tranquilizers.

22.4.6. Aside from the biologic plausibility that general anesthesia and Alzheimer's disease both have sensorial effects, there is no explicatory mechanism.

22.4.7. Because Lyme disease has been found in places remote from Eastern Connecticut, the two events are not distinctively related. The visit to Eastern Connecticut might have been important as an etiologic hint before the causal organism became identified, but a positive association between Eastern Connecticut and Lyme disease would have little scientific value today.

Answer 22.5. Individual reports to be submitted.

Answer 22.6. Adverse effects of dioxin, Agent Orange, and living near Love Canal. As the public has become increasingly frightened by frequent reports of hazards associated with events of everyday life (e.g., aspirin, fluoridation of water, etc.), people are highly anxious and predisposed to believe any kind of accusation as soon as it is brought up. By the time a scientific study is mounted, the toxic relationship may be regarded as well established.

Chapter 23

Answer 23.1. Answers depend on individual studies.

Answer 23.2.

23.2.1. Protopathic bias. As the cancer develops, it produces unpleasant oral sensations that the patient tries to relieve by using mouthwash.

23.2.2. Protopathic bias. The initial cholesterol level is reduced by an undetected cancer.

23.2.3. Susceptibility bias. Digitalis treatment is given to the patients with conditions that make them particularly likely to die early.

23.2.4. Protopathic bias. The retroperitoneal fibrosis produces hypertension that is treated with the beta blockers.

23.2.5. Protopathic bias. The cimetidine is given to treat an ulcer that is an undiagnosed or misdiagnosed gastric cancer.

Answer 23.3. The results may have the co-manifestation and co-morbidity biases that can arise from diagnostic procedure frameworks. From the large reservoir of existing but frequently undetected gallstones, patients usually come to diagnostic detection if they develop characteristic symptoms of pain or jaundice due to stones that become impacted in the cystic or hepatic duct. Because exodus from the gallbladder and impaction in a duct is more readily accomplished by small stones than by larger ones, the benign gallbladder disease group may contain a disproportionately high content of patients with stones alone. This problem would produce a falsely high odds ratio. To adjust for this type of manifestation-induced detection bias in the control group, stratify the results and examine odds ratios in the case and control groups separately for patients who did or did not present with characteristic clinical manifestations of gallstone impaction. The cogent value would be the one determined in patients *without* the characteristic manifestations.

To adjust for co-morbidity bias, check the odds ratios that are found when patients who simultaneously have both small and large stones are eliminated from the tabulations.

A separate problem, analogous to co-morbidity bias, can arise because patients with small stones in a duct but with large stones in the gallbladder were counted only in the *large* group. This decision might artificially inflate the number of *large* people in the benign gallbladder disease group, and would reduce the true magnitude of the odds ratio. To adjust for this problem, check the odds ratios that are found for large stones alone versus small stones alone, after eliminating patients with both small and large stones from the case group and the control group.

Answer 23.4. Perhaps the most overt problem to be considered is the unexamined effect of detection bias. If smokers are more likely than nonsmokers to develop a distressing cough, the increased diagnostic surveillance would lead to more frequent and intensive tests for lung cancer. The problem could be managed by sampling through a diagnostic test (such as chest films and sputum Pap smears) or by stratifying the patients according to a medical surveillance index (based on frequency of clinical tests and examinations). Other potential problems that were not considered in the research are susceptibility bias (in family history), performance bias (in occupational exposure), and the possibility that the amount of smoking was overestimated by an exposure definition based on "most recent amount smoked." At the time of the study, when people did not believe cigarette smoking was harmful, a recent increase in smoking may have led to the symptoms responsible for detection of the disease.

Answer 23.5. Detection bias is an important problem here because asymptomatic women with gallbladder disease are more likely, if under medical surveillance because of oral contraceptives, to receive a suitable diagnostic procedure than women who do not use oral agents and do not receive surveillance. The problem can be avoided by using a diagnostic procedure framework. In a suitable age group of women who received cholecystograms or ultrasonograms of the gallbladder (or both tests), the cases would consist of people with abnormal tests showing stones or convincing nonvisualization of the gallbladder. The remaining women, with normal tests, would become the pool of potential controls who could be matched (by age, race, and date of admission) to the case group.

Answer 23.6. Individual answers to be submitted.

Answer 23.7. Individual answers to be submitted.

Answer 23.8. Individual answers to be submitted.

Answer 23.9. Individual answers to be submitted.

Chapter 24

Answer 24.1. In Figure 24–2, why is there no legend to indicate which countries are represented by the abbreviations? In Figure 24–3, why are milk, margarine, and sugar shown in the first graph but not the second? Why are coffee and cigarette smoking shown in the second but not the first? Why is cigarette smoking shown only for women? What are the units of ischemic heart disease mortality? Why has it not risen in women concomitant with their rise in cigarette smoking?

Answer 24.2.

    24.2.1. Detection bias. Because cancer of the colon is often a silent or minimally symptomatic disease, it will be discovered more often in people who receive more medical care. The increased medical attention and detection may occur with increased income.

    24.2.2. Detection bias. Are the defects more likely to be diagnosed for city dwellers because the births occur in municipal hospitals that have more diagnostically alert cardiologists? Are the defects found more often in summer because cardiac fellows, distrusting the new interns, check all births themselves? (Regardless of what alternative explanation may be offered, the observed relationship has been contradicted by subsequent data, reported in letters that followed the original publication.)

    24.2.3. Detection bias. Lymphomas may be more likely to be diagnosed in people in rich countries that have better diagnostic technology and that can also afford to eat more bovine protein than poor countries.

    24.2.4. Whatever explanation you want to offer is acceptable. The results have subsequently been contradicted by other heterodemic data.

Answer 24.3. The first scientific steps would be to see whether the problem really exists or is an epidemiologic artefact. Several sources of artefact can be suspected:

    1. If cancer rates are ranked for 50 states, one of the states is bound to be highest and another lowest. Because the chance of being highest is 1/50, or P = 0.02, the rank may appear to be statistically significant, but it may not be quantitatively menacing. What are the cancer rates in the three or four next highest states, and how much different are they from New Jersey's?

    2. What are the patterns of cancer detection, medical care, and diagnostic nomenclature in New Jersey? Are the cancers being found as an artefact of detection bias because of good medical care and thorough usage of technologic methods of diagnosis throughout the state?

    3. Is the rate of cancer consistently high throughout the state, and how do these rates compare with those of similar regions (having similar medical care patterns) in other states? For example, how do the rates in purely rural regions compare with those of purely rural regions elsewhere?

    4. The two most populous cities in New Jersey are Newark and Jersey City, both of which have good municipal hospital facilities and both of which have had a heavy influx of black in-migration. If most of the fatal cancers in blacks are being medically identified, but if all the blacks are not being counted in the census, the occurrence rates for cancer can be falsely elevated because of the spuriously low denominators.

Answer 24.4. In view of the considerable previous inconsistencies and fluctuations in statistical coding of deaths caused by asthma, the investigators for the prosecution have been remarkably credulous about accepting the stated rates of death as correct. The investigators also seem remarkably complacent in accepting the death certificate numerators without examining a denominator of cases with asthma to see whether case fatality rates have indeed changed. Finally, shouldn't we rule out the possibility that moribund people received powerful broncho-dilators because they were moribund rather than vice versa?

Answer 24.5. Individual reports to be submitted.

Answer 24.6. The ones that seem reasonably unequivocal are: "Abortive and Still Born," "Drowned," "Kil'd by Several Accident," "Made Away Themselves," and "Murthered" in Graunt's list; and "Stillborn," "Abortive," "Accidents & Violence," "Apoplexy," "Suddenly," and "Scald Head" in Forbes' list. All others may be diagnosed in different terms today or may represent entities different from what we now associate with the terms today. *Example:* Several centuries ago "fever" often referred to a rapid heartbeat. "Smallpox" was probably used for chickenpox and many other rashes besides today's smallpox.

Answer 24.7. Debility; Consumption; Convulsions; Age; Inflammation; Dropsy; Fevers; Insane, Lunatic; Coroner's Warrant. Today's death certificates would also be more specific about distinguishing among asthma, chest diseases, lung diseases, heart diseases, and liver diseases.

Note that the top five categories (Debility through Inflammation) encompassed 1953 (43%) of the 4513 deaths. All of these conditions were available in the 19th century to provide rises for the incidence rates of 20th century "diseases."

Answer 24.8. I do not recall any. I do not recall any. Yes. Lectures can be included as part of epidemiology–public health–biostatistics instruction. Also, clinical clerks can be asked to fill out a "mock" death certificate for any patient who dies. Attending M.D. must check the mock certificates. (Who checks the attending M.D.?)

Answer 24.9. The answers below are verbatim copies of statements for each of these cases, cited as illustrative examples in either the Coding Manuals or Nosology Guidelines issued by the NCHS. You may or may not agree with the answers, and you also may or may not be occasionally shocked by the decisions.

(1) *Select* chronic alcoholism. Chronic alcoholism is accepted as the cause of both conditions entered above it.

(2) *Select* cirrhosis of liver. The *general rule* is not applicable. The *reported* sequence terminating in the condition first entered on the certificate is esophageal varices due to cirrhosis of liver.

(3) *Select* rheumatic heart disease. There is no *reported* sequence.

(4) *Select* diabetes. There is no *reported* sequence.

(5) *Code to* renal failure. Heart failure, selected by the *general rule,* is ignored.

(6) *Select* and *code* cleft palate by the *general rule.* Rule 6 is *not* applicable because the trivial condition is reported as the cause of a more serious *related* condition.

(7) *Code to* late effects of rickets.

(8) *Code to* paralysis agitans. This category includes parkinsonism due to arteriosclerosis.

(9) *Code to* general arteriosclerosis according to the general rule. No linkage, because the arteriosclerosis is not stated as the underlying cause of the parkinsonism.

(10) *Code: Generalized ischemic cerebrovascular disease without mention of hypertension.* The General Rule. Cerebral arteriosclerosis is accepted as the cause of the pneumonia as well as the aspiration of food. This is also regarded as a properly completed certificate where there is one condition to a line in an ascending causal order of sequence. Aspiration of milk or other food due to a disease that presumably affects the ability to control the process of swallowing is regarded as a causal sequence.

(11) *Code: Chronic nephritis.* The General Rule. Chronic interstitial nephritis entered alone on the lowest used line in Part I is accepted as the cause of all the conditions entered above it. The General Rule is applied in such cases even though the durations on I(a) and I(b) indicate the conditions were not entered on the certificate in the correct causal relationship.

(12) *Code: Cholelithiasis.* The General Rule. Cholelithiasis is accepted as the cause of the conditions reported above it.

(13) *Code: Diabetes mellitus without mention of acidosis or coma.* The General Rule. Diabetes entered alone on the lowest used line in Part I is accepted as the cause of all conditions entered above it.

(14) *Code: Hemiplegia.* The General Rule. Hemiplegia is accepted as the cause of all the conditions reported above it.

(15) *Code: Other and unspecified fall.* Selection Rule 1, Reported sequence terminating in the condition first entered on the certificate. The underlying cause of the *reported* sequence is fracture of hip. The coded category includes fracture(s) of any site when the external cause of the fracture(s) is not reported.

(16) *Code: Accident caused by cutting or piercing instrument.* This category includes cuts from falling on certain cutting machines such as powered hand tools and metal-cutting machines.

(17) *Code: Chronic nephritis.* The General Rule and Modification Rule 7, Linkage. Hypertensive vascular disease is selected because it is entered alone on the lowest used line in Part I and may give rise to all the conditions entered above it. There is a conflict in linkages. The chronic renal disease would have been selected by Rules 1 and 3 if the hypertension had not been reported. Therefore hypertension is linked with chronic renal disease for the code assignment of chronic nephritis.

(18) *Code: Other heart disease specified as rheumatic.* The General Rule. Bacterial endocarditis (acute) (chronic) (subacute) is classified elsewhere whether or not there is indication that a specific valve was involved. When bacterial endocarditis is superimposed on a rheumatic heart disease, the bacterial endocarditis is not considered as specifying the part of the heart affected by the rheumatic process. Also, the bacterial endocarditis does not specify the rheumatic process as active at the time of death.

(19) *Code: Influenza with pneumonia.* The General Rule and Modification Rule 7, Linkage. Influenza links with any form of pneumonia for this category.

(20) *Code: Unspecified mental retardation.* The General Rule and Modification Rule 5, Ill-defined condition. Vomiting (784.1) is selected as the cause of dehydration (788.0). The "days" in the column for approximate interval between onset and death is not interpreted to mean that the vomiting was pernicious, persistent, or uncontrolled. In accordance with Modification Rule 5, a condition on the certificate classifiable elsewhere than to 780–796 takes preference over conditions classifiable to 784.1 and 788.0. Therefore, classification is to the mental deficiency.

(21) *Code: Chronic ischemic heart disease.* Selection Rule 1. The underlying cause of the first reported sequence terminating in the condition first entered on the certificate is selected. No special preference is given to the surgical procedure.

(22) *Code: Disease of knee joint.* Selection Rule 1. A reported sequence terminating in the condition first entered on the certificate. Without further qualification, surgery of a site is assigned to disease of that site. In this case, it is assumed that the knee surgery was performed for a disease of the knee joint.

Chapter 25

Answer 25.1. If we start with 10,000 school-aged children, of whom 4% are physically abused, the fourfold table will show

	Confirmed Condition		
Physical Exam	*Abused*	*Not Abused*	**Total**
Positive	384	768	1152
Negative	16	8832	8848
Total	400	9600	10,000

Of the 400 abused children, 96% (384) are detected by the physical exam; of the 9600 nonabused, 8% (768) have false-positive exams. Consequently, nosologic sensitivity = 96% (384/400); nosologic specificity = 92% (8832/9600), and diagnostic sensitivity (positive predictive accuracy) = 33% (384/1152).

Answer 25.2. Individual reports to be submitted.

Answer 25.3. There is no easy solution to the dilemma of the gold standard. Several possible diagnostic substitutes can be tried: (1) Ask an expert panel of gastroenterologists to review all of the clinical data at the time of the patient's clinical presentation and to provide a consensus diagnosis of pancreatitis. (This single-state assessment should not include the amylase clearance ratio); (2) perform the same consensus review of all the clinical data during the patient's hospitalization, so that information on the clinical course is added to data on the initial clinical presentation (this multi-state assessment should also exclude data on the amylase clearance ratio); (3) change the endpoint of the evaluation to a management decision, such as whether to perform an abdominal laparotomy. The last approach would attempt to study the management efficacy, rather than the diagnostic efficacy, of the amylase clearance ratio.

As a diagnostic challenge, suitable patients must represent the full spectrum of disease severity, including not only patients with severe pancreatitis but also patients with mild disease who have abdominal pain but little evidence of peritoneal irritation or severe volume loss. The test should also be challenged by appropriate co-morbid diseases (e.g., biliary stone, alcoholic liver disease) and by conditions that might cause false-positive or -negative test results (e.g., renal disease or diabetic ketoacidosis).

Answer 25.4. The complete probability table is as follows:

Roth Spots	**Endocarditis**	**No Endocarditis**	**Row Totals**
Present	0.001	0	0.001
Absent	0.199	0.8	0.999
Column Totals	0.2	0.8	1.00

a. This answer, given in the statement of the exercise, is 0.005.
b. This answer, also given in the statement of the exercise, is 0.
c. The fourfold table is constructed by multiplying 0.2×1.00 to get the total prevalence

proportion for endocarditis. The prevalence of no endocarditis is then 0.8. Multiplying 0.005×0.2 gives us 0.001 for the cell in the upper left corner. Because nosologic specificity is cited as 1 in the statement of the problem, we can now fill in the "No Endocarditis" column vertically as 0 and 0.8. The rest of the numbers are constructed by appropriate additions and subtractions. From these numbers, the probability that a patient with Roth spots has endocarditis is $0.001/0.001 = 1.0$. (This answer is also predictable, however, from the statement of the exercise, without any calculations. If the sign has perfect specificity, the disease is always present if the sign is present.)

d. This answer is the only one of the four that requires calculations. The result is $0.199/0.999 = 0.199$. On the other hand, by thinking about the specified clinical details, you could have estimated that the result should be very close to 0.2—and it is.

Answer 25.5.

a. The target disease should have reasonably high prevalence and importance, from the viewpoints of morbidity, mortality, and cost.

b. The test must have a high sensitivity for detecting the disease and must be simple to administer, acceptable to the screened population, and of low cost.

c. There should be evidence that treatment of early identified risk or disease will significantly reduce adverse outcomes and that the therapy can be implemented successfully on a wide-scale basis.

d. The specificity of the test should be high enough so that the number of false positive results does not become a nuisance.

Answer 25.6. Individual reports to be submitted.

Chapter 26

Answer 26.1. Individual reports to be submitted.

Chapter 27

Answer 27.1.

27.1.1. Many factors in this study could have obscured a positive relationship between process and outcome. In spectrum of challenges, the patient group as a whole may have been relatively easy to care for, offering too limited a scope for adequate assessment. In the procedures chosen to represent process, many of the selected activities (e.g., recording of smoking history) would be unlikely to affect control of blood pressure; and the most powerful procedure—aggressive antihypertensive therapy—may not have been defined in a way that would show a correlation with blood pressure control. In collection of data, many desirable procedures performed by the clinicians may have been rated as inadequate because they were not recorded; and the investigators' variability (or bias) in obtaining and rating the data was not studied. (Widely random imprecisions in these observations would tend to reduce a positive process-outcome correlation.)

The outcome event may not have been chosen suitably for a sensitive indication of degree of blood pressure control. Arbitrary levels of blood pressure were rated as *good*, *fair*, or *poor* rather than according to degree or proportion of reduction for the originally elevated level of pressure; and some of the selected levels may have been clinically inappropriate (e.g., the BP of a healthy octogenarian might be adequately controlled at 160/100).

Statistically, poor outcome events were relatively uncommon (only 14/130 patients had poor BP control); and the total group size was relatively small (138), so that impressive statistical correlations would be difficult to demonstrate.

27.1.2. No. Presentation of P values gives no information about the magnitude of the associations, which would be better displayed as correlation (or regression) coefficients.

27.1.3. The stratification was presumably done to control for baseline severity of hypertension, under the assumption that higher initial BPs are more difficult to lower. Although partly related to initial height, susceptibility to lowering of BP is also related to other variables (e.g., etiology, end-organ damage) that were not taken into account.

Furthermore, the arbitrary partitioning of a dimensional variable reduces the opportunity to show statistically significant correlations, particularly when the outcome variable is also an arbitrarily partitioned dimension.

Answer 27.2.

27.2.1. Emergency room visits. This is an unsatisfactory unit of analysis in the study, because the results of closely spaced sequential visits for individual patients can hardly be considered as independent events, either in terms of the care given or the outcomes experienced. This problem was particularly significant because 54/177 visits were return visits.

27.2.2. No. The process criteria were aimed at evaluating treatment for physiologic derangements; but the outcome criteria had a much broader scope. It included not only breathlessness but also patient satisfaction and patient education. Because of the dissociation between the two sets of criteria, it is somewhat surprising that a correlation was found in this study.

27.2.3. As noted on page 688 of the published paper, 51% of the group was assessed at 24 hours and 49% of the group was assessed at seven days. These are low rates of participation. The results could have been substantially biased if the studied group was distorted by patients who were reached for follow-up only because they had particularly good or particularly bad outcomes. It seems plausible that the patients with good outcomes would be more easy to reach and more willing to cooperate than patients with poor outcomes.

27.2.4. Although statistically significant, these coefficients are not quantitatively impressive. For example, the coefficient of 0.35 for both hospitals indicates that only 12% of the variance in outcomes was explained by variability in process. Because the acute care delivered in emergency rooms would be expected to have very short-term effects, particularly in the absence of follow-up, it is not surprising that the correlation between process and outcome was reduced for the seven-day outcome score.

Answer 27.3.

27.3.1. Not really. The authors have prepared a series of clusters of clinical phenomena and have developed appropriate process criteria for each cluster. The criteria thus have a flexibility and cogency that is not contained in a "laundry list" of individual items—but the criteria do not show the sequence of input/decision/response, followed by new decisions and new responses, that occurs in customary clinical activities. The data noted in emergency room encounter forms cannot show a truly sequential branching scheme of clinical logic.

27.3.2. The study by Nobrega and coworkers used the "laundry list" approach, in which each of the cited process items was rated for each patient's care—regardless of the pertinence of those items for individual patients. The criteria-mapping technique provides a more direct approach to the clinical distinctions of individual patients, but the criteria are more complex and more difficult to create and to apply. Each approach may have been best for the type of clinical situation to which it was addressed.

27.3.3. The patients who were admitted presumably had a worse prognosis (e.g., strongly suspected or definite myocardial infarction) than those who were discharged. Accordingly, the outcomes might be substantially different in the discharged and admitted patients and might not correlate well with the process. A patient who was inappropriately admitted with a minor ailment might have a good outcome; and a patient who was appropriately admitted with a lethal myocardial infarction might have a poor outcome. The authors, aware of this distinction, investigated the records of the admitted patients and found that 74% (78/105) had unequivocally justified admissions and that the remainder were at high risk for myocardial infarction. In the group discharged from the emergency room, however, the process criteria may not be a true measure of adequate care. In view of the selected negative outcome event—death or subsequent hospitalization within 21 days—the process criteria may simply reflect their prognostic ability to distinguish groups with relatively high or low risk for a negative outcome. Although an important component of care, prognostication alone may not be an adequate measure of care.

Answer 27.4.

27.4.1. One principal difficulty is that outcomes were assessed too long after presentation of the mild, self-limited illnesses that were studied. This excessively long interval might lead to an insensitive detection of poor outcomes that resolved spontaneously and nonspecific detection of bad outcomes that occurred long after the illness and that were erroneously attributed to the illness and its care. A second difficulty is that outcomes such as anxiety and limitation of activity seem inappropriate for the relatively minor investigated illnesses, which tend to create minimal anxiety and minimal limitations of activity.

27.4.2. Because the desired outcome of care must occur both frequently and soon after the care is delivered, the approach is not suitable for studying low-incidence, long-latency outcomes, which are the targets of many types of care for chronic diseases. In addition, because the focus is on *desired* outcomes, this method does not deal with undesired adverse outcomes. A separate problem is that the method may avoid the limitations of medical record data, but it assesses only the outcome events. The remediable inadequate elements of process must still be discerned from medical records. Finally, in eliminating the arbitrariness and irrelevancies of many types of process criteria, the investigators create a new set of criteria for desirable outcome events. Not all reviewers may agree with these arbitrary new criteria.

Answer 27.5. Before accepting the information as evidence of successful quality assurance, wouldn't you like to know the secular trend for data showing whether the blood was being given for suitable clinical indications and in suitable quantities? These questions are not answered by statistics for the proportions of transfusions that were given as packed cells or whole blood.

Chapter 28

Answers 28.1 and 28.2. Individual reports to be submitted.

Chapter 29

Answer 29.1. Individual reports to be submitted.
Answer 29.2. Individual reports to be submitted.
Answer 29.3.
    29.3.1. Two significant problems may arise in detection bias. Because the trial was not conducted blindly, a problem in cause-specific mortality rates would occur if physicians are affected by a knowledge of treatment when assigning a diagnostic cause for deaths whose exact origin is uncertain or ambiguous. A problem in morbidity rates would occur because the stepped-care patients were examined more frequently than the other group, thus allowing detection of many morbid events that might otherwise be unnoticed.
    29.3.2. The mortality-bias problem could be avoided by having all causes of deaths assigned blindly from a suitably prepared excerpt of each patient's case record. The morbidity problem is more difficult to deal with, because an equal frequency of medical visits in both groups would alter the basic design of the study. To get around this problem, both groups of patients could receive telephone calls or self-administered questionnaires at the same regular intervals. The only morbid events to be counted in both groups would be the events cited by the patients spontaneously in these conversations or questionnaires. (Phenomena noted only by physicians at medical visits would be excluded.)
Answer 29.4.
    29.4.1. Because a nasogastric tube was inserted in both groups of patients, the original therapeutic question was altered. We are comparing antacids versus no antacids in patients with nasogastric tubes. Because the tube itself may cause erosions and evidence of gastrointestinal bleeding, we will not answer the original therapeutic question; and the rate of GI bleeding may be elevated by the tube.
    29.4.2. The patients could be stratified into those who *clinically* require a nasogastric tube and those who do not. In the former stratum, the protocol could remain unchanged. In the latter stratum, antacids could be compared against nothing, without a nasogastric tube being inserted in either group.
    29.4.3. Are we trying to prevent gastrointestinal bleeding or a positive result in the stool guaiac test? Because a positive result in the latter can arise from many clinically insignificant causes, does this trial have a suitable focus in its outcome event? We are measuring microscopic evidence of blood rather than clinically important episodes of GI bleeding.

Subject Index

Note: Page numbers in italics refer to illustrations; page numbers followed by t refer to tables.

Author Index

All references in the text are listed by first author's name at the end of each chapter. A complete alphabetical list of all references, accompanied by indication of the chapters in which they are cited, appears on pages 732–750. The authors in the list that follows are mentioned by name in the text on the cited pages.

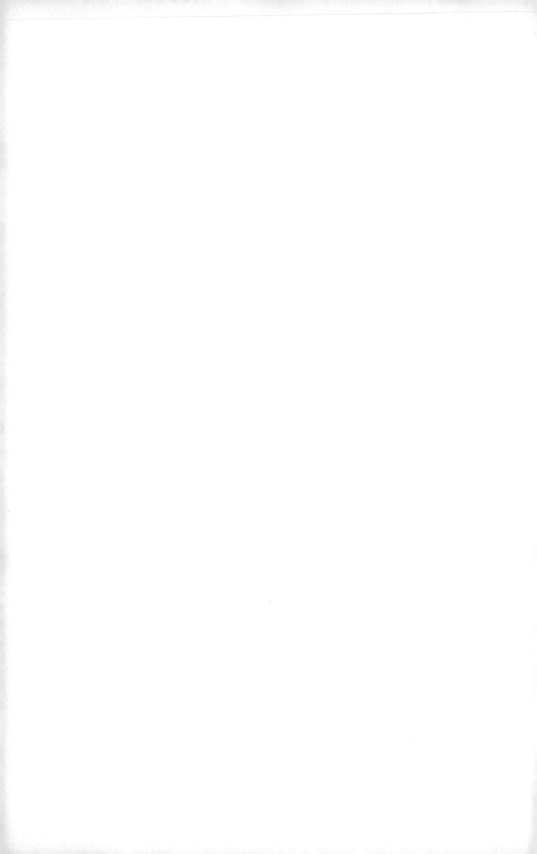